INTEGRATIVE RHEUM.

Concepts, Perspectives, Algorithms, and Protocols
Second Edition 2007

The art of creating wellness while effectively managing acute and chronic musculoskeletal disorders

ALEX VASQUEZ, D.C., N.D.

- Private practice of chiropractic and naturopathic medicine in Seattle, Washington (2000-2001) and Houston, Texas (2001-2006)

- Former Adjunct Professor of Orthopedics (2000), Radiographic Interpretation 1 (2000), and Rheumatology (2001) for the Naturopathic Medicine program at Bastyr University in Kenmore, Washington

- Forum Consultant (2003-present) and Former Adjunct Faculty (2004-2005), The Institute for Functional Medicine in Gig Harbor, Washington

- Editor, *Naturopathy Digest*

- Columnist, *Nutritional Wellness*

- Doctor of Chiropractic, graduate of Western States Chiropractic College. Licensed Doctor of Chiropractic, Washington (1996-2002) and Texas (2002-present)

- Doctor of Naturopathic Medicine, graduate of Bastyr University, Licensed Naturopathic Physician with Additional Prescriptive Authority in Washington (2000-present), Licensed Naturopathic Physician in Oregon (2004-present)

- Author of numerous articles and letters published in *Annals of Pharmacotherapy, The Lancet, Nutritional Perspectives, British Medical Journal, Journal of Manipulative and Physiological Therapeutics, JAMA: Journal of the American Medical Association, The Original Internist, Integrative Medicine: A Clinician's Journal, Holistic Primary Care, Nutritional Wellness, Dynamic Chiropractic, Alternative Therapies in Health and Medicine, Journal of the American Osteopathic Association, Evidence-based Complementary and Alternative Medicine,* and *Arthritis & Rheumatism: Official Journal of the American College of Rheumatology*

OPTIMALHEALTHRESEARCH.COM

Dr. Alex Vasquez

Integrative and Biological Medicine Research and Consulting, LLC
150 Boland Street, Suite 150
Fort Worth, Texas 76017

See website for updated contact information:
www.OptimalHealthResearch.com

ISBN-13: 978-0-9752858-7-9

Vasquez A. Integrative Rheumatology: Concepts, Perspectives, Algorithms, and Therapeutics. The art of creating wellness while effectively managing acute and chronic musculoskeletal disorders. Volume 1: Autoimmune Disorders. Fort Worth, TX; Integrative and Biological Medicine Research and Consulting, LLC: 2007

Dedications: I dedicate this book to the following people in appreciation for their works, their direct and indirect support of this work, and for their contributions to the advancement of authentic healthcare.

- **To the students and practitioners of chiropractic and naturopathic medicine**, those who continue to learn so that they can provide the best possible care to their patients

- **To the researchers** whose works are cited in this text

- **To Drs William Gould, Keith Innes, Alan Gaby, Jeffrey Bland, Ronald LeFebvre, and Gilbert Manso,** my most memorable and influential professors and mentors

- **To Dr Bruce Ames[1] and the late Dr Roger Williams[2],** for helping us to view our individuality as biochemically unique

- **To Dr Chester Wilk[3,4] and countless others** for documenting and resisting the organized oppression of natural, non-pharmaceutical, non-surgical healthcare[5,6,7]

- **To Jorge Strunz and Ardeshir Farah,** for artistic inspiration

Acknowledgements for Peer and Editorial Review: Acknowledgement here does not imply that the reviewer fully agrees with or endorses the material in this text but rather that they were willing to review specific sections of the book for clinical applicability and clarity and to make suggestions to their own level of satisfaction. Credit for improvements and refinements to this text are due in part to these reviewers; responsibility for oversights remains that of the author.

- <u>2007 Edition of *Integrative Orthopedics*</u>: Barry Morgan MD, Dennis Harris DC, Richard Brown DC (DACBI candidate), Ron Mariotti ND, Patrick Makarewich MBA, Reena Singh (SCNM ND4), Zachary Watkins DC, Charles Novak MS DC, Marnie Loomis ND, James Bogash DC, Sara Croteau DC, Kris Young DC, Joshua Levitt ND, Jack Powell III MD, Chad Kessler MD, Amy Neuzil ND

- <u>2006 Edition of *Integrative Rheumatology*</u>: Amy Neuzil ND, Cathryn Harbor MD, Julian Vickers DC, Tamara Sachs MD, Bob Sager BSc MD, DABFM (Clinical Instructor in the Department of Family Medicine, University of Kansas), Ron Mariotti ND, Titus Chiu (DC4), Zachary Watkins (DC4), Gilbert Manso MD, Bruce Milliman ND, William Groskopp DC, Robert Silverman DC, Matthew Breske (DC4), Dean Neary ND, Thomas Walton DC, Fraser Smith ND, Ladd Carlston DC, David Jones MD, Joshua Levitt ND

- <u>2004 Edition of *Integrative Orthopedics*</u>: Peter Knight ND, Kent Littleton ND MS, Barry Morgan MD, Ron Hobbs ND, Joshua Levitt ND, John Neustadt (Bastyr ND4), Allison Gandre BS (Bastyr ND4), Peter Kimble ND, Jack Powell III MD, Chad Kessler MD, Mike Gruber MD, Deirdre O'Neill ND, Mary Webb ND, Leslie Charles ND, Amy Neuzil ND

---

[1] Ames BN, Elson-Schwab I, Silver EA. High-dose vitamin therapy stimulates variant enzymes with decreased coenzyme binding affinity (increased K(m)): relevance to genetic disease and polymorphisms. *Am J Clin Nutr.* 2002 Apr;75(4):616-58 http://www.ajcn.org/cgi/content/full/75/4/616
[2] Williams RJ. <u>Biochemical Individuality: The Basis for the Genetotrophic Concept</u>. Austin and London: University of Texas Press; 1956
[3] Wilk CA. <u>Medicine, Monopolies, and Malice: How the Medical Establishment Tried to Destroy Chiropractic</u>. Garden City Park: Avery, 1996
[4] Getzendanner S. Permanent injunction order against AMA. *JAMA.* 1988 Jan 1;259(1):81-2 http://optimalhealthresearch.com/archives/wilk.html
[5] Carter JP. <u>Racketeering in Medicine: The Suppression of Alternatives</u>. Norfolk: Hampton Roads Pub; 1993
[6] Morley J, Rosner AL, Redwood D. A case study of misrepresentation of the scientific literature: recent reviews of chiropractic. *J Altern Complement Med.* 2001 Feb;7(1):65-78
[7] Terrett AG. Misuse of the literature by medical authors in discussing spinal manipulative therapy injury. *J Manipulative Physiol Ther.* 1995 May;18(4):203-10

Format and Layout: The format and layout of this book is designed to efficiently take the reader though the clinically relevant spectrum of considerations for each condition that is detailed. Important topics are given their own section within each chapter, while other less important or less common conditions are only described briefly in terms of the four "clinical essentials" of 1) definition/pathophysiology, 2) clinical presentation, 3) assessment/diagnosis, and 4) treatment/management. Each expanded section which details the more important/common conditions maintains a consistent format, taking the reader through the spectrum of primary clinical considerations: definition/pathophysiology, clinical presentations, differential diagnoses, assessments (physical examination, laboratory, imaging), complications, management, and treatment.

References and Citations: Major references to texts and articles are listed along with each section; these references are "recommended reading" and form the foundation for the clinical approach delineated in the text. Citations to articles, abstracts, texts, and personal communications are footnoted throughout the text to provide supporting information and to provide interested readers the resources to find additional information. Many of the cited articles are available on-line for free, and when possible I have included the website addresses so that readers can access the complete article.

Language, Semantics, and Perspective: As a diligent student who previously aspired to be an English professor, I have written this text with great (though inevitably imperfect) attention to detail. Individual words were chosen with care. With regard to the he/she and him/her debacle of the English language, I've mixed singular and plural pronouns for the sake of being efficient and so that the images remain gender-neutral to the extent reasonable. The subtitle *The art of creating wellness while effectively managing acute and chronic musculoskeletal disorders* was chosen to emphasize the intentional creation of wellness rather than a limited focus on disease treatment and symptom suppression. *Managing* was chosen to emphasize the importance of treating-monitoring-referring-reassessing, rather than merely *treating*. *Disorders* was chosen to reflect the fact that a distinguishing characteristic of **life** is the ability to habitually create *organized structure* and *higher order* from chaos and *disorder*. For example, plants organize the randomly moving molecules of air and water into the organized structure of biomolecules and plant structure. Similarly, the human body creates organized structure of increased complexity from consumed plants and other foods; molecules ingested and inhaled from the environment are organized into specific biochemicals and tissue structures with distinct characteristics and definite functions. Injury and disease *result in* or *result from* a lack of order, hence my use of the word "disorders" to characterize human illness and disease. A motor vehicle accident that results in bodily injury, for example, is an example of an external chaotic force, which, when imparted upon human body tissues, results in a disruption (disorder) of the normal structure and organization that previously defined and characterized the now-damaged tissues of the body. Likewise, an autoimmune disease process that results in tissue destruction is an anti-evolutionary process that takes molecules of higher complexity and reverts them to simpler, fragmented, and non-functional forms. From the perspective of "health" as *organized structure and meaningful function* and "disease" as *the reversion to chaos, destruction of structure, and the loss of function*, the task of healthcare providers is essentially to restore order, and to acutely reduce and proactively prevent/eliminate clinical-biochemical-biomechanical-emotional chaos insofar as it adversely affects the patient's life experience as an individual and our collective experience as an interdependent society.

Integrity and Creativity: I have endeavored to accurately represent the facts as they have been presented in texts and research, and to specifically resist any temptation to embellish or misrepresent data as others have done.[8,9] Conversely, I have not endeavored to make this book "normal" or "average." Rather I have allowed this text to be unique in format, content, and style, so that the personality of this text can be contrasted with that of the instructor and reader, thus enabling the learner to at least benefit from an intentionally different – though altogether honest – perspective and approach. Students using this text with the guidance of a qualified professor will benefit from the experience of "two teachers" rather than just one.

---

[8] Vasquez A. Zinc treatment for reduction of hyperplasia of prostate. *Townsend Letter for Doctors and Patients* 1996; January: 100

[9] Broad W, Wade N. Betrayers of the Truth: Fraud and Deceit in the Halls of Science. New York: Simon and Schuster; 1982

Peer-review and Quality Control: Peer-review is essential to help ensure accuracy and clinical applicability of health-related information. Consistent with the importance of our goals, I have employed several "checks and balances" to increase the accuracy and applicability of the information within my textbooks:

- Reliance upon authoritative references: Nearly all important statements are referenced to peer-reviewed biomedical journals or authoritative texts, such as *The Merck Manual* and *Current Medical Diagnosis and Treatment*. Each citation is provided by a footnote at the bottom of each page so that readers will know quickly and easily exactly where the information came from.

- Extensive cross-referencing: Readers will notice, if not be overwhelmed by, the number of references and citations. Many important statements have several references. Many references (especially textbooks) are referenced several times even on the same page. The purpose of this extensive referencing is three-fold: 1) to guide you to additional information, 2) to help me (the writer) stay organized, and 3) to help you and me (the practicing physicians) employ this information with confidence.

- Periodic revision: The book is updated and revised on a regular basis. New information is added; superfluous information removed. Inspired by the popular text *Current Medical Diagnosis and Treatment* which is updated every year, I want *Integrative Orthopedics* and *Integrative Rheumatology* to be accurate, timely, and in pace with the ever-growing literature on natural medicine. Any significant errors that are brought to my attention will be posted at www.OptimalHealthResearch.com/updates; please check this page periodically to ensure that you are working with the most accurate information of which I am aware.

- Peer-review: The peer-review process for *Integrative Orthopedics* and *Integrative Rheumatology* takes two forms. First, select colleagues are invited to review new and revised sections of the text before publication; every section of the book that you are holding has been independently reviewed by chiropractic and naturopathic students and/or practicing clinicians from various backgrounds: allopathic, chiropractic, osteopathic, naturopathic. Second, you - the reader - are invited to provide feedback about the information in the book, typographical errors, syntax, case reports, new research, etc. If your ideas truly change the nature of the material, I will be glad to acknowledge you in the text (with your permission, of course). If your contribution is hugely significant, such as reviewing three or more chapters or helping in some important way, I will be glad to not only acknowledge you, but to also send you the next edition at a discount or courtesy when your ideas take effect. By implementing these quality control steps, I hope to create a useful text and advance our professions and our practices by improving the quality of care that we deliver to our patients. Readers with ideas, suggestions, or corrections can email me from the website at http://OptimalHealthResearch.com/corrections.

How to Use This Book Safely and Most Effectively: Readers are encouraged to complete chapters 1, 2, and 3 of *Integrative Orthopedics* and Chapters 1-5 of *Integrative Rheumatology* before reading and using the information in the region- and condition-specific chapters that follow these introductory and conceptual chapters. Ideally, these books should be read cover-to-cover within a context of coursework that is supervised by an experienced professor. For post-graduate professionals, they might consider forming a local "book club" and meeting for weekly or monthly discussions to check their understandings and share their clinical experiences to refine the application of clinical knowledge, perceptions, and skills. Virtual groups and internet forums—such as the forum hosted by the Institute for Functional Medicine at www.FunctionalMedicine.org—can provide access to an international group of professional peers where sharing of clinical experience and questions is synergistic. Throughout this book, references are amply provided and are often footnoted with hyperlinks providing full-text access. This book is intended for licensed doctorate-level healthcare professionals with graduate and post-graduate training.

Notice: The intention and scope of this text are to provide the reader with clinically useful information and a familiarity with available research and resources pertinent to the management of patients with musculoskeletal disorders in a holistic primary care setting. Specifically, the information in this book is intended to be used by licensed healthcare professionals who have received hands-on clinical training and supervision at accredited chiropractic/naturopathic colleges. Additionally, information in this book should be confirmed and used in conjunction with other resources, texts, and in combination with the clinician's best judgment with the intention to "first do no harm" and second to provide effective healthcare. Information and treatments applicable to a specific *condition* may not be appropriate for or applicable to a specific *patient* in your office; this is especially true for patients with concomitant illnesses and those taking pharmaceutical medications.

Throughout this text, I describe treatments—manual, dietary, nutritional, botanical, and pharmacologic—and their research support for the clinical conditions being discussed; each practitioner must determine appropriateness of these treatments for his/her individual patient and with consideration of the doctor's scope of practice, education, training, skill, and possible "off label" use of medications and treatments. This book has been carefully written and checked for accuracy by the author and professional colleagues. However, in view of the possibility of human error and new discoveries in the biomedical sciences, neither the author nor any party associated in any way with this text warrants that this text is perfect, accurate, or complete in every way, and we disclaim responsibility for harm or loss associated with the application of the material herein. With all conditions/treatments described herein, each physician must be sure to consider the balance between what is best for the patient and the physician's own level of ability, expertise, and experience. When in doubt, or if the physician is not a specialist in the treatment of a given severe condition, referral is appropriate. These notes are written with the routine "outpatient" in mind and are not tailored to severely injured patients or emergency or "playing field" or "emergency response" situations. Consult your First Aid and Emergency Response texts and course materials for appropriate information. These notes represent the author's perspective based on academic education, experience, and post-graduate continuing education and are not inclusive of every fact that a clinician may need to know. Consult other texts, references, and articles for additional information and perspectives. This is not an "entry level" book except when used in an academic setting with a knowledgeable professor who can explain the abbreviations, tests, physical exam procedures, and treatments. This book requires a certain level of knowledge from the reader and familiarity with clinical concepts, laboratory assessments, and physical examination procedures.

Important Updates and Corrections: When omissions, errata, and the need for important updates become clear to me, I will post these at the website: www.OptimalHealthResearch.com/updates. Be sure to access this page periodically to ensure that you are informed of any corrections that might have clinical relevance. This book consists not only of the text in the printed pages you are holding, but also the footnotes and any updates at the website.

Bon Voyage: All artists, and scientists—regardless of genre—grapple with the divergent goals of 1) perfecting their work and 2) completing their work; the former is impossible, while the latter is the only means by which the effort can become useful. At some point, we must all agree that it is "good enough" and that it contains the essence of what needs to be communicated. While neither this nor any future edition of this book is likely to be "perfect", I am content with the literature reviewed, presented, and the new conclusions and implications which are described—many for the first time ever—in this text. Particularly for *Integrative Rheumatology*, each chapter in the book is a paradigm shift which distances us further from the simplistic pharmacocentric model and toward one which authentically empowers both practitioners and patients. I hope you are able to implement these conclusions and research findings into your own life and into the treatment plans for your patients.

Thank you, and I wish you and your patients the best in health,

[signature]

Alex Vasquez, D.C., N.D.
March 25, 2007

"He who would learn one day to *fly* must first learn *standing*
and *walking*
and *running*
and *climbing*
and *dancing*.

One cannot *fly* into flying."

Friedrich Nietzsche[10]

[10] Nietzsche FW. [Translated from German by Kaufmann W]. Thus Spoke Zarathustra: A Book for None and All. 1892. New York; Viking Penguin: 1954, page 195

<u>Topics:</u>
- **Musculoskeletal Medicine: The Goal is *Wellness***
- **Clinical Assessments**
  - History taking
  - Physical examination
  - Orthopedic/musculoskeletal examination: Concepts and goals
  - Neurologic assessment: Review
  - Laboratory assessments: General considerations of commonly used tests
    i. CRP
    ii. ESR
    iii. CBC
    iv. Chemistry/metabolic panel
    v. Complements C3 and C4
    vi. Ferritin
    vii. Serum 25(OH)-vitamin D
    viii. TSH: Thyroid stimulating hormone
    ix. ANA: Antinuclear antibodies
    x. ANCA: Antineutrophilic cytoplasmic antibodies
    xi. RF: Rheumatoid factor
    xii. CCP: Cyclic citrullinated protein antibodies; anticitrullinated protein antibodies
    xiii. HLA-B27
    xiv. Lactulose-mannitol assay
    xv. Comprehensive stool analysis and comprehensive parasitology
- **High-Risk Pain Patients**
- **Concepts**
  - Not all injury-related problems are injury-related problems
  - Safe patient + safe treatment = safe outcome
  - Four clues to underlying problems
  - Special considerations in the evaluation of children
  - No errors allowed: Differences between primary healthcare and spectator sports
  - "Disease treatment" is different from "patient management"
- **Musculoskeletal Emergencies**
  - Acute compartment syndrome
  - Acute red eye, including acute iritis and scleritis
  - Atlantoaxial subluxation and instability
  - Cauda equina syndrome
  - Giant cell arteritis, temporal arteritis
  - Myelopathy, spinal cord compression
  - Neuropsychiatric lupus
  - Osteomyelitis
  - Septic arthritis, acute nontraumatic monoarthritis
- **Naturopathic Principles**
  - Naturopathic model of illness and healing
  - Naturopathic principles, concepts & the healing power of nature (*Vis Medicatrix Naturae*)
  - Hierarchy of Therapeutics
- **Chiropractic: Overview of History and Current Science**
- **Osteopathic Medicine**

Core Competencies:

- You must know how to test and grade muscle reflexes and muscle strength.
- You must be able to explain and apply the "principle of neurologic localization" in conjunction with your comprehensive neurologic examination.
- You must know how to rapidly diagnose and effectively manage the following musculoskeletal emergencies:
    - Acute compartment syndrome
    - Acute red eye, including acute iritis and scleritis
    - Atlantoaxial subluxation and instability
    - Cauda equina syndrome
    - Giant cell arteritis, temporal arteritis
    - Myelopathy, spinal cord compression
    - Neuropsychiatric lupus
    - Osteomyelitis
    - Septic arthritis, acute nontraumatic monoarthritis
- Regarding acute monoarthritis, what are the main differential diagnoses and what (beyond routine history and physical examination) is the single most important diagnostic procedure?
- You must demonstrate competency in the correlative and differential interpretation of the following routine blood tests:
    - ANA
    - CBC
    - CCP antibodies
    - Chemistry/metabolic panel
    - CRP
    - ESR
    - Ferritin
    - Serum 25(OH)D
    - TSH

Sample questions about laboratory test interpretation:
- What is the diagnostic difference between "elevated CRP with a normal ferritin" and "elevated CRP with elevated ferritin"?
- What is the standard of care when you find that your adult asymptomatic patient has a ferritin less than 20 mcg/L?
- What is the proper management of an asymptomatic patient with a ferritin > 300 mcg/L (male) or > 200 mcg/L (female)?
- Name two common nutritional deficiencies that would be correlated with a MCV > 95 fL; also name the corresponding treatments and appropriate doses.
- What are the six most common causes of an elevated lactulose-mannitol ratio and how are these differentially diagnosed?
- Name six causes of hypercalcemia and means for assessing each.
- Describe the two components of "composite seropositivity" and describe the patient management for 1) a young patient who is asymptomatic, and 2) a middle-aged patient with peripheral polyarthropathy and recent onset of hyperreflexia, iritis, and visual changes.

Integrative Musculoskeletal Medicine: the Goal is *Wellness*

Since **approximately 1 of every 7 (14% of total) visits to a primary healthcare provider is for the treatment of musculoskeletal pain or dysfunction**[1], every healthcare provider needs to have 1) knowledge of important concepts related to musculoskeletal medicine, 2) the ability to recognize urgent and emergency conditions, 3) the ability to competently perform orthopedic examination procedures and interpret laboratory assessments, and 4) the knowledge and ability to design and implement effective treatment plans and to coordinate patient management. Written for students and experienced clinicians, this chapter introduces and reviews many new and common terms, procedures, and concepts relevant to the management of patients with musculoskeletal disorders. Especially for students, the reading of this chapter is essential to understanding the extensive material in this book and will facilitate the clinical assessment and management of patients with musculoskeletal disorders.

Healthcare is currently in a time of significant fluctuation and is ready for changes in the balance of power and the paradigms which direct our therapeutic interventions. For nearly a century, allopathic medicine has hailed itself as "the gold standard", and other professions have either submitted to or been crushed by their ongoing political/scientific manipulations and their continual proclamation of intellectual and therapeutic superiority[2,3,4,5,6,7,8,9,10,11,12,13,14] despite 180,000-220,000 iatrogenic *medically-induced* deaths per year (500-600 iatrogenic deaths per day)[15,16] and consistent documentation that most medical/allopathic physicians are unable to provide accurate musculoskeletal diagnoses due to pervasive inadequacies in medical training.[17,18,19,20] Increasing disenchantment with allopathic "neoHeroic" medicine and its adverse outcomes of inefficacy, exorbitant expenses, and unnecessary death are fostering change, such that allopathic medicine has been dethroned as the leading paradigm among American patients, who spend the majority of their volitional healthcare dollars on consultations and treatments provided by "alternative" healthcare providers.[21,22] With the ever-increasing utilization of chiropractic, naturopathic, and osteopathic medical services, we must see that our paradigms and interventions keep pace with the evolving research literature and our increasing professional responsibilities so that we can deliver the highest possible quality of care.

In allopathic medicine, the goal of musculoskeletal treatment is to address the patient's injury or disorder by alleviating pain with the use of drugs, preventing further injury, and returning the patient to his/her previous status and activities. The most commonly employed interventions are 1) rest and "watchful waiting", 2) non-steroidal anti-inflammatory drugs (NSAIDS) and cyclooxygenase-2-inhibitors ("coxibs"), and 3) surgery. Chiropractic, naturopathic, and osteopathic physicians criticize this approach because, although avoidance of and "rest" from damaging activities is reasonable and valuable, too much rest without an emphasis on active preventive rehabilitation encourages patient passivity, assumption of the sick role, fails to actively promote tissue healing, and fails to address the underlying proprioceptive deficits that are common in patients with chronic musculoskeletal pain and recurrent injuries.[23,24,25] **NSAIDs are considered "first line" therapy for**

[1] American College of Rheumatology Ad Hoc Committee on Clinical Guidelines. Guidelines for the initial evaluation of the adult patient with acute musculoskeletal symptoms. *Arthritis Rheum.* 1996 Jan;39(1):1-8 See also: Vasquez A. Musculoskeletal disorders and iron overload disease: comment on the American College of Rheumatology guidelines. *Arthritis Rheum* 1996;39: 1767-8
[2] Wilk CA. Medicine, Monopolies, and Malice: How the Medical Establishment Tried to Destroy Chiropractic. Garden City Park: Avery, 1996
[3] Getzendanner S. Permanent injunction order against AMA. *JAMA.* 1988 Jan 1;259(1):81-2 http://optimalhealthresearch.com/archives/wilk.html
[4] Carter JP. Racketeering in Medicine: The Suppression of Alternatives. Norfolk: Hampton Roads Pub; 1993
[5] Morley J, Rosner AL, Redwood D. A case study of misrepresentation of the scientific literature: recent reviews of chiropractic. *J Altern Complement Med.* 2001 Feb;7(1):65-78
[6] Terrett AG. Misuse of the literature by medical authors in discussing spinal manipulative therapy injury. *J Manipulative Physiol Ther.* 1995 May;18(4):203-10
[7] National Alliance of Professional Psychology Providers. AMA Seeks To Control and Restrict Psychologist's Scope of Practice. http://www.nappp.org/scope.pdf Accessed November 25, 2006
[8] "In an effort to marshal the medical community's resources against the growing threat of expanding scope of practice for allied health professionals, the AMA has formed a national partnership to confront such initiatives nationwide… The committee will use $25,000..." Daly R, American Psychiatric Association. AMA Forms Coalition to Thwart Non-M.D. Practice Expansion. *Psychiatric News* 2006 March; 41: 17 http://pn.psychiatryonline.org/cgi/content/full/41/5/17-a?eaf Accessed November 25, 2006
[9] Spivak JL. The Medical Trust Unmasked. Louis S. Siegfried Publishers; New York: 1961
[10] Trever W. In the Public Interest. Los Angeles; Scriptures Unlimited; 1972. This is probably the most authoritative documentation of the illegal actions of the AMA up to 1972; contains numerous photocopies of actual AMA documents and minutes of official meetings with overt intentionality of destroying Americans' healthcare options so that the AMA and related organizations would have a monopoly in national healthcare.
[11] Wenban AB. Inappropriate use of the title 'chiropractor' and term 'chiropractic manipulation' in the peer-reviewed biomedical literature. *Chiropr Osteopat.* 2006;14:16 http://chiroandosteo.com/content/14/1/16
[12] Orme-Johnson DW, Herron RE. An innovative approach to reducing medical care utilization and expenditures. *Am J Manag Care.* 1997 Jan;3:135-44 http://www.ajmc.com/Article.cfm?Menu=1&ID=2154
[13] van der Steen WJ, Ho VK. Drugs versus diets: disillusions with Dutch health care. *Acta Biotheor.* 2001;49(2):125-40
[14] Texas Medical Association. Physicians Ask Court to Protect Patients From Illegal Chiropractic Activities. http://www.texmed.org/Template.aspx?id=5259 Accessed February 20, 2007
[15] Starfield B. Is US health really the best in the world? *JAMA.* 2000 Jul 26;284(4):483-5
[16] "Recent estimates suggest that each year more than 1 million patients are injured while in the hospital and approximately 180,000 die because of these injuries. Furthermore, drug-related morbidity and mortality are common and are estimated to cost more than $136 billion a year." Holland EG, Degruy FV. Drug-induced disorders. *Am Fam Physician.* 1997;56(7):1781-8, 1791-2
[17] Freedman KB, Bernstein J. The adequacy of medical school education in musculoskeletal medicine. *J Bone Joint Surg Am.* 1998;80(10):1421-7
[18] Freedman KB, Bernstein J. Educational deficiencies in musculoskeletal medicine. *J Bone Joint Surg Am.* 2002;84-A(4):604-8
[19] Matzkin E, Smith ME, Freccero CD, Richardson AB. Adequacy of education in musculoskeletal medicine. *J Bone Joint Surg Am.* 2005 Feb;87-A(2):310-4
[20] Schmale GA. More evidence of educational inadequacies in musculoskeletal medicine. *Clin Orthop Relat Res.* 2005 Aug;(437):251-9
[21] "...Americans made an estimated 425 million visits to providers of unconventional therapy. This number exceeds the number of visits to all U.S. primary care physicians (388 million)." Eisenberg DM, Kessler RC, Foster C, Norlock FE, Calkins DR, Delbanco TL. Unconventional medicine in the United States. Prevalence, costs, and patterns of use. *N Engl J Med.* 1993 Jan 28;328(4):246-52
[22] "Estimated expenditures for alternative medicine professional services increased 45.2% between 1990 and 1997 and were conservatively estimated at $21.2 billion in 1997, with at least $12.2 billion paid out-of-pocket. This exceeds the 1997 out-of-pocket expenditures for all US hospitalizations." Eisenberg DM, Davis RB, Ettner SL, Appel S, Wilkey S, Van Rompay M, Kessler RC. Trends in alternative medicine use in the United States, 1990-1997: results of a follow-up national survey. *JAMA.* 1998 Nov 11;280(18):1569-75
[23] McPartland JM, Brodeur RR, Hallgren RC. Chronic neck pain, standing balance, and suboccipital muscle atrophy--a pilot study. *J Manipulative Physiol Ther.* 1997;20(1):24-9
[24] Bullock-Saxton JE, Janda V, Bullock MI. Reflex activation of gluteal muscles in walking. An approach to restoration of muscle function for patients with low-back pain. *Spine* 1993 May;18(6):704-8
[25] Sinaki M, Brey RH, Hughes CA, Larson DR, Kaufman KR.Significant reduction in risk of falls and back pain in osteoporotic-kyphotic women through a Spinal Proprioceptive Extension Exercise Dynamic (SPEED) program. *Mayo Clin Proc.* 2005 Jul;80(7):849-55

musculoskeletal disorders by allopaths despite the data showing that "**There is no evidence that widely used NSAIDs have any long-term benefit on osteoarthritis.**"[26] What is worse than this lack of efficacy is the evidence showing that NSAIDs *exacerbate* musculoskeletal disease (rather than *cure* it). **NSAIDs are known to inhibit cartilage formation and to promote bone necrosis and joint degradation with long-term use**[27,28,29,30] and **NSAIDs are responsible for more than 16,000 gastrohemorrhagic deaths and 100,000 hospitalizations each year.**[31] The "coxibs" were supposed to provide anti-inflammatory benefits with an enhanced safety profile, but the gastrocentric focus of these drug developers failed to appreciate that COX-2 is necessary for the formation of prostacyclin, a prostaglandin created from arachidonic acid via COX-2 that plays an important role in vasodilation and antithrombosis; not surprisingly therefore, use of COX-2-inhibiting drugs has consistently been associated with increased risk for adverse cardiovascular effects including myocardial infarction, unstable angina, cardiac thrombus, resuscitated cardiac arrest, sudden or unexplained death, ischemic stroke, and transient ischemic attacks.[32] Additionally, the use of a COX-2 inhibiting treatment in patients who overconsume

> "...only about 15% of medical interventions are supported by solid scientific evidence..."
>
> Smith R. Where is the wisdom...? The poverty of medical evidence. *BMJ.* 1991 Oct 5;303:798-9

arachidonic acid (i.e., most people in America and other industrialized nations[33]) would be expected to shunt bioavailable arachidonate into the formation of leukotrienes, a group of inflammatory mediators now known to contribute directly to atherogenesis.[34] Thus, it was entirely predictable that overuse of COX-2 inhibitors would create a catastrophe of iatrogenic cardiovascular death, and this is exactly what was allowed to occur—clearly indicating independent but synergistic failures on the part of pharmaceutical companies, the FDA, and the medical profession.[35,36,37,38] According to David J. Graham, MD, MPH, (Associate Director for Science, Office of Drug Safety, FDA) **an estimated 139,000 Americans who took Vioxx suffered serious complications including stroke or myocardial infarction; between 26,000 and 55,000 Americans died as a result of their doctors' prescribing Vioxx.**[39] Furthermore, the surgical procedures employed by allopaths for the treatment of musculoskeletal pain do not consistently show evidence of efficacy, safety, or cost-effectiveness. Arthroscopic surgery for osteoarthritis of the knee, for example, costs thousands of dollars to each individual and billions of dollars to the American healthcare system but is no more effective than placebo.[40,41,42] In a review which also noted that only 15% of medical procedures are supported by literature references and that only 1% of such references are deemed scientifically valid, Rosner[43] showed that the risks of serious injury (i.e., cauda equina syndrome or vertebral artery dissection) associated with spinal manipulation are "*400 times lower* than the death rates observed from gastrointestinal bleeding due to the use of nonsteroidal anti-inflammatory drugs and *700 times lower* than the overall mortality rate for spinal surgery."

In chiropractic, osteopathic, and naturopathic medicine, the goal and means of musculoskeletal treatment is to address the patient's injury or disorder by simultaneously alleviating pain with the use of natural, noninvasive, low-cost, and low-risk interventions while improving the patient's overall health, preventing future health problems, and "upgrading" the patient's overall paradigm of health maintenance and disease prevention from one that is passive and reactive to one that is empowered and pro-active. Commonly employed therapeutics include spinal manipulation[44,45,46], exercise[47] and the use of nutritional supplements and botanical medicines[48] which have been demonstrated in peer-reviewed clinical trials to be safe and effective for the treatment of

---

[26] Beers MH, Berkow R (eds). The Merck Manual. 17th Edition. Whitehouse Station; Merck Research Laboratories 1999 page 451

[27] "At...concentrations comparable to those... in the synovial fluid of patients treated with the drug, several NSAIDs suppress proteoglycan synthesis... These NSAID-related effects on chondrocyte metabolism ... are much more profound in osteoarthritic cartilage than in normal cartilage, due to enhanced uptake of NSAIDs by the osteoarthritic cartilage." Brandt KD. Effects of nonsteroidal anti-inflammatory drugs on chondrocyte metabolism in vitro and in vivo. Am J Med. 1987 Nov 20; 83(5A): 29-34

[28] "The case of a young healthy man, who developed avascular necrosis of head of femur after prolonged administration of indomethacin, is reported here." Prathapkumar KR, Smith I, Attara GA. Indomethacin induced avascular necrosis of head of femur. Postgrad Med J. 2000 Sep; 76(899): 574-5

[29] "This highly significant association between NSAID use and acetabular destruction gives cause for concern, not least because of the difficulty in achieving satisfactory hip replacements in patients with severely damaged acetabula." Newman NM, Ling RS. Acetabular bone destruction related to non-steroidal anti-inflammatory drugs. Lancet. 1985 Jul 6; 2(8445): 11-4

[30] Vidal y Plana RR, Bizzarri D, Rovati AL. Articular cartilage pharmacology: I. In vitro studies on glucosamine and non steroidal antiinflammatory drugs. Pharmacol Res Commun. 1978 Jun;10(6):557-69

[31] Singh G. Recent considerations in nonsteroidal anti-inflammatory drug gastropathy. Am J Med. 1998;105(1B):31S-38S

[32] Mukherjee D, Nissen SE, Topol EJ. Risk of cardiovascular events associated with selective COX-2 inhibitors. JAMA. 2001 Aug 22-29;286(8):954-9

[33] Seaman DR. The diet-induced proinflammatory state: a cause of chronic pain and other degenerative diseases? J Manipulative Physiol Ther. 2002 Mar-Apr;25(3):168-79

[34] Dwyer JH, Allayee H, Dwyer KM, Fan J, Wu H, Mar R, Lusis AJ, Mehrabian M. Arachidonate 5-lipoxygenase promoter genotype, dietary arachidonic acid, and atherosclerosis. N Engl J Med. 2004 Jan 1;350(1):29-37

[35] Topol EJ. Arthritis medicines and cardiovascular events--"house of coxibs". JAMA. 2004 Jan 19;293(3):366-8. Epub 2004 Dec 28

[36] Ray WA, Griffin MR, Stein CM. Cardiovascular toxicity of valdecoxib. N Engl J Med. 2004 Dec 23;351(26):2767. Epub 2004 Dec 17

[37] Topol EJ. Failing the public health--rofecoxib, Merck, and the FDA. N Engl J Med. 2004 Oct 21;351(17):1707-9

[38] Horton R. Vioxx, the implosion of Merck, and aftershocks at the FDA. Lancet. 2004 Dec 4-10;364(9450):1995-6

[39] David J. Graham, MD, MPH, (Associate Director for Science, Office of Drug Safety, US FDA) estimated that 139,000 Americans who took Vioxx suffered serious side effects; he estimated that the drug killed between 26,000 and 55,000 people. http://www.commondreams.org/views05/0223-35.htm http://www.fda.gov/cder/drug/infopage/vioxx/vioxxgraham.pdf Accessed November 25, 2006

[40] Gina Kolata. A Knee Surgery for Arthritis Is Called Sham. The New York Times, July 11, 2002

[41] Moseley JB, O'Malley K, Petersen NJ, Menke TJ, Brody BA, Kuykendall DH, Hollingsworth JC, Ashton CM, Wray NP. A controlled trial of arthroscopic surgery for osteoarthritis of the knee. N Engl J Med. 2002;347:81-8

[42] Bernstein J, Quach T. A perspective on the study of Moseley et al: questioning the value of arthroscopic knee surgery for osteoarthritis. Cleve Clin J Med. 2003;70(5):401, 405-6, 408-10

[43] Rosner AL. Evidence-based clinical guidelines for the management of acute low-back pain: response to the guidelines prepared for the Australian Medical Health and Research Council. J Manipulative Physiol Ther. 2001;24(3):214-20

[44] Manga P, Angus D, Papadopoulos C, et al. The Effectiveness and Cost-Effectiveness of Chiropractic Management of Low-Back Pain. Richmond Hill, Ontario: Kenilworth Publishing; 1993

[45] Meade TW, Dyer S, Browne W, Townsend J, Frank AO. Low-back pain of mechanical origin: randomised comparison of chiropractic and hospital outpatient treatment. BMJ. 1990;300(6737):1431-7

[46] Meade TW, Dyer S, Browne W, Frank AO. Randomised comparison of chiropractic and hospital outpatient management for low-back pain: results from extended follow up. BMJ. 1995;311(7001):349-5

[47] Harold Elrick, MD. Exercise is Medicine. The Physician and Sportsmedicine - Volume 24 - No. 2 - February 1996

[48] Vasquez A. Reducing pain and inflammation naturally - Part 3: Improving overall health while safely and effectively treating musculoskeletal pain. Nutr Perspect 2005; 28: 34-38, 40-42 http://optimalhealthresearch.com/part3

musculoskeletal pain. More specifically, chiropractic and naturopathic physicians are well versed in the clinical utilization of such treatments as niacinamide[49], glucosamine and chondroitin sulfates[50], vitamin D[51], vitamin B-12[52], balanced and complete fatty acid therapy[53,54], anti-inflammatory diets[55,56,57], proteolytic/pancreatic enzymes[58], and botanical medicines such as *Boswellia*[59], *Harpagophytum*[60], *Uncaria*, and willow bark[61,62]—each of these interventions has been validated in peer-reviewed research for safety and effectiveness.[63] Furthermore, from the perspective of integrative chiropractic and naturopathic medicine, aiming for such a limited accomplishment as mere "returning the patient to previous status and activities" would be considered substandard, since the patient's overall health was neither addressed nor improved and since returning the patient to his/her previous status and activities would be a direct invitation for the problem to recur indefinitely. Chiropractic and naturopathic physicians appreciate that, especially regarding chronic health problems, any treatment plan that allows the patient to resume his/her previous lifestyle is by definition doomed to fail because a return to the patient's previous lifestyle and activities that allowed the onset of the disease/disorder in the first place will most certainly result in the perpetuation and recurrence of the illness or disorder. **Stated more directly: for *healing* to truly be effective, the comprehensive treatment plan must generally result in a permanent and profound change in the patient's lifestyle and emotional climate, which are the primary modifiable determinants of either health or disease.**

While we all readily acknowledge the importance of emergency care for emergency situations, those of us who advocate and practice a more complete approach to healthcare and life readily see the shortcomings of a limited and mechanical approach to healthcare, and we aspire to do more than simply fix problems. The implementation of *multidimensional* (i.e., *comprehensive* and *multifaceted*) treatment plans that address many aspects of pathophysiologic phenomena is a huge step forward in creating improved health and preventing future illness in the patients who seek our professional assistance.

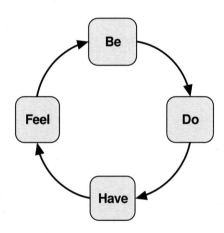

However, even complete multidimensional treatment plans still fall short of the goal of creating wellness, if for no other reasons than 1) they are still disease- and problem-oriented, rather than health-oriented, 2) they are prescribed from outside ("The doctor told me to do it.") rather than originating internally and spontaneously by the patient's own direction and affirmation ("I *do* this because I *am* this."), and, finally and most difficult to relay, 3) they are mechanistic rather than organic, they can do no better than the sum of their parts, they flow exclusively from the mind ("do") and not also from the body-soul ("am"). The art of creating wellness takes time to understand, longer to implement clinically, and even longer to apply to one's own life. Wellness is a state of being rather than a checklist of activities in a "preventive health program." The subtle differences that distinguish "wellness" from any "program" or "prescription" are the differences between *leading* versus *following* and *flowing* versus *performing*. **Wellness is multidimensional self-actualization, full integration of one's life— present, past, and future; physical, mental, emotional, spiritual, biochemical—one's shadow[64], work[65], feelings, thoughts, and goals into a cohesive living whole – "a wheel rolling from its own center."[66]**

[49] Kaufman W. Niacinamide therapy for joint mobility. Therapeutic reversal of a common clinical manifestation of the "normal" aging process. *Conn State Med J* 1953;17:584-591
[50] Reginster JY, Deroisy R, Rovati LC, Lee RL, Lejeune E, Bruyere O, Giacovelli G, Henrotin Y, Dacre JE, Gossett C. Long-term effects of glucosamine sulphate on osteoarthritis progression: a randomised, placebo-controlled clinical trial. *Lancet*. 2001;357(9252):251-6
[51] Vasquez A, Manso G, Cannell J. The clinical importance of vitamin D: a paradigm shift with implications for all healthcare providers. *Altern Ther Health Med* 2004;10:28-36 http://optimalhealthresearch.com/monograph04
[52] Mauro GL, Martorana U, Cataldo P, Brancato G, Letizia G. Vitamin B12 in low back pain: a randomised, double-blind, placebo-controlled study. *Eur Rev Med Pharmacol Sci*. 2000 May-Jun;4(3):53-8
[53] Vasquez A. Reducing Pain and Inflammation Naturally. Part 1: New Insights into Fatty Acid Biochemistry and the Influence of Diet. *Nutritional Perspectives* 2004; October: 5, 7-10, 12, 14 http://optimalhealthresearch.com/part1
[54] Vasquez A. Reducing Pain and Inflammation Naturally. Part 2: New Insights into Fatty Acid Supplementation and Its Effect on Eicosanoid Production and Genetic Expression. *Nutritional Perspectives* 2005; January: 5-16 http://optimalhealthresearch.com/part2
[55] Seaman DR. The diet-induced proinflammatory state: a cause of chronic pain and other degenerative diseases? *J Manipulative Physiol Ther*. 2002 Mar-Apr;25(3):168-7
[56] Vasquez A. Integrative Orthopedics: Concepts, Algorithms, and Therapeutics. The art of creating wellness while effectively managing acute and chronic musculoskeletal disorders. Natural Health Consulting Corporation: www.OptimalHealthResearch.com 2004, Revised edition August 2004, Second Edition 2007
[57] Vasquez A. Reducing Pain and Inflammation Naturally. Part 1: New Insights into Fatty Acid Biochemistry and the Influence of Diet. *Nutritional Perspectives* 2004; October: 5, 7-10, 12, 14 http://optimalhealthresearch.com/part1
[58] Trickett P. Proteolytic enzymes in treatment of athletic injuries. *Appl Ther*. 1964;30:647-52
[59] Kimmatkar N, Thawani V, Hingorani L, Khiyani R. Efficacy and tolerability of Boswellia serrata extract in treatment of osteoarthritis of knee--a randomized double blind placebo controlled trial. *Phytomedicine*. 2003 Jan;10(1):3-7
[60] "...subgroup analyses suggested that the effect was confined to patients with more severe and radiating pain accompanied by neurological deficit. ...a slightly different picture, with the benefits seeming, if anything, to be greatest in the H600 group and in patients without more severe pain, radiation or neurological deficit." Chrubasik S, Junck H, Breitschwerdt H, Conradt C, Zappe H. Effectiveness of Harpagophytum extract WS 1531 in the treatment of exacerbation of low-back pain: a randomized, placebo-controlled, double-blind study. *Eur J Anaesthesiol* 1999 Feb;16(2):118-29
[61] Chrubasik S, Eisenberg E, Balan E, Weinberger T, Luzzati R, Conradt C. Treatment of low-back pain exacerbations with willow bark extract: a randomized double-blind study. *Am J Med*. 2000;109:9-14
[62] Vasquez A, Muanza DN. Comment: Evaluation of Presence of Aspirin-Related Warnings with Willow Bark. *Ann Pharmacotherapy* 2005 Aug 30; [Epub ahead of print]
[63] Vasquez A. Reducing pain and inflammation naturally - Part 3: Improving overall health while safely and effectively treating musculoskeletal pain. *Nutritional Perspectives* 2005; 28: 34-38, 40-42 http://optimalhealthresearch.com/part3
[64] Robert Bly. The Human Shadow. Sound Horizons, New York 1991 [ISBN: 1879323001] and Bly R. A Little Book on the Human Shadow.[ISBN: 0062548476]
[65] Rick Jarow. Creating the Work You Love: Courage, Commitment and Career; Inner Traditions Intl Ltd; (December 1995) [ISBN: 0892815426]
[66] Walter Kaufmann (Translator), Friedrich Wilhelm Nietzsche. Thus Spoke Zarathustra. Penguin USA; 1978, page 27

Clinical Assessments

The clinical assessments reviewed in the following sections are history-taking, orthopedic/musculoskeletal, and neurologic examinations, and commonly used laboratory tests.

History taking is the art of conducting an *informative* and *collaborative* patient interview.

The role of the doctor during the interview process is not merely that of a data-collecting machine, spewing out questions and receiving responses. Patient interviews can be a creative, enjoyable, comforting opportunity to build rapport and to establish meaningful connection with another human being. Patients are not simply people with health problems – they are first and foremost our fellow human beings, not so dissimilar from ourselves perhaps, and always full of complexity. Our task is not to fully understand their complexity nor to solve all of their mysteries, but rather to help orchestrate these dynamics into a coordinated if not unified direction that promotes health and healing.

Patient Care: History, Comprehensive Assessment, Diagnosis, Treatment, and Management

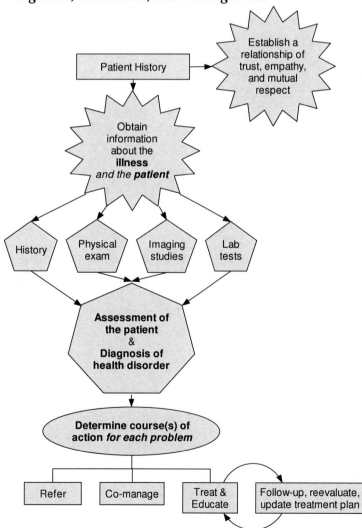

Patient History: Main Considerations
• **History of the primary complaint**: "D.O.P.P. Q.R.S.T."
o Description/location
o Onset
o Provocation: exacerbates
o Palliation: alleviates
o Quality
o Radiation of pain
o Severity
o Timing
• **Associated complaints**
o Additional manifestations
o Concomitant diseases
• **Review of systems**
o Head-to-toe inventory of health status, associated health problems, and complications
• **Past health history**
o Surgeries
o Hospitalizations
o Traumas
o Vaccinations and medications
o Successful and failed treatments for the current complaint(s)
• **Family health history**
o Genotropic illnesses and predispositions
o Lifestyle patterns
o Emotional expectations about health
• **Social history**
o Hobbies
o Relationships and emotional experiences
o Interpersonal support
o Occupation and work
o Malpractice litigation
• **Health Habits**
o Diet: appropriate intake of protein, fruits, vegetables, fats, sugars
o Sleep
o Stress management
o Exercise / Sedentary Lifestyle
o Spirituality / Centeredness
o Caffeine and tobacco
o Ethanol and recreational drugs
• **Medication and supplements**
o Reason, doses, duration, cost
o Side-effects
o Interactions
• **Responsibility and Compliance**
o Ability and willingness to comply with prescribed treatment plan and to incorporate the necessary diet-exercise-relationship-emotional-lifestyle modifications
o *Internal* versus *external* locus of control

Components of a Complete Patient History: "D.O.P.P. Q.R.S.T."

Category	Application and considerations
Description & Location: Always start with open-ended questions	• *What is it like for you?* • *What do you experience?* • *What are you feeling?* • *Where is the pain/sensation/problem)?* • Ask about specifics: **Pain, numbness, weakness, tingling,** fatigue, recent or chronic infections, burning, aching, dull, sharp, cramping, stretching, pins and needles, weakness, changes in function (i.e., bowel and bladder continence).
Onset	• *When did it begin?* • *Have you ever had anything like this before?* • *Was there a specific event associated with the onset of the problem, such as an injury or an illness, or did the problem start gradually or insidiously?* • *How has it changed over time?* • *Prior injuries to site?* • *Why are you seeking care for this now (rather than last week or last month)?* • *What has changed? How is the pain/problem developing over time—getting worse or getting better?*
Palliation	• *How have you tried treating it? Does anything make it go away?* • *What makes it better? What relieves the pain?* • Ask about prior and current treatments, radiographs, medications, supplements (herbs, vitamins, minerals), injections, surgery, massage, manipulation, counseling. • Knowing response/resistance to previous treatments can provide clinical insight.
Provocation	• *Are your symptoms constant, or does the problem come and go?* • *What makes it worse? What makes the pain worse?* • *When during the day/week/month/year are your symptoms the worst?*
Quality	• *Can you describe the pain to me?* • *What does it feel like?* • *What do you experience?* • Get a clear understanding of the type of sensation(s): stabbing, shooting pain, pins and needles, sharp pain, electric sensation, numbness, burning, aching, throbbing, weakness, tingling, gel phenomenon, dizziness, confusion, fatigue, shortness of breath.
Radiation	• *Does the pain stay localized or does it move to your arm/leg/head/face?* • *Do you feel pain in other areas of your body?*
Severity	• *How bad is it? How would you rate it on a scale of one to ten if one were almost no pain and ten was the worst pain you could imagine?* Use the validated VAS—visual analog scale—to quantify the level of pain and impairment. • *Does this problem prevent you from engaging in your daily activities, such as work, exercise, or hobbies?* This is a very important question for determining functional impairment and internal consistency; if the patient is "too injured to work" yet is still able to fully participate in recreational activities that are physically challenging, then malingering needs to be strongly considered.
Timing	• *When do you notice this problem?* • *Is it constant, or does it come and go?* • *Is it worse in the morning, or worse in the evening?* • *Worse during the week, or on the weekends?* • *Is it constant, or are there times when you notice that it is gone?* • *Where are you when you notice it the most?* • *Does anyone else in your [home/office/worksite] have this same problem?* • *What times of the day or what days of the week is it the worst?*

Category	Application and considerations
Associated manifestations and constitutional symptoms	• *Have you noticed any other problems associated with this problem?* • *Fatigue?* • *Fever?* • *Weight loss? Weight gain?* • *Night sweats?* • *Diarrhea? Constipation?* • *Weakness?* • *Nausea?* • *Bowel or bladder difficulties or changes? Difficulty with sexual function?* These could be related to hormonal imbalances, drug side-effects, relationship problems, nutritional deficiencies, nerve compression, and/or depression • *Change in sensation near your anus/genitals?* Cauda equina syndrome is an important consideration in patients with low-back pain • *Loss of appetite?* • *Difficulty sleeping?* • *Skin rash or change in pigmentation?*
ROS: review of systems	• <u>General constitution</u>: fatigue, malaise, fever, chills, weight gain/loss… • *"Now we are going to conduct a head-to-toe inventory just to make sure that we have covered everything."* • <u>Head</u>: headaches, head pain, pressure inside head, difficulty concentrating, difficulty remembering, mental function • <u>Ears</u>: ringing in ears, dizziness, hearing loss, hypersensitivity to noise, ear pain, discharge from ear, pressure in ears • <u>Eyes</u>: eye pain, loss of vision or decreased vision or ability to focus, redness or irritation, seeing flashing lights or spots, double vision • <u>Nose</u>: sinus problems, chronically stuffy nose, difficulty smelling things, nose bleeds, change or decrease in sense of smell or taste • <u>Mouth</u>, teeth, TMJ, pain or sores in mouth, difficulty chewing, sensitive teeth, bleeding gums, pain in jaw joint, change or decrease in sense of taste • <u>Neck</u>: pain at the base of skull, pain in neck, stiffness • <u>Throat</u>: difficulty swallowing, pain in throat, feeling like things get stuck in throat, change in voice, difficulty getting air or food in or out • <u>Chest and breasts</u>: any chest pain, difficult breathing, wheezing, coughing, pain, lumps, or discharge from nipple • <u>Shoulders</u>: pain or aching in your shoulders, restricted motion or stiffness • <u>Arms, elbows, hands</u>: pain or problems with your arms, elbows, hands, …in the joints or the muscles…, numbness, tingling, weakness, swelling, changes in fingernails, cold hands? • <u>Stomach, abdomen, pelvis, genitals, urinary tract, rectum, </u>: pain in stomach or abdomen, difficulty with digestion, gas, bloating, regurgitation, ulcer, any problems lower down in your abdomen—near your lower intestines? Pain, lumps, swelling, difficulty passing stool, pain or itching near your anus, genitalia; any genital pain, burning, discharge, redness, irritation, sexual dysfunction or impotence, loss of bowel or bladder control? Diarrhea or constipation? How often do you have a bowel movement? • <u>Hips, legs, knees, ankles, feet</u>: numbness, weakness, pain or tingling in the hips, knees, ankles, or feet; pain in calves with walking, swelling of ankles, cold feet • *Is there anything that I did not ask about that you think I should know in order to help you?*

Components of a Complete Patient History—*continued*

Category	Application and considerations

Medical history	• *Are you taking any **medications**? What medications have you taken in the past few years?* Finding out that your new patient recently discontinued his 20-year regimen of valproic acid, lithium, and risperidone may significantly change your interpretation of the clinical interview
	• *Have you been **treated for any medical conditions** or health problems?*
	• *Have you ever been **hospitalized**?*
	• *Have you ever had **surgery**?*
	• *Have you ever been **diagnosed with any health problems** such as high blood pressure or diabetes?*
	• Investigate for specific problems in the past health history that would be a major oversight to miss:
	   o Cancer
	   o Diabetes
	   o Allergies and arthritis
	   o Hypertension or high cholesterol
	   o Medications, especially corticosteroids
	   o Surgeries
	   o Hospitalizations
	   o Infections
	   o Trauma or previous injuries
	   o Mental illness

Social history	• **Work**—*What do you do for work? Are you exposed to chemicals or fumes at your workplace?* • **Hobbies**—*What do you do for recreation or hobbies? Are you exposed to chemicals or fumes at home or with your hobbies (e.g., painting, gardening)?* • **Eat**—*Tell me about your breakfast, lunch, dinner, snacks… Do you consume foods or drinks that contain NutraSweet/aspartame* (linked to increased incidence of brain tumors[67]) *or carrageenan* (possibly linked to increased risk of breast cancer and inflammatory bowel disease[68,69])? • **Exercise**—*What do you do for exercise or physical activity?* • **Drink**—*Do you **drink alcohol**? Coffee/caffeine? Water?* • **Drugs**—*Do you use recreational **drugs**? **Now or in the past?*** • **Smoke**—*Do you **smoke**?* • **Sex**—*Are you **sexually active**? If so, do you practice safer sex practices? For premenopausal women: Is there any chance you could be pregnant right now?* • **Emotional support** • **Family contact and relationships**
Family health history	• *Does anyone in your family have any health problems, especially your parents and siblings?* • *Do you have any children? Do they have any health problems?* • *Do any diseases "run in the family" such as cancer, diabetes, arthritis, heart disease?*
Additional questions	• *Do you have any other information for me?* • *Is there anything that I did not ask?* • *What is your opinion as to why you are having this health problem?* • *Are you in litigation for your illness or injuries?*

---

[67] "In the past two decades brain tumor rates have risen in several industrialized countries, including the United States... Compared to other environmental factors putatively linked to brain tumors, the artificial sweetener aspartame is a promising candidate to explain the recent increase in incidence and degree of malignancy of brain tumors." Olney JW, Farber NB, Spitznagel E, Robins LN. Increasing brain tumor rates: is there a link to aspartame? *J Neuropathol Exp Neurol* 1996 Nov;55(11):1115-23
[68] Tobacman JK. Review of harmful gastrointestinal effects of carrageenan in animal experiments. *Environ Health Perspect.* 2001 Oct;109(10):983-94
[69] "However, the gum carrageenan which is comprised of linked, sulfated galactose residues has potent biological activity and undergoes acid hydrolysis to poligeenan, an acknowledged carcinogen." Tobacman JK, Wallace RB, Zimmerman MB. Consumption of carrageenan and other water-soluble polymers used as food additives and incidence of mammary carcinoma. *Med Hypotheses.* 2001 May;56(5):589-98

Physical Examination

Goals and purpose of the orthopedic/musculoskeletal examination:
1. **To establish an accurate diagnosis (or diagnoses)**
2. **To assess the patient's functional status**
3. **To assess for concomitant and/or underlying and preexisting problems**
4. **To rule out emergency situations**
- *Example*: If your patient presents with low back and leg pain, and you determine that his fall off a horse resulted in ischial bursitis, have you also excluded a lumbar compression fracture? You can send the patient home with anti-inflammatories and ice packs for the bursitis; but if you missed the spinal fracture, your patient could suffer neurologic injury resultant from your "failure to diagnose." **Don't assume that the patient has only one problem until you have proven with your history and examination that other likely problems do not exist.**

Functional assessment: When working with patients with acute injuries and systemic diseases, **take a wider view of the patient than simply diagnosing the problem.**
- *Will she be able to return to work?*
- *Will he be able to drive home safely?*
- *Will she need help with activities of daily living?*
- *Is there an occult disease, infection, malignancy, or toxic exposure that is causing these problems?*

Neurologic examination: One of the most important areas to assess when a patient presents with a musculoskeletal complaint is the neurologic system, especially if the complaint is related to a recent traumatic injury. Blood circulation is essential for life; but lack of circulation is only a major consideration in a small number of injuries, and it is usually readily apparent when severe because the problem will become acute quickly. Nerve injuries, however, can be subtle and insidious. All patients with spine (neck, thoracic, low back) pain must be questioned thoroughly for evidence of neurologic compromise. Nerve injuries can be painless, can progress rapidly, and can lead to permanent functional disability from muscle weakness or paralysis. **Every patient with pain, weakness, or recent trauma must be evaluated for neurologic deficits before the patient is treated and released from care.** Neurologic examinations are briefly reviewed in the pages that follow; citations can be used for sources of additional information.

Resources for neurologic assessment:
- Goldberg S. The Four-Minute Neurologic Exam. Medmaster http://www.medmaster.net/
- http://www.neuroexam.com Information and free on-line videos of a neurologic exam
- http://rad.usuhs.mil/rad/eye_simulator/eyesimulator.html Excellent interactive simulation of assessment of extraocular muscles in a neurologic examination; important for visualizing the combination of lesions and the subtlety of clinical presentation
- http://www.pennhealth.com/health_info/animationplayer/ Many health-related animations
- http://www.emedicine.com/neuro/topic632.htm This is an excellent review, noteworthy for its description of a "+5" level of reflex grading that denotes sustained clonus; most textbooks use a 0-4 scale

Resources for neuroanatomy review:
- Fix JD. Neuroanatomy. Third Edition. BRS: Board Review Series. Lippincott Williams & Wilkins; 3rd edition (January 15, 2002); ISBN: 0781728290
- Goldberg S. Clinical Neuroanatomy Made Ridiculously Simple. Medmaster www.medmaster.net
- http://library.med.utah.edu/kw/animations/hyperbrain/pathways/index.html
- http://www9.biostr.washington.edu/da.html Excellent interactive neuroanatomy review
- http://www.neuroanatomy.wisc.edu/coursebook.html
- http://anatomy.med.umich.edu/bnb/Autonomics.html Animated review of the autonomic nervous system

Orthopedic Musculoskeletal Examination: Concepts and Goals

Orthopedic tests are detailed or reviewed in each respective chapter of <u>*Integrative Orthopedics*</u>[70] (i.e., shoulder exams are in the chapter on shoulders, knee exams in the chapter on knees). This section reviews the concepts and goals that provide the rationale for performing these tests. **Orthopedic tests are designed to place particular types of stress on specific body tissues.** Types of stress include tension/distraction, compression/pressure, shear force, vibration, friction, and percussion. Each type of stress is applied to elicit specific information about the exact tissue or structure that is being tested. **If you understand the reason for the type of stress that you are applying, and you are aware of the tissue/structure that you are testing, then you will find it much easier to perform the dozens of tests that are required in clinical practice.**

If you understand the "how" and the "why" then you won't be overwhelmed with named tests that otherwise appear illogical or superfluous. Except for certain tests that all doctors need to know, illogical and superfluous tests have intentionally been omitted from this text. The tests that are described here meet at least one of the following two criteria: 1) it is a common test that all doctors know and which you will need to know for the sake of communication and for passing your academic and licensing examinations, or 2) it is going to be a useful test in your clinical practice.

Type of stress	General application
Tension, traction	To provoke pain from injured/compromised tissues: tendons, muscles, ligaments, and nerves
Compression, pressure	To provoke pain from inflamed tissues; also used to assess for swelling and fluid accumulation in subcutaneous tissue, bursa, and joint spaces such as the knee
Shearing force	To test the integrity of ligaments and intervertebral discs
Vibration	To assess vibration sense (neurologic: peripheral nerves and dorsal columns) and screen for broken bones (orthopedic)
Friction, grinding	To elicit pain from injured tissues (cross-fiber friction) and articular surfaces (grinding tests)
Percussion, over bone and discs	To assess for bone fractures, bone infections, and acute disc injuries
Percussion, over peripheral nerves	To assess hypesthesia/tingling suggesting reduced threshold for depolarization secondary to nerve irritation or compression, i.e., Tinel's sign
Fulcrum tests	To assess for bone fractures: commonly the doctor's arm or a firm object is placed centrally under the bone in question and increasingly firm downward stress is applied to both ends of the bone to test for occult fracture
Torque, twisting	To test joint integrity (restriction or laxity) or for occult bone fracture (particularly of the digits)

Always remember that abnormalities found during the physical examination—particularly the neurologic examination—are often indicative of an underlying *nonmusculoskeletal* problem that must be identified or—at the very least—considered and then excluded by additional testing. For example, a patient **shoulder pain** and neurologic deficits found during the neuromusculoskeletal portion of your examination could have a **herniated cervical disc** as the underlying cause; but the cause could also be **syringomyelia**, or an **apical lung tumor** that is invading local bone and destroying the nerves of the brachial plexus.[71]

As a clinician, the successful management and treatment of your patients depends in large part on the following: ❶ **knowledge**: your ability to conceptualize broadly and to consider many *functional* and *pathologic* causes of your patient's complaints, ❷ **tact**: the efficiency and accuracy with which you assess, accept, and exclude the various differential diagnoses into your final working diagnosis from which your treatment, management, referral, and co-management decisions are made, ❸ **art**: your ability to create the changes in your patient's outlook, lifestyle, biochemistry, biomechanics/anatomy, and physiology to effect the desired outcome.

[70] Vasquez A. <u>Integrative Orthopedics: Concepts, Algorithms, and Therapeutics</u>. <u>www.OptimalHealthResearch.com</u>
[71] "Pancoast tumor has long been implicated as a cause of brachial plexopathy...The possibility of Pancoast lesion should be considered not only in the presence of brachial plexopathy, but also when C8 or T1 radiculopathy is found." Vargo MM, Flood KM. Pancoast tumor presenting as cervical radiculopathy. *Arch Phys Med Rehabil.* 1990 Jul;71(8):606-9

Neurologic Assessment

Clinical neurology is a complex area of study. However, for most doctors, knowledge of clinical neurology hinges on answering three questions:
- **Is this patient's presentation normal or abnormal?**
- **If it is abnormal, does it indicate a specific disease or lesion?**
- **Does this condition require referral to a specialist or emergency care?**

Every clinician needs thorough training in anatomy and clinical neurology to be competent in the management of patients, because even common problems such as "pain" and "fatigue" and "headache" may herald devastating neurologic illness that must be assessed accurately and managed skillfully. While a complete review of clinical neurology is beyond the scope of this text, the following section provides a basic review of the clinical essentials. Clinicians needing an efficient refresher course in clinical neurology are encouraged to read the concise review texts by Goldberg.[72,73]

<u>**Reliable indicators of organic neurologic disease**</u>: These cannot be feigned and must be assumed to reveal organic neurologic illness that **must be evaluated by a neurologist**:
- **Significant asymmetry of pupillary light reflex**
- **Ocular divergence**
- **Papilledema**
- **Marked nystagmus**
- **Muscle atrophy and fasciculation**
- **Muscle weakness with neurologic deficit**; upper motor neuron lesions (UMNL) indicate a CNS lesion and need to be fully evaluated, probably by a neurologist; the need for referral is less necessary in cases of chronic neuropathy of known cause

<u>**Purpose of Neurologic Examination and *Principle of Neurologic Localization***</u>:
The purpose of the neurologic examination is to qualify ("yes" or "no") the presence of a neurologic deficit, and—if present—to localize the lesion so that it can be further assessed with the proper laboratory, imaging, electrodiagnostic, or biopsy techniques. The following 9-point summary of localized lesions does not supplant independent studies of neurology and neuroanatomy but is useful for a quick clinically-relevant review.
1. **Cerebral cortex and internal capsule**: Neurologic deficit depends on location of lesion but is typically a combination of sensory/motor deficit and impaired higher neurologic function such as comprehension (superior temporal gyrus) or socially appropriate behavior (frontal lobe, ventral frontal gyri)
2. **Basal ganglia and striatal system**: Athetosis (lentiform nucleus: putamen and globus pallidus), (hemi)ballism (subthalamic nucleus), chorea (putamen), akinesia, bradykinesia, hypokinesia (lack of nigrostriatal dopamine)
3. **Cerebellum**: Ataxia, awkward clumsy execution of *intentional* motions; may have nystagmus, hypotonia
4. **Brainstem**: Cranial nerve deficit(s) with contralateral distal sensory and/or UMN motor deficits
5. **Spinal cord**: Cranial nerves and higher cortical functions are intact; lesion can be a combination of sensory and motor (UMN and LMN) deficits and the pattern distal to lesion may be a complete or incomplete pattern of sensory and motor deficits on one or both sides of body depending on area of spinal cord affected
6. **Nerve root**: Segmental unilateral motor deficit; dermatomal distribution pain or sensory disturbance
7. **Peripheral nerve**: Localized combination of sensory and motor deficits; may be bilateral or unilateral
8. **Neurmuscular junction**: Painless weakness and "fatigable weakness": weakness that *worsens* with repeated testing; typically involves cranial nerves first in myasthenia gravis; also consider Eaton-Lambert Syndrome (ELS: autoimmune neuromuscular junction disorder associated with occult malignancy; contrasts with myasthenia gravis in that ELS strength *increases* with repeated testing)
9. **Muscle disease**: Painless weakness, typically involving proximal hip/shoulder muscles first; elevated serum aldolase and (phospho)creatine kinase

---

[72] Goldberg S. <u>Clinical Neuroanatomy Made Ridiculously Simple</u>. Miami, Medimaster, Inc, 1990. Now in a third edition with interactive CD.
[73] Goldberg S. <u>The Four-Minute Neurologic Exam</u>. Miami, Medimaster, Inc, 1992

Cortex	Cerebellum
• <u>Orientation</u>: Person, place, time, situation. • <u>Mood and cooperation</u> • <u>Level of consciousness</u>: Alert, lethargic, stupor, coma (indirect assessment of reticular system in brainstem) • <u>Memory</u>: Remember objects or numbers; *recent* memory is most commonly affected by brain lesions: *What day of the month is it? How did you get here?* • <u>Mentation</u>: *Count backward from 100 by 7's.* • <u>Spelling</u>: *Spell the word "hand" backwards.* • <u>Stereognosis</u>: Identify by touch a familiar object such as a key or coin. • <u>Hoffman's reflex</u>: Doctor rapidly extends DIP of patient's middle finger and watches for patient's hand to perform grasp reflex; this test is performed for motor tract lesions involving the cerebral cortex, cerebellum, and upper motor neurons of the spinal cord. • <u>Pronator drift</u>: Supinated hands and arms outstretched forward for 30 seconds; doctor taps on palms; falling of hands and arms into pronation suggests UMNL. • <u>Babinski reflex</u>: Scraping the bottom of the foot results in splaying and flexing of the toes and extension (dorsiflexion) of the big toe; normal in infants.	• <u>Gait</u> (lesion: ataxia) • <u>Heel-to-toe walk</u> • <u>Tandem gait</u> • <u>Hand flip</u>, <u>foot tap</u> (lesion: dysdiadochokinesia) • <u>Finger-to-nose</u>: Patient reaches out to doctor's finger, then patient touches patient nose, then back to new location of doctor's finger. • <u>Heel-to-shin</u>: Slide heel along shin. • <u>Walk in circle around chair</u> • <u>Move eyes in a rapid "figure 8"</u>: Technique for provoking latent nystagmus • <u>Rhomberg's test</u>: Patient stands with feet close together and eyes closed; tests proprioception (peripheral nerves, dorsal columns, spinocerebellar tracts); vision (eyes open tests optic righting reflex) and coordinated motor activity (cerebellum).

Several of the above '"cerebral" deficits may also result from intoxicative, nutritional, or metabolic disorders rather than an organic irreversible physical lesion. Likewise "cerebellar" deficits may also result from lesion of the brainstem tracts/nuclei and cerebellar peduncles, rather than the cerebellum itself.

Deep tendon reflexes are summarized below and on the following page. Hyperreflexia is noted with upper motor neuron lesions (UMNL) in the cortex, subcortical nuclei, brainstem, or corticospinal tracts of the spinal cord, whereas hyporeflexia can result from lesions of lower motor neurons (LMNL) in spinal cord, peripheral nerves, as well as from sensory/afferent defects including diabetic neuropathy, vitamin B-12 deficiency, and Guillain-Barre disorder. Muscle strength should always be "five over five" to be considered normal, whereas in the testing of reflexes, symmetry/asymmetry is generally more important than the grade of response (except with sustained clonus). **Asymmetry of reflex or strength (especially when seen together) is never normal and requires clinical correlation and investigation.**

Deep tendon reflexes	*Muscle strength*
+5 <u>Hyperreflexia *with sustained clonus*</u>: Sustained clonus strongly suggests UMNL and requires investigation; most textbooks use a 0-4 scale, yet this 0-5 scale facilitates clear communication of observed lesions[74]	5/5 <u>*Normal*</u>: **Full strength: able to withstand gravity and full resistance**
+4 <u>Marked hyperreflexia</u>: Up to 4 beats of *unsustained* clonus may be normal[75]; suggests UMNL but may be caused by medications, electrolyte disturbances, etc.	4/5 <u>Partial strength</u>: Able to withstand gravity and partial resistance
+3 <u>Hyperreflexia</u>: More than normal	3/5 <u>Partial strength</u>: Only able to resist gravity
+2 <u>*Normal*</u>: **Neither hyporeflexia nor hyperreflexia**	2/5 <u>Partial strength</u>: Able to contract muscle but unable to resist gravity
+1 <u>Hyporeflexia</u>: Less than normal	1/5 <u>Slight flicker of muscle contraction</u>: Does not result in joint movement
0 <u>No reflex</u>: Requires clinical correlation for lesion of sensory receptors, peripheral nerve, spinal cord, anterior horn, or neuromuscular junction; this is a common finding in normal individuals	0/5 <u>No clinically detectable contraction</u>: Correlate with lesion of peripheral nerve, cord, cerebrum, anterior horn, or neuromuscular junction

---

[74] Oommen K, edited by Berman SA, et al. Neurological History and Physical Examination. Last Updated: October 4, 2006. *eMedicine* http://www.emedicine.com/neuro/topic632.htm
[75] "…three to four beats of clonus can be elicited at the ankles in some normal individuals." Waxman SG. <u>Clinical Neuroanatomy 25th Edition</u>. McGraw Hill Medical, New York, 2003, p 325

Brainstem and Cranial Nerves	**Spinal Cord, Roots, Nerves**

Brainstem and Cranial Nerves

1. Olfactory: **smell**
   - Smell: Test with strong and common odors such as coffee; do not use ammonia or other irritants which are perceived via trigeminal nerve (cranial nerve 5)
   - This is a worthwhile test in patients with recent head trauma (direct or indirect) such as from motor vehicle accidents (MVA); any violent motion of the head may result in injury to the olfactory fibers passing through the cribiform plate; patients may have associated anosmia or altered sense of flavor; frontal lobe disorders such as altered social behavior may be noted in lesioned patients

2. Ophthalmic: **reading, peripheral vision, fundoscopic**
   - Snellen chart for far vision, Rosenbaum card for near vision
   - Peripheral vision
   - Fundoscopic examination

3. Oculomotor: **move eyes and constrict pupils**
   - Eye motion in cardinal fields of gaze
   - Pupil contraction to light
   - Pupil contraction to accommodation

4. Trochlear: **motor to superior oblique**
   - Look "down and in" toward nose

5. Trigeminal: **bite, sensory to face and eyes**
   - Bite (motor to muscles of mastication)
   - Feel (sensory to face, eyes, and tongue)

6. Abducens: **motor to lateral rectus**
   - Looks laterally to the ear

7. Facial: **face muscles and taste to anterior tongue**
   - Furrow forehead
   - Close eyes
   - Smile and frown
   - Taste to anterior tongue

8. Vestibulocochlear: **hearing and balance**
   - Hearing and Rinne-Weber tests, useful if hearing loss is present[76]
   - Balance: observe gait and Romberg test

9. Glossopharyngeal: **swallowing, and gag reflex**
   - Swallow
   - Gag reflex (sensory component)

10. Vagus: **motor to palate**
    - Say "ahh" to raise uvula
    - Gag reflex (motor component)

11. Spinal accessory: **motor to SCM and trapezius**
    - Raise your shoulders (against resistance)
    - Turn your head (against resistance)

12. Hypoglossal: **motor to tongue**
    - Stick out tongue to front

Spinal Cord, Roots, Nerves

Motor and reflex
   - Strength: Specific muscles are tested and rated 0-5
   - Plantar (Babinski) reflex: Signifies UMNL
   - Abdominal reflexes: "Present" or "absent" (not rated 0-4); superficial reflexes are lost (rather than hyperactive) with UMNL
       o Upper abdominal: T8-10
       o Lower abdominal: T10-12
   - Anal reflex: Cauda equina and sacral nerve roots
   - Reflexes: Rate 0-4; asymmetric reflexes are more significant than finding absent or hyperactive (+3) reflexes; +4 reflex with sustained clonus is almost always pathologic and requires neurologist referral. Deep tendon reflexes with main spinal root levels are as follows:
       o Biceps: C5
       o Brachioradialis: C6
       o Triceps: C7
       o Patellar: L3-L4
       o Hamstring: L5
       o Achilles: S1

Sensory
   - Light touch
   - Two-point discrimination
   - Vibration (tested with 128 Hz tuning fork)
   - Joint position sense and proprioception (eyes closed, locate position of joint)
   - Sharp and dull
   - Hot and cold
   - Sensory loss mapping (if deficits are found)
   - Romberg (peripheral nerves, dorsal columns, vestibular, cerebellar)
   - Nerve root tension tests such as straight leg raising
   - *Subjective pain and discomfort can be indicated on pain diagrams and VAS (visual analog scale) as shown on the following page*

---

[76] "The Rinne and Weber tuning fork tests are the most important tools in distinguishing between conductive and sensorineural hearing loss." Ruckenstein MJ. Hearing loss. A plan for individualized management. *Postgrad Med.* 1995 Oct;98(4):197-200, 203, 206

Patients can be asked to <u>localize</u> and <u>describe</u> their pain/discomfort on drawings such as these.
Examples of descriptions:

- Numb
- Hypersensitive
- Tingling

- Shooting pain
- Electrical pain
- Stabbing pain

- Burning pain
- Dull ache
- Muscle weakness

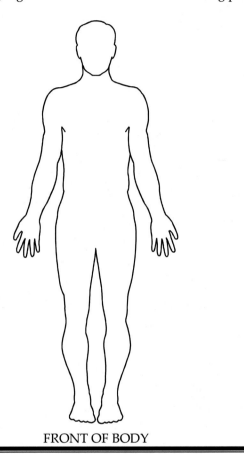

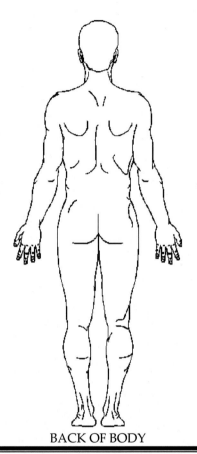

FRONT OF BODY   BACK OF BODY

On the lines below, indicate which pain/discomfort you are referring to and then quantify it by placing an "X" on the line.

Location of pain:_____

|—————————————————————————————————————|

No pain at all   Worst pain imaginable

Location of pain:_____

|—————————————————————————————————————|

No pain at all   Worst pain imaginable

Laboratory Assessments: General Considerations of Commonly Used Tests

"The laboratory evaluation of patients with rheumatic disease is often informative but rarely definitive."[77]

Laboratory tests are immensely important in evaluating patients with musculoskeletal pain, as these tests allow you to 1) assess for infection (e.g., subacute osteomyelitis), 2) quantify the degree of inflammation (i.e., with CRP or ESR), 3) assess or exclude other disease processes that may be the cause of pain or dysfunction, and 4) assess for concomitant diseases (e.g., septic arthritis complicating rheumatoid arthritis). Additionally, 5) these tests open the door to more complete patient care and holistic management of the whole person because they allow for a more comprehensive and complete understanding of the patient's underlying physiology. **The recommended routine is to use the following panel of tests when assessing patients with musculoskeletal pain: 1) CBC, 2) CRP, 3) chemistry/metabolic panel, and preferably also 4) ferritin, 5) 25(OH)-vitamin D, and 6) thyroid assessment, minimally including TSH** and optimally including free T4 and anti-thyroid antibodies. The use of this screening evaluation on a routine basis helps identify patients with occult diseases and also allows for more comprehensive management of the patient's overall health. Other tests are indicated in specific situations. *Orthopedics* relies heavily upon physical examination and imaging, whereas *rheumatology* relies more heavily upon laboratory analysis. In orthopedics, laboratory tests are used mainly for the purposes of discovering or excluding rheumatic and systemic diseases. In rheumatolgy, lab tests are used to specifically identify the type of illness, quantify the severity of the condition, and to assess for concomitant illnesses and complications.

Overview of Commonly Used Screening Laboratory Tests in the Evaluation of Patients with Musculoskeletal Complaints

Essential Tests: These Tests are Required for Basic Patient Assessment

Test	Purpose	Clinical application
CRP (or ESR)	Screening for **infection, inflammation**, and possibly **cancer**; if inflammation is present, then these tests allow for a generalized quantification of severity.	**Useful in all new patients** for helping to differentiate systemic/inflammatory disorders from those which are noninflammatory and mechanical. Also very helpful as a general "barometer" of health since higher values correlate with increased risk for diabetes mellitus and cardiovascular disease; thus this test helps bridge the gap between acute care and wellness promotion.
CBC	Screening for **anemia, infection**, certain cancers (namely **leukemia**).	Useful in any patient with **nontraumatic musculoskeletal pain** or **systemic manifestations**, especially **fever or weight loss;** commonly detects occult B-12 and folate deficiencies.
Chemistry panel	Screening for **diabetes, liver disease, kidney failure**, bone lesions (alkaline phosphatase), **electrolyte disturbances,** adrenal insufficiency (hyponatremia with hyperkalemia), **hyperparathyroidism, hypercalcemia.**	Any patient with **nontraumatic musculoskeletal pain** or **systemic manifestations**; all patients with **hypertension, diabetes**, or who use **medications** that cause **hepatotoxicity, nephrotoxicity,** etc.

---

[77] Klippel JH (ed). Primer on the Rheumatic Diseases. 11th Edition. Atlanta: Arthritis Foundation. 1997 page 94

Overview of Important Tests: Common Components of Routine Evaluation

Test	Purpose	Clinical Application
Ferritin	Important for assessing for **iron overload** (e.g., hemochromatoic polyarthropathy), and **iron deficiency** (e.g., low back pain due to colon cancer metastasis). Ferritin values less than 20 or greater than 200 in women and 300 in men necessitate evaluation and effective treatment.	Ferritin is the ideal test for both iron overload and iron deficiency. All patients should be screened for hemochromatosis and other hereditary forms of iron overload regardless of age, gender, or ethnicity.[78] Iron deficiency—particularly in adults—may be the first clue to gastric/colon cancer and generally necessitates referral to gastroenterologist.
25(OH)D	**Vitamin D deficiency is a common cause of musculoskeletal pain and inflammation**[79,80], and vitamin D deficiency is a significant risk factor for cancer and other serious health problems.[81,82,83]	Measurement of serum 25(OH) vitamin D (or empiric treatment with 2,000 – 4,000 IU vitamin D3 per day for adults) is indicated in patients with chronic musculoskeletal pain.[84,85] Optimal vitamin D status correlates with serum 25(OH)D levels of 40 – 65 ng/mL (100 - 160 nmol/L).[86]
TSH	Hypothyroidism is a common problem and is an often overlooked cause of musculoskeletal pain.[87]	This is a reasonable test for any patient with fatigue, cold extremities, depression, "arthritis", muscle pain, hypercholesterolemia, or other manifestations of hypothyroidism.
ANA	Sensitive for the detection of several autoimmune diseases, especially systemic lupus erythematosus.	This test is particularly valuable for assessing patients with polyarthropathy, facial rash, and/or fatigue.
Rheumatoid factor (RF)	The primary value of this test is in supporting a diagnosis of rheumatoid arthritis; specificity is low.	RF may be positive in normal health, iron overload, chronic infections, hepatitis, sarcoidosis, and bacterial endocarditis.
Citrullinated protein antibodies (CPA)	Citrullinated protein antibodies become present before the clinical onset of rheumatoid arthritis.	Citrullinated protein antibodies are rapidly becoming *the test* for diagnosing and confirming rheumatoid arthritis; used with RF for highly specific "conjugate seropositivity."
Lactulose-mannitol assay	Assesses for malabsorption and excess intestinal permeability—"leaky gut."	Diagnostic test for intestinal damage; screening test for pathology or pathophysiology
Comprehensive parasitology, stool analysis	Identification and quantification of intestinal yeast, bacteria, and other microbes.	Extremely valuable test when working with patients with chronic fatigue syndromes or autoimmunity; see Chapter 4 of *Integrative Rheumatology*.

[78] Vasquez A. Musculoskeletal disorders and iron overload disease: comment on the American College of Rheumatology guidelines for the initial evaluation of the adult patient with acute musculoskeletal symptoms. *Arthritis Rheum* 1996;39: 1767-8
[79] Masood H, Narang AP, Bhat IA, Shah GN. Persistent limb pain and raised serum alkaline phosphatase the earliest markers of subclinical hypovitaminosis D in Kashmir. *Indian J Physiol Pharmacol.* 1989 Oct-Dec;33(4):259-61
[80] Al Faraj S, Al Mutairi K. Vitamin D deficiency and chronic low back pain in Saudi Arabia. *Spine.* 2003 Jan 15;28(2):177-9
[81] Grant WB. An estimate of premature cancer mortality in the U.S. due to inadequate doses of solar ultraviolet-B radiation. *Cancer.* 2002 Mar 15;94(6):1867-75
[82] Zittermannn A. Vitamin D in preventive medicine: are we ignoring the evidence? *Br J Nutr.* 2003 May;89(5):552-72
[83] Holick MF. Vitamin D: importance in the prevention of cancers, type 1 diabetes, heart disease, and osteoporosis. *Am J Clin Nutr.* 2004 Mar;79(3):362-71
[84] Plotnikoff GA, Quigley JM. Prevalence of severe hypovitaminosis D in patients with persistent, nonspecific musculoskeletal pain. *Mayo Clin Proc.* 2003 Dec;78(12):1463-70
[85] Al Faraj S, Al Mutairi K. Vitamin D deficiency and chronic low back pain in Saudi Arabia. *Spine.* 2003 Jan 15;28(2):177-9
[86] Vasquez A, Manso G, Cannell J. The Clinical Importance of Vitamin D (Cholecalciferol): A Paradigm Shift with Implications for All Healthcare Providers. *Alternative Therapies in Health and Medicine* 2004; 10: 28-37. Also published in *Integrative Medicine: A Clinician's Journal* 2004; 3: 44-54. See www.optimalhealthresearch.com/monograph04
[87] "Hypothyroidism is frequently accompanied by musculoskeletal manifestations ranging from myalgias and arthralgias to true myopathy and arthritis." McLean RM, Podell DN. Bone and joint manifestations of hypothyroidism. *Semin Arthritis Rheum.* 1995 Feb;24(4):282-90

CRP: C-reactive protein

Overview and interpretation:	- CRP is a protein made by the liver in response to the immunologic activation characteristic of infectious and inflammatory conditions. Generally, any tissue injury or inflammatory process especially that involves the immune system's increased production of IL-6 will result in increased production of CRP.[88] High sensitivity CRP (hsCRP) is preferred over normal CRP due to its greater sensitivity and use in assessing cardiovascular risk.
	
	- Elevated values are seen with:
	  - <u>Infections</u>: Bacterial, fungal, parasitic, viral diseases; some patients with dysbiosis[89] will have mildly-moderately elevated CRP
	  - <u>Inflammatory bowel disease</u>: Crohn's disease and ulcerative colitis (higher in CD than UC)
	  - <u>Autoimmune disease</u>: Rheumatoid arthritis, polymyalgia rheumatica, giant cell arteritis, polyarteritis nodosa, (not always SLE)
	  - <u>Acute myocardial infarction or other tissue ischemia</u>
	  - <u>Organ transplant rejection</u>: Renal, (NOT cardiac)
	  - <u>Trauma</u>: Burns, surgery
	  - <u>Obesity</u>: Leads to modest elevations in CRP

Advantages:	- This is an excellent screening test for differentiating "serious problems" (e.g., inflammatory and infectious arthropathy) from "benign problems" such as osteoarthritis. - Since higher values of CRP are a well-recognized risk factor for cardiovascular disease, screening "musculoskeletal patients" with hsCRP provides data for cardiovascular risk assessment and a more comprehensive and holistic treatment approach, thus bridging the gap between acute care and preventive care.
Limitations:	- Elevations in CRP are completely nonspecific, requiring clinical investigation to determine the underlying cause of the immune activation. - CRP may be normal in some patients with severe systemic diseases (such as lupus or cancer), and therefore a normal CRP does not entirely exclude the presence of significant illness.
Comments:	- Writing in *The New England Journal of Medicine*, authors Gabay and Kushner[90] note that measurements of plasma or serum **C-reactive protein can help differentiate inflammatory from non-inflammatory conditions and are useful in managing the patient's disease, since "the concentration often reflects the response to and the need for therapeutic intervention."** Additionally, they note, "Most normal subjects have plasma C-reactive protein concentrations of 2 mg per liter or less, but some have concentrations as high as 10 mg per liter." Deodhar[91] noted that **"Any clinical disease characterized by tissue injury and/or inflammation is accompanied by significant elevation of serum CRP…"** and that **CRP should replace ESR as a method of laboratory evaluation.** Deodhar also noted that **some patients with severe SLE will have normal CRP levels.**

[88] Deodhar SD. C-reactive protein: the best laboratory indicator available for monitoring disease activity. *Cleve Clin J Med* 1989 Mar-Apr;56(2):126-30
[89] See Chapter 4 of *Integrative Rheumatology* and Vasquez A. Reducing Pain and Inflammation Naturally. Part 6: Nutritional and Botanical Treatments Against "Silent Infections" and Gastrointestinal Dysbiosis, Commonly Overlooked Causes of Neuromusculoskeletal Inflammation and Chronic Health Problems. *Nutr Perspect* 2006; Jan http://optimalhealthresearch.com/part6
[90] Gabay C, Kushner I. Acute-phase proteins and other systemic responses to inflammation. *N Engl J Med.* 1999 Feb 11;340(6):448-54
[91] Deodhar SD. C-reactive protein: the best laboratory indicator available for monitoring disease activity. *Cleve Clin J Med* 1989 Mar-Apr;56(2):126-30

ESR: erythrocyte sedimentation rate

Overview and interpretation:	▪ Values may be elevated even when no pathology is present because ESR increases with anemia and with age.
	
	▪ Much more sensitive than WBC count when screening for infection.[92]
	
	▪ May be normal in about 10% of patients who have pathology such as **giant cell arteritis** and **polymyalgia rheumatica** (conditions where it is generally the only lab abnormality); may also be normal in several other diseases.
	
	▪ **May be normal in patients with septic arthritis and patients with crystal-induced arthritis: joint aspiration for synovial fluid analysis is indicated if septic arthritis is suspected.**[93]
	
	▪ Increased with age, anemia, inflammation; higher in women than men. Age-adjusted normal ranges: any value over 25 is considered high in young people, or 40 in elderly women.
	
	▪ Age-related adjustments for men and women are as follows:
	   ○ MEN: age divided by 2
	   ○ WOMEN: (age + 10) divided by 2

Advantages:	▪ Inexpensive and easy to perform—use the same lavender-topped tube that you use for CBC. ▪ Provides a quick screen for infection, inflammation, and multiple myeloma—the most common primary bone tumor in adults. ▪ In patients with elevated levels, ESR can be used to monitor progression of disease and response to treatment.[94] However, a negative/normal test result does not exclude the presence of significant disease; some noteworthy examples include the following: 1) elderly—due to diminished ability to mount an inflammatory response, 2) patients taking anti-inflammatory drugs and immunosuppressants, 3) a significant proportion of patients with lupus will have normal ESR despite aggressive disease, and 4) many cancer patients with clinically significant tumor burden will not show signs of systemic inflammation. ▪ **ESR may be more reliable than CRP for multiple myeloma.**[95]
Limitations:	▪ ESR may be normal in a subset of patients with clinically significant infection or inflammation. ▪ Values are elevated in the elderly and patients with anemia and are thus not necessarily indicative of disease in these populations.
Comments:	▪ **This test is generally considered *outdated* and has been replaced in most circumstances by CRP for the evaluation of inflammation and infection.** ▪ **The only time I use this test clinically is when I am highly suspicious of inflammation and the CRP is normal. Further, this test may be preferred when assessing for temporal arteritis and for multiple myeloma, two conditions which are classically associated with elevated ESR.**

[92] Shaw BA, Gerardi JA, Hennrikus WL. How to avoid orthopedic pitfalls in children. *Patient Care* 1999; Feb 28: 95-116
[93] Klippel JH (ed). Primer on the Rheumatic Diseases. 11ᵗʰ Edition. Atlanta: Arthritis Foundation. 1997 page 94
[94] Shojania K. Rheumatology: 2. What laboratory tests are needed? *CMAJ*. 2000 Apr 18;162(8):1157-63 http://www.cmaj.ca/cgi/content/full/162/8/1157
[95] "We conclude that ESR, a simple and easily performed marker, was found to be an independent prognostic factor for survival in patients with multiple myeloma." Alexandrakis MG, Passam FH, Ganotakis ES, Sfiridaki K, Xilouri I, Perisinakis K, Kyriakou DS. The clinical and prognostic significance of erythrocyte sedimentation rate (ESR), serum interleukin-6 (IL-6) and acute phase protein levels in multiple myeloma. *Clin Lab Haematol*. 2003 Feb;25(1):41-6

CBC: complete blood count

Overview and interpretation:	This test measures numbers and indices of white and red blood cells and platelets:
	
	• WBC (white blood cells): The primary value of the WBC count in patients with musculoskeletal pain is that it allows screening assessment for 1) infection and 2) hematologic malignancies such as leukemia. **However, relying on the WBC count for the assessment of infection is potentially problematic since it is elevated in less than 50% of patients with acute and chronic musculoskeletal infections.** *"Therefore, it is helpful when it is high, but potentially misleading when it is normal."*[96] Be alert to the possibility of gaining additional information by assessing quantitative WBC indices associated with neutrophils, lymphocytes, and eosinophils, elevations of which may suggest bacterial infections, viral infections, or allergic or parasitic conditions, respectively.
	
	• RBC (red blood cells and associated indices): In most clinical situations you are looking for anemia, which may be related to:
	
	  o Nutritional deficiency of B-12 or folate: My approach is to critique the MCV and to interpret MCV values greater than 90 with an increased suspicion of folate and/or B-12 deficiency. Clinical experience has shown that MCV values greater than 95 correlate with increased homocysteine levels, and a clinical response (improvement in mood, energy, and a reduction in MCV) is commonly seen following three months of nutritional supplementation. Deficiency of vitamin B-12 can easily be treated with oral administration of 2,000 mcg per day of vitamin B-12.[97] I generally rely on 5-20 mg per day of oral folate for the treatment of probable or documented folic acid deficiency since such a modest dose is clearly effective for correcting folate insufficiency while also being safe for most patients (excluding those on antiepileptic drugs).[98] B-12 and folic acid *function together* and should be *administered together*.
	
	  o Iron deficiency (confirmed with assessment of serum ferritin): While inadequate intake, malabsorption, or menstrual bleeding may cause iron deficiency, **adult patients with iron deficiency are at higher probability for gastrointestinal pathology and should therefore be evaluated with endoscopy or other comprehensive assessment** *beyond fecal occult-blood testing* to rule out **gastrointestinal disease.**[99,100] **The standard of care for all healthcare professionals is that adult patients with iron deficiency are referred for gastroenterological evaluation to evaluate for occult gastric or colon cancer.**
	
	  o **The anemia of chronic disease:** Generally associated with a corresponding disease history such as long-term rheumatoid arthritis and often associated with increased ESR/CRP and ferritin. **Do not assume that an anemic patient has iron deficiency until proven with measurement of serum ferritin.**

Advantages:	• Inexpensive and easy to perform. • Allows a quick screen for leukemia, infection, and for provisional evidence of B-12/folate and iron deficiencies.
Limitations:	• WBC count may be normal even in patients with serious infections. • RBC indices may be normal in people with clinically significant nutritional deficiencies. Ferritin should be used to confirm iron deficiency—*I have seen many patients with no evidence of anemia on the CBC, yet they have ferritin values less than 6 mcg/L, clearly indicating iron deficiency.*
Comments:	• This test is part of a routine assessment for all new patients.

[96] Shaw BA, Gerardi JA, Hennrikus WL. How to avoid orthopedic pitfalls in children. *Patient Care* 1999; Feb 28: 95-116
[97] "In cobalamin deficiency, 2 mg of cyanocobalamin administered orally on a daily basis was as effective as 1 mg administered intramuscularly on a monthly basis and may be superior." Kuzminski AM, Del Giacco EJ, Allen RH, Stabler SP, Lindenbaum J. Effective treatment of cobalamin deficiency with oral cobalamin. *Blood* 1998 Aug 15;92(4):1191-8 http://www.bloodjournal.org/cgi/content/full/92/4/1191
[98] "PGA administered in doses up to 1,000 mg orally a day… The folate was well absorbed, as reflected by marked increases in the serum and erythrocyte folate concentrations… There was no evidence of clinical or laboratory toxicity at these high doses of folate." Boss GR, Ragsdale RA, Zettner A, Seegmiller JE. Failure of folic acid (pteroylglutamic acid) to affect hyperuricemia. *J Lab Clin Med* 1980 Nov;96(5):783-9
[99] Rockey DC, Cello JP. Evaluation of the gastrointestinal tract in patients with iron-deficiency anemia. *N Engl J Med.* 1993;329(23):1691-5
[100] "Endoscopy revealed a clinically important lesion in 23 (12%) of 186 patients. … CONCLUSIONS: Endoscopy yields important findings in premenopausal women with iron deficiency anemia, which should not be attributed solely to menstrual blood loss." Bini EJ, Micale PL, Weinshel EH. Evaluation of the gastrointestinal tract in premenopausal women with iron deficiency anemia. *Am J Med.* 1998 Oct;105(4):281-6

Chemistry/metabolic panel	
Overview and interpretation:	▪ Measures glucose, electrolytes, markers for kidney and liver function, and other parameters. ▪ Requires knowledge and pattern-recognition by the doctor to translate numbers into differential diagnoses that are correlated with the clinical presentation, examination and imaging findings to arrive at probable diagnoses.
Advantages:	▪ Inexpensive and easy to perform—use serum separator tube. ▪ Provides a quick screen for diabetes, hepatitis, renal insufficiency, alcohol abuse, hyperparathyroidism, and other problems.

Limitation and considerations:	▪ <u>Liver enzymes</u>: may be normal in patients with chronic viral hepatitis, hemochromatosis, or other cause of ongoing liver damage.
	▪ <u>Hypercalcemia</u>: some of the more common causes in clinical practice are:
	   1) <u>Calcium-sparing diuretics</u>: Such as hydrochlorothiazide
	   2) <u>Hyperparathyroidism</u>: Assess by measuring parathyroid hormone
	   3) <u>Sarcoidosis</u>: Begin investigation with lab evaluation and chest radiograph
	   4) <u>Vitamin D excess</u>: Measure 25-OH-vitamin D
	   5) <u>Multiple myeloma</u>: ESR and serum electrophoresis
	   6) <u>Lymphoma or cancer</u>: Assess with imaging, lab tests, clinical correlation, referral
	▪ <u>BUN and creatinine</u>: may be normal in patients with early kidney failure—always assess with urinalysis if renal insufficiency is suspected, such as in diabetic or hypertensive patients. Conversely, BUN and creatinine may be significantly elevated—mimicking renal failure—simply by dehydration.

Comments:	▪ Abnormalities need to be pursued—repeat test within 2-4 weeks as part of routine follow-up along with additional investigation. ▪ Many ill patients (such as those with chronic fatigue syndrome, fibromyalgia, etc) will have normal results with the metabolic panel. Therefore, normal results do not ensure that the patient is healthy.

Complement C3 and C4	
Overview and interpretation:	▪ Complement proteins are consumed in the complement cascades (typically activated by immune complexes) and thus low levels of complement proteins provide indirect evidence of extensive consumption due to immune complex-mediated inflammation. **Low levels of complement are seen with immune complex disorders (such as SLE, vasculitis, mixed cryoglobulinemia, rheumatoid vasculitis, glomerulonephritis) and inherited complement deficiencies.** ▪ 10%–15% of Caucasian patients with SLE have an inherited complement deficiency.[101]
Advantages:	▪ Low complement levels provide indirect evidence of immune complex-mediated inflammation.
Limitations:	▪ Some patients have a hereditary absence of complement proteins and thus their levels are always abnormally low; obviously the test cannot be used in these patients for monitoring inflammatory disease.

---

[101] Shojania K. Rheumatology: 2. What laboratory tests are needed? *CMAJ.* 2000 Apr 18;162(8):1157-63 http://www.cmaj.ca/cgi/content/full/162/8/1157

Ferritin	
Overview and interpretation:	▪ Ferritin levels are directly proportional to body iron stores, except in patients with inflammation, infection, hepatitis, or cancer. Therefore, **measuring ferritin allows assessment for iron deficiency (as a cause of fatigue, or early manifestation of colon cancer) and allows for assessment of iron overload (as a cause of joint pain and arthropathy).** This test should be performed in all African Americans[102,103], white men over age 30 years[104], diabetics[105], and patients with peripheral arthropathy[106] (i.e., pain in one or more joints, such as the hands, wrists, knees, hips, shoulders, shoulders, elbows, ankles, or feet), and exercise-associated joint pain[107,108] The research also justifies testing children[109], women[110], young adults[111] and the general asymptomatic public.[112] ▪ Low ferritin = iron deficiency ▪ High ferritin = iron overload, cancer, inflammation, infection, and/or hepatitis (viral, alcoholic, or toxic)
Advantages:	▪ Reliable screening test for iron overload when used in conjunction with patient assessment and evidence (e.g., normal CRP) of no infection or acute phase response. ▪ This is the blood test of choice for iron deficiency *and* iron overload.
Limitations:	▪ Iron-deficient patients with an acute phase response may have a falsely normal level of ferritin since ferritin is an acute phase reactant and will be elevated *disproportionate to iron status* during inflammation. ▪ Elevations of ferritin (i.e., >200 mcg/L in women and >300 mcg/L in men) need to be retested along with CRP (to rule out false elevation due to excessive inflammation) before making the presumptive diagnosis of iron overload. **In the absence of significant inflammation, ferritin values >200 mcg/L in women and >300 mcg/L in men indicate iron overload and the need for treatment regardless of the absence of symptoms or end-stage complications.**[113]
Comments:	▪ Note that since ferritin is an acute-phase reactant, a high level of serum ferritin by itself does not allow differentiation between iron overload, infection, and the inflammation associated with tissue injury or metastatic disease. Ferritin must be evaluated within the context of the patient's clinical condition and the assessment of at least one other marker for inflammation such as CRP. If the patient is not acutely ill or has not recently suffered tissue injury (e.g., myocardial infarction) and the CRP is normal, then an elevated ferritin value indicates iron overload until proven otherwise with diagnostic phlebotomy, which is safer and less expensive than liver biopsy or MRI. ▪ Transferrin saturation can also be measured when the interpretation of ferritin is unclear. By itself, serum iron is unreliable.

[102] Barton JC, Edwards CQ, Bertoli LF, Shroyer TW, Hudson SL. Iron overload in African Americans. *Am J Med.* 1995 Dec;99(6):616-23
[103] Wurapa RK, Gordeuk VR, Brittenham GM, Khiyami A, Schechter GP, Edwards CQ. Primary iron overload in African Americans. *Am J Med.* 1996;101(1):9-18
[104] Baer DM, Simons JL, Staples RL, Rumore GJ, Morton CJ. Hemochromatosis screening in asymptomatic ambulatory men 30 years of age and older. *Am J Med.* 1995 May;98(5):464-8
[105] Phelps G, Chapman I, Hall P, Braund W, Mackinnon M. Prevalence of genetic haemochromatosis among diabetic patients. *Lancet* 1989; 2: 233-4
[106] Olynyk J, Hall P, Ahern M, KwiatekR, MackinnonM. Screening for hemochromatosis in a rheumatology clinic. *Aust NZ J Med* 1994; 24: 22-5
[107] McCurdie I, Perry JD. Haemochromatosis and exercise related joint pains. *BMJ.* 1999 Feb 13;318(7181):449-5
[108] "RESULTS: Our findings indicate a high prevalence of HFE gene mutations in this population (49.2%) compared with sedentary controls (33.5%). No association was detected in the athletes between mutations and blood iron markers. CONCLUSIONS: The findings support the need to assess regularly iron stores in elite endurance athletes." Chicharro JL, Hoyos J, Gomez-Gallego F, Villa JG, Bandres F, Celaya P, Jimenez F, Alonso JM, Cordova A, Lucia A. Mutations in the hereditary haemochromatosis gene HFE in professional endurance athletes. *Br J Sports Med.* 2004 Aug;38(4):418-21. Erratum in: *Br J Sports Med.* 2004 Dec;38(6):793 http://bjsm.bmjjournals.com/cgi/content/full/38/4/418 Accessed September 12, 2005
[109] Kaikov Y, Wadsworth LD, Hassall E, Dimmick JE, Rogers PCJ. Primary hemochromatosis in children: report of three newly diagnosed cases and review of the pediatric literature. *Pediatrics* 1992; 90: 37-42
[110] Edwards CQ, Kushner JP. Screening for hemochromatosis. *N Engl J Med* 1993; 328: 1616-20
[111] Gushusrt TP, Triest WE. Diagnosis and management of precirrhotic hemochromatosis. *W Virginia Med J* 1990; 86: 91-5
[112] Balan V, Baldus W, Fairbanks V, et al. Screening for hemochromatosis: a cost-effectiveness study based on 12, 258 patients. *Gastroenterology* 1994; 107: 453-9
[113] Barton JC, McDonnell SM, Adams PC, Brissot P, Powell LW, Edwards CQ, Cook JD, Kowdley KV. Management of hemochromatosis. Hemochromatosis Management Working Group. *Ann Intern Med.* 1998 Dec 1;129(11):932-9

Ferritin—*Interpretation of serum levels*	
Serum levels	*Categorization and management*
≥ 800 mcg/L	**Practically diagnostic of iron overload**[114,115]: Repeat tests; rule out inflammation or occult pathology. Initiate phlebotomy and consider liver biopsy or MRI
≥ 300 mcg/L	**Probable iron overload**[116]: Repeat tests; rule out inflammation or occult pathology. In men, initiate phlebotomy and consider liver biopsy or MRI[117]
≥ 200 mcg/L	*In women*: **Suggestive of iron overload**[118]: Repeat tests, rule out inflammation or occult pathology. In women, initiate phlebotomy and consider liver biopsy or MRI[119] *In men*: **High-normal *unhealthy* iron status with increased risk of myocardial infarction**[120]: Rule out inflammation or occult pathology. No follow-up is mandated, yet blood donation and/or abstention from dietary iron are strongly recommended preventative healthcare measures
≥ 160 mcg/L	*In women*: **Abnormal iron status**[121]: Repeat tests, rule out inflammation or occult pathology. Consider phlebotomy and liver biopsy or MRI
≥80-120 mcg/L	**High-normal unhealthy iron status**[122,123]: No follow-up is mandated; blood donation and abstention from dietary iron are suggested preventative healthcare measures
40-70 mcg/L	**Optimal iron status**[124,125]
< 20 mcg/L	**Iron deficiency:** Search for occult gastrointestinal blood loss with endoscopy or imaging assessments in adults; refer to gastroenterologist[126,127]

Ferritin is an acute-phase reactant, which means that its production is increased during the acute phase of inflammatory and/or infectious disorders. Therefore the numeric value and hence its clinical meaning can be interpreted only within a context that also includes assessment of the patient's inflammatory status, which is best assessed with either ESR or CRP. If CRP/ESR is high, then the physician might assume that the ferritin value is "falsely elevated"—disproportionately elevated with respect to body iron stores. *Common clinical examples requiring use and skillful interpretation of ferritin*:

- **Elderly or arthritic patient with iron deficiency despite normal serum ferritin**: An elderly patient with normal ferritin and elevated CRP/ESR is probably iron deficient; retesting of ferritin and measurement of transferrin saturation and CBC should be performed promptly. If iron deficiency is confirmed or cannot be excluded, referral for endoscopic examination must be implemented. In a patient with known inflammatory arthropathy, the ferritin may appear normal even though the patient is iron deficient and in need of supplementation and endoscopy.
- **Non-anemic iron deficiency**: A middle-aged patient (commonly a premenopausal woman) presents with fatigue and during the course of evaluation is found to have a normal CBC. Do not let the normal CBC prevent you from assessing ferritin; many of these patients are completely iron deficient with ferritin values of 4-6 mcg/L and are in need of iron replacement and gastrointestinal evaluation.

[114] Milman N, Albeck MJ. Distinction between homozygous and heterozygous subjects with hemochromatosis using iron status markers and receiver operating characteristic (ROC) analysis. *Eur J Clin Biochem* 1995; 33: 95-8
[115] MilmanN.Iron status markers in hereditary hemochromatosis:distinction between individuals beinghomozygous and heterozygous for the hemochromatosis allele.*EurJHaematol*1991;47:292-8
[116] Olynyk JK, Bacon BR. Hereditary hemochromatosis: detecting and correcting iron overload. *Postgrad Med* 1994;96: 151-65
[117] "Therapeutic phlebotomy is used to remove excess iron and maintain low normal body iron stores, … initiated in men with serum ferritin levels of 300 microg/L or more and in women with serum ferritin levels of 200 microg/L or more, regardless of the presence or absence of symptoms." Barton JC, McDonnell SM, Adams PC, Brissot P, Powell LW, Edwards CQ, Cook JD, Kowdley KV. Management of hemochromatosis. Hemochromatosis Management Working Group. *Ann Intern Med.* 1998 Dec 1;129(11):932-9
[118] Barton JC, Edwards CQ, Bertoli LF, Shroyer TW, Hudson SL. Iron overload in African Americans. *Am J Med* 1995; 99: 616-23
[119] Barton JC, McDonnell SM, Adams PC, Brissot P, Powell LW, Edwards CQ, Cook JD, Kowdley KV. Management of hemochromatosis. Hemochromatosis Management Working Group. *Ann Intern Med.* 1998 Dec 1;129(11):932-9
[120] Salonen JT, Nyyssonen K, Korpela H, Tuomilehto J, Seppanen R, Salonen R. High stored iron levels are associated with excess risk of myocardial infarction in eastern Finnish men. *Circulation* 1992; 86: 803-11
[121] Nicoll D. Therapeutic drug monitoring and laboratory reference ranges. In: Tierney LM, McPhee SJ, Papadakis MA. Current Medical Diagnosis and Treatment 1996 (35th Edition). Stamford: Appleton and Lange, 1996: 1442
[122] Lauffer, RB. Iron and Your Heart. New York: St. Martin's Press, 1991: 79-8, 83-88, 162
[123] Sullivan JL. Iron and the sex difference in heart disease risk. *Lancet.* 1981 Jun 13;1(8233):1293-4
[124] Lauffer, RB. Iron and Your Heart. New York: St. Martin's Press, 1991: 79-8, 83-88, 162
[125] Vasquez A. High body iron stores: causes, effects, diagnosis, and treatment. *Nutritional Perspectives* 1994; 17: 13, 15-7, 19, 21, 28 and Vasquez A. Men's Health: Iron in men: why men store this nutrient in their bodies and the harm that it does. *MEN Magazine* 1997; January: 11, 21-23 http://www.vix.com/menmag/alexiron.htm
[126] Rockey DC, Cello JP. Evaluation of the gastrointestinal tract in patients with iron-deficiency anemia. *N Engl J Med.* 1993;329(23):1691-5
[127] "Endoscopy revealed a clinically important lesion in 23 (12%) of 186 patients. … CONCLUSIONS: Endoscopy yields important findings in premenopausal women with iron deficiency anemia, which should not be attributed solely to menstrual blood loss." Bini EJ, Micale PL, Weinshel EH. Evaluation of the gastrointestinal tract in premenopausal women with iron deficiency anemia. *Am J Med.* 1998 Oct;105(4):281-6

Algorithm for the Comprehensive Assessment of Iron Status

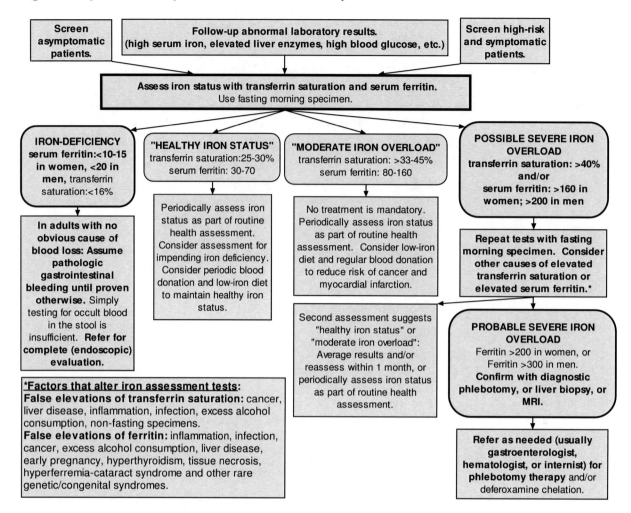

Basic treatment of severe iron overload:

- **Iron-removal therapy is mandatory:** Phlebotomy therapy is generally performed weekly or twice-weekly; deferoxamine chelation is reserved for patients who do not withstand phlebotomy (due to cardiomyopathy, severe anemia, or hypoproteinemia) or may be used concurrently with phlebotomy in some patients. Periodically assess hematologic and iron indexes. Continue with weekly iron removal therapy until patient reaches mild iron-deficiency anemia, then decrease frequency and continue phlebotomy as needed (e.g., 4 times per year).
- **Laboratory tests and physical examination:** Assess general physical condition and hepatic, cardiac, endocrine, and general health status.
- **Confirm diagnosis:** Liver biopsy ("gold standard") or diagnostic phlebotomy; perhaps MRI.
- **Assess liver status:** Liver biopsy ("gold standard") or perhaps MRI. Cirrhosis indicates increased risk of hepatocellular carcinoma and reduced life expectancy. Consider liver ultrasound, serum liver enzyme measurement, and serum alpha-fetoprotein to screen for hepatocellular carcinoma every 6 months. Hepatoma surveillance is mandatory in cirrhotic patients.
- **Implement dietary modifications and nutritional therapies:** Avoid iron supplements, multivitamin supplements with iron, iron-fortified foods, liver, beef, pork, alcohol, and excess vitamin C. Ensure adequate protein intake to replace protein lost during phlebotomy. Diet modifications are not substitutes for iron removal therapy. Consider antioxidant therapy.
- **Screen all blood relatives of patients with primary iron overload**. *Mandatory!*
- **Monitor patient condition, and compliance** with lifelong phlebotomy therapy
- **Assess and address psychoemotional issues/concerns**

25(OH)D: serum 25(OH) vitamin D

Overview and interpretation:	▪ **Vitamin D deficiency is a common cause of musculoskeletal pain**[128,129,130], and vitamin D deficiency is a significant risk factor for cancer and other serious health problems.[131,132,133]
	
	▪ **The mechanism by which vitamin D deficiency causes skeletal pain has been clearly elucidated:**
	   1. Vitamin D deficiency causes a reduction in calcium absorption,
	   2. Production of parathyroid hormone (PTH) is increased to maintain blood calcium levels,
	   3. PTH results in increased urinary excretion of phosphorus, which leads to hypophosphatemia,
	   4. Insufficient calcium phosphate results in deposition of unmineralized collagen matrix on the endosteal (inside) and periosteal (outside) surfaces of bones,
	   5. When the unmineralized collagen matrix hydrates and swells, it causes pressure on the sensory-innervated periosteum resulting in pain.[134]
	
	▪ Measurement of serum 25(OH) vitamin D (or empiric treatment with 2,000 – 4,000 IU vitamin D3 per day for adults) is indicated in patients with chronic musculoskeletal pain, particularly low-back pain.[135] Optimal vitamin D status correlates with serum 25(OH)D levels of 40 – 65 ng/mL (100 - 160 nmol/L)—see our review article for more details[136]; 25(OH)D levels greater than 80 ng/mL are not necessarily indicative of toxicity; however levels greater than 100 ng/mL are unnecessary and increase the risk of hypercalcemia.
	
	Normal and optimal ranges for serum 25(OH)D levels
	
	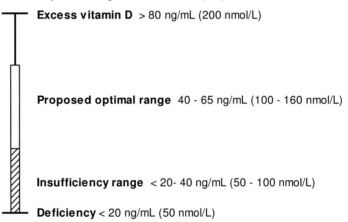
	Excess vitamin D > 80 ng/mL (200 nmol/L)
	Proposed optimal range 40 - 65 ng/mL (100 - 160 nmol/L)
	Insufficiency range < 20- 40 ng/mL (50 - 100 nmol/L)
	Deficiency < 20 ng/mL (50 nmol/L)

Advantages:	▪ Accurate assessment of vitamin D status.
Limitations:	▪ Patients with certain granulomatous conditions such as sarcoidosis or Crohn's disease and patients taking certain drugs such as thiazide diuretics (hydrochlorothiazide) can develop hypercalcemia due to "vitamin D hypersensitivity" or drug side effects—these patients require frequent monitoring of serum calcium while taking vitamin D supplements.
Comments:	▪ Routine measurement and/or empiric treatment with vitamin D3 needs to become a routine component of patient care.[137] ▪ Periodic assessment of 25(OH)D and serum calcium are required to ensure effectiveness and safety of treatment, respectively.

[128] Masood H, Narang AP, Bhat IA, Shah GN. Persistent limb pain and raised serum alkaline phosphatase the earliest markers of subclinical hypovitaminosis D in Kashmir. *Indian J Physiol Pharmacol.* 1989 Oct-Dec;33(4):259-61

[129] Al Faraj S, Al Mutairi K. Vitamin D deficiency and chronic low back pain in Saudi Arabia. *Spine.* 2003 Jan 15;28(2):177-9

[130] Plotnikoff GA, Quigley JM. Prevalence of severe hypovitaminosis D in patients with persistent, nonspecific musculoskeletal pain. *Mayo Clin Proc.* 2003 Dec;78(12):1463-70

[131] Grant WB. An estimate of premature cancer mortality in the U.S. due to inadequate doses of solar ultraviolet-B radiation. *Cancer.* 2002 Mar 15;94(6):1867-75

[132] Zittermannn A. Vitamin D in preventive medicine: are we ignoring the evidence? *Br J Nutr.* 2003 May;89(5):552-72

[133] Holick MF. Vitamin D: importance in the prevention of cancers, type 1 diabetes, heart disease, and osteoporosis. *Am J Clin Nutr.* 2004 Mar;79(3):362-71

[134] Holick MF. Vitamin D deficiency: what a pain it is. *Mayo Clin Proc.* 2003 Dec;78(12):1457-9

[135] Al Faraj S, Al Mutairi K. Vitamin D deficiency and chronic low back pain in Saudi Arabia. *Spine.* 2003 Jan 15;28(2):177-9

[136] **Vasquez A, Manso G, Cannell J. The Clinical Importance of Vitamin D (Cholecalciferol): A Paradigm Shift with Implications for All Healthcare Providers. *Alternative Therapies in Health and Medicine** 2004; 10: 28-37. Also published in *Integrative Medicine: A Clinician's Journal* 2004; 3: 44-54. See www.optimalhealthresearch.com/monograph04

[137] Heaney RP. Vitamin D, nutritional deficiency, and the medical paradigm. *J Clin Endocrinol Metab.* 2003 Nov;88(11):5107-8 http://jcem.endojournals.org/cgi/content/full/88/11/5107

TSH: thyroid stimulating hormone

Overview and interpretation:	■ TSH is produced by the anterior pituitary to stimulate the thyroid gland to produce T4 and T3. If the thyroid gland begins to fail, then TSH levels increase as the body attempts to stimulate production of thyroid hormones from a failing gland. Thyroid hormones have many different functions in the body, and their chief effect is contributing to the control of the basal metabolic rate, or the "speed" of reactions and the "temperature" of the body. For reasons that are not entirely clear, some people do not make enough thyroid hormone to function optimally.[138] Williams[139] noted that "a wide variation in thyroid activity exists among 'normal' human beings." ■ TSH values greater than 2 represent a disturbance of the thyroid-pituitary axis and an increased risk for future thyroid problems[140], and the American Association of Clinical Endocrinologists encourages doctors to consider treatment for patients who test outside the boundaries of a narrower margin based on a target TSH level of 0.3 to 3.0.[141] It appears reasonable to implement a therapeutic trial of thyroid hormone treatment in patients who are clinically hypothyroid even if they are biochemically euthyroid provided that treatment is implemented cautiously, in appropriately selected patients, and patients are appropriately informed.[142,143] ■ This is a routine test for general health assessment in asymptomatic patients, especially women and those with clinical manifestations of hypothyroidism which can include: fatigue, depression, dry skin, constipation, menstrual irregularities, infertility, PMS, uterine fibroids, excess menstrual bleeding, low body temperature, cold hands and feet, weak fingernails, increased need for sleep (hypersomnia), slow heart rate (bradycardia), overweight, gain weight easily, difficulty loosing weight, high cholesterol, slow healing, decreased memory and concentration, muscle weakness or myopathy, sleep apnea, frog-like husky voice, low libido, recurrent infections, high blood pressure, poor digestion, acid reflux, and delayed Achilles return.
Advantages:	■ A quick and inexpensive screening test for hypothyroidism.
Limitations:	■ Some patients will have a completely normal TSH value but a low free T4 or low free T3. Thus, even a properly interpreted TSH test may overlook problems of T4 production or conversion to active T3. Additionally, in some patients, all of these tests are normal but they may have thyroid autoimmunity (i.e., thyroid peroxidase antibodies, anti-TPO) and should receive treatment with thyroid hormone[144] or some other corrective treatment (e.g., selenium supplementation[145,146] and a gluten-free diet[147]) to normalize thyroid status.
Comments:	■ The combination of T3 and T4 (as in the prescription Liotrix/Thyrolar or Armour thyroid) appears to have similar safety to T4 alone (Levothyroxine, Synthroid) and results in greater improvements in mood and neuropsychological function.[148] ■ Glandular thyroid supplements and Armour thyroid should *not* be used in patients with thyroid autoimmunity or Hashimoto's Thyroiditis because the bovine/porcine antigens will exacerbate the anti-thyroid immune response as evidenced by increased anti-TPO antibodies.

[138] Broda Barnes MD, Lawrence Galton, Hypothyroidism: The Unsuspected Illness. Ty Crowell Co; 1976

[139] Williams RJ. Biochemical Individuality : The Basis for the Genetotrophic Concept. Austin and London: University of Texas Press, 1956 page 82

[140] Weetman AP. Fortnightly review: Hypothyroidism: screening and subclinical disease. BMJ: British Medical Journal 1997;314: 1175

[141] American Association of Clinical Endocrinologists: "Until November 2002, doctors had relied on a normal TSH level ranging from 0.5 to 5.0 to diagnose and treat patients with a thyroid disorder who tested outside the boundaries of that range . Now AACE encourages doctors to consider treatment for patients who test outside the boundaries of a narrower margin based on a target TSH level of 0.3 to 3.04. AACE believes the new range will result in proper diagnosis for millions of Americans who suffer from a mild thyroid disorder, but have gone untreated until now." Available at http://www.aace.com/pub/tam2003/press.php on January 2004. For more current information, see "The target TSH level should be between 0.3 and 3.0 µIU/mL." American Association of Clinical Endocrinologists Medical Guidelines for Clinical Practice for the Evaluation and Treatment of Hyperthyroidism and Hypothyroidism. http://www.aace.com/pub/pdf/guidelines/hypo_hyper.pdf December 20,2005

[142] Skinner GR, Thomas R, Taylor M, Sellarajah M, Bolt S, Krett S, Wright A. Thyroxine should be tried in clinically hypothyroid but biochemically euthyroid patients. BMJ: British Medical Journal 1997 Jun 14; 314(7096): 1764

[143] McLaren EH, Kelly CJ, Pollack MA. Trial of thyroxine treatment for biochemically euthyroid patients has been approved. BMJ 1997 Nov 29; 315(7120): 1463

[144] Beers MH, Berkow R (eds). The Merck Manual. 17th Edition. Whitehouse Station; Merck Research Laboratories 1999 page 96

[145] Duntas LH, Mantzou E, Koutras DA. Effects of a six month treatment with selenomethionine in patients with autoimmune thyroiditis. Eur J Endocrinol. 2003 Apr;148(4):389-93 http://eje-online.org/cgi/reprint/148/4/389

[146] "We recently conducted a prospective, placebo-controlled clinical study, where we could demonstrate, that a substitution of 200 wg sodium selenite for three months in patients with autoimmune thyroiditis reduced thyroid peroxidase antibody (TPO-Ab) concentrations significantly." Gartner R, Gasnier BC. Selenium in the treatment of autoimmune thyroiditis. Biofactors. 2003;19(3-4):165-70

[147] Sategna-Guidetti C, Volta U, Ciacci C, Usai P, Carlino A, De Franceschi L, Camera A, Pelli A, Brossa C. Prevalence of thyroid disorders in untreated adult celiac disease patients and effect of gluten withdrawal: an Italian multicenter study. Am J Gastroenterol. 2001 Mar;96(3):751-7

[148] "CONCLUSIONS: In patients with hypothyroidism, partial substitution of triiodothyronine for thyroxine may improve mood and neuropsychological function; this finding suggests a specific effect of the triiodothyronine normally secreted by the thyroid gland." Bunevicius R, Kazanavicius G, Zalinkevicius R, Prange AJ Jr. Effects of thyroxine as compared with thyroxine plus triiodothyronine in patients with hypothyroidism. N Engl J Med. 1999 Feb 11;340(6):424-9

Antinuclear antibody: ANA

Overview and interpretation:	■ **Good screening test for autoimmune conditions**: SLE, Sjogren's syndrome, and various other connective tissue diseases. ■ Good and "highly sensitive" for initial assessment of SLE; positive in 95-98% of SLE patients; **negative result strongly suggests against diagnosis of SLE**.[149] Only 2% of patients with SLE have a negative ANA test—these patients may be identified by testing with anti-RO antibodies and CH50 (complement levels). ■ This test measures for the presence of antibodies that react to nucleoproteins. Some labs report titers of 1:20 or 1:40 as "positive"; however, low levels of ANA are common in the general population. Not specific for any one disease; may be positive in SLE, RA, scleroderma, Sjogren's, also seen with elderly, infected patients, cancer, and certain medications. ■ **Titers less than 1:160 should be interpreted cautiously as they may not indicate the presence of *clinical* autoimmunity.**[150] ■ **Titers greater than 1:320 are considered indicative of clinically significant autoimmunity.**

Methodologies, subtypes, and patterns reported for ANA results may be irrelevant or clinically meaningful; the most common descriptors are provided here:

ANA patterns and descriptions[151,152]	*Clinical correlation*
Homogeneous	Nonspecific
Speckled	Nonspecific
Anti-centromere: selective staining of the centromeres of nuclei in metaphase	Highly specific for the limited scleroderma subtype associated with CREST syndrome
Nucleolar	Suggests diffuse scleroderma
Rim	Suggests SLE and warrants assessment for anti-dsDNA, which is specific for lupus
FANA: fluorescent ANA	The standard ANA test in the US
Anti-Sm: anti-Smith[153]	Highly specific for SLE; low sensitivity: only positive in 20-30% of SLE patients
Anti-dsDNA: anti-double stranded DNA	Highly specific for SLE and indicative of an increased likelihood of poor prognosis with major organ involvement[154]
Anti-Ro (SSA)	Correlates with SLE, Sjögren's syndrome, and neonatal SLE
Anti-La (SSB)	Sjögren's syndrome, SLE
Anti-RNP	SLE and/or MCTD
Anti-Jo-1	Specific but not sensitive for polymyositis/dermatomyositis
Antihistone	SLE and especially drug-induced SLE
Antitopoisomerase (Scl-70)	Correlates with diffuse scleroderma, especially with interstitial lung disease

---

[149] Shojania K. Rheumatology: 2. What laboratory tests are needed? *CMAJ*. 2000 Apr 18;162(8):1157-63 http://www.cmaj.ca/cgi/content/full/162/8/1157
[150] Hardin JG, Waterman J, Labson LH. Rheumatic disease: Which diagnostic tests are useful? *Patient Care* 1999; March 15: 83-102
[151] Shojania K. Rheumatology: 2. What laboratory tests are needed? *CMAJ*. 2000 Apr 18;162(8):1157-63 http://www.cmaj.ca/cgi/content/full/162/8/1157
[152] Ward MM. Laboratory testing for systemic rheumatic diseases. *Postgrad Med.* 1998 Feb;103(2):93-100.
[153] Lane SK, Gravel JW Jr. Clinical utility of common serum rheumatologic tests. *Am Fam Physician.* 2002 Mar 15;65(6):1073-80 http://www.aafp.org/afp/20020315/1073.html
[154] Shojania K. Rheumatology: 2. What laboratory tests are needed? *CMAJ*. 2000 Apr 18;162(8):1157-63 http://www.cmaj.ca/cgi/content/full/162/8/1157

Antinuclear antibody: ANA—*continued*

Advantages:	▪ ANA has 98% sensitivity and 90% specificity for SLE in an unselected population. ▪ The negative predictive value in an unselected population is greater than 99%. ANA is therefore an excellent test for *excluding* the diagnosis of SLE.
Limitations:	▪ The positive predictive value in an unselected population is about 30%; **only 30% of unselected people with a positive result will have SLE**—this fact underscores the importance of patient selection and judicious interpretation of this test. ▪ Positive ANA is seen in patients with conditions other than SLE, including rheumatoid arthritis, Sjogren's syndrome, scleroderma, polymyositis, vasculitis, juvenile rheumatoid arthritis (JRA), and infectious diseases.
Comments:	▪ ANA is most often used to support the diagnosis of SLE in a patient with multisystemic illness and a clinical picture compatible with SLE. Nearly all patients with SLE will have positive ANA. However, a positive ANA does not mean that the patient necessarily has SLE. ▪ I view any "positive ANA" as an indicator of poor health in general and immune dysfunction in particular. The goal, then, is to restore health. I have seen ANA show a trend toward normalization or completely normalize with effective health restoration as detailed in *Integrative Rheumatology* (chapter 4). I realize that my experience in this regard contrasts sharply with the allopathic view that serial measurements of ANA are worthless because the result never normalizes once a patient is ANA-positive[155]; I consider this evidence of the effectiveness of my naturopathic approach and the comparable failure of the allopathic approach.

Antineutrophilic cytoplasmic antibodies: ANCA

Overview:	▪ ANCA are autoantibodies to the cytoplasmic constituents of granulocytes and are characteristically found in vasculitic syndromes and also in (Chinese) patients with inflammatory bowel disease[156] and nearly all patients with hepatic amebiasis due to *Entamoeba histolytica.*[157] Two types: ▪ Cytoplasmic ANCA (C-ANCA): classically seen in **Wegener's granulomatosis**; also seen in some types of glomerulonephritis and vasculitis; this test is highly sensitive and specific for these conditions. In fact, a positive C-ANCA result can replace biopsy in a patient with a clinical picture of **Wegener's granulomatosis.**[158] ▪ Perinuclear ANCA (P-ANCA): considered a nonspecific finding[159] that correlates with SLE, drug induced lupus, and some types of glomerulonephritis and vasculitis. Shojania[160] stated that this test must be confirmed with antimyeloperoxidase antibodies to evaluate for Churg–Strauss syndrome, crescentic glomerulonephritis, and microscopic polyarteritis.
Advantages, limitations, and comments	▪ Obviates biopsy in a patient with clinical Wegener's granulomatosis. ▪ Not to be used as a screening test, except in patients with idiopathic vasculitis or glomerulonephritis. ▪ The fact that hepatic amebiasis due to *Entamoeba histolytica* induces production of C-ANCA antibodies in nearly 100% of infected patients may support the hypothesis that autoimmunity can be induced or exacerbated by parasitic infections.

---

[155] Shojania K. Rheumatology: 2. What laboratory tests are needed? *CMAJ.* 2000 Apr 18;162(8):1157-63 http://www.cmaj.ca/cgi/content/full/162/8/1157
[156] "Fourteen patients (73.5%) were positive, of which six (31.5%) showed a perinuclear staining pattern and eight (42%) demonstrated a cytoplasmic pattern." Sung JY, Chan KL, Hsu R, Liew CT, Lawton JW. Ulcerative colitis and antineutrophil cytoplasmic antibodies in Hong Kong Chinese. *Am J Gastroenterol.* 1993 Jun;88(6):864-9
[157] "ANCA was detected in 97.4% of amoebic sera; the pattern of staining was cytoplasmic, homogeneous, without central accentuation (C-ANCA)." Pudifin DJ, Duursma J, Gathiram V, Jackson TF. Invasive amoebiasis is associated with the development of anti-neutrophil cytoplasmic antibody. *Clin Exp Immunol.* 1994 Jul;97(1):48-5
[158] Shojania K. Rheumatology: 2. What laboratory tests are needed? *CMAJ.* 2000 Apr 18;162(8):1157-63 http://www.cmaj.ca/cgi/content/full/162/8/1157
[159] Shojania K. Rheumatology: 2. What laboratory tests are needed? *CMAJ.* 2000 Apr 18;162(8):1157-63 http://www.cmaj.ca/cgi/content/full/162/8/1157
[160] Shojania K. Rheumatology: 2. What laboratory tests are needed? *CMAJ.* 2000 Apr 18;162(8):1157-63 http://www.cmaj.ca/cgi/content/full/162/8/1157

RF: Rheumatoid Factor

Overview and interpretation:	• Rheumatoid factor—"anti-IgG antibodies"—are antibodies directed to the Fc portion of the patient's own IgG. Rheumatoid factors are anti-immunoglobulin antibodies, classically anti-IgG IgM. RF are found in low levels in most patients, and despite the "rheumatoid" name, RF is not specific for rheumatoid arthritis.[161] Current tests (latex fixation or nephelometry) detect IgM anti-immunoglobulin antibodies; however IgA-RF appears to have clinical superiority over other forms of RF because it correlates more strongly with clinical status.[162] • This test is most commonly used to support the diagnosis of rheumatoid arthritis in a patient with a compelling clinical picture: peripheral polyarthritis lasting >6 weeks.[163] A negative result with a compelling clinical presentation of RA is termed "seronegative rheumatoid arthritis" by allopathic textbooks whereas a more appropriate term might be oligoarthritis, a condition described as "idiopathic" by allopathic text books despite the clear evidence that the majority of patients have one or more subsets of multifocal dysbiosis.[164] • **Titers (latex fixation) of 1:160 are considered clinically significant, favoring the diagnosis of RA.**[165] However the positive predictive value is low—only 20-34% of people in an unselected population with a positive test result actually have RA.[166,167] • The test has a relatively high sensitivity with a low specificity.
Advantages:	• Supports the diagnosis of rheumatoid arthritis: about 60-85% positive/sensitive in patients with rheumatoid arthritis (RA).[168,169] • Quantitative titers of RF correlate with prognosis: a very high RF value portends a poor prognosis.[170]
Limitations:	• **Positive findings are common in the following conditions: rheumatoid arthritis, viral hepatitis, Sjögren's syndrome, endocarditis, scleroderma, mycobacteria diseases, polymyositis and dermatomyositis, syphilis, systemic lupus erythematosus, old age, mixed connective tissue disease, sarcoidosis**; positive results may also been noted in: **cryoglobulinemia, parasitic infection, interstitial lung disease, asymptomatic relatives of people with autoimmune diseases.** • Febrile patients with arthralgia are more likely to have endocarditis than RA.[171] • Patients with iron overload present with a similar clinical picture (i.e., polyarthropathy with systemic complaints) and may have a positive RF. Thus, patients with positive RF and polyarthropathy should be tested for iron overload; use serum ferritin.[172,173]
Comments:	• This test should only be used to confirm the diagnosis of rheumatoid arthritis in patients with a compelling clinical picture of the disease: inflammatory peripheral polyarthropathy with systemic complaints for > 6 weeks. A negative result does not mean that the patient *does not* have rheumatoid arthritis; a positive result does not mean that the patient *does* have rheumatoid arthritis.[174] • CCP (cyclic citrullinated protein) antibodies appear to be more specific and sensitive for RA and is becoming the test of choice for RA as described on the following page.

[161] Shojania K. Rheumatology: 2. What laboratory tests are needed? *CMAJ.* 2000 Apr 18;162(8):1157-63 http://www.cmaj.ca/cgi/content/full/162/8/1157
[162] Jonsson T, Valdimarsson H. What about IgA rheumatoid factor in rheumatoid arthritis? *Ann Rheum Dis.* 1998 Jan;57(1):63-4 http://ard.bmjjournals.com/cgi/content/full/57/1/63
[163] Shojania K. Rheumatology: 2. What laboratory tests are needed? *CMAJ.* 2000 Apr 18;162(8):1157-63 http://www.cmaj.ca/cgi/content/full/162/8/1157
[164] See Chapter 4 of *Integrative Rheumatology* and Vasquez A. Reducing Pain and Inflammation Naturally. Part 6: Nutritional and Botanical Treatments Against "Silent Infections" and Gastrointestinal Dysbiosis, Commonly Overlooked Causes of Neuromusculoskeletal Inflammation and Chronic Health Problems. *Nutr Perspect* 2006; Jan http://optimalhealthresearch.com/part6
[165] Beers MH, Berkow R (eds). The Merck Manual. Seventeenth Edition. Whitehouse Station; Merck Research Laboratories 1999 Page 417
[166] Ward MM. Laboratory testing for systemic rheumatic diseases. *Postgrad Med.* 1998 Feb;103(2):93-100.
[167] Shojania K. Rheumatology: 2. What laboratory tests are needed? *CMAJ.* 2000 Apr 18;162(8):1157-63 http://www.cmaj.ca/cgi/content/full/162/8/1157
[168] Tierney ML. McPhee SJ, Papadakis MA (eds). Current Medical Diagnosis and Treatment 2002, 41st Edition. New York: Lange Medical Books, 2002 Page 854
[169] Shojania K. Rheumatology: 2. What laboratory tests are needed? *CMAJ.* 2000 Apr 18;162(8):1157-63 http://www.cmaj.ca/cgi/content/full/162/8/1157
[170] Shojania K. Rheumatology: 2. What laboratory tests are needed? *CMAJ.* 2000 Apr 18;162(8):1157-63 http://www.cmaj.ca/cgi/content/full/162/8/1157
[171] Klippel JH (ed). Primer on the Rheumatic Diseases. 11th Edition. Atlanta: Arthritis Foundation. 1997 page 96
[172] Bensen WG, Laskin CA, Little HA, Fam AG. Hemochromatoic arthropathy mimicking rheumatoid arthritis. A case with subcutaneous nodules, tenosynovitis, and bursitis. *Arthritis Rheum* 1978; 21: 844-8
[173] Vasquez A. Musculoskeletal disorders and iron overload disease: comment on the American College of Rheumatology guidelines for the initial evaluation of the adult patient with acute musculoskeletal symptoms. *Arthritis Rheum* 1996;39: 1767-8
[174] Shojania K. Rheumatology: 2. What laboratory tests are needed? *CMAJ.* 2000 Apr 18;162(8):1157-63 http://www.cmaj.ca/cgi/content/full/162/8/1157

CCP: Cyclic citrullinated protein antibody; Citrullinated protein antibodies (CPA); anti-CCP antibodies: anticyclic citrullinated peptide antibody

Overview and interpretation:	<ul><li>CCP—cyclic citrullinated protein antibodies; anticitrullinated protein antibodies: this is a relatively new auto-antibody marker that shows great promise and specificity for the early diagnosis of rheumatoid arthritis (RA). The test often becomes positive/present in asymptomatic patients years before the onset of clinical manifestations of RA.</li><li>As of the first inclusion of this information in my books in December 2006, the information on anti-CCP antibodies is so new that it is not even included in most 2006-edition medical and rheumatology reference textbooks; nonetheless, doctors nationwide are already starting to use this test for the early diagnosis of RA. This may be particularly important because some research has shown that *early* and *aggressive* treatment of RA has an important impact on long-term prognosis[175]; however, the importance of early intervention is debatable.[176]</li><li>anti-CCP antibodies are directed toward several native proteins (e.g., filaggrin, fibrinogen, and vimentin) that have become posttranslationally modified by a uncharged citrulline in contrast to the normal positively charged arginine. This "citrullination" is catalyzed by a calcium-dependent enzyme, peptidylarginine deiminase (PAD). These changes in protein charge and sequence make the native protein a target of auto-antibody attack by IgG antibodies in RA.[177] However, this does not necessarily imply that citrullination of native proteins is "the cause" of RA because citrullination of native proteins can also occur *de novo* in inflamed joints, which are then further targeted for inflammatory destruction. Until more information is available, we should withhold final judgment as to the ultimate role and origin of anti-CCP antibodies and in the meanwhile view them as a very strong and sensitive association with RA that facilitates the early diagnosis of this disease.</li></ul>
Advantages:	<ul><li>Anti-CCP antibodies have 98% specificity for RA[178] and is likely to become the future laboratory standard in the diagnosis and prognosis of RA.[179]</li><li>Anti-CCP antibodies with a positive rheumatoid factor (RF) is termed "composite seropositivity" and appears to be more specific than isolated anti-CCP antibodies or RF.[180]</li></ul>
Limitations:	<ul><li>**The best current data indicates that anti-CCP antibodies are sensitive and specific for RA[181], and clinicians should use this test to diagnose and confirm RA**; however, continue to monitor research on this test as its value is verified or questioned in future reports.</li></ul>
Comments:	<ul><li>Healthy people do not generally have anti-CCP antibodies. Asymptomatic patients with anti-CCP antibodies are at increased risk for clinical RA and are probably *en route* to the manifestation of clinical autoimmunity—RA, Sjogren's disease, or SLE. *Holistically intervene.*</li><li>Given that the test is still somewhat new, clinicians should periodically survey the news and literature on this test to see if perspectives change either positively or negatively in the next few years as clinical experience with this marker accumulates. We must also recall however the speed with which laboratory markers can rise from obscurity to fame; take for example CRP, which was still very new to most clinicians in 1999 and by 2001—only 2 years later—the test had rapidly become a daily component of clinical care.</li><li>I hypothesize that PAD may become upregulated in synovial joints exposed to allergens, xenobiotics, bacterial debris/toxins/lipopolysaccharides and that the subsequent citrullination of joint proteins may lead to an autoimmune arthropathy that persists, perhaps despite removal of the inciting immunogen. More obviously, given that PAD is calcium-dependent, it may be upregulated secondary to intracellular hypercalcinosis secondary to vitamin D deficiency, magnesium deficiency, or fatty acid imbalance.[182]</li></ul>

---

[175] "CONCLUSION: An initial 6-month cycle of intensive combination treatment that includes high-dose corticosteroids results in sustained suppression of the rate of radiologic progression in patients with early RA, independent of subsequent antirheumatic therapy." Landewe RB, Boers M, Verhoeven AC, Westhovens R, van de Laar MA, Markusse HM, van Denderen JC, Westedt ML, Peeters AJ, Dijkmans BA, Jacobs P, Boonen A, van der Heijde DM, van der Linden S. COBRA combination therapy in patients with early rheumatoid arthritis: long-term structural benefits of a brief intervention. *Arthritis Rheum.* 2002 Feb;46(2):347-56

[176] "By 5 years patients receiving early DMARDs had similar disease activity and comparable health assessment questionnaire scores to patients who received DMARDs later in their disease course." Scott DL. Evidence for early disease-modifying drugs in rheumatoid arthritis. *Arthritis Res Ther.* 2004;6(1):15-18 http://arthritis-research.com/content/6/1/15

[177] Hill J, Cairns E, Bell DA. The joy of citrulline: new insights into the diagnosis, pathogenesis, and treatment of rheumatoid arthritis. *J Rheumatol.* 2004 Aug;31(8):1471-3 http://www.jrheum.com/subscribers/04/08/1471.html

[178] Hill J, Cairns E, Bell DA. The joy of citrulline: new insights into the diagnosis, pathogenesis, and treatment of rheumatoid arthritis. *J Rheumatol.* 2004 Aug;31(8):1471-3

[179] "We conclude that, at present, the antibody response directed to citrullinated antigens has the most valuable diagnostic and prognostic potential for RA." van Boekel MA, Vossenaar ER, van den Hoogen FH, van Venrooij WJ. Autoantibody systems in rheumatoid arthritis: specificity, sensitivity and diagnostic value. *Arthritis Res.* 2002;4(2):87-93 http://arthritis-research.com/content/4/2/87

[180] "…our findings suggest that a positive anti-CCP antibody result does not necessarily exclude SLE in African American patients presenting with inflammatory arthritis. In such patients, the additional assessment of IgA-RF or IgM-RF isotypes may be of added value since composite seropositivity appears to be nearly exclusive to patients with RA." Mikuls TR, Holers VM, Parrish L, Kuhn KA, Conn DL, Gilkeson G, Smith EA, Kamen DL, Jonas BL, Callahan LF, Alarcon GS, Howard G, Moreland LW, Bridges SL Jr. Anti-cyclic citrullinated peptide antibody and rheumatoid factor isotypes in African Americans with early rheumatoid arthritis. *Arthritis Rheum.* 2006 Sep;54(9):3057-9

[181] "Serum antibodies reactive with citrullinated proteins/peptides are a very sensitive and specific marker for rheumatoid arthritis." Migliorini P, Pratesi F, Tommasi C, Anzilotti C. The immune response to citrullinated antigens in autoimmune diseases. *Autoimmun Rev.* 2005 Nov;4(8):561-4

[182] See http://optimalhealthresearch.com/archives/intracellular-hypercalcinosis and www.naturopathydigest.com/archives/2006/sep/vasquez.php for additional discussion

HLA-B27: Human leukocyte antigen B-27	
Overview and interpretation:	▪ A common (5-10% of general population) genetic marker strongly associated with seronegative* spondyloarthropathy (all of which occur more commonly in men[183]): 　　o Ankylosing spondylitis (90-95% of 'whites' and 50% of 'blacks')[184] 　　o Reiter's syndrome (85%) 　　o Enteropathic spondyloarthropathy 　　o Psoriatic spondylitis (<60%) * Recall that "seronegative" in this context implies that the *rheumatoid factor is negative, even though the HLA-B27 may be positive.*
Advantages: *Limitations:* *Comments:*	▪ *From a diagnostic perspective*: The clinical application and significance of this test is of limited value. All of the above-listed conditions are better assessed with the combination of clinical assessment and radiographs. In a patient with early and mild disease, this test may add evidence either supporting or refuting the diagnosis; but the test itself is not diagnostic of anything other than a genetic/histologic marker associated with various types of infection-induced arthropathy and autoimmunity (dysbiotic arthropathy[185]). ▪ *From an integrative/functional medicine perspective*: This test can be of some value if the result is positive and the patient has evidence of a systemic inflammatory/autoimmune disorder since it therefore more strongly suggests that a dysbiotic locus is the cause of disease.[186] 　　o A consistent theme in the rheumatology literature is that of "molecular mimicry"—the phenomenon by which structural similarities between human and microbial structures lead to targeting of human tissues by immune responses aimed at microbial antigens. This topic is explored in considerable detail in the section on multifocal dysbiosis in *Integrative Rheumatology*. The important link between microbe-induced autoimmunity and HLA-B27 is that many dysbiotic bacteria produce an HLA-B27-like molecule that appears to trigger an immune response which then erroneously affects human tissues, leading to the clinical picture of autoimmune inflammation. Many of these HLA-B27-producing bacteria colonize the gastrointestinal and genitourinary tracts, promoting musculoskeletal inflammation via molecular mimicry and other mechanisms.[187,188] A strong and growing body of research shows that HLA-B27 is a risk factor for microbe-induced autoimmunity. "Autoimmune" patients positive for HLA-B27 are presumed to have an occult infection—especially gastrointestinal, genitourinary, or sinorespiratory—until proven otherwise. ▪ **Keep in mind that HLA-B27 itself is not a disease** and therefore a "positive" result merely means that the patient has this particular human leukocyte antigen; this test is not and will never be diagnostic of a specific disease—it simply correlates with increased propensity toward dysbiotic arthropathy and suggests the need for dysbiosis testing and the (re)establishment of eubiosis.[189]

[183] "The major diseases associated with HLA-B27 (Reiter's disease, ankylosing spondylitis, acute anterior uveitis, and psoriatic arthritis) all occur much more commonly in men." James WH. Sex ratios and hormones in HLA related rheumatic diseases. *Ann Rheum Dis.* 1991 Jun;50(6):401-4

[184] Shojania K. Rheumatology: 2. What laboratory tests are needed? *CMAJ.* 2000 Apr 18;162(8):1157-63 http://www.cmaj.ca/cgi/content/full/162/8/1157

[185] See Chapter 4 of *Integrative Rheumatology* and Vasquez A. Reducing Pain and Inflammation Naturally. Part 6: Nutritional and Botanical Treatments Against "Silent Infections" and Gastrointestinal Dysbiosis, Commonly Overlooked Causes of Neuromusculoskeletal Inflammation and Chronic Health Problems. *Nutr Perspect* 2006; Jan http://optimalhealthresearch.com/part6

[186] "The association between HLA-B27 and reactive arthritis (ReA) has also been well established... In a similar way, microbiological and immunological studies have revealed an association between Klebsiella pneumoniae in AS and Proteus mirabilis in RA." Ebringer A, Wilson C. HLA molecules, bacteria and autoimmunity. *J Med Microbiol.* 2000 Apr;49(4):305-11

[187] **Inman RD. Antigens, the gastrointestinal tract, and arthritis.** *Rheum Dis Clin North Am.* **1991 May;17(2):309-21**

[188] **Hunter JO. Food allergy--or enterometabolic disorder?** *Lancet.* **1991 Aug 24;338(8765):495-6**

[189] Dysbiotic arthropathy—joint inflammation and destruction as a result of a neuroimmune inflammatory response to microorganisms. Phrase coined by Alex Vasquez on December 15, 2005. No matching term on Medline or Google search. See Chapter 4 of *Integrative Rheumatology* and Vasquez A. Reducing Pain and Inflammation Naturally. Part 6: Nutritional and Botanical Treatments Against "Silent Infections" and Gastrointestinal Dysbiosis, Commonly Overlooked Causes of Neuromusculoskeletal Inflammation and Chronic Health Problems. *Nutr Perspect* 2006; Jan http://optimalhealthresearch.com/part6

Lactulose-mannitol assay: assessment for intestinal hyperpermeability and malabsorption	
Overview and interpretation:	▪ The lactulose-mannitol assay is a highly validated assessment for the accurate determination of small intestine permeability. This test is used to diagnose "leaky gut", which is a common problem and contributor to systemic inflammation in patients with inflammation and immune dysfunction—see Chapter 4 of *Integrative Rheumatology*. Intestinal hyperpermeability reflects inflammation of and damage to the small intestine mucosa and is seen in patients with parasite infections, food allergies, celiac disease, malnutrition, bacterial infections, systemic ischemia or inflammation, ankylosing spondylitis, Crohn's disease, eczema, psoriasis, and those who consume enterotoxins such as NSAIDs and excess ethanol.[190] ▪ Elevations of lactulose indicate increased paracellular permeability caused by intestinal damage and are diagnostic of "leaky gut." *Clinical pearl*: remember that the "L" in *lactulose* rhymes with *leaky*. ▪ Decrements in mannitol suggest impaired transcellular absorption and suggest malabsorption in general and villous atrophy in particular. *Clinical pearl*: remember that the "M" in *mannitol* rhymes with *malabsorption*. ▪ Classically, in patients with damaged intestinal mucosa, we generally see a combined ***increase in transcellular*** permeability (measured with lactulose) and a ***reduction in paracellular*** transport (measured with mannitol). These divergent effects result in an increased lactulose-to-mannitol ratio, which is reliable indicator of mucosal damage and relative malabsorption.[191]

Advantages:	**This test is safe and affordable for the assessment of small intestine mucosal integrity. Abnormal results—"leaky gut" and/or malabsorption—generally indicate one or more of following:**
	    1. <u>**Malnutrition**</u>**: may be due to poor intake, catabolism, or malabsorption.**
	    2. <u>**Enterotoxins**</u>**: generally NSAIDs or ethanol**
	    3. <u>**Food allergies**</u>**: including celiac disease**
	    4. <u>**"Parasites"**</u>**: including yeast, bacteria, protozoa, amebas, worms, etc.** [192]
	    5. <u>**Systemic inflammation**</u>**: tissue hypoxia, trauma, recent surgery, etc.**
	    6. <u>**Genetic predisposition toward enteropathy**</u>**: check family history for IBD**

Limitations:	▪ Abnormalities and the identification of "leaky gut" are nonspecific and do not point to a specific or single diagnosis or treatment.
Comments:	▪ The value of this test is two-fold: 1) as a screening test for the above-mentioned disorders, and 2) as a method for determining the efficacy of treatment once the cause of the problem has been putatively identified and treated. ▪ This test can be used to promote compliance and to encourage the use of additional testing in patients who are otherwise prone to noncompliance or who resist other tests, such as stool testing. In other words, the clinician can gain an advantage by showing the patient an objective abnormality which then validates the need for treatment and additional testing. ▪ I only use this test on rare occasions because I more commonly either assume that a patient has leaky gut if he/she has one of the aforementioned conditions or we move directly to stool testing and comprehensive parasitology—clearly one of the most valuable tests in the management and treatment of systemic inflammation and immune dysfunction—otherwise known as "autoimmunity" and "allergy."

[190] Miller AL. The Pathogenesis, Clinical Implications, and Treatment of Intestinal Hyperpermeability. *Alt Med Rev 1997*;2(5):330-345 http://www.thorne.com/pdf/journal/2-5/intestinalhyperpermiability.pdf
[191] Uil JJ, van Elburg RM, van Overbeek FM, Mulder CJ, VanBerge-Henegouwen GP, Heymans HS.Clinical implications of the sugar absorption test: intestinal permeability test to assess mucosal barrier function. *Scand J Gastroenterol* Suppl. 1997;223:70-8
[192] See Chapter 4 of *Integrative Rheumatology* and Vasquez A. Reducing Pain and Inflammation Naturally. Part 6: Nutritional and Botanical Treatments Against "Silent Infections" and Gastrointestinal Dysbiosis, Commonly Overlooked Causes of Neuromusculoskeletal Inflammation and Chronic Health Problems. *Nutr Perspect* 2006; Jan http://optimalhealthresearch.com/part6

Comprehensive stool analysis and comprehensive parasitology

Overview and interpretation:

- **This is clearly one of the most valuable tests in clinical practice when working with patients with chronic fatigue, systemic inflammation, and autoimmunity. Second only to routine laboratory assessments such as CBC, chemistry panel, and CRP, the importance of stool testing and comprehensive parasitology assessments must be appreciated by progressive clinicians of all disciplines.**
- Stool testing must be performed by a specialty laboratory because the quality of testing provided by most standard "medical labs" and hospitals is completely inadequate. Initial samples should be collected on three separate occasions by the patient and each sample should be analyzed separately by the laboratory.
- Important qualitative and quantitative markers include the following:
    - <u>**Beneficial bacteria (" probiotics")**</u>: Microbiological testing should quantify and identify various beneficial bacteria, which should be present at "+4" levels on a 0-4 scale.
    - <u>**Harmful and potentially harmful bacteria, protozoans, amebas, etc**</u>.: Questionable or harmful microbes should be eradicated even if they are not identified as true pathogens in the paleo-classic Pasteurian/Kochian sense.[193]
    - <u>**Yeast and mycology**</u>: At least two tests must be performed for a complete assessment: 1) yeast culture, and 2) microscopic examination for yeast elements. Both tests are necessary because some patients—perhaps those with the most severe symptomatology and the most favorable response to anti-yeast treatment—will have a negative yeast culture and positive findings on the microscopic examination. In other words, these patients have intestinal yeast that contributes to their disease/symptomatology but which does not grow on culture despite being clearly visible with microscopy; a similar pattern (using a swab of the rectal mucosa rather than microscopy) is referred to as "negative culture with positive smear."[194]
    - <u>**Microbial sensitivity testing**</u>: An important component to parasitology testing is the determination of which anti-microbial agents (natural and synthetic) the microbe is sensitive to. This helps to guide and enhance the effectiveness of anti-microbial therapy.
    - <u>**Secretory IgA**</u>: SIgA levels are elevated in patients who are having an immune response to either food or microbial antigens.[195] Thus, in a patient with minimal dysbiosis, say for example with *Candida albicans*, an elevated sIgA can indicate that the patient is having a hypersensitivity reaction to an otherwise benign microbe—in this case, eradication of the microbe is warranted and may result in a positive clinical response. Low sIgA suggests either primary or secondary immune defect such as selective sIgA deficiency[196] or malnutrition, stress, prednisone/corticosteroids, or possibly mycotoxicosis (immunosuppression due to fungal immunotoxins). In addition to addressing any systemic causative factors, a low sIgA may be addressed with the administration of bovine colostrum, glutamine, vitamin A, and *Saccharomyces boulardii*; the following doses may be considered for use in adults with proportionately smaller doses for children:
        - Bovine colostrum: 2.4 – 3.6 grams per day in divided doses for adults. No drug interactions are known. Side effects may include increased energy, insomnia, and stimulation. One study in particular used very large doses of 10 grams per day for four days in children and found no adverse effects[197]; another case report of a child involved the use of 50 grams per day for at least two weeks and showed no adverse effects.[198]

[193] **Vasquez A. Reducing Pain and Inflammation Naturally. Part 6: Nutritional and Botanical Treatments Against "Silent Infections" and Gastrointestinal Dysbiosis, Commonly Overlooked Causes of Neuromusculoskeletal Inflammation and Chronic Health Problems.** *Nutr Perspect* 2006; Jan http://optimalhealthresearch.com/part6

[194] "According to Galland, the best predictor of who will respond to anticandida medication is a negative stool culture combined with a positive smear of the rectal mucosa (for the identification of intracellular hyphal forms of the organism); however, even that test is not 100% reliable." Gaby AR. Before you order that lab test: part 2. *Townsend Letter for Doctors and Patients.* 2004; January http://www.findarticles.com/p/articles/mi_m0ISW/is_246/ai_112728028

[195] Quig DW, Higley M. Noninvasive assessment of intestinal inflammation: inflammatory bowel disease vs. irritable bowel syndrome. *Townsend Letter for Doctors and Patients* 2006;Jan:74-5

[196] "Selective IgA deficiency is the most common form of immunodeficiency. Certain select populations, including allergic individuals, patients with autoimmune and gastrointestinal tract disease and patients with recurrent upper respiratory tract illnesses, have an increased incidence of this disorder." Burks AW Jr, Steele RW. Selective IgA deficiency. *Ann Allergy.* 1986;57:3-13

[197] "In this double blind placebo-controlled trial, 80 children with rotavirus diarrhea were randomly assigned to receive orally either 10 g of IIBC (containing 3.6 g of antirotavirus antibodies) daily for 4 days or the same amount of a placebo preparation." Sarker SA, Casswall TH, Mahalanabis D, Alam NH, Albert MJ, Brussow H, Fuchs GJ, Hammarstrom L. Successful treatment of rotavirus diarrhea in children with immunoglobulin from immunized bovine colostrum. *Pediatr Infect Dis J.* 1998 Dec;17(12):1149-54

[198] Lactobin-R is a commercial hyperimmune bovine colostrum with some specificity for cryptosporidiosis; administration to a 4 year old child with AIDS and severe diarrhea resulted in significant clinical improvement in the diarrhea and "permanent elimination of the parasite from the gut as assessed through serial jejunal biopsy and stool specimens." Shield J, Melville C, Novelli V, Anderson G, Scheimberg I, Gibb D, Milla P. Bovine colostrum immunoglobulin concentrate for cryptosporidiosis in AIDS. *Arch Dis Child.* 1993 Oct;69(4):451-3

- - **Glutamine:** 6 grams 3 times per day (18 grams per day) is a common dosage with significant literature support.
  - **Vitamin A:** Correction of subclinical vitamin A deficiency improves mucosal integrity and increases sIgA production in humans.[199] Common doses used by integrative clinicians are in the range of 200,000 IU to 300,000 for a limited amount of time, generally 1-4 weeks; thereafter the dose is tapered. Patients are educated as to manifestations of toxicity (see the chapter on *Therapeutics* toward the end of this book) and the importance of limited duration of treatment.
  - *Saccharomyces boulardii:* Common dose for adults is 250 mg thrice daily; ability of this treatment to increase sIgA levels and its anti-infective efficacy have been documented in human and animal studies.
  - **Short-chain fatty acids:** These are produced by intestinal bacteria. Quantitative excess indicates bacterial overgrowth of the intestines, while insufficiency indicates a lack of probiotics or an insufficiency of dietary substrate, i.e., soluble fiber. Abnormal patterns of individual short-chain fatty acids indicate qualitative/quantitative abnormalities in gastrointestinal microflora, particularly anaerobic bacteria that cannot be identified with routine bacterial cultures.
  - **Beta-glucuronidase:** This is an enzyme produced by several different intestinal bacteria. High levels of beta-glucuronidase in the intestinal lumen serve to nullify the benefits of detoxification (specifically glucuronidation) by cleaving the toxicant from its glucuronide conjugate. This can result in re-absorption of the toxicant through the intestinal mucosa which then re-exposes the patient to the toxin that was previously detoxified ("enterohepatic recirculation" or "enterohepatic recycling"[200]). This is an exemplary aspect of "auto-intoxication" that results in chronic fatigue and upregulation of Phase 1 detoxification systems (chapter 4 of *Integrative Rheumatology*).
  - **Lactoferrin:** The iron-binding glycoprotein lactoferrin is an inflammatory marker that helps distinguish functional disorders (i.e., IBS) from more serious diseases (i.e., IBD). Approximate values are as follows:
    - Healthy and IBS: 2 mcg/ml
    - Severe dysbiosis: up to 120 mcg/ml
    - Inactive IBD: 60-250 mcg/ml
    - Active IBD: > 400 mcg/ml.
  - **Lysozyme:** Elevated in proportion to intestinal inflammation in dysbiosis and IBD.
  - **Other markers:** Other markers of digestion, inflammation, and absorption are reported with the more comprehensive panels performed on stool samples. These tests are not always necessary, but such additional information is always helpful when working with complex patients. These markers are relatively self-explanatory and/or are described on the results of the test by the laboratory.

Advantages:	- **Stool analysis in general and parasitology assessments in particular provide supremely valuable information in the comprehensive assessment and treatment of patients with complex illnesses such as chronic fatigue, irritable bowel syndrome, fibromyalgia, and all of the autoimmune/rheumatic diseases**
Limitations:	- Tests vary in price from about $250-$400 - Anaerobic bacteria are difficult to culture - Specialty examinations, such as for *Helicobacter pylori* antigen and enterohemorrhagic *E. coli* cytotoxin, must be requested specifically at additional cost
Comments:	- I have found stool testing to be the single most powerful diagnostic tool for helping chronically ill patients to attain improved health. Insights from stool/parasitology testing can be used to implement powerfully effective treatments. The value of this test in the treatment of patients with rheumatic disease must be appreciated and is extensively detailed in chapter 4 of *Integrative Rheumatology*

---

[199] "It can increase resistance to infection by increasing mucosal integrity, increasing surface immunoglobulin A (sIgA) and enhancing adequate neutrophil function. If infection occurs, vitamin A can act as an immune enhancer, increasing the adequacy of natural killer (NK) cells and increasing antibody production." Faisel H, Pittrof R. Vitamin A and causes of maternal mortality: association and biological plausibility. *Public Health Nutr.* 2000 Sep;3(3):321-7
[200] Parker RJ, Hirom PC, Millburn P.Enterohepatic recycling of phenolphthalein, morphine, lysergic acid diethylamide (LSD) and diphenylacetic acid in the rat. Hydrolysis of glucuronic acid conjugates in the gut lumen. *Xenobiotica.* 1980 Sep;10(9):689-70

High-risk Pain Patients:

When a patient has musculoskeletal pain and any of the following characteristics, radiographs should be considered as an appropriate component of comprehensive evaluation. These considerations are particularly—though not exclusively—relevant for spine and low-back pain.[201]

1. **More than 50 years of age**
2. **Physical trauma** (accident, fall, etc.)
3. **Pain at night**
4. **Back pain not relieved by lying supine**
5. **Neurologic deficits** (motor or sensory)
6. **Unexplained weight loss**
7. **Documentation or suspicion of inflammatory arthropathy**[202]
   - **Ankylosing spondylitis**
   - **Lupus**
   - **Rheumatoid arthritis**
   - **Juvenile rheumatoid arthritis**
   - **Psoriatic arthritis**
8. **Drug or alcohol abuse** (increased risk of infection, nutritional deficiencies, anesthesia)
9. **History of cancer**
10. **Intravenous drug use**
11. **Immunosuppression, due to illness (e.g., HIV) or medications (e.g., steroids or cyclosporine)**
12. **History of corticosteroid use** (causes osteoporosis and increased risk for infection)
13. **Fever above 100° F or suspicion of septic arthritis or osteomyelitis**
14. **Diabetes** (increased risk of infection, nutritional deficiencies, anesthesia)
15. **Hypertension** (abdominal aneurysm: low back pain, nausea, pulsatile abdominal mass)
16. **Recent visit for same problem and not improved**
17. **Patient seeking compensation for pain/ injury** (increased need for documentation)
18. **Skin lesion** (psoriasis, melanoma, dermatomyositis, the butterfly rash of lupus, scars from previous surgery, accident, etc....)
19. **Deformity or immobility**
20. **Lymphadenopathy** (suggests cancer or infection)
21. **Elevated ESR/CRP** (cancer, infection, inflammatory disorder)
22. **Elevated WBC count**
23. **Elevated alkaline phosphatase** (bone lesions, metabolic bone disease, hepatopathy)
24. **Elevated acid phosphatase** (occasionally used to monitor prostate cancer)
25. **Positive rheumatoid factor and/or CCP—cyclic citrullinated protein antibodies**
26. **Positive HLA-B27** (propensity for inflammatory arthropathies)
27. **Serum gammopathy** (multiple myeloma is the most common primary bone tumor)
28. **"High-risk for disease"** *examples:*
    - Long-term heavy smoking of cigarettes
    - Long-term exposure to radiation
    - Obesity
29. **Strong family history of inflammatory, musculoskeletal, or malignant disease**
30. **Others:** _____
    _____
    _____

---

[201] Remember that metastasis often travel first from the primary site to bone, therefore bone pain may be an early manifestation of occult cancer. Most of the above are from "Table 1: The high-risk patient: clinical indications for radiography in low back pain patients." J Taylor, DC, DACBR, D Resnick, MD. Imaging decisions in the management of low back pain. Advances in Chiropractic. Mosby Year Book. 1994; 1-28

[202] Radiographs are often essential for diagnosis or to rule out complications of the disease. For example, in patients with inflammatory arthropathies such as these, spontaneous rupture of the transverse ligament (at the odontoid process) has been reported; although rare, this complication could be life-threatening if mismanaged or undiagnosed.

Concept: Not all "Injury-related Problems" are "Injury-related Problems"

In the case of most acute injuries, the underlying problem is often the injury itself. However, the physician must conduct a thorough history and examination to assess for possible underling pathologies that cause or contribute to the problem that "appears" to be injury-related. Congenital anomalies, underlying pathology, previous injury, occult infections, and psychoemotional disorders may have been present *before* the "injury." Just because the patient reports a problem such as pain following an injury does not mean that the injury is the *sole* cause of the pain. *Do not let a biased history lead you down the wrong path.*

> **"Pediatric infections and neoplasms are notorious for masquerading as sport injuries.** ...Take the relevant history directly from the patient, and keep tumors and infections high on your list of differential diagnoses... For example, about 15% of children with leukemia present with musculoskeletal complaints..."
>
> Shaw BA, Gerardi JA, Hennrikus WL.
> How to avoid orthopedic pitfalls in children.
> *Patient Care* 1999; Feb 28: 95-116

In children and young adults, 5% of "sports-related" injuries are associated with preexisting infection, anomalies, or other conditions. In adult women, "...between 9% and 20% of women with breast cancer attribute their symptoms to previous trauma to the breast. In these cases, the association of the breast mass with a traumatic event resulted in a delay in diagnosis ranging from four months to one year."[203]

When treating children, be very careful to get an accurate history—this is difficult since your two sources of information are not very reliable: parents often think that they already have the problem figured out, and so their history will be biased toward convincing you of what they think is the problem and solution; children are often not good historians and can form illogical relationships between events that can be misleading.

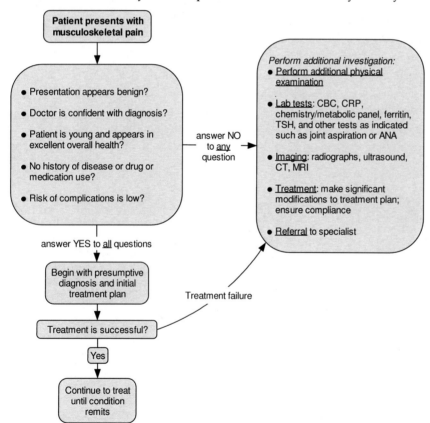

A group of German physicians describe a man who presented with a soft-tissue pain following a soccer game; he was later diagnosed with a malignant tumor—synovial sarcoma.[204] Similarly, Wakeshima and Ellen[205] describe a young athletic woman who presented with chronic hip pain. The woman's history was significant for ulcerative colitis, but otherwise her radiographs were normal and her history and examination lead to a diagnosis of trochanteric bursitis.

However, the patient's condition did not respond to routine treatment, and additional investigation over several months lead to a diagnosis of giant cell carcinoma. The authors concluded, "This case shows **the importance of repeat radiographic studies in patients whose joint pain does not respond or responds slowly to conservative therapy, despite initial normal findings.**"

---

[203] Seifert S. Medical Illness Simulating Trauma (MIST) syndrome: case reports and discussion of syndrome. *Fam Med* 1993 Apr;25(4):273-6
[204] Engel C, Kelm J, Olinger A. Blunt trauma in soccer. The initial manifestation of synovial sarcoma. [Article in German] *Zentralbl Chir* 2001 Jan;126(1):68-71
[205] Wakeshima Y, Ellen MI. Atypical hip pain origin in a young athletic woman: a case report of giant cell carcinoma. *Arch Phys Med Rehabil* 2001 Oct;82(10):1472-5

What you expect to find and hear when taking a trauma-related history is that **1) a healthy patient** with no previous health concerns was **2) exposed to a traumatic event**, the history and consequences of which perfectly coincide with the injury you are assessing in your office, and that **3) your physical examination findings are all consistent** and lead to a specific diagnosis, which then **4) responds to your treatment**. **If you find discrepancies between the history of the injury and your physical examination findings (e.g., fever after a "sports-related" injury), if the patient appears unhealthy in disproportion to the presenting complaint, or if the patient does not respond to your treatment, then you must consider the possibility of preexisting or concomitant disease.** Astute doctors search for and rule out preexisting and underlying pathology before ascribing the problem to the "obvious cause." Always assess for consistency between the history, examination findings, and response to treatment—inconsistencies suggest the need for additional assessment.

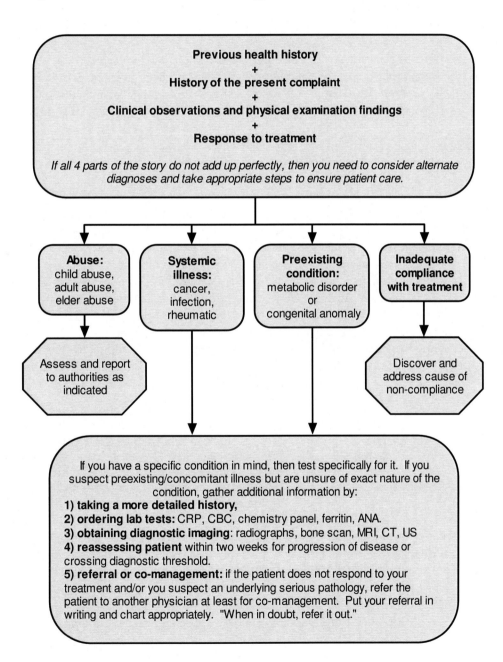

Previous health history
+
History of the present complaint
+
Clinical observations and physical examination findings
+
Response to treatment

If all 4 parts of the story do not add up perfectly, then you need to consider alternate diagnoses and take appropriate steps to ensure patient care.

Abuse:
child abuse, adult abuse, elder abuse

Systemic illness:
cancer, infection, rheumatic

Preexisting condition:
metabolic disorder or congenital anomaly

Inadequate compliance with treatment

Assess and report to authorities as indicated

Discover and address cause of non-compliance

If you have a specific condition in mind, then test specifically for it. If you suspect preexisting/concomitant illness but are unsure of exact nature of the condition, gather additional information by:
1) taking a more detailed history,
2) ordering lab tests: CRP, CBC, chemistry panel, ferritin, ANA.
3) obtaining diagnostic imaging: radiographs, bone scan, MRI, CT, US
4) reassessing patient within two weeks for progression of disease or crossing diagnostic threshold.
5) referral or co-management: if the patient does not respond to your treatment and/or you suspect an underlying serious pathology, refer the patient to another physician at least for co-management. Put your referral in writing and chart appropriately. "When in doubt, refer it out."

Concept: Safe Patient + Safe Treatment = Safe Outcome

The purpose of performing the history and physical examination on a new *or established* patient is to determine their current health status—including their mental and emotional health and their physical health, particularly as this relates to important and life-threatening possibilities such as cancer, infections, fractures, systemic diseases, and neurologic compromise. The questions that lead this investigation are: "**What is this patient's current status?**" "**Does this patient have a serious disease, neurologic injury, or are they at high risk for developing a serious complication in the near future that can be prevented with appropriate care** *now*?"

"Is this patient safe?"
- The question to ask yourself is, "Is this patient's health problem or current complaint/exacerbation a manifestation of an underlying condition that could result in a negative outcome?
- If a patient comes to you with a headache, and you neglect to find that their blood pressure is 230/130, then you missed the opportunity to help them avoid the stroke that they could have after leaving your office.
- If a patient comes to you with a complaint of low back pain, and you neglect to perform a neurologic examination to find that *the patient already has a neurologic deficit even before you treated them*, then you have lost the opportunity to defend yourself in court when the patient later claims that *your* treatment and *your* management of their case is the reason that they now have a permanent neurologic deficit.

Is your treatment safe?

Have you been perfectly clear with the patient about the risks and benefits of your treatment plan? **Have you obtained informed consent**? Have you charted "**PAR-B**" to indicate that you have discussed the **P**rocedures, **A**lternatives, **R**isks, and **B**enefits of your treatment plan? Have you been clear about the duration of treatment and the need for appropriate follow-up? If you are prescribing nutrition or botanical medicines, have you informed the patient about the duration of treatment? **Have you looked for contraindications to your otherwise brilliant treatment plan**? What about the fact that this patient was on corticosteroids for the past 15 years and only discontinued prednisone 2 months before arriving at your office? *The patient may have steroid-induced osteoporosis even though he is no longer on prednisone.* When you recommend that your patient take 100,000 IU of vitamin A to treat her throat infection, what happens when she presents to your office 8 months later with signs of vitamin A toxicity because she continued her treatment plan indefinitely rather than using it only for 7 days as you had intended? *Be sure to put a time limit on your treatment plans.* Every treatment plan should be 1) given to the patient in legible print and clear statements, 2) be copied for the chart, 3) include "what to do if things get worse" in the event of adverse treatment effect or exacerbation of problem, and 4) include patient's responsibility for returning to office/clinic for follow-up and reassessment.

> Double-check to ensure that your patient is safe (no forthcoming complications or predictable emergencies) and that your treatment is safe (appropriate, effective, clearly communicated, and time-limited with instructions to return for office visit).

Informed consent:

From a legal standpoint, doctors can only treat a patient after the patient has given *consent to treatment*. Patients can only authoritatively consent to treatment after they have been fully educated about the treatment—thus they can provide *informed consent*. Full disclosure about the treatment plan includes informing the patient of the Procedures—what will take place; Alternatives—what options are available; Risks—what risks are involved, and (optionally) Benefits—what benefits can be expected. This is commonly charted as "**PAR—no questions**" or "**PAR—questions answered**" once the patient gives consent to treatment.

Concept: Four Clues to Discovering Underlying Problems

When I taught Orthopedics at Bastyr University I encouraged students to search for specific **sets of clues** when evaluating patients. These clues—often insignificant in isolation but meaningful in combination—were often the "red flags" that could help make the difference between an accurate diagnosis and a missed diagnosis. These four categories can be recalled with the mnemonic *"S.C.I.N."* or *"S.C.I.M."* These four areas of assessment/safety emphasis differ from the *"vindicates"* mnemonic which is used for differential diagnosis.

- **Systemic symptoms and signs**: We specifically search for systemic signs and symptoms such as fever, weight loss, lymphadenopathy, or skin rash in patients who present with pain because these "whole body" manifestations might indicate an underlying or concomitant disease that deserves attention, either independently from the musculoskeletal pain, or as a cause of the musculoskeletal pain. For example, "headache" may appear benign, whereas "headache with fever and skin rash" suggests meningitis—a medical emergency. "Low-back pain" is a common occurrence; yet "low-back pain with weight loss and fever" might suggest occult malignancy, osteomyelitis, or other systemic disease.

- **Complications:** We ask about and look for already existing complications, such as "numbness, weakness, tingling in the arms or hands, legs or feet" to rapidly screen for neurologic deficits and we follow this up with screening assessments such as "squat and rise", toe walk, heel walk, and reflexes for spinal cord and lower extremity neuromuscular integrity. Additionally, when dealing with patients with spine-related complaints or injuries, we also ask about changes or loss of function in bowel and bladder control and numbness near the anus or genitals, which may be the *only* clinical clues to cauda equina syndrome—a medical emergency. Ask about effects of the condition on ADL (activities of daily living) to attain a more comprehensive view of the condition and to ensure that the patient's story is consistent.

- **Indicators from the history**: We look for specific "red flags" and "yellow flags" such as trauma, risk factors (such as smoking, prednisone, alcohol), or a positive history of chronic infections or cancer. Nonmechanical musculoskeletal pain in a patient with a history of cancer is highly suspicious and mandates thorough investigation.

- **Non-mechanical pain**: Non-mechanical pain suggests a pathologic etiology rather than simple joint dysfunction. Pain at night, pain that occurs without an inciting injury, pain that is not strongly affected by motion and is not powerfully provoked by your physical examination assessments suggests the possibility of underlying disorder such as cancer, neuropathy, or infection. However, the ability to elicit an exacerbation of pain with "mechanical" maneuvers does not indicate that the pain is "mechanical" and therefore "non-pathologic." Mechanical pain can still be pathologic pain, such as the exquisite pain felt by patients with spinal fractures—they may be neurologically intact, they do have pain worse with motion, but they are not safe to manipulate, and they require appropriate treatment and referral on an urgent basis.

Vindicates: a popular mnemonic for differential diagnosis	
V	Vascular
	Visceral referral
I	Infectious
	Inflammatory
	Immunologic
N	Neurologic
	Nutritional
	New growth: neoplasia or pregnancy
D	Deficiency
	Degenerative
I	Iatrogenic (drug related)
	Intoxication
	Idiosyncratic
C	Congenital
	Cardiac or circulatory
A	Allergy / Autoimmune
	Abuse: drugs, alcohol, physical
T	Trauma
	Toxicity
E	Endocrine
	Exposure
S	Subluxation
	Somatic dysfunction
	Structural
	Stress
	Secondary gain

> Keeping these four assessment categories in mind can serve as a useful "checkpoint" to ensure that your patient is safe, and that your treatment is appropriate and therefore safe, too.

Concept: Special Considerations in the Evaluation of Children

> "Pediatric infections and neoplasms are notorious for masquerading as sport injuries. … There is only one way to avoid this trap: Take the relevant history directly from the patient, and keep tumors and infections high on your list of differential diagnoses."[206]

- **Consider the possibility of child abuse when a child presents with an injury:** As a non-naïve physician, you always have to consider the possibility of child abuse when a child presents with an injury. Be detailed in your history taking, and be sure to search for discrepancies between 1) the child's version of the incident, 2) the adult's version of the incident, and 3) what is realistic (based on your practical life experience and clinical training). As a primary care physician, you are obligated to report your *suspicion* of child abuse to law enforcement agencies and/or child protective services.
- **Children heal quickly:** This rapid healing is good as long as tissues are approximated. But if a fractured bone is displaced and not correctly replaced, then problematic malunion deformities may result *within days*.
- **Children are more susceptible to rapidly progressing infections than are adults:** Soft tissue, joint, and bone infections need to be diagnosed expeditiously and treated aggressively.
- **Children are radiographically different from adults:** Make sure that your radiographs are interpreted by a competent radiologist with experience in the interpretation of *pediatric radiographs*. Radiographic considerations specific to children include:
  - **Epiphyseal growth plates**
  - **Secondary ossification centers**
  - **Variants in trabecular patterns and bone densities**
  - **Specific conditions that happen only in children, such as slipped capital femoral epiphysis**
  - **Congenital anomalies**
  - **Difficulty following directions with positioning** (applies to some adults, too!)
  - **Bone scans can be difficult to interpret in children:** Bone scans derive their value from the demonstration of a focal increase in uptake of radioactive isotopes, which demonstrates and localizes an area of increased metabolic activity. In adults, this increased and localized activity generally indicates pathology, especially malignant disease in bone (primary or metastatic) and recent fracture. In children, however, since their bones are already highly metabolically active due to the normal growth process, bone scans are difficult to interpret and are not highly reliable for the demonstration of focal lesions.

Always consider the possibility of abuse, cancer, infection, or congenital anomaly as a cause of musculoskeletal pain in children, even if the injury appears to be related to injury or trauma. Strongly consider lab tests, as well as radiographs (interpreted by a pediatric radiologist). When in doubt, refer for second opinion. If you suspect abuse, you have a legal and ethical obligation to report your *suspicion*.

---

[206] Shaw BA, Gerardi JA, Hennrikus WL. How to avoid orthopedic pitfalls in children. *Patient Care* 1999; Feb 28: 95-116

Concept: Differences between Primary Healthcare and Spectator Sports

In baseball, "errors" have been defined as "a defensive mistake that allows a batter to stay at the plate or reach first base, or that advances a base runner."[207] In baseball, a few errors can make the difference between winning and losing a particular game or season. However, a few errors in a game are to be expected, and ultimately the team can start over at the next game or season and try to do better.

Healthcare, however, is not a game, and even relatively minor errors such as the doctor's forgetting to ask a particular question or perform a specific test can result in a patient's catastrophic injury or death. In healthcare, when we are dealing with serious injuries and illnesses, even a single "error" is not allowed. "Failure to diagnose" is one of the biggest reasons for malpractice claims against doctors; such judgments often result in loss of licensure and awards of hundreds of thousands of dollars. "Failure to treat" results when the patient is injured because the

> While your compassion for human suffering and your love of nutrition and exercise may have directed you into healthcare, your professional success and survival will depend in large part on your ability to manage the technical and defensive aspects of clinical practice.
>
> Neuromusculoskeletal disorders and autoimmune diseases are "big league" clinical problems, and they need to be taken seriously.

doctor failed to effectively treat the patient or when the doctor failed to provide the appropriate referral to a specialist in a timely manner. Such failures are not only capable of destroying a physician's career and forcing the liquidation of his/her possessions, but such cases can also greatly damage the integrity of whole professions, especially the naturopathic and chiropractic professions which are generally guilty until proven innocent due to the double standards imposed by those adherent to the "always right" dogma of the medical paradigm.[208] Stated differently, **if the doctor does not ask the right questions and perform the right tests, then the doctor may miss an emergency diagnosis. Missing an emergency diagnosis can result in patient death. Patient death may result in litigation, loss of license for the doctor, and irreparable harm to the profession.**

The upcoming section on **Musculoskeletal Emergencies** represents *core competencies* that every clinician must keep present in his/her mind during each interaction with a patient with musculoskeletal complaints, especially patients who are elderly, on medications such as prednisone, and those with known autoimmune or immunosuppressive disorders.

Concept: "Disease Treatment" is Different from "Patient Management"

> "The key to successful intervention for orthopedic problems in a primary care practice is to know what conditions to refer and when and to whom to refer the refractory patient."[209]

Treating a problem is one thing, managing a patient is something different. "Problems" such as "low back pain" are abstract concepts, and we automatically form mental lists of treatments for problems that are irrespective of the patient who has the condition. However this list may be of only very limited applicability to the individual patient with whom you are working. Management of patients includes ❶ assessing and reassessing the differential diagnoses, ❷ monitoring compliance with treatments, including the treatments of other healthcare providers, ❸ co-treating with other healthcare providers, ❹ assessing for contraindications, ❺ monitoring patient status and effectiveness of treatments, and also ❻ the office-related tasks of charting, documentation, billing, and correspondence.

The management of emergency conditions often involves transport to the nearest hospital. In some situations, the patient will be able to drive himself/herself without difficulty. In other situations, the patient should be driven by friend, family, or taxi. In the most extreme, the patient should be transported by ambulance. When in doubt about the mode of transport, do not hesitate to call 911 for an ambulance. If the taxi driver gets lost on the way to the hospital, or your patient goes into shock while being driven by a friend, the liability will come back to haunt the *doctor*, not the *friend* or the *taxi driver*.

---

[207] http://www.nocryinginbaseball.com/glossary/glossary.html Accessed November 11, 2006
[208] Micozzi MS. Double standards and double jeopardy for CAM research. *J Altern Complement Med*. 2001 Feb;7(1):13-4
[209] Brier S. Primary Care Orthopedics. St. Louis: Mosby, 1999 page ix

Concept: Clinical Practice Involves Much More than "Diagnosis and Treatment"

Emergency room and hospital-based physicians are appropriately able to focus solely on diagnosis and treatment as their primary spheres of activity and interaction with patients. However, those of us in private practice learn that *healthcare* involves much more than simply being a "good doctor." From an integrative perspective we have to go beyond diagnosis and treatment *for each health disorder* with each patient. Beyond *diagnosis* and *treatment* are *understanding* and *integration*. Orchestrating all of this into a treatment plan that the patient can actually implement requires creativity, resourcefulness, and the ability to enroll patients in the process of *redesigning*—often *rebuilding*—their lives.

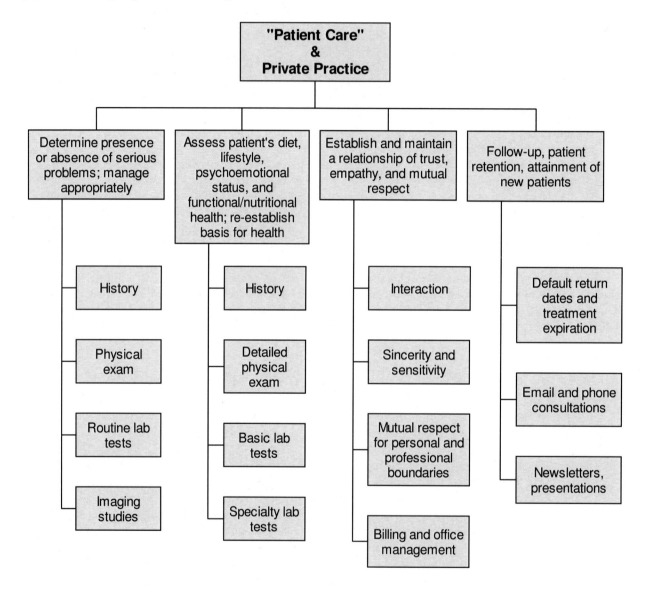

Recall that **28% of malpractice claims involve mistakes made by medical office staff**; this includes unreturned phone calls which can culminate in malpractice by way of "patient abandonment." Similarly, inability to get a timely consultation may result in sufficient "sense of harm" that a patient may decide to sue; this is a factor in 10% of malpractice cases.[210]

---

[210] James R. Hall, Ph.D., L.Psych.,FABMP, FGICPP. Departments of Internal Medicine and Psychology, UNT Health Science Center at Fort Worth. "Communication and Medico-Legal Issues." October 19, 2006

Musculoskeletal Emergencies

These are some of the "core competencies" that clinicians can never afford to miss, and these are pertinent to patients with musculoskeletal disorders, whether structural/orthopedic or metabolic/rheumatic. With these conditions, clinicians are wise to err on the side of caution— *"When in doubt, refer out"*—and implement the appropriate referral on an expedient basis. These are organized in a clinical/logical manner rather than listed alphabetically.

Neurovascular Disorders

Problem	*Presentation*	*Assessment*	*Management*
Neuropsychiatric lupus	▪ Psychosis ▪ Seizures ▪ Transient ischemic attacks ▪ Severe depression ▪ Delirium, confusion	▪ Neuropsychiatric manifestations with history of lupus	▪ Emergency or prompt referral as indicated
Giant cell arteritis, Temporal arteritis: Considered a medical emergency since it may rapidly progress to blindness due to associated involvement of the ophthalmic artery: *"Loss of vision is the most feared manifestation and occurs quite commonly."*[211]	Presentation typically includes the following: ▪ Headache, scalp tenderness ▪ Jaw claudication ▪ Changes in vision ▪ Systemic manifestations of rheumatic disease: fever, weight loss, muscle aches	▪ Palpation of the temporal artery may reveal a "cord-like" artery ▪ Elevated ESR ▪ CBC may show anemia ▪ Temporal artery biopsy is diagnostic	▪ Standard medical treatment is with immediate prednisone ▪ Implement treatment that is immediately effective or refer patient for medical treatment
Acute red eye: General term including acute iritis and scleritis; despite the name of this condition, redness may actually be rather minimal, and it is typically accompanied by cloudy changes in region of the iris and lens	▪ Eye pain and redness ▪ May have facial pain ▪ May be the presenting manifestation of rheumatic disease	▪ Red eye ▪ Photophobia ▪ Reduced vision ▪ May have fixed pupil ▪ Differential diagnosis includes acute glaucoma, bacterial/amebic/viral conjunctivitis or keratitis, allergy, and irritation due to contact lens	▪ "The **acute** onset of a **painful, red** eye, even in the absence of visual upset, should be regarded primarily as an ophthalmological emergency."[212] ▪ **Granulomatous uveitis** occurs in 15% of patients with sarcoidosis and can result in bilateral blindness—this must be managed as a medically urgent condition

---

[211] Tierney ML. McPhee SJ, Papadakis MA (eds). Current Medical Diagnosis and Treatment, 41st Edition. New York: Lange Medical Books; 2002. Page 999-1005
[212] McInnes I, Sturrock R. Rheumatological emergencies. *Practitioner*. 1994 Mar;238(1536):220-4

Musculoskeletal Emergencies—*continued*
Neural canal compression

Problem	Presentation	Assessment	Management
Atlantoaxial instability: Excess mobility between the atlas and axis (commonly due to lesion of the dens or transverse ligament) makes the spinal cord vulnerable to compressive injury when the atlas translates anteriorly on the axis especially during cervical flexion; may progress to neurologic compromise including respiratory and somatic paralysis	▪ Post-traumatic neck injury ▪ Down's syndrome ▪ May present spontaneously (without trauma) in patients with inflammatory rheumatic disease, especially rheumatoid arthritis and ankylosing spondylitis ▪ May have gradual or sudden onset of myelopathy: upper motor neuron lesion (UMNL) signs (e.g., spastic weakness), changes in bowel-bladder function, numbness	▪ Clinical suspicion is followed by lateral cervical and APOM (anteroposterior open mouth) radiographs to assess ADI (atlantodental interval) and dens ▪ MRI should be performed in patients with suspected myelopathy ▪ Neurologic examination of the upper and lower extremities ▪ Do not force neck flexion; do not perform the Soto Hall test	▪ **Urgent neurosurgical consultation is recommended** ▪ **Stabilizing surgery is the best option for the prevention of neurologic catastrophes**[213] ▪ Onset of myelopathy mandates referral to ER and/or neurosurgeon; immobilize with spine board or hard cervical collar and transport appropriately ▪ Asymptomatic and mild increases in ADI (< 5mm) might be managed conservatively with activity restriction, exercises, and bracing/collars) ▪ PAR discussion and referral for surgical consultation is necessary for informed consent and safe management
Myelopathy, spinal cord compression or lesion: May occur due to infection, edema, tumor, spinal fracture, stenosis, or inflammatory disease	▪ **Spastic weakness** ▪ Bowel-bladder dysfunction ▪ Numbness ▪ Problems are distal to cord lesion	▪ Hyperreflexia ▪ Rigidity ▪ Muscle weakness ▪ MRI (with and without contrast) should be performed in patients with suspected myelopathy; CT may also be indicated	▪ Obtain MRI to confirm diagnosis ▪ Immobilize spine and transport if necessary ▪ Acute myelopathy is a medical emergency that can result in rapid-onset paralysis
Cauda equina syndrome: Compression of the sacral nerve roots due to lumbar disc herniation **Cauda equina syndrome is a surgical emergency.**	▪ History of sciatic low back pain ▪ Urinary retention, perineal numbness, and fecal incontinence are common ▪ May have lower extremity weakness	▪ Assess for bladder distention ▪ Assess anal sphincter strength with rectal exam ▪ Lower extremity neurologic examination	▪ Urgent referral for CT/MRI to confirm diagnosis ▪ If diagnosis is confirmed or strongly suspected clinically, urgent referral for surgical decompression is mandatory

---

[213] "When atlantoaxial stability is lost...it is thought that surgical stabilisation of the atlantoaxial joint is more reasonable and beneficial than conservative management. Minimal trauma of an unstable atlantoaxial joint can lead to serious neurological injury." Moon MS, Choi WT, Moon YW, Moon JL, Kim SS. Brooks' posterior stabilization surgery for atlantoaxial instability: review of 54 cases. *J Orthop Surg* (Hong Kong). 2002 Dec;10(2):160-4. http://www.josonline.org/PDF/v10i2p160.pdf

Musculoskeletal Emergencies—*continued*
Acute peripheral nerve compression

Problem	Presentation	Assessment	Management
Acute compartment syndrome: acute compartment syndromes are characterized by acute onset of *potentially irreversible* muscle and/or nerve compression injury due to inflammation, swelling, or bleeding within a fascial compartment **Acute compartment syndrome is a surgical emergency.**	▪ Most commonly occurs in the anterior leg; may also occur in the posterior leg as well as forearm—these are the areas most notable anatomically for the investment of muscle in tight and resilient fascial sheaths ▪ Onset generally follows strenuous exercise that leads to reactive hyperemia and secondary edema ▪ May occur following trauma or fracture	Assess for: ▪ Pulslessness ▪ Palor ▪ Painful passive stretch ▪ Weakness ▪ **Numbness** ▪ Assessment and treatment should be performed on an emergency basis since irreversible nerve damage begins within 6 hours of intracompartmental hypertension	▪ Decompressive fasciotomy is the standard treatment for acute compartment syndrome that could result in permanent muscle necrosis and/or permanent nerve death ▪ Acute compartment syndrome can be fatal if rhabdomyolysis precipitates renal failure[214]

Musculoskeletal infections

Problem	Presentation	Assessment	Management
Septic arthritis: intraarticular bacterial infection; complications of septic arthritis are 1) articular destruction and 2) **death in 5-10% of patients**[215] **Septic arthritis is a medical emergency**	▪ **Febrile** patient has **acute/subacute mono/oligo-arthritis** ▪ Some patients may not have fever ▪ Other possible findings: Immuno-suppression due to medications, concomitant disease (RA, DM), elderly ▪ In some patients with concomitant disease or medications, the clinical picture can be blurred	▪ **Warm, swollen, tender joint** ▪ Clinical assessment with **immediate referral for joint aspiration**, which reveals manifestations of infection such as WBC's and bacteria ▪ Differential diagnosis includes trauma, gout, CPPD, hemochromatosis	▪ **Immediate referral for joint aspiration** ▪ **An aggressive and prolonged course of IV and oral antimicrobials** ▪ "Immune support" such as vitamin A and glutamine and general measures to improve health and prevent recurrence
Osteomyelitis, infectious discitis: considered a medical emergency[216] **Osteomyelitis—especially vertebral osteomyelitis—is a medical emergency**	▪ Febrile patient with bone pain ▪ Assess for constitutional manifestations such as weight loss, night sweats, and malaise	▪ Exacerbation of bone pain when stress/percussion is applied to the bone ▪ Lab: CRP & WBC may be elevated ▪ MRI is more sensitive than CT, bone scan, or radiography[217]	▪ Emergency referral for vertebral osteomyelitis, since **up to 15% of patients will develop nerve lesions or cord compression**[218] ▪ Urgent referral for other types of osteomyelitis

[214] Paula R. Compartment Syndrome, Extremity. *eMedicine* June 22, 2006 http://www.emedicine.com/emerg/topic739.htm Accessed November 26, 2006
[215] Tierney ML. McPhee SJ, Papadakis MA. Current Medical Diagnosis and Treatment. 35th edition. Stamford: Appleton & Lange, 1996 page 759
[216] American College of Rheumatology Ad Hoc Committee on Clinical Guidelines. Guidelines for the initial evaluation of the adult patient with acute musculoskeletal symptoms. *Arthritis Rheum*. 1996;39(1):1-8
[217] Tierney ML. McPhee SJ, Papadakis MA (eds). Current Medical Diagnosis and Treatment 2002, 41st Edition. New York: Lange Medical Books; 2002. Page 883
[218] King RW, Johnson D. Osteomyelitis. Updated July 13, 2006. *eMedicine* http://www.emedicine.com/emerg/topic349.htm Accessed December 24, 2006

Acute Nontraumatic Monoarthritis and Septic Arthritis

- "Acute monoarthritis is a potential medical emergency that must be investigated and treated promptly."[219]
- "Monoarthropathies should initially be investigated to exclude sepsis." "Diagnostic joint aspiration … should be carried out immediately."[220]
- "In acute monoarthritis, it is essential that infection of a joint be diagnosed or excluded, and this can only be done by joint aspiration and synovial fluid culture."[221]
- "Acute monoarthritis should be considered infectious until proven otherwise."[222]

> The primary goal of this section is to solidify your awareness of septic arthritis, its differential diagnoses, and the method and importance of assertive diagnosis and management.
>
> Septic arthritis is a medical emergency, and some authoritative textbooks report a mortality rate of 5-10%.
>
> Septic arthritis must diagnosed urgently with joint aspiration, and it must be treated with antibiotics in order to preserve the joint and prevent spread of the infection.

<u>Clinical presentations</u>:
- Patient presents with acute joint pain in one joint (occasionally more than one joint may be involved).
- May or may not have fever and other systemic manifestations of infection.

Major Differential Diagnoses for Nontraumatic Monoarthritis

Problem	Presentation	Assessment	Management
Septic arthritis: intraarticular bacterial infection; complications of septic arthritis are 1) articular destruction and 2) **death in 5-10% of patients**[223]	▪ **Febrile** patient has **acute/subacute mono/oligo-arthritis** ▪ **Onset over hours or days** Other possible findings: ▪ Immuno-suppression due to medications, concomitant disease (RA, DM), elderly ▪ Some patients may not have fever ▪ In some patients with a previous or concomitant disease process, the clinical picture can be blurred	▪ **Warm, swollen, red, painful joint** ▪ Clinical assessment with **immediate referral for <u>joint aspiration</u>**, which reveals characteristic manifestations of infection such as WBCs and bacteria	▪ **Immediate joint aspiration** ▪ An aggressive and prolonged course of IV and oral antimicrobials ▪ "Immune support" and general measures to improve health and prevent recurrence

> **"Septic arthritis is still a life-threatening disease with a mortality of 2–5% and high morbidity."**
>
> Zacher J, Gursche A. Regional musculoskeletal conditions: 'hip' pain. *Best Practice & Research Clinical Rheumatology.* 2003 Feb;17:71-85

---

[219] Cibere J. Rheumatology: 4. Acute monoarthritis. CMAJ (*Canadian Medical Association Journal*). 2000;162(11):1577-83 http://www.cmaj.ca/cgi/content/full/162/11/1577 January 24, 2004
[220] McInnes I, Sturrock R. Rheumatological emergencies. Practitioner. 1994 Mar;238(1536):220-4
[221] American College of Rheumatology Ad Hoc Committee on Clinical Guidelines. Guidelines for the initial evaluation of the adult patient with acute musculoskeletal symptoms. *Arthritis Rheum.* 1996 Jan;39(1):1-8
[222] Cibere J. Rheumatology: 4. Acute monoarthritis. CMAJ (*Canadian Medical Association Journal*). 2000;162(11):1577-83 http://www.cmaj.ca/cgi/content/full/162/11/1577 January 24, 2004
[223] Tierney ML. McPhee SJ, Papadakis MA. <u>Current Medical Diagnosis and Treatment. 35th edition</u>. Stamford: Appleton and Lange, 1996 page 759

Major differential diagnoses for non-traumatic monoarthritis—*continued*

Problem	Presentation	Assessment	Management
Osteochondritis dissecans: A disorder of unclear etiology (trauma and/or avascular necrosis) which results in the death and subsequent fragmentation of subchondral bone[224]	<ul><li>Primarily affects ages 10-30 years</li><li>**Most common in the knees and elbows**</li><li>Locking and crepitus due to intraarticular loose bodies ("joint mice")</li><li>Some patients are almost asymptomatic, while others have acute pain</li><li>Swelling of the affected joint</li></ul>	<ul><li>Radiographs— consider to assess both knees as the condition is bilateral in 30%</li><li>MRI is used to assess severity and need for surgical intervention</li></ul>	<ul><li>Stable and nondisplaced lesions may be managed nonsurgically; larger and displaced fragments require surgical repair to reduce long-term complications[225]</li></ul>
Transient synovitis, irritable hip: Non-specific short-term inflammation and effusion of the hip joint	<ul><li>Acute onset of painful hip and limp</li><li>Decreased pain with hip in flexion and abduction</li><li>Considered the most common cause of hip pain in children[226]</li><li>More common in boys, age 3-6 years and generally younger than 10 years</li><li>May have recent history of viral infection, and some children (1.5-10%) eventually manifest RA or AVN[227]</li></ul>	<ul><li>May have slight elevation of ESR</li><li>Normal WBC</li><li>No fever; the child appears healthy</li><li>"…radiography is indicated to exclude osseous pathological conditions…"[228]</li><li>**Joint aspiration is indicated if septic arthritis is suspected**[229]</li></ul>	<ul><li>Conservative treatment, restricted exertion and weight-bearing for several weeks</li></ul>
Avascular necrosis (AVN) of the femoral head, osteonecrosis: Ischemic necrosis of the femoral head **Legg-Calve-Perthe's disease**: Idiopathic ischemic necrosis of the femoral head occurring in children	Perthe's disease:<ul><li>80% occur in children generally between ages of 4-9 years; more common in boys; may present with hip pain or knee pain</li></ul>AVN:<ul><li>Ages 20-40 years</li><li>Unilateral hip pain</li><li>May have knee pain</li><li>May have limp</li><li>History of trauma is common</li></ul>AVN associations:<ul><li>Steroid use, prednisone</li><li>Hyperlipidemia</li><li>Alcoholism</li><li>Pancreatitis</li><li>Hemoglobinopathies</li><li>Smoking</li><li>Fatty liver disease: "fat globules from the liver"[230]</li></ul>	<ul><li>Limited ROM</li><li>**Radiographs**; if normal and clinical suspicion is high order MRI or bone scan</li></ul>	<ul><li>**Crutches**</li><li>**Orthopedic referral is recommended** although not all patients will require surgery and some may be managed conservatively[231]</li></ul>

[224] Tatum R. Osteochondritis dissecans of the knee: a radiology case report. *J Manipulative Physiol Ther* 2000 Jun;23(5):347-51
[225] Browne RF, Murphy SM, Torreggiani WC, Munk PL, Marchinkow LO. Radiology for the surgeon: musculoskeletal case 30. Osteochondritis dissecans of the medial femoral condyle. *Can J Surg*. 2003 Oct;46(5):361-3 http://www.cma.ca/multimedia/staticContent/HTML/N0/l2/cjs/vol-46/issue-5/pdf/pg361.pdf
[226] Maroo S. Diagnosis of hip pain in children. *Hosp Med* 1999 Nov;60(11):788-93
[227] Souza TA. Differential Diagnosis for the Chiropractor: Protocols and Algorithms. Gaithersberg, Maryland: Aspen Publications. 1997 page 265
[228] Maroo S. Diagnosis of hip pain in children. *Hosp Med* 1999 Nov;60(11):788-93
[229] Maroo S. Diagnosis of hip pain in children. *Hosp Med* 1999 Nov;60(11):788-93
[230] Skinner HB, Scherger JE. Identifying structural hip and knee problems. Patient age, history, and limited examination may be all that's needed. *Postgrad Med* 1999;106(7):51-2, 55-6, 61-4
[231] Souza TA. Differential Diagnosis for the Chiropractor: Protocols and Algorithms. Gaithersberg, Maryland: Aspen Publications. 1997 page 263

Major differential diagnoses for non-traumatic monoarthritis—*continued*

Problem	Presentation	Assessment	Management
Gout	▪ **Febrile** patient has **acute/subacute mono/oligo-arthritis** ▪ **Onset over hours or days** ▪ "A history of discreet attacks, usually affecting one joint, that precede the onset of fixed symmetric arthritis is the major clue."[232]	▪ May have fever, chills, tachycardia, leukocytosis—just like septic arthritis ▪ Clinical presentation may be sufficient for DX; however septic arthritis should be excluded ▪ Serum uric acid is generally meaningless for the diagnosis of gout since many gout patients will have normal serum uric acid	▪ Medical treatment is rest, NSAID's, and allopurinol ▪ Fluid loading: >3 liters per day; monitor for electrolyte imbalances and hyponatremia as needed ▪ Integrative assessment and treatment for insulin resistance, hormonal imbalances, and nutritional deficiencies
CPPD: Calcium pyrophosphate dihydrate deposition disease	▪ Idiopathic ▪ May be caused by iron overload in some patients ▪ Presentation may be acute or subacute	▪ Medical diagnosis is by synovial biopsy ▪ Radiographs reveal chondrocalcinosis	▪ Allopathic treatment is NSAIDs; phytonutritional anti-inflammatory treatments may also be used (see Chapter 3) ▪ Oral colchicine 0.5 to 1.5 mg per day prevents attacks[233]
Hemarthrosis: Generally associated with trauma, anticoagulation (i.e., coumadin), leukemia, hemophilia	▪ Monoarthralgia with limited motion ▪ May follow direct trauma ▪ Nontraumatic hemarthrosis may be due to anticoagulation, leukemia, hemophilia	▪ Synovial fluid analysis reveals blood	▪ Treatment of underlying disorder; refer as indicated
Slipped capital femoral epiphysis (SCFE): The most common cause of hip pain in adolescents[234]	▪ Seen in adolescents generally 8-17 years of age ▪ Classic presentation is a tall overweight boy with **hip pain**, knee pain, and/or a painful limp: *"Slipped femoral capital epiphysis is a developmental injury that must be considered in any adolescent who presents with hip pain."*[235]	▪ **Radiographs** of both hips (bilateral SCFE in 40%): "**AP and frog lateral views are recommended in all children over age of 9 years with hip pain.**"[236]	▪ Orthopedic referral—*"…the patient should be referred immediately to an orthopedist for surgical stabilization."* [237]

[232] Hardin JG, Waterman J, Labson LH. Rheumatic disease: Which diagnostic tests are useful? *Patient Care* 1999; March 15: 83-102
[233] Beers MH, Berkow R (eds). The Merck Manual. Seventeenth Edition. Whitehouse Station; Merck Research Laboratories 1999 Page
[234] Maroo S. Diagnosis of hip pain in children. *Hosp Med* 1999 Nov;60(11):788-93
[235] O'Kane JW. Anterior hip pain. *Am Fam Physician* 1999 Oct 15;60(6):1687-96
[236] Maroo S. Diagnosis of hip pain in children. *Hosp Med* 1999 Nov;60(11):788-93
[237] O'Kane JW. Anterior hip pain. *Am Fam Physician* 1999 Oct 15;60(6):1687-96

<u>Clinical assessment</u>:
- History and orthopedic assessment of the joint
- Laboratory tests must be performed if you have a suspicion of infection

<u>History/subjective</u>:
- Acute or subacute joint pain with or without systemic manifestations and fever.
- History or may not be significant; other than the obvious risk factor of immunosuppression, septic arthritis can occur with impressive spontaneity and randomness

<u>Differential physical examination and objective findings</u>:
- **Septic arthritis**: pain and limitation of motion, swelling, redness; patient may have systemic symptoms of fever and malaise
- **Gout**: pain and limitation of motion, swelling, redness; patient may have systemic symptoms of fever and malaise
- **Pseudogout and calcium pyrophosphate dihydrate deposition disease (CPDD/CPPD)**: pain and limitation of motion, swelling, redness; patient may have systemic symptoms of fever and malaise
- **Ischemic necrosis**: pain and limitation of motion; swelling, redness and systemic symptoms are less likely.
- **Hemarthrosis**: pain and limitation of motion; often associated with trauma, use of anticoagulant medications[238], or hemophilia and other hematologic abnormalities[239]
- **Tumor**: assess with history, imaging, and biopsy if possible
- **Injury**: Meniscal injury, fracture, ligament injury; physical examination procedures are described in the chapters that follow

<u>Imaging and laboratory assessments</u>:
- **Septic arthritis**: joint aspiration; STAT CBC (for WBC count) and CRP
- **Gout**: joint aspiration; CBC (for WBC count) and CRP
- **Pseudogout and PPDD**: rule out septic arthritis with joint aspiration, CBC, and CRP; radiographs often show chondrocalcinosis
- **Ischemic necrosis**: radiographs are diagnostic
- **Hemarthrosis**: joint aspiration and assessment for underlying disease or medication, especially if the condition was not trauma-induced
- **Tumor**: assess with radiographs
- **Injury**: rule out infection; consider imaging with radiography or MRI

<u>Establishing the diagnosis</u>:
- The aforementioned examinations and lab assessments should establish the exact diagnosis. **The priorities are 1) first exclude life-threatening illness (i.e., septic arthritis), then 2) to exclude serious injury or illness,** and finally 3) to help manage the exact problem

<u>Complications</u>:
- **Septic arthritis can result in death 5-10% of patients. "Five to 10 percent of patients with an infected joint die, chiefly from respiratory complications of sepsis. The mortality rate is 30% for patients with polyarticular sepsis. Bony ankylosis and articular destruction commonly also occur if the treatment is delayed or inadequate."[240]** Complications vary per location, infecting organism, severity, and patient

<u>Clinical management</u>:
- **Suspected septic arthritis requires referral for joint aspiration and antimicrobial drugs**
- Referral if clinical outcome is unsatisfactory or if serious complications are evident
- Treatment of other conditions that cause acute monoarthritis (such as gout and calcium pyrophosphate dihydrate deposition disease) is based on the problem and individual patient

<u>Treatments</u>:
- <u>**Septic arthritis requires IV/oral antimicrobial drugs:**</u> Intravenous antibiotics are generally started before culture results are available. After results and culture from synovial fluid analysis have been considered, the dose, combination, and administration of antibiotics can be fine-tuned. Frequently, antibiotics are administered intravenously for at least 3-4 weeks. Surgical/endoscopic drainage/debridement and immobilization during the acute phase may also be implemented[241]

[238] Riley SA, Spencer GE. Destructive monarticular arthritis secondary to anticoagulant therapy. *Clin Orthop.* 1987 Oct;(223):247-51
[239] Jean-Baptiste G, De Ceulaer K. Osteoarticular disorders of haematological origin. *Baillieres Best Pract Res Clin Rheumatol.* 2000 Jun;14(2):307-23
[240] Tierney ML. McPhee SJ, Papadakis MA. <u>Current Medical Diagnosis and Treatment.</u> 35th edition. Stamford: Appleton & Lange, 1996 page 759
[241] Brusch JL. Septic Arthritis (Last Updated: October 18, 2005). *eMedicine.* http://www.emedicine.com/med/topic3394.htm Accessed November 25, 2006

- **Immunonutrition:** Immunonutritional considerations are listed below; doses listed are for adults. Although studies have not been performed specifically in patients with bone/joint infections, general benefits derived from the use of immunonutrition are reductions in severity/frequency/duration of major infections, abbreviated hospitalization (i.e., early discharge due to expedited healing and recovery), reductions in the need for medications, significant improvements in survival, and hospital savings.[242,243,244,245,246,247,248]
  - <u>Paleo-Mediterranean diet</u>: as detailed later in this text and elsewhere[249,250]
  - <u>Vitamin and mineral supplementation</u>: anti-infective benefits shown in elderly diabetics[251]
  - <u>High-dose vitamin A</u>: Vitamin A shows potent immunosupportive benefits, and vitamin A stores are depleted by the stress of infection and injury. Consider 200,000-300,000 IU per day of retinol palmitate for 1-4 weeks, then taper; reduce dose or discontinue with onset of toxicity symptoms such as skin problems (dry skin, flaking skin, chapped or split lips, red skin rash, hair loss), joint pain, bone pain, headaches, anorexia (loss of appetite), edema (water retention, weight gain, swollen ankles, difficulty breathing), fatigue, and/or liver damage.
  - <u>Arginine</u>: Dose for adults is in the range of 5-10 grams daily
  - <u>Fatty acid supplementation</u>: In contrast to the higher doses used to provide an anti-inflammatory effect in patients with autoimmune/inflammatory disorders, doses used for immunosupportive treatments should be kept rather modest to avoid the *relative* immunosuppression that has been controversially reported in patients treated with EPA and DHA. Reasonable doses are in the following ranges for adults: EPA+DHA: 500-1,500, and GLA: 300-500 mg.
  - <u>Glutamine</u>: Glutamine enhances bacterial killing by neutrophils[252], and administration of 18 grams per day in divided doses to patients in intensive care units was shown to improve survival, expedite hospital discharge, and reduce total healthcare costs.[253] Another study using glutamine 12-18 grams per day showed no benefit in overall mortality but significant benefits in terms of reduced healthcare costs (-30%) and significantly reduced need for medical interventions.[254] After administering glutamine 26 grams/d to severely burned patients, Garrel et al[255] concluded that glutamine reduced the risk of infection by 3-fold and that oral glutamine "may be a life-saving intervention" in patients with severe burns. A dose of 30 grams/d was used in a recent clinical trial showing hemodynamic benefit in patients with sickle cell anemia.[256] The highest glutamine dose that the current author is aware of is the study by Scheltinga et al[257] who used 0.57 gm/kg/day in cancer patients following chemotherapy administration; for a 220-lb-pt, this would be approximately 57 grams of glutamine per day.
  - <u>Melatonin</u>: 20-40 mg hs (*hora somni*—Latin: sleep time). Immunostimulatory anti-infective action of melatonin was demonstrated in a small clinical trial wherein septic newborns administered 20 mg melatonin showed significantly increased survival over nontreated controls.[258]

[242] "To evaluate the metabolic and immune effects of dietary arginine, glutamine and omega-3 fatty acids (fish oil) supplementation, we performed a prospective study... CONCLUSIONS: The feeding of Neomune in critically injured patients was well tolerated as Traumacal and significant improvement was observed in serum protein. Shorten ICU stay and wean-off respirator day may benefit from using the immunonutrient formula." Chuntrasakul C, Siltham S, Sarasombath S, Sittapairochana C, Leowattana W, Chockvivatanavanit S, Bunnak A. Comparison of a immunonutrition formula enriched arginine, glutamine and omega-3 fatty acid, with a currently high-enriched enteral nutrition for trauma patients. *J Med Assoc Thai.* 2003 Jun;86(6):552-6

[243] "CONCLUSIONS: In conclusion, arginine-enhanced formula improves fistula rates in postoperative head and neck cancer patients and decreases length of stay." de Luis DA, Izaola O, Cuellar L, Terroba MC, Aller R. Randomized clinical trial with an enteral arginine-enhanced formula in early postsurgical head and neck cancer patients. *Eur J Clin Nutr.* 2004;58(11):1505-8

[244] "In this prospective, randomised, double-blind, placebo-controlled study, we randomly assigned 50 patients who were scheduled to undergo coronary artery bypass to receive either an oral immune-enhancing nutritional supplement containing L-arginine, omega3 polyunsaturated fatty acids, and yeast RNA (n=25), or a control (n=25) for a minimum of 5 days... Intake of an oral immune-enhancing nutritional supplement for a minimum of 5 days before surgery can improve outlook in high-risk patients who are undergoing elective cardiac surgery." Tepaske R, Velthuis H, Oudemans-van Straaten HM, Heisterkamp SH, van Deventer SJ, Ince C, Eysman L, Kesecioglu J. Effect of preoperative oral immune-enhancing nutritional supplement on patients at high risk of infection after cardiac surgery: a randomised placebo-controlled trial. *Lancet.* 2001 Sep 1;358(9283):696-701

[245] "The feeding of IMMUNE FORMULA was well tolerated and significant improvement was observed in nutritional and immunologic parameters as in other immunoenhancing diets. Further clinical trials of prospective double-blind randomized design are necessary to address the so that the necessity of using immunonutrition in critically ill patients will be clarified." Chuntrasakul C, Siltharm S, Sarasombath S, Sittapairochana C, Leowattana W, Chockvivatanavanit S, Bunnak A. Metabolic and immune effects of dietary arginine, glutamine and omega-3 fatty acids supplementation in immunocompromised patients. *J Med Assoc Thai.* 1998 May;81(5):334-43

[246] "enteral diet supplemented with arginine, dietary nucleotides, and omega-3 fatty acids (IMPACT, Sandoz Nutrition, Bern, Switzerland)" Senkal M, Mumme A, Eickhoff U, Geier B, Spath G, Wulfert D, Joosten U, Frei A, Kemen M. Early postoperative enteral immunonutrition: clinical outcome and cost-comparison analysis in surgical patients. *Crit Care Med* 1997;25(9):1489-96

[247] "supplemented diet with glutamine, arginine and omega-3-fatty acids... It was clearly established in this trial that early postoperative enteral feeding is safe in patients who have undergone major operations for gastrointestinal cancer. Supplementation of enteral nutrition with glutamine, arginine, and omega-3-fatty acids positively modulated postsurgical immunosuppressive and inflammatory responses." Wu GH, Zhang YW, Wu ZH. Modulation of postoperative immune and inflammatory response by immune-enhancing enteral diet in gastrointestinal cancer patients. *World J Gastroenterol.* 2001 Jun;7(3):357-62 http://www.wjgnet.com/1007-9327/7/357.pdf

[248] "using a formula supplemented with arginine, mRNA, and omega-3 fatty acids from fish oil (Impact)... CONCLUSIONS: Immune-enhancing enteral nutrition resulted in a significant reduction in the mortality rate and infection rate in septic patients admitted to the ICU. These reductions were greater for patients with less severe illness." Galban C, Montejo JC, Mesejo A, Marco P, Celaya S, Sanchez-Segura JM, Farre M, Bryg DJ. An immune-enhancing enteral diet reduces mortality rate and episodes of bacteremia in septic intensive care unit patients. *Crit Care Med.* 2000 Mar;28(3):643-8

[249] Vasquez A. A Five-Part Nutritional Protocol that Produces Consistently Positive Results. *Nutritional Wellness* 2005 September http://www.nutritionalwellness.com/archives/2005/sep/09_vasquez.php

[250] Vasquez A. Implementing the Five-Part Nutritional Wellness Protocol for the Treatment of Various Health Problems. *Nutritional Wellness* 2005 November. http://www.nutritionalwellness.com/archives/2005/nov/11_vasquez.php

[251] "CONCLUSIONS: A multivitamin and mineral supplement reduced the incidence of participant-reported infection and related absenteeism in a sample of participants with type 2 diabetes mellitus and a high prevalence of subclinical micronutrient deficiency." Barringer TA, Kirk JK, Santaniello AC, Foley KL, Michielutte R. Effect of a multivitamin and mineral supplement on infection and quality of life. A randomized, double-blind, placebo-controlled trial. *Ann Intern Med.* 2003 Mar 4;138(5):365-71 http://jn.nutrition.com/cgi/reprint/138/5/365

[252] Furukawa S, Saito H, Fukatsu K, Hashiguchi Y, Inaba T, Lin MT, Inoue T, Han I, Matsuda T, Muto T. Glutamine-enhanced bacterial killing by neutrophils from postoperative patients. *Nutrition* 1997;13(10):863-9. *In vitro* study.

[253] Griffiths RD, Jones C, Palmer TE. Six-month outcome of critically ill patients given glutamine-supplemented parenteral nutrition. *Nutrition* 1997 Apr;13(4):295-302

[254] "There was no mortality difference between those patients receiving glutamine-containing enteral feed and the controls. However, there was a significant reduction in the median postintervention ICU and hospital patient costs in the glutamine recipients $23 000 versus $30 900 in the control patients." Jones C, Palmer TE, Griffiths RD. Randomized clinical outcome study of critically ill patients given glutamine-supplemented enteral nutrition. *Nutrition.* 1999 Feb;15(2):108-15

[255] The glutamine dose in this study was "a total of 26 g/day" administered in four divided doses. CONCLUSION: "The results of this prospective randomized clinical trial show that enteral G reduces blood culture positivity, particularly with P. aeruginosa, in adults with severe burns and may be a life-saving intervention." Garrel D, Patenaude J, Nedelec B, Samson L, Dorais J, Champoux J, D'Elia M, Bernier J. Decreased mortality and infectious morbidity in adult burn patients given enteral glutamine supplements: a prospective, controlled, randomized clinical trial. *Crit Care Med.* 2003 Oct;31(10):2444-9

[256] Niihara Y, Matsui NM, Shen YM, Akiyama DA, Johnson CS, Sunga MA, Magpayo J, Embury SH, Kalra VK, Cho SH, Tanaka KR. L-glutamine therapy reduces endothelial adhesion of sickle red blood cells to human umbilical vein endothelial cells. *BMC Blood Disord.* 2005 Jul 25;5:4 http://www.biomedcentral.com.proxy.hsc.unt.edu/1471-2326/5/4

[257] "Subjects with hematologic malignancies in remission underwent a standard treatment of high-dose chemotherapy and total body irradiation before bone marrow transplantation. After completion of this regimen, they were randomized to receive either standard parenteral nutrition (STD, n = 10) or an isocaloric, isonitrogenous nutrient solution enriched with crystalline L-glutamine (0.57 g/kg/day, GLN, n = 10)." Scheltinga MR, Young LS, Benfell K, Bye RL, Ziegler TR, Santos AA, Antin JH, Schloerb PR, Wilmore DW. Glutamine-enriched intravenous feedings attenuate extracellular fluid expansion after a standard stress. *Ann Surg.* 1991 Oct;214(4):385-93; discussion 393-5 http://www.pubmedcentral.nih.gov/articlerender.fcgi?tool=pubmed&pubmedid=1953094 For additional review, see Ziegler TR. Glutamine supplementation in cancer patients receiving bone marrow transplantation and high dose chemotherapy. *J Nutr.* 2001 Sep;131(9 Suppl):2578S-84S http://jn.nutrition.org/cgi/content/full/131/9/2578S

[258] Gitto E, Karbownik M, Reiter RJ, Tan DX, Cuzzocrea S, Chiurazzi P, Cordaro S, Corona G, Trimarchi G, Barberi I. Effects of melatonin treatment in septic newborns. *Pediatr Res.* 2001 Dec;50(6):756-60 http://www.pedresearch.org/cgi/content/full/50/6/756

Naturopathic Model of Wellness, Illness, and Healing

"The work of the naturopathic physician is to elicit healing by helping patients to create or recreate conditions for health to exist within them. Health will occur where the conditions for health exist. Disease is the product of conditions which allow for it." *Jared Zeff, ND*[259]

The diagram to the right is derived from the monograph by Zeff published in 1997 in *Journal of Naturopathic Medicine* entitled "The process of healing: a unifying theory of naturopathic medicine." By my interpretation, the diagram is important for at least three reasons. First, whereas the allopathic profession describes the genesis of most diseases as *idiopathic* and therefore serviceable by drugs and surgery, the naturopathic profession describes disease processes as *multifactorial* and *logical* and therefore treatable by the skilled discovery and treatment of the underlying causes. Such underlying causes, which nearly always occur as a plurality, may vary mildly or significantly even within a group of patients with the same "diagnosis." Second, the diagram shows that the development of disease and the restoration of health are both *processes*. The restoration and retention of health requires *intentionality* and *tenacity* in lieu of the simplistic *miracle cures* and *silver bullets* proffered by the pharmaceutical industry. Chronic disease does not arrive from outside without first exploiting some internal imbalance; illness is the result of manifold internal imbalances that culminate in the accumulation of physiologic insults which compromise function to the point that organ systems begin to fail—"disease." Likewise, health is restored through a progressive and stepwise program that addresses as many facets of the illness as possible while vigorously supporting optimal physiologic function. Third, the fact that Zeff considered the discharge or "healing crisis" so important that it merited inclusion in this diagram shows, indirectly, the naturopathic emphasis on

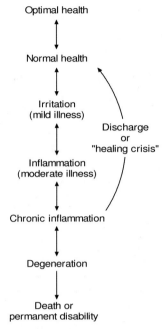

detoxification and the eradication of dysbiosis. Both in the treatment of toxic metal/chemical exposure and in the treatment of chronic infections, patients often go through an acute or subacute phase of feeling quite ill before experiencing a dramatic alleviation of symptoms; the fact that symptoms may temporarily "get worse before getting better" has been referred to as the "healing crisis." This can occur for at least three reasons. First, in the elimination of chemicals and metals from the body, they must first be released from the tissues; the transition from tissues to blood is similar to an acute re-exposure which triggers symptoms of toxicity until the toxin is excreted via sweat, urine, or bile. Similarly, improvement in nutritional status—a cornerstone of all naturopathic interventions—expedites physiologic processes that have been relatively dormant due to lack of enzymatic cofactors such as vitamins and minerals; optimization of nutritional status provides an opportunity for these pathways to function again at which time they must "catch up" on work that has not been performed during the time of nutritional deficiency, namely detoxification of stored xenobiotics. The activation of these pathways is an essential step toward health restoration but results in an initial upregulation of hepatic phase-1/oxidative biotransformation which often results in the formation of reactive intermediates that temporarily impair physiologic processes and cause an initial exacerbation of symptoms. Third, whether through immunorestoration or the use of botanical/pharmacologic antimicrobial agents, the symptom-exacerbating "die off" reaction—classically called the Jarisch-Herxheimer reaction in the context of treating syphilis—is a result of increased (endo)toxin production/release by bacteria/microbes in response effective antimicrobial processes, whether physiologic or pharmacologic.

Modern naturopathic medicine has grown from deeply rooted European healing traditions reaching back several centuries; naturopathic physicians have unwaveringly demonstrated respect, love, and appreciation for the healing powers of nature and the process of life itself.[260] Following their coursework in the basic biomedical sciences, naturopathic physicians are trained in urology, oncology, neurology, pediatrics, obstetrics and gynecology, urology, manual physical manipulation (including spinal manipulation), minor surgery, medical procedures, professional ethics, therapeutic diets, clinical and interventional nutrition, botanical medicines, psychological counseling, environmental medicine, and other modalities. Licensed naturopathic physicians commonly practice as generalists and family doctors.[261,262,263,264]

---

[259] Zeff JL. The process of healing: a unifying theory of naturopathic medicine. *Journal of Naturopathic Medicine* 1997; 7: 122-5

[260] Kirchfeld F, Boyle W. <u>Nature Doctors: Pioneers in Naturopathic Medicine</u>. Portland, Oregon; Medicina Biologica (Buckeye Naturopathic Press, East Palestine, Ohio), 1994

[261] Boon HS, Cherkin DC, Erro J, Sherman KJ, Milliman B, Booker J, Cramer EH, Smith MJ, Deyo RA, Eisenberg DM. Practice patterns of naturopathic physicians: results from a random survey of licensed practitioners in two US States. *BMC Complement Altern Med.* 2004;4(1):14

[262] Smith MJ, Logan AC. Naturopathy. *Med Clin North Am.* 2002 Jan;86(1):173-84

[263] Cherkin DC, Deyo RA, Sherman KJ, et al. Characteristics of visits to licensed acupuncturists, chiropractors, massage therapists, and naturopathic physicians. *J Am Board Fam Pract.* 2002 Nov-Dec;15(6):463-72

[264] Cherkin DC, Deyo RA, Sherman KJ, et al. Characteristics of licensed acupuncturists, chiropractors, massage therapists, and naturopathic physicians. *J Am Board Fam Pract.* 2002 Sep-Oct;15(5):378-90

Naturopathic Principles, Concepts, & the *Vis Medicatrix Naturae*

"The healing power of nature is the inherent self-organizing and healing process of living systems... It is the naturopathic physician's role to support, facilitate and augment this process by identifying and removing obstacles to health and recovery, and by supporting the creation of a healthy internal and external environment."[265]

Identify and Treat the Causes *(Tolle Causam)*: *"Illness does not occur without cause."*
- Naturopathic physicians focus on identifying and addressing the underlying deficiency, toxicity, impairment, or imbalance that is the cause of the health problem or disease.

Treat the Whole Person: *"The multifactorial nature of health and disease requires a personalized and comprehensive approach to diagnosis and treatment."*
- On some occasions the illness does take precedence over the person who has it—such as with emergency situations like acute onset myelopathy, septic arthritis, acute red eye, and atlantoaxial instability. In these cases, the *situation* must be managed appropriately, and these situations are not immediately amenable to long-term lifestyle changes—they require immediate treatment. However, the vast majority of cases in routine clinical practice will require detailed and *bipartite* attention to the facets of *both* **the disease process** and **the person who has the illness**. Our focus on the individual patient is what sets our healing professions apart from others that focus exclusively on the disease and do not consider the manifold intricacies of the individual patient.

The Healing Power of Nature: *Vis Medicatrix Naturae*
- Naturopathic medicine recognizes an inherent self-healing process in the person that is ordered and intelligent. The body has many highly efficient mechanisms for sustaining and regaining health. These mechanisms have their specific and necessary components (e.g., nutrients) and means by which they can be impaired (e.g., xenobiotic immunosuppression). Poor health and disease can result from impairment of these self-healing processes and biologic mechanisms, and thus the body's inherent, natural, self-healing mechanisms—the "healing power of nature"—can be diminished to the state of ineffectiveness or harm (e.g., autoimmunity). Recognizing that the body has this inherent goal of and movement toward self-healing, naturopathic physicians start by identifying and removing "obstacles to cure" rather than ignoring these factors and masking the manifestations of dysfunction with symptom-suppressing drugs.

First Do No Harm *(Primum Non Nocere)*
- Naturopathic physicians use good judgment and compassion to ensure that the treatment does not cause the patient harm. This contrasts with the effects of allopathic treatment, which collectively kill more than 180,000-220,000 patients per year: 500-600 American patients per day.[266]

Prevention
- Healthy lifestyle and emotional hygiene go a long way toward preventing (and treating) many conditions. Specific conditions have specific risk factors and causes that have to be considered per patient and condition.

Doctor As Teacher *(Docere)*
- Explain the situation and your proposed solution to your patient so that they are empowered with understanding and the comfort of knowing what has happened and what is happening.
- Let your own life be a model for your patients. This does not mean that you have to feign perfection—people who demand perfection from you have their own issues to work on; your task is to live the best and most conscious life that you can, to be present with your emotions, qualities, and faults and to treat yourself with respect and acceptance. You can exemplify health (rather than perfection) to your patients by being who you are and can thus facilitate their own acceptance of their current health situation, which is a prerequisite to self-initiated change.

> **"Physician, heal thyself.**
> Thus you help your patient, too.
> Let this be his best medicine that he beholds with his eyes: the doctor who heals himself."
>
> Nietzsche FW. Thus Spoke Zarathustra (1892). [Kaufmann W, translator]. Viking Penguin: 1954, page 77

---

[265] Quoted from the American Association of Naturopathic Physicians website http://aanp.net/Basics/h.naturo.philo.html on February 4, 2001. Other italicized quotes in this section are from the same source. This website has since been replaced by http://naturopathic.org/
[266] "Recent estimates suggest that each year more than 1 million patients are injured while in the hospital and approximately 180,000 die because of these injuries. Furthermore, drug-related morbidity and mortality are common and are estimated to cost more than $136 billion a year." Holland EG, Degruy FV. Drug-induced disorders. *Am Fam Physician*. 1997;56(7):1781-8, 1791-2

<u>Re-Establish the Foundation for Health</u>: An overview of this important naturopathic concept is provided below and is extensively detailed in Chapter 2 of this text.

- **Nutritious, balanced, diverse, fruit- and vegetable-rich, organic, whole foods diet**
    - The Paleo-Mediterranean diet is a diet that emphasizes reliance upon fresh fruits, vegetables, nuts, seeds and lean protein such as soy, whey, fish, poultry[267,268]
    - Vegetarian diets are particularly helpful in the treatment of autoimmune disorders and cancer
- **Basic supplementation**
    - Multivitamin/multimineral supplementation[269]
    - Complete, balanced fatty acid supplementation containing ALA (alpha-linolenic acid), GLA (gamma-linolenic acid), EPA (eicosapentaenoic acid), DHA (docosahexaenoic acid), and oleic acid[270]
    - Physiologic doses of vitamin D3: 1,000 IU for infants; 2,000 IU for children; 4,000 IU for adults[271,272,273]
    - Probiotics (and elimination of dysbiosis)
- **Removing obstacles to cure:** *examples*
    - Toxic exposures, medication side-effects
    - Toxic relationships, emotional obstacles, past events, unfulfilling occupation,
    - Social isolation: the typical American has only two friends no-one in whom to confide[274]
    - Diet with excess fat, arachidonate, sugar, additives, colorants, and insufficiency of protein, fiber, phytonutrients, and health-promoting fatty acids: ALA, GLA, EPA, DHA, and oleic acid
    - Sedentary lifestyle, lack of exercise
    - Weight gain/loss as necessary for weight optimization
    - Epidemic exposure to mercury, lead, and xenobiotics
- **Immune support**
    - Sleep and rest
    - Diet and avoidance of simple sugars[275]
    - Botanical and nutritional medicine
    - Acupuncture[276]
    - Constitutional/contrast hydrotherapy[277]
    - Emotional work and counseling
    - Spinal health and spinal manipulation[278,279]
- **Detoxification and Hydrotherapy**
    - Hyperthermia, sauna
    - Exercise
    - Hydration, and nutritional and botanical medicine to promote hepatic detoxification and excretion[280]
    - Bowel cleansing and enemas[281] to promote bile flow[282] and to reduce intestinal toxicity/putrefaction/dysbiosis[283] for the alleviation of chronic illness[284]
    - Alkalinization: for urinary retention of minerals and enhanced xenobiotic excretion[285]

[267] Vasquez A. A Five-Part Nutritional Protocol that Produces Consistently Positive Results. *Nutritional Wellness* 2005 Sept http://optimalhealthresearch.com/protocol
[268] Vasquez A. Implementing the Five-Part Nutritional Wellness Protocol for Treatment of Various Health Problems. *Nutritional Wellness* 2005 Nov http://optimalhealthresearch.com/protocol
[269] Fletcher RH, Fairfield KM. Vitamins for chronic disease prevention in adults: clinical applications. *JAMA* 2002 Jun 19;287(23):3127-9
[270] Vasquez A. Reducing Pain and Inflammation Naturally. Part 2: New Insights into Fatty Acid Supplementation and Its Effect on Eicosanoid Production and Genetic Expression. *Nutritional Perspectives* 2005; January: 5-16 http://optimalhealthresearch.com/part2
[271] Vasquez A, Cannell J. Calcium and vitamin D in preventing fractures: data are not sufficient to show inefficacy. [letter] *BMJ: British Medical Journal* 2005;331:108-9
[272] Vasquez A. Reducing pain and inflammation naturally - Part 3: Improving overall health while safely and effectively treating musculoskeletal pain. *Nutritional Perspectives* 2005; 28: 34-38, 40-42 http://optimalhealthresearch.com/part3
[273] Vasquez A, Manso G, Cannell J. The clinical importance of vitamin D (cholecalciferol): a paradigm shift with implications for all healthcare providers. *Altern Ther Health Med*. 2004 Sep-Oct;10(5):28-36 http://optimalhealthresearch.com/monograph04
[274] McPherson M, Smith-Lovin L, Brashears ME. Social Isolation in America: Changes in Core Discussion Networks over Two Decades. *American Sociological Review* 2006; 71: 353-75 http://www.asanet.org/galleries/default-file/June06ASRFeature.pdf
[275] "Oral 100-g portions of carbohydrate from glucose, fructose, sucrose, honey, or orange juice all significantly decreased the capacity of neutrophils to engulf bacteria ... The greatest effects occurred between 1 and 2 hr postprandial, but the values were still significantly below the fasting control values 5 hr after feeding." Sanchez A, Reeser JL, Lau HS, Yahiku PY, Willard RE, McMillan PJ, Cho SY, Magie AR, Register UD. Role of sugars in human neutrophilic phagocytosis. *Am J Clin Nutr*. 1973 Nov;26(11):1180-4
[276] "Analysis of the individual patients indicated that the peripheral blood leucocyte and lymphocyte counts differed insignificantly after needling, while the body temperature, rate of respiration, pulse, blood pressure and acupoint temperature all dropped, with a simultaneous increase in the percentage of T-lymphocytes". Tan D. Treatment of fever due to exopathic wind-cold by rapid acupuncture. *J Tradit Chin Med*. 1992 Dec;12(4):267-71
[277] "These results indicate that acute cold exposure has immunostimulating effects and that, with thermal clamping, pretreatment with physical exercise can enhance this response." Brenner IK, Castellani JW, Gabaree C, Young AJ, Zamecnik J, Shephard RJ, Shek PN. Immune changes in humans during cold exposure: effects of prior heating and exercise. *J Appl Physiol*. 1999 Aug;87(2):699-710
[278] Brennan PC, Triano JJ, McGregor M, Kokjohn K, Hondras MA, Brennan DC. Enhanced neutrophil respiratory burst as a biological marker for manipulation forces: duration of the effect and association with substance P and tumor necrosis factor. *J Manipulative Physiol Ther*. 1992 Feb;15(2):83-9
[279] Brennan PC, Kokjohn K, Kaltinger CJ, Lohr GE, Glendening C, Hondras MA, McGregor M, Triano JJ. Enhanced phagocytic cell respiratory burst induced by spinal manipulation: potential role of substance P. *J Manipulative Physiol Ther*. 1991 Sep;14(7):399-408
[280] Crinnion WJ. Results of a decade of naturopathic treatment for environmental illness: a review of clinical records. *J Naturopathic Med* 1997;7:21-27
[281] Bastedo WA. Colon irrigations: their administration, therapeutic applications, and dangers. *Journal of the American Medical Association* 1932; 98(9): 734-6
[282] Garbat AL, Jacobi HG. Secretion of Bile in Response to Rectal Installations. *Arch Intern Med* 1929; 44: 455-462
[283] Snyder RG. The value of colonic irrigations in countering auto-intoxication of intestinal origin. *Medical Clinics of North America* 1939; May: 781-788. See Chapter 4 of ***Integrative Rheumatology*** (www.OptimalHealthResearch.com) for more details.
[284] Crinnion WJ. Results of a decade of naturopathic treatment for environmental illness: a review of clinical records. *J Naturopathic Med* 1997;7:21-27

Hierarchy of Therapeutics: This naturopathic concept articulates the importance of addressing *the underlying cause* rather than simply focusing on *the presenting problem*, which is the *symptom of the cause*. Further, interventions are *prioritized*, for example:

- Patient-implemented *before* doctor-implemented
- Removal of harming agent *before* addition of a therapeutic agent: e.g., stop smoking *before* investing in respiratory therapy; implement healthy diet and exercise before higher-risk and higher-cost drugs for hypertension and hypercholesterolemia
- Low-force interventions *before* high-force interventions
- Diet *before* nutritional supplements; nutrients *before* botanicals; botanicals *before* drugs; modulatory drugs *before* suppressive/inhibitory drugs; integrative care *before* surgery

Reestablish the foundation for health

- Mental/emotional/spiritual health
- Meditation, freeze-frame, "time out"
- Relaxation
- Positive visualization, positive expectation, affirmation
- Counseling, social contact, group work[286]
- Family contact and resolution
- Dietary intake and nutritional health which addresses the patient's biochemical individuality[287] and correction of deficiencies or excesses
- Identification and elimination of food allergies and food sensitivities
- Reduce toxin exposure, promote detoxification
- Identification and elimination of exposure to gastrointestinal and inhalant xenobiotics
- Remove or reduce specific "obstacles to cure"

Stimulation of the "healing power of nature" and the "vital force"

- Constitutional hydrotherapy
- Homeopathy
- Exercise
- Acupuncture
- Spinal manipulation
- Meditation
- Tai Chi
- Qigong: "energy-cultivation"

Tonification of weakened systems:

- Botanical medicines and other supplements to help restore normal tissue function
- Spinal manipulation to address the primary somatovisceral dysfunction and/or secondary musculoskeletal disorders
- Hormonal supplementation
- Nutritional supplementation
- Exercise
- Physiotherapy

Correction of structural integrity:

- Spinal manipulation to address the primary somatovisceral dysfunction and/or secondary musculoskeletal disorders
- Deep tissue massage, visceral manipulation, lymphatic pump to promote immune surveillance[288]
- Stretching, balancing, muscle strengthening, and proprioceptive retraining
- Surgery, as a last resort

---

[285] Proudfoot AT, Krenzelok EP, Vale JA. Position Paper on urine alkalinization. *J Toxicol Clin Toxicol*. 2004;42(1):1-26. See Chapter 4 of *Integrative Rheumatology* (www.OptimalHealthResearch.com) for more details on the importance and implementation of alkalinization.
[286] See http://www.mkp.org and www.WomanWithin.org for examples.
[287] Williams RJ. Biochemical Individuality: The Basis for the Genetotrophic Concept. Austin and London: University of Texas Press, 1956
[288] "Lymph flow in the thoracic duct increased from 1.57±0.20 mL·min-1 to a peak TDF of 4.80±1.73 mL·min-1 during abdominal pump, and from 1.20±0.41 mL·min-1 to 3.45±1.61 mL·min-1 during thoracic pump." Knott EM, Tune JD, Stoll ST, Downey HF. Increased lymphatic flow in the thoracic duct during manipulative intervention. *J Am Osteopath Assoc*. 2005 Oct;105(10):447-56 http://www.jaoa.org/cgi/content/full/105/10/447

Chiropractic: Overview of History and Current Science

"Doctors of Chiropractic are physicians who consider man as an integrated being and give special attention to the physiological and biochemical aspects including structural, spinal, musculoskeletal, neurological, vascular, nutritional, emotional and environmental relationships." *American Chiropractic Association*[289]

"The human body represents the actions of three laws—spiritual, mechanical, and chemical—united as one triune. As long as there is perfect union of these three, there is health." *Daniel David Palmer, founder of the modern chiropractic profession*[290]

The basic philosophical paradigm which is taught in many chiropractic colleges is to envision health, disease, and patient care from a conceptual model named the "triad of health" which gives its attention to the three fundamental foundations for well-being: namely, the physical/structural, mental/emotional, and biochemical/nutritional/hormonal aspects of health. Revolutionary at the time of its inception in the early 1900's, this model now forms the foundation for the increasingly dominant and very popular paradigm of "holistic medicine." It remains a powerful contrast and an attractive alternative to the reductionistic allopathic approach, which generally approaches the human body as if it were simply a conglomerate of independent organ systems that have little or no functional relationship to each other.[291]

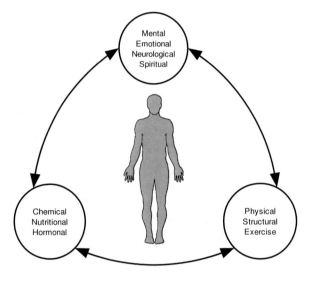

Using the state of the sciences before the year 1910, chiropractic was founded with a profound appreciation of the integrated nature of health and the therapeutic focus was on spinal manipulation. In describing the chiropractic model of health, DD Palmer[292] wrote, "The human body represents the actions of three laws—spiritual, mechanical, and chemical—united as one triune. As long as there is perfect union of these three, there is health." While the therapeutic focus of the profession has been spinal manipulation, from its inception the chiropractic profession has emphasized a holistic, integrative model of therapeutic intervention, health, and disease, and chiropractic was the first healthcare profession in America to specifically claim that the optimization of health requires attention to spiritual-emotional-psychological, mechanical-physical-structural, and biochemical-nutritional-hormonal-chemical considerations. Accordingly, these cornerstones are fundamental to the modern definition of the chiropractic profession recently articulated by the American Chiropractic Association[293]: "Doctors of Chiropractic are physicians who consider man as an integrated being and give special attention to the physiological and biochemical aspects including structural, spinal, musculoskeletal, neurological, vascular, nutritional, emotional, and environmental relationships."

From its inception, chiropractic was a philosophy of healing that considered the entire health of the patient by addressing the interconnected aspects of our chemical-spiritual-physical being. Later, intraprofessional factions polarized between holistic and vitalistic paradigms; the latter has been presumed to be the philosophy of the entire profession by organizations such as the American Medical Association[294] that have sought to

[289] American Chiropractic Association. http://www.amerchiro.org/media/whatis/ Accessed March 13, 2004
[290] Palmer DD. The Science, Art, and Phiosphy, of Chiropractic. Portland, OR; Portland Printing House Company, 1910: 107
[291] Beckman JF, Fernandez CE, Coulter ID. A systems model of health care: a proposal. *J Manipulative Physiol Ther*. 1996 Mar-Apr; 19(3): 208-15
[292] Palmer DD. The Science, Art, and Phiosophy, of Chiropractic. Portland, OR; Portland Printing House Company, 1910: 107
[293] American Chiropractic Association. What is Chiropractic? http://amerchiro.org/media/whatis/ Accessed January 9, 2005
[294] American Medical Association. Report 12 of the Council on Scientific Affairs (A-97) Full Text. http://www.ama-assn.org/ama/pub/category/13638.html Accessed September 10, 2005.

contain and eliminate chiropractic and other forms of natural healthcare[295] by falsifying research[296,297], intentionally misleading the public and manipulating politicians[298,299,300], , arriving at illogical conclusions which support the medical paradigm and refute the value of manual therapies[301], and exploiting weaknesses within the profession for its own financial profitability and political advantage.[302] Intentional misrepresentation and defamation of chiropractic continues to occur today, as documented by the 2006 review by Wenban.[303]

Chiropractic Training and Clinical Benefits

In addition to the basic sciences and foundational skills of laboratory and clinical diagnosis, chiropractic physicians receive extensive training in manual physical manipulation, rehabilitation, therapeutic exercise, and clinical nutrition. According to data with hundreds of medical students and allopathic clinicians, medical school preparation in musculoskeletal medicine is inadequate, and the vast majority of medical graduates are incompetent in basic musculoskeletal diagnosis and management[304,305,306,307,308,309]; conversely, according to limited data with 123 chiropractic students and 10 chiropractic doctors, chiropractic training in musculoskeletal medicine is significantly superior to allopathic and osteopathic musculoskeletal training.[310] In accord with this comprehensive training in musculoskeletal management, numerous sources of evidence demonstrate that chiropractic management is much safer and less expensive than allopathic medical treatment, particularly for treatment of low-back pain. In their extensive review of the literature, Manga et al[311] published in 1993 that chiropractic management of low-back pain is superior to allopathic medical management in terms of greater safety, greater effectiveness, and reduced cost; they concluded, "There is an overwhelming body of evidence indicating that chiropractic management of low-back pain is more cost-effective than medical management" and "There would be highly significant cost savings if more management of LBP [low-back pain] was transferred from medical physicians to chiropractors." In a randomized trial involving 741 patients, Meade et al[312] showed, "**Chiropractic treatment was more effective than hospital outpatient management, mainly for patients with chronic or severe back pain**... The benefit of chiropractic treatment became more evident throughout the follow up period. Secondary outcome measures also showed that chiropractic was more beneficial." A 3-year follow-up study by these same authors[313] in 1995 showed, "At three years the results confirm the findings of an earlier report that when chiropractic or hospital therapists treat patients with low-back pain as they would in day to day practice, **those treated by chiropractic derive more benefit and long term satisfaction than those treated by hospitals**." More recently, in 2004 Legorreta et al[314] reported that the availability of chiropractic care was associated with significant cost savings among 700,000 patients with chiropractic coverage compared to 1 million patients whose insurance coverage was limited to allopathic medical treatments. Simple extrapolation of the average savings per patient in this study ($208 annual savings associated with chiropractic coverage) to the US population (295 million citizens in 2005[315]) suggests that, if fully implemented in a nation-wide basis, America could save $61,360,000,000 (more than $61 billion per year) in healthcare annual expenses by ensuring chiropractic for all citizens in contrast to failing to provide such coverage; obviously extrapolations such as this should consider other variables, such as the relatively higher

[295] Getzendanner S. Permanent injunction order against AMA. *JAMA*. 1988 Jan 1;259(1):81-2 http://www.optimalhealthresearch.com/archives/wilk-ama-judgement.pdf

[296] Terrett AG. Misuse of the literature by medical authors in discussing spinal manipulative therapy injury. *J Manipulative Physiol Ther*. 1995 May;18(4):203-10

[297] Morley J, Rosner AL, Redwood D. A case study of misrepresentation of the scientific literature: recent reviews of chiropractic. *J Altern Complement Med*. 2001 Feb;7(1):65-78

[298] Spivak JL. The Medical Trust Unmasked. Louis S. Siegfried Publishers; New York: 1961

[299] Trever W. In the Public Interest. Los Angeles; Scriptures Unlimited; 1972. This is probably the most authoritative documentation of the illegal actions of the AMA up to 1972; contains numerous photocopies of actual AMA documents and minutes of official meetings with overt intentionality of destroying Americans' healthcare options so that the AMA and related organizations would have a monopoly in healthcare.

[300] Wolinsky H, Brune T. The Serpent on the Staff: The Unhealthy Politics of the American Medical Association. GP Putnam and Sons, New York, 1994

[301] Mein EA, Greenman PE, McMillin DL, Richards DG, Nelson CD. Manual medicine diversity: research pitfalls and the emerging medical paradigm. *J Am Osteopath Assoc*. 2001 Aug;101(8):441-4

[302] Wilk CA. Medicine, Monopolies, and Malice: How the Medical Establishment Tried to Destroy Chiropractic. Garden City Park: Avery, 1996

[303] Wenban AB. Inappropriate use of the title 'chiropractor' and term 'chiropractic manipulation' in the peer-reviewed biomedical literature. *Chiropr Osteopat*. 2006;14:16 http://chiroandosteo.com/content/14/1/16

[304] Freedman KB, Bernstein J. The adequacy of medical school education in musculoskeletal medicine. *J Bone Joint Surg Am*. 1998;80(10):1421-7

[305] Freedman KB, Bernstein J. Educational deficiencies in musculoskeletal medicine. *J Bone Joint Surg Am*. 2002;84-A(4):604-8

[306] Joy EA, Hala SV. Musculoskeletal Curricula in Medical Education: Filling In the Missing Pieces. *The Physician and Sportsmedicine*. 2004; 32: 42-45

[307] Matzkin E, Smith ME, Freccero CD, Richardson AB. Adequacy of education in musculoskeletal medicine. *J Bone Joint Surg Am*. 2005 Feb;87-A(2):310-4

[308] Schmale GA. More evidence of educational inadequacies in musculoskeletal medicine. *Clin Orthop Relat Res*. 2005 Aug;(437):251-9

[309] Stockard AR, Allen TW. Competence levels in musculoskeletal medicine: comparison of osteopathic and allopathic medical graduates. *J Am Osteopath Assoc*. 2006 Jun;106(6):350-5

[310] **Humphreys BK, Sulkowski A, McIntyre K, Kasiban M, Patrick AN. An examination of musculoskeletal cognitive competency in chiropractic interns. *J Manipulative Physiol Ther*. 2007;30(1):44-9**

[311] Manga P, Angus D, Papadopoulos C, et al. The Effectiveness and Cost-Effectiveness of Chiropractic Management of Low-Back Pain. Richmond Hill, Ontario: Kenilworth Publishing; 1993

[312] Meade TW, Dyer S, Browne W, Townsend J, Frank AO. Low-back pain of mechanical origin: randomised comparison of chiropractic and hospital outpatient treatment. *BMJ*. 1990;300(6737):1431-7

[313] Meade TW, Dyer S, Browne W, Frank AO. Randomised comparison of chiropractic and hospital outpatient management for low-back pain: results from extended follow up. *BMJ*. 1995;311(7001):349-5

[314] **Legorreta AP, Metz RD, Nelson CF, Ray S, Chernicoff HO, Dinubile NA. Comparative analysis of individuals with and without chiropractic coverage: patient characteristics, utilization, and costs. *Arch Intern Med*. 2004;164:1985-92**

[315] US Census Bureau http://factfinder.census.gov/home/saff/main.html?_lang=en Accessed January 12, 2005

prevalence of injury and death among patients treated with drugs and surgery.[316,317] Furthermore, whether the cost savings associated with chiropractic availability are due to 1) improved overall health and reduced need for pharmacosurgical intervention, 2) greater safety and lower cost of chiropractic treatment versus pharmacosurgical treatment, and/or 3) self-selection by wellness-oriented and higher-income patients, remains to be determined. A literature review by Dabbs and Lauretti[318] showed that spinal manipulation is safer than the use of NSAIDs in the treatment of neck pain. Contrasting the rates of manipulation-associated cerebrovascular accidents to the dangers of medical and surgical treatments for spinal disorders, Rosner[319] noted, "These rates are 400 times lower than the death rates observed from gastrointestinal bleeding due to the use of nonsteroidal anti-inflammatory drugs and 700 times lower than the overall mortality rate for spinal surgery." Similarly, in his review of the literature comparing the safety of chiropractic manipulation in patients with low-back pain associated with lumbar disc herniation, Oliphant[320] showed that, "The apparent safety of spinal manipulation, especially when compared with other [medically] accepted treatments for [lumbar disk herniation], should stimulate its use in the conservative treatment plan of [lumbar disk herniation]."

The clinical benefits and cost-effectiveness of chiropractic management of musculoskeletal conditions is extensively documented, and that spinal manipulation generally shows superior safety to drug and surgical treatment of back and neck pain is also well established.[321,322,323,324,325,326,327] Adjunctive therapies such as post-isometric relaxation[328] and correction of myofascial dysfunction[329] can lead to tremendous and rapid reductions in musculoskeletal pain without the hazards and expense associated with pharmaceutical drugs. Nonmusculoskeletal benefits of musculoskeletal/spinal manipulation include improved pulmonary function and/or quality of life in patients with asthma[330,331,332,333] and improvement or restoration of vision in patients with post-traumatic visual loss.[334,335,336,337,338,339,340,341] More research is required to quantify the potential benefits of spinal manipulation in patients with wide-ranging conditions such as epilepsy[342,343], attention-deficit hyperactivity disorder[344,345], and Parkinson's disease.[346] Given that most pharmaceutical drugs work on single biochemical pathways, spinal manipulation is discordant with the medical/drug paradigm because its effects are numerous (rather than singular) and physical and physiological (rather than biochemical). Thus, when

[316] Rosner AL. Evidence-based clinical guidelines for the management of acute low-back pain: response to the guidelines prepared for the Australian Medical Health and Research Council. *J Manipulative Physiol Ther.* 2001;24(3):214-20

[317] Topol EJ. Failing the public health--rofecoxib, Merck, and the FDA. *N Engl J Med.* 2004 Oct 21;351(17):1707-9

[318] Dabbs V, Lauretti WJ. A risk assessment of cervical manipulation vs. NSAIDs for the treatment of neck pain. *J Manipulative Physiol Ther.* 1995;18:530-6

[319] Rosner AL. Evidence-based clinical guidelines for the management of acute low-back pain: response to the guidelines prepared for the Australian Medical Health and Research Council. *J Manipulative Physiol Ther.* 2001;24(3):214-20

[320] Oliphant D. Safety of spinal manipulation in the treatment of lumbar disk herniations: a systematic review and risk assessment. *J Manipulative Physiol Ther.* 2004;27:197-210

[321] Dabbs V, Lauretti WJ. A risk assessment of cervical manipulation vs. NSAIDs for the treatment of neck pain. *J Manipulative Physiol Ther.* 1995;18:530-6

[322] Rosner AL. Evidence-based clinical guidelines for the management of acute low-back pain: response to the guidelines prepared for the Australian Medical Health and Research Council. *J Manipulative Physiol Ther.* 2001 Mar-Apr;24(3):214-20

[323] Oliphant D. Safety of spinal manipulation in the treatment of lumbar disk herniations: a systematic review and risk assessment. *J Manipulative Physiol Ther.* 2004;27:197-210

[324] Meade TW, Dyer S, Browne W, Townsend J, Frank AO. Low-back pain of mechanical origin: randomised comparison of chiropractic and hospital outpatient treatment. *BMJ.* 1990;300(6737):1431-7

[325] Meade TW, Dyer S, Browne W, Frank AO. Randomised comparison of chiropractic and hospital outpatient management for low-back pain: results from extended follow up. *BMJ.* 1995;311(7001):349-5

[326] Manga P, Angus D, Papadopoulos C, et al. The Effectiveness and Cost-Effectiveness of Chiropractic Management of Low-Back Pain. Richmond Hill, Ontario: Kenilworth Publishing; 1993

[327] Legorreta AP, Metz RD, Nelson CF, Ray S, Chernicoff HO, Dinubile NA. Comparative analysis of individuals with and without chiropractic coverage: patient characteristics, utilization, and costs. *Arch Intern Med.* 2004;164:1985-92

[328] Lewit K, Simons DG. Myofascial pain: relief by post-isometric relaxation. *Arch Phys Med Rehabil.* 1984;65(8):452-6

[329] Ingber RS. Iliopsoas myofascial dysfunction: a treatable cause of "failed" low-back syndrome. *Arch Phys Med Rehabil.* 1989 May;70(5):382-6

[330] Nielson NH, Bronfort G, Bendix T, Madsen F, Wecke B. Chronic asthma and chiropractic spinal manipulation: a randomized clinical trial. *Clin Exp Allergy* 1995;25:80-8

[331] Mein EA, Greenman PE, McMillin DL, Richards DG, Nelson CD. Manual medicine diversity: research pitfalls and the emerging medical paradigm. *J Am Osteopath Assoc.* 2001 Aug;101(8):441-4

[332] "There were small increases (7 to 12 liters per minute) in peak expiratory flow in the morning and the evening in both treatment groups,… Symptoms of asthma and use of beta-agonists decreased and the quality of life increased in both groups, with no significant differences between the groups." Balon J, Aker PD, Crowther ER, Danielson C, Cox PG, O'Shaughnessy D, Walker C, Goldsmith CH, Duku E, Sears MR. A comparison of active and simulated chiropractic manipulation as adjunctive treatment for childhood asthma. *N Engl J Med.* 1998 Oct 8;339(15):1013-20

[333] Bronfort G, Evans RL, Kubic P, Filkin P. Chronic pediatric asthma and chiropractic spinal manipulation: a prospective clinical series and randomized clinical pilot study. *J Manipulative Physiol Ther.* 2001 Jul-Aug;24(6):369-77

[334] Stephens D, Pollard H, Bilton D, Thomson P, Gorman F. Bilateral simultaneous optic nerve dysfunction after periorbital trauma: recovery of vision in association with chiropractic spinal manipulation therapy. *J Manipulative Physiol Ther.* 1999 Nov-Dec;22(9):615-21

[335] Stephens D, Gorman F, Bilton D. The step phenomenon in the recovery of vision with spinal manipulation: a report on two 13-yr-olds treated together. *J Manipulative Physiol Ther.* 1997;20(9):628-33

[336] Stephens D, Gorman F. The association between visual incompetence and spinal derangement: an instructive case history. *J Manipulative Physiol Ther.* 1997 Jun;20(5):343-50.

[337] Stephens D, Gorman RF. Does 'normal' vision improve with spinal manipulation? *J Manipulative Physiol Ther.* 1996 Jul-Aug;19(6):415-8

[338] Gorman RF. Monocular scotomata and spinal manipulation: the step phenomenon. *J Manipulative Physiol Ther.* 1996 Jun;19(5):344-9

[339] Gorman RF. Monocular visual loss after closed head trauma: immediate resolution associated with spinal manipulation. *J Manipulative Physiol Ther.* 1995 Jun;18(5):308-14

[340] Gorman RF. The treatment of presumptive optic nerve ischemia by spinal manipulation. *J Manipulative Physiol Ther.* 1995;18(3):172-7

[341] Gorman RF. Automated static perimetry in chiropractic. *J Manipulative Physiol Ther.* 1993 Sep;16(7):481-7

[342] Elster EL. Treatment of bipolar, seizure, and sleep disorders and migraine headaches utilizing a chiropractic technique. *J Manipulative Physiol* Ther. 2004 Mar-Apr;27(3):E5

[343] Alcantara J, Heschong R, Plaugher G, Alcantara J. Chiropractic management of a patient with subluxations, low-back pain and epileptic seizures. *J Manipulative Physiol Ther.* 1998;21(6):410-8

[344] Giesen JM, Center DB, Leach RA. An evaluation of chiropractic manipulation as a treatment of hyperactivity in children. *J Manipulative Physiol Ther.* 1989 Oct;12(5):353-63

[345] Bastecki AV, Harrison DE, Haas JW. Cervical kyphosis is a possible link to attention-deficit/hyperactivity disorder. *J Manipulative Physiol Ther.* 2004 Oct;27(8):e14

[346] Elster EL. Upper cervical chiropractic management of a patient with Parkinson's disease: a case report. *J Manipulative Physiol Ther.* 2000 Oct;23(8):573-7

viewed through the allopathic/pharmaceutical lens, spinal manipulation (like acupuncture and other physical modalities), will be viewed as "unscientific" and "does not make sense." In this case, the fault lies with the viewer and the lens, not with the object.

Research documenting the systemic and "nonmusculoskeletal" benefits of spinal manipulation mandates that our concept of "musculoskeletal" must be expanded to appreciate that **musculoskeletal interventions benefit nonmusculoskeletal body systems and physiologic processes**. This conceptual expansion applies also to soft tissue therapeutics such as massage, which can reduce adolescent aggression[347], improve outcome in preterm infants[348], alleviate premenstrual syndrome[349], and increase serotonin and dopamine levels in patients with low-back pain.[350] Studies also suggest benefit in the treatment of non-musculoskeletal complaints[351] with notable research having been performed in the treatment of asthma[352,353], post-traumatic visual loss[354,355,356,357,358,359,360,361], and modulation of immune function.[362,363]

Spinal Manipulation: Mechanistic Considerations

Applied to either the spine or peripheral joints, high-velocity low-amplitude joint manipulation appears to have numerous physical and physiological effects, including but not limited to the following:

1. Releasing entrapped intraarticular menisci and synovial folds,
2. Acutely reducing intradiscal pressure, thus promoting replacement of decentralized disc material,
3. Stretching of deep periarticular muscles to break the cycle of chronic autonomous muscle contraction by lengthening the muscles and thereby releasing excessive actin-myosin binding,
4. Promoting restoration of proper kinesthesia and proprioception,
5. Promoting relaxation of paraspinal muscles by stretching facet joint capsules,
6. Promoting relaxation of paraspinal muscles via "postactivation depression", which is the temporary depletion of contractile neurotransmitters,
7. Temporarily elevating plasma beta-endorphin,
8. Temporarily enhancing phagocytic ability of neutrophils and monocytes, and
9. Activation of the diffuse descending pain inhibitory system located in the periaqueductal gray matter—this is an important aspect of nociceptive inhibition by intense sensory/mechanoreceptor stimulation, which will be discussed in a following section for its relevance to neurogenic inflammation.
10. Improving neurotransmitter balance and reducing pain (soft-tissue manipulation).[364]

While the above list of mechanisms-of-action is certainly not complete, for purposes of this paper it is sufficient to have established that, indeed, joint manipulation in general and spinal manipulation in particular have objective mechanistic effects that correlate with their clinical benefits. Additional details are provided in

[347] Diego MA, Field T, Hernandez-Reif M, Shaw JA, Rothe EM, Castellanos D, Mesner L. Aggressive adolescents benefit from massage therapy. *Adolescence* 2002 Fall;37(147):597-607
[348] Mainous RO. Infant massage as a component of developmental care: past, present, and future. *Holist Nurs Pract* 2002 Oct;16(5):1-7
[349] Hernandez-Reif M, Martinez A, Field T, Quintero O, Hart S, Burman I. Premenstrual symptoms are relieved by massage therapy. *J Psychosom Obstet Gynaecol* 2000 Mar;21(1):9-15
[350] "RESULTS: By the end of the study, the massage therapy group, as compared to the relaxation group, reported experiencing less pain, depression, anxiety and improved sleep. They also showed improved trunk and pain flexion performance, and their serotonin and dopamine levels were higher." Hernandez-Reif M, Field T, Krasnegor J, Theakston H. Lower back pain is reduced and range of motion increased after massage therapy. *Int J Neurosci* 2001;106(3-4):131-45
[351] Leboeuf-Yde C, Axen I, Ahlefeldt G, Lidefelt P, Rosenbaum A, Thurnherr T. The types and frequencies of improved nonmusculoskeletal symptoms reported after chiropractic spinal manipulative therapy. *J Manipulative Physiol Ther*. 1999 Nov-Dec;22(9):559-64
[352] Mein EA, Greenman PE, McMillin DL, Richards DG, Nelson CD. Manual medicine diversity: research pitfalls and the emerging medical paradigm. *J Am Osteopath Assoc*. 2001 Aug;101(8):441-4
[353] "There were small increases (7 to 12 liters per minute) in peak expiratory flow in the morning and the evening in both treatment groups,... Symptoms of asthma and use of beta-agonists decreased and the quality of life increased in both groups, with no significant differences between the groups." Balon J, Aker PD, Crowther ER, Danielson C, Cox PG, O'Shaughnessy D, Walker C, Goldsmith CH, Duku E, Sears MR. A comparison of active and simulated chiropractic manipulation as adjunctive treatment for childhood asthma. *N Engl J Med*. 1998 Oct 8;339(15):1013-20
[354] Stephens D, Pollard H, Bilton D, Thomson P, Gorman F. Bilateral simultaneous optic nerve dysfunction after periorbital trauma: recovery of vision in association with chiropractic spinal manipulation therapy. *J Manipulative Physiol Ther*. 1999 Nov-Dec;22(9):615-21
[355] Stephens D, Gorman F, Bilton D. The step phenomenon in the recovery of vision with spinal manipulation: a report on two 13-yr-olds treated together. *J Manipulative Physiol Ther*. 1997;20(9):628-33
[356] Stephens D, Gorman F. The association between visual incompetence and spinal derangement: an instructive case history. *J Manipulative Physiol Ther*. 1997 Jun;20(5):343-50.
[357] Stephens D, Gorman RF. Does 'normal' vision improve with spinal manipulation? *J Manipulative Physiol Ther*. 1996 Jul-Aug;19(6):415-8
[358] Gorman RF. Monocular scotomata and spinal manipulation: the step phenomenon. *J Manipulative Physiol Ther*. 1996 Jun;19(5):344-9
[359] Gorman RF. Monocular visual loss after closed head trauma: immediate resolution associated with spinal manipulation. *J Manipulative Physiol Ther*. 1995 Jun;18(5):308-14
[360] Gorman RF. The treatment of presumptive optic nerve ischemia by spinal manipulation. *J Manipulative Physiol Ther*. 1995;18(3):172-7
[361] Gorman RF. Automated static perimetry in chiropractic. *J Manipulative Physiol Ther*. 1993 Sep;16(7):481-7
[362] Brennan PC, Triano JJ, McGregor M, Kokjohn K, Hondras MA, Brennan DC. Enhanced neutrophil respiratory burst as a biological marker for manipulation forces: duration of the effect and association with substance P and tumor necrosis factor. *J Manipulative Physiol Ther*. 1992 Feb;15(2):83-9
[363] Brennan PC, Kokjohn K, Kaltinger CJ, Lohr GE, Glendening C, Hondras MA, McGregor M, Triano JJ. Enhanced phagocytic cell respiratory burst induced by spinal manipulation: potential role of substance P. *J Manipulative Physiol Ther*. 1991 Sep;14(7):399-408
[364] "RESULTS: By the end of the study, the massage therapy group, as compared to the relaxation group, reported experiencing less pain, depression, anxiety and improved sleep. They also showed improved trunk and pain flexion performance, and their serotonin and dopamine levels were higher." Hernandez-Reif M, Field T, Krasnegor J, Theakston H. Lower back pain is reduced and range of motion increased after massage therapy. *Int J Neurosci* 2001;106(3-4):131-45

numerous published reviews and primary research[365,366,367,368,369,370,371] and by Leach[372], whose extensive description of the mechanisms of action of spinal manipulative therapy is unsurpassed. Given such a wide base of experimental and clinical support published in peer-reviewed journals and widely-available textbooks, denigrations directed toward spinal manipulation on the grounds that it is "unscientific" or "unsupported by research" are unfounded and are indicative of selective ignorance.

Mechanoreceptor-Mediated Inhibition of Neurogenic Inflammation: A Possible Mechanism of Action of Spinal Manipulation

Neurogenic inflammation causes catabolism of articular structures and thus promotes joint destruction[373,374], a phenomena that the current author has termed "neurogenic chondrolysis."[375] The biologic and scientific basis for this concept rests on the following sequence of events which ultimately form a self-perpetuating and multisystem cycle:

1. Using joint pain as an example, we know that acute or chronic joint injury results in the release of inflammatory mediators in local tissues as **immunogenic inflammation,**

2. Nociceptive input is received centrally and results in release of inflammatory mediators *from sensory neurons* termed **neurogenic inflammation**[376] and results in a neurologically-mediated catabolic effect in articular cartilage[377,378] termed **neurogenic chondrolysis,**

3. As immunogenic and neurogenic inflammation synergize to promote joint destruction, pain from degenerating joints further increases nociceptive afferent transmission to further increase neurogenic and thus immunogenic inflammation. Thus, a *positive feedback* vicious cycle of immunogenic and neurogenic inflammation promotes and perpetuates joint destruction,

4. Further complicating this *regional* cycle of neurogenic-immunogenic inflammation and tissue destruction would be any pain or inflammation *in distant parts of the body*, since pain in one part of the body can exacerbate neurogenic inflammation in another part of the body via **neurogenic switching**[379,380] and immunologic reactivity such as allergy or autoimmunity in one part of the body may be transmitted *via the nervous system* to cause immunogenic inflammation in another part of the body via **immunogenic switching.**[381]

The clinical relevance of neurogenic inflammation and immunogenic switching is that they provide a means *beyond biochemistry* by which to understand how and why inflammation *transmitted and perpetuated by the nervous system* must be treated on a body-wide *holistic* basis.

The current author is the first to propose the concept of **mechanoreceptor-mediated inhibition of neurogenic inflammation.**[382] Since neurogenic chondrolysis is inhibited by interference with C-fiber (type IV) mediated afferent transmission[383] and since chiropractic high-velocity low-amplitude (HVLA) manipulation appears to

[365] Maigne JY, Vautravers P. Mechanism of action of spinal manipulative therapy. *Joint Bone Spine.* 2003;70(5):336-41

[366] Brennan PC, Triano JJ, McGregor M, Kokjohn K, Hondras MA, Brennan DC. Enhanced neutrophil respiratory burst as a biological marker for manipulation forces: duration of the effect and association with substance P and tumor necrosis factor. *J Manipulative Physiol Ther.* 1992 Feb;15(2):83-9

[367] Brennan PC, Kokjohn K, Kaltinger CJ, Lohr GE, Glendening C, Hondras MA, McGregor M, Triano JJ. Enhanced phagocytic cell respiratory burst induced by spinal manipulation: potential role of substance P. *J Manipulative Physiol Ther.* 1991 Sep;14(7):399-408

[368] Heikkila H, Johansson M, Wenngren BI. Effects of acupuncture, cervical manipulation and NSAID therapy on dizziness and impaired head repositioning of suspected cervical origin: a pilot study. *Man Ther.* 2000 Aug;5(3):151-7

[369] Rogers RG. The effects of spinal manipulation on cervical kinesthesia in patients with chronic neck pain: a pilot study. *J Manipulative Physiol Ther.* 1997;20(2):80-5

[370] Bergman, Peterson, Lawrence. Chiropractic Technique. New York: Churchill Livingstone 1993. An updated edition is now availabe published by Mosby.

[371] Herzog WH. Mechanical and physiological responses to spinal manipulative treatments. *JNMS: J Neuromusculoskeltal System* 1995; 3: 1-9

[372] Leach RA. (ed). The Chiropractic Theories: A Textbook of Scientific Research, Fourth Edition. Baltimore: Lippincott, Williams & Wilkins, 2004

[373] Gouze-Decaris E, Philippe L, Minn A, Haouzi P, Gillet P, Netter P, Terlain B. Neurophysiological basis for neurogenic-mediated articular cartilage anabolism alteration. *Am J Physiol Regul Integr Comp Physiol.* 2001;280(1):R115-22

[374] Decaris E, Guingamp C, Chat M, Philippe L, Grillasca JP, Abid A, Minn A, Gillet P, Netter P, Terlain B. Evidence for neurogenic transmission inducing degenerative cartilage damage distant from local inflammation. *Arthritis Rheum.* 1999;42(9):1951-60

[375] Vasquez A. *Integrative Orthopedics: Exploring the Structural Aspect of the Matrix.* Applying Functional Medicine in Clinical Practice. Tampa, Florida November 29-December 4, 2004. Hosted by the Institute for Functional Medicine: www.FunctionalMedicine.org

[376] Meggs WJ.Mechanisms of allergy and chemical sensitivity. *Toxicol Health.* 1999 Apr-Jun;15(3-4):331-8

[377] Gouze-Decaris E, Philippe L, Minn A, Haouzi P, Gillet P, Netter P, Terlain B. Neurophysiological basis for neurogenic-mediated articular cartilage anabolism alteration. *Am J Physiol Regul Integr Comp Physiol.* 2001;280(1):R115-22

[378] Decaris E, Guingamp C, Chat M, Philippe L, Grillasca JP, Abid A, Minn A, Gillet P, Netter P, Terlain B. Evidence for neurogenic transmission inducing degenerative cartilage damage distant from local inflammation. *Arthritis Rheum.* 1999;42(9):1951-60

[379] Meggs WJ. Neurogenic Switching: A Hypothesis for a Mechanism for Shifting the Site of Inflammation in Allergy and Chemical Sensitivity. *Environ Health Perspect* 1995; 103:54-56

[380] Meggs WJ. Mechanisms of allergy and chemical sensitivity. *Toxicol Ind Health.* 1999 Apr-Jun;15(3-4):331-8

[381] "…—immunogenic switching—… In this scenario, the afferent stimulation from the cranial vasculature, which is inflamed during a migraine because of neurogenic processes, is rerouted by the CNS to produce immunogenic inflammation at the nose and sinuses." Cady RK, Schreiber CP. Sinus headache or migraine? Considerations in making a differential diagnosis. *Neurology.* 2002;58(9 Suppl 6):S10-4

[382] Vasquez A. *Integrative Orthopedics: Exploring the Structural Aspect of the Matrix.* Applying Functional Medicine in Clinical Practice. Tampa, Florida November 29-December 4, 2004. Hosted by the Institute for Functional Medicine: www.FunctionalMedicine.org

[383] Gouze-Decaris E, Philippe L, Minn A, Haouzi P, Gillet P, Netter P, Terlain B. Neurophysiological basis for neurogenic-mediated articular cartilage anabolism alteration. *Am J Physiol Regul Integr Comp Physiol.* 2001;280(1):R115-22

inhibit C-fiber mediated nociception[384,385], then chiropractic HVLA manipulation may reduce neurogenic inflammation and may promote articular integrity by inhibiting neurogenic chondrolysis. Further, mechanoreceptor-mediated inhibition of neurogenic inflammation would, for example, help explain the benefits of spinal manipulation in the treatment of asthma[386,387,388], since asthma is known to be mediated in large part by neurogenic inflammation.[389,390] Thus, spinal manipulation appears to provide a means *in addition to other anti-inflammatory interventions such as diet, lifestyle and phytonutritional interventions* by which pain and inflammation can be treated naturally.

A science-based comprehensive protocol can be implemented against pain and inflammation by using ❶ an anti-inflammatory diet, ❷ frequent exercise, ❸ lifestyle and bodyweight optimization, ❹ nutritional supplementation, ❺ botanical supplementation[391,392] ❻ spinal manipulation (with its kinesthetic, analgesic, *directly* and *indirectly* anti-inflammatory, and *probably* piezoelectric benefits[393]), ❼ stress reduction[394,395], ❽ anti-dysbiosis protocols[396], ❾ hormonal correction ("orthoendocrinology"), and ❿ ancillary treatments such as acupuncture[397,398]; additional details and citations for these interventions are provided throughout the text and especially Chapters 2, 3, and the chapter on *Therapeutics*. Pain and inflammation are self-perpetuating vicious cycles, perfectly suited to intervention with comprehensive and multicomponent treatment plans profiled above and detailed in *Integrative Orthopedics* and *Integrative Rheumatology*.

[384] Gillette, R. A speculative argument for the coactivation of diverse somatic receptor populations by forceful chiropractic adjustments. *Man Med* 1987; 3:1-14

[385] Boal RW, Gillette RG. Central neuronal plasticity, low-back pain and spinal manipulative therapy. *J Manipulative Physiol Ther.* 2004;27(5):314-26

[386] Nielson NH, Bronfort G, Bendix T, Madsen F, Wecke B. Chronic asthma and chiropractic spinal manipulation: a randomized clinical trial. *Clin Exp Allergy* 1995;25:80-8

[387] "There were small increases (7 to 12 liters per minute) in peak expiratory flow in the morning and the evening in both treatment groups,... Symptoms of asthma and use of beta-agonists decreased and the quality of life increased in both groups, with no significant differences between the groups." Balon J, Aker PD, Crowther ER, Danielson C, Cox PG, O'Shaughnessy D, Walker C, Goldsmith CH, Duku E, Sears MR. A comparison of active and simulated chiropractic manipulation as adjunctive treatment for childhood asthma. *N Engl J Med.* 1998 Oct 8;339(15):1013-20

[388] Bronfort G, Evans RL, Kubic P, Filkin P. Chronic pediatric asthma and chiropractic spinal manipulation: a prospective clinical series and randomized clinical pilot study. *J Manipulative Physiol Ther.* 2001 Jul-Aug;24(6):369-77

[389] Renz H. Neurotrophins in bronchial asthma. *Respir Res.* 2001;2(5):265-8

[390] Groneberg DA, Quarcoo D, Frossard N, Fischer A. Neurogenic mechanisms in bronchial inflammatory diseases. *Allergy.* 2004 Nov; 59(11): 1139-52

[391] Jancso N, Jancso-Gabor A, Szolcsanyi J. Direct evidence for neurogenic inflammation and its prevention by denervation and by pretreatment with capsaicin. *Br J Pharmacol.* 1967 Sep;31(1):138-51

[392] Miller MJ, Vergnolle N, McKnight W, Musah RA, Davison CA, Trentacosti AM, Thompson JH, Sandoval M, Wallace JL. Inhibition of neurogenic inflammation by the Amazonian herbal medicine sangre de grado. *J Invest Dermatol.* 2001;117(3):725-30

[393] Lipinski B. Biological significance of piezoelectricity in relation to acupuncture, Hatha Yoga, osteopathic medicine and action of air ions. *Med Hypotheses.* 1977;3(1):9-12 See also: Athenstaedt H. Pyroelectric and piezoelectric properties of vertebrates. *Ann N Y Acad Sci.* 1974;238:68-94 See also: Athenstaedt H. "Functional polarity" of the spinal cord caused by its longitudinal electric dipole moment. *Am J Physiol.* 1984;247(3 Pt 2):R482-7

[394] Lutgendorf S, Logan H, Kirchner HL, Rothrock N, Svengalis S, Iverson K, Lubaroff D. Effects of relaxation and stress on the capsaicin-induced local inflammatory response. *Psychosom Med.* 2000;62:524-34

[395] "Couples who demonstrated consistently higher levels of hostile behaviors across both their interactions healed at 60% of the rate of low-hostile couples. High-hostile couples also produced relatively larger increases in plasma IL-6 and tumor necrosis factor alpha..." Kiecolt-Glaser JK, Loving TJ, Stowell JR, Malarkey WB, Lemeshow S, Dickinson SL, Glaser R. Hostile marital interactions, proinflammatory cytokine production, and wound healing. *Arch Gen Psychiatry.* 2005 Dec;62(12):1377-84

[396] Chapter 4 of Integrative Rheumatology and Vasquez A. Reducing Pain and Inflammation Naturally. Part 6: Nutritional and Botanical Treatments Against "Silent Infections" and Gastrointestinal Dysbiosis, Commonly Overlooked Causes of Neuromusculoskeletal Inflammation and Chronic Health Problems. *Nutr Perspect* 2006; Jan http://optimalhealthresearch.com/part6

[397] Joos S, Brinkhaus B, Maluche C, Maupai N, Kohnen R, Kraehmer N, Hahn EG, Schuppan D. Acupuncture and moxibustion in the treatment of active Crohn's disease: a randomized controlled study. *Digestion.* 2004;69(3):131-9

[398] "These results demonstrate an unorthodox new type of neurohumoral regulatory mechanism of sensory fibres and provide a possible mode of action for the anti-inflammatory effect of counter-irritation and acupuncture." Pinter E, Szolcsanyi J. Systemic anti-inflammatory effect induced by antidromic stimulation of the dorsal roots in the rat. *Neurosci Lett.* 1996;212(1):33-6

Osteopathic Medicine

Osteopathic medicine and chiropractic are American-born healthcare professions and paradigms that started at nearly the same time in history and from many of the same foundational principles. Both professions were started in the late 1900's and early 20th century and were founded upon the philosophical premise that the body functioned as a whole and that therefore medicine in general and therapeutic interventions in particular needed to be comprehensive in scope and multifaceted in their application. Further, both professions emphasized the importance of structural integrity as a foundational component of health and thus embraced manual manipulative therapy and spinal manipulation.

From their common origins, subtle differences and chance historic events shaped and further separated these professions from each other. Osteopathy was founded by Andrew Taylor Still, a medical doctor who sought to reform what was then called the "Heroic" paradigm of medicine, which embraced bloodletting and the administration of leeches, purgatives, emetics, and poisons such as mercury as means for "rebalancing" what were perceived to be internal causes of disease, namely the "four humours" of the body which were thought to be blood, phlegm, black bile, and yellow bile. In part because of his training within and identification with the medical profession, Still sought to *reform* rather than *directly oppose* the "mainstream medicine" of his day; in contrast, chiropractic's founder Daniel David Palmer was more strongly opposed to the horrific medicine of his time and thus was more *revolutionary* than *evolutionary* in his approach to forging a new paradigm of health and healthcare. Still's willingness to align with the medical profession and increasingly powerful and influential pharmaceutical industry unquestionably helped his fledgling profession survive the extinction that would have otherwise been swift at the hands of allopathic groups such as the American Medical Association (AMA), which labeled osteopathic physicians as "cultists" and systematically restricted inclusion of the osteopathic profession into mainstream healthcare by proclamation in 1953 that "...all voluntary associations with osteopaths are unethical." When osteopathic resistance mounted, the AMA and its co-conspirators, who were later found guilty of violating the nation's antitrust laws by illegally suppressing competition and attempting to build a medical monopoly[399], acquiesced and accepted osteopaths into its ranks—a strategy which the medical profession believed would eventually destroy the osteopathic profession by forcing it to resign its ideals and identity. In his review of osteopathic history, Gevitz[400] writes, "...the M.D.'s gradually came to believe that the only way to destroy osteopathy was through the absorption of D.O.'s, much as the homeopaths and eclectics [naturopaths] had been swallowed up early in the century." Even today, the AMA continues to list osteopathic medicine under "alternative medicine"[401] although several osteopathic medical colleges have consistently provided training that is superior to most "conventional" medical schools.[402] Today, osteopathic physicians practice in most ways similarly to allopaths—i.e., with unlimited scope of practice in all 50 states, full access to the use of drugs and surgery, and with a very pharmacosurgical paradigm of disease and healthcare. Osteopathic medicine is one of the fastest growing healthcare professions in America.

Osteopathic Manipulative Medicine

Osteopathic manipulative medicine (OMM) is similar to and yet distinct from chiropractic manipulation, while true to its eclectic roots, the naturopathic profession incorporates techniques from all professions. In contrast to chiropractic, OMM terminology and therapeutics focus much more on soft tissues, and the osteopathic lesion—"somatic dysfunction"—is clearly originated from soft tissues in contrast to the chiropractic lesion—the "vertebral subluxation"—which obviously originates from spinal articulations. Whereas the chiropractic intent of correcting or "adjusting" the "subluxation" was historically to improve function of the nervous system, the osteopathic lesion is addressed to more fully improve not only function of the nervous system but also of the vascular, lymphatic, and myofascial systems, too.[403] With regard to the latter, the osteopathic profession has

---

[399] Getzendanner S. Permanent injuction order against AMA. *JAMA*. 1988 Jan 1;259(1):81-2
[400] Gevitz N. The D.O.'s: Osteopathic Medicine in America. Johns Hopkins University Press; 1991; pages 100-103
[401] American Medical Association. Report 12 of the Council on Scientific Affairs (A-97) Full Text http://www.ama-assn.org/ama/pub/category/13638.html Accessed November 23, 2006
[402] Special report. America's best graduate schools. Schools of Medicine. The top schools: primary care. *US News World Rep*. 2004 Apr 12;136(12):74
[403] Williams N. Managing back pain in general practice--is osteopathy the new paradigm? *Br J Gen Pract*. 1997 Oct;47(423):653-5
http://www.pubmedcentral.nih.gov/articlerender.fcgi?tool=pubmed&pubmedid=9474832

always emphasized the importance of fascia in the genesis of "somatic dysfunction." Indeed, fascia appears to play an important and dynamic (not passive) role in neuromusculoskeletal health, particularly as it is a major contributor to proprioception and may also have a more direct effect through the recently described ability of fascia to actively contract in a smooth-muscle-like manner.[404]

From this author's perspective, an unfortunate consequence of the broadness of osteopathic manipulative conceptualizations (i.e., vertebral, skeletal, vascular, lymphatic, myofascial,…) is the relative lack (compared to chiropractic) of modernization and sophistication and development of its terminology and training textbooks; two of the most widely used osteopathic texts—*Osteopathic Principles in Practice* (1994) by Kuchera and Kuchera[405], and *Outline of Osteopathic Manipulative Procedures* (2006) by Kimberly[406]—both leave very much to be desired with respect to their clarity, terminology, clinical applicability, and referencing to the scientific literature. *Manipulation of the Spine, Thorax and Pelvis: An Osteopathic Perspective* (2006) by Gibbons and Tehan[407] is much more accessible and clinically applicable; however the text focuses exclusively on high-velocity low-amplitude (HVLA) techniques and therefore does not provide sufficient background and training for students in the very techniques that distinguish osteopathic from chiropractic techniques, namely heightened attention to the myofascial dysfunction that underlies the osteopathic lesion.

Ironically, the very growth and "allopathicization" of the profession that has threatened the profession's adherence to its holistic tenets has caused a reflexive re-affirmation of these tenets, and the profession has responded with a well-funded and intentional directive to scientifically investigate the mechanisms and efficacy of osteopathic manipulative medicine.[408,409] Recent findings include improved function and reduced pain in patients treated with a comprehensive manipulative technique for the shoulder[410], as well as the significant efficacy of ankle manipulation for patients with recent ankle injuries.[411] Further, OMM treatment of patients medicated for depression was found to triple the effectiveness of drug monotherapy.[412] Other studies affirmed the effectiveness of OMM in the treatment of geriatric pneumonia[413], pediatric asthma[414], carpal tunnel syndrome[415], low-back pain[416], and recovery from cardiac bypass surgery.[417]

---

[404] "…the existence of an active fascial contractility could have interesting implications for the understanding of musculoskeletal pathologies with an increased or decreased myofascial tonus. It may also offer new insights and a deeper understanding of treatments directed at fascia, such as manual myofascial release therapies or acupuncture." Schleip R, Klingler W, Lehmann-Horn F. Active fascial contractility: Fascia may be able to contract in a smooth muscle-like manner and thereby influence musculoskeletal dynamics. *Med Hypotheses*. 2005;65(2):273-7

[405] Kuchera WA, Kuchera ML. *Osteopathic Principles In Practice, revised second edition*. Kirksville, MO, KCOM Press; 1994

[406] Kimberly PE. *Outline of Osteopathic Manipulative Procedures. The Kimberly Manual 2006*. Kirksville College of Osteopathic Medicine. Walsworth Publishing Company Marceline, Mo

[407] Gibbons P, Tehan P. *Manipulation of the Spine, Thorax and Pelvis: An Osteopathic Perspective*. Churchill Livingstone; 2006. Isbn: 044310039X

[408] Wisnioski SW 3rd. "Circle Turns Round" to "Allopathic Osteopathy." *J Am Osteopath Assoc* 2006; 106: 423-4 http://www.jaoa.org/cgi/content/full/106/7/423

[409] Teitelbaum HS, Bunn WE 2nd, Brown SA, Burchett AW. Osteopathic medical education: renaissance or rhetoric? *J Am Osteopath Assoc*. 2003 Oct;103(10):489-90 http://www.jaoa.org/cgi/reprint/103/10/489

[410] The "seven stages of Spencer" is an organized technique of range-of-motion exercises and post-isometric stretching to improve functionality of the shoulder. This clinical trial showed improved shoulder function in a group of elderly patients treated with this technique. Knebl JA, Shores JH, Gamber RG, Gray WT, Herron KM. Improving functional ability in the elderly via the Spencer technique, an osteopathic manipulative treatment: a randomized, controlled trial. *J Am Osteopath Assoc*. 2002 Jul;102(7):387-96 http://www.jaoa.org/cgi/reprint/102/7/387 See also "CONCLUSION: Manipulative therapy for the shoulder girdle in addition to usual medical care accelerates recovery of shoulder symptoms." Bergman GJ, Winters JC, Groenier KH, Pool JJ, Meyboom-de Jong B, Postema K, van der Heijden GJ. Manipulative therapy in addition to usual medical care for patients with shoulder dysfunction and pain: a randomized, controlled trial. *Ann Intern Med*. 2004 Sep 21;141(6):432-9 http://www.annals.org/cgi/reprint/141/6/432.pdf

[411] This study shows the rapid onset and benefit of manipulative medicine for the treatment of acute ankle sprains: Eisenhart AW, Gaeta TJ, Yens DP. Osteopathic manipulative treatment in the emergency department for patients with acute ankle injuries. *J Am Osteopath Assoc*. 2003 Sep;103(9):417-21 http://www.jaoa.org/cgi/reprint/103/9/417

[412] This study impressively showed that musculoskeletal manipulation improved treatment effectiveness for depression from 33% to 100%. "After 8 weeks, 100% of the OMT treatment group and 33% of the control group tested normal by psychometric evaluation. ... The findings of this pilot study indicate that OMT may be a useful adjunctive treatment for alleviating depression in women." Plotkin BJ, Rodos JJ, Kappler R, Schrage M, Freydl K, Hasegawa S, Hennegan E, Hilchie-Schmidt C, Hines D, Iwata J, Mok C, Raffaelli D. Adjunctive osteopathic manipulative treatment in women with depression: a pilot study. *J Am Osteopath Assoc*. 2001 Sep;101(9):517-23 http://www.jaoa.org/cgi/reprint/101/9/517

[413] This study showed improved clinical outcomes and reduced antibiotic use in elderly patients with pneumonia when treated with manipulative medicine: "The treatment group had a significantly shorter duration of intravenous antibiotic treatment and a shorter hospital stay." Noll DR, Shores JH, Gamber RG, Herron KM, Swift J Jr. Benefits of osteopathic manipulative treatment for hospitalized elderly patients with pneumonia. *J Am Osteopath Assoc*. 2000 Dec;100(12):776-82 http://www.jaoa.org/cgi/reprint/100/12/776

[414] Osteopathic manipulation improved pulmonary function in pediatric patients with asthma: "With a confidence level of 95%, results for the OMT group showed a statistically significant improvement of 7 L per minute to 9 L per minute for peak expiratory flow rates. These results suggest that OMT has a therapeutic effect among this patient population." Guiney PA, Chou R, Vianna A, Lovenheim J. Effects of osteopathic manipulative treatment on pediatric patients with asthma: a randomized controlled trial. *J Am Osteopath Assoc*. 2005 Jan;105(1):7-12 http://www.jaoa.org/cgi/content/full/105/1/7

[415] Sucher BM, Hinrichs RN, Welcher RL, Quiroz LD, St Laurent BF, Morrison BJ. Manipulative treatment of carpal tunnel syndrome: biomechanical and osteopathic intervention to increase the length of the transverse carpal ligament: part 2. Effect of sex differences and manipulative "priming". *J Am Osteopath Assoc*. 2005 Mar;105(3):135-43. Erratum in: J Am Osteopath Assoc. 2005 May;105(5):238 http://www.jaoa.org/cgi/content/full/105/3/135

[416] "CONCLUSION: OMT significantly reduces low back pain. The level of pain reduction is greater than expected from placebo effects alone and persists for at least three months." Licciardone JC, Brimhall AK, King LN. Osteopathic manipulative treatment for low back pain: a systematic review and meta-analysis of randomized controlled trials. *BMC Musculoskelet Disord*. 2005 Aug 4;6:43 http://www.biomedcentral.com/1471-2474/6/43

[417] This study showed benefit from osteopathic manipulation administered immediately after coronary artery bypass graft surgery: "The observed changes in cardiac function and perfusion indicated that OMT had a beneficial effect on the recovery of patients after CABG surgery. The authors conclude that OMT has immediate, beneficial hemodynamic effects after CABG surgery when administered while the patient is sedated and pharmacologically paralyzed." O-Yurvati AH, Carnes MS, Clearfield MB, Stoll ST, McConathy WJ. Hemodynamic effects of osteopathic manipulative treatment immediately after coronary artery bypass graft surgery. *J Am Osteopath Assoc*. 2005 Oct;105(10):475-81 http://www.jaoa.org/cgi/content/full/105/10/475

<u>**Topics:**</u>
- **Introduction**
- **Re-establishing the Foundation for Health**
  - **Daily living**
    - Lifestyle habits
    - Motivation: background and clinical applications
    - Exceptional living: the key to exceptional results
    - Recognize and affirm individual uniqueness
    - Individuation & conscious living: alternatives to common paradigms
    - Quality and quantity of sleep: concepts and clinical applications
    - Exercise
    - Obesity, BMI, and the proinflammatory activity of adipose tissue
  - **Diet is a powerful tool for the prevention and treatment of disease**
    - Make "whole foods" the foundation of the diet
    - Increase consumption of fruits and vegetables
    - Phytochemicals: food-derived anti-inflammatory nutrients
    - Eat the right amount of protein
    - Benefits of complex carbohydrates
    - Reducing consumption of sugars: exceptions for supercompensation
    - Avoiding artificial sweeteners, colors, and other additives
    - Reducing or eliminating caffeine
    - To the extent possible, eat "organic" foods
    - Recognize the importance of avoiding food allergens
    - Supplement your healthy diet with specific vitamins, minerals, and fatty acids
    - Putting it all together: *the supplemented Paleo-Mediterranean diet*
  - **Advanced concepts in nutrition**
    - "Biochemical Individuality" and "Orthomolecular Medicine"
    - Nutrigenomics: Nutritional Genomics
    - General guidelines for the safe use of nutritional supplements
  - **Emotional, mental, and social health**
    - Stress management and authentic living
    - Stress always has a biochemical/physiologic component
    - The body functions as a whole
    - Healing past experiences
    - Autonomization, intradependence, emotional literacy, corrective experience
  - **Environmental health**
    - Environmental exposures and the importance of detoxification
    - Avoid unnecessary chemical medications and medical procedures
    - Intestinal health, bowel function, and introduction to dysbiosis
- **Preventive health screening**
- **Natural holistic healthcare contrasted to standard medical treatment**
- **Opposite influences of health promotion vs. disease promotion**

---

* Date of printing, update, or revision: March 25, 2007

Introduction to Chapter 2

The *Foundation for Health* refers to the lifestyle and nutrition **basics** that need to be attended to in order for a person to have a chance at being truly healthy. Without a basic, healthy foundation, *survival* is possible, but *long-term health*—let alone *wellness*—is not possible. Indeed, **many so-called "diseases" may be effectively treated with comprehensive lifestyle improvements** and *without disease-specific treatments*. The research literature on the management of chronic illnesses is replete with documentation supporting the effectiveness of non-drug non-surgical healthcare; yet these natural treatments continue to be labeled as "unscientific" and "unproven" and are cast aside in favor of "medical" treatments simply because the latter conform to the financially-leveraged nationally-televised medical paradigm[1,2] of patient passivity, medicalization, surgery, and superfluous technological sophistication.[3] One of the most thoroughly documented conditions responsive to lifestyle interventions is heart disease. The work of Dr. Dean Ornish[4,5] has shown that coronary atherosclerosis can be reversed with intensive lifestyle intervention; previous to his pioneering research, patients were forced to submit to expensive/hazardous drugs and invasive surgery as their only treatment options. **Atherosclerosis, hypertension, and hypercholesterolemia are virtually unknown in societies that follow healthy diets and lifestyles[6], yet each of these is a multibillion-dollar medical business in industrialized nations.**[7] The safest and most effective treatments for chronic hypertension ever documented—short-term fasting[8,9,10], supplemented protein-sparing caloric restriction for obese and type-2 diabetic hypertensives[11,12,13], and nutritional supplementation as with coenzyme Q-10[14,15,16] and vitamin D3[17]—are unknown to and underutilized by most allopathic cardiologists and are not offered to most hypertensive patients who must then resort to dependence upon chemical drugs that are inaccurately prescribed 40% of the time.[18] Meanwhile, the nation's only doctorate-level healthcare providers with graduate-level training in diet therapy and clinical nutrition—*the chiropractic and naturopathic physicians*—are excluded from full participation in the national healthcare system despite clear evidence that such integration has the potential to address the nation's healthcare crisis with effectiveness, safety, and major cost savings.[19,20,21,22]

---

[1] "…many ads may be targeted specifically at women and older viewers. Our findings suggest that Americans who watch average amounts of television may be exposed to more than 30 hours of direct-to-consumer drug advertisements each year, far surpassing their exposure to other forms of health communication." Brownfield ED, Bernhardt JM, Phan JL, Williams MV, Parker RM. Direct-to-consumer drug advertisements on network television: an exploration of quantity, frequency, and placement. *J Health Commun.* 2004 Nov-Dec;9(6):491-7

[2] Kaphingst KA, DeJong W, Rudd RE, Daltroy LH. A content analysis of direct-to-consumer television prescription drug advertisements. *J Health Commun.* 2004 Nov-Dec;9(6):515-2

[3] "…**despite lush advertisements from companies with obvious vested interests, and authoritative testimonials from biased investigators who presumably believe in their own work to the point of straining credulity and denying common sense… (translate: economic improvement, not biological superiority)**." Stevens CW, Glatstein E. Beware the Medical-Industrial Complex. *Oncologist* 1996;1(4):IV-V   http://theoncologist.alphamedpress.org/cgi/reprint/1/4/190-iv.pdf on July 4, 2004

[4] "More regression of coronary atherosclerosis occurred after 5 years… In contrast, in the control group, coronary atherosclerosis continued to progress and more than twice as many cardiac events occurred." Ornish D, et al. Intensive lifestyle changes for reversal of coronary heart disease. *JAMA.* 1998 Dec 16;280(23):2001-7

[5] Ornish D. Dr. Dean Ornish's Program for Reversing Heart Disease: The Only System Scientifically Proven to Reverse Heart Disease Without Drugs or Surgery. Ballentine; 1990

[6] O'Keefe JH, Cordain L, Harris, WH, Moe RM, Vogel R. Optimal low-density lipoprotein is 50 to 70 mg/dl. Lower is better and physiologically normal. *J Am Coll Cardiol* 2004;43: 2142-6

[7] "The economic impact of hypertension is enormous, representing $US23.74 billion in the US …and hypertension represents one of the 3 leading causes of visits to primary healthcare centres." Pardell H, et al. Pharmacoeconomic considerations in the management of hypertension. *Drugs.* 2000;59 Suppl 2:13-20; discussion 39-40

[8] Goldhamer A, et al. Medically supervised water-only fasting in the treatment of hypertension. *J Manipulative Physiol Ther* 2001 Jun;24(5):335-9

[9] Goldhamer AC, et al. Medically supervised water-only fasting in the treatment of borderline hypertension. *J Altern Complement Med.* 2002 Oct;8(5):643-50

[10] Goldhamer AC. Initial cost of care results in medically supervised water-only fasting for treating high blood pressure and diabetes. *J Altern Complement Med.* 2002 Dec;8(6):696-7

[11] Vertes V, Genuth SM, Hazelton IM. Supplemented fasting as a large-scale outpatient program. *JAMA.* 1977 Nov 14;238(20):2151-3

[12] Bauman WA, Schwartz E, Rose HG, Eisenstein HN, Johnson DW. Early and long-term effects of acute caloric deprivation in obese diabetic patients. *Am J Med.* 1988 Jul;85(1):38-46

[13] "Average weight loss was 63.9 kg... Concomitant with weight reduction, there were significant decrements in blood pressure... This study demonstrates that massively obese persons can achieve marked weight reduction, even normalization of weight, without hospitalization, surgery, or pharmacologic intervention." Kempner W, Newborg BC, Peschel RL, Skyler JS. Treatment of massive obesity with rice/reduction diet program. An analysis of 106 patients with at least a 45-kg weight loss. *Arch Intern Med.* 1975 Dec;135(12):1575-84

[14] "RESULTS: The mean reduction in systolic blood pressure of the CoQ-treated group was 17.8 +/- 7.3 mm Hg (mean +/- SEM). None of the patients exhibited orthostatic blood pressure changes. CONCLUSIONS: Our results suggest CoQ may be safely offered to hypertensive patients as an alternative treatment option." Burke BE, Neuenschwander R, Olson RD. Randomized, double-blind, placebo-controlled trial of coenzyme Q10 in isolated systolic hypertension. *South Med J.* 2001 Nov;94(11):1112-7

[15] "These findings indicate that treatment with coenzyme Q10 decreases blood pressure possibly by decreasing oxidative stress and insulin response in patients with known hypertension receiving conventional antihypertensive drugs." Singh RB, Niaz MA, Rastogi SS, Shukla PK, Thakur AS. Effect of hydrosoluble coenzyme Q10 on blood pressures and insulin resistance in hypertensive patients with coronary artery disease. *J Hum Hypertens.* 1999 Mar;13(3):203-8

[16] "…51% of patients came completely off of between one and three antihypertensive drugs at an average of 4.4 months after starting CoQ10." Langsjoen P, Langsjoen P, Willis R, Folkers K. Treatment of essential hypertension with coenzyme Q10. *Mol Aspects Med.* 1994;15 Suppl:S265-72

[17] "..supplementation with vitamin D(3) and calcium resulted in…a decrease in systolic blood pressure (SBP) of 9.3% (P = 0.02), and a decrease in heart rate of 5.4% (P = 0.02)… Inadequate vitamin D(3) and calcium intake could play a contributory role in the pathogenesis and progression of hypertension and cardiovascular disease in elderly women." Pfeifer M, Begerow B, Minne HW, Nachtigall D, Hansen C. Effects of a short-term vitamin D(3) and calcium supplementation on blood pressure and parathyroid hormone levels in elderly women. *J Clin Endocrinol Metab.* 2001 Apr;86(4):1633-7

[18] "We identified 815,316 prescriptions (40%) for which an alternative regimen appeared more appropriate according to evidence-based recommendations. Such changes would have reduced the costs to payers in 2001 by 11.6 million dollars (nearly a quarter of program spending on antihypertensive medications), as well as being more clinically appropriate overall." Fischer MA, Avorn J. Economic implications of evidence-based prescribing for hypertension: can better care cost less? *JAMA* 2004 Apr 21;291(15):1850-6

[19] "Systematic access to managed chiropractic care not only may prove to be clinically beneficial but also may reduce overall health care costs." Legorreta A, Metz D, Nelson C, Ray S, Chernicoff H, DiNubile N. Comparative Analysis of Individuals With and Without Chiropractic Coverage. *Archives of Internal Medicine* 2004; 164: 1985-1992

[20] Orme-Johnson DW, Herron RE. An innovative approach to reducing medical care utilization and expenditures. *Am J Manag Care.* 1997 Jan;3(1):135-44 http://www.ajmc.com/Article.cfm?Menu=1&ID=2154

[21] Goldhamer A, et al. Medically supervised water-only fasting in the treatment of hypertension. *J Manipulative Physiol Ther* 2001 Jun;24(5):335-9

[22] Herron R, Schneider RH, Mandarino JV, Alexander CN, Walton KG. Cost-effective hypertension management: Comparison of drug therapies with an alternative program. *American Journal of Managed Care* 1996; 2(4): 427-437 http://www.ajmc.com/article.cfm?ID=2345

Preventive research by Orme-Johnson and Herron[23] utilizing a "multicomponent prevention program" that included 1) twice-daily meditation, 2) daily yoga, 3) herbal dietary supplements, and 4) "recommendations for diet and daily routine" documented that total medical expenses were reduced by 59% over 4 years and by 63% over 11 years compared to outcomes obtained by patients relegated to standard allopathic medical treatment. Hospital admission rates were reduced 11.4-fold for cardiovascular disease, 3.3-fold for cancer, and 6.7-fold for mental health and substance abuse. Based on these and other illustrative examples described later in this text, we might reasonably conclude that American healthcare would be more effective, more affordable, and safer if **chiropractic and naturopathic physicians** were fully integrated into the healthcare system rather than being politically excluded (e.g., restrictive licensure laws[24]) or functionally excluded (e.g., discriminatory CPT codes and HMO policies[25]) by a system of drug- and surgery-based healthcare that financially depletes the people[26], business[27], and communities of our nation[28,29] while failing to deliver consistently competent healthcare[30,31,32] and cost-effective nationwide health improvements[33] that are proportional to the continuous increase in spending.[34]

Patients are people with health problems, and they have their health problems because some event (e.g., injury or other trauma) **or group of events and processes** (chronic stress, dysbiosis, chemical exposure, metabolic disease) **has disrupted their physiology to such an extent that they are functionally compromised and have developed symptoms** (pain, fatigue, depression, anxiety), **signs** (inflammation from conditions such as arthritis, lupus, bursitis, colitis), **or loss of organ function** (diabetes, weakness). In pursuit of relief from their ailment(s), they come to doctors for advice and treatment. However, the advice that they get varies tremendously in safety, effectiveness, and method of delivery depending upon the paradigm of the provider and the sociopolitical context in which the patient has come to view reality and healthcare options.

Since patients have been indoctrinated into the passive medical model of disease treatment[35,36], which relies on abdication and passivity rather than empowerment and personal responsibility, they generally come to doctors for the wrong answer to the wrong question. The question that people generally ask is, "What can *you* do to solve *my problem*?" This question implies that the doctor does the work, the patient does nothing other than implementing a rather minor interventional plan, and that the problem is rather simple, linear, and one-dimensional. Patients have been taught to think this way by the dominant

---

[23] Orme-Johnson DW, Herron RE. An innovative approach to reducing medical care utilization and expenditures. *Am J Manag Care*. 1997 Jan;3(1):135-44

[24] **Getzendanner S. Permanent injunction order against AMA.** *JAMA.* **1988 Jan 1;259(1):81-2** http://optimalhealthresearch.com/archives/wilk-ama-judgement.pdf

[25] "The Solla plaintiffs argued that each HMO defendant is "by itself a combination in restraint of trade, and that there is no concerted action requirement for an illegal combination." Solla Case DISMISSED! *Dynamic Chiropractic*; August 24, 1998, Volume 16, Issue 18 http://www.chiroweb.com/archives/16/18/22.html on July 12, 2004

[26] "A national study released today reports 20 million American families — or one in seven families — faced hardships paying medical bills last year, which forced many to choose between getting medical attention or paying rent or buying food…" Freeman, Liz. 'Working poor' struggle to afford health care. Naples Daily News. Published in Naples, Florida and online at http://www.naplesnews.com/npdn/news/article/0,2071,NPDN_14940_3000546,00.html Accessed July 28, 2004

[27] "The USA's 5.8 million small companies… Health care costs are rising about 15% this year for those with fewer than 200 workers vs. 13.5% for those with 500 or more… But many small employers cite increases of 20% or more. That's made insurance the No. 1 small business problem…" Jim Hopkins. Health care tops taxes as small business cost drain. USA TODAY. http://www.usatoday.com/news/health/2003-04-20-small-business-costs_x.htm. Accessed July 28, 2004

[28] "In 1994, we spent $1 trillion on health care in the US, or, more accurately, we spent most of this astounding sum on disease treatment. …Corporations now spend an incredible 48% of their after-tax profits on health care, …." Pizzorno JE. Total Wellness. Rocklin: Prima; 1996 page 7

[29] "Though the U.S. has slightly fewer doctors per capita than the typical developed nation, we have almost twice as many MRI machines and perform vastly more angioplasties. …at least 31 percent of all the incremental income we'll earn between 1999 and 2010 will go to health care." Pat Regnier, *Money Magazine*. Healthcare myth: We spend too much. October 13, 2003: 11:29 AM EDT http://money.cnn.com/2003/10/08/pf/health_myths_1/ Accessed Monday, July 12, 2004

[30] "Although they spend more on health care than patients in any other industrialized nation, Americans receive the right treatment less than 60 percent of the time, resulting in unnecessary pain, expense and even death…" Ceci Connolly. U.S. Patients Spend More but Don't Get More, Study Finds: Even in Advantaged Areas, Americans Often Receive Inadequate Health Care. Washington Post, May 5, 2004; Page A15. On-line at http://www.washingtonpost.com/ac2/wp-dyn/A1875-2004May4 accessed on July 28, 2004

[31] "Participants received 54.9 percent (95 percent confidence interval, 54.3 to 55.5) of recommended care...CONCLUSIONS: **The deficits we have identified in adherence to recommended processes for basic care pose serious threats to the health of the American public**." McGlynn EA, Asch SM, Adams J, Keesey J, Hicks J, DeCristofaro A, Kerr EA. The quality of health care delivered to adults in the United States. *N Engl J Med*. 2003 Jun 26;348(26):2635-45

[32] "CONCLUSIONS: There is a substantial amount of injury to patients from medical management, and many injuries are the result of substandard care." Brennan TA, Leape LL, Laird NM, Hebert L, Localio AR, Lawthers AG, Newhouse JP, Weiler PC, Hiatt HH. Incidence of adverse events and negligence in hospitalized patients: results of the Harvard Medical Practice Study I. 1991. *Qual Saf Health Care*. 2004 Apr;13(2):145-51; discussion 151-2

[33] "Basically, you die earlier and spend more time disabled if you're an American rather than a member of most other advanced countries." Christopher Murray MD PhD, Director of World Health Organization's Global Program on Evidence for Health Policy http://www.who.int/inf-pr-2000/en/pr2000-life.html Accessed July 12, 2004

[34] "The results of the study demonstrate that, over the past four decades, the United States has been spending more and accomplishing less when compared with other industrialized nations." Shi L. Health care spending, delivery, and outcome in developed countries: a cross-national comparison. *Am J Med Qual* 1997;12(2):83-93

[35] "…many ads may be targeted specifically at women and older viewers. Our findings suggest that Americans who watch average amounts of television may be exposed to more than 30 hours of direct-to-consumer drug advertisements each year, far surpassing their exposure to other forms of health communication." Brownfield ED, Bernhardt JM, Phan JL, Williams MV, Parker RM. Direct-to-consumer drug advertisements on network television: an exploration of quantity, frequency, and placement. *J Health Commun*. 2004 Nov-Dec;9(6):491-7

[36] Kaphingst KA, DeJong W, Rudd RE, Daltroy LH. A content analysis of direct-to-consumer television prescription drug advertisements. *J Health Commun*. 2004 Nov-Dec;9(6):515-22

medical-drug system[37] that can function most profitably if patients are convinced that they are powerless to effect significant self-directed improvements in their health status and if they are convinced that low-cost simple natural treatments are "**unscientific**" (which implies that they do not follow logic), "**unconventional**" (which implies that they are radical and unpredictable), and "**alternative**" (which implies that they are of secondary quality, presumably behind drugs and surgery). The answer that patients have been conditioned to accept is, "*Take this drug, and it will solve your problem. You don't have to do anything else.*" Patients like this answer because, when the focus remains on an external treatment, the implication is that they are exonerated from personal responsibility for their health problems even though their lifestyle and dietary choices may have caused the problem in the first place. Patients and doctors are creatures of habit in both thought and action; getting them to appreciate and implement lifestyle change for the prevention and treatment of disease is a major challenge—yet it offers our best opportunity for improving health outcomes on an individual basis as well as on a national level.

Patients ask for care in different ways depending on the specifics of their current health. They want a doctor to "give me a treatment" that will "relieve my pain," "lower my cholesterol" or "help me feel better." Most patients have no concept of wellness and the health possibilities that are available to them and the level of self-reliance, self-direction, and self-development that are necessary for them to attain optimal functioning in all aspects of their lives—physical, emotional, spiritual, and social. For practical reasons, we have to start from where they are, take care of the major problems and then move them toward optimal health after they are stabilized and have re-attained normal health. However the latter statement implies that *the promotion and attainment of optimal health* and *the treatment of problems* are distinct, while often they are connected and interdependent. Many times in clinical practice, for a patient to attain sufficient improvement with their primary complaint, we must look *beyond the problem* to the environment, diet, lifestyle, attitudes, beliefs, activities, habits, and emotional landscape (intrapersonal and interpersonal) that set the stage for the problem to have developed in the first place.

Healthcare is delivered along a continuum that ranges from reductionistic to holistic, from micromanagement to macromanagement, from "solving problems" to "healing lives." The latter is generally inclusive of the former, but ending at the "accomplishment" of problem-solving never attains the larger goal of healing of an entire person. For practical purposes as clinicians, we have to begin with a problem-oriented model of healthcare and ensure that major, life-threatening problems are addressed before moving on to more subtle—yet still highly important—problems such as poor lifestyle habits and self-defeating behavior. If a patient comes to you with back pain, and you overlook their *cauda equina syndrome* for the sake of dealing with their *unrecognized childhood issues* and *poor diet*, you are more likely to find yourself out of a career than praised for your holistic approach, no matter how good your intentions. Even the best holistic physicians with the broadest perspectives and most comprehensive wellness-promoting goals must utilize effective micromanagement strategies for acute and life-threatening problems. Thus, with **recognition of the importance of *simultaneous* problem management *and* wellness promotion**, we begin this chapter that provides minimal and elemental building blocks for the restoration of health and the attainment of optimal wellness.

---

[37] Mintzes B, Barer ML, Kravitz RL, Kazanjian A, Bassett K, Lexchin J, Evans RG, Pan R, Marion SA. Influence of direct to consumer pharmaceutical advertising and patients' requests on prescribing decisions: two site cross sectional survey. *BMJ*. 2002 Feb 2; 324(7332): 278-9

Re-establishing the Foundation for Health

"The work of the naturopathic physician is to elicit healing by helping patients to create or recreate conditions for health to exist within them.
Health will occur where the conditions for health exist.
Disease is the product of conditions which allow for it."   *Jared Zeff, N.D.*[38]

One of the most important concepts within the philosophy and practice of naturopathic medicine is that of "re-establishing the foundation for health." This means that instead of first looking to a specific treatment or "magic bullet" to solve a health problem, we first look at the environment in which the problem arose to determine if the patient's environment has initiated or perpetuated the problem. The term *environment* as used here means much more than the patient's immediate surroundings at home and work; it is used as a term to include all modifiable factors that may have an effect on the patient's health, such as lifestyle, diet, exercise, supplementation, chronic and situational stress, exposure to toxicants and microbes, nutritionally-modifiable genetic factors[39], emotions, feelings, and unconscious assumptions[40], and many other considerations.

"Virtually all human diseases result from the interaction of genetic susceptibility factors and modifiable environmental factors, broadly defined to include infectious, chemical, physical, nutritional, and behavioral factors."   *Centers for Disease Control and Prevention (CDC)*[41]

"Optimal health" does not *and never will* come in a pill or tonic—the human body and the interactions that we each have between our genes, outlooks, environments, and lifestyles are far too complex to ever be addressed wholly and completely by a simplistic paradigm or single treatment. Even a superficial observation of the complexity of human physiology and the complexity of our environments (including noise, toxins such as benzene from pollution, chemicals such as formaldehyde from building materials, work stress and multitasking, radiation exposure, microwaves) shows that **our modern lifestyles subject the human body to many more "stressors" than ever before in the history of human existence.** Each of these stressors depletes our psychic and physiologic reserves, such that daily replenishment and protection are necessary.

Research in nutrition and physiology is revealing the mechanisms by which "simple" lifestyle practices and dietary interventions exert their powerful benefits. For example, whole foods such as fruits and vegetables contain over 8,000 phytochemicals with different physiologic effects[42], and simple practices such as meditation and massage can significantly alter hormone and neurotransmitter levels.[43,44] On the surface, a simple practice such as consumption of fruits and vegetables and a multivitamin/multimineral supplement may seem to be a way to provide merely "good nutrition"; however the clinical effects can include antidepressant[45] and anti-inflammatory benefits[46], by enhancing the efficiency of biochemical reactions[47] and by reducing excess activity of NF-kappaB[48], respectively. The power of interventional

---

[38] Zeff JL. The process of healing: a unifying theory of naturopathic medicine. *Journal of Naturopathic Medicine* 1997; 7: 122-5
[39] Kaput J, Rodriguez LR. Nutritional genomics: the next frontier in the postgenomic era. *Physiol Genomics* 16: 166–177 http://physiolgenomics.physiology.org/cgi/content/full/16/2/166
[40] Miller A. The truth will set you free: overcoming emotional blindness and finding your true adult self. New York: Basic Books; 2001
[41] Gene-Environment Interaction Fact Sheet by the Centers for Disease Control and Prevention, August 2000
[42] "We propose that the additive and synergistic effects of phytochemicals in fruit and vegetables are responsible for their potent antioxidant and anticancer activities, and that the benefit of a diet rich in fruit and vegetables is attributed to the complex mixture of phytochemicals present in whole foods." Liu RH. Health benefits of fruit and vegetables are from additive and synergistic combinations of phytochemicals. *Am J Clin Nutr.* 2003 Sep;78(3 Suppl):517S-520S
[43] "The significant decrease of the catecholamine metabolite VMA (vanillic-mandelic acid) in meditators, that is associated with a reciprocal increase of 5-HIAA supports as a feedback necessity the "rest and fulfillment response" versus "fight and flight"." Bujatti M, Riederer P. Serotonin, noradrenaline, dopamine metabolites in transcendental meditation-technique. *J Neural Transm.* 1976;39(3):257-67
[44] "By the end of the study, the massage therapy group, as compared to the relaxation group, reported experiencing less pain, depression, anxiety and improved sleep. They also showed improved trunk and pain flexion performance, and their serotonin and dopamine levels were higher." Hernandez-Reif M, Field T, Krasnegor J, Theakston H. Lower back pain is reduced and range of motion increased after massage therapy. *Int J Neurosci* 2001;106(3-4):131-45
[45] Benton D, Haller J, Fordy J. Vitamin supplementation for 1 year improves mood. *Neuropsychobiology.* 1995;32(2):98-105
[46] Church TS, Earnest CP, Wood KA, Kampert JB. Reduction of C-reactive protein levels through use of a multivitamin. *Am J Med.* 2003 Dec 15;115(9):702-7
[47] Ames BN, Elson-Schwab I, Silver EA. High-dose vitamin therapy stimulates variant enzymes with decreased coenzyme binding affinity (increased K(m)): relevance to genetic disease and polymorphisms. *Am J Clin Nutr.* 2002 Apr;75(4):616-58 http://www.ajcn.org/cgi/content/full/75/4/616

nutrition utilizing high-doses and/or synergistic formulations of nutraceuticals and phytonutraceuticals becomes much more clinically apparent when patients first (re)establish a healthy foundation of diet and lifestyle practices upon which these additive treatments can be added; I estimate that the effectiveness of treatments for complex illness such as inflammatory diseases and cancer is *at least* doubled when patients implement these lifestyle changes in addition to specific natural treatments rather than relying on natural treatments alone without a healthy supportive lifestyle. In other words, "*foundation for health* + natural treatments" is much more effective than "*unhealthy lifestyle* + natural treatments." This explains, in part, the discrepancy between the relatively lackluster response seen in single intervention clinical trials* compared to the better results that we attain clinically when using a holistic approach characterized by multicomponent treatment plans. The biochemical and "scientific" reasons for this positive/negative synergism will become clear during the course of this chapter in particular and this textbook in general.

*Single intervention clinical trials (i.e., clinical trials that utilize only one treatment) are the "gold standard" in allopathic drug-based research because their goal is to quantify and qualify the nature of positive and negative responses. However, this approach loses much of its luster in clinical settings where neither patients nor lifestyles and treatment plans can be standardized due to the unique constitution, lifestyle, history, and treatment plan of each patient. Single intervention clinical trials have a place in the researching of all treatments, including natural interventions. However, clinicians—especially recent graduates—must pry themselves away from this research tool when it comes to treating individual patients in clinical practice, where **single interventions are the antithesis of holistic treatment**.

Additional notes:

_____
_____
_____
_____
_____
_____
_____
_____
_____
_____
_____
_____
_____
_____
_____
_____
_____
_____
_____

[48] Vasquez A. Reducing pain and inflammation naturally - part 4: nutritional and botanical inhibition of NF-kappaB, the major intracellular amplifier of the inflammatory cascade. A practical clinical strategy exemplifying anti-inflammatory nutrigenomics. *Nutritional Perspectives*, July 2005:5-12. www.OptimalHealthResearch.com/part4

Daily Living

> Realize that the choices that are made on a daily basis greatly influence whether or not we will be healthy in the future. Doctors and patients should choose a healthy diet, appropriate supplementation, healthy relationships, and physical activity rather than junk foods, toxic relationships, and physical inactivity.

Life occurs on a moment-to-moment and daily basis. Choices that we make in relationships, occupations, exercise, and diet have profound and powerful influence over the course of our lives—particularly our health and happiness. Despite the previous and ongoing obfuscation of health information by allopathic groups[49,50,51,52,53] and the pharmaceutical industry[54,55], enough valid information and common sense is available to doctors and the public such that **ignorance is no longer a viable excuse for deferring responsibility for lifestyle-induced disease and misery.**[56] Eating too much sugar and fat while not eating enough fruits and vegetables is making a choice to have an increased probability of developing diabetes, cancer, heart disease, arthritis, and obesity. Exercising regularly, eating a healthy diet, and supplementing the diet with high-quality nutrients and botanicals is making the choice to greatly reduce your risk of health problems[57,58] and to nurture your life and your body so that you can make the most of your life experience and enjoy your life, your hobbies, life purpose(s), and time with friends and family.

When we were children, we looked to other people to provide for us and to "take care of us." **As adults, we have to assume responsibility for the course of our own lives, to make decisions based on long-term considerations rather than instant gratification and selective ignorance.** Of course, this does not mean that we have to abandon enjoyment; but it does mean that we can make decisions based on priorities, and if health is a priority then it follows that we should take steps to attain and maintain it. For people who have chosen to make their health a priority, sugar- and fat-laden food begins to lose its appeal, and exploring new adventures in healthy cooking becomes an activity that can be transformed into an art—one that is particularly amenable to building relationships and connections with other people. **The improved sense of wellbeing and improved physical and intellectual performance obtained from consumption of a health-promoting Paleo-Mediterranean diet (described later) supercedes any short-term gratification from the disease-promoting diet commonly referred to as the Standard American Diet (SAD).** When people want to be healthy, exercising and spending enjoyable time outdoors becomes more fun than the inactivity and passivity of watching television. When we consider that the average American watches 3-4 hours of television per day then it is no surprise that, with such inactive lifestyles, Americans show increasingly high rates of obesity, cancer, heart disease, and diabetes. Such an inactive lifestyle also affects our children: on average, each American child watches more than 23 hours of television per week[59]—a national habit that unquestionably contributes to the high levels of obesity and (social) illiteracy demonstrated by America's youth. Adults who watch average amounts of television are exposed to (indoctrinated by) more than 2.5 hours of direct-to-consumer drug advertisements each month—more than 30 hours of drug advertisements per year—far exceeding their exposure to other, potentially more authentic, health-promoting information.[60] Not only does television siphon time and energy that could be used more productively, more socially, or more enjoyably, but at a cost of $540 to $900 per year ($45-75 per month), **cable television subtracts from the available resources (i.e., time, money, attention/focus) that could be directed toward health-promoting choices.** Cable television is only one of

[49] Wolinsky H, Brune T. The Serpent on the Staff: The Unhealthy Politics of the American Medical Association. GP Putnam and Sons, New York, 1994
[50] Wilk CA. Medicine, Monopolies, and Malice: How the Medical Establishment Tried to Destroy Chiropractic. Garden City Park: Avery, 1996
[51] Carter JP. Racketeering in Medicine: The Suppression of Alternatives. Norfolk: Hampton Roads Pub; 1993
[52] National Alliance of Professional Psychology Providers. AMA Seeks To Control and Restrict Psychologist's Scope of Practice. http://www.nappp.org/scope.pdf Accessed November 25, 2006
[53] "In an effort to marshal the medical community's resources against the growing threat of expanding scope of practice for allied health professionals, the AMA has formed a national partnership to confront such initiatives nationwide… The committee will use $25,000…" Daly R, American Psychiatric Association. AMA Forms Coalition to Thwart Non-M.D. Practice Expansion. *Psychiatric News* 2006 March; 41: 17 http://pn.psychiatryonline.org/cgi/content/full/41/5/17-a?eaf Accessed November 25, 2006
[54] Angell M. The Truth About the Drug Companies: How They Deceive Us and What to Do About it. Random House; August 2004
[55] "**It begins on the first day of medical school… It starts slowly and insidiously, like an addiction, and can end up influencing the very nature of medical decision-making and practice… Attempts to influence the judgment of doctors by commercial interests serving the medical industrial complex are nothing if not thorough.**" Editorial. Drug-company influence on medical education in USA. *Lancet*. 2000 Sep 2;356(9232):781
[56] "Error is not blindness, error is cowardice. Every acquisition, every step forward in knowledge is the result of courage, of severity towards oneself, of cleanliness with respect to oneself." Nietzsche FW. Ecce Homo: How One Becomes What One Is. [Translated by Hollingdale RJ] Penguin Books: 1979, page 34
[57] Orme-Johnson DW, Herron RE. An innovative approach to reducing medical care utilization and expenditures. *Am J Manag Care*. 1997 Jan;3(1):135-44
[58] Vasquez A. A Five-Part Nutritional Protocol that Produces Consistently Positive Results. *Nutritional Wellness* 2005Sept. http://nutritionalwellness.com/archives/2005/sep/09_vasquez.php and http://optimalhealthresearch.com/reprints/vasquez-nutritional-wellness-5-part-protocol-2005-sept.pdf
[59] "American children view over 23 hours of television per week. * Teenagers view an average of 21 to 22 hours of television per week. * By the time today's children reach age 70, they will have spent 7 to 10 years of their lives watching television." American Academy of Pediatrics http://www.aapca1.org/aapca1/tv.html accessed September 30, 2003
[60] "…many ads may be targeted specifically at women and older viewers. Our findings suggest that Americans who watch average amounts of television may be exposed to more than 30 hours of direct-to-consumer drug advertisements each year, far surpassing their exposure to other forms of health communication." Brownfield ED, Bernhardt JM, Phan JL, Williams MV, Parker RM. Direct-to-consumer drug advertisements on network television: an exploration of quantity, frequency, and placement. *J Health Commun*. 2004 Nov-Dec;9(6):491-7

many examples of how everyday choices can have an impact on long-term health. **Encourage your patients to become mindful of their choices and the impact these choices have on long-term health and vitality.**

Lifestyle habits: Without the conscious decision that **health is a priority** and the realization that **optimal health has to be earned rather than taken for granted**, patients and doctors alike can fall into the belief that healthcare and health maintenance are *burdens* and *inconveniences* rather than opportunities for fulfillment and self-care. Taking an **empowered** and **pro-active** role in one's healthcare may include a coordinated program of diet changes (such as eating certain foods, while avoiding others), regular exercise, nutritional supplementation, stress reduction, and relationship improvement. Unhealthy habits such as eating junk foods, using tobacco, and watching too much television rob people of the time, energy, motivation, and financial resources that could otherwise be used to improve health and prevent unnecessary illness. As described later in this chapter, the choices that are made on a daily basis from this point forward are the most powerful predictors of future health and are generally more powerful than past habits or genetic inheritance. We can all greatly increase our probability of enjoying a future of high-energy health rather than painful illness by consistently choosing health-promoting options instead of foods, behaviors, and emotional states that promote illness.

While prevention of lung cancer and heart disease are important enough, smoking cessation has taken on new importance recently now that **the connection between tobacco smoking and the induction of autoimmunity—rheumatoid arthritis and systemic lupus erythematosus—is becoming increasingly well established**. Patients with any form of autoimmunity should not smoke tobacco and should minimize any exposure to second-hand smoke.[61]

One hour of time per day and/or about $2 - $8 per day:

Active self-care	Benefits	Distraction	Result
1. Meditation 2. Yoga, stretching 3. Walking, jogging, biking, no-cost calisthenics 4. Martial arts, Tai Chi 5. Hot bath 6. Cooking new healthy meals 7. Herbal teas (especially green tea) provide anti-inflammatory, anticancer, and antioxidant benefits 8. Basic nutritional supplementation (less than $2 per day): 1) High-potency multivitamin and multimineral supplement, 2) Complete balanced, fatty acid supplementation, 3) 2,000 – 4,000 IU vitamin D per day for adults, 4) probiotics and/or synbiotics. *At $2 per day for meditation, stretching, calisthenics, (etc.) and basic supplementation, the total comes to $730 per year.*	1. Increased flexibility and joint mobility 2. Reduction in blood pressure 3. Reduced risk for cancer 4. Increased strength 5. Improved cognitive function 6. New and enjoyable meals 7. Relaxation 8. New life skills 9. Improved heart health 10. The opportunity to develop social skills and more friends and a better social support network 11. Reduced risk for Alzheimer's and Parkinson's diseases	1. Cable television ($1.50 - $2.50 per day) 2. 1 pack of cigarettes per day ($3 per day) 3. Grande Café Latte ($3 per day) *At $8 per day for cable television, designer coffee, and cigarettes, the total comes to approximately $3,000 per year.*	1. Watching an hour of television may or may not contribute significantly to life and long-term goals. (Cable television costs between $600 and $800 per year.) 2. One pack of cigarettes per day at $2.88 per pack equals $1,051 per year for increased risk of cancer and heart disease. 3. Grande Café Latte at $3.05 per day costs $1,113 per year for 7-per-week and $793 per year for 5-per-week.

---

[61] "Counseling against smoking should be mandatory in rheumatological practice both to patients and to their relatives. Studies on the mechanisms whereby smoking triggers rheumatoid arthritis and systemic lupus erythematosus may provide fundamental new knowledge about the cause and molecular pathogenesis of these diseases." Klareskog L, Padyukov L, Alfredsson L. Smoking as a trigger for inflammatory rheumatic diseases. *Curr Opin Rheumatol.* 2007 Jan;19(1):49-54

Motivation: We all have a combination of reasons, feelings, inclinations, and unconscious influences that support and perpetuate our health behaviors[62,63]; getting in touch with those motivations can help us to better understand the healthy/functional (health-promoting) and unhealthy/dysfunctional (illness-promoting) aspects of our psyches. Uncovering and "upgrading" these motivations can help us and our patients to develop more authentic lives and improved health. Self-defeating behaviors, such as 1) a willingness to remain ignorant of factors which influence health, 2) a willingness to frequently consume disease-promoting processed and "fast foods", and 3) submission to confinement within the boundaries of one's insurance coverage (which often confines one to drugs and surgery as the only treatment options), reflect—*at best*—the willingness to settle for mediocrity and—*at worst*—an unconscious movement in the direction of illness and early death—masochism and suicide by lifestyle. Conversely, an unencumbered drive toward health will create the greatest opportunity for wellness. Since **actions originate from beliefs and goals**, we can surmise much about undisclosed beliefs and goals in others and ourselves simply by observing outward behavior. Effectively changing actions (such as diet and lifestyle choices) therefore must include not only behavior modification but also careful examination and reconsideration of largely unconscious goals and beliefs that motivate and underlie those behaviors. **When a fully empowered motivation toward health is matched with accurate informational insight, we have the** *potential* **for health-promoting change**—*potential* **which only becomes** *manifest* **after the habitual application of appropriate action.** Patients and doctors alike can benefit from considering the factors that incline them *toward* or *away* from behaviors that promote health or disease.

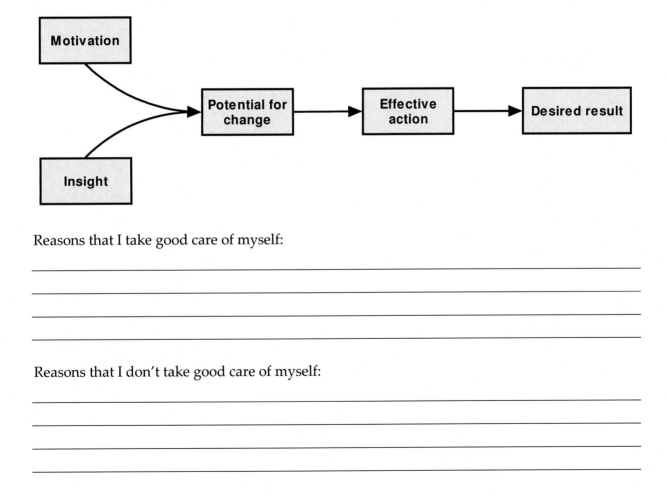

Reasons that I take good care of myself:

_____

_____

_____

_____

Reasons that I don't take good care of myself:

_____

_____

_____

_____

[62] Bradshaw J. Healing the Shame that Binds You [Audio Cassette (April 1990) Health Communications Audio; ISBN: 1558740430]
[63] Miller A. The Drama of the Gifted Child: The Search for the True Self. Basic Books: 1981

Motivation: moving from theory to practice: Many recently-graduated doctors start with the erroneous assumption that all patients actually want to become healthier, and furthermore, that all the doctor has to do is "enlighten" them to the error of their ways and the patient will be dutifully compliant unto the attainment of his or her health-related goals. In reality, many people are indifferent about their health. Many people do not care if they are 30 lbs overweight or have hypertension or will die early as a result of their lifestyle; they often have to be encouraged to begin to *consider* making positive changes.

At our 2004 Functional Medicine Symposium, Dr. James Prochaska[64] elucidated the different stages of patient preparedness, and we note that each of these five levels of thought and action produces specific results and requires different types of support from the doctor. I have paraphrased, translated, and embellished Dr. Prochaska's lecture in the following table; for additional information and insights, obtain his lecture from the Institute for Functional Medicine or his book *Changing for Good*.[65]

Level of preparedness and readiness for change

Stage/level	*Doctor's interventions and social support*
1. **Pre-contemplation**: "I am not seriously thinking about making a change to be healthier."	▪ Outreach ▪ Retainment
2. **Contemplation**: "I am thinking about making a change, but I am not ready for action."	▪ Resolve resistance ▪ Emphasize benefits ▪ Address ambivalence
3. **Preparation**: "I am getting ready to make a change, but I am not taking effective action yet."	▪ Ensure adequate preparation ▪ Prevent relapse following initial action
4. **Action**: "I am beginning to make changes to become healthier."	▪ Support (group support is best) ▪ Encouragement ▪ Reward system
5. **Maintenance**: "I take action every day and on a consistent basis to reach my goals."	▪ Continued provision for continuation of health changes: facilities, supplements, social support, affirmation

Recognizing the different levels of patient preparedness and addressing individual patients with a customized approach not only for their *disease* but also for their *level of preparedness* for action can help doctors deliver more effective healthcare. Also, patients may have different levels of preparedness for different aspects of their treatment plans. He/she may be ready for **action** with regard to exercise, in **preparation** for dietary change, but in **precontemplation** for the use of supplements and botanicals.

---

[64] Prochaska JO. Changing for good: motivating diabetic patients. The Coming Storm: Reversing the Rising Pandemic of Diabetes and Metabolic Syndrome. The Eleventh International Symposium on Functional Medicine. May 13-15, 2004 in Vancouver, British Columbia, Canada. Pages 173-180. Presented by the Institute for Functional Medicine in Gig Harbor, Washington. www.FunctionalMedicine.org
[65] Prochaska, JO, Norcross, JC, and DiClemente, CC (1994). Changing for Good: A Revolutionary Six-Stage Program for Overcoming Bad Habits and Moving Your Life. NY, William Morrow and Company; 1994

Here is the secret to being exceptionally healthy: *You have to live in an exceptional way*. We cannot expect to achieve the goal of being vibrantly healthy or exceptionally happy if we live in the same way as everyone else, particularly when our fellow citizens are likely to be overweight, depressed, unhealthy, taking multiple pharmaceutical medications[66], and experiencing a state of progressively declining health.[67]

> **"Basically, you die earlier and spend more time disabled if you're an American rather than a member of most other advanced countries."**
>
> Christopher Murray MD PhD, *Director of World Health Organization's Global Program on Evidence for Health Policy* June 2000
> http://www.who.int/inf-pr-2000/en/pr2000-life.html

Healthy lifestyle not only includes the basics of adequate sleep, healthy whole-foods diet, supportive relationships, and regular exercise, but it also includes preventive medicine and pro-active healthcare. **Despite the fact that we as a nation spend more on medical treatments than any other country in the world, Americans have the worst health outcomes of all the major industrialized countries.**[68,69,70] This is largely because *American medicine* is centered on a *disease-oriented model of medicine* which means that instead of having a healthcare system and social structure that proactively promotes health and prevents disease before it happens, our systems are *reactive*—treating disease *after* it occurs rather than emphasizing the prevention of disease *before* it occurs. It is also reductionistic: focusing on the small problem (micromanagement) rather than the big picture (macromanagement). The problem is compounded by the use of expensive pharmaceutical drugs which carry high rates of inefficacy (50-70%[71]) and which can exacerbate the diseases they are designed to treat or which result in adverse health effects that outweigh the purported benefits.[72,73,74,75,76,77,,78,79,80,81,82,83,84,85,86] **Every year "medication errors" kill over 7,000 people in America**[87]**, and at least 180,000 Americans (493 patients per day) die due to "hospital errors."**[88] Drug-related morbidity and mortality cost America more than $136 billion a year.[89]

---

[66] "According to the latest available data, total health care costs reached $1.3 trillion in 2000. This represents a per capita health care expenditure of $4,637. The total prescription drug expenditure in 2000 was $121.8 billion, or approximately $430 per person." Presentation to the U.S. Senate Commerce Committee April 23, 2002 "Drug Pricing & Consumer Costs" Kathleen D. Jaeger, R.Ph., J.D. http://commerce.senate.gov/hearings/042302jaegar.pdf

[67] Zack MM, Moriarty DG, Stroup DF, Ford ES, Mokdad AH. Worsening trends in adult health-related quality of life and self-rated health-United States, 1993-2001. *Public Health Rep*. 2004 Sep-Oct;119(5):493-505 http://www.pubmedcentral.nih.gov/articlerender.fcgi?tool=pubmed&pubmedid=15313113

[68] "[America] also has the fewest hospital days per capita, the highest hospital expenditures per day, and substantially higher physician incomes than the other OECD countries. On the available outcome measures, the United States is generally in the bottom half, and its relative ranking has been declining since 1960." Anderson GF, Poullier JP. Health spending, access, and outcomes: trends in industrialized countries. *Health Aff* (Millwood) 1999 May-Jun;18(3):178-92 http://content.healthaffairs.org/cgi/reprint/18/3/178.pdf

[69] "However, on outcomes indicators such as life expectancy and infant mortality, the United States is frequently in the bottom quartile among the twenty-nine industrialized countries, and its relative ranking has been declining since 1960." Anderson GF. In search of value: an international comparison of cost, access, and outcomes. *Health Aff* 1997 Nov-Dec;16(6):163-71

[70] "Basically, you die earlier and spend more time disabled if you're an American rather than a member of most other advanced countries," says Christopher Murray, M.D., Ph.D., Director of WHO's Global Program on Evidence for Health Policy. http://www.who.int/inf-pr-2000/en/pr2000-life.html

[71] "The vast majority of drugs - more than 90 percent - only work in 30 or 50 percent of the people." Allen Roses, M.D., worldwide vice-president of genetics at GlaxoSmithKline. http://commondreams.org/headlines03/1208-02.htm

[72] Whitaker R. **The case against antipsychotic drugs: a 50-year record of doing more harm than good**. *Med Hypotheses*. 2004;62(1):5-13

[73] Titier K, Canal M, Deridet E, Abouelfath A, Gromb S, Molimard M, Moore N. Determination of myocardium to plasma concentration ratios of five antipsychotic drugs: comparison with their ability to induce arrhythmia and sudden death in clinical practice. *Toxicol Appl Pharmacol*. 2004;199(1):52-60

[74] Ray WA, Meredith S, Thapa PB, Meador KG, Hall K, Murray KT. **Antipsychotics and the risk of sudden cardiac death**. *Arch Gen Psychiatry*. 2001;58(12):1161-7

[75] Straus SM, Bleumink GS, Dieleman JP, van der Lei J, 't Jong GW, Kingma JH, Sturkenboom MC, Stricker BH. **Antipsychotics and the risk of sudden cardiac death**. *Arch Intern Med*. 2004 Jun 28;164(12):1293-7

[76] Ray WA, Meredith S, Thapa PB, Hall K, Murray KT. **Cyclic antidepressants and the risk of sudden cardiac death**. *Clin Pharmacol Ther*. 2004;75(3):234-41

[77] Relling MV, Rubnitz JE, Rivera GK, Boyett JM, Hancock ML, Felix CA, Kun LE, Walter AW, Evans WE, Pui CH. High incidence of secondary brain tumours after radiotherapy and antimetabolites. *Lancet*. 1999 Jul 3;354(9172):34-9

[78] "The leukemia risk associated with partial-body radiotherapy for uterine corpus cancer was small; about 14 excess leukemia cases were due to radiation per 10,000 women followed for 10 years." Curtis RE, Boice JD Jr, Stovall M, Bernstein L, Holowaty E, Karjalainen S, Langmark F, Nasca PC, Schwartz AG, Schymura MJ, et al. Relationship of leukemia risk to radiation dose following cancer of the uterine corpus. J Natl Cancer Inst. 1994 Sep 7;86(17):1315-24

[79] "Platinum-based treatment of ovarian cancer increases the risk of secondary leukemia." Travis LB, Holowaty EJ, Bergfeldt K, Lynch CF, Kohler BA, Wiklund T, Curtis RE, Hall P, Andersson M, Pukkala E, Sturgeon J, Stovall M. Risk of leukemia after platinum-based chemotherapy for ovarian cancer. *N Engl J Med*. 1999 Feb 4;340(5):351-7

[80] Zhang F, Chen Y, Pisha E, Shen L, Xiong Y, van Breemen RB, Bolton JL. **The major metabolite of equilin, 4-hydroxyequilin, autoxidizes to an o-quinone which isomerizes to the potent cytotoxin 4-hydroxyequilenin-o-quinone**. *Chem Res Toxicol*. 1999 Feb;12(2):204-13

[81] Pisha E, Lui X, Constantinou AI, Bolton JL. **Evidence that a metabolite of equine estrogens, 4-hydroxyequilenin, induces cellular transformation in vitro**. *Chem Res Toxicol*. 2001;14(1):82-90

[82] Zhang F, Swanson SM, van Breemen RB, Liu X, Yang Y, Gu C, Bolton JL. Equine estrogen metabolite 4-hydroxyequilenin induces DNA damage in the rat mammary tissues: formation of single-strand breaks, apurinic sites, stable adducts, and oxidized bases. *Chem Res Toxicol*. 2001 Dec;14(12):1654-9

[83] "At...concentrations comparable to those... in the synovial fluid of patients treated with the drug, several NSAIDs suppress proteoglycan synthesis... **These NSAID-related effects on chondrocyte metabolism ... are much more profound in osteoarthritic cartilage than in normal cartilage, due to enhanced uptake of NSAIDs by the osteoarthritic cartilage**." Brandt KD. Effects of nonsteroidal anti-inflammatory drugs on chondrocyte metabolism in vitro and in vivo. *Am J Med*. 1987 Nov 20; 83(5A): 29-34

[84] "The case of a young healthy man, who developed avascular necrosis of head of femur after prolonged administration of indomethacin, is reported here." Prathapkumar KR, Smith I, Attara GA. Indomethacin induced avascular necrosis of head of femur. *Postgrad Med J*. 2000 Sep; 76(899): 574-5

[85] "This highly significant association between **NSAID use and acetabular destruction** gives cause for concern, not least because of the difficulty in achieving satisfactory hip replacements in patients with severely damaged acetabula." Newman NM, Ling RS. Acetabular bone destruction related to non-steroidal anti-inflammatory drugs. *Lancet*. 1985 Jul 6; 2(8445): 11-4

[86] Vidal y Plana RR, Bizzarri D, Rovati AL. Articular cartilage pharmacology: I. In vitro studies on glucosamine and non steroidal antiinflammatory drugs. *Pharmacol Res Commun*. 1978 Jun;10(6):557-69

[87] "In 1983, 2876 people died from medication errors. ... By 1993, this number had risen to 7,391 - a 2.57-fold increase." Phillips DP, Christenfeld N, Glynn LM. Increase in US medication-error deaths between 1983 and 1993. *Lancet*. 1998 Feb 28;351(9103):643-4

[88] "Recent estimates suggest that each year more than 1 million patients are injured while in the hospital and approximately 180,000 die because of these injuries. Furthermore, drug-related morbidity and mortality are common and are estimated to cost more than $136 billion a year." Holland EG, Degruy FV. Drug-induced disorders. *Am Fam Physician*. 1997;56:1781-8, 1791-2

[89] "Recent estimates suggest that each year more than 1 million patients are injured while in the hospital and approximately 180,000 die because of these injuries. Furthermore, drug-related morbidity and mortality are common and are estimated to cost more than $136 billion a year." Holland EG, Degruy FV. Drug-induced disorders. *Am Fam Physician*. 1997;56:1781-8, 1791-2

Examples of allopathic iatrogenesis abound, and some of the more notable problems will be cited here:

- Many non-steroidal anti-inflammatory drugs for arthritis actually exacerbate joint destruction.[90,91,92]

- A recent study evaluating arthroscopic knee surgery found it to be no more effective than placebo[93], yet it continues to be used "on at least 225,000 middle-age and older Americans each year at a cost of more than a billion dollars to Medicare, the Department of Veterans Affairs and private insurers."[94]

- The so-called "safer" new COX-2 inhibitors, which cost seven times the price of other analgesics with no improvement in efficacy over older medications[95], increase the risk for heart attack, stroke, other cardiovascular events including sudden unexplained death[96], and hypertension.[97]

- Several antidepressant drugs *increase* the risk of suicide in children[98] as well as adults.[99]

- Long-term use of so-called antipsychotic medications is clinically unsatisfying[100] and may worsen long-term outcomes in a large percentage of patients.[101]

- Although adenoidectomy for the treatment of recurrent ear infections in children is no more effective than placebo[102], it is routinely performed at a cost of approximately $4,000 per procedure.[103] Naturopathic treatment is safer, more effective, and more cost-effective.[104]

- As a final example, some authors have argued that reliance upon mammography (e.g., diagnostic radiation) as a "cancer preventive" may be inefficacious and possibly unsafe[105,106] especially when emphasis on mammography supercedes emphasis on a cancer-preventing diet and lifestyle.[107]

Clearly, the most effective method for avoiding expensive and potentially dangerous medical procedures and drug treatments is for us as a nation and as individuals to shift our thinking from a *disease treatment* model of healthcare to a more logical program of aggressive *disease prevention* and *wellness promotion* via the use of safe natural treatments rather than heroic interventions.[108,109] Of course, this means that our concept and view of health and healthcare will have to change. As noted by Shi[110], "**Redesigning the**

---

[90] Dingle JT. The effects of NSAID on the matrix of human articular cartilages. *Z Rheumatol* 1999 Jun;58(3):125-9

[91] Hugenberg ST, Brandt KD, Cole CA. Effect of sodium salicylate, aspirin, and ibuprofen on enzymes required by the chondrocyte for synthesis of chondroitin sulfate. *J Rheumatol* 1993 Dec;20(12):2128-33

[92] Fujii K, et al. Effects of nonsteroidal antiinflammatory drugs on collagen biosynthesis of cultured chondrocytes. *Semin Arthritis Rheum* 1989 Feb;18(3 Suppl 1):16-8

[93] Moseley JB, O'Malley K, Petersen NJ, Menke TJ, Brody BA, Kuykendall DH, Hollingsworth JC, Ashton CM, Wray NP. A controlled trial of arthroscopic surgery for osteoarthritis of the knee. *N Engl J Med* 2002 Jul 11;347(2):81-8

[94] Gina Kolata. A Knee Surgery for Arthritis Is Called Sham. *The New York Times*, July 11, 2002

[95] "In these trials rofecoxib 12.5-25 mg/day was no more effective than the comparators (ibuprofen or diclofenac) used at maximal recommended doses." Rofecoxib: new preparation. A disappointing NSAID analgesic. *Prescrire Int* 2000 Dec;9(50):166-7, 169

[96] "The results from VIGOR showed that the relative risk of developing a confirmed adjudicated thrombotic cardiovascular event (myocardial infarction, unstable angina, cardiac thrombus, resuscitated cardiac arrest, sudden or unexplained death, ischemic stroke, and transient ischemic attacks) with rofecoxib treatment compared with naproxen was 2.38." Mukherjee D, Nissen SE, Topol EJ. Risk of cardiovascular events associated with selective COX-2 inhibitors. *JAMA* 2001; 286(8):954-9

[97] "Systolic blood pressure increased significantly in 17% of rofecoxib- compared with 11% of celecoxib-treated patients (P = 0.032) at any study time point." Whelton A, Fort JG, Puma JA, Normandin D, Bello AE, Verburg KM; SUCCESS VI Study Group.Cyclooxygenase-2--specific inhibitors and cardiorenal function: a randomized, controlled trial of celecoxib and rofecoxib in older hypertensive osteoarthritis patients. *Am J Ther* 2001 Mar-Apr;8(2):85-95

[98] "In addition, the pooled results showed that suicidal thoughts, suicide attempts and episodes of self-harm were more frequent among the paroxetine users (5.3% of 378 children) than among those in the placebo group (2.8% of 285 children)." Wooltorton E. Paroxetine (Paxil, Seroxat): increased risk of suicide in pediatric patients. *CMAJ*. 2003 Sep 2;169(5):446 http://www.cmaj.ca/cgi/content/full/169/5/446 on July 4, 2004

[99] "Similarly for fatal suicide, the RR among patients who were first prescribed an antidepressant within 1 to 9 days before their index date was 38.0... **The risk of suicidal behavior is increased in the first month after starting antidepressants**, especially during the first 1 to 9 days." Jick H, Kaye JA, Jick SS. Antidepressants and the risk of suicidal behaviors. *JAMA*. 2004 Jul 21;292(3):338-43

[100] "CONCLUSIONS: The majority of patients in each group discontinued their assigned treatment owing to inefficacy or intolerable side effects or for other reasons." Lieberman JA, Stroup TS, McEvoy JP, Swartz MS, Rosenheck RA, Perkins DO, Keefe RS, Davis SM, Davis CE, Lebowitz BD, Severe J, Hsiao JK; Clinical Antipsychotic Trials of Intervention Effectiveness (CATIE) Investigators. Effectiveness of antipsychotic drugs in patients with chronic schizophrenia. *N Engl J Med*. 2005 Sep 22;353(12):1209-23. Epub 2005 Sep 19

[101] "...standard of care in developed countries is to maintain schizophrenia patients on neuroleptics, this practice is not supported by the 50-year research record for the drugs. ...this paradigm of care worsens long-term outcomes, ... 40% of all schizophrenia patients would fare better if they were not so medicated." Whitaker R. The case against antipsychotic drugs: a 50-year record of doing more harm than good. *Med Hypotheses*. 2004;62(1):5-1

[102] "Adenoidectomy, as the first surgical treatment of children aged 10 to 24 months with recurrent acute otitis media, is not effective in preventing further episodes. It cannot be recommended as the primary method of prophylaxis." Koivunen P, Uhari M, Luotonen J, Kristo A, Raski R, Pokka T, Alho OP.Adenoidectomy versus chemoprophylaxis and placebo for recurrent acute otitis media in children aged under 2 years: randomised controlled trial. *BMJ*. 2004 Feb 28;328(7438):487

[103] See cost estimations at http://www.healthcentral.com/peds/top/003011.cfm#Cost: July 4, 2004

[104] Sarrell EM, Cohen HA, Kahan E. Naturopathic treatment for ear pain in children. *Pediatrics*. 2003 May;111(5 Pt 1):e574-9

[105] "INTERPRETATION: Screening for breast cancer with mammography is unjustified. If the Swedish trials are judged to be unbiased, the data show that for every 1000 women screened biennially throughout 12 years, one breast-cancer death is avoided whereas the total number of deaths is increased by six." Gotzsche PC, Olsen O. Is screening for breast cancer with mammography justifiable? *Lancet*. 2000 Jan 8;355(9198):129-34

[106] "...no large study has shown the effectiveness of breast cancer screening by either CBE or mammography for women whose risk of breast cancer is higher than the general population." *Patient Care Archive* January 15, 1998

[107] Sellman S. Breast cancer awareness: seeing deception is your only protection. *Alternative Medicine* November 2001, pages 68-74 See also: "...mammography improves early cancer detection and survival in post-menopausal women, no such benefit is demonstrable for younger women." "Mammograms increase the risk for developing breast cancer and raise the risk of spreading or metastasizing an existing growth," says Dr. Charles Simone, former clinical associate in immunology and pharmacology at NCI. Sellman S. Seeing Deception is your Only Protection: The Breast Cancer Awareness Month Story. Available at http://www.mercola.com/2000/oct/29/breast_cancer_awareness.htm on July 4, 2004

[108] "Systematic access to managed chiropractic care not only may prove to be clinically beneficial but also may reduce overall health care costs." Legorreta A, Metz D, Nelson C, Ray S, Chernicoff H, DiNubile N. Comparative Analysis of Individuals With and Without Chiropractic Coverage. *Archives of Internal Medicine* 2004; 164: 1985-1992

[109] Orme-Johnson DW, Herron RE. An innovative approach to reducing medical care utilization and expenditures. *Am J Manag Care*. 1997 Jan;3(1):135-44

[110] Shi L. Health care spending, delivery, and outcome in developed countries: a cross-national comparison. *Am J Med Qual* 1997;12(2):83-93

system of health care delivery in the United States may be the only viable option to improve the quality of health care." In the meantime, while we work for change on a national level, we are wise to change our personal habits and healthcare choices in favor of natural and preventive healthcare.

<u>**Recognize and affirm that you are a unique individual with unique needs**</u>: Your "personality" extends far beyond and far deeper than your sense of humor and your choice of clothing; you are also very unique on a physiologic and biochemical level as well. So-called *normal* and *apparently healthy* individuals vary greatly in their biochemical efficiency and nutritional needs. This is the concept of "biochemical individuality" which was first detailed in 1956 by the renowned scientist Roger J Williams from the University of Texas. In his historic work, Dr. Williams[111] reviews research that conclusively proves that among *apparently healthy* individuals, we can objectively determine great differences in physiology, organ efficiency, enzyme function, and nutritional needs. For example, variables that promote health include increased enzyme efficiency and efficient digestion and assimilation of nutrients, while internal factors that reduce health can include inadequate digestion, inefficient absorption, increased excretion of nutrients, impaired detoxification, nutritional deficiencies, poor enzyme function and "partial genetic blocks"—a term now understood to imply single nucleotide polymorphisms[112] and related enzyme defects, which result in **supradietary requirements for specific vitamins and minerals** for the prevention of disease and maintenance of health.[113] What this means for us as doctors and for our patients in practical terms is that in order for us to become as healthy as possible, we will almost certainly have to give attention to each person's unique abilities/disabilities in order to maximize the function of the various body systems and to optimize genetic expression.[114] This means that what works for your neighbor, spouse, or best friend in terms of exercise, diet and nutrition may not work for your unique physiology. Have the courage to affirm that, in order for you to attain your goal of better health, you will have to learn about how your body works and will have to learn to make changes in your lifestyle and daily routine which reflect and honor your body's way of working. This may mean modifying work, sleep, and exercise schedules, avoiding some foods and eating others, and customizing nutrient intake to meet the body's needs as they are *in the present*. The process of learning how a person's body works requires time, patience, and the process of trial and error—from patient and doctor—but achieving the goal of improved health and increased energy are well worth the effort.

<u>**Individuation and the practice of conscious living**</u>: Our visions of reality are influenced by religious institutions, large corporations, advertising networks[115], corporate-owned mass media[116], and what Professors Stevens and Glatstein called "the medical-industrial complex."[117] Some of the paradigms that are advocated are both *unhistorical* (having no historical precedent) and *antihistorical* (contrary to the available historical precedent, which includes sustainability). Some of these companies and organizations offer us a view of reality and vision of our individual potentials that is fashioned in such a way as to promote the financial and political interests of the company or organization. Conversely, the actualization of our true physical, emotional, intellectual, and spiritual potentials may require that we separate from or at least attain a conscious appreciation of the (pseudo)reality that we have been advised

---

[111] Williams RJ. <u>Biochemical Individuality : The Basis for the Genetotrophic Concept</u>. Austin and London: University of Texas Press, 1956
[112] Ames BN. Cancer prevention and diet: help from single nucleotide polymorphisms. *Proc Natl Acad Sci U S A*. 1999 Oct 26;96(22):12216-8
[113] Ames BN, Elson-Schwab I, Silver EA. High-dose vitamin therapy stimulates variant enzymes with decreased coenzyme binding affinity (increased K(m)): relevance to genetic disease and polymorphisms. *Am J Clin Nutr*. 2002 Apr;75(4):616-58 http://www.ajcn.org/cgi/content/full/75/4/616
[114] "The combination of biochemical individuality and known functional utilities of allelic variants should converge to create a situation in which nutritional optima can be specified as part of comprehensive lifestyle prescriptions tailored to the needs of each person." Eckhardt RB. Genetic research and nutritional individuality. *J Nutr* 2001;131(2):336S-9S
[115] "Patients' requests for medicines are a powerful driver of prescribing decisions. In most cases physicians prescribed requested medicines but were often ambivalent about the choice of treatment. If physicians prescribe requested drugs despite personal reservations, sales may increase but appropriateness of prescribing may suffer." Mintzes B, Barer ML, Kravitz RL, Kazanjian A, Bassett K, Lexchin J, Evans RG, Pan R, Marion SA. Influence of direct to consumer pharmaceutical advertising and patients' requests on prescribing decisions: two site cross sectional survey. *BMJ*. 2002 Feb 2; 324(7332): 278-9
[116] <u>Manufacturing Consent: Noam Chomsky and the Media</u>. Movie directed by Mark Achbar and Peter Wintonick. 1992. See www.imdb.com/title/tt0104810/ and www.zeitgeistfilms.com
[117] "…despite lush advertisements from companies with obvious vested interests, and authoritative testimonials from biased investigators who presumably believe in their own work to the point of straining credulity and denying common sense… (translate: economic improvement, not biological superiority)." Stevens CW, Glatstein E. Beware the Medical-Industrial Complex. *Oncologist* 1996;1(4):IV-V http://theoncologist.alphamedpress.org/cgi/reprint/1/4/190-iv.pdf on July 4, 2004

to follow.[118,119] Critiques of and reasonable alternatives to our current paradigms of school[120], work[121], and money[122] have been discussed elsewhere and are worthy of consideration. Becoming mindful of the paradigms and assumptions under which we live is the first step in true individuation, characterized by choosing (creating the best option: freedom) rather than deciding (selecting one of the offered options: the illusion of freedom). Different "layers of illusions" create our "working reality" which represents the way that we see things and the paradigm by which we *act in* and *interact with* the larger world. These layers come from our own families, schools, teachers, churches, companies, friends, parents, and ourselves—our previous interpretations and misinterpretations of ourselves and events. Becoming conscious of these illusions allows us the opportunity to discard those views that are inaccurate, dysfunctional, and harmful and to accept a truer reality based on what we experience, feel, and know to be real. Once we are freed from *unreality*, we can live true to ourselves in a way that is authentically responsible to our own needs *and* the needs of our communities so that we can simultaneously sustain our obligations to society[123,124] while being free to be unique individuals.[125]

Examples of commonly accepted paradigms and their reasonable alternatives

Commonly advocated/accepted paradigms ↳ *Implication and effect*	*Alternate paradigm* ↳ *Implication and effect*
It is OK to be irresponsible in daily choices and then blame health problems on bad luck, bad genes, or both. ↳ Many people fail to take responsibility for their lives and thereby become victims of circumstances—negative circumstances that they themselves helped to create.	**Lifestyle, especially diet and nutrition, is the most powerful influence on health outcomes. Therefore, an educated patient is empowered to direct his/her health destiny.** ↳ Optimal health *per individual* is attained when people take responsibility for their lives, seek health information, and then incorporate this information into their daily lives in the form of healthy living: healthy lifestyle, healthy eating, healthy exercise, healthy supplementation, healthy relationships, and healthy occupational and social activities, including socio-political involvement to protect the environment and resist the privatization of life and the spoliation of the environment in which we live and upon which our lives and health depend.[126,127]
In general, chemical medications are the answer to nearly all health problems. ↳ The belief in medications as the primary treatment of disease creates a patient population that is apathetic, disempowered, and dependent upon the medical-pharmaceutical industry, which grows richer and more powerful despite so-called 'earnest' attempts at cost containment.[128]	**Many acute and chronic problems can be more effectively managed in terms of prevention, safety, efficacy, and cost-effectiveness when phytonutritional interventions are either used as primary therapy or, when necessary, used in conjunction with medications.** ↳ A reduction in disease prevalence via health-promoting diet and lifestyle along with integrative treatments offers the best opportunity for benefit to patients, doctors, and third-party payers.[129]

[118] Breton D, Largent C. The Paradigm Conspiracy: Why Our Social Systems Violate Human Potential-And How We Can Change Them. Center City; Hazelden: 1996
[119] Pearce JC. Exploring the Crack in the Cosmic Egg: Split Minds and Meta-Realities. New York: Washington Square Press; 1974
[120] Gatto JT. Dumbing us down: the hidden curriculum of compulsory education. Gabriola Island, Canada; New Society Publishers: 2005
[121] "No one should ever work. In order to stop suffering, we have to stop working. That doesn't mean we have to stop doing things. It does mean creating a new way of life based on play..." Black B. The abolition of work and other essays. Port Townsend: Loompanics Unlimited; 1985, pages 17-33
[122] Dominguez JR. Transforming Your Relationship With Money. Sounds True; Book and Cassette edition: 2001 Audio tape.
[123] Bly R. The Sibling Society. Vintage Books USA; Reprint edition (June 1, 1997) ISBN: 0679781285 (Abridged audio edition (May 1, 1996), ASIN: 0679451609)
[124] Bly R. Where have all the parents gone? A talk on the Sibling Society. New York: Sound Horizons, 1996 Highly recommended.
[125] Rick Jarow. Creating the Work You Love: Courage, Commitment and Career; Inner Traditions Intl Ltd; 1995 [ISBN: 0892815426]
[126] "**Your lack of interest in the past, your lack of involvement, your unwillingness to develop coherent strategies, your unwillingness to challenge authority - these have created a vacuum in decision-making, that has been filled by professional groups with close relationships with the chemical industries...**" Samuel Epstein MD, 1993. Professor of Occupational and Environmental Medicine at the School of Public Health, University of Illinois Medical Center Chicago. http://www.converge.org.nz/pirm/pestican.htm accessed September 11, 2004
[127] Kristin S. Schafer, Margaret Reeves, Skip Spitzer, Susan E. Kegley. Chemical Trespass: Pesticides in Our Bodies and Corporate Accountability. Pesticide Action Network North America. May 2004 Available at http://www.panna.org/campaigns/docsTrespass/chemicalTrespass2004.dv.html on August 1, 2004
[128] "In this paper I offer four hypotheses to help explain why use of pharmaceuticals has continued to grow even as managed care and other cost containment efforts have flourished." Berndt ER. The U.S. pharmaceutical industry: why major growth in times of cost containment? Health Aff (Millwood). 2001 Mar-Apr;20(2):100-14
[129] "Hospital admission rates in the control group were 11.4 times higher than those in the MVAH group for cardiovascular disease, 3.3 times higher for cancer, and 6.7 times higher for mental health and substance abuse. ...MVAH patients older than age 45...had 88% fewer total patients days compared with control patients." Orme-Johnson DW, Herron RE. An innovative approach to reducing medical care utilization and expenditures. Am J Manag Care. 1997 Jan;3(1):135-44

Examples of commonly accepted paradigms and their reasonable alternatives—*continued*

Commonly advocated/accepted paradigms ↳ *Implication and effect*	Alternate paradigm ↳ *Implication and effect*
Work ethic: a belief that "hard work" has moral value and makes a person "better." ↳ Belief in the principle of "work ethic" encourages people to mindlessly engage in work for the sake of engaging in work without considering the implications of their actions or other alternatives that might produce a more beneficial outcome.[130]	**Work is the means rather than an end unto itself (except when the "work" is enjoyable, in which case it is no longer "work").** ↳ Occupations and professions can be designed for the enhancement of life (health, pleasure, relationships, the environment, care of the poor) rather than as an end to themselves at the expense of the individual, society, and the environment.
It is "normal" for adults to give 10.5-12 hours per day 5 days per week to work. ↳ In most corporate environments, employee's work at least 8.5 hours per day, with 1 additional hour spent in commuting[131] and another hour spent in preparation, transportation, and maintenance of work-related clothing, preparing work-related meals, maintaining the auto that is used for work-related tasks. With 10.5 hours given directly to work, 0.5-1 additional hours are needed for recuperation from work-related stress ("daily decompression"); thus the average amount of time given to work-related activities is much larger than commonly believed.[132] Because of the time and energies devoted to "work" the vast majority of people feel that they do not have sufficient time for themselves, their families and friends, their creativity, learning about the world, political involvement, and other more important aspects of life. "Not enough time" is the most common reason given by patients for not exercising.	**A paradigm of a 4-day workweek is just as valid and perhaps more so than one that advocates a 5-day workweek. A paradigm of a 6-hour workday is at least as valid as one of an 8-10 hour workday.** ↳ Many people in our culture are chronically overworked, undernourished, tired and suffer from an insufficiency of time to simply be in community, to rest, to be creative. It is no surprise that they then behave addictively (e.g., drugs, alcohol) and destructively (e.g., over-eating, alcohol, sugar, fat)—their behaviors are simply frustrated and maladaptive coping strategies to combat the stress caused by a damaging, unnatural paradigm from which they cannot escape.[133] Redesigning our societal structures and expectations in ways that conform to our natural humanity and biologic, nutritional, and emotional needs is more rational than forcing *en masse* all of humanity to contort and conform to an artificial posture and cadence of performance, productivity, professionalism, and other unnatural expectations. Less time dedicated to "work" and all that it entails leaves more time for 1) healthy cooking, 2) relaxed, conscious, and enjoyable eating, 3) exercise, 4) creativity and hobbies, 5) keeping informed of and involved with political change, and 6) participation in social relationships.[134]

---

[130] "Conventional wisdom is the habitual, the unexamined life, absorbed into the culture and the fashion of the time, lost in the mad rush of accumulation, lulled to sleep by the easy lies of political hacks and newspaper scribblers, or by priests who wouldn't know a god if they met one." Nisker W. Crazy Wisdom. Berkeley; Ten Speed Press: 1990, page 7
[131] Monday, September 8, 2003 -- The average daily one-way commute to work in the United States takes just over 26 minutes, according to the Bureau of Transportation Statistics' Omnibus Household Survey. Omnibus Household Survey Shows Americans' Average Commuting Time is Just Over 26 Minutes. http://www.bts.gov/press_releases/2003/bts020_03/html/bts020_03.html on August 3, 2004
[132] Dominguez JR. Transforming Your Relationship With Money. Sounds True; Book and Cassette edition: 2001
[133] Breton D and Largent C. The Paradigm Conspiracy: Why Our Social Systems Violate Human Potential-And How We Can Change Them. Hazelden: 1998
[134] TAKE BACK YOUR TIME is a major U.S./Canadian initiative to challenge the epidemic of overwork, over-scheduling and time famine that now threatens our health, our families and relationships, our communities and our environment. http://www.simpleliving.net/timeday/ on August 3, 2004

Quality and quantity of sleep: Anything less than 8 hours of solid sleep each and every night is insufficient for the vast majority of people, and many people feel their best with 9 hours of sleep. Not only is it important to get a sufficient *quantity* of sleep, but we need to ensure that the *quality* of the sleep receives appropriate attention, as well. Sleep should be mostly continuous, not "broken" or interrupted for extended periods of time. Some experts believe that people should be able to recall their dreams at night, as this may be a sign of proper neurotransmitter status, especially with regard to serotonin, which is affected by pyridoxine[135] as well as other factors. Going to bed at a regular hour (not later than 10 or 11 at night) helps to synchronize the daily schedule with the body's inherent hormonal rhythms and "physiological clock" which expects one to be in deep sleep by midnight and to be waking at approximately 8 o'clock in the morning. Recent research has shown that **sleep deprivation causes a systemic inflammatory response manifested objectively by increases in high-sensitivity C-reactive protein**.[136] Correspondingly, sleep apnea, a condition associated with repetitive sleep disturbances, is also associated with an elevation of CRP[137], and effective treatment of sleep apnea results in a normalization of CRP levels.[138]   We could therefore conclude that **sleep deprivation creates a proinflammatory condition**. Furthermore, **sleep deprivation has been proven to impair intellectual functioning, emotional state, and immune function**, with abnormalities in immune status already evident the morning after sleep deprivation.[139] Wakefulness and exposure to light at night result in a suppression of melatonin production and may therefore contribute to cancer development since melatonin has anticancer actions that would be abrogated by its reduced production.[140,141] Limited evidence also suggests that melatonin production is altered in patients with the inflammatory conditions eczema[142] and psoriasis[143] and that this sleep-related hormone has anti-rheumatic/anti-autoimmune benefits that may be relevant for the suppression of inflammatory diseases such as multiple sclerosis[144] and sarcoidosis.[145]

> *In summary*: Regulation of sleep-wake cycles and the regular satisfaction of sleep needs are important for preservation of immune function, intellectual performance, emotional stability, and the internal regulation of the body's inflammatory tendency.

---

[135] "…a significant difference in dream-salience scores (this is a composite score containing measures on vividness, bizarreness, emotionality, and color) between the 250-mg condition and placebo over the first three days of each treatment… An hypothesis is presented involving the role of B-6 in the conversion of tryptophan to serotonin." Ebben M, Lequerica A, Spielman A. Effects of pyridoxine on dreaming: a preliminary study. *Percept Mot Skills* 2002 Feb;94(1):135-40

[136] "CONCLUSIONS: Both acute total and short-term partial sleep deprivation resulted in elevated high-sensitivity CRP concentrations… We propose that sleep loss may be one of the ways that inflammatory processes are activated and contribute to the association of sleep complaints, short sleep duration, and cardiovascular morbidity observed in epidemiologic surveys." Meier-Ewert HK, Ridker PM, et al. Effect of sleep loss on C-reactive protein, an inflammatory marker of cardiovascular risk. *J Am Coll Cardiol.* 2004 Feb 18;43(4):678-83

[137] "OSA is associated with elevated levels of CRP, a marker of inflammation and of cardiovascular risk. The severity of OSA is proportional to the CRP level." Shamsuzzaman AS, Winnicki M, Lanfranchi P, Wolk R, Kara T, Accurso V, Somers VK. Elevated C-reactive protein in patients with obstructive sleep apnea. *Circulation.* 2002 May 28;105(21):2462-4

[138] "CONCLUSIONS: Levels of CRP and IL-6 and spontaneous production of IL-6 by monocytes are elevated in patients with OSAS but are decreased by nCPAP." Yokoe T, Minoguchi K, Matsuo H, Oda N, Minoguchi H, Yoshino G, Hirano T, Adachi M. Elevated levels of C-reactive protein and interleukin-6 in patients with obstructive sleep apnea syndrome are decreased by nasal continuous positive airway pressure. *Circulation.* 2003 Mar 4;107(8):1129-34 Available on-line at http://circ.ahajournals.org/cgi/reprint/107/8/1129.pdf on August 2, 2004

[139] "Taken together, SD induced a deterioration of both mood and ability to work, which was most prominent in the evening after SD, while the maximal alterations of the host defence system could be found twelve hours earlier, i.e., already in the morning following SD." Heiser P, Dickhaus B, Opper C, Hemmeter U, Remschmidt H, Wesemann W, Krieg JC, Schreiber W. Alterations of host defense system after sleep deprivation are followed by impaired mood and psychosocial functioning. *World J Biol Psychiatry* 2001 Apr;2(2):89-94

[140] "Observational studies support an association between night work and cancer risk. We hypothesise that the potential primary culprit for this observed association is the lack of melatonin, a cancer-protective agent whose production is severely diminished in people exposed to light at night." Schernhammer ES, Schulmeister K. Melatonin and cancer risk: does light at night compromise physiologic cancer protection by lowering serum melatonin levels? *Br J Cancer.* 2004 Mar 8;90(5):941-3

[141] "This is the first biological evidence for a potential link between constant light exposure and increased human breast oncogenesis involving MLT suppression and stimulation of tumor LA metabolism." Blask DE, Dauchy RT, Sauer LA, Krause JA, Brainard GC. Growth and fatty acid metabolism of human breast cancer (MCF-7) xenografts in nude rats: impact of constant light-induced nocturnal melatonin suppression. *Breast Cancer Res Treat.* 2003 Jun;79(3):313-20

[142] "In 6 patients exhibiting low serum levels of melatonin, the circadian melatonin rhythm was found to be abolished. In 8 patients a diminished nocturnal melatonin increase was observed compared with the controls (n = 40)." Schwarz W, Birau N, Hornstein OP, Heubeck B, Schonberger A, Meyer C, Gottschalk J. Alterations of melatonin secretion in atopic eczema. *Acta Derm Venereol.* 1988;68(3):224-9

[143] "Our results show that psoriatic patients had lost the nocturnal peak and usual circadian rhythm of melatonin secretion." Mozzanica N, Tadini G, Radaelli A, Negri M, Pigatto P, Morelli M, Frigerio U, Finzi A, Esposti G, Rossi D, et al. Plasma melatonin levels in psoriasis. *Acta Derm Venereol.* 1988;68(4):312-6

[144] "This hypothesis is supported by the observation that administration of melatonin (3 mg, orally) at 2:00 p.m., when the patient experienced severe blurring of vision, resulted within 15 minutes in a dramatic improvement in visual acuity and in normalization of the visual evoked potential latency after stimulation of the left eye." Sandyk R. Diurnal variations in vision and relations to circadian melatonin secretion in multiple sclerosis. *Int J Neurosci.* 1995 Nov;83(1-2):1-6

[145] Cagnoni ML, Lombardi A, Cerinic MC, Dedola GL, Pignone A. Melatonin for treatment of chronic refractory sarcoidosis. *Lancet.* 1995 Nov 4;346(8984):1229-30

Helping patients improve quality and quantity of sleep

- Reduce intake of stimulants such as caffeine, tobacco, and aspartame. Some patients will need to reduce intake only in the evening, while others will need to reduce intake even in the morning in order to have improved quality and quantity of sleep later at night.

- Exercise early in the day (morning or early afternoon) to promote restful sleep at night.[146]

- Avoid aggressive or arousing physical activity in the evening to avoid increases in norepinephrine, epinephrine, and cortisol, which can discourage sleep.

- Dim lights at night to promote melatonin production. Beginning one to two hours before bedtime, turn off bright lights and use only dim lighting. Bright lights reduce melatonin secretion and stimulate neocortical activity and thereby inhibit sleep.

- Have an evening ritual/pattern that helps the psyche recognize that the time for sleep has arrived. Such practices can include relaxing warm tea, meditation, prayer, and daily reflection.

- For patients with a pattern of falling asleep and then waking approximately 4-6 hours later with feelings of hunger or anxiety (nocturnal hypoglycemia), they should eat a small meal or snack of complex carbohydrates, protein, and fat before going to bed. For example, the combination of nuts (or nut butter) with whole fruit such as apples provides protein, fat, and complex carbohydrate with a low glycemic index to provide sustenance throughout the night. Protein powders and other sources of "predigested" amino acids should generally be avoided late at night because an excess consumption of high protein foods can reduce tryptophan entry into the brain and thus reduce serotonin and melatonin synthesis. Most amino acid-derived neurotransmitters such as dopamine, glutamate, and norepinephrine are excitatory/stimulatory in nature.

- Vitamin and mineral supplementation is commonly beneficial, particularly with thiamine[147], methylcobalamin (weak evidence[148]), and magnesium (particularly sleep disturbance associated with restless leg syndrome[149]). Vitamins should be taken earlier in the day (with breakfast and lunch; not before bed); however calcium and magnesium can be taken before bed.

- Earplugs, window covers, and a quiet, snore-free environment are generally conducive to better sleep.

- For patients with difficulty falling asleep, consider 5-hydroxytryptophan consumed with simple carbohydrate (50-200 mg for adults, up to 2 mg/kg[150] for children), melatonin (0.5-10 mg), valerian-hops tea or capsules[151] 60-90 minutes before bedtime.

---

[146] "This is the first report to demonstrate that low intensity activity in an elderly population can increase deep sleep and improve memory functioning." Naylor E, Penev PD, Orbeta L, Janssen I, Ortiz R, Colecchia EF, Keng M, Finkel S, Zee PC. Daily social and physical activity increases slow-wave sleep and daytime neuropsychological performance in the elderly. *Sleep.* 2000 Feb 1;23(1):87-95

[147] Wilkinson TJ, Hanger HC, Elmslie J, George PM, Sainsbury R. The response to treatment of subclinical thiamine deficiency in the elderly. *Am J Clin Nutr.* 1997;66(4):925-8

[148] "However, because the percentage of improvement was low and significant improvement was inconsistent, Met-12 might be considered to have a low therapeutic potency and possible use as a booster for other treatment methods of the disorders." Takahashi K, et al. Double-blind test on the efficacy of methylcobalamin on sleep-wake rhythm disorders. *Psychiatry Clin Neurosci.* 1999 Apr;53(2):211-3

[149] "Our study indicates that magnesium treatment may be a useful alternative therapy in patients with mild or moderate RLS-or PLMS-related insomnia." Hornyak M, Voderholzer U, et al. Magnesium therapy for periodic leg movements-related insomnia and restless legs syndrome: an open pilot study. *Sleep.* 1998 Aug 1;21(5):501-5

[150] Bruni O, Ferri R, Miano S, Verrillo E. 1-5-Hydroxytryptophan treatment of sleep terrors in children. *Eur J Pediatr.* 2004 May 14

[151] "Sleep improvements with a valerian-hops combination are associated with improved quality of life. Both treatments appear safe and did not produce rebound insomnia upon discontinuation during this study. Overall, these findings indicate that a valerian-hops combination and diphenhydramine might be useful adjuncts in the treatment of mild insomnia." Morin CM, Koetter U, Bastien C, Ware JC, Wooten V. Valerian-hops combination and diphenhydramine for treating insomnia: a randomized placebo-controlled clinical trial. *Sleep.* 2005 Nov 1;28(11):1465-71

Exercise:

"The health rewards of exercise extend far beyond its benefits for specific diseases." Exercise reduces blood clotting, lowers blood pressure, lowers cholesterol, improves glucose tolerance and insulin sensitivity, enhances self-image, elevates mood, reduces stress, creates a feeling of well-being, reinforces other positive life-style changes, stimulates creative thinking, increases muscle mass, increases basal metabolic rate, promotes improved sleep, stimulates healthy intestinal function, promotes weight loss, and enhances appearance. "Furthermore, **the ability of exercise to restore function to organs, muscles, joints, and bones is not shared by drugs or surgery.**"[152]

Human existence has changed radically over the past few millennia, centuries, and decades, and one of the most profound changes has been in our relationship to physical activity. Paleologists and historical scientists agree that physical activity among humans is at its all-time historical low, and that levels of exertion that we now call "vigorous and frequent exercise" would have been *completely normal* in the daily lives of our ancestors, who engaged in at least four times more physical activity than their modern-day progeny.[153] It is interesting to fathom a time in which physical activity was such a normal part of daily life that there was no word for "exercise."

"Although modern technology has made physical exertion optional, it is still important to exercise as though our survival depended on it, and in a different way it still does. **We are genetically adapted to live an extremely physically active lifestyle.**"[154]

Our current mode of compulsory primary and secondary education prioritizes "being still" over physical exertion and physical expression for the vast majority of students' time. Thus having been separated from their inherent tendency to be physically active and emotionally expressive, many children grow into adults who have to be *retaught to inhabit their bodies* and to engage in physical activity on a daily basis. Basic science has proven that this is true: when animals are restrained, they show less activity when freed and no longer tied down. Conversely, when animals are rigorously exercised, they show higher levels of *spontaneous physical activity* when left to their own discretion. A probable sociological parallel is at work in human cultures where, under the guise of *work* and *entertainment*, people are corralled into lifestyles of physical inactivity in a wide range of apparently divergent activities. Watching television, driving a car, seeing a movie, doing computer/desk work at the office, attending a sports event or educational lecture, seeing the opera—all of these are simply different forms of *sitting*, of physical inactivity. Changing our social structure in a way that prioritizes *life* over *work*, such as moving toward a 4-day work week and/or a 6-hour work day, would allow people more time to live their lives, to pursue healthy diets and relationships, to be creative, and to engage in more physical activity; thus, "escape entertainment" such as fiction books and movies and processed "fast foods"—the latter of which are inherently unhealthy[155]—would become less necessary and less attractive.

Inactivity	Minimally active	Active	Healthy	Athletic
• Bed-ridden • Chair-ridden • Minimal activity, such as walking to car or bathroom or to buy groceries • Activity in this category is equivalent to or barely above that which is necessary to sustain life	• The performance of more activity than the minimal needed to sustain life, such as walking around the block after dinner, or taking a brief stroll at a park or at the beach	• Regular performance of low/moderate levels of activity at work or leisure, at least 30-60 minutes of physical activity per day	• 60-120 minutes of vigorous activity such as running, swimming, or cycling 4-7 days per week	• More than 2 hours devoted to conditioning, strengthening, and skill-building 4-7 days per week

[152] Harold Elrick, MD. Exercise is Medicine. *The Physician and Sportsmedicine* - Volume 24 - No. 2 - February 1996
[153] Eaton SB, Cordain L, Eaton SB. An evolutionary foundation for health promotion. *World Rev Nutr Diet* 2001; 90:5-12
[154] O'Keefe JH Jr, Cordain L. Cardiovascular disease resulting from a diet and lifestyle at odds with our Paleolithic genome: how to become a 21st-century hunter-gatherer. *Mayo Clin Proc.* 2004 Jan;79(1):101-8. Available on-line at http://www.thepaleodiet.com/articles/Hunter-Gatherer%20Mayo.pdf on May 19, 2004
[155] For an additional perspective see movie by Morgan Spurlock (director). Super Size Me. www.supersizeme.com released in 2004

At least 30-45 minutes of exercise four days per week is the *absolute minimum*. Following a health assessment, patients who have been previously sedentary for many years can start slowly with their new exercise program, gradually increasing the duration and intensity. **With the simple addition of regular exercise to their routine, patients will have significantly reduced risk for problems such as depression, chronic pain, cancer, coronary artery disease, stroke, hypertension, diabetes, arthritis, osteoporosis, dyslipidemia, obesity, chronic obstructive pulmonary disease, constipation, and other problems.**[156] Furthermore, successful prevention and treatment of health problems with exercise and lifestyle modifications reduces dependency on pharmaceutical drugs, thereby further saving lives. O'Keefe and Cordain[157] report that **during the hunter-gatherer period, humans averaged 5-10 miles of daily running *and walking*.** Additionally, **other physical activities such as heavy lifting, digging, and climbing would have been considered "normal" aspects of daily life rather than "exercise"—an achievement for which modern people seek recognition.** Thus, when sedentary patients achieve the first-step goal of walking around the block after dinner, we can commend them for making a significant stride forward in ultimately attaining better health, but we cannot stop there nor delude them into believing that this is adequate.

Common physical activities and exercises

- **Walking**: easy, accessible, virtually free; allows for conversation and exploration; allows for time outdoors
- **Jogging and running**: easy, accessible, virtually free; allows for conversation and exploration; increases endorphin production and promotes a sense of well-being
- **Hiking**: virtually free of expense; allows for conversation, exploration, and time in nature; mountains required
- **Swimming**: requires access to a pool or suitable body of water; excellent for promoting fitness in a way that is generally easy on joints and muscles and is without impact; requires and thus promotes coordination and timing
- **Indoor aerobics**: excellent for cardiovascular fitness and weight loss, requires and thus promotes coordination and timing
- **Indoor cycling**: excellent for cardiovascular fitness and weight loss, easy on the joints; accessible during inclement weather
- **Outdoor cycling (road)**: same as above with added bonus of being outdoors; promotes independence from automobiles and petroleum products – thereby reducing pollution and sustaining the environment
- **Outdoor cycling (mountain and trail)**: same as above; requires more balance and coordination
- **Weight lifting, bodybuilding, and powerlifting**: excellent for increasing lean body mass – one of the primary determinants of basal metabolic rate; promotes bone strengthening
- **Tennis and racket sports**: requires more balance, coordination, timing, strategy, endurance; the rapid stops, starts, and turns can be hard on joints; upper body exertion is asymmetric and can promote muscle imbalance
- **Aerobic machines such as elliptical runners and stair-climbing machines**: easy on joints; accessible during inclement weather; easy to integrate with weight-lifting which is commonly available at the same facility
- **Rock-climbing (indoor and outdoor)**: requires upper body and grip strength; promotes agility, resourcefulness, courage, and trust; good for building stronger relationships; carries some inherent risk
- **Volleyball**: good team activity; not highly exertional in terms of either aerobic fitness nor strength acquisition
- **Baseball**: requires some skill in throwing and batting, but otherwise this is a very inactive sport
- **Football**: much of the game is spent in inactivity; most of the fitness comes from preparation for the game, not the game itself; high impact activity wherein injuries are expected
- **Soccer**: excellent for lower-body conditioning, teamwork, and coordination, the rapid stops and turns can be hard on joints
- **Yoga, Pilates, Calisthenics**: inexpensive, can be done alone or in groups; does not require much/any equipment
- **Martial arts**: requires more balance, coordination, timing, strategy, endurance; injuries are to be expected
- **Surfing**: paddling requires upper body endurance and strength; some leg strength is required but is not strongly developed during the riding portion of surfing, which is mostly technique and "style"; excellent proprioceptive training
- **Kayaking and canoeing**: excellent combination of relaxation and exertion; develops upper body strength and balance

[156] Harold Elrick, MD. Exercise is Medicine. *The Physician and Sportsmedicine* - Volume 24 - No. 2 - February 1996
[157] O'Keefe JH Jr, Cordain L. Cardiovascular disease resulting from a diet and lifestyle at odds with our Paleolithic genome: how to become a 21st-century hunter-gatherer. *Mayo Clin Proc.* 2004 Jan;79(1):101-8. Available on line at http://www.thepaleodiet.com/articles/Hunter-Gatherer%20Mayo.pdf on May 19, 2004

Obesity:

Obesity is a major risk factor for cardiovascular disease, cancer, diabetes, depression, and joint pain. Obese people also commonly report difficulties with performing daily activities, and they also report higher rates of depression and social isolation than do people of normal weight.

> "The magnitude of the problem in the United States is perhaps greater than in any other country. Estimates of the number of overweight Americans range from 50 million to 200 million. **The average American is said to have 20 to 30 lb of excess body fat.**"[158]

To calculate the "Body Mass Index" simply chart height and weight to determine the BMI number. Numbers greater than 25 correlate with being "overweight" while numbers greater than 30 meet the criteria for "obesity." BMI determinations may not be reflective of disease risk for people who are pregnant, highly muscular, or for young children or the frail elderly.

BODY MASS INDEX interpretation

- ❏ Underweight: Under 18.5
- ❏ Normal: 18.5-24
- ❏ Overweight: 25-29
- ❏ Obese: 30 and over

WEIGHT in pounds

HEIGHT	100	110	120	130	140	150	160	170	180	190	200	210	220	230	240	250
5'0"	20	21	23	25	27	29	31	33	35	37	39	41	43	45	47	49
5'1"	19	21	23	25	26	28	30	32	34	36	38	40	42	43	45	47
5'2"	18	20	22	24	26	27	29	31	33	35	37	38	40	42	44	46
5'3"	18	19	21	23	25	27	28	30	32	34	35	37	39	41	43	44
5'4"	17	19	21	22	24	26	27	29	31	33	34	36	38	39	41	43
5'5"	17	18	20	22	23	25	27	28	30	32	33	35	37	38	40	42
5'6"	16	18	19	21	23	24	26	27	29	31	32	34	36	37	39	40
5'7"	16	17	19	20	22	23	25	27	28	30	31	33	34	36	38	39
5'8"	15	17	18	20	21	23	24	26	27	29	30	32	33	35	36	38
5'9"	15	16	18	19	21	22	24	25	27	28	30	31	32	34	35	37
5'10"	14	16	17	19	20	22	23	24	26	27	29	30	32	33	34	36
5'11"	14	15	17	18	20	21	22	24	25	26	27	28	30	32	33	35
6'0"	14	15	16	18	19	20	22	23	24	26	27	28	30	31	33	34
6'1"	13	15	16	17	18	20	21	22	24	25	26	28	29	30	32	33
6'2"	13	14	15	17	18	19	21	22	23	24	26	27	28	30	31	32
6'3"	12	14	15	16	17	19	20	21	22	24	25	26	27	29	30	31
6'4"	12	13	15	16	17	18	19	21	22	23	24	26	27	28	29	30

---

[158] Harold Elrick, MD. Exercise is Medicine. *The Physician and Sportsmedicine* - Volume 24 - No. 2 - February 1996

Overview of the Proinflammatory and Endocrinologic Activity of Adipose Tissue

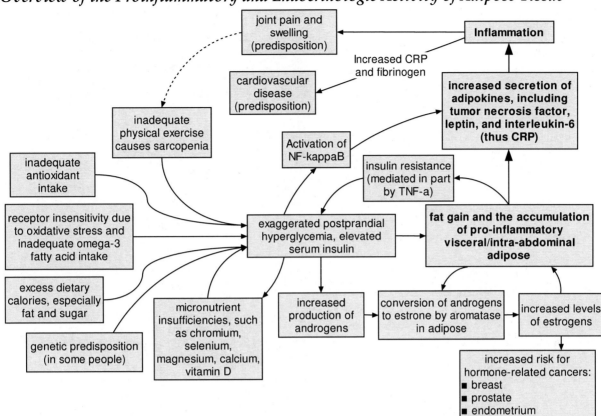

The old paradigm of fat (adipose) tissue as merely serving as an inert and inactive depot for lipid/energy storage is now replaced with the view that adipose tissue is biologically-active tissue that influences overall health via complex mechanisms that are biochemical-inflammatory-endocrinologic and not merely mechanical (i.e., excess weight, excess mass).[159] **Excess fat tissue creates a systemic proinflammatory state** evidenced most readily by elevations in C-reactive protein commonly seen in patients with obesity and the metabolic syndrome.[160] Adipokines are cytokines secreted by adipose tissue and include tumor necrosis factor-alpha, interleukin-6, adiponectin, and leptin—a cytokine derived from fat cells that promotes inflammation and immune activation; levels are higher in obese patients and decrease after weight loss. Obese patients also appear to have "leptin resistance" with regard to the suppression of appetite by leptin. **Adipose creates excess estrogens;** concomitant hyperglycemia increases androgen production[161], and these androgens are subsequently converted to estrogens by aromatase in the adipose tissue. For example, the adrenal gland makes androstenedione, which can be converted by aromatase in adipose tissue into estrone.[162] These proinflammatory and hormonal perturbations manifest clinically as an increased risk for breast, prostate, endometrial, colon and gallbladder cancers, and cardiovascular disease. This pattern of inflammation, reduced testosterone, and elevated estrogen is also a predisposition toward the development of autoimmune/inflammatory disease.

[159] "The fat cell is a true endocrine cell that secretes a variety of factors, including metabolites such as lactate, fatty acids, prostaglandin derivatives and a variety of peptides, including cytokines (leptin, tumor necrosis factor, interleukin-1 and -6, adiponectin), angiotensinogen, complement D (adipsin), plasminogen activator inhibitor-1 and undoubtedly many others." Bray GA. The underlying basis for obesity: relationship to cancer. *J Nutr*. 2002 Nov;132(11 Suppl):3451S-3455S

[160] "Our results indicate a strong relationship between adipocytokines and inflammatory markers, and suggest that cytokines secreted by adipose tissue could play a role in increased inflammatory proteins secretion by the liver." Maachi M, Pieroni L, Bruckert E, Jardel C, Fellahi S, Hainque B, Capeau J, Bastard JP. Systemic low-grade inflammation is related to both circulating and adipose tissue TNFalpha, leptin and IL-6 levels in obese women. *Int J Obes Relat Metab Disord*. 2004 Aug;28(8):993-7

[161] Christensen L, Hagen C, Henriksen JE, Haug E. Elevated levels of sex hormones and sex hormone binding globulin in male patients with insulin dependent diabetes mellitus. Effect of improved blood glucose regulation. *Dan Med Bull*. 1997 Nov;44(5):547-50

[162] "The conversion of androstenedione secreted by the adrenal gland into estrone by aromatase in adipose tissue stroma provides an important source of estrogen for the postmenopausal woman. This estrogen may play an important role in the development of endometrial and breast cancer." Bray GA. The underlying basis for obesity: relationship to cancer. *J Nutr*. 2002 Nov;132(11 Suppl):3451S-3455S

Diet is a Powerful Intervention for the Prevention and Treatment of Disease

Make "whole foods" the foundation of the diet— emphasize whole fruits, vegetables, and lean meats. "Whole foods" are foods that are found in nature, and they should be eaten as closely as possible to their natural state—preferably *unprocessed* and *raw*. Creating a diet based on whole, natural foods by emphasizing the consumption of fruits, vegetables, and lean meats and excluding high-fat factory meats, high-sugar foods like white potatoes, and milled grains like wheat and corn is essential for our efforts of promoting health by matching the human *diet* with the human *genome*.[163] Our genetic make-up was co-created over a period of more than 2.6 million years with an environment that mandated daily physical activity and a diet that was exclusively composed of 1) fresh fruits, 2) fresh vegetables (mostly uncooked), 3) nuts, seeds, berries, roots, and 4) generous portions of lean meat that was rich in omega-3 fatty acids from free-living

> My conclusion after reading several hundred articles on epidemiology, nutritional biochemistry, and dietary intervention studies is that the Paleo-Mediterranean pesco-vegetarian diet is the single most healthy dietary regimen for the broadest range of patients and for the prevention of the widest range of diseases— including cancer, hypertension, diabetes, dermatitis, depression, obesity, arthritis and all inflammatory and autoimmune diseases. By definition, this is a diet that helps patients increase their intake of fruits and vegetables (fiber and antioxidants), increases their intake of fish (for the anti-inflammatory omega-3 fats EPA and DHA) while reducing intake of the pro-cancer and pro-inflammatory omega-6 fats) and it is naturally low in sugars and cholesterol (for reducing high cholesterol and high blood sugar). It helps patients avoid grains, particularly wheat (a common allergen), and it reduces the intake of the high-fermentation carbohydrates in breads, pasta, pastries, potatoes, and sucrose which promote overgrowth of bacteria and yeast in the intestines. Supplementing this pesco-vegetarian diet with vitamins, minerals, fatty acids such as fish oil and GLA (from borage oil), and protein from soy and whey makes this diet effective for both the treatment and prevention of many conditions; I call this "**the Supplemented Paleo-Mediterranean Diet.**"

animals. Humans have deviated from this original diet for the sake of ease, conformity, and short-term satisfaction at the expense of health, power, and longevity. Peoples who consume traditional, natural diets have dramatically lower incidences *major* health disasters such as cancer, cardiovascular disease, diabetes, obesity and also suffer much less from *milder* problems such as acne, psoriasis, cavities, oral malocclusion, and chronic sinus congestion. Societies that are free of these disorders become overwhelmed with them—*within only one or two generations*—as soon as they adopt the American/Western style of eating. These facts were conclusively documented by Weston Price in his famous 1945 masterpiece *Nutrition and Physical Degeneration*[164] and have been reiterated recently in an excellent review by O'Keefe and Cordain in *Mayo Clinic Proceedings*.[165]

Most patients (and doctors) need to increase consumption of fruits and vegetables: Encourage consumption of collard greens, broccoli, kale, spinach, chard, lettuce, onions, red peppers, green beans, carrots, apples, oranges, nuts, blueberries and other fruits and vegetables. Patients can find or make a good low-carbohydrate dressing (such as lemon garlic tahini[166]) to make these vegetables taste great. Fresh fruits and vegetables are best; but frozen fruits and vegetables are acceptable. Patients can buy a package of (organic) frozen vegetables; then when they are ready for a healthy-and-fast meal, simply warm/steam the vegetables on the stovetop. In just a few minutes and with only minimal effort, by regularly eating vegetables, they will have significantly reduced their risk for heart disease, diabetes, cancer, hemorrhoids, constipation, and many other chronic health problems. Using frozen vegetables and eating vegetables only twice per day is not *optimal*—it is *minimal*. For many patients, consuming two servings of vegetables per day is a major lifestyle change. *Ultimately, the goal is for fresh fruits and vegetables to form a major portion of the diet*, to be the main course rather than simply a side dish. A diet based on fruits and vegetables is a powerful nutritional strategy for reducing the risk for cancer, heart disease, and autoimmune and inflammatory disorders.[167]

---

[163] O'Keefe JH Jr, Cordain L. Cardiovascular disease resulting from a diet and lifestyle at odds with our Paleolithic genome: how to become a 21st-century hunter-gatherer. *Mayo Clin Proc.* 2004 Jan;79(1):101-8. Available on line at http://www.thepaleodiet.com/articles/Hunter-Gatherer%20Mayo.pdf on May 19, 2004
[164] Price WA. Nutrition and Physical Degeneration: A Comparison of Primitive and Modern Diets and Their Effects. Santa Monica; Price-Pottinger Nutrition Foundation: 1945
[165] O'Keefe JH Jr, Cordain L. Cardiovascular disease resulting from a diet and lifestyle at odds with our Paleolithic genome: how to become a 21st-century hunter-gatherer. *Mayo Clin Proc.* 2004 Jan;79(1):101-8
[166] Mollie Katzen. The New Moosewood Cookbook Ten Speed Press; page 103
[167] "...one of the most consistent research findings is that those who consume higher amounts of fruits and vegetables have lower rates of heart disease and stroke as well as cancer..." Seaman DR. The diet-induced proinflammatory state: a cause of chronic pain and other degenerative diseases? *J Manipulative Physiol Ther.* 2002;25(3):168-79

Phytochemicals—important antioxidant and anti-inflammatory nutrients from fruits and vegetables: While we have all commonly thought of the benefits of fruits and vegetables as being derived from the vitamins, minerals, and fiber, we are learning from new research that many if not most of the health-promoting benefits of fruits and vegetables come from the phenolic chemicals that they contain. For example, while in the past we might have thought of the benefits of eating apples as being derived from the vitamin C content, we now know that vitamin C only provides 0.4% of the antioxidant action contained

VEGETABLES	
Phenolic content	**Antioxidant capacity**
1) Broccoli	1. Red pepper
2) Spinach	2. Broccoli
3) Yellow onion	3. Carrot
4) Red pepper	4. Spinach
5) Carrot	5. Cabbage
6) Cabbage	6. Yellow onion
7) Potato	7. Celery
8) Lettuce	8. Potato
9) Celery	9. Lettuce
10) Cucumber	10. Cucumber

within a whole apple—obviously the other components of the apple, namely the phenolic compounds are responsible for most of an apple's antioxidant activity.[168] Recent research has shown that cranberries, apples, red grapes, and strawberries have the most antioxidant power of the fruits[169], while red peppers, broccoli, carrots, and spinach are the best antioxidant vegetables.[170] This is a very important concept to appreciate and remember: **the benefits derived from fruits and vegetables are not derived principally from the vitamins and therefore can never be obtained from the use of multivitamin pills as a substitute for whole foods. Multivitamin and multimineral supplements are valuable and worthwhile _supplements_ to a whole-foods diet but should not be used as _substitutes_ for a whole-foods diet.**

Fruits and vegetables contain more than 8,000 phytochemicals, most of which have anti-inflammatory, anti-proliferative, and anti-cancer benefits[171]—the best and only way to benefit from these chemicals is to change the diet in favor of relying principally on fruits and vegetables as the major component of the diet, and the easiest way to do this is to eliminate carbohydrate-rich antioxidant-poor foods such as bread, pasta, rice, sweets, crackers, chips and "junk foods."

Different fruits and vegetables contain different types, quantities, and ratios of vitamins, minerals, and phytochemicals, and *dietary diversity* will therefore help patients to obtain a broad spectrum of and maximum benefit from these different nutrients. The revelation that, in order to be as healthy as possible, we have to consume a diet that is derived principally from fruits and vegetables in order to obtain the diverse phytochemicals contained therein is somewhat problematic for at least two reasons. In the healthcare world, our policies, politics, and paradigms

FRUITS	
Phenolic content	**Antioxidant capacity**
1. Cranberry	1. Cranberry
2. Apple	2. Apple
3. Red grape	3. Red grape
4. Strawberry	4. Strawberry
5. Pineapple	5. Peach
6. Banana	6. Lemon
7. Peach	7. Pear
8. Lemon	8. Banana
9. Orange	9. Orange
10. Pear	10. Grapefruit
11. Grapefruit	11. Pineapple

are centered around the pharmaceutical "silver bullet" model—the belief that single-drug interventions hold the promise to health. The reasons that this paradigm has dominated the American healthcare scene for the past 100 years are that 1) it is profitable for doctors and drug companies, and 2) because it exonerates patients from taking personal responsibly for their health by changing their lifestyles. Taking appropriate action with the data that a fruit/vegetable-based diet has powerful health-promoting benefits means that we as doctors and patients have to change our lifestyles with regard to how we plan our meals, what we buy, what we prepare, and what we eat. Behavior modification is a tremendous challenge for people, especially those who lack sufficient motivation or insight. This text is providing the *insight*—the data, references, and concepts. But without *motivation*—from doctors to help their patients attain the highest levels of health, and from patients to change their lifestyles to become as healthy as possible—the research itself does little to promote health. When

[168] "We propose that the additive and synergistic effects of phytochemicals in fruit and vegetables are responsible for their potent antioxidant and anticancer activities, and that the benefit of a diet rich in fruit and vegetables is attributed to the complex mixture of phytochemicals present in whole foods." Liu RH. Health benefits of fruit and vegetables are from additive and synergistic combinations of phytochemicals. *Am J Clin Nutr.* 2003 Sep;78(3 Suppl):517S-520S
[169] "Cranberry had the highest total antioxidant activity (177.0 +/- 4.3 micromol of vitamin C equiv/g of fruit), followed by apple, red grape, strawberry, peach, lemon, pear, banana, orange, grapefruit, and pineapple." Sun J, Chu YF, Wu X, Liu RH. Antioxidant and antiproliferative activities of common fruits. *J Agric Food Chem.* 2002 Dec 4;50(25):7449-54
[170] "Red pepper had the highest total antioxidant activity, followed by broccoli, carrot, spinach, cabbage, yellow onion, celery, potato, lettuce, and cucumber." Chu YF, Sun J, Wu X, Liu RH. Antioxidant and antiproliferative activities of common vegetables. *J Agric Food Chem.* 2002 Nov 6;50(23):6910-6
[171] Liu RH. Health benefits of fruit and vegetables are from additive and synergistic combinations of phytochemicals. *Am J Clin Nutr.* 2003 Sep;78(3 Suppl):517S-520S

insight is combined with *motivation* we have the *potential for change*, but the potential for change is meaningless until it is manifested into the world with *persistent, effective action.*

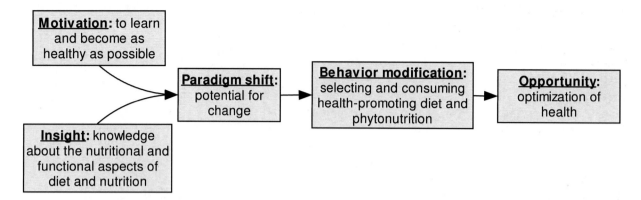

Eat the right amount of protein: Dietary protein is eaten to provide the body with amino acids, which are the building blocks that the body uses to create new tissues, heal wounds, fight off infections, grow hair and fingernails, and to create specific hormones and neurotransmitters. Meats, eggs, and milk contain the types and amounts of essential amino acids that the human body requires and are thus said to provide more "complete protein" than do vegetable proteins. For most people (without kidney or liver problems) the goal should be ½ to ¾ gram of protein per pound of lean body weight, depending on activity level. Sufficient dietary protein is essential for patients with musculoskeletal injuries because tissue healing relies on the constant availability of amino acids and micronutrients[172], which should be supplied by a healthy, balanced, whole-foods diet that may be supplemented with specific nutraceuticals, as discussed later in this text. Low-protein diets suppress immune function, reduce muscle mass, and impair healing[173,174], whereas intakes of higher amounts of protein safely facilitate healing and the maintenance of muscle mass. Increased protein intake does not adversely affect bone health as long as dietary calcium intake is adequate.[175] According to the recent review by Lemon[176]:

> "Those involved in strength training might need to consume as much as …1.7 g protein x kg(-1) x day(-1)…while those undergoing endurance training might need about 1.2 to 1.6 g x kg(-1) x day(-1)… **…there is no evidence that protein intakes in the range suggested will have adverse effects in healthy individuals."**

For patients who are completely sedentary: multiply body weight in pounds by 0.4 and this will give the number of grams of protein that should be eaten each day.[177]

For patients who are very active (frequent weight lifting, or competitive athlete): multiply body weight in pounds by 0.7-0.9 and this will give the number of grams of protein that should be eaten each day.

Again, compared with sedentary people, *sick people, injured people,* **and** *athletes* **need more protein** to maintain weight, fight infections, repair injuries, and build and maintain muscle. Not only can insufficient protein intake cause muscle weakness and loss of weight, but recent articles have also suggested that low-protein diets can cause suppression of the immune system[178] and impairment of healing after injury or surgery.[179]

[172] "Supplementation with protein and vitamins, specifically arginine and vitamins A, B, and C, provides optimum nutrient support of the healing wound." Meyer NA, Muller MJ, Herndon DN. Nutrient support of the healing wound. *New Horiz* 1994 May;2(2):202-14
[173] Castaneda C, Charnley JM, Evans WJ, Crim MC. Elderly women accommodate to a low-protein diet with losses of body cell mass, muscle function, and immune response. *Am J Clin Nutr* 1995 Jul;62(1):30-9 http://www.ajcn.org/cgi/reprint/62/1/30
[174] [No author listed]. Vegetarians and healing. *JAMA* 1995; 273: 910
[175] Heaney RP. Excess dietary protein may not adversely affect bone. *J Nutr* 1998 Jun;128(6):1054-7
[176] Lemon PW. Effects of exercise on dietary protein requirements. *Int J Sport Nutr* 1998 Dec;8(4):426-47
[177] Pellet PL. Protein requirements in humans. *Am J Clin Nutr* 1990 May;51(5):723-37
[178] Castaneda C, Charnley JM, Evans WJ, Crim MC. Elderly women accommodate to a low-protein diet with losses of body cell mass, muscle function, and immune response. *Am J Clin Nutr* 1995 Jul;62(1):30-9
[179] Vegetarians and healing. *Journal of the American Medical Association* 1995; 273: 910

Recommended <u>Grams of Protein</u> Per <u>Pound of Body Weight</u> Per Day[180]	
Infants and children ages 1-6 years[181]	0.68-0.45
RDA for sedentary adult and children ages 6-18 years[182]	0.4
Adult recreational exerciser	**0.5-0.75**
Adult competitive athlete	0.6-0.9
Adult building muscle mass	0.7-0.9
Dieting athlete	0.7-1.0
Growing teenage athlete	0.9-1.0
Pregnant women need additional protein	Add 15-30 grams/day[183]

For example, in most instances, a person weighing 120 pounds should aim for at least 60 grams of protein per day, or 90 grams of protein per day if he/she is more physically active, ill, or injured. A can of tuna has 30 grams of protein; one egg has 6 grams of protein. If she is going to eat eggs as a source of protein for a meal, she might have to eat as many as five eggs to reach a target of 30 grams of protein per meal. When eating meat, visualize the amount of meat in a can of tuna to estimate the amount of protein being eaten—for example, if the portion of meat at a given meal is about the size of a half can of tuna, then we can estimate that the serving contains 15-20 grams of high-quality protein. By knowing the "target intake" for the day, and by estimating the amount of protein eaten with each meal, patients will be able to modify their protein intake to ensure that they reach their target intake.

Protein supplements can be used *in conjunction with a healthy diet.* Patients using a protein supplement should eat a healthy diet and then add protein supplements between regular meals. If they substitute a protein supplement for a regular meal, then they may not actually increase protein intake. Whole *real* foods should form the foundation for the diet—patients should not rely too heavily on *protein supplements* when patients can get better results *and improved overall health* with *whole foods.* Whey, casein, and lactalbumin are proteins from milk and dairy products, and may therefore be allergenic in people allergic to milk. Soy protein is safe and a source of high-quality protein for adults[184], and recent research indicates that consumption of soy protein can help reduce the risk of cancer and heart disease[185]; however, I do not recommend the use of large quantities of supplemental soy protein for pregnant women, or for children due to the potential for disrupting endocrine function. Patients may have to experiment with different products until they find one that "works" with regard to taste, texture, digestibility, hypoallergenicity, nutritional effects, and affordability.

Recall again that the goal is *improved health*, not simply *adequate protein intake.* If we focus solely on "grams of protein" then we might overlook adverse effects that are associated with certain protein sources. Cow's milk is a high quality protein, but it is commonly allergenic and can exacerbate joint pain in sensitive individuals.[186] Beef, liver, pork and other land animal meats are excellent sources of protein, but they are also rich sources of arachidonic acid[187] and iron[188], both of which have been shown to exacerbate joint pain and inflammation. Fish is an excellent source of protein, but fish are often poisoned with mercury and other toxicants, which are then ingested by humans with adverse effects.[189,190]

---

[180] Slightly modified from Nancy Clark, MS, RD. The Power of Protein. *The Physician and Sportsmedicine* 1996, volume 24, number 4

[181] 1.5-1 g/kg/d (0.68-0.45 grams per pound of body weight. Younger people need proportionately more protein.) Brown ML (ed). <u>Present Knowledge in Nutrition. Sixth Edition.</u> Washington DC: International Life Sciences Institute Nutrition Foundation; 1990 page 68

[182] 0.83 g.kg-1.d-1 (equivalent to 0.37 grams per pound of body weight) Pellet PL. Protein requirements in humans. *Am J Clin Nutr* 1990 May;51(5):723-37

[183] Weinsier RL, Morgan SL (eds). <u>Fundamentals of Clinical Nutrition.</u> St. Louis: Mosby, 1993 page 50

[184] "These results indicate that for healthy adults, the isolated soy protein is of high nutritional quality, comparable to that of animal protein sources, and that the methionine content is not limiting for adult protein maintenance." Young VR, Puig M, Queiroz E, Scrimshaw NS, Rand WM. Evaluation of the protein quality of an isolated soy protein in young men: relative nitrogen requirements and effect of methionine supplementation. *Am J Clin Nutr.* 1984 Jan;39(1):16-24

[185] Lissin LW, Cooke JP. Phytoestrogens and cardiovascular health. *J Am Coll Cardiol.* 2000 May;35(6):1403-10

[186] Golding DN. Is there an allergic synovitis? *J R Soc Med* 1990 May;83(5):312-4

[187] Adam O, Beringer C, Kless T, Lemmen C, Adam A, Wiseman M, Adam P, Klimmek R, Forth W. Anti-inflammatory effects of a low arachidonic acid diet and fish oil in patients with rheumatoid arthritis. *Rheumatol Int* 2003 Jan;23(1):27-36

[188] Dabbagh AJ, Trenam CW, Morris CJ, Blake DR. Iron in joint inflammation. *Ann Rheum Dis* 1993; 52:67-73

[189] "These fish often harbor high levels of methylmercury, a potent human neurotoxin." Evans EC. The FDA recommendations on fish intake during pregnancy. *J Obstet Gynecol Neonatal Nurs* 2002 Nov-Dec;31(6):715-20

Eat complex carbohydrates to stabilize blood sugar, mood, and energy: Choose items with a "low glycemic index"[191] to stabilize blood sugar and—for many people—to lower triglycerides and cholesterol levels. Foods with a low Glycemic Index (GI < 55)[192] include yogurt, apple (36), whole orange (43), peach (28), legumes, lentils (28), and soybeans (18), cherries, dried apricots, nuts, most meats, and most vegetables. **Healthy foods that have both a low *glycemic index* as well as a low *glycemic load* include: apples, carrots, chick peas, grapes, green peas, kidney beans, oranges, peaches, peanuts, pears, pinto beans, red lentils, and strawberries.[193]**

Reduce or eliminate simple sugars from the diet (as necessary): Nearly everyone should minimize intake of table sugar (sucrose), fructose and high-fructose corn syrup, and all artificial sweeteners. Chronic overconsumption of refined carbohydrates promotes disease by 1) increasing urinary excretion of magnesium and calcium, 2) inducing oxidative stress, 3) promoting fat deposition and obesity, which then generally leads to insulin resistance and hyperinsulinemia with an increase in production of cholesterol, triglycerides, and proinflammatory adipokines[194], and 4) reducing function of leukocytes.[195] Among sweeteners, honey is the best choice since it is the only natural sweetener available with a wide range of health-promoting benefits including anti-inflammatory, anticancer, antibacterial, antioxidant and anti-allergy effects. Also consider the herb *Stevia* as a non-caloric and nutritive sweetener. Occasional intake of sweets is likely to be of little consequence for people who are generally healthy and who are willing to sustain relatively short-term endothelial dysfunction[196], oxidative stress[197], increased LDL oxidation[198], and activation of proinflammatory and oncogenic NF-kappaB[199] as a result of their iatrogenic hyperglycemia. Postexertional hyperglycemia can be used to enhance athletic performance by sustaining and inducing glycogen storage following and during exercise (i.e., carbohydrate loading for glycogen "supercompensation"[200,201]). Similarly, consumption of "simple" carbohydrate without protein can be used to promote entry of tryptophan across the blood-brain barrier and into the brain to promote serotonin synthesis.[202] In summary, *habitual overconsumption* of simple carbohydrates promotes disease by oxidative and proinflammatory mechanisms, while conversely *periodic consumption* of simple carbohydrates can be used to promote athletic performance and to increase intracerebral serotonin synthesis for the promotion of enhanced mood and cognitive performance and for the regulation of food intake.

Avoid artificial sweeteners, colors and other additives: Absolutely never use **aspartame**—this is a synthetic chemical that is easily converted to the toxin formaldehyde.[203] Aspartame causes cancer in animals and is strongly linked to brain tumors in humans.[204,205] **Sodium benzoate** is a food preservative that can cause

[190] "Geometric mean mercury levels were almost 4-fold higher among women who ate 3 or more servings of fish in the past 30 days compared with women who ate no fish in that period.." Schober SE, Sinks TH, Jones RL, Bolger PM, McDowell M, Osterloh J, Garrett ES, Canady RA, Dillon CF, Sun Y, Joseph CB, Mahaffey KR. Blood mercury levels in US children and women of childbearing age, 1999-2000. *JAMA* 2003 Apr 2;289(13):1667-74

[191] For more information on glycemic index, consult a nutrition book or website such as http://www.stanford.edu/~dep/gilists.htm last accessed August 16, 2003

[192] Janette Brand-Miller, Kaye Foster-Powell. Diets with a low glycemic index: from theory to practice. *Nutrition Today* 1999 March. Accessed on-line at: http://www.findarticles.com/cf_dls/m0841/2_34/54654508/p1/article.jhtml on August 16, 2003.

[193] Mendosa D. Glycemic Values of Common American Foods http://www.mendosa.com/common_foods.htm Accessed on August 4, 2004

[194] "Because visceral and subcutaneous adipose tissues are the major sources of cytokines (adipokines), increased adipose tissue mass is associated with alteration in adipokine production (eg, overexpression of tumor necrosis factor-a, interleukin-6, plasminogen activator inhibitor-1, and underexpression of adiponectin in adipose tissue)." Aldhahi W, Hamdy O. Adipokines, inflammation, and the endothelium in diabetes. *Curr Diab Rep.* 2003 Aug;3(4):293-8

[195] Sanchez A, Reeser JL, Lau HS, Yahiku PY, Willard RE, McMillan PJ, Cho SY, Magie AR, Register UD. Role of sugars in human neutrophilic phagocytosis. *Am J Clin Nutr.* 1973 Nov;26(11):1180-4

[196] "Modest hyperinsulinemia, mimicking fasting hyperinsulinemia of insulin-resistant states, abrogates endothelium-dependent vasodilation in large conduit arteries, probably by increasing oxidant stress. These data may provide a novel pathophysiological basis to the epidemiological link between hyperinsulinemia/insulin-resistance and atherosclerosis in humans." Arcaro G, Cretti A, Balzano S, Lechi A, Muggeo M, Bonora E, Bonadonna RC. Insulin causes endothelial dysfunction in humans: sites and mechanisms. *Circulation.* 2002 Feb 5;105(5):576-82

[197] "Hyperglycemia increased plasma MDA concentrations, but the activities of GSH-Px and SOD were significantly higher after a larger dose of glucose only. Plasma catecholamines were unchanged. These results indicate that the transient increase of plasma catecholamine and insulin concentrations did not induce oxidative damage, while glucose already in the low dose was an important triggering factor for oxidative stress." Koska J, Blazicek P, Marko M, Grna JD, Kvetnansky R, Vigas M. Insulin, catecholamines, glucose and antioxidant enzymes in oxidative damage during different loads in healthy humans. *Physiol Res.* 2000;49 Suppl 1:S95-100

[198] "In conclusion, insulin at physiological doses is associated with increased LDL peroxidation independent of the presence of hyperglycemia." Quinones-Galvan A, Sironi AM, Baldi S, Galetta F, Garbin U, Fratta-Pasini A, Cominacini L, Ferrannini E. Evidence that acute insulin administration enhances LDL cholesterol susceptibility to oxidation in healthy humans. *Arterioscler Thromb Vasc Biol.* 1999 Dec;19(12):2928-32

[199] "These data show that the intake of a mixed meal results in significant inflammatory changes characterized by a decrease in IkappaBalpha and an increase in NF-kappaB binding, plasma CRP, and the expression of IKKalpha, IKKbeta, and p47(phox) subunit." Aljada A, Mohanty P, Ghanim H, Abdo T, Tripathy D, Chaudhuri A, Dandona P. Increase in intranuclear nuclear factor kappaB and decrease in inhibitor kappaB in mononuclear cells after a mixed meal: evidence for a proinflammatory effect. *Am J Clin Nutr.* 2004 Apr;79(4):682-90

[200] "A significant glycogen sparing, as well as supercompensation within 24 h of recovery, was observed after [carbohydrate] supplementation." Brouns F, Saris WH, Beckers E, Adlercreutz H, van der Vusse GJ, Keizer HA, Kuipers H, Menheere P, Wagenmakers AJ, ten Hoor F. Metabolic changes induced by sustained exhaustive cycling and diet manipulation. *Int J Sports Med.* 1989 May;10 Suppl 1:S49-62

[201] "The accepted method of increasing muscle glycogen stores is by 'glycogen loading,' which classically involves depletion of muscle glycogen, usually by exercise, followed by consumption of a high-CHO diet for several days (e.g., 3, 39). ...increase muscle glycogen concentrations ([glycogen]) to between 150 and 200% of normal resting levels." Robinson TM, Sewell DA, Hultman E, Greenhaff PL. Role of submaximal exercise in promoting creatine and glycogen accumulation in human skeletal muscle. *J Appl Physiol.* 1999 Aug;87(2):598-604

[202] "Our results suggest that high-carbohydrate meals have an influence on serotonin synthesis. We predict that carbohydrates with a high glycemic index would have a greater serotoninergic effect than carbohydrates with a low glycemic index." Lyons PM, Truswell AS. Serotonin precursor influenced by type of carbohydrate meal in healthy adults. *Am J Clin Nutr.* 1988 Mar;47(3):433-9

[203] Trocho C, Pardo R, Rafecas I, Virgili J, Remesar X, Fernandez-Lopez JA, Alemany M. Formaldehyde derived from dietary aspartame binds to tissue components in vivo. *Life Sci.* 1998;63(5):337-4949

[204] Compared to other environmental factors putatively linked to brain tumors, the artificial sweetener aspartame is a promising candidate to explain the recent increase in incidence and degree of malignancy of brain tumors. ...exceedingly high incidence of brain tumors in aspartame-fed rats compared to no brain tumors in concurrent controls..." Olney JW, Farber NB, Spitznagel E, Robins LN. Increasing brain tumor rates: is there a link to aspartame? *J Neuropathol Exp Neurol* 1996;55(11):1115-23

asthma[206] and skin rashes[207] in sensitive individuals. **Tartrazine (yellow dye #5)** is a food/drug coloring agent that can cause asthma and skin rashes in sensitive individuals.[208] **Carrageenan** is a naturally-occurring carbohydrate extracted from red seaweed. Common sources of carrageenan are certain brands of "rice milk" and "soy milk." In addition to suppressing immune function[209], carrageenan causes intestinal ulcers and inflammatory bowel disease in animals[210] and some research indicates that carrageenan consumption is associated with an increased risk for cancer in humans.[211,212]

Consider reducing or eliminating caffeine: This is especially important for people with reactive hypoglycemia, insomnia, anxiety, hypertension, low-back pain, and for women with fibrocystic breast disease. For people who are in good health, 1-3 servings of caffeine per day is not harmful. Herbal teas and green tea have many significant health-promoting effects.

To the extent possible, eat "organic" foods rather than industrially-produced foods: Organic foods (i.e., foods which are *naturally grown* rather than being treated with insect poisons, synthetic fertilizers, and chemicals to enhance shelf-life) tend to cost more than chemically-produced foods; but the increased phytonutrient content justifies the cost. Organic foods contain more nutrients than do chemically-produced foods.[213] More importantly, recent research has also indicated that organic foods are better able to prevent the genetic damage that can lead to cancer than are foods that have been grown in an environment of artificial fertilizers and pesticides.[214]

Recognize the importance of avoiding food allergens: Biomedical research has established that adverse food reactions, regardless of the underlying mechanisms or classification of allergy, intolerance, or sensitivity, can exacerbate a wide range of human illnesses, including thyroid disease[215], mental depression[216,217], asthma, rhinitis,[218] recurrent otitis media[219], migraine[220,221,222], attention deficit and hyperactivity disorders[223], epilepsy[224,225,226], gastrointestinal inflammation[227], hypertension[228], joint pain and inflammation[229,230,231,232,233,234,235,236] and a wide range of other health problems. Any program of health promotion and health maintenance must include consideration of food allergies, food intolerances, and food sensitivities.

---

[205] Russell Blaylock MD. Excitotoxins. Health Press; December 1996 [ISBN: 0929173252] Pages 211-214

[206] "Adverse reactions to benzoate in this patient required avoidance of some drugs, some of those classically prescribed under the form of syrups in asthma." Petrus M, Bonaz S, Causse E, Rhabbour M, Moulie N, Netter JC, Bildstein G. [Asthma and intolerance to benzoates] [Article in French] *Arch Pediatr.* 1996 Oct;3(10):984-7

[207] Munoz FJ, Bellido J, Moyano JC, Alvarez M, Fonseca JL. Perioral contact urticaria from sodium benzoate in a toothpaste. *Contact Dermatitis.* 1996 Jul;35(1):51

[208] "Tartrazine sensitivity is most frequently manifested by urticaria and asthma... Vasculitis, purpura and contact dermatitis infrequently occur as manifestations of tartrazine sensitivity." Dipalma JR. Tartrazine sensitivity. *Am Fam Physician.* 1990 Nov;42(5):1347-50

[209] "Impairment of complement activity and humoral responses to T-dependent antigens, depression of cell-mediated immunity, prolongation of graft survival and potentiation of tumour growth by carrageenans have been reported." Thomson AW, Fowler EF. Carrageenan: a review of its effects on the immune system. *Agents Actions.* 1981;11(3):265-73

[210] Watt J, Marcus R. Experimental ulcerative disease of the colon. *Methods Achiev Exp Pathol.* 1975;7:56-71

[211] Tobacman JK. Review of harmful gastrointestinal effects of carrageenan in animal experiments. *Environ Health Perspect.* 2001 Oct;109(10):983-94

[212] "However, the gum carrageenan which is comprised of linked, sulfated galactose residues has potent biological activity and undergoes acid hydrolysis to poligeenan, an acknowledged carcinogen." Tobacman JK, Wallace RB, Zimmerman MB. Consumption of carrageenan and other water-soluble polymers used as food additives and incidence of mammary carcinoma. *Med Hypotheses.* 2001 May;56(5):589-98

[213] Smith B. Organic Foods versus Supermarket Foods: element levels. *Journal of Applied Nutrition* 1993; 45(1), p35-9

[214] "Against BaP, three species of OC vegetables showed 30-57% antimutagenecity, while GC ones did only 5-30%." Ren H, Endo H, Hayashi T. The superiority of organically cultivated vegetables to general ones regarding antimutagative activities. *Mutat Res.* 2001 Sep 20;496(1-2):83-8

[215] Sategna-Guidetti C, Volta U, Ciacci C, Usai P, Carlino A, De Franceschi L, Camera A, Pelli A, Brossa C. Prevalence of thyroid disorders in untreated adult celiac disease patients and effect of gluten withdrawal: an Italian multicenter study. *Am J Gastroenterol.* 2001 Mar;96(3):751-7

[216] "The detection and treatment of psychological dysfunction related to food intolerance with particular reference to the problem of objective evaluation is discussed... Long-term follow-up revealed maintenance of marked improvements in psychological and physical functioning." Mills N. Depression and food intolerance: a single case study. *Hum Nutr Appl Nutr.* 1986 Apr;40(2):141-5

[217] "OBJECTIVE: To describe a patient with food intolerance probably contributing to depressive symptoms, intolerance to psychotropic medication and treatment resistance... RESULTS: The patient's course improved considerably with an elimination diet." Parker G, Watkins T. Treatment-resistant depression: when antidepressant drug intolerance may indicate food intolerance. *Aust N Z J Psychiatry.* 2002 Apr;36(2):263-5

[218] Speer F. The allergic child. *Am Fam Physician.* 1975 Feb;11(2):88-94

[219] Juntti H, Tikkanen S, Kokkonen J, Alho OP, Niinimaki A. Cow's milk allergy is associated with recurrent otitis media during childhood. *Acta Otolaryngol.* 1999;119(8):867-73

[220] "Foods which provoked migraine in 9 patients with severe migraine refractory to drug therapy were identified... These observations confirm that a food-allergic reaction is the cause of migraine in this group of patients." Monro J, Carini C, Brostoff J. Migraine is a food-allergic disease. *Lancet.* 1984 Sep 29;2(8405):719-21

[221] Egger J, Carter CM, Wilson J, et al. Is migraine food allergy? A double-blind controlled trial of oligoantigenic diet treatment. *Lancet.* 1983 Oct 15;2(8355):865-9

[222] Monro J, Brostoff J, Carini C, Zilkha K. Food allergy in migraine. Study of dietary exclusion and RAST. *Lancet.* 1980 Jul 5;2(8184):1-4

[223] Boris M, Mandel FS. Foods and additives are common causes of the attention deficit hyperactive disorder in children. *Ann Allergy.* 1994 May;72(5):462-8

[224] Egger J, Carter CM, Soothill JF, Wilson J. Oligoantigenic diet treatment of children with epilepsy and migraine. *J Pediatr.* 1989;114(1):51-8

[225] Pelliccia A, Lucarelli S, Frediani T, D'Ambrini G, Cerminara C, Barbato M, Vagnucci B, Cardi E. Partial cryptogenetic epilepsy and food allergy/intolerance. A causal or a chance relationship? Reflections on three clinical cases. *Minerva Pediatr.* 1999 May;51(5):153-7

[226] Frediani T, Lucarelli S, Pelliccia A, Vagnucci B, et al. Allergy and childhood epilepsy: a close relationship? *Acta Neurol Scand.* 2001 Dec;104(6):349-52

[227] Marr HY, Chen WC, Lin LH. Food protein-induced enterocolitis syndrome: report of one case. *Acta Paediatr Taiwan.* 2001;42(1):49-52

[228] Grant EC. Food allergies and migraine. *Lancet.* 1979 May 5;1(8123):966-9

[229] "Food allergy appeared to be responsible for the joint symptoms in three patients and in one it was possible to precipitate swelling of a knee due to synovitis with effusion by drinking milk a few hours beforehand, the synovial fluid having mildly inflammatory features and a relatively high eosinophil count." Golding DN. Is there an allergic synovitis? *J R Soc Med.* 1990 May;83(5):312-4

[230] Panush RS. Food induced ("allergic") arthritis: clinical and serologic studies. *J Rheumatol.* 1990 Mar;17(3):291-4

[231] Pacor ML, Lunardi C, Di Lorenzo G, Biasi D, Corrocher R. Food allergy and seronegative arthritis: report of two cases. *Clin Rheumatol.* 2001;20(4):279-81

[232] Schrander JJ, Marcelis C, de Vries MP, van Santen-Hoeufft HM. Does food intolerance play a role in juvenile chronic arthritis? *Br J Rheumatol.* 1997 Aug;36(8):905-8

[233] van de Laar MA, van der Korst JK. Food intolerance in rheumatoid arthritis. I. A double blind, controlled trial of the clinical effects of elimination of milk allergens and azo dyes. *Ann Rheum Dis.* 1992 Mar;51(3):298-302

[234] Haugen MA, Kjeldsen-Kragh J, Forre O. A pilot study of the effect of an elemental diet in the management of rheumatoid arthritis. *Clin Exp Rheumatol.* 1994;12(3):275-9

[235] van de Laar MA, Aalbers M, Bruins FG, et al. Food intolerance in rheumatoid arthritis. II. Clinical and histological aspects. *Ann Rheum Dis.* 1992 Mar;51(3):303-6

[236] Panush RS, Stroud RM, Webster EM. Food-induced (allergic) arthritis. Inflammatory arthritis exacerbated by milk. *Arthritis Rheum.* 1986 Feb; 29(2): 220-6

<u>Supplement your healthy diet with specific vitamins, minerals, and fatty acids</u>:   Despite the fact that America is one of the richest nations on earth, and that we produce more than enough food to feed ourselves and many other nations with a healthy diet, Americans tend to have poor dietary habits and inadequate levels of nutritional intake that do not meet the minimal standards, such as the Recommended Daily Allowance (RDA, now Daily Reference Intake (DRI)).[237] Many people are under the misperception that if they appear healthy or are even overweight then they could not possibly have nutritional deficiencies. The truths of this matter are that 1) gross/obvious nutritional deficiencies are common among "apparently healthy" individuals, 2) common situations like stress, poor diets, and use of medications predispose people to nutritional deficiencies, 3) hereditary/genetic disorders affect a large portion of the population and lead to an increased need for nutritional intake which can generally only be met with supplementation in addition to a healthy whole-foods diet. Taking a "one-a-day" multivitamin is insufficient for people who truly desire significant benefit from supplementation. These one-a-day preparations generally only provide the minimum daily allowance—this dose is not large enough to provide truly preventive medicine results.

For people still not convinced of the importance of a multi-vitamin/mineral supplement as part of the basic foundation of the health plan, please consider the following data from the medical research:

- Many people think that eating a "healthy diet" will supply them with the nutrients that they need and that they do not need to take a vitamin supplement. This may have been true 200 years ago, but today's industrially produced "foods" are generally stripped of much of their nutritional value long before they leave the factory. Industrially-produced fruits and vegetables contain less nutrients than naturally raised "organic" produce. [238]
- The reason that people can be of normal weight or can even be overweight and obese and still have nutrient deficiencies is that the body lowers the metabolic rate when the intake of vitamins and minerals is low. This is referred to as the "physiologic adaptation to marginal malnutrition." Even though people may eat enough calories and protein, they can still suffer from growth retardation and behavioral problems as a result of malnutrition, even though they *appear* nourished.[239]
- Most nutrition-oriented doctors will agree that magnesium is one of the most important nutrients, especially for helping prevent heart attack and stroke. **Magnesium deficiency is an epidemic in so-called "developed" nations, with 20-40% of different populations showing objective serologic/cytologic evidence of magnesium deficiency**.[240,241,242,243]
- Add to the above that every day we are confronted with more chronic emotional stress and toxic chemicals than has ever before existed on the planet, and it becomes easy to see that basic nutritional support and an organic whole foods diet is just the start of attaining improved health.

<u>Putting it all together with "the supplemented Paleo-Mediterranean diet"</u>:

The health-promoting diet of choice for the majority of people is a diet based on abundant consumption of fruits, vegetables, seeds, nuts, omega-3 and monounsaturated fatty acids, and lean sources of protein such as lean meats, fatty cold-water fish, soy and whey proteins. This diet prohibits and obviates overconsumption of chemical preservatives, artificial sweeteners, and carbohydrate-dominant foods such as candies, pastries, breads, potatoes, grains, and other foods with a high glycemic load and high glycemic index. This "Paleo-Mediterranean Diet" is a combination of the "Paleolithic" or "Paleo diet" and the well-known "Mediterranean diet", both of which are well described in peer-reviewed journals and the lay press. The Mediterranean diet is characterized by increased proportions of legumes, nuts, seeds, whole grain products, fruits, vegetables (including potatoes), fish and lean meats, and monounsaturated and n-3 fatty acids.[244] Consumption of this diet is consistently associated with improvements in insulin sensitivity and reductions in cardiovascular

[237] "Most people do not consume an optimal amount of all vitamins by diet alone. Pending strong evidence of effectiveness from randomized trials, it appears prudent for all adults to take vitamin supplements." Fletcher RH, Fairfield KM. Vitamins for chronic disease prevention in adults: clinical applications. *JAMA* 2002 Jun 19;287(23):3127-9
[238] Smith B. Organic Foods versus Supermarket Foods: element levels. *Journal of Applied Nutrition* 1993; 45(1), p35-9. I recently found that this article is also available on-line at http://journeytoforever.org/farm_library/bobsmith.html as of June 19, 2004
[239] Allen LH. The nutrition CRSP: what is marginal malnutrition, and does it affect human function? *Nutr Rev* 1993 Sep;51(9):255-67
[240] "The American diet is low in magnesium, and with modern water systems, very little is ingested in the drinking water." Innerarity S. Hypomagnesemia in acute and chronic illness. *Crit Care Nurs Q*. 2000 Aug;23(2):1-19
[241] "Altogether 43% of 113 trauma patients had low magnesium levels compared to 30% of noninjured cohorts." Frankel H, Haskell R, Lee SY, Miller D, Rotondo M, Schwab CW. Hypomagnesemia in trauma patients. *World J Surg*. 1999 Sep;23(9):966-9
[242] "There was a 20% overall prevalence of hypomagnesemia among this predominantly female, African American population." Fox CH, Ramsoomair D, Mahoney MC, Carter C, Young B, Graham R. An investigation of hypomagnesemia among ambulatory urban African Americans. *J Fam Pract*. 1999 Aug;48(8):636-9
[243] "Suboptimal levels were detected in 33.7 per cent of the population under study. These data clearly demonstrate that the Mg supply of the German population needs increased attention." Schimatschek HF, Rempis R. Prevalence of hypomagnesemia in an unselected German population of 16,000 individuals. *Magnes Res*. 2001 Dec;14(4):283-90
[244] Curtis BM, O'Keefe JH Jr. Understanding the Mediterranean diet. Could this be the new "gold standard" for heart disease prevention? *Postgrad Med*. 2002 Aug;112(2):35-8, 41-5 http://www.postgradmed.com/issues/2002/08_02/curtis.htm

disease, diabetes, cancer, and all-cause mortality.[245]   The Paleolithic diet detailed by collaborators Eaton[246], O'Keefe[247], and Cordain[248] is similar to the Mediterranean diet except for stronger emphasis on fruits and vegetables (preferably raw or minimally cooked), omega-3-rich lean meats, and reduced consumption of starchy foods such as potatoes and grains, the latter of which were not staples in the human diet until the last few thousand years.   Emphasizing the olive oil and red wine of the Mediterranean diet and the absence of grains and potatoes per the Paleo diet appears to be the way to get the best of both dietary worlds; the remaining diet is characterized by fresh whole fruits, vegetables, nuts (especially almonds), seeds, olive oil, lean meats rich in n-3 fatty acids, and red wine in moderation.   In sum, this dietary plan along with the inclusion of garlic and dark chocolate (a rich source of cardioprotective, antioxidative, and anti-inflammatory polyphenolic flavonoids[249,250]) is expected to reduce adverse cardiovascular events by more than 76%.[251] Biochemical justification for this type of diet is ample and is well supported by numerous long-term studies in humans wherein both Mediterranean and Paleolithic diets result in dramatic reductions in disease-specific and all-cause mortality.[252,253,254,255]   Diets rich in fruits and vegetables are sources of more than 5,000 phytochemicals, many of which have antioxidant, anti-inflammatory, and anti-cancer properties.[256]   Oleic acid, squalene, and phenolics in olive oil and phenolics and resveratrol in red wine have antioxidant, anti-inflammatory, and anti-cancer properties and also protect against cardiovascular disease.[257]   N-3 fatty acids have numerous health benefits via multiple mechanisms as described in the sections that follow.   Increased intake of dietary fiber from fruits and vegetable favorably modifies gut flora, promotes xenobiotic elimination (via flora modification, laxation, and overall reductions in enterohepatic recirculation), and is associated with reductions in morbidity and mortality.   Such a "Paleolithic diet" can also lead to urinary alkalinization (average urine pH of ≥ 7.5 according to Sebastian et al[258]) which increases renal *retention of minerals* for improved musculoskeletal health[259,260,261] and which increases *urinary elimination of many toxicants and xenobiotics* for a tremendous reduction in serum levels and thus adverse effects from chemical exposure or drug overdose.[262]   Furthermore, therapeutic alkalinization was recently shown in an open trial with 82 patients to reduce symptoms and disability associated with low-back pain and to increase intracellular magnesium concentrations by 11%.[263] **Ample intake of amino acids via dietary proteins supports phase-2 detoxification** (amino acid and sulfate conjugation) for proper xenobiotic elimination[264,265], **provides amino acid precursors for neurotransmitter synthesis** and maintenance of mood, memory, and cognitive performance[266,267,268,269], **and prevents the**

[245] Knoops KT, de Groot LC, Kromhout D, Perrin AE, Moreiras-Varela O, Menotti A, van Staveren WA. Mediterranean diet, lifestyle factors, and 10-year mortality in elderly European men and women: the HALE project. *JAMA.* 2004 Sep 22;292(12):1433-9

[246] Eaton SB, Shostak M, Konner M. The Paleolithic Prescription: A program of diet & exercise and a design for living, New York: Harper & Row, 1988

[247] O'Keefe JH Jr, Cordain L. Cardiovascular disease resulting from a diet and lifestyle at odds with our Paleolithic genome: how to become a 21st-century hunter-gatherer. *Mayo Clin Proc.* 2004 Jan;79(1):101-8

[248] Cordain L. The Paleo Diet: Lose Weight and Get Healthy by Eating the Food You Were Designed to Eat. Indianapolis; John Wiley and Sons, 2002

[249] Schramm DD, Wang JF, Holt RR, Ensunsa JL, Gonsalves JL, Lazarus SA, Schmitz HH, German JB, Keen CL. Chocolate procyanidins decrease the leukotriene-prostacyclin ratio in humans and human aortic endothelial cells. *Am J Clin Nutr.* 2001;73(1):36-40

[250] Engler MB, Engler MM, Chen CY, et al. Flavonoid-rich dark chocolate improves endothelial function and increases plasma epicatechin concentrations in healthy adults. *J Am Coll Nutr.* 2004;23(3):197-204

[251] Franco OH, Bonneux L, de Laet C, Peeters A, Steyerberg EW, Mackenbach JP. The Polymeal: a more natural, safer, and probably tastier (than the Polypill) strategy to reduce cardiovascular disease by more than 75%. *BMJ.* 2004;329(7480):1447-50

[252] de Lorgeril M, Salen P, Martin JL, Monjaud I, Boucher P, Mamelle N. Mediterranean dietary pattern in a randomized trial: prolonged survival and possible reduced cancer rate. *Arch Intern Med.* 1998 Jun 8;158(11):1181-7

[253] Knoops KT, de Groot LC, Kromhout D, Perrin AE, Moreiras-Varela O, Menotti A, van Staveren WA. Mediterranean diet, lifestyle factors, and 10-year mortality in elderly European men and women: the HALE project. *JAMA.* 2004 Sep 22;292(12):1433-9

[254] Lindeberg S, Cordain L, and Eaton SB. Biological and clinical potential of a Paleolithic diet. *J Nutri Environ Med* 2003; 13:149-160

[255] O'Keefe JH Jr, Cordain L, Harris WH, Moe RM, Vogel R. Optimal low-density lipoprotein is 50 to 70 mg/dl: lower is better and physiologically normal. *J Am Coll Cardiol.* 2004 Jun 2;43(11):2142-6

[256] Liu RH. Health benefits of fruit and vegetables are from additive and synergistic combinations of phytochemicals. *Am J Clin Nutr.* 2003 Sep;78(3 Suppl):517S-520S

[257] Alarcon de la Lastra C, Barranco MD, Motilva V, Herrerias JM. Mediterranean diet and health: biological importance of olive oil. *Curr Pharm Des.* 2001;7:933-50

[258] Sebastian A, Frassetto LA, Sellmeyer DE, Merriam RL, Morris RC Jr. Estimation of the net acid load of the diet of ancestral preagricultural Homo sapiens and their hominid ancestors. *Am J Clin Nutr* 2002;76:1308-16

[259] Sebastian A, Harris ST, Ottaway JH, Todd KM, Morris RC Jr. Improved mineral balance and skeletal metabolism in postmenopausal women treated with potassium bicarbonate. *N Engl J Med.* 1994;330(25):1776-81

[260] Tucker KL, Hannan MT, Chen H, Cupples LA, Wilson PW, Kiel DP. Potassium, magnesium, and fruit and vegetable intakes are associated with greater bone mineral density in elderly men and women. *Am J Clin Nutr.* 1999;69(4):727-36

[261] Whiting SJ, Boyle JL, Thompson A, Mirwald RL, Faulkner RA. Dietary protein, phosphorus and potassium are beneficial to bone mineral density in adult men consuming adequate dietary calcium. *J Am Coll Nutr.* 2002;21(5):402-9

[262] Proudfoot AT, Krenzelok EP, Vale JA. Position Paper on urine alkalinization. *J Toxicol Clin Toxicol.* 2004;42(1):1-26

[263] "The results show that a disturbed acid-base balance may contribute to the symptoms of low back pain. The simple and safe addition of an alkaline multimineral preparate was able to reduce the pain symptoms in these patients with chronic low back pain." Vormann J,Worlitschek M,Goedecke T,Silver B. Supplementation with alkaline minerals reduces symptoms in patients with chronic low back pain. J Trace Elem Med Biol. 2001;15(2-3):179-83

[264] Liska DJ. The detoxification enzyme systems. *Altern Med Rev.* 1998;3:187-9

[265] Anderson KE, Kappas A. Dietary regulation of cytochrome P450. *Annu Rev Nutr.* 1991;11:141-67

[266] Rogers RD, Tunbridge EM, Bhagwagar Z, Drevets WC, Sahakian BJ, Carter CS. Tryptophan depletion alters the decision-making of healthy volunteers through altered processing of reward cues. *Neuropsychopharmacology.* 2003;28:153-62 Accessed at http://www.acnp.org/sciweb/journal/Npp062402336/default.htm on November 10, 2004

[267] Arnulf I, Quintin P, Alvarez JC, Vigil L, Touitou Y, Lebre AS, Bellenger A, Varoquaux O, Derenne JP, Allilaire JF, Benkelfat C, Leboyer M. Mid-morning tryptophan depletion delays REM sleep onset in healthy subjects. *Neuropsychopharmacology.* 2002;27(5):843-51 Accessed at http://www.acnp.org/sciweb/journal/Npp042502293/default.htm on November 10, 2004

[268] Thomas JR, Lockwood PA, Singh A, Deuster PA. Tyrosine improves working memory in a multitasking environment. *Pharmacol Biochem Behav.* 1999;64:495-500

[269] Markus CR, Olivier B, Panhuysen GE, Van Der Gugten J, Alles MS, Tuiten A, Westenberg HG, Fekkes D, Koppeschaar HF, de Haan EE. The bovine protein alpha-lactalbumin increases the plasma ratio of tryptophan to the other large neutral amino acids, and in vulnerable subjects raises brain serotonin activity, reduces cortisol concentration, and improves mood under stress. *Am J Clin Nutr.* 2000;71:1536-44

immunosuppression and decrements in musculoskeletal status caused by low-protein diets.[270] Described originally by the current author[271], the "supplemented Paleo-Mediterranean diet" provides patients the best of current knowledge in nutrition by relying on a foundational diet plan of fresh nuts, seeds, fruits, vegetables, fish, and lean meats which is adorned with olive oil for its squalene, phenolic antioxidant/anti-inflammatory and monounsaturated fatty acid content. Inclusive of medical foods such as red wine, garlic, and dark chocolate which may synergize to effect at least a 76% reduction in cardiovascular disease[272], this diet also reduces the risk for cancer[273] and can be an integral component of a health-promoting lifestyle.[274] Competitive athletes are allowed increased carbohydrate consumption before and after training and competition.[275]

Profile of The Supplemented Paleo-Mediterranean Diet[276]

Foods to consume: whole, natural, minimally processed foods include:	_Foods to avoid: factory products, high-sugar foods, and chemicals_
☺ **Lean sources of protein** • <u>Fish</u> (avoiding tuna which is commonly loaded with mercury) • <u>Chicken</u> • <u>Turkey</u> • <u>Lean cuts of free-range grass-fed meats</u>: beef, buffalo, lamb are occasionally acceptable • <u>Soy</u>[277] • <u>Whey</u>[278,279] ☺ **Fruits** ☺ **Vegetables** ☺ **Nuts, seeds, berries** ☺ **Generous use of olive oil**: On sautéed vegetables and fresh salads ☺ **Daily vitamin/mineral supplementation**: With a high-potency broad-spectrum multivitamin and multimineral supplement[280] ☺ **Sun exposure or vitamin D3 supplementation**: To ensure provision of 2,000-5,000 IU of vitamin D3 per day for adults[281] ☺ **Balanced broad-spectrum fatty acid supplementation**: With ALA, GLA, EPA, and DHA[282] ☺ **Water, tea, fruit and vegetable juices**: Commercial vegetable juices are commonly loaded with sodium chloride; choose appropriately. Fruit juices can be loaded with natural and superfluous sugars. Herbal teas can be selected based on the medicinal properties of the plant that is used.	☒ **Avoid as much as possible fat-laden arachidonate-rich meats like beef, liver, pork, and lamb, as well as high-fat cream and other dairy products with emulsified, readily absorbed saturated fats and arachidonic acid** ☒ **High-sugar pseudofoods**: • Corn syrup • Cola and soda • Donuts, candy, etc...."junk food" ☒ **Grains such as wheat, rye, barley**: These have only existed in the human diet for less than 10,000 years and are consistently associated with increased prevalence of degenerative diseases due to the allergic response they invoke and because of their high glycemic load and high glycemic index. ☒ **Potatoes and rice**: High in sugar, low in phytonutrients ☒ **Avoid allergens**: Determined per individual ☒ **Chemicals**: • <u>Pesticides, Herbicides, Fungicides</u> • <u>Carcinogenic sweeteners</u>: aspartame[283] • <u>Artificial flavors</u> • <u>Artificial colors</u>: tartrazine • <u>Preservatives</u>: benzoate • <u>Flavor enhancers</u>: carrageenan and monosodium glutamate

[270] Castaneda C, Charnley JM, Evans WJ, Crim MC. Elderly women accommodate to a low-protein diet with losses of body cell mass, muscle function, and immune response. *Am J Clin Nutr.* 1995;62:30-9

[271] Vasquez A. A Five-Part Nutritional Protocol that Produces Consistently Positive Results. *Nutritional Wellness* 2005Sept. http://nutritionalwellness.com/archives/2005/sep/09_vasquez.php and http://optimalhealthresearch.com/protocol

[272] Franco OH, Bonneux L, de Laet C, Peeters A, Steyerberg EW, Mackenbach JP. The Polymeal: a more natural, safer, and probably tastier (than the Polypill) strategy to reduce cardiovascular disease by more than 75%. *BMJ.* 2004;329(7480):1447-50

[273] "The combination of 4 low risk factors lowered the all-cause mortality rate to 0.35 (95% CI, 0.28-0.44). In total, lack of adherence to this low-risk pattern was associated with a population attributable risk of 60% of all deaths, 64% of deaths from coronary heart disease, 61% from cardiovascular diseases, and 60% from cancer." Knoops KT, de Groot LC, Kromhout D, et al. Mediterranean diet, lifestyle factors, and 10-year mortality in elderly European men and women: the HALE project. *JAMA.* 2004 Sep 22;292(12):1433-9

[274] Orme-Johnson DW, Herron RE. An innovative approach to reducing medical care utilization and expenditures. *Am J Manag Care.* 1997 Jan;3(1):135-44

[275] Cordain L, Friel J. <u>The Paleo Diet for Athletes : A Nutritional Formula for Peak Athletic Performance</u>: Rodale Books (September 23, 2005)

[276] Vasquez A. A Five-Part Nutritional Protocol that Produces Consistently Positive Results. *Nutritional Wellness* 2005Sept. http://nutritionalwellness.com/archives/2005/sep/09_vasquez.php and http://optimalhealthresearch.com/protocol

[277] "These results indicate that for healthy adults, the isolated soy protein is of high nutritional quality, comparable to that of animal protein sources, and that the methionine content is not limiting for adult protein maintenance." Young VR, Puig M, Queiroz E, Scrimshaw NS, Rand WM. Evaluation of the protein quality of an isolated soy protein in young men: relative nitrogen requirements and effect of methionine supplementation. *Am J Clin Nutr.* 1984 Jan;39(1):16-24

[278] Bounous G. Whey protein concentrate (WPC) and glutathione modulation in cancer treatment. *Anticancer Res.* 2000 Nov-Dec;20(6C):4785-92

[279] Markus CR, Olivier B, Panhuysen GE, Van Der Gugten J, Alles MS, Tuiten A, Westenberg HG, Fekkes D, Koppeschaar HF, de Haan EE. The bovine protein alpha-lactalbumin increases the plasma ratio of tryptophan to the other large neutral amino acids, and in vulnerable subjects raises brain serotonin activity, reduces cortisol concentration, and improves mood under stress. *Am J Clin Nutr.* 2000 Jun;71(6):1536-44 http://www.ajcn.org/cgi/content/full/71/6/1536

[280] "Most people do not consume an optimal amount of all vitamins by diet alone. ...it appears prudent for all adults to take vitamin supplements."Fletcher RH, Fairfield KM. Vitamins for chronic disease prevention in adults: clinical applications. *JAMA.* 2002;287:3127-9

[281] Vasquez A, Manso G, Cannell J. The clinical importance of vitamin D (cholecalciferol): a paradigm shift with implications for all healthcare providers. *Altern Ther Health Med.* 2004 Sep-Oct;10(5):28-36 http://optimalhealthresearch.com/monograph04

Biochemical Individuality and Orthomolecular Medicine

> "About 50 human genetic dis-eases due to defective enzymes can be remedied or ameliorated by the administration of high doses of the vitamin component of the corresponding coenzyme, which at least partially restores enzymatic activity."   *Bruce Ames, et al.*[284]

"**Biochemical individuality**" was the term coined by biochemist Dr. Roger Williams of the University of Texas[285] to describe the genetic and physiologic variations in human beings that produced different nutritional needs among individuals. Because we all have different genes, each of our bodies therefore creates different protein enzymes, and many of these enzymes—which are essential for proper cellular function—are adversely affected by defects in their construction (i.e., amino acid sequence) that reduce their efficiency. Dr. Linus Pauling[286] noted that single amino acid substitutions could produce dramatic alterations in protein function. Pauling discovered that sickle cell disease was caused by a single amino acid substitution in the hemoglobin molecule, and for this discovery he won the Nobel Prize in Chemistry in 1954.[287] With recognition of the importance of individual molecules in determining health or disease, Pauling coined the phrase "**orthomolecular medicine**" based on his thesis that many diseases could be effectively prevented and treated if we used the "**right molecules**" to correct abnormal physiologic function. Pauling contrasted the clinical use of nutrients for the improvement of physiologic function (orthomolecular medicine) with the use of chemical drugs, which generally work by interfering with normal physiology (toximolecular medicine). Since nutrients are the fundamental elements of the human body from which all enzymes, chemicals, and cellular structures are formed, Pauling advocated that the use of customized nutrition and nutritional supplements could promote optimal health by optimizing cellular function and efficiency. More recently, Dr. Bruce Ames has thoroughly documented the science of the orthomolecular precepts[288] and has advocated **optimal diets along with nutritional supplementation** as a highly efficient and cost-effective method for preventing disease and optimizing health.[289,290] In sum, we see that 1) the foundational diet must be formed from whole foods such as fruits, nuts, seeds, vegetables, and lean meats, 2) processed and artificial foods should be avoided, and 3) the use of nutritional supplements is necessary to provide sufficiently high levels of nutrition to overcome defects in enzymatic activity.

Orthomolecular precepts
- The functions of the body are dependent upon thousands of enzymes. Because of genetic defects that are common in the general population, some of these enzymes are commonly defective – even if only slightly – in large portions of the human population.
- Enzyme defects reduce the function and efficiency of important chemical reactions. Because enzymes are so important for normal function and the prevention of disease, defects in enzyme function can result in disruptions in physiology and the creation of what later manifests as "disease."
- Rather than treating these diseases with synthetic chemical drugs, it is commonly possible to prevent and treat disease with high-doses of vitamins, minerals, and other nutrients to compensate for or bypass defects in metabolic dysfunctions, thus allowing for the promotion of optimal health by promoting optimal physiologic function.

---

[282] Vasquez A. Reducing Pain and Inflammation Naturally. Part 2: New Insights into Fatty Acid Supplementation and Its Effect on Eicosanoid Production and Genetic Expression. *Nutritional Perspectives* 2005; January: 5-16 www.optimalhealthresearch.com/part2
[283] "In the past two decades brain tumor rates have risen in several industrialized countries, including the United States... Compared to other environmental factors putatively linked to brain tumors, the artificial sweetener aspartame is a promising candidate to explain the recent increase in incidence and degree of malignancy of brain tumors." Olney JW, Farber NB, Spitznagel E, Robins LN. Increasing brain tumor rates: is there a link to aspartame? *J Neuropathol Exp Neurol* 1996 Nov;55(11):1115-23
[284] Ames BN, Elson-Schwab I, Silver EA. High-dose vitamin therapy stimulates variant enzymes with decreased coenzyme binding affinity (increased K(m)): relevance to genetic disease and polymorphisms. *Am J Clin Nutr*. 2002 Apr;75(4):616-58
[285] "Every individual organism that has a distinctive genetic background has distinctive nutritional needs which must be met for optimal well-being. ...[N]utrition applied with due concern for individual genetic variations...offers the solution to many baffling health problems." Williams RJ. Biochemical Individuality : The Basis for the Genetotrophic Concept. Austin and London: University of Texas Press, 1956. Page x
[286] "...the concentration of coenzyme [vitamins and minerals] needed to produce the amount of active enzyme required for optimum health may well be somewhat different for different individuals. ...many individuals may require a considerably higher concentration of one or more coenzymes than other people do for optimum health..." Pauling L. On the Orthomolecular Environment of the Mind: Orthomolecular Theory. In: Williams RJ, Kalita DK. A Physician's Handbook on Orthomolecular Medicine. New Cannan; Keats Publishing: 1977. Page 76
[287] http://www.nobel.se/chemistry/laureates/1954/pauling-bio.html on April 4, 2004
[288] "About 50 human genetic dis-eases due to defective enzymes can be remedied or ameliorated by the administration of high doses of the vitamin component of the corresponding coenzyme, which at least partially restores enzymatic activity." Ames BN, Elson-Schwab I, Silver EA. High-dose vitamin therapy stimulates variant enzymes with decreased coenzyme binding affinity (increased K(m)): relevance to genetic disease and polymorphisms. *Am J Clin Nutr*. 2002 Apr;75(4):616-58
[289] "An optimum intake of micronutrients and metabolites, which varies with age and genetic constitution, would tune up metabolism and give a marked increase in health, particularly for the poor and elderly, at little cost." Ames BN. The metabolic tune-up: metabolic harmony and disease prevention. *J Nutr*. 2003 May;133(5 Suppl 1):1544S-8S
[290] "Optimizing micronutrient intake [through better diets, fortification of foods, or multivitamin-mineral pills] can have a major impact on public health at low cost." Ames BN. Cancer prevention and diet: help from single nucleotide polymorphisms. *Proc Natl Acad Sci U S A*. 1999 Oct 26;96(22):12216-8

Nutrigenomics: Nutritional Genomics

"The fundamental concepts of [nutrigenomics] are that **the progression from a healthy phenotype to a chronic disease phenotype must occur by changes in gene expression** or by differences in activities of proteins and enzymes and that **dietary chemicals directly or indirectly regulate the expression of genomic information.**"[291]

"Genome" refers to all of the genetic material in an organism, and "genomics" is the field of study of this information. The field of nutritional genomics—nutrigenomics—refers to the clinical synthesis of 1) research on the human genome (e.g., the Human Genome Project[292]), and 2) the advancing science of clinical nutrition, including research on nutraceuticals (nutritional medicines) and phytomedicinals (botanical medicines). Nutrigenomics represents a major advance in our understanding of the underlying biochemical and physiologic mechanisms of the effects of nutrition. Nutrition is far more than "fuel" for our biophysiologic machine; we know now that nutrition—the consumption of specific proteins, amino acids, vitamins, minerals, fatty acids, and phytochemicals—can alter genetic expression and can thus either promote health or disease at the very fundamental level of genetic expression. The commonly employed excuse that many patients use—"I just have bad genes"—now takes on a whole new meaning; it may be that these patients suffer from the expression of "bad genes" *because of the food that they eat*. The concept and phenomenon of nutrigenomics can be described by saying that each of us has the genes for health, as well as the genes for disease; what largely determines our level of health is how we treat our genes with environmental inputs, especially nutrition. We appear able, to a large extent, to "turn on" disease-promoting genes with poor nutrition and a pro-inflammatory lifestyle[293,294], while, to a lesser extent, we are able to activate or "turn on" health-promoting genes with a healthy diet[295] and with proper nutritional supplementation.[296,297]

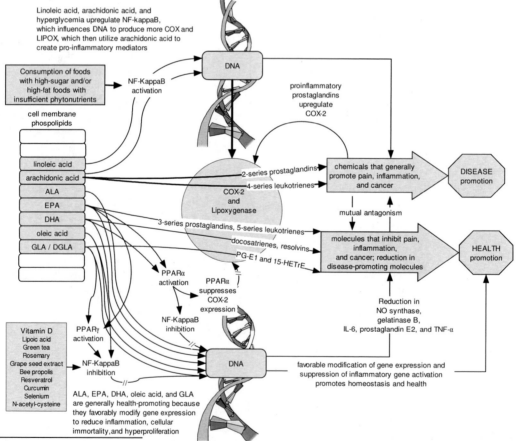

[291] Kaput J, Rodriguez LR. Nutritional genomics: the next frontier in the postgenomic era. *Physiol Genomics* 16: 166–177 http://physiolgenomics.physiology.org/cgi/content/full/16/2/166
[292] "Begun formally in 1990, the U.S. Human Genome Project is a 13-year effort coordinated by the U.S. Department of Energy and the National Institutes of Health. The project originally was planned to last 15 years, but rapid technological advances have accelerated the expected completion date to 2003. Project goals are to identify all the approximate 30,000 genes in human DNA..." See the official Human Genome website at http://www.ornl.gov/sci/techresources/Human_Genome/home.shtml
[293] Rusyn I, Bradham CA, Cohn L, Schoonhoven R, Swenberg JA, Brenner DA, Thurman RG. Corn oil rapidly activates nuclear factor-kappaB in hepatic Kupffer cells by oxidant-dependent mechanisms. *Carcinogenesis*. 1999 Nov;20(11):2095-100 http://carcin.oxfordjournals.org/cgi/content/full/20/11/2095
[294] Aljada A, Mohanty P, Ghanim H, Abdo T, Tripathy D, Chaudhuri A, Dandona P. Increase in intranuclear nuclear factor kappaB and decrease in inhibitor kappaB in mononuclear cells after a mixed meal: evidence for a proinflammatory effect. *Am J Clin Nutr*. 2004 Apr;79(4):682-90
[295] O'Keefe JH Jr, Cordain L. Cardiovascular disease resulting from a diet and lifestyle at odds with our Paleolithic genome. *Mayo Clin Proc*. 2004 Jan;79(1):101-8
[296] "About 50 human genetic dis-eases due to defective enzymes can be remedied or ameliorated by the administration of high doses of the vitamin component of the corresponding coenzyme, which at least partially restores enzymatic activity." Ames BN, Elson-Schwab I, Silver EA. High-dose vitamin therapy stimulates variant enzymes with decreased coenzyme binding affinity (increased K(m)): relevance to genetic disease and polymorphisms. *Am J Clin Nutr*. 2002 Apr;75(4):616-58 http://www.ajcn.org/cgi/content/full/75/4/616
[297] Kaput J, Rodriguez LR. Nutritional genomics: the next frontier in the postgenomic era. *Physiol Genomics* 16: 166–177 http://physiolgenomics.physiology.org/cgi/content/full/16/2/166

General Guidelines for the Safe Use of Nutritional Supplements

Supplementation with vitamins and minerals is generally safe, especially if the following guidelines are followed:

- **Iron is potentially harmful**: Iron promotes the formation of "free radicals" and is thus implicated in several diseases, such as infections, cancer, liver disease, diabetes, and cardiovascular disease. Iron supplements should not be consumed except by people who have been definitively diagnosed with iron deficiency by measurement of serum ferritin.

- **Vitamins and minerals should generally be taken with food in order to eliminate the possibility of nausea and to increase absorption**: Most vitamins and other supplements should be taken with food so that nausea is avoided.

- **Vitamin A is one of the only vitamins with the potential for serious toxicity even at low doses**: Attention should be given to vitamin A intake so that toxicity is avoided. Add vitamin A amounts from all sources—foods, fish oils, and vitamin supplements. Manifestations of vitamin A toxicity include: skin problems (dry skin, flaking skin, chapped or split lips, red skin rash, hair loss), joint pain, bone pain, headaches, anorexia (loss of appetite), edema (water retention, weight gain, swollen ankles, difficulty breathing), fatigue, and/or liver damage.

  - Adults: Women who are pregnant or might become pregnant and who are planning to carry the baby to full term delivery should not ingest more than 10,000 IU of vitamin A per day. Vitamin A toxicity is seen with chronic ingestion of therapeutic doses (for example: 25,000 IU per day for 6 years, or 100,000 IU per day for 2.5 years[298]). Most patients should not consume more than 20,000 IU of vitamin A per day for more than 2 months without express supervision by a healthcare provider. Vitamin A is present in some multivitamins, in cod liver oil, and in other supplements—read labels to ensure that the total daily intake is not greater than 20,000 IU per day.

  - Infants and Children: Different studies have used either daily or monthly schedules of vitamin A supplementation. In a study with extremely low-birth weight infants, 5,000 IU of vitamin A per day for 28 days was safely used.[299] In another study conducted in sick children, those aged less than 12 months received 100,000 IU on two consecutive days, while children between ages 12-60 months received a larger dose of 200,000 IU on two consecutive days.[300]

- **Preexisting kidney problems (such as renal failure) increase the risks associated with nutritional supplementation**: Supplementation with vitamins and minerals does not cause kidney damage. However, if a patient already has kidney problems, then vitamin/mineral/protein supplementation may become hazardous. Assessment of renal function with serum or urine tests is encouraged before beginning an aggressive plan of supplementation. Conditions which cause kidney damage include:

  - Use of medications that promote kidney failure—acetaminophen, aspirin, others
  - Hypertension, high blood pressure
  - Diabetes mellitus
  - Use of recreational drugs, such as cocaine[301]
  - Certain health disorders, such as lupus (SLE)

---

[298] "The smallest continuous daily consumption leading to cirrhosis was 25,000 IU during 6 years, whereas higher daily doses (greater than or equal to 100,000 IU) taken during 2 1/2 years resulted in similar histological lesions. ... The data also indicate that prolonged and continuous consumption of doses in the low "therapeutic" range can result in life-threatening liver damage." Geubel AP, De Galocsy C, Alves N, Rahier J, Dive C. Liver damage caused by therapeutic vitamin A administration: estimate of dose-related toxicity in 41 cases. *Gastroenterology*. 1991 Jun;100(6):1701-9

[299] "Infants with birth weight < 1000 g were randomised at birth to receive oral vitamin A supplementation (5000 IU/day) or placebo for 28 days." Wardle SP, Hughes A, Chen S, Shaw NJ. Randomised controlled trial of oral vitamin A supplementation in preterm infants to prevent chronic lung disease. *Arch Dis Child Fetal Neonatal Ed*. 2001 Jan;84(1):F9-F13 Available on-line at http://adc.bmjjournals.com/cgi/content/full/fetalneonatal%3b84/1/F9

[300] "Children were assigned to oral doses of 200 000 IU vitamin A (half that dose if <12 months) or placebo on the day of admission, a second dose on the following day, and third and fourth doses at 4 and 8 months after discharge from the hospital, respectively." Villamor E, Mbise R, Spiegelman D, Hertzmark E, Fataki M, Peterson KE, Ndossi G, Fawzi WW. Vitamin A supplements ameliorate the adverse effect of HIV-1, malaria, and diarrheal infections on child growth. *Pediatrics*. 2002 Jan;109(1):E6

[301] Horowitz BZ, Panacek EA, Jouriles NJ. Severe rhabdomyolysis with renal failure after intranasal cocaine use. *J Emerg Med*. 1997 Nov-Dec;15(6):833-7

- **Several drugs/medications may adversely interact with vitamin/mineral supplements and with botanical medicines**: Vitamins/minerals may reduce the effectiveness of some prescription medications. For example, taking certain antibiotics such as Cipro or tetracycline with calcium reduces absorption of the drugs, therefore rendering the drugs much less effective. Taking botanical medicines with medications may make the drugs dangerously less effective (such as when St. John's Wort is combined with protease inhibitor drugs[302]) or may make the drug dangerously more effective (such when Kava is combined with the anti-anxiety drug alprazolam[303]). If vitamin D is used in doses greater than 800 IU/d in patients taking hydrochlorothiazide or other calcium-retaining drugs, serum calcium should be monitored at least monthly until safety (i.e., lack of hypercalcemia) has been established per patient.[304] Patients should not combine nutritional or botanical medicines with chemical/synthetic drugs without specific advice from a knowledgeable doctor. Do not increase vitamin K consumption from supplements or dietary improvements in patients taking coumadin/warfarin. A reasonable recommendation is that nutritional supplements be taken 2 hours away from pharmaceutical medications to avoid complications such as intraintestinal drug-nutrient binding.
- **Pre-existing medical conditions may make supplementation unsafe**: A few rare medical conditions may cause nutritional supplementation to be unsafe, including severe liver disease, renal failure, electrolyte imbalances, hyperparathyroidism and other vitamin D hypersensitivity syndromes.

Notes:

_____
_____
_____
_____
_____
_____
_____
_____
_____
_____
_____
_____
_____
_____
_____
_____
_____
_____
_____
_____
_____
_____
_____
_____
_____
_____

[302] Piscitelli SC, Burstein AH, Chaitt D, Alfaro RM, Falloon J. Indinavir concentrations and St John's wort. *Lancet*. 2000 Feb 12;355(9203):547-8
[303] Almeida JC, Grimsley EW. Coma from the health food store: interaction between kava and alprazolam. *Ann Intern Med*. 1996 Dec 1;125(11):940-1
[304] Vasquez A, Manso G, Cannell J. The clinical importance of vitamin D (cholecalciferol): a paradigm shift with implications for all healthcare providers. *Altern Ther Health Med*. 2004 Sep-Oct;10(5):28-36 http://optimalhealthresearch.com/monograph04

Emotional, Mental, and Social Health

Stress management and authentic living

Mental, emotional, and physical "stress" describes any unpleasant living condition which can lead to negative effects on health, such as increased blood pressure, depression, apathy, increased muscle tension, and, according to some research, increased risk of serious health problems such as early death from cardiovascular disease and cancer. Many people find that their modern lives are characterized by excess amounts of multitasking, job responsibilities, family responsibilities, commuter traffic, expenses and an insufficient amount of relaxation, sleep, community support, exercise, time in nature, healthy nutrition, and time to simply *be* rather than *do*. Stress comes in many different forms and includes malnutrition, trauma, insufficient exercise (epidemic), excess exercise (rare), sleep deprivation, emotional turmoil, and exposure to chemicals and radiation. When most people talk about "stress" they are referring to either chronic anxiety (such as with high-pressure work situations or dysfunctional interpersonal relationships) or the acute stress reaction that is typical of unpredictable rapid-onset events such as an injury, accident, or other physically threatening situation. These **"different types of stress" are not separate from each other**; emotional stress causes nutritional depletion[305]; sleep deprivation alters immune response[306], chemical exposure can disrupt endocrine function.[307] Therefore, **any type of stress can cause other types of stress**. Avoiding stressful situations is, of course, an effective way to avoid being bothered or harmed by them. If work-related stress is the problem, then finding a new position or occupation is certainly an option worth considering and implementing. High-stress jobs are often high-paying jobs; but if in the process of making money, a person ruins her health and loses years from her life, then no one would ever say, "It was worth it." Money, success, and freedom only have value for the person alive and healthy to enjoy them. *Toxic relationships*, whether at home or work, are relationships that cause more harm than good by re-injuring

> **"Good relationships make you feel loved, wanted, and cared for."**
>
> Malcolm LL. Health Style. London; Thorsons: 2001, p 133

old emotional wounds and by creating new emotional injuries. We can all benefit from affirming our right to a happy and healthy life by minimizing/eliminating contact with people who cause emotional harm to us—this requires conscious effort[308]; Engel[309] provides a clear articulation and description of abusive relationships, along with checklists for their recognition and exercises for their remediation.

	Mental/emotional	*Physical*	*Nutritional/biochemical*
Therapeutic considerations	• Social support • Re-parenting • Conversational style[310] • Meditation, prayer • Healthy boundaries • Books, tapes, groups • Expressive writing[311] • Time to simply experience and otherwise "do nothing"	• Yoga • Massage • Exercise • Stretching • Swimming • Resting • Biking • Hiking • Affection	• Vitamins, including vitamin C[312] • Fish oil[313] • Hormones, cytokines, neurotransmitters, and eicosanoids • Botanical medicines such as *kava*[314], *Ashwaganda*, and *Eleutherococcus*

---

[305] Ingenbleek Y, Bernstein L. The stressful condition as a nutritionally dependent adaptive dichotomy. *Nutrition* 1999 Apr;15(4):305-20

[306] Heiser P, Dickhaus B, Opper C, Hemmeter U, Remschmidt H, Wesemann W, Krieg JC, Schreiber W. Alterations of host defense system after sleep deprivation are followed by impaired mood and psychosocial functioning. *World J Biol Psychiatry* 2001 Apr;2(2):89-94

[307] "Evidence suggests that environmental exposure to some anthropogenic chemicals may result in disruption of endocrine systems in human and wildlife populations." http://www.epa.gov/endocrine on March 7, 2004

[308] Bryn C. Collins. **How to Recognize Emotional Unavailability and Make Healthier Relationship Choices**. [Mjf Books; ISBN: 1567313442] Recently reprinted as: Emotional Unavailability: Recognizing It, Understanding It, and Avoiding Its Trap [McGraw Hill - NTC (April 1998); ISBN: 0809229145]

[309] Engel B. **The Emotionally Abusive Relationship: How to Stop Being Abused and How to Stop Abusing**. Wiley Publishers: 2003

[310] Rick Brinkman ND and Rick Kirschner ND. How to Deal With Difficult People [Audio Cassette. Career Track, 1995]

[311] Smyth JM, Stone AA, Hurewitz A, Kaell A. Effects of writing about stressful experiences on symptom reduction in patients with asthma or rheumatoid arthritis: a randomized trial. *JAMA*. 1999 Apr 14;281(14):1304-9

[312] Brody S, Preut R, Schommer K, Schurmeyer TH. A randomized controlled trial of high dose ascorbic acid for reduction of blood pressure, cortisol, and subjective responses to psychological stress. *Psychopharmacology* (Berl). 2002 Jan;159(3):319-24

[313] Hamazaki T, Itomura M, Sawazaki S, Nagao Y. Anti-stress effects of DHA. *Biofactors*. 2000;13(1-4):41-5

[314] Cagnacci A, et al. Kava-Kava administration reduces anxiety in perimenopausal women. *Maturitas*. 2003 Feb 25;44(2):103-9

Stress is a whole-body phenomenon; its amelioration must likewise be multifaceted

Stress affects the whole body.

Therefore, a complete stress management program must address the whole body:

Physical
Structural

Biochemical
Hormonal
Nutritional

Mental
Emotional
Spiritual

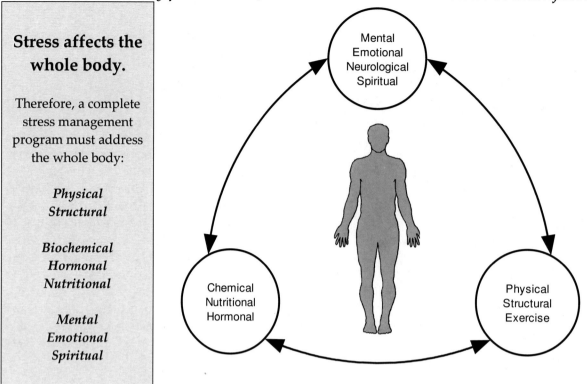

An important concept is that **stress is a "whole body" phenomenon**: affecting the mind, the brain, emotional state, the physical body (including musculoskeletal, immune, and cardiovascular systems), as well as the nutritional status of the individual. The adverse effects of stress can be reduced with an integrated combination of therapeutics that addresses each of the major body systems affected by stress, which are 1) mental/emotional, 2) physical, and 3) nutritional/biochemical.

Sometimes a stressful situation can be modified into one that is less stressful or dysfunctional, so that the benefits are retained, yet the negative aspects are reduced. Of course, the best example of this is interpersonal relationships, which easily lend themselves to improvement with the application of conscious effort. Many audiotapes, books, and seminars are available for people interested in having improved interpersonal relationships.

- <u>Men & Women: Talking Together</u> by Deborah Tannen and Robert Bly [Sound Horizons, 1992. ISBN: 1879323095] A lively discussion of the different communication and relationship styles of men and women by two respected experts in their fields.

- <u>How to Deal with Difficult People</u> by Drs. Rick Brinkman and Rick Kirschner. [Audio Cassette. Career Track, 1995] An entertaining format with solutions to common workplace and situational difficulties. Authored and performed by two naturopathic physicians.

- <u>Men are From Mars, Women are From Venus</u> by John Gray. [Audio Cassette and Books]. Phenomenally popular concepts in understanding, accepting, and effectively integrating the differences between men and women.

- <u>The ManKind Project</u> (<u>www.mkp.org</u>). An international organization hosting events for men and women. The men's events, formats, and groups are authentic, clear, and healthy. The ManKind Project has an organization for women called The WomanWithin (<u>www.womanwithin.org</u>). No book or tape can substitute for the dynamics and personal attention that can be experienced by a conscious, empowered, and well-intended group.

When "the problem" cannot be avoided, and the interaction/relationship with the problem cannot be improved, a remaining option is to supplement the internal environment so that it is somewhat "strengthened" to deal with the stress of the bothersome event or situation. For example, when dealing with emotional stress, we can use counseling, support groups, or various relaxation techniques.[315] If we determine that the emotional stress has a biochemical component, then we can use specific botanical and nutritional supplementation to safely and naturally support and restore normal function. Moving deeper into the issue of "stress management" requires that we ask why a person is in a stressful situation to begin with. Of course, with *random acts of chaos* like car accidents, we cannot always ascribe the problem to the person, unless the accident resulted from their own negligence. But **when people are chronically stressed and unhappy about their jobs and/or relationships, then we need to employ more than stress reduction techniques,** and as clinicians we need to offer more than the latest adaptogen. **We have to ask why a person would subject himself/herself to such a situation, and what fears or limitations (self-imposed and/or externally applied) keep him/her from breaking free into a life that works.**[316,317,318,319]

Stress always has a biochemical/physiologic component: Regardless of its origins, stress always takes a toll on the body—*the whole body*. Well-documented effects of stress include:

1. Increased levels of cortisol—higher levels are associated with osteoporosis, memory loss, slow healing
2. Reduced function of thyroid hormones[320]
3. Reduced levels of testosterone (in men)
4. Increased intestinal permeability and "leaky gut"[321]
5. Increased excretion of minerals in the urine
6. Increased need for vitamins and amino acids
7. Suppression of immune function and of natural killer cells that fight viral infections and tumors
8. Decreased production of sIgA—the main defense of the lungs, gastrointestinal tract, and genitourinary tract
9. Increased populations of harmful bacteria in the intestines and an associated increased rate of lung and upper respiratory tract infections
10. Increased incidence of food allergies[322]
11. Sleep disturbance

The body functions as a whole—not as independent, autonomous organ systems: Problems with one aspect of health create problems in other aspects of health. Treatment of disease and promotion of wellness must therefore improve overall health and functioning while simultaneously addressing the disease or presenting complaint.

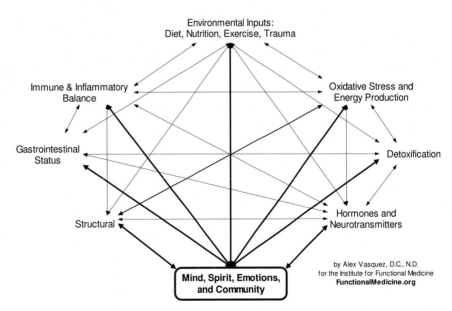

Environmental Inputs: Diet, Nutrition, Exercise, Trauma

Immune & Inflammatory Balance

Oxidative Stress and Energy Production

Gastrointestinal Status

Detoxification

Structural

Hormones and Neurotransmitters

Mind, Spirit, Emotions, and Community

by Alex Vasquez, D.C., N.D. for the Institute for Functional Medicine **FunctionalMedicine.org**

[315] Martha Davis PhD, Matthew McKay MSW, Elizabeth Robbins Eshelman PhD. The Relaxation & Stress Reduction Workbook 5th edition. New Harbinger Publishers; 2000. [ISBN: 1572242140]
[316] Rick Jarow. Creating the Work You Love: Courage, Commitment and Career; Inner Traditions Intl Ltd; 1995 [ISBN: 0892815426]
[317] Breton D and Largent C. The Paradigm Conspiracy: Why Our Social Systems Violate Human Potential-And How We Can Change Them. Hazelden: 1998
[318] Dominguez JR. Transforming Your Relationship With Money. Sounds True; Book and Cassette edition: 2001 Audio tape.
[319] Gatto JT. Dumbing us down: the hidden curriculum of compulsory education. Gabriola Island, Canada; New Society Publishers: 2005
[320] Ingenbleek Y, Bernstein L. The stressful condition as a nutritionally dependent adaptive dichotomy. *Nutrition* 1999 Apr;15(4):305-20
[321] Hart A, Kamm MA. Review article: mechanisms of initiation and perpetuation of gut inflammation by stress. *Aliment Pharmacol Ther* 2002;16(12):2017-28
[322] Anderzen I, Arnetz BB, Soderstrom T, Soderman E. Stress and sensitization in children: a controlled prospective psychophysiological study of children exposed to international relocation. *Journal of Psychosomatic Research* 1997; 43: 259-69

Autonomization, intradependence, emotional literacy, corrective experience:

> "None of us are completely developed people when we reach adulthood.
> We are each incomplete in our own way."   *Merle Fossum*[323]

Consciousness-raising is a keystone gift that holistic physicians can impart to their patients and one which may be necessary for true healing to be manifested and maintained. Healthcare providers are quick to enlighten their patients to the details of diet, exercise, nutrition, medications, surgeries, and other *biomechanical* and *biochemical* aspects of health, but are routinely negligent when it comes to sharing with patients the emotional tools that may be necessary to repair or construct the "self" which is supposed to implement the treatment plan that the doctor has designed. Passivity and ignorance are not hindrances to the success of the *medical paradigm*, which requires that patients are "compliant" rather than self-directed; however, for *authentic, holistic healthcare* to be successful, it must empower the patient sufficiently such that he/she attains/regains appropriate *autonomy*—an "internal locus of control"—sufficient for lifelong internally-driven health maintenance. Health implications of autonomy (or its absence) are obvious and intuitive. For example, patients with an underdeveloped internal locus of control appear to experience greater degrees of social stress which can lead to hypercortisolemia and hippocampal atrophy.[324] Additionally, internal locus of control correlates strongly with the success of weight-loss programs, and for nonautonomous patients it is necessary to encourage the development of autonomous self-care behavior in addition to the provision of information about diet and exercise.[325]

Completely formed internal identities are the natural result of the *continuum* of positive childhood experiences (inclusive of stability, "unconditional love", healthy parenting, and active, conscious intergenerational social contact) which are ideally segued into adolescent and adulthood experiences of success, acceptance, inclusion, independence, interdependence, and intradependence with the end result being a socially-conscious adult with an internal locus of control. Where the patient has experienced a relative absence of these natural and expected prerequisites, there can only exist a truncated self. This largely explains why so many adult patients feign that they are incapable of action, "can't exercise", and "can't leave" their abusive jobs and relationships, and "can't resist" the dietary habits which daily contribute to their physical and psychoemotional decline. Thus, for more than a few patients, a therapeutic path must be explored which helps to re-create the foundation from which an autonomous adult and authentic self can grow—it is a *process* (not an event) of **emotional recovery**.[326] To this extent, interventional or therapeutic *autonomization* resembles a *recovery program* that can include various forms of conscious action, including goal-setting, positive reinforcement, developing **emotional literacy**[327] and **emotional intelligence**[328], and consciousness-raising experiences such as therapy and group work—all of which serve to intentionally (re)create the necessary climate for selfhood. Therewith, the patient can accept challenges to further develop an *empowered self* by participating in exercises of intentional intradependence (self-reliance)—situations in which the ability to decide, choose, and act responsibly and appropriately are reinforced to eventually become second nature, replacing passivity, inaction, and ineffectiveness.[329]

[323] Fossum M. Catching Fire: Men Coming Alive in Recovery. New York; Harper/Hazelden: 1989, 4-7

[324] "Cumulative exposure to high levels of cortisol over the lifetime is known to be related to hippocampal atrophy... Self-esteem and internal locus of control were significantly correlated with hippocampal volume in both young and elderly subjects." Pruessner JC, Baldwin MW, Dedovic K, Renwick R, Mahani NK, Lord C, Meaney M, Lupien S. Self-esteem, locus of control, hippocampal volume, and cortisol regulation in young and old adulthood. *Neuroimage*. 2005 Jul 13; [Epub ahead of print]

[325] "Their weight loss was significant and associated with an internal locus of control orientation (P < 0.05)... Participants with an internal orientation could be offered a standard weight reduction programme. Others, with a more external locus of control orientation, could be offered an adapted programme, which also focused on and encouraged the participants' internal orientation." Adolfsson B, Andersson I, Elofsson S, Rossner S, Unden AL. Locus of control and weight reduction. *Patient Educ Couns*. 2005 Jan;56(1):55-61

[326] Bradshaw J. Healing the Shame that Binds You [Audio Cassette (April 1990) Health Communications Audio; ISBN: 1558740430]

[327] Dayton T. Trauma and Addiction: Ending the Cycle of Pain Through Emotional Literacy. Deerfield Beach; Health Communications, 2000

[328] Goleman D. Emotional Intelligence. New York; Bantam Books: 1995. Although the book as a whole was considered pioneering for its time, and the book continues to make a valuable contribution, a few of the concepts and author's personal stories are embarrassingly simplistic.

[329] Gatto JT. A Schooling Is Not An Education: interview by Barbara Dunlop. http://www.johntaylorgatto.com/bookstore/index.htm

"Empowerment" can only be authentic if it is built on the foundation of a developed self. Thus while *recovery* and *empowerment* are separate spheres of activity and attention, they are not mutually exclusive and indeed are synergistic. However, *empowerment* cannot succeed without *recovery* because otherwise so-called "empowerment" is simply a complex defense mechanism that "protects" against pain and thereby blocks the development of an authentic self. In the words of Janov[330], "**Anything that builds a stronger defense system deepens the neurosis.**"

Primary, secondary, and tertiary means for developing an autonomous, authentic self: Ideally, positive childhood experiences (A) segue into adolescent and adult experiences of confidence and maturity (B) for the development of a true adult (C). If A or B are lacking or insufficient, the result is an incomplete self often incapable of *effective* and *appropriate* action. **Corrective experiences must then be pursued to re-establish the foundation from which an authentic self can arise.**

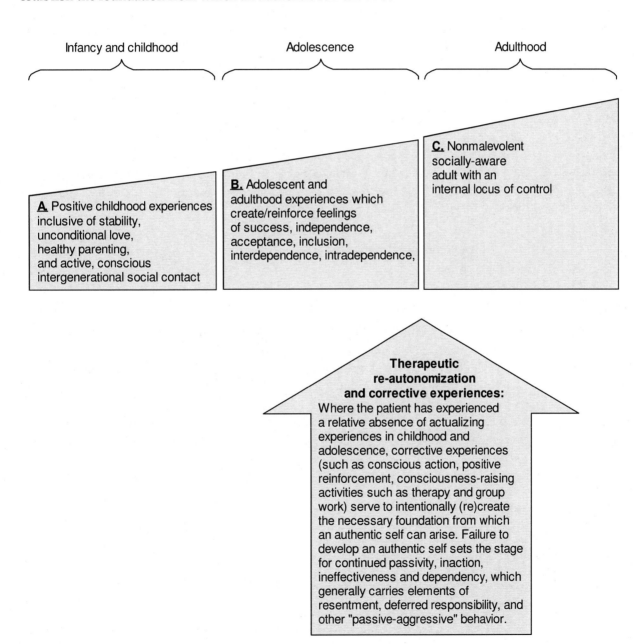

Infancy and childhood   Adolescence   Adulthood

A. Positive childhood experiences inclusive of stability, unconditional love, healthy parenting, and active, conscious intergenerational social contact

B. Adolescent and adulthood experiences which create/reinforce feelings of success, independence, acceptance, inclusion, interdependence, intradependence,

C. Nonmalevolent socially-aware adult with an internal locus of control

Therapeutic re-autonomization and corrective experiences: Where the patient has experienced a relative absence of actualizing experiences in childhood and adolescence, corrective experiences (such as conscious action, positive reinforcement, consciousness-raising activities such as therapy and group work) serve to intentionally (re)create the necessary foundation from which an authentic self can arise. Failure to develop an authentic self sets the stage for continued passivity, inaction, ineffectiveness and dependency, which generally carries elements of resentment, deferred responsibility, and other "passive-aggressive" behavior.

---

[330] Janov A. The Primal Scream. New York; GP Putnam's Sons: 1970, page 20

> "The object of healing is...to move closer to wholeness."
>
> *Albert Kreinheder, PhD, Jungian analyst*[331]

Patients lacking an internal locus of control are much more likely to succumb to the tantalizing barrage of direct-to-consumer drug advertising[332] which infantilizes patients by 1) oversimplifying diseases, their causes, and treatments, 2) telling them that the disease is not their fault, and 3) encouraging a dependent, passively receptive role by telling patients that they have no proactive role other than to "ask your doctor if a prescription is right for you." It is no accident that Americans consume more prescription and OTC medications per capita than people in any other country.[333,334] With the combined and synergistic effects of 1) the dissolution of first the extended family and now the nuclear family[335], 2) a society-wide famine of mentors, elders, and community[336,337,338], 3) a dearth of autonomous, genuine exploration from childhood to adulthood, and 4) primary and secondary "educational" institutions designed to squelch independence and autonomy in favor of the more efficient, predictable, and controllable conformity and "standardization"[339,340], **industrialized societies have raised generations of people who lack completely formed internal identities.** Lacking an internal locus of control and identity from which to think independently and critically, these "adults" are easy prey for slick and flashy drug advertisements that promise the illusion of perfect health in exchange for passivity, abdication, and lifelong medicalization. It's bad enough that on average each American watches 4 hours of television per day[341] but what's worse is that "Americans who watch average amounts of television may be exposed to more than 30 hours of direct-to-consumer drug advertisements each year, far surpassing their exposure to other forms of health communication."[342] Thus, the pharmaceutical companies are the main source of "health education" for Americans, and—as we would expect—the solutions they propose for all health problems is drugs, drugs, drugs. It is obvious that if we are to wean our suckling culture from undue dependence on the pharmaceutical industry, we have to address our patient population directly and transform them from *passive, nonautonomous, and ignorant about health and disease* to pro-active, autonomous, and well-informed about health and the means required to obtain and sustain it.

> "...like most prospective consumers of therapy, I made up a bunch of excuses for why I could handle this on my own...
> I was smiling like an idiot..."
>
> *Jeffrey Kottler, The Compleat Therapist*[343]

Insight into a patient's internal dynamic can provide the clinician with an understanding that explains the phenomena of *non-compliance* and *disease identification*. Rather than seeing non-compliance as "weakness of will", non-compliance as a form of "disobedience" may be a reflection of the patient's unconscious need to wrestle with and resolve parental introjects. For example, if a patient had a rejecting, nonaffirming parent, he/she may need to find another rejecting authority figure in order to continue playing the role of the child; by assuming this role and "setting the stage", the patient is unconsciously attempting to create a situation wherein the primary relationship can be healed.[344] Complicating this is *disease identification*—in which patients use their disease as a source of identity and secondary gain for martyrdom, social support, group participation, acceptance, admiration, purpose, excitement, and drama.

[331] Kreinheder A. Body and soul: the other side of illness. Toronto, Canada; Inner City Books: 1991, page 38
[332] Aronson E. The Social Animal. San Fransisco; WH Freeman and company: 1972: 21-22, 53
[333] America the medicated. http://www.cbsnews.com/stories/2005/04/21/health/printable689997.shtml and http://www.msnbc.msn.com/id/7503122/ . See also http://usgovinfo.about.com/od/healthcare/a/usmedicated.htm Accessed September 17, 2005.
[334] Kivel P.You Call This a Democracy? Apex Press (August, 2004). ISBN: 1891843265 http://www.paulkivel.com/
[335] Bly R. Iron John. Reading, Mass.: Addison Wesley, 1990
[336] Bly R. The Sibling Society. Vintage Books USA; Reprint edition (June 1, 1997) ISBN: 0679781285 (Abridged audio edition (May 1, 1996), ASIN: 0679451609)
[337] Bly R. Where have all the parents gone? A talk on the Sibling Society. New York: Sound Horizons, 1996 Highly recommended.
[338] Bly R, Hillman J, Meade M. Men and the Life of Desire. Oral Tradition Archives. ISBN: 1880155001. Audio Cassette
[339] Gatto JT. Dumbing Us Down: the Hidden Curriculum of Compulsory Education. Gabriola Island, Canada; New Society Publishers: 2005
[340] Gatto JT. The Paradox of Extended Childhood. [From a presentation in Cambridge, Mass. October 2000] http://www.johntaylorgatto.com/bookstore/index.htm
[341] "American children view over 23 hours of television per week. * Teenagers view an average of 21 to 22 hours of television per week. * By the time today's children reach age 70, they will have spent 7 to 10 years of their lives watching television." American Academy of Pediatrics http://www.aapca1.org/aapca1/tv.html See also TV-Turnoff Network. Facts and Figures About our TV Habit http://www.tvturnoff.org/factsheets.htm Accessed September 17, 2005
[342] Brownfield ED, Bernhardt JM, Phan JL, Williams MV, Parker RM. Direct-to-consumer drug advertisements on network television: an exploration of quantity, frequency, and placement. J Health Commun. 2004 Nov-Dec;9(6):491-7
[343] Kottler JA. The Compleat Therapist. San Francisco; Jossey-Bass publishers; 1991, pages 2-3
[344] Miller A. The Drama of the Gifted Child: The Search for the True Self. Basic Books: 1981, page 88

Helping Patients (Re)Create Themselves:
Practical Applications, Exercises, and Concepts

An absent or underdeveloped locus of control is the key problem that underlies many anxiety disorders, addictive behavioral traits such as overeating, overworking, codependency, as well as chronic ineffectiveness in the pursuit of one's goals. The solutions to this problem are logical, practical, and accessible to everyone; the major costs associated with each are open-mindedness, attentiveness, discipline and persistence. There is scant mention of this concept and its intervention in the biomedical literature; however, it is well described in the psychological literature, particularly that which focuses on various types of "recovery" such as that from addiction, co-dependence, and low self-esteem, the latter two of which are virtually synonymous with an insufficient internal locus of control.

There is no single path here. There are many paths. The goal is not to choose the right path; rather the goal is to travel several paths to the degree necessary, implement what has been learned, travel other paths, and return to the same path again to retrace one's steps in new ways. The process is similar to that of *ceremonial initiation*, the purpose of which is to formally mark the *beginning* of a process that is *ongoing* and *infinite*.[345] Each path and each process has its gifts, significance, and limitations. However, the ultimate goal of each must be a tangible and positive change in the ways which the patient either feels and/or behaves in and interacts with the world on a day-to-day basis.

In no particular order (since the proper sequence will have to be customized to the situation and willingness of the patient), the following are some of the more commonly cited exercises, processes, and sources of additional information:

Apprenticeship and Mentoring: books, tapes, and lectures: Children and non-autonomous adults are pulled into authentic adulthood by mentors, elders, and true adults. The therapeutic encounters thus provided—whether interpersonal or vicarious in the form of lectures, books, or audiotapes— serve as sources of information from which new possibilities can be gleaned, and these therefore serve as infinitely valuable resources for expanding the narrow horizons that characterize an underdeveloped internal locus of control. In essence, books, tapes, and lectures allow the patient to become a student and to choose a vicarious mentor. *Advantages*: Books and tapes allow access to many of the best minds in psychology; books and tapes are inexpensive; allow patients to explore and benefit from many different perspectives; books and tapes are always available and are therefore amenable to various schedules of work and responsibility. *Disadvantages*: Books and tapes do not re-create the interpersonal bridge which is essential for authentic recovery; do not provide a direct and objective means of accountably, thus potentially allowing patients to delude themselves about the effectiveness (or lack thereof) of their recovery process. Examples of better-known books, tapes and recorded lectures on the *process* of emotional recovery:
- ***Healing the Shame that Binds You*** by John Bradshaw [Audio Cassette (April 1990) Health Communications Audio; ISBN: 1558740430] Available as book and cassette with identical titles and different content.
- ***A Little Book on the Human Shadow*** by Robert Bly. Certainly among the most concise, accessible, and complete books ever written on the processes involved in losing and recovering the self.
- ***The Drama of the Gifted Child*** by Alice Miller. This internationally acclaimed book is considered a true classic among therapists and patients alike. Available as book and a brilliantly performed audio cassette.
- ***You Can Heal Your Life*** by Louise Hay. Another standard for recovery; very "new age."
- ***Codependent No More: How to Stop Controlling Others and Start Caring for Yourself*** by Melody Beattie. Pioneering for its time.
- ***The Artist's Date Book*** by Julia Cameron.   Each page has a new creative idea for creative expression and "creative recovery."

---

[345] Hillman J, Meade M, Some M. Images of initiation. Oral Tradition Archives; 1992

Therapy: _"Therapy is a conversation that matters."_ Therapy in this context specifically means face-to-face, active interaction, either one-on-one or in a group setting, with the specific intention to give and/or provide support for personal growth. Whether 12-step groups such as Codependents Anonymous qualify as a form of therapy depends entirely upon the level of engagement of the participant; sitting in a room while _other people_ do _their_ work provides slow or no benefit for the passive observer. **Recovery is an active process, which is why it is antithetical to depression, which is a _passive_ state of being.** Patients should go in knowing that this is a _process_ and to not expect to be "fixed" after the first hour or even the first month. **_Advantages_**: Therapists can provide crucial support and insight while the client wrestles with undecipherable and convoluted emotional and psychic data. Therapists can help the client set goals ("stretches" and "homework") by which the client reaches beyond his/her comfort zone to attain the next expansion in being and experience. Therapists must create a safe space or "container" in which ideas and feelings can be brought forth to intermingle and be consciously appreciated. **_Disadvantages_**: Requires a flexible and disciplined schedule; costs money; bad therapists can do more harm than good if they misdirect their clients away from volatile and core issues and authentic expression.[346,347,348,349] Therapy can be disempowering if the patient continues to project his/her locus of control onto the therapist.

Some of the more commonly used tools of the psychotherapeutic trade include:

- **_Active listening_**
- **_Insight, explanation of events_**: their origins, reasons, and significance
- **_Reminders_** of previous conclusions and stories
- **_Challenge old ideas and habits_**: Therapy that generally or completely lacks confrontation and accountability is ineffective.
- **_Encourage exploration and new modes of being and interacting_**
- **_Creating a safe container wherein the client can review the details, significance, and feelings associated with past events_**
- **_Modeling the expression of feeling_**
- **_Defining goals and helping the client focus on what is significant_**
- **_Correcting distortions of reality_**
- **_Asking patients to get in touch with and then express their feelings_**
- **_Support and encourage clients to take calculated risks for the sake of self-expansion_**
- **_Pointing out errors in logic_**
- **_Coaching patients in the proper and responsible use of emotional language_**
- **_Discouraging evasiveness; requiring accountability_**[350]

Creativity: All types of self-expression reinforce and validate the patient's sense of self. Creative self-expression, such as writing about thoughts and feelings about significant experiences, can reduce symptomatology in patients with rheumatoid arthritis and asthma.[351]

Experiential: Corrective experiences can be obtained in therapy, with friends and family, in integration groups, and during "experiential" retreats. **_Advantages_**: Experiential events orchestrated by therapists and various groups such as ManKind Project (mkp.org) and WomanWithin.org can rapidly facilitate personal growth while also providing an ongoing container and support system that encourages self-development rather than the ego-inflation that accompanies short-term events. **_Disadvantages_**: "Adventures" like driving across the nation or climbing a mountain are unconscious and largely impotent attempts at self-initiation; authentic initiation has always been supervised by community elders. However, once a well-founded initiation has taken place, preferably with an on-going community that facilitates continued refinement and self-exploration, then "adventures" can be undertaken consciously to maintain and reinforce the experience of autonomy and competent selfhood. Eventually, transformative and sustentative experiences can be integrated and created in the daily life experience so that dramatic adventures become unnecessary for the continued renewal and "recharging" of the self.

---

[346] Lee J. Expressing Your Anger Appropriately (Audio Cassette). Sounds True (June 1, 1990); ISBN: 1564550338

[347] Bradshaw J. Healing the Shame that Binds You [Audio Cassette (April 1990) Health Communications Audio; ISBN: 1558740430]

[348] Miller A. The Drama of the Gifted Child: The Search for the True Self. Basic Books: 1981

[349] Miller A. The truth will set you free: overcoming emotional blindness and finding your true adult self. New York: Basic Books; 2001

[350] Kottler JA. The Compleat Therapist. San Francisco; Jossey-Bass publishers; 1991, pages 134-174

[351] Smyth JM, Stone AA, Hurewitz A, Kaell A. Effects of writing about stressful experiences on symptom reduction in patients with asthma or rheumatoid arthritis: a randomized trial. _JAMA._ 1999 Apr 14;281(14):1304-9

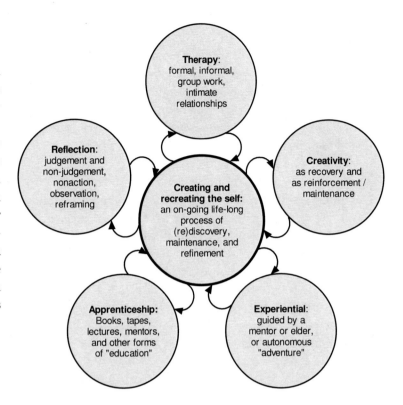

Creating and Re-creating the Self: An on-going process that involves various types of "therapy" such as healthy formal/informal interpersonal and group relationships, creative expression and exploration, the periodic infusion of new ideas from teachers and mentors, attendance in workshops and seminars (or other forms of on-going consciousness-raising), reflection, and the integration of transformative and sustentative significance into everyday life, in such a way that daily life itself becomes *therapeutic* and *affirmative*.

Sequence of events for effective, lasting, and authentic autonomization

The caterpillar does not blossom into a butterfly without spending time in its cocoon. The airborne seed descends into the earth for its nourishment before it sprouts and searches for the sun. Similarly, gratification of our ascentionist and impatient ego must be deferred for the sake of allowing the *time* and *descent* that provide the "grounding" that allows the formation of a solid foundation from which authentic growth can arise. The Western view of "personal development" idealizes a life course of constant ascension that is generally inconsistent with living in a real world fraught with imperfections; two of the major complications arising from such a perfectionistic paradigm are 1) that it causes people to feel anxious and ashamed when confronted with otherwise *normal* delays and failures, and 2) that it biases people into believing that improvement comes only from *advancement* rather than also from the *return* and short-term *regression* that are characteristic of nearly all authentic healing traditions. With modification of the stepwise model proposed by Bradshaw[352], here I propose the following sequence:

1. *Short-term behavior modification*: For people whose behavior is acutely dysfunctional or harmful to themselves or others, they must stop the "acting out" that is the symptom of the underlying emotional injury or schism. Accepting abuse—at work or home—is a form of **acting out** that perpetuates old wounds and saps the strength required for recovery.

2. *Emotional recovery*: Complete healing is only possible when consciously pursued, and conscious healing can only be pursued after one has become conscious of the wounds, injuries, absences, dynamics, and events that lead to the current state. This process of recovery is referred to mythologically as the "descent" or the time of "eating ashes" that is a recurrent theme in various fairy tales ("Cinderella" literally means "ash girl") and cultural-religious histories (such as Jesus' descent into the tomb).[353] The biggest blockades to this process are 1) the ego, which prefers to ascend and to deny intrapersonal "negativity"[354], and 2) the challenge in finding elders and mentors in a society that constantly perpetuates and encourages immaturity, materialism, and superficiality.[355] In the words of

---

[352] Bradshaw J. Healing the Shame that Binds You [Audio Cassette (April 1990) Health Communications Audio; ISBN: 1558740430]
[353] Bly R, Hillman J, Meade M. Men and the Life of Desire. Oral Tradition Archives. ISBN: 1880155001
[354] Robert Bly. The Human Shadow. Sound Horizons, New York 1991 [ISBN: 1879323001] and Bly R. A Little Book on the Human Shadow.[ISBN: 0062548476]
[355] Bly R. Where have all the parents gone? A talk on the Sibling Society. New York: Sound Horizons, 1996

famed psychologist Carl Gustav Jung, "One does not become enlightened by imagining figures of light, but by making the darkness *conscious*. The latter procedure, however, is disagreeable, and therefore unpopular." Recovery and the courage to relinquish the illusion of control must be an active process, often portrayed in ancient myths as "the hero's journey."[356]

3. *Long-term behavior modification and integration*: Insight allows for an illumination of the internal mental-emotional landscape, and effective insight must then be manifested externally by changes/modifications in behavior, habits, and interaction in the world. **Externalized behaviors simultaneously reflect and reinforce thoughts and feelings.** According to Grieneeks[357], patients (and their healthcare providers!) can "*think their way into new ways of acting*" and "*act their way into new ways of thinking*." Eventually, a consciously designed life can be created so that actions, interactions, thoughts, and feelings are melded together in such ways that everyday life itself becomes simultaneously *therapeutic, affirmative, sustentative*, and *empowering*. In this way, the person and his/her life are unified in such ways as to become self-perpetuating and self-sustaining cycles of ascents and descents, thought-feeling and action, reflection and courage, independence and interdependence—in sum: "a wheel rolling from its own center."[358] At this point the self is established, though it must be maintained and developed with the continuous application of conscious effort, reflection, and effective action.

4. *Metapersonal involvement in community, religion, spirituality, and the world*: Many people are tempted to move from a state of woundedness, relative incompleteness and the feelings of shame and impotence to a state of *perfection, enlightenment* and *omnipotence* without doing the requisite hard work that makes personal growth possible. People with unhealed emotional wounds often seek to camouflage those deficiencies by becoming pious and projecting an image of completeness and of "having it all figured out" and "having it all together"; religion and the acquisition of power are often misused for this purpose. Many people are successful in wearing this mask for many years; but its crumbling—often manifested as the "midlife crisis"—heralds an opportunity for personal growth if not medicated with anti-depressants, vacations, or the purchase of a sports car and flashy clothes.[359] The temptation to bypass Steps 2 [emotional recovery] and 3 [integration] and leapfrog to Step 4 [spirituality] should be resisted because the religion or spirituality is then used as a shield *against authenticity* and as a tool for illusory control. Religion can be misused in this way by providing an "identity" and sense of redemption for people with incompletely formed identities and for those with incompletely reconciled shadows and unresolved childhood-parental introjects.[360,361,362] Nietzsche's[363] response to this problem was to encourage self-knowledge and self-reconciliation as prerequisites to religious devotion, hence his admonition, "By all means love your neighbor as yourself – but *first* be such that you love yourself." Historical and recent events remind us of how religion can be misused for misanthropic ends.[364] What is commonly referred to as "spiritual development"—a level of resolution, reconciliation, and autonomy that allows for compassionate interdependence with people, the planet and the larger "world"—is synergistic with and can be supported by religion; but the latter is not a substitute for the former.[365,366] Religion and other forms of metapersonal involvement (e.g., community participation and social generosity) are *important* and *necessary* extensions of self-development. In order for personal development to blossom from the germ of necessary narcissism into its flower of functional completeness, it must eventually manifest in the larger community and the world.

---

[356] Campbell J with Moyers B. Joseph Campbell and the Power of Myth. The Hero's Adventure. Published in various years as book, audiotape, CD, and DVD.
[357] Keith Grieneeks PhD. "Psychological Assessment" taught in 1998 at Bastyr University.
[358] Friedrich Wilhelm Nietzsche, Walter Kaufmann (Translator). Thus Spoke Zarathustra. Penguin USA; 1978, page 27
[359] Robinson JC. Death of a Hero, Birth of a Soul: Answering the Call of Midlife. Council Oak Books, March 1997 ISBN: 1571780432
[360] Bradshaw J. Healing the Shame that Binds You [Audio Cassette (April 1990) Health Communications Audio; ISBN: 1558740430]
[361] Miller A. The Drama of the Gifted Child: The Search for the True Self. Basic Books; 1981
[362] Miller A. The truth will set you free: overcoming emotional blindness and finding your true adult self. New York: Basic Books; 2001
[363] Nietzsche N. Thus spoke Zarathustra. Read by Jon Cartwright and Alex Jennings. Naxos AudioBooks: http://www.naxosaudiobooks.com/nabusa/pages/432512.htm
[364] Bonhoeffer. (movie documentary by director/writer Martin Doblmeier) http://www.bonhoeffer.com/
[365] Lozoff B. It's a Meaningful Life : It Just Takes Practice. March 1, 2001. ISBN: 0140196242
[366] Bradshaw J. Healing the Shame that Binds You [Audio Cassette (April 1990) Health Communications Audio; ISBN: 1558740430]

5. <u>*Acceptance of mortality and death*</u>: No individual person or any system of thought, whether scientific or religious, can feign completeness without accounting for the end of life and incorporating this account into its overarching paradigm. The event is too significant, and the fear and concerns it provokes are too weighty to not be addressed directly and held in consciousness on a frequent basis. This topic is of practical importance, too, not only in our own lives and those of our friends and family, but also to the national healthcare system, which currently spends the bulk of its money and resources vainly attempting to preserve life in the last few years and months after which disease or age call unrelentingly for the end of life; perhaps if we as individuals and as part of the healthcare system could accept and deal with our own deaths, then we would not have to panic and participate in such superfluous expenditures of time, energy, emotion, and money when death arrives, either for our patients, our friends and family, or ourselves.

> **"The event of death is not a tragedy**—to rabbit, fox or man. But **the *concept* of death *is* a tragedy**, for man, and *indirectly* for poor fox, rabbit, bush, bird, just anything and everything in man's path."
>
> Pearce JC, Exploring the Crack in the Cosmic Egg. Washington Square Press; 1974, page 59

Proximal to the panic and aversion that characterizes the West's relationship to death is the "subclinical" panic and aversion that infiltrate the lives, practices, and policies that we experience every day. Surely, many unconscious events and subconscious influences contribute to the "lives of quiet desperation"[367] and "universal anxiety"[368] that subtly yet powerfully afflict most people; surely, lack of reconciliation with death is a major contributor. Especially in western cultures, death is commonly seen as some type of failure or shortcoming, either on behalf of the patient or his/her doctors, and the most common questions asked on the topic of death are "*how can this be avoided?*" before the event and "*who is to blame?*" after the event. Other cultures accept death as a natural part of life, and indeed, people are seen to have an obligation to die so that the next generations can have their turn in the cycle of life. Alternatives to western hysteria are founded on acceptance of death, and the prerequisites for the acceptance of death are 1) the dedication of sufficient time for its consideration (most people would rather watch a bad movie or attend spectator sports), 2) reframing the event in terms of its being a natural part of our lives, certainly nothing to be ashamed of (discussed below), 3) making necessary logistical preparations (e.g., writing of wills, providing for dependents, and other obvious technicalities), and 4) living as completely, consciously, compassionately, effectively, and authentically as possible so that remorse can be minimized, perhaps completely mitigated. Reframing the event of death begins with its description in general terms so that its enigma, from which its power over the hearts and minds of humanity is derived, can be deciphered and thus deflated. The main characteristics of death which precipitate its fear are 1) the unpredictability of its arrival, 2) the duration of the dying process, and 3) the quality of that process, for example whether it is painful or associated with or precipitated by severe illness or injury. The first characteristic of *timeliness*—the unpredictability of its arrival—stresses people because of their inadequate preparation and the feeling that they have only recently begun to live or have not quite yet begun to live their authentic lives. These concerns are allayed by preparation, both logistical and intrapersonal. Each of us has the responsibility to "become authentically whole" so that we do not inflict our incompleteness onto others, either directly through various forms of transference or deprivation[369] or indirectly though the more subtle means of politics and cultural mores. If a person can live with vitality, authenticity, compassion and effectiveness then little is left to want, and fears of death and its untimely arrival are diminished. The remaining variables are both controllable and uncontrollable; they are uncontrollable to the extent that we are all subject to chaos and accidents, whether in cars, planes, or bathtubs. *Duration* and *quality* are both controllable on an inpatient setting to the extent that palliative care[370] and voluntary euthanasia are sufficiently available.[371]

---

[367] Throreau HD, (Thomas O, ed). Walden and Civil Disobedience. New York: WW Norton and Company; 1966, page 5
[368] Becker E. The Denial of Death. New York: Free Press; 1973, pages 11 and 21
[369] Miller A. The Drama of the Gifted Child: The Search for the True Self. Basic Books: 1981
[370] "Failure to give an effective therapy to seriously ill patients, either adults or children, violates the core principles of both medicine and ethics... Therefore, in the patient's best interest, patients and parents/surrogates, have the right to request medical marijuana under certain circumstances and physicians have the duty to disclose medical marijuana as an option and prescribe it when appropriate." Clark PA. Medical marijuana: should minors have the same rights as adults? *Med Sci Monit*.2003;9:ET1-9 www.medscimonit.com/pub/vol_9/no_6/3640.pdf
[371] Steinbrook R. Medical marijuana, physician-assisted suicide, and the Controlled Substances Act. N Engl J Med. 2004 Sep 30;351(14):1380-3

"Once accepted, death is an integral component of every event, as the left hand to the right. The cultural death concept could only be instilled in a mind split from its own life flow."

Joseph Chilton Pearce[372]

Life can only be authentically and completely experienced after one has created an authentic self and has thereafter accepted life *as it is*. Since death is part of life, the full engagement of life requires *acceptance of* and *reconciliation with* death. Acceptance of death does not necessarily entail that life becomes permeated with nihilistic resignation; on the contrary, it infuses daily events with significance and makes all experiences rare and unique.

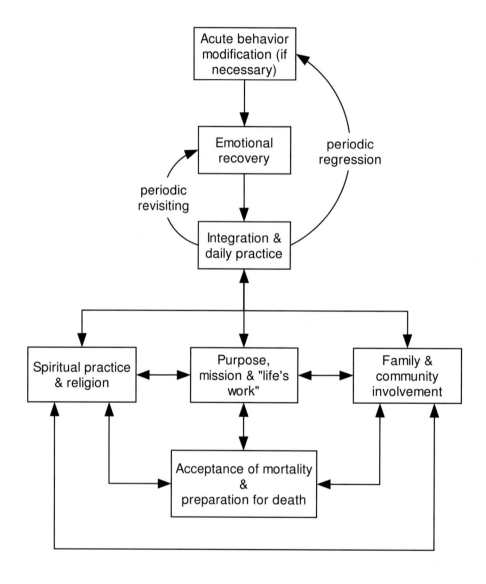

"They say there's no future for us. They're right, which is fine with us."

Rumi[373]

[372] Pearce JC. Exploring the Crack in the Cosmic Egg: Split Minds and Meta-Realities. New York: Washington Square Press; 1974, page 59
[373] Rumi in Barks C (translator). The Essential Rumi. HarperSanFransisco: 1995, page 2

Environmental Health: Tribute to Rachel Carson[374] and Walter Crinnion, ND[375]

> "Man's attitude toward nature is today critically important simply because we have now acquired a fateful power to alter and destroy nature. But man is a part of nature, and his war against nature is inevitably a war against himself."
>
> *Rachel Carson[376]*

Environmental exposures to chemicals and toxic substances:

Studies using blood tests and tissue samples from Americans across the nation have consistently shown that **all** Americans have toxic chemical **accumulation** whether or not they work in chemical factories or are exposed at home or work.[377,378] **The recent report from the CDC found toxic chemicals such as pesticides in all Americans, especially minorities, women, and children.**[379] Nearly all of these chemicals are known to contribute to health problems in humans—problems such as cancer, fatigue, poor memory, endocrinopathy, subfertility/infertility, Parkinson's disease, autoimmune diseases like lupus, and many other serious conditions. Therefore, *detoxification programs are a necessity—not a luxury*.

Examples of common toxicants found in Americans

Environmental pollutant (population frequency with elevated levels)	Biologic effects as quoted from HSDB: Hazardous Substances Data Bank. National Library of Medicine, NIH[380] or other reference as noted
DDE (99% of Americans):DDE is the main metabolite of DDT, a pesticide that was presumably banned in the US in 1972	<ul><li>DDT is known to be immunosuppressive in animals. A study published in 2004 showed that increasing levels of DDE in African-American male farmers in North Carolina correlated with a higher prevalence of antinuclear antibodies and up to 50% reductions in serum IgG.[381]</li><li>Other studies in humans have suggested an estrogenic or anti-androgenic effect.[382]</li><li>All women have evidence of DDT accumulation. Women with higher levels of DDT show pregnancy and childbirth complications and have higher rates of infant mortality.[383]</li></ul>
2,4-dichlorophenol (87% of Americans): pesticide	<ul><li>Human Toxicity Excerpts: same as for 2,5-dichlorophenol</li><li>In males, significant increases in relative risk ratios for lung cancer, rectal cancer, and soft tissue sarcomas were reported; in females, there were increases in the relative risk of cervical cancer.</li></ul>

---

[374] Rachel Carson. Silent Spring. Boston, Houghton Mifflin Company (2002). ISBN: 0395683297

[375] Crinnion W. Results of a Decade of Naturopathic Treatment for Environmental Illnesses: A Review of Clinical Records. *Journal of Naturopathic Medicine* vol. 7, # 2. p 21-27

[376] Rachel Carson Dies of Cancer; 'Silent Spring' Author Was 56. New York Times 1956. http://www.rachelcarson.org/ on August 1, 2004

[377] "The average concentration of 2,3,7,8-tetrachlorodibenzo-p-dioxin in the adipose tissue of the US population was 5.38 pg/g, increasing from 1.98 pg/g in children under 14 years of age to 9.40 pg/g in adults over 45." Orban JE, Stanley JS, Schwemberger JG, Remmers JC. Dioxins and dibenzofurans in adipose tissue of the general US population and selected subpopulations. *Am J Public Health* 1994 Mar;84(3):439-45

[378] "Although the use of HCB as a fungicide has virtually been eliminated, detectable levels of HCB are still found in nearly all people in the USA." Robinson PE, Leczynski BA, Kutz FW, Remmers JC. An evaluation of hexachlorobenzene body-burden levels in the general population of the USA. *IARC Sci Publ* 1986;(77):183-92

[379] "Many of the pesticides found in the test subjects have been linked to serious short- and long-term health effects including infertility, birth defects and childhood and adult cancers." http://www.panna.org/campaigns/docsTrespass/chemicalTrespass2004.dv.html July 25, 2004

[380] Primary source for this data is the Hazardous Substances Data Bank. National Library of Medicine, National Institutes of Health: http://toxnet.nlm.nih.gov/cgi-bin/sis/htmlgen?HSDB accessed on August 1, 2004

[381] Cooper GS, Martin SA, Longnecker MP, Sandler DP, Germolec DR. Associations between plasma DDE levels and immunologic measures in African-American farmers in North Carolina. *Environ Health Perspect.* 2004 Jul;112(10):1080-4

[382] Dalvie MA, Myers JE, Lou Thompson M, Dyer S, Robins TG, Omar S, Riebow J, Molekwa J, Kruger P, Millar R. The hormonal effects of long-term DDT exposure on malaria vector-control workers in Limpopo Province, South Africa. *Environ Res.* 2004 Sep;96(1):9-19

[383] "The findings strongly suggest that DDT use increases preterm births, which is a major contributor to infant mortality. If this association is causal, it should be included in any assessment of the costs and benefits of vector control with DDT." Longnecker MP, Klebanoff MA, Zhou H, Brock JW. Association between maternal serum concentration of the DDT metabolite DDE and preterm and small-for-gestational-age babies at birth. *Lancet.* 2001 Jul 14;358(9276):110-4

Examples of common toxicants found in Americans—*continued*

Environmental pollutant (population frequency)	*Biologic effects as quoted from HSDB: Hazardous Substances Data Bank. National Library of Medicine, NIH[384] or other reference as noted*
2,5-dichlorophenol (88% nationally and up to 96% in select children populations): Dichlorophenols can occur in tap water as a result of standard chlorination treatment; general population may be exposed to 2,5-dichlorophenol through oral consumption or dermal contact with chlorinated tap water; 2,5-Dichlorophenol was identified in 96% of the urine samples of children residing in Arkansas near a herbicide plant at concentrations of 4-1,200 ppb. The sole manufacturer for herbicide use is Sandoz (Clariant Corporation).	▪ Human Toxicity Excerpts: 1. Burning pain in mouth and throat. White necrotic lesions in mouth, esophagus, and stomach. Abdominal pain, vomiting ... and bloody diarrhea. 2. Pallor, sweating, weakness, headache, dizziness, tinnitus. 3. Shock: Weak irregular pulse, hypotension, shallow respirations, cyanosis, pallor, and a profound fall in body temperature. 4. Possibly fleeting excitement and confusion, followed by unconsciousness. ... 5. Stentorous breathing, mucous rales, rhonchi, frothing at nose and mouth and other signs of pulmonary edema are sometimes seen. Characteristic odor of phenol on the breath. 6. Scanty, dark-colored ... urine ... moderately severe renal insufficiency may appear. 7. Methemoglobinemia, Heinz body hemolytic anemia and hyperbilirubinemia have been reported. ... 8. Death from respiratory, circulatory or cardiac failure. 9. If spilled on skin, pain is followed promptly by numbness. The skin becomes blanched, and a dry opaque eschar forms over the burn. When the eschar sloughs off, a brown stain remains.
Chlorpyrifos (93% of Americans): insecticide used on corn and cotton and for termite control. Conservative estimates hold that 80% of the chlorpyrifos in the US was produced directly or indirectly by Dow Chemical Corporation.[385] This pesticide is routinely used in schools and is thus found in blood and tissue samples of nearly all American children.	▪ Toxic if inhaled, in contact with skin and if swallowed. ▪ All the organophosphorus insecticides have a cumulative effect by progressive inhibition of cholinesterase. ▪ The symptoms of chronic poisoning due to organophosphorus pesticides include headache, weakness, feeling of heaviness in head, decline of memory, quick onset of **fatigue**, **disturbed sleep**, loss of appetite, and loss of orientation. **Psychic disorders**, nystagmus, trembling of the hands and other nervous system disorders can be observed in certain cases. Sometimes neuritis and paralysis develop. Other manifestations of accumulation include **tension, anxiety, restlessness, insomnia, headache, emotional instability, fatigue**... ▪ Chlorpyrifos is a suspected endocrine disruptor.[386]
Mercury (8% of American women of reproductive age have mercury levels high enough to cause brain damage to their fetuses)	▪ Mercury is a well-known neurotoxin, with damaging and deadly effects in adults and especially in children. ▪ A recent study published by the American Medical Association[387] noted that "**Humans are exposed to methylmercury, a well-established neurotoxin**, through fish consumption. The fetus is most sensitive to the adverse effects of exposure. ... **approximately 8% of women had concentrations higher than the US EPA's recommended reference dose (5.8 microg/L),** below which exposures are considered to be without adverse effects." The most obvious interpretation of this data published in *JAMA* is that 8% of American women have mercury poisoning—poisoning in this case refers specifically to elevated blood levels of a known toxicant that consistently demonstrates adverse effects on human health. Logical deduction holds that such a high level of human poisoning should be unacceptable and should lead directly to legislative restrictions on corporate emissions to protect and salvage the health of the public.

[384] Primary source for this data is the Hazardous Substances Data Bank, National Institutes of Health: http://toxnet.nlm.nih.gov/cgi-bin/sis/htmlgen?HSDB accessed on August 1, 2004
[385] Kristin S. Schafer, Margaret Reeves, Skip Spitzer, Susan E. Kegley. Chemical Trespass: Pesticides in Our Bodies and Corporate Accountability. Pesticide Action Network North America. May 2004 Available at http://www.panna.org/campaigns/docsTrespass/chemicalTrespass2004.dv.html on August 1, 2004
[386] http://www.panna.org/resources/documents/factsChlorpyrifos.dv.html accessed August 1, 2004
[387] Schober SE, Sinks TH, Jones RL, Bolger PM, McDowell M, Osterloh J, Garrett ES, Canady RA, Dillon CF, Sun Y, Joseph CB, Mahaffey KR. Blood mercury levels in US children and women of childbearing age, 1999-2000. *JAMA*. 2003 Apr 2;289(13):1667-74

Though a detailed clinical explanation of detoxification procedures will not be included here (see Chapter 4 of *Integrative Rheumatology*), the general concepts for detoxification are as follows:

1. *Avoidance*: reduced exposure = reduced problem
   a. If there were less chemical pollution, then our environment would be less toxic and therefore we would not have such problems with environmental poisoning.
   b. Limit or eliminate exposure to paint fumes, car exhaust, new carpet, solvents, adhesives, artificial foods, synthetic chemical drugs, copier fumes, pesticides, herbicides, chemical fertilizers, etc.

2. *Depuration*: "The act or process of freeing from foreign or impure matter"[388]
   a. Exercise and sauna
   b. Bowel cleansing, fiber, probiotics, antibiotics, laxatives
   c. Liver and bile stimulators
   d. Cofactors for phase 1 oxidation and phase 2 conjugation
   e. Chelation for heavy metals
   f. Urine alkalinization

3. *Damage control*: managing the consequences of chemical and heavy metal toxicity
   a. Hormone replacement
   b. Antioxidant therapy
   c. Occupational and rehabilitative training
   d. Management of resultant diseases, particularly autoimmune diseases

4. *Political and social action*: Due in large part to corporate influence and government deregulation, environmental contamination with pesticides from American corporations has increased to such an extent over the past few decades that now all Americans show evidence of pesticide accumulation in their bodies. Failure to hold corporations to tight regulatory standards has jeopardized the future of humanity. Voter passivity combined with collusion between multinational corporations and government officials is the underlying problem. Political action is the solution. The past and recent history on this topic is clear and well documented for those who wish to access the facts.[389,390,391,392,393,394,395,396,397]

"Your lack of interest in the past, your lack of involvement, your unwillingness to develop coherent strategies, your unwillingness to challenge authority - these have created a vacuum in decision-making, that has been filled by professional groups with close relationships with the chemical industries..." *Samuel Epstein, M.D.* [398]

---

[388] Webster's 1913 Dictionary
[389] Robert Van den Bosch. The pesticide conspiracy. Garden City, NY: Doubleday, 1978. ISBN: 0385133847
[390] "Monsanto Corporation is widely known for its production of the herbicide Roundup and genetically engineered Roundup-ready crops… altered to survive a dousing of the toxic herbicide. …glyphosate, is known to cause eye soreness, headaches, diarrhea, and other flu-like symptoms, and has been linked to non-Hodgkin's lymphoma." Bush Names Former Monsanto Executive as EPA Deputy Administrator. Daily News Archive From March 29, 2001 http://www.beyondpesticides.org/NEWS/daily_news_archive/2001/03_29_01.htm accessed on August 1, 2004
[391] "They pointed to budgets cuts for research and enforcement, to steep declines in the number of cases filed against polluters, to efforts to relax portions of the Clean Air Act, to an acceleration of federal approvals for the spraying of restricted pesticides and more." Patricia Sullivan. Anne Gorsuch Burford, 62, Dies; Reagan EPA Director. *Washington Post*. Thursday, July 22, 2004; Page B06 http://www.washingtonpost.com/wp-dyn/articles/A3418-2004Jul21.html on August 2, 2004
[392] "In fact, amongst the crimes of Reagan and Bush which will go down in history are their emasculation of Federal regulatory apparatus... But in 1988, under the Bush administration, the EPA - illegally, in our view - revoked the Dellaney Law..." Samuel Epstein MD, 1993. Professor of Occupational and Environmental Medicine at the School of Public Health, University of Illinois Medical Center Chicago. http://www.converge.org.nz/pirm/pestican.htm accessed August 1, 2004
[393] "The Environmental Protection Agency will be free to approve pesticides without consulting wildlife agencies to determine if the chemical might harm plants and animals protected by the Endangered Species Act, according to new Bush administration rules…. It also is intended to head off future lawsuits, the officials said." Associated Press. Bush Eases Pesticide Laws http://www.cbsnews.com/stories/2004/07/29/tech/main633009.shtml accessed August 1, 2004
[394] "The new policy also could bolster pesticide makers' contention that federal labeling insulates them from suits alleging that their products cause illness or environmental damage, Olson says. 'It . . . could really be disastrous for public health.'" Bush Exempts Pesticide Companies from Lawsuits. Law on Pesticides Reinterpreted: Government Alters Policy in Effort to Protect Manufacturers. Peter Eisler. USA TODAY. October 6, 2003 http://www.organicconsumers.org/foodsafety/bushpesticides100703.cfm Accessed August 1, 2004
[395] WASHINGTON (AP) — "The Environmental Protection Agency will be free to approve pesticides without consulting wildlife agencies to determine if the chemical might harm plants and animals protected by the Endangered Species Act, according to new Bush administration rules." Bush eases pesticide reviews for endangered species. http://www.usatoday.com/news/washington/2004-07-29-epa-pesticides_x.htm?csp=34 accessed on August 1, 2004
[396] "It is simply intolerable that the EPA, instead of providing an example for open scientific discussion, has continuously violated key environmental legislation, stifling legitimate dissent. The failure of EPA to properly encourage and protect whistleblowing has undermined the ability of the EPA and state environmental agencies to enforce environmental laws." Letter to Carol Browner, Administrator U.S. Environmental Protection Agency from Stephen Kohn, Chair National Whistleblower Center Board of Directors dated March 23, 1999. Availble at http://www.whistleblowers.org/statements.htm on October 10, 2004
[397] "The Bush administration has imposed a gag order on the U.S. Environmental Protection Agency from publicly discussing perchlorate pollution, even as two new studies reveal high levels of the rocket-fuel component may be contaminating the nation's lettuce supply." Peter Waldman. Rocket Fuel Residues Found in Lettuce: Bush administration issues gag order on EPA discussions of possible rocket fuel tainted lettuce. *THE WALL STREET JOURNAL*. See http://www.organicconsumers.org/toxic/lettuce042903.cfm http://www.rhinoed.com/epa's_gag_order.htm http://www.peer.org/press/508.html http://yubanet.com/artman/publish/article_13637.shtml
[398] Samuel Epstein MD, 1993. Professor of Occupational and Environmental Medicine at the School of Public Health, University of Illinois Medical Center Chicago. http://www.converge.org.nz/pirm/pestican.htm accessed September 11, 2004

The recent findings that mercury poisoning can result from once-weekly consumption of tuna[399] and that the average American has 13 pesticides in his/her body[400] should be seen as an indication of how dangerously toxic our environment has become, largely due to irresponsible corporate and government policies that value profitability over sustainability. "Detoxification" is the micromanagment band-aid for the problem, and it is professionally and ethically inappropriate for healthcare professionals to limit their attention to clinical detoxification when the real problem is manifest on a much wider—national and worldwide—level. Focusing on *detoxification* only benefits a minute section of the population, namely those with the worst symptoms and/or the most money, leaving huge sections of the population untreated, unserved, and unrepresented.

Personal plans for taking responsible action and avoiding political/social passivity that has created the opportunity for regulatory failure and corporate exploitation of the environment that threatens the sustainability of the human species:

_____
_____
_____
_____
_____
_____
_____
_____
_____
_____
_____
_____
_____
_____
_____
_____
_____
_____
_____
_____
_____
_____
_____
_____
_____

[399] "The neurobehavioral performance of subjects who consumed tuna fish regularly was significantly worse on color word reaction time, digit symbol reaction time and finger tapping speed (FT)." Carta P, Flore C, Alinovi R, Ibba A, Tocco MG, Aru G, Carta R, Girei E, Mutti A, Lucchini R, Randaccio FS. Sub-clinical neurobehavioral abnormalities associated with low level of mercury exposure through fish consumption. *Neurotoxicology*. 2003 Aug;24(4-5):617-23

[400] "A comprehensive survey of more than 1,300 Americans has found traces of weed- and bug-killers in the bodies of everyone tested, …. The survey, conducted by the U.S. Centers for Disease Control and Prevention, found that the body of the average American contained 13 of these chemicals." Martin Millelstaedt. 13 pesticides in body of average American. *The Globe and Mail*. Friday, May 21, 2004 - Page A17   Available on-line at http://www.theglobeandmail.com/servlet/ArticleNews/TPStory/LAC/20040521/HPEST21/TPEnvironment/ on August 6, 2004

Overview of Toxicant Exposure and Detoxification/Depuration

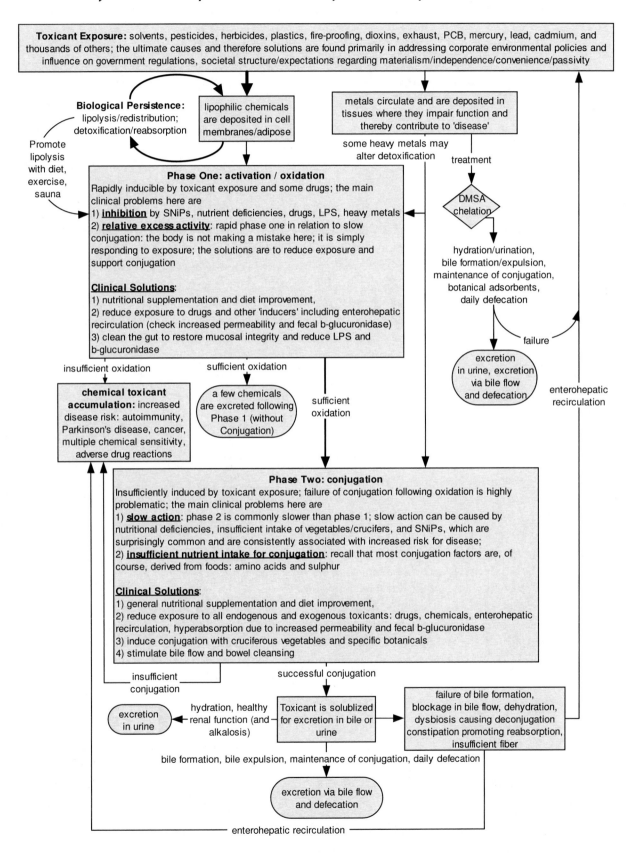

Avoid chemical medications and medical procedures to the greatest extent possible

"In 1983, 2876 people died from medication errors... By 1993, this number had risen to 7,391 - a 2.57-fold increase."[401]

"Recent estimates suggest that **each year more than 1 million patients are injured while in the hospital and approximately 180,000 die because of these injuries**. Furthermore, drug-related morbidity and mortality are common and are estimated to cost more than $136 billion a year."[402]

"There is a substantial amount of injury to patients from medical management, and many injuries are the result of substandard care."[403]

Adverse effects of chemical medications and surgical procedures are a major cause of death and disability in America.[406] **Choose your drugs carefully**, and whenever possible choose natural treatments, which are generally safer, less expensive, and more effective for the long-term management and prevention of chronic health problems.[407] Chemical-pharmaceutical drugs are a significant cause of death in America[408], perhaps because they generally function by inhibiting or blocking the body's natural processes, e.g., calcium channel *blockers*, serotonin *antagonists*[409], HMG-CoA reductase *inhibitors*[410], and angiotensin converting enzyme (ACE) *inhibitors*. Chemical drugs are often necessary for patients with acute and life-threatening problems; but on a more frequent basis they are unnecessary and/or obfuscate true healthcare. In contrast to the illusion of efficacy portrayed by the medical-pharmaceutical industry, it is commonly appreciated that most pharmaceutical drugs are only partially effective or are almost ineffective for the conditions they are claimed to treat, as demonstrated in the table.

Health condition[404]	Drug efficacy*
Asthma	60%
Cardiac arrhythmias	60%
Depression (SSRI)	62%
Diabetes	57%
Hepatitis C (HCV)	47%
Migraine (prophylaxis)	50%
Oncology	25%
Rheumatoid arthritis	50%
Schizophrenia[405]	60%

*** Drug efficacy percentage**: Note that a drug is generally considered "effective" if it elicits a "response"—most commonly *alleviation of symptoms* rather than *correction of the underlying problem*. However, from a naturopathic perspective, we would often consider this a treatment *failure* since the underlying problem has not been addressed, the patient's overall health has not been improved, the patient has been disempowered and is now reliant upon a drug treatment when other integrative options may have well produced better long-term results at lower cost and would have retained or established the patient's autonomy. For life-threatening emergencies and conditions for which there are no natural effective treatments, pharmaceutical drugs are, of course, valuable.

[401] Phillips DP, Christenfeld N, Glynn LM. Increase in US medication-error deaths between 1983 and 1993. *Lancet*. 1998 Feb 28;351(9103):643-4

[402] Holland EG, Degruy FV. Drug-induced disorders. *Am Fam Physician*. 1997 Nov 1;56(7):1781-8, 1791-2. http://aafp.org/afp/971101ap/holland.html

[403] Brennan TA, Leape LL, Laird NM, Hebert L, Localio AR, Lawthers AG, Newhouse JP, Weiler PC, Hiatt HH. Incidence of adverse events and negligence in hospitalized patients: results of the Harvard Medical Practice Study I. 1991. *Qual Saf Health Care*. 2004 Apr;13(2):145-51; discussion 151-2

[404] "A senior executive with Britain's biggest drugs company has admitted that most prescription medicines do not work on most people who take them. Allen Roses, worldwide vice-president of genetics at GlaxoSmithKline, said fewer than half of the patients prescribed some of the most expensive drugs actually derived any benefit from them." Connor S. Glaxo Chief: Our Drugs Do Not Work on Most Patients. Published on Monday, December 8, 2003 by the Independent/UK. Available on-line at http://www.commondreams.org/headlines03/1208-02.htm on July 4, 2004

[405] See also: Whitaker R. The case against antipsychotic drugs: a 50-year record of doing more harm than good. *Med Hypotheses*. 2004;62(1):5-13

[406] Holland EG, Degruy FV. Drug-induced disorders. *Am Fam Physician*. 1997 Nov 1;56(7):1781-8, 1791-2. http://aafp.org/afp/971101ap/holland.html

[407] Orme-Johnson DW, Herron RE. An innovative approach to reducing medical care utilization and expenditures. *Am J Manag Care* 1997 Jan;3(1):135-44

[408] Phillips DP, Christenfeld N, Glynn LM. Increase in US medication-error deaths between 1983 and 1993. *Lancet*. 1998 Feb 28;351(9103):643-4

[409] "Lotronex was an early example of a new class of drug for irritable bowel, the 5-HT3 antagonists... At least five people had died after taking the drug... There had been 49 cases of ischemic colitis and ... 34 patients had required admission to hospital and ten needed surgery." Horton R. Lotronex and the FDA: a fatal erosion of integrity. *Lancet*. 2001 May 19;357(9268):1544-5

[410] "FDA has received reports of 31 U.S. deaths due to severe rhabdomyolysis associated with use of Baycol, 12 of which involved concomitant gemfibrozil use." US Food and Drug Administration. Bayer voluntarily withdraws Baycol. http://www.fda.gov/bbs/topics/ANSWERS/2001/ANS01095.html March 14, 2004

Intestinal Health and Bowel Function:

We are not simply talking about the quantity of bowel movements (which must never average less than one per day, and should be at least 2 per day). Chronic constipation increases the circulation of toxins in the blood and may predispose to "minor" problems like fatigue and headaches while possibly contributing to an increased risk of colon cancer, too.[411] A study published in *The American Journal of Public Health* showed that women with mild constipation had an increased incidence of breast cancer.[412] More recently, research has shown and increased risk for Parkinson's disease in people with a life-long history of constipation; researchers have proposed that chronic constipation may contribute to neurodegeneration via toxins from the gut being absorbed into the vagus nerve and thereby transported directly into the central nervous system.[413,414] Additionally, we need to talk about the quality of digestion, absorption, and the presence or absence of harmful bacteria, yeasts, and parasites.

> "They also hypothesize that some yet undefined toxins break through the mucosal barrier of the intestine and are incorporated into the axon terminal of the vagus nerve and transported in a retrograde manner to the vagus nucleus [in the central nervous system]."
>
> Ueki A, Otsuka M. Life style risks of Parkinson's disease: association between decreased water intake and constipation. *J Neurol.* 2004 Oct;251 Suppl 7:vII18-23

- **Poor digestion—insufficient stomach acid or insufficient pancreatic enzymes**: For reasons that are not always clear, some people do not make enough stomach acid and pepsin[415] (this is especially true of older adults), and as a result they are not able to properly/completely digest their foods and they are less able to sterilize the foods that enter their intestines. As a result, people with low stomach acid often have nutritional deficiencies and excessive growth of bacteria and yeast in the intestines. It is well established that medications used to mask the symptom of gastrointestinal reflux disease by blocking acid production can cause such a severe degree of impaired digestion and bacterial overgrowth that vitamin deficiencies result.[416] Recent studies have shown that impairment of acid secretion by the use of antacid medications promotes bacterial overgrowth of the small bowel[417], exacerbation of nutritional deficiencies[418], and the development of food allergies (animal study).[419]

- **Malabsorption**: Once the food is digested, it must be absorbed into the body. Intestinal absorption can be assessed quantitatively with the lactulose-mannitol assay, as well as measuring fecal fat levels.

- **Harmful yeast, bacteria, and other parasites**: If you think parasites are rare, think again: in my own clinical practice I find patients with "parasites" (harmful gastrointestinal microorganisms) on a routine basis, even in patients with no specific or obvious gastrointestinal complaints such as nausea, constipation, or diarrhea. A study of 197 patients published in *American Journal of Gastroenterology*[420] reported that 48% of people with irritable bowel syndrome (which affects an estimated 35 million Americans—more than 10% of the US population) and other chronic digestive complaints were infected with the parasite *Giardia lamblia*—getting rid of the parasite cured 90% of patients. Gastrointestinal infections with microbes such as *Blastocystis hominis* and *Entamoeba histolytica* can produce manifestations similar to irritable bowel syndrome, rheumatoid arthritis, fibromyalgia, food allergy, endogenous mental depression, chronic fatigue syndrome, or multiple chemical sensitivity and can exacerbate HIV infection.[421] While many of these people could probably benefit from other treatments as well, in many cases the most important treatment that they needed was a specific treatment to get rid of their parasites—treating the cause of the problem is always the most effective way to obtain health improvements for people with specific health complaints. Presence of intestinal overgrowth of harmful yeast, bacteria, and other "parasites" is currently referred to as dysbiosis and was previously referred to in the medical literature as "autointoxication"[422]; this critically important topic is detailed in *Integrative Rheumatology* within the context of treating systemic autoimmune diseases such as rheumatoid arthritis.

[411] Talley NJ. Definitions, epidemiology, and impact of chronic constipation. *Rev Gastroenterol Disord.* 2004;4 Suppl 2:S3-S10 http://www.medreviews.com/pdfs/articles/RIGD_4Suppl2_S3.pdf on July 4, 2004

[412] Micozzi MS, Carter CL, Albanes D, Taylor PR, Licitra LM. Bowel function and breast cancer in US women. *Am J Public Health* 1989 Jan;79(1):73-5

[413] "The present results support previous findings that constipation precedes the onset of motor dysfunction in PD." Ueki A, Otsuka M. Life style risks of Parkinson's disease: association between decreased water intake and constipation. *J Neurol.* 2004 Oct;251 Suppl 7:vII18-23

[414] "...the disorder might originate outside of the central nervous system, caused by a yet unidentified pathogen that is capable of passing the mucosal barrier of the gastrointestinal tract and, via postganglionic enteric neurons, entering the central nervous system along unmyelinated praeganglionic fibers generated from the visceromotor projection cells of the vagus nerve." Braak H, Rub U, Gai WP, Del Tredici K. Idiopathic Parkinson's disease: possible routes by which vulnerable neuronal types may be subject to neuroinvasion by an unknown pathogen. *J Neural Transm.* 2003 May;110(5):517-36

[415] Williams RJ. Biochemical Individuality : The Basis for the Genetotrophic Concept. Austin/London: University of Texas Press, 1956 pages 60-61

[416] Ruscin JM, Page RL 2nd, Valuck RJ. Vitamin B(12) deficiency associated with histamine(2)-receptor antagonists and a proton-pump inhibitor. *Ann Pharmacother* 2002 May;36(5):812-6

[417] "CONCLUSION: Drug-induced hypochlorhydria causes high duodenal bacterial counts in the elderly but, in the short term, this bacterial overgrowth is not associated with malabsorption." Pereira SP, Gainsborough N, Dowling RH. Drug-induced hypochlorhydria causes high duodenal bacterial counts in the elderly. *Aliment Pharmacol Ther.* 1998 Jan;12(1):99-104

[418] Force RW, Nahata MC. Effect of histamine H2-receptor antagonists on vitamin B12 absorption. *Ann Pharmacother.* 1992 Oct;26(10):1283-6

[419] "CONCLUSIONS: When antacid medication impairs the gastric digestion, IgE synthesis toward novel dietary proteins is promoted, leading to food allergy." Untersmayr E, Scholl I, Swoboda I, Beil WJ, Forster-Waldl E, Walter F, Riemer A, Kraml G, Kinaciyan T, Spitzauer S, Boltz-Nitulescu G, Scheiner O, Jensen-Jarolim E. Antacid medication inhibits digestion of dietary proteins and causes food allergy: a fish allergy model in BALB/c mice. *J Allergy Clin Immunol.* 2003 Sep;112(3):616-23

[420] Galland L, Lee M. #170 High frequency of giardiasis in patients with chronic digestive complaints. *Am J Gastroenterol* 1989;84:1181

[421] Galland L. Intestinal protozoan infection is a common unsuspected cause of chronic illness. *J Advancement Med.* 1989;2: 539-552

[422] "The writer has observed numerous cases suffering from such conditions as chronic arthritis, hypertension, coronary disease, chronic abdominal distention, constipation, and colitis, in which the element of constipation, auto-intoxication and possible colon infection seemed to play a prominent part, which responded very satisfactorily to colonic irrigations after failure to improve following the usual forms of medical treatment." Snyder RG. The value of colonic irrigations in countering auto-intoxication of intestinal origin. *Medical Clinics of North America* 1939; May: 781-788

Preventive Health Screening: General Recommendations[423]

ALL GROUPS	• Height and weight • Blood pressure measurement at least every 1-2 years • Regular dental care • Periodic eye examinations • Dietary advice; smoking cessation; limited alcohol consumption
19 months to 6 years	• Eye examination for strabismus • Consider hearing tests; consider testing for lead poisoning
7-18 years: office visit every 3-5 years	• Physical examination for normal physical development • Screening assessments including: cholesterol, blood glucose, and electrolytes; kidney and liver function should be performed at least once • Sexually active adolescents should begin receiving periodic clinical examinations and blood tests to assess for STDs; additionally, sexually active females should receive a pelvic examination with Pap smear. Young men should be taught to perform self-testicular examination to assess for testicular cancer.
19-39 years: office visit every 2-3 years	• Screening assessments including: cholesterol, blood glucose, and electrolytes, kidney and liver function should be performed at least every five years; men and women with high risk for or concern about cardiovascular disease should consider comprehensive risk factor analysis. • Clinical skin examination • MEN: All men over age 30 years should be tested for iron overload[424]; monthly testicular self-examination, and annual clinical testicular examination. • WOMEN: monthly breast self-examination; clinical breast examination every 1-3 years beginning at age 30; annual pelvic examination with Pap smear beginning at age 18; consider assessments for developing osteoporosis.
40-64 years: office visits at least every 1-2 years	• Screening assessments including: cholesterol, blood glucose, and electrolytes, kidney and liver function; men and women with high risk for or concern about cardiovascular disease should consider comprehensive risk factor analysis • Clinical skin examination • Cardiac assessment (ECG) can be considered for persons 1) with two or more risk factors for cardiovascular disease, 2) who are considering exercise after a long period of sedentary lifestyle, and 3) whose health affects public safety (e.g., pilots, police officers). • Beginning at age 50: annual testing for blood in the feces (a sign of colon cancer); begin sigmoidoscopy every 5 years. • WOMEN: Annual clinical breast examination; mammogram every 1-2 years until age 50, annual mammogram between age 50-70 (controversial[425]: "…no large study has shown the effectiveness of breast cancer screening by either CBE or mammography for women whose risk of breast cancer is higher than the general population."[426]); assessments for osteoporosis are strongly recommended; thyroid hormone assessment every 5 years. • MEN: consider annual digital examination of the prostate and baseline PSA.

Wear your seatbelt. ♦ Don't smoke tobacco. ♦ Eat fruit/vegetables every day. ♦ Get regular exercise. ♦ Have people in your life who support you and listen to you. ♦ Get a massage. ♦ Practice safe sex. ♦ Brush and floss your teeth. ♦ Wear eye and ear protection when operating machinery. ♦ Get plenty of sleep.

[423] *American Family Physician* 1992; 45: 1917 et al; *Patient Care Archive* January 15, 1998; *Cleveland Clin J Med* 2000; 67: 521-30
[424] Baer DM, Simons JL, et al. Hemochromatosis screening in asymptomatic ambulatory men 30 years of age and older. *Am J Med.* 1995 May;98(5):464-8.
[425] Sellman S. Breast cancer awareness: seeing deception is your only protection. *Alternative Medicine* November 2001, pages 68-74
[426] *Patient Care Archive* January 15, 1998

Natural holistic healthcare empowers patients with the ability to understand and effectively participate in the course of their life and health

Allopathic chemical medicine	Paradigm	Holistic natural healthcare
• Doctor as "savior" and indifferent observer	*Role of the doctor*	• Doctor as "teacher" and active partner
• Helpless victim, disempowered, dependent	*Role of the patient*	• Active participant, empowered, responsible
• Illness is impossibly complex, and treating this with natural means is impossible • Treatment is simple: you have this disease, and you need to take a drug for every problem • You can change your diet and lifestyle but it won't make a big difference	*Nature of illness*	• Multifactorial: involving many different aspects of lifestyle, diet, exercise, genetic inheritance, and environment • Many causes allows for many different treatment approaches and different ways of attaining health • Illness can be modified via selective dietary and lifestyle changes and a custom-tailored treatment plan
• Disease-centered, drug-centered	*Viewpoint*	• Patient-centered, wellness-centered
• Drugs, including chemotherapy • Surgery • Radiation • Electroconvulsive treatment	*Treatment and options*	• Diet and lifestyle improvement • Relationship/emotional work • Botanical and nutritional medicines • Physical medicine, chiropractic, exercise • Acupuncture • *Selective* rather than *wanton* use of pharmaceuticals and medical procedures
• Symptom suppression • Drug side-effects are a significant cause of death in the US • Only *treats disease*, does not *promote health*; cannot reach optimal health by only reactively treating established health problems • Enormous expense	*Long-term outcome*	• Improved health • Potential for successful prevention, treatment or eradication of chronic disease • Potential to become optimally healthy • Proven cost-reduction
• For the most part, drugs are chemicals that have action in the body by interfering with the way that they body works • Every drug has side-effects, some of which can be life-threatening • Surgery causes irreparable changes to the body, many times for the worse. • Radiation and chemotherapy can cause a secondary cancer to develop	*Risks*	• Minimal, since most of the botanical treatments and all of the nutritional medicines have been a major part of the human diet for centuries/millennia and have proven safety • Most treatments are not fast-acting enough to be of value in traumatic or acutely life-threatening situations • Patients must be willing to discard unhealthy lifestyles.
• Allows a doctor to see many patients within a short amount of time, thus increasing profitability • Since drugs do not cure problems, patients must return for lifelong prescription renewals • Therapeutic passivity: minimal action or effort required by patient and doctor • The doctor holds all the power, and the patient is completely dependent on the doctor for treatment	*Benefits*	• Improved short-term and long-term health • Empowerment • Understanding of body processes as well as healthcare directions and goals • Options

Opposite Influences of Health Promotion vs. Disease Promotion: Concept Summary

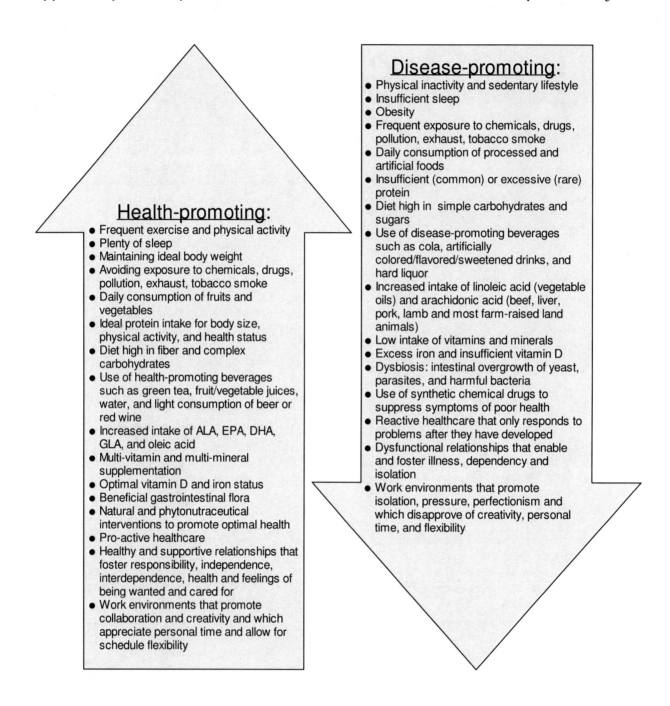

Health-promoting:
- Frequent exercise and physical activity
- Plenty of sleep
- Maintaining ideal body weight
- Avoiding exposure to chemicals, drugs, pollution, exhaust, tobacco smoke
- Daily consumption of fruits and vegetables
- Ideal protein intake for body size, physical activity, and health status
- Diet high in fiber and complex carbohydrates
- Use of health-promoting beverages such as green tea, fruit/vegetable juices, water, and light consumption of beer or red wine
- Increased intake of ALA, EPA, DHA, GLA, and oleic acid
- Multi-vitamin and multi-mineral supplementation
- Optimal vitamin D and iron status
- Beneficial gastrointestinal flora
- Natural and phytonutraceutical interventions to promote optimal health
- Pro-active healthcare
- Healthy and supportive relationships that foster responsibility, independence, interdependence, health and feelings of being wanted and cared for
- Work environments that promote collaboration and creativity and which appreciate personal time and allow for schedule flexibility

Disease-promoting:
- Physical inactivity and sedentary lifestyle
- Insufficient sleep
- Obesity
- Frequent exposure to chemicals, drugs, pollution, exhaust, tobacco smoke
- Daily consumption of processed and artificial foods
- Insufficient (common) or excessive (rare) protein
- Diet high in simple carbohydrates and sugars
- Use of disease-promoting beverages such as cola, artificially colored/flavored/sweetened drinks, and hard liquor
- Increased intake of linoleic acid (vegetable oils) and arachidonic acid (beef, liver, pork, lamb and most farm-raised land animals)
- Low intake of vitamins and minerals
- Excess iron and insufficient vitamin D
- Dysbiosis: intestinal overgrowth of yeast, parasites, and harmful bacteria
- Use of synthetic chemical drugs to suppress symptoms of poor health
- Reactive healthcare that only responds to problems after they have developed
- Dysfunctional relationships that enable and foster illness, dependency and isolation
- Work environments that promote isolation, pressure, perfectionism and which disapprove of creativity, personal time, and flexibility

Maximize factors that promote health ♦ Minimize factors that promote disease

Improved clinical outcomes will be attained when doctors and patients attend to both **prescription of health-promoting activities** and **proscription of disease-promoting activities**. Indeed, attention needs to be given to the **ratio** of these disparate and opposing forces, which ultimately influence genetic expression and physiologic function of many organ systems.

<u>Topics:</u>
- **Comprehensive Musculoskeletal Care**
    - Protect, prevent re-injury
    - Relative rest
    - Ice/heat, individualize treatment
    - Compression
    - Elevation, establish treatment program
    - Anti-inflammatory & analgesic treatments
    - Treat with physical/manual medicine
    - Uncover the underlying problem
    - Re-educate, rehabilitate, resourcefulness, return to active life, refer to specialist
    - Nutrition, diet, and supplements
- **Myofascial trigger points (MFTP): diagnosis and treatment**
- **Musculoskeletal Manipulative Manual Medicine**
- **Proprioceptive retraining/rehabilitation**
- **Reasons to avoid the use of nonsteroidal anti-inflammatory drugs (NSAIDs) and COX-2 inhibitors (coxibs)**

<u>Core Competencies</u>:
- Provide one example from each letter of the "p.r.i.c.e. a. t.u.r.n." and/or "b.e.n.d. s.t.e.m.s." mnemonic acronyms for holistic and comprehensive acute care for musculoskeletal injuries.
- List at least 6 of the 10 mechanisms of action of spinal manipulative therapy.
- List the two most common clinical findings associated with myofascial trigger points and describe appropriate physical/manual and nutritional treatments.
- Describe plans for low-back and ankle proprioceptive retraining/rehabilitation for a patient who has no exercise equipment.
- Describe the effects of stereotypic NSAIDs on chrondrocyte metabolism and the long-term effects on joint structure.
- Name four biochemical/physiologic mechanisms by which COX-2 inhibiting drugs predispose to cardiovascular death.
- By the time you finish reading this chapter (if necessary, see additional information in the chapter on *Therapeutics*), you should be able to describe 1) indications, 2) contraindications, 3) drug interactions, 4) adult doses and administration, and 5) molecular/physiologic mechanisms of action for each of the following commonly employed therapeutics:
    - Flaxseed oil: Alpha-linolenic acid (ALA)
    - Fish oil: Eicosapentaenoic acid (EPA), Docosahexaenoic acid (DHA)
    - Gamma-linolenic acid (GLA)
    - Vitamin D3: Cholecalciferol
    - Vitamin E: Alpha-tocopherol, beta-tocopherol, delta-tocopherol, gamma-tocopherol
    - Niacinamide
    - Glucosamine sulfate and Chondroitin Sulfate
    - Pancreatin, bromelain, papain, trypsin and alpha-chymotrypsin: "proteolytic enzymes" and "pancreatic enzymes"
    - *Zingiber officinale*, Ginger
    - *Uncaria tomentosa, Uncaria guianensis*, "Cat's claw", "una de gato"
    - *Salix alba*, Willow Bark
    - *Capsicum annuum, Capsicum frutescens*, Cayenne pepper, hot chili pepper
    - *Boswellia serrata*, Frankincense, Salai guggal
    - *Harpagophytum procumbens*, Devil's claw

Introduction: Whether dealing with a *recent and acutely painful injury* or an *exacerbation of a chronic injury or musculoskeletal disease,* all integrative clinicians are wise to have at their disposal a comprehensive protocol for the management of acute and subacute pain and exacerbations of joint inflammation. Incompetence in musculoskeletal medicine, which is common among allopathic physicians[1,2,3,4,5], forces doctors to overuse simplistic and dangerous treatments (i.e., pharmaceutical drugs) because they are unaware of better options.[6] Failure to understand how to arrive at an accurate diagnosis and subsequent failure to know how to manage musculoskeletal pain leaves doctors *and thus their patients* with no other option than the overuse of so-called anti-inflammatory drugs such as non-steroidal anti-inflammatory drugs (NSAIDs, such as aspirin), which kill at least 17,000 patients per year[7], and the cyclooxygenase-2 inhibiting drugs (COX-2 inhibitors, coxibs, such as Vioxx and Celebrex) which have killed tens of thousands of patients.[8,9,10,11]

Previously, any medical treatment that was non-surgical was commonly described as "conservative" simply because it was *non-invasive/non-surgical*. However, many so-called "conservative" drug treatments are dangerously lethal and expensive, as the coxibs, with their lethality and high costs, have demonstrated. Further, "conservative" has become such a confusing term in modern politics that even people who identify themselves as such are often at a loss for an accurate definition of the term. Thus, I have replaced the previous "holistic conservative care" with the current "comprehensive acute care" to indicate the consideration and selective implementation of the treatments described in this chapter.

Throughout the other chapters this text, when the phrase **"comprehensive musculoskeletal care"** is included in the list of therapeutic considerations, readers should understand that this implies these treatments for musculoskeletal problems *in addition to reestablishing the foundation for health,* which was detailed in Chapter 2. While all of us are familiar with the components of basic care for injuries—"*rice*": rest, ice, compression, elevation—I have expanded this list to include protect, prevent re-injury, relative rest, ice, individualize treatment, compression, elevation, establish treatment program, anti-inflammatory and analgesic treatments, treat with physical/manual medicine, uncover the underlying problem, re-educate, rehabilitate, retrain, resourcefulness, return to active life, and nutrition including diet and nutritional and botanical supplements. The mnemonic acronym spells "*price a turn*" which is cumbersome but perhaps easy to remember and therefore useful. The major point is to think outside of the "rice" box; as integrative clinicians, we have much more to offer our patients than rest, ice, compression, and elevation.

Understanding the shorthand that is conveyed by *comprehensive musculoskeletal care* is important for grasping the important differences between our medicine and the myopic and pharmacocentric allopathic approach. Whereas the allopathic approach stops with minimal disease treatment and provides essentially nothing in terms of prevention or comprehensive patient management—let alone promotion of optimal health—the holistic and integrative approach is centered on the *patient* and seeks to help him/her attain optimal health while being treated for the musculoskeletal disorder. We can and must help our patients attain optimal health while effectively managing their acute and chronic musculoskeletal problems.[12,13,14] **Indeed, since for many patients their only interaction with the healthcare system is when they are injured, we must seize upon this opportunity to enroll patients in preventive and pro-active healthcare.**

[1] Joy EA, Hala SV. Musculoskeletal Curricula in Medical Education: Filling In the Missing Pieces. *The Physician and Sportsmedicine.* 2004; 32: 42-45
[2] Freedman KB, Bernstein J. The adequacy of medical school education in musculoskeletal medicine. *J Bone Joint Surg Am.* 1998;80(10):1421-7
[3] Freedman KB, Bernstein J. Educational deficiencies in musculoskeletal medicine. *J Bone Joint Surg Am.* 2002;84-A(4):604-8
[4] Matzkin E, Smith ME, Freccero CD, Richardson AB. Adequacy of education in musculoskeletal medicine. *J Bone Joint Surg Am.* 2005 Feb;87-A(2):310-4
[5] Schmale GA. More evidence of educational inadequacies in musculoskeletal medicine. *Clin Orthop Relat Res.* 2005 Aug;(437):251-9
[6] Vasquez A. The Importance of Integrative Chiropractic Health Care in Treating Musculoskeletal Pain and Reducing the Nationwide Burden of Medical Expenses and Iatrogenic Injury and Death: Concise Review of Current Research and Implications for Clinical Practice and Healthcare Policy. *The Original Internist* 2005;12:159-182 www.optimalhealthresearch.com/monograph06
[7] Singh G. Recent considerations in nonsteroidal anti-inflammatory drug gastropathy. *Am J Med.* 1998;105(1B):31S-38S
[8] "The results from VIGOR showed that the relative risk of developing a confirmed adjudicated thrombotic cardiovascular event (myocardial infarction, unstable angina, cardiac thrombus, resuscitated cardiac arrest, sudden or unexplained death, ischemic stroke, and transient ischemic attacks) with rofecoxib treatment compared with naproxen was 2.38." Mukherjee D, Nissen SE, Topol EJ. Risk of cardiovascular events associated with selective COX-2 inhibitors. *JAMA.* 2001 Aug 22-29;286(8):954-9
[9] Topol EJ. Failing the public health--rofecoxib, Merck, and the FDA. *N Engl J Med.* 2004 Oct 21;351(17):1707-9
[10] Ray WA, Griffin MR, Stein CM. Cardiovascular toxicity of valdecoxib. *N Engl J Med.* 2004;351(26):2767
[11] "Patients in the clinical trial taking 400 mg. of Celebrex twice daily had a 3.4 times greater risk of CV events compared to placebo. For patients in the trial taking 200 mg. of Celebrex twice daily, the risk was 2.5 times greater. The average duration of treatment in the trial was 33 months." FDA Statement on the Halting of a Clinical Trial of the cox-2 Inhibitor Celebrex. http://www.fda.gov/bbs/topics/news/2004/NEW01144.html Available on January 4, 2005
[12] Vasquez A. Reducing Pain and Inflammation Naturally. Part 2: New Insights into Fatty Acid Supplementation and Its Effect on Eicosanoid Production and Genetic Expression. *Nutritional Perspectives* 2005; January: 5-16 www.optimalhealthresearch.com/part2
[13] Vasquez A. Reducing pain and inflammation naturally - Part 3: Improving overall health while safely and effectively treating musculoskeletal pain. *Nutritional Perspectives* 2005; 28: 34-38, 40-42 http://optimalhealthresearch.com/part3
[14] Vasquez A. The Importance of Integrative Chiropractic Health Care in Treating Musculoskeletal Pain and Reducing the Nationwide Burden of Medical Expenses and Iatrogenic Injury and Death: A Concise Review of Current Research and Implications for Clinical Practice and Healthcare Policy. *The Original Internist* 2005; 12(4): 159-182

Basic Treatment Concepts and Commonly Employed Therapeutics

The following pages summarize the basic therapeutics most commonly employed by integrative physicians in the treatment of acute and chronic musculoskeletal conditions. Knowledge of some of the clinical skills relied upon in orthopedics[15] is necessary when treating rheumatic musculoskeletal problems[16] because an acutely inflamed joint associated with a *chronic* and *systemic* disorder may need to be treated as if it were a *recent* and *focal* injury.

Orthopedics generally centers on the clinical management of 1) **acute injuries** (e.g., whiplash), 2) **chronic injuries** (tendonitis and myofasciitis/myofascitis), and 3) **congenital/developmental anomalies**, (odontoid hypoplasia and scoliosis). For most clinicians, management of congenital anomalies centers on accurate diagnosis and then either observation or appropriate referral. For the treatment of common acute and chronic injuries encountered in general practice, **comprehensive acute care** can include the facets described in the following section, modified for the clinical situation and individual patient. Although *rheumatology* is generally concerned with the treatment of *non-traumatic* disorders of an inflammatory or autoimmune nature, knowledge of orthopedics is necessary during the course of evaluating and treating patients with autoimmunity because differential diagnosis, qualification/quantification, and comanagement of joint disorders *within the same patient* are commonly necessary. For example, a patient with rheumatoid arthritis (chronic autoimmune disease) affecting the knees and hips may also develop carpal tunnel syndrome (orthopedic problem) and later present with neck pain and leg spasticity secondary to atlantoaxial instability (neuro-orthopedic emergency).

Generally, different types and locations of injuries can be treated from a common framework of interventions that are then customized for the three following primary considerations:

1) <u>Location</u>: The specific location and associated functional considerations, e.g., lower extremity injuries may require crutches while upper extremity injuries may benefit from a brace or sling,

2) <u>Tissue</u>: The type of tissue that is injured—i.e., muscle, cartilage, tendons, or ligaments—may respond to a particular nutritional and rehabilitative protocol,

3) <u>Patient</u>: The specific goals, needs, comorbidities, medications, occupation, recreational activities, age, and other characteristics of the individual patient.

Protect & prevent re-injury:

- **Avoid motions and activities that cause significant pain, as pain indicates that damaged/inflamed tissues are being stressed.** The goals are 1) to allow healing of injured tissues, and 2) to promote maximal physical restoration and functional ability. An excess of rest promotes functional disability, muscle atrophy, and psychological dysfunction (e.g., iatrogenic neurosis, inaccurate perception of patient being permanently damaged or defective, loss of confidence, loss of social contact [especially for children, and adults for whom physical activity is important]). Returning to activities and work too quickly may not allow time for sufficient healing and may thus promote re-injury, temporary exacerbation, progression from mild to severe injury, and/or progression to repetitive strain injury.
- **Use bracing, taping, bandages, wrapping, canes, crutches, and walkers as needed.**[17,18]

Relative rest:

- **"Relative rest" simply means to take time away from the activities that either promote additional injury or that unnecessarily drain energies which could otherwise be used for healing and recuperation.** For some patients, this means avoiding certain exercises during a workout, while for other patients this may mean using a crutch or taking days off from work.
- "Bed rest" is generally to be avoided since it promotes muscle atrophy, intraarticular adhesions, loss of neuromuscular coordination, constipation, and patients' assumption of the sick role.[19]

[15] Vasquez A. <u>Integrative Orthopedics</u>. http://optimalhealthresearch.com/orthopedics.html
[16] Vasquez A. <u>Integrative Rheumatology</u>. http://www.optimalhealthresearch.com/rheumatology.html
[17] Van Hook FW, Demonbreun D, Weiss BD. Ambulatory devices for chronic gait disorders in the elderly. *Am Fam Physician*. 2003 Apr 15;67(8):1717-24 http://www.aafp.org/afp/20030415/1717.html and http://www.aafp.org/afp/20030415/1717.pdf Accessed July 23, 2006
[18] Joyce BM, Kirby RL. Canes, crutches and walkers. *Am Fam Physician*. 1991 Feb;43(2):535-42
[19] "Glucose intolerance, anorexia, constipation, and pressure sores might develop. Central nervous system changes could affect balance and coordination and lead to increasing dependence on caregivers." Teasell R, Dittmer DK. Complications of immobilization and bed rest. Part 2: Other complications. *Can Fam Physician*. 1993 Jun;39:1440-2, 1445-6

Ice/heat:

- **First 48-72 hours after injury: Apply ice or cold pack for 10 minutes each 30-60 minutes for reduction in pain and inflammation.** The best protocol appears to be interrupted application of ice to maximize deep cooling of tissues while minimizing cold-induced damage to the skin.[20] Ice massage is more effective than stationary application of ice or an ice bag.[21] Intraarticular temperatures can be lowered with topical application of ice[22], and immersion into ice water appears to be the best method for reducing intraarticular temperature according to an animal study.[23] Greater skin thickness due to subcutaneous adipose increases the amount of time needed to achieve clinically significant cooling of deep tissues.[24] Avoid frostbite and cold injuries to skin and superficial nerves. Use caution in patients with decreased skin sensitivity, circulatory insufficiency, and/or suboptimal ability to follow directions and employ good judgment.
- **After 48-72 hours post-injury: Apply gentle heat as needed for the relief of pain and reduction in muscle spasm and to promote healing by increasing circulation.** Avoid heat injuries to skin. Use caution in patients with decreased skin sensitivity (e.g., diabetics and the elderly) or suboptimal ability to follow directions and employ good judgment.

Individualize treatment:

- **The cornerstone of effective holistic and integrative treatment is to design treatment plans that simultaneously 1) address "the problem" while also 2) improving the patient's overall health.** Often, serious and so-called "untreatable" diseases can be ameliorated or eradicated simply with general, non-specific, overall health improvement even when these conditions repeatedly fail to respond to specific "disease-targeting" medical treatments.

Compression:

- Snug bandages/wraps may help to reduce swelling and can provide support for injured tissues and weakened joints. Care must be utilized to avoid arterial, venous, or lymphatic obstruction.

Educate, establish treatment program, elevation:

- Educate patient about the injury.
- Educate patient about the need for appropriate follow-up office visits for reexamination, reassessment, and treatment.
- Estimate the amount of time during which most recovery will take place.
- Estimate the extent of return to previous status.
- Elevate the injured part to minimize swelling and edema.

Anti-inflammatory & analgesic treatments:

- Anti-inflammation versus hemostasis: Anti-inflammatory/analgesic medications that impair coagulation (e.g., aspirin) are contraindicated in patients with possible internal bleeding such as severe hematoma, hemarthrosis, spleen injury, intracranial hemorrhage (i.e., subdural hematoma following a whiplash injury) and in patients about to undergo surgery. Caution should also be used with nutritional/botanical supplements that have anti-coagulant effects, such as ginkgo biloba[25] and garlic.[26]
- Avoidance of pro-inflammatory foods: **Arachidonic acid** (high in cow's milk, beef, liver, pork, and lamb) is the direct precursor to pro-inflammatory prostaglandins and leukotrienes[27] and pain-

[20] "The evidence from this systematic review suggests that melting iced water applied through a wet towel for repeated periods of 10 minutes is most effective." MacAuley DC. Ice therapy: how good is the evidence? *Int J Sports Med.* 2001 Jul;22(5):379-84

[21] Zemke JE, Andersen JC, Guion WK, McMillan J, Joyner AB. Intramuscular temperature responses in the human leg to two forms of cryotherapy: ice massage and ice bag. *J Orthop Sports Phys Ther.* 1998 Apr;27(4):301-7

[22] Martin SS, Spindler KP, Tarter JW, Detwiler K, Petersen HA. Cryotherapy: an effective modality for decreasing intraarticular temperature after knee arthroscopy. *Am J Sports Med.* 2001 May-Jun;29(3):288-91

[23] Bocobo C, Fast A, Kingery W, Kaplan M. The effect of ice on intra-articular temperature in the knee of the dog. *Am J Phys Med Rehabil.* 1991 Aug;70(4):181-5

[24] Otte JW, Merrick MA, Ingersoll CD, Cordova ML. Subcutaneous adipose tissue thickness alters cooling time during cryotherapy. *Arch Phys Med Rehabil.* 2002 Nov;83(11):1501-5

[25] "A structured assessment of published case reports suggests a possible causal association between using ginkgo and bleeding events… Patients using ginkgo, particularly those with known bleeding risks, should be counseled about a possible increase in bleeding risk." Bent S, Goldberg H, Padula A, Avins AL. Spontaneous bleeding associated with ginkgo biloba: a case report and systematic review of the literature: a case report and systematic review of the literature. *J Gen Intern Med.* 2005 Jul;20(7):657-61 http://www.pubmedcentral.gov/picrender.fcgi?artid=1490168&blobtype=pdf

[26] "The authors report a case of spontaneous spinal epidural hematoma causing paraplegia secondary to a qualitative platelet disorder from excessive garlic ingestion." Rose KD, Croissant PD, Parliament CF, Levin MB. Spontaneous spinal epidural hematoma with associated platelet dysfunction from excessive garlic ingestion: a case report. *Neurosurgery.* 1990 May;26(5):880-2

[27] Vasquez A. Reducing Pain and Inflammation Naturally. Part 2: New Insights into Fatty Acid Supplementation and Its Effect on Eicosanoid Production and Genetic Expression. *Nutritional Perspectives* 2005; January: 5-16 www.optimalhealthresearch.com/part2

promoting isoprostanes.[28]   **Saturated fats** promote inflammation by activating/enabling pro-inflammatory Toll-like receptors, which are otherwise "specific" for inducing pro-inflammatory responses to microorganisms.[29]   Consumption of saturated fat in the form of **cream** creates marked oxidative stress and lipid peroxidation that lasts for at least 3 hours postprandially.[30]   **Corn oil** rapidly activates NF-kappaB (in hepatic Kupffer cells) for a pro-inflammatory effect[31]; similarly, consumption of PUFA and linoleic acid promotes intracellular antioxidant depletion and may thus promote oxidation-mediated inflammation via activation of NF-kappaB.   **Linoleic acid** causes intracellular oxidative stress and calcium influx and results in increased NF-kappaB-stimulated transcription of pro-inflammatory genes.[32]   **High glycemic foods** cause oxidative stress[33,34] and inflammation via activation of NF-kappaB and other mechanisms—e.g., *white bread causes inflammation*[35] as **does** *a high-fat high-carbohydrate fast-food breakfast.*[36]   **High glycemic foods** suppress immune function[37,38] and thus promote the development of infection/dysbiosis.[39]   Delivery of a **high carbohydrate load** to the gastrointestinal lumen promotes bacterial overgrowth[40,41], which is inherently pro-inflammatory[42,43] and which appears to be myalgenic in humans[44] at least in part due to the ability of endotoxin to impair muscle function.[45]   Overconsumption of high-carbohydrate low-phytonutrient **grains, potatoes, and manufactured foods** displaces phytonutrient-dense foods such as fruits, vegetables, nuts, seeds, and berries which contain more than 8,000 phytonutrients, many of which have antioxidant and thus anti-inflammatory actions.[46,47]

- Anti-inflammatory diet, the "supplemented Paleo-Mediterranean diet": The health-promoting diet of choice for the majority of people is a diet based on **abundant consumption of fruits, vegetables, seeds, nuts, berries, omega-3 and monounsaturated fatty acids, and lean sources of protein such as lean meats, fatty cold-water fish, soy and whey proteins.** This diet obviates overconsumption of chemical preservatives, artificial sweeteners, and carbohydrate-dominant foods such as candies, pastries, breads, potatoes, grains, and other foods with a high glycemic load and high glycemic index. This "Paleo-Mediterranean Diet" is a combination of the "Paleolithic" or "Paleo diet" and the well-known "Mediterranean diet", both of which are well described in peer-reviewed journals and the lay

[28] Evans AR, Junger H, Southall MD, Nicol GD, Sorkin LS, Broome JT, Bailey TW, Vasko MR. Isoprostanes, novel eicosanoids that produce nociception and sensitize rat sensory neurons. *J Pharmacol Exp Ther*. 2000 Jun;293(3):912-20

[29] Lee JY, Sohn KH, Rhee SH, Hwang D. Saturated fatty acids, but not unsaturated fatty acids, induce the expression of cyclooxygenase-2 mediated through Toll-like receptor 4. *J Biol Chem*. 2001 May 18;276(20):16683-9. Epub 2001 Mar 2 http://www.jbc.org/cgi/content/full/276/20/16683

[30] "CONCLUSIONS: Both fat and protein intakes stimulate ROS generation. The increase in ROS generation lasted 3 h after cream intake and 1 h after protein intake. Cream intake also caused a significant and prolonged increase in lipid peroxidation." Mohanty P, Ghanim H, Hamouda W, Aljada A, Garg R, Dandona P. Both lipid and protein intakes stimulate increased generation of reactive oxygen species by polymorphonuclear leukocytes and mononuclear cells. *Am J Clin Nutr*. 2002 Apr;75(4):767-72 http://www.ajcn.org/cgi/content/full/75/4/767

[31] Rusyn I, Bradham CA, Cohn L, Schoonhoven R, Swenberg JA, Brenner DA, Thurman RG. Corn oil rapidly activates nuclear factor-kappaB in hepatic Kupffer cells by oxidant-dependent mechanisms. *Carcinogenesis*. 1999 Nov;20(11):2095-100 http://carcin.oxfordjournals.org/cgi/content/full/20/11/2095

[32] "Exposing endothelial cells to 90 micromol linoleic acid/L for 6 h resulted in a significant increase in lipid hydroperoxides that coincided wih an increase in intracellular calcium concentrations." Hennig B, Toborek M, Joshi-Barve S, Barger SW, Barve S, Mattson MP, McClain CJ. Linoleic acid activates nuclear transcription factor-kappa B (NF-kappa B) and induces NF-kappa B-dependent transcription in cultured endothelial cells. *Am J Clin Nutr*. 1996 Mar;63(3):322-8 http://www.ajcn.org/cgi/reprint/63/3/322

[33] Mohanty P, Hamouda W, Garg R, Aljada A, Ghanim H, Dandona P. Glucose challenge stimulates reactive oxygen species (ROS) generation by leucocytes. *J Clin Endocrinol Metab*. 2000 Aug;85(8):2970-3 http://jcem.endojournals.org/cgi/content/full/85/8/2970   Glucose/carbohydrate and saturated fat consumption appear to be the two biggest offenders in the food-stimulated production of oxidative stress. The effect by protein is much less. "CONCLUSIONS: Both fat and protein intakes stimulate ROS generation. The increase in ROS generation lasted 3 h after cream intake and 1 h after protein intake. Cream intake also caused a significant and prolonged increase in lipid peroxidation." Mohanty P, Ghanim H, Hamouda W, Aljada A, Garg R, Dandona P. Both lipid and protein intakes stimulate increased generation of reactive oxygen species by polymorphonuclear leukocytes and mononuclear cells. *Am J Clin Nutr*. 2002 Apr;75(4):767-72 http://www.ajcn.org/cgi/content/full/75/4/767

[34] Koska J, Blazicek P, Marko M, Grna JD, Kvetnansky R, Vigas M. Insulin, catecholamines, glucose and antioxidant enzymes in oxidative damage during different loads in healthy humans. *Physiol Res*. 2000;49 Suppl 1:S95-100 http://www.biomed.cas.cz/physiolres/pdf/2000/49_S95.pdf

[35] "Conclusion - The present study shows that high GI carbohydrate, but not low GI carbohydrate, mediates an acute proinflammatory process as measured by NF-kappaB activity." Dickinson S, Hancock DP, Petocz P, Brand-Miller JC..High glycemic index carbohydrate mediates an acute proinflammatory process as measured by NF-kappaB activation. *Asia Pac J Clin Nutr*. 2005;14 Suppl:S120

[36] Aljada A, Mohanty P, Ghanim H, Abdo T, Tripathy D, Chaudhuri A, Dandona P. Increase in intranuclear nuclear factor kappaB and decrease in inhibitor kappaB in mononuclear cells after a mixed meal: evidence for a proinflammatory effect. *Am J Clin Nutr*. 2004 Apr;79(4):682-90 http://www.ajcn.org/cgi/content/full/79/4/682

[37] Sanchez A, Reeser JL, Lau HS, et al. Role of sugars in human neutrophilic phagocytosis. *Am J Clin Nutr*. 1973 Nov;26(11):1180-4

[38] "Postoperative infusion of carbohydrate solution leads to moderate fall in the serum concentration of inorganic phosphate. ... The hypophosphatemia was associated with significant reduction of neutrophil phagocytosis, intracellular killing, consumption of oxygen and generation of superoxide during phagocytosis." Rasmussen A, Segel E, Hessov I, Borregaard N. Reduced function of neutrophils during routine postoperative glucose infusion. *Acta Chir Scand*. 1988 Jul-Aug;154(7-8):429-33

[39] Vasquez A. Reducing Pain and Inflammation Naturally. Part 6: Nutritional and Botanical Treatments Against "Silent Infections" and Gastrointestinal Dysbiosis, Commonly Overlooked Causes of Neuromusculoskeletal Inflammation and Chronic Health Problems. *Nutritional Perspectives* 2006; January http://optimalhealthresearch.com/part6

[40] Ramakrishnan T, Stokes P. Beneficial effects of fasting and low carbohydrate diet in D-lactic acidosis associated with short-bowel syndrome. *JPEN J Parenter Enteral Nutr*. 1985 May-Jun;9(3):361-3

[41] Gottschall E. Breaking the Vicious Cycle: Intestinal Health Through Diet. Kirkton Press; Rev edition (August 1, 1994)

[42] Lin HC. Small intestinal bacterial overgrowth: a framework for understanding irritable bowel syndrome. *JAMA*. 2004 Aug 18;292(7):852-8

[43] Lichtman SN, Wang J, Sartor RB, Zhang C, Bender D, Dalldorf FG, Schwab JH. Reactivation of arthritis induced by small bowel bacterial overgrowth in rats: role of cytokines, bacteria, and bacterial polymers. *Infect Immun*. 1995 Jun;63(6):2295-301

[44] Pimentel M, et al. A link between irritable bowel syndrome and fibromyalgia may be related to findings on lactulose breath testing. *Ann Rheum Dis*. 2004 Apr;63(4):450-2

[45] Bundgaard H, Kjeldsen K, Suarez Krabbe K, van Hall G, Simonsen L, Qvist J, Hansen CM, Moller K, Fonsmark L, Lav Madsen P, Klarlund Pedersen B. Endotoxemia stimulates skeletal muscle Na+-K+-ATPase and raises blood lactate under aerobic conditions in humans. *Am J Physiol Heart Circ Physiol*. 2003 Mar;284(3):H1028-34. Epub 2002 Nov 21 http://ajpheart.physiology.org/cgi/reprint/284/3/H1028

[46] "We propose that the additive and synergistic effects of phytochemicals in fruit and vegetables are responsible for their potent antioxidant and anticancer activities, and that the benefit of a diet rich in fruit and vegetables is attributed to the complex mixture of phytochemicals present in whole foods." Liu RH. Health benefits of fruit and vegetables are from additive and synergistic combinations of phytochemicals. *Am J Clin Nutr*. 2003 Sep;78(3 Suppl):517S-520S

[47] **Seaman DR. The diet-induced proinflammatory state: a cause of chronic pain and other degenerative diseases?** *J Manipulative Physiol Ther*. 2002;25(3):168-79

press, particularly by Eaton[48], O'Keefe[49], and Cordain.[50] See Chapter 2 and my other reviews[51,52] for details. This diet is the most nutrient-dense diet available, and its benefits are further enhanced by supplementation with vitamins, minerals, probiotics, and the health-promoting polyunsaturated fatty acids: ALA, GLA, EPA, DHA.

- Anti-inflammatory nutrients and botanicals: Nutritional and botanical therapeutics are prescribed *per patient* and *per condition*. Select botanicals and therapeutics are detailed later in this book. Doses listed are for adults and can be reduced when numerous interventions are simultaneously applied.

  o Fish oil, EPA with DHA: Three grams per day (3,000 mg/d) of combined EPA and DHA is a reasonable therapeutic dose[53] and is generally supplied in one tablespoon of liquid fish oil. Encapsulated fish oil supplements vary tremendously in their concentration of EPA and DHA and may require consumption of as few as five and as many as 21 capsules per day to achieve the same dosage and of EPA+DHA found in one tablespoon of liquid fish oil; encapsulated fish oil supplements also generally cost significantly more than do liquid fish oil supplements. The routine use of eicosapentaenoic acid (EPA) and docosahexaenoic acid (DHA) supplements is justified based on the following data:

    1. Most modern diets are profoundly deficient in omega-3 fatty acids.[54]
    2. Dietary/supplemental intake of omega-3 fatty acids is a necessary prerequisite to reducing the pro-inflammatory effects of omega-6 fatty acids.[55]
    3. Supplementation with EPA+DHA is safe and reduces all-cause mortality.[56]
    4. Supplementation with EPA+DHA consistently provides clinically significant benefits in the treatment of a wide range of inflammatory conditions.[57,58]

  o GLA, Gamma-linolenic acid: Approximately 500 mg per day is the common anti-inflammatory dose[59] although higher doses of 2.8 grams per day have been safely used in patients with rheumatoid arthritis.[60] Except in the rarest circumstances (perhaps including temporal lobe epilepsy[61]), **GLA (most concentrated in borage oil) should always be co-administered with EPA and DHA (from fish oil) in order to obtain maximal benefit and avoid the increased formation of arachidonic acid that occurs when GLA is administered alone and the reduction in GLA/DGLA that occurs when fish oil is administered alone**. For more details on fatty acid metabolism, see the final chapter in this text on *Therapeutics* and the 2005 fatty acid review published by Vasquez available on-line.[62]

  o *Uncaria guianensis* and *Uncaria tomentosa* ("cat's claw", "una de gato"): A double-blind placebo-controlled study using 100 mg daily of highly-concentrated freeze-dried aqueous extract of *Uncaria tomentosa* found significant pain relief (reduction by 36%) and minimal adverse effects after 4 weeks of treatment in 30 male patients with osteoarthritis of the knees, a benefit mediated via antioxidant activities and inhibition of NF-kappaB, TNFα, COX-2, and PGE-2 production.[63] Inhibition of NF-kappaB and iNOS are of primary importance in the

[48] Eaton SB, Shostak M, Konner M. The Paleolithic Prescription: A program of diet & exercise and a design for living. New York: Harper & Row, 1988
[49] O'Keefe JH Jr, Cordain L. Cardiovascular disease resulting from a diet and lifestyle at odds with our Paleolithic genome: how to become a 21st-century hunter-gatherer. *Mayo Clin Proc.* 2004 Jan;79(1):101-8
[50] Cordain L. The Paleo Diet: Lose Weight and Get Healthy by Eating the Food You Were Designed to Eat. Indianapolis; John Wiley and Sons, 2002
[51] **Vasquez A. A Five-Part Nutritional Protocol that Produces Consistently Positive Results.** *Nutritional Wellness* **2005 September Available in the printed version and on-line at** http://www.nutritionalwellness.com/archives/2005/sep/09_vasquez.php **and** http://optimalhealthresearch.com/protocol
[52] **Vasquez A. Implementing the Five-Part Nutritional Wellness Protocol for the Treatment of Various Health Problems.** *Nutritional Wellness* **2005 November. Available on-line at** http://www.nutritionalwellness.com/archives/2005/nov/11_vasquez.php **and** http://optimalhealthresearch.com/protocol
[53] "...clinical benefits of the n-3 fatty acids were not apparent until they were consumed for > or =12 wk. It appears that a minimum daily dose of 3 g eicosapentaenoic and docosahexaenoic acids is necessary to derive the expected benefits [in patients with rheumatoid arthritis]." Kremer JM. n-3 fatty acid supplements in rheumatoid arthritis. *AmJ Clin Nutr.* 2000;71(1Suppl):349S-51S
[54] Simopoulos AP. Essential fatty acids in health and chronic disease. *Am J Clin Nutr.* 1999 Sep;70(3 Suppl):560S-569S
[55] Rubin D, Laposata M. Cellular interactions between n-6 and n-3 fatty acids: a mass analysis of fatty acid elongation/desaturation, distribution among complex lipids, and conversion to eicosanoids. *J Lipid Res.* 1992 Oct;33(10):1431-40.
[56] "The recent GISSI (Gruppo Italiano per lo Studio della Sopravvivenza nell'Infarto miocardico)-Prevention study of 11,324 patients showed a 45% decrease in risk of sudden cardiac death and a 20% reduction in all-cause mortality in the group taking 850 mg/d of omega-3 fatty acids. These fatty acids have potent anti-inflammatory effects and may also be antiatherogenic." O'Keefe JH Jr, Harris WS. From Inuit to implementation: omega-3 fatty acids come of age. *Mayo Clin Proc.* 2000 Jun;75(6):607-14
[57] "Many of the placebo-controlled trials of fish oil in chronic inflammatory diseases reveal significant benefit, including decreased disease activity and a lowered use of anti-inflammatory drugs." Simopoulos AP. Omega-3 fatty acids in inflammation and autoimmune diseases. *J Am Coll Nutr.* 2002 Dec;21(6):495-505
[58] **Vasquez A. Reducing Pain and Inflammation Naturally. Part 2: New Insights into Fatty Acid Supplementation and Its Effect on Eicosanoid Production and Genetic Expression.** *Nutritional Perspectives* **2005; January: 5-16** www.optimalhealthresearch.com/part2
[59] "Forty patients with rheumatoid arthritis and upper gastrointestinal lesions due to non-steroidal anti-inflammatory drugs entered a prospective 6-month double-blind placebo controlled study of dietary supplementation with gamma-linolenic acid 540 mg/day..." Brzeski M, Madhok R, Capell HA. Evening primrose oil in patients with rheumatoid arthritis and side-effects of non-steroidal anti-inflammatory drugs. *Br J Rheumatol.* 1991 Oct;30(5):370-2
[60] Zurier RB, Rossetti RG, Jacobson EW, DeMarco DM, Liu NY, Temming JE, White BM, Laposata M. gamma-Linolenic acid treatment of rheumatoid arthritis. A randomized, placebo-controlled trial. *Arthritis Rheum.* 1996 Nov;39(11):1808-17
[61] "Three long-stay, hospitalised schizophrenics who had failed to respond adequately to conventional drug therapy were treated with gamma-linolenic acid and linoleic acid in the form of evening primrose oil. They became substantially worse and electroencephalographic features of temporal lobe epilepsy became apparent." Vaddadi KS. The use of gamma-linolenic acid and linoleic acid to differentiate between temporal lobe epilepsy and schizophrenia. *Prostaglandins Med.* 1981 Apr;6(4):375-9
[62] Vasquez A. Reducing Pain and Inflammation Naturally. Part 2: New Insights into Fatty Acid Supplementation and Its Effect on Eicosanoid Production and Genetic Expression. *Nutritional Perspectives* 2005; January: 5-16 www.optimalhealthresearch.com/part2
[63] Piscoya J, Rodriguez Z, Bustamante SA, Okuhama NN, Miller MJ, Sandoval M. Efficacy and safety of freeze-dried cat's claw in osteoarthritis of the knee: mechanisms of action of the species Uncaria guianensis. *Inflamm Res.* 2001 Sep;50(9):442-8

treatment of inflammatory conditions.[64] A year-long study of patients with active rheumatoid arthritis (RA) treated with sulfasalazine or hydroxychloroquine showed "relative safety and modest benefit" of coadministration of *Uncaria tomentosa*.[65] Other studies with *Uncaria tomentosa* have shown enhancement of post-vaccination immunity[66] and enhancement of DNA repair in humans.[67] Traditional uses have included the use of the herb as a contraceptive and as treatment for gastrointestinal ulcers.

o <u>Topical application of *Capsicum annuum, Capsicum frutescens* (Cayenne pepper, hot chili pepper)</u>: Controlled clinical trials have conclusively demonstrated capsaicin's ability to deplete sensory fibers of substance P to thus reduce pain. Capsaicin also blocks transport and de-novo synthesis of substance P. Topical capsaicin alleviates diabetic neuropathy[68], chronic low back pain[69], chronic neck pain[70], osteoarthritis[71], rheumatoid arthritis[72], notalgia paresthetica[73], reflex sympathetic dystrophy[74], and cluster headache (intranasal application).[75,76,77] Doctors should experiment on themselves with this treatment before administering to patients in order to gain understanding by experience.

o *Boswellia serrata*: *Boswellia* inhibits 5-lipoxygenase[78] with no apparent effect on cyclooxygenase[79] and has been shown effective in the treatment of osteoarthritis of the knees[80] as well as asthma[81] and ulcerative colitis.[82] When used as monotherapy, the target dose is approximately 150 mg of boswellic acids TID.

o *Zingiber officinale* (Ginger): Ginger is a well known spice and food with a long history of use as an anti-inflammatory, anti-nausea, and gastroprotective agent[83], and components of ginger have been shown to reduce production of the leukotriene LTB4 by inhibiting 5-lipoxygenase and to reduce production of the prostaglandin PGE2 by inhibiting cyclooxygenase.[84,85] With its dual reduction in the formation of pro-inflammatory prostaglandins and leukotrienes, ginger has been shown to safely reduce nonspecific musculoskeletal pain[86,87] and to provide relief from osteoarthritis of the knees[88] and migraine headaches.[89] Ginger can be consumed somewhat liberally as a supplement or as whole food, and it is safe for use in pregnancy up to one gram per day.[90]

o *Harpagophytum procumbens* (Devil's claw): The safety and effectiveness of *Harpagophytum* has been established in patients with hip pain, low-back pain, and knee pain.[91,92,93] The

[64] Sandoval-Chacon M, Thompson JH, Zhang XJ, Liu X, Mannick EE, Sadowska-Krowicka H, Charbonnet RM, Clark DA, Miller MJ. Antiinflammatory actions of cat's claw: the role of NF-kappaB. *Aliment Pharmacol Ther*. 1998 Dec;12(12):1279-89

[65] "This small preliminary study demonstrates relative safety and modest benefit to the tender joint count of a highly purified extract from the pentacyclic chemotype of UT in patients with active RA taking sulfasalazine or hydroxychloroquine." Mur E, Hartig F, Eibl G, Schirmer M. Randomized double blind trial of an extract from the pentacyclic alkaloid-chemotype of uncaria tomentosa for the treatment of rheumatoid arthritis. *J Rheumatol*. 2002 Apr;29(4):678-81

[66] "...Uncaria tomentosa or Cat's Claw which is known to possess immune enhancing and antiinflammatory properties in animals. There were no toxic side effects observed as judged by medical examination, clinical chemistry and blood cell analysis. However, statistically significant immune enhancement for the individuals on C-Med-100 supplement was observed..." Lamm S, Sheng Y, Pero RW. Persistent response to pneumococcal vaccine in individuals supplemented with a novel water soluble extract of Uncaria tomentosa, C-Med-100. *Phytomedicine*. 2001;8(4):267-74

[67] Sheng Y, Li L, Holmgren K, Pero RW. DNA repair enhancement of aqueous extracts of Uncaria tomentosa in a human volunteer study. *Phytomedicine*. 2001 Jul;8(4):275-82

[68] "Study results suggest that topical capsaicin cream is safe and effective in treating painful diabetic neuropathy. "[No author listed] Treatment of painful diabetic neuropathy with topical capsaicin. A multicenter, double-blind, vehicle-controlled study. The Capsaicin Study Group. *Arch Intern Med*. 1991 Nov;151(11):2225-9

[69] Keitel W, Frerick H, Kuhn U, Schmidt U, Kuhlmann M, Bredehorst A. Capsicum pain plaster in chronic non-specific low back pain. *Arzneimittelforschung*. 2001 Nov;51(11):896-903

[70] Mathias BJ, Dillingham TR, Zeigler DN, Chang AS, Belandres PV. Topical capsaicin for chronic neck pain. A pilot study. *Am J Phys Med Rehabil* 1995 Jan-Feb;74(1):39-44

[71] McCarthy GM, McCarty DJ. Effect of topical capsaicin in the therapy of painful osteoarthritis of the hands. *J Rheumatol*. 1992;19(4):604-7

[72] Deal CL, Schnitzer TJ, Lipstein E, Seibold JR, Stevens RM, Levy MD, Albert D, Renold F. Treatment of arthritis with topical capsaicin: a double-blind trial. *Clin Ther*. 1991 May-Jun;13(3):383-95

[73] Leibsohn E. Treatment of notalgia paresthetica with capsaicin. *Cutis* 1992 May;49(5):335-6

[74] "Capsaicin is effective for psoriasis, pruritus, and cluster headache; it is often helpful for the itching and pain of postmastectomy pain syndrome, oral mucositis, cutaneous allergy, loin pain/hematuria syndrome, neck pain, amputation stump pain, and skin tumor; and it may be beneficial for neural dysfunction (detrusor hyperreflexia, reflex sympathetic dystrophy, and rhinopathy)." Hautkappe M, Roizen MF, Toledano A, Roth S, Jeffries JA, Ostermeier AM. Review of the effectiveness of capsaicin for painful cutaneous disorders and neural dysfunction. *Clin J Pain* 1998 Jun;14(2):97-106

[75] "Capsaicin application to human nasal mucosa was found to induce painful sensation, sneezing, and nasal secretion. All of these factors exhibit desensitization upon repeated applications." Sicuteri F, Fusco BM, Marabini S, Campagnolo V, Maggi CA, Geppetti P, Fanciullacci M. Beneficial effect of capsaicin application to the nasal mucosa in cluster headache. *Clin J Pain*. 1989;5(1):49-53

[76] "The efficacy of repeated nasal applications of capsaicin in cluster headache is congruent with previous reports on the therapeutic effect of capsaicin in other pain syndromes (post-herpetic neuralgia, diabetic neuropathy, trigeminal neuralgia) and supports the use of the drug to produce a selective analgesia." Fusco BM, Marabini S, Maggi CA, Fiore G, Geppetti P. Preventative effect of repeated nasal applications of capsaicin in cluster headache. *Pain*. 1994 Dec;59(3):321-5

[77] "These results indicate that intranasal capsaicin may provide a new therapeutic option for the treatment of this disease." Marks DR, Rapoport A, Padla D, Weeks R, Rosum R, Sheftell F, Arrowsmith F. A double-blind placebo-controlled trial of intranasal capsaicin for cluster headache. *Cephalalgia*. 1993 Apr;13(2):114-6

[78] Wildfeuer A, Neu IS, Safayhi H, Metzger G, Wehrmann M, Vogel U, Ammon HP. Effects of boswellic acids extracted from a herbal medicine on the biosynthesis of leukotrienes and the course of experimental autoimmune encephalomyelitis. *Arzneimittelforschung* 1998 Jun;48(6):668-74

[79] Safayhi H, Mack T, Sabieraj J, Anazodo MI, Subramanian LR, Ammon HP. Boswellic acids: novel, specific, nonredox inhibitors of 5-lipoxygenase. *J Pharmacol Exp Ther* 1992 Jun;261(3):1143-6

[80] Kimmatkar N, Thawani V, Hingorani L, Khiyani R. Efficacy and tolerability of Boswellia serrata extract in treatment of osteoarthritis of knee--a randomized double blind placebo controlled trial. *Phytomedicine*. 2003 Jan;10(1):3-7

[81] Gupta I, Gupta V, Parihar A, Gupta S, Ludtke R, Safayhi H, Ammon HP. Effects of Boswellia serrata gum resin in patients with bronchial asthma: results of a double-blind, placebo-controlled, 6-week clinical study. *Eur J Med Res*. 1998 Nov 17;3(11):511-4

[82] Gupta I, Parihar A, Malhotra P, Singh GB, Ludtke R, Safayhi H, Ammon HP. Effects of Boswellia serrata gum resin in patients with ulcerative colitis. *Eur J Med Res*. 1997 Jan;2(1):37-43

[83] Langner E, Greifenberg S, Gruenwald J. Ginger: history and use. *Adv Ther* 1998 Jan-Feb; 15(1):25-44

[84] Kiuchi F, Iwakami S, Shibuya M, Hanaoka F, Sankawa U. Inhibition of prostaglandin and leukotriene biosynthesis by gingerols and diarylheptanoids. *Chem Pharm Bull* (Tokyo) 1992 Feb;40(2):387-91

[85] Tjendraputra E, Tran VH, Liu-Brennan D, Roufogalis BD, Duke CC. Effect of ginger constituents and synthetic analogues on cyclooxygenase-2 enzyme in intact cells. *Bioorg Chem* 2001 Jun;29(3):156-63

[86] Srivastava KC, Mustafa T. Ginger (Zingiber officinale) in rheumatism and musculoskeletal disorders. *Med Hypotheses*. 1992 Dec;39(4):342-8

[87] Srivastava KC, Mustafa T. Ginger (Zingiber officinale) and rheumatic disorders. *Med Hypotheses*. 1989 May;29(1):25-8

[88] Altman RD, Marcussen KC. Effects of a ginger extract on knee pain in patients with osteoarthritis. *Arthritis Rheum*. 2001 Nov;44(11):2531-8

[89] Mustafa T, Srivastava KC. Ginger (Zingiber officinale) in migraine headache. *J Ethnopharmacol*. 1990 Jul;29(3):267-73

[90] "...oral ginger 1 g per day... No adverse effect of ginger on pregnancy outcome was detected." Vutyavanich T, Kraisarin T, Ruangsri R. Ginger for nausea and vomiting in pregnancy: randomized, double-masked, placebo-controlled trial. *Obstet Gynecol* 2001 Apr;97(4):577-82.

[91] Chrubasik S, Thanner J, Kunzel O, Conradt C, Black A, Pollak S. Comparison of outcome measures during treatment with the proprietary Harpagophytum extract doloteffin in patients with pain in the lower back, knee or hip. *Phytomedicine* 2002 Apr;9(3):181-94

mechanisms of action include weak anti-inflammatory effects and a stronger analgesic effect.[94,95] Research suggests that *Harpagophytum* is an effective analgesic for low back pain[96], including low back pain with radiculitis and radiculopathy.[97] The common dose is 60 mg harpagoside per day.[98]

- *Willow bark (Salix spp)*: In a double-blind placebo-controlled clinical trial in 210 patients with moderate/severe low-back pain (20% of patients had positive straight-leg raising test), willow bark extract showed a dose-dependent analgesic effect with benefits beginning in the first week of treatment.[99] In a head-to-head study of 228 patients comparing willow bark (standardized for 240 mg salicin) with Vioxx (rofecoxib), treatments were equally effective yet willow bark was safer and 40% less expensive.[100] Because willow bark's salicylates were the original source for the chemical manufacture of acetylsalicylic acid (aspirin), researchers and clinicians have erroneously mistaken willow bark to be synonymous with aspirin; this is certainly inaccurate and therefore clarification of willow's mechanism of action will be provided here. Aspirin has two primary effects via three primary mechanisms of action: 1) anticoagulant effects mediated by the acetylation and permanent inactivation of thromboxane-A synthase, which is the enzyme that makes the powerfully proaggregatory thromboxane-A2; 2) antiprostaglandin action via acetylation of both isoforms of cyclooxygenase (COX-1 inhibition 25-166x more than COX-2) with widespread inhibition of prostaglandin formation, and 3) antiprostaglandin formation via retroconversion of acetylsalicylate into salicylic acid which then inhibits cyclooxygenase-2 gene transcription.[101] Notice that the acetylation reactions are specific to aspirin and thus actions #1 and #2 are not seen with willow bark; whereas #3—inhibition of COX-2 transcription by salicylates—appears to be the major mechanism of action of willow bark extract. Proof of this principle is supported by the lack of adverse effects associated with willow bark in the research literature. If willow bark were pharmacodynamically synonymous with aspirin, then we would expect case reports of gastric ulceration, hemorrhage, and Reye's syndrome to permeate the research literature; this is not the case and therefore—**with the exception of possible allergic reactions in patients previously allergic/anaphylactic to aspirin and salicylates—extensive "warnings" on willow bark products[102] are unnecessary.**[103] Salicylates are widely present in fruits, vegetables, herbs and spices and are partly responsible for the anti-cancer, anti-inflammatory, and health-promoting benefits of fruit and vegetable consumption.[104,105] With willow bark products, the daily dose should not exceed 240 mg of salicin, and products should include other components of the whole plant. **Except for rare allergy in patients previously sensitized to aspirin or salicylates, no adverse effects are known**; to be on the medicolegal safe side, use is discouraged during pregnancy, before surgery, or when anti-coagulant medications are being used.

Treat with physical/manual medicine:

- <u>Massage</u>: Gentle massage provides comfort, increases circulation, reduces edema, and promotes healing. After the acute phase, deeper massage may help restore range of motion by breaking adhesions and reducing the feeling of vulnerability that may occur after injury. Research indicates

[92] Chantre P, Cappelaere A, Leblan D, Guedon D, Vandermander J, Fournie B. Efficacy and tolerance of Harpagophytum procumbens versus diacerhein in treatment of osteoarthritis. *Phytomedicine* 2000 Jun;7(3):177-83

[93] Leblan D, Chantre P, Fournie B. Harpagophytum procumbens in the treatment of knee and hip osteoarthritis. Four-month results of a prospective, multicenter, double-blind trial versus diacerhein. *Joint Bone Spine* 2000;67(5):462-7

[94] Whitehouse LW, Znamirowska M, Paul CJ. Devil's Claw (Harpagophytum procumbens): no evidence for anti-inflammatory activity in the treatment of arthritic disease. *Can Med Assoc J* 1983 Aug 1;129(3):249-51

[95] Moussard C, Alber D, Toubin MM, Thevenon N, Henry JC. A drug used in traditional medicine, harpagophytum procumbens: no evidence for NSAID-like effect on whole blood eicosanoid production in human. *Prostaglandins Leukot Essent Fatty Acids* 1992 Aug;46(4):283-6

[96] Chrubasik S, Model A, Black A, Pollak S. A randomized double-blind pilot study comparing Doloteffin and Vioxx in the treatment of low back pain. *Rheumatology* (Oxford). 2003 Jan;42(1):141-8

[97] "The majority of responders' were patients who had suffered less than 42 days of pain, and subgroup analyses suggested that the effect was confined to patients with more severe and radiating pain accompanied by neurological deficit... There was no evidence for Harpagophytum-related side-effects, except possibly for mild and infrequent gastrointestinal symptoms." Chrubasik S, Junck H, Breitschwerdt H, Conradt C, Zappe H. Effectiveness of Harpagophytum extract WS 1531 in the treatment of exacerbation of low back pain: a randomized, placebo-controlled, double-blind study. *Eur J Anaesthesiol* 1999 Feb;16(2):118-29

[98] "They took an 8-week course of Doloteffin at a dose providing 60 mg harpagoside per day... Doloteffin is well worth considering for osteoarthritic knee and hip pain and nonspecific low back pain." Chrubasik S, Thanner J, Kunzel O, Conradt C, Black A, Pollak S. Comparison of outcome measures during treatment with the proprietary Harpagophytum extract doloteffin in patients with pain in the lower back, knee or hip. *Phytomedicine* 2002 Apr;9(3):181-94

[99] Chrubasik S, Eisenberg E, Balan E, Weinberger T, Luzzati R, Conradt C. Treatment of low-back pain exacerbations with willow bark extract: a randomized double-blind study. *Am J Med.* 2000;109:9-14

[100] Chrubasik S, Kunzel O, Model A, Conradt C, Black A. Treatment of low-back pain with a herbal or synthetic anti-rheumatic: a randomized controlled study. Willow bark extract for low-back pain. *Rheumatology* (Oxford). 2001;40:1388-93

[101] Hare LG, Woodside JV, Young IS. Dietary salicylates. *J Clin Pathol* 2003 Sep;56(9):649-50 http://jcp.bmj.com/cgi/content/full/56/9/649

[102] Clauson KA, Santamarina ML, Buettner CM, Cauffield JS. Evaluation of Presence of Aspirin-Related Warnings with Willow Bark (July/August). *Ann Pharmacother.* 2005 May 31; [Epub ahead of print]

[103] **Vasquez A, Muanza DN. Evaluation of Presence of Aspirin-Related Warnings with Willow Bark: Comment on the Article by Clauson et al. *Ann Pharmacotherapy* 2005 Oct;39(10):1763**

[104] Lawrence JR, Peter R, Baxter GJ, Robson J, Graham AB, Paterson JR. Urinary excretion of salicyluric and salicylic acids by non-vegetarians, vegetarians, and patients taking low dose aspirin. *J Clin Pathol.* 2003 Sep;56(9):651-3

[105] Paterson JR, Lawrence JR. Salicylic acid: a link between aspirin, diet and the prevention of colorectal cancer. *QJM.* 2001 Aug;94(8):445-8 http://qjmed.oxfordjournals.org/cgi/content/full/94/8/445

that massage can reduce adolescent aggression[106], improve outcome in preterm infants[107], alleviate premenstrual syndrome[108], improve flexibility, reduce pain, increase serotonin and dopamine in patients with low back pain[109], and improve function and alleviate depression in patients with Parkinson's disease (Alexander technique).[110]

- <u>Joint mobilization and manipulation</u> as appropriate (after contraindications have been excluded) and to the level of patient comfort. Mechanisms of action are listed later in this section.
- <u>Treatment of associated muscle spasm and myofascial trigger points (MFTP)</u>: Such treatment can increase range of motion and decrease pain. See notes on the diagnosis and treatment of MFTP in the following section in this chapter.
- <u>Consider physiotherapy</u>: As appropriate.[111]

Uncover the underlying problem:

- In the case of most acute injuries, the underlying problem is often the injury itself. However, the physician must not be overly naïve and must conduct a thorough history and examination to assess for possible underlying pathologies that cause or contribute to the problem that "appears" to be injury related. Congenital anomalies, underlying pathology, previous injury, and psychoemotional disorders may have been present before the "injury."
  - o **In children and young adults, 5% of "sports-related" injuries are associated with preexisting infection, anomalies, or other conditions.**
  - o In adult women: "In three cases of carcinoma, the breast mass was not noticed until after the [auto accident] and was initially thought by the patient to have been caused by the trauma. **Indeed between 9% and 20% of women with breast cancer attribute their symptoms to previous trauma to the breast.**"[112]
- Look for leg length inequalities and biomechanical faults such as hyperpronation and pelvic torque.
- Assess and correct poor posture, poor ergonomics, lack of flexibility, muscle strength imbalances, and proprioceptive/coordination deficits.
- Patients may experience a reduction in pain—particularly low-back pain and osteoarthritis pain—when they eliminate coffee/caffeine, food allergens, and/or specific foods to which they are sensitive, most notably the *Solanaceae*/nightshade family—eggplant, tobacco, tomatoes, potatoes, and bell peppers. Foods in the *Solanaceae* family contain anti-acetylcholinesterases[113] that may effect increased synaptic transmission of afferent pain sensations, particularly via NMDA receptors.
- Correction of **diet-induced chronic metabolic acidosis** with the use of alkalinizing diets/supplements[114] can alleviate musculoskeletal pain[115], at least in part by raising/normalizing intracellular magnesium levels and by reducing intracellular calcium levels. Additional benefits of alkalinization include increased mineral retention, reduced bone resorption[116] and enhanced clearance of toxic xenobiotics[117], especially many pesticides and pharmacologic agents.

---

[106] Diego MA, Field T, Hernandez-Reif M, Shaw JA, Rothe EM, Castellanos D, Mesner L. Aggressive adolescents benefit from massage therapy. *Adolescence* 2002 Fall;37(147):597-607

[107] Mainous RO. Infant massage as a component of developmental care: past, present, and future. *Holist Nurs Pract* 2002 Oct;16(5):1-7

[108] Hernandez-Reif M, Martinez A, Field T, Quintero O, Hart S, Burman I. Premenstrual symptoms are relieved by massage therapy. *J Psychosom Obstet Gynaecol* 2000 Mar;21(1):9-15

[109] "RESULTS: By the end of the study, the massage therapy group, as compared to the relaxation group, reported experiencing less pain, depression, anxiety and improved sleep. They also showed improved trunk and pain flexion performance, and their serotonin and dopamine levels were higher." Hernandez-Reif M, Field T, Krasnegor J, Theakston H. Lower back pain is reduced and range of motion increased after massage therapy. *Int J Neurosci* 2001;106(3-4):131-45

[110] Stallibrass C, Sissons P, Chalmers C. Randomized controlled trial of the Alexander technique for idiopathic Parkinson's disease. *Clin Rehabil* 2002 Nov;16(7):695-708

[111] Download the free notes at http://www.OptimalHealthResearch.com/physiotherapy

[112] Seifert S. Medical Illness Simulating Trauma (MIST) syndrome: case reports and discussion of syndrome. *Fam Med* 1993 Apr;25(2):273-6

[113] Krasowski MD, McGehee DS, Moss J. Natural inhibitors of cholinesterases: implications for adverse drug reactions. *Can J Anaesth*. 1997 May;44(5 Pt 1):525-34 www.cja-jca.org/cgi/reprint/44/5/525.pdf

[114] For long-term out-patient treatment of patients who do not achieve alkalinization with diet alone, oral administration of potassium citrate and/or sodium bicarbonate can be implemented. See the following article for concepts: "Urine alkalinization is a treatment regimen that increases poison elimination by the administration of intravenous sodium bicarbonate to produce urine with a pH > or = 7.5." Proudfoot AT, Krenzelok EP, Vale JA. Position Paper on urine alkalinization. *J Toxicol Clin Toxicol*. 2004;42:1-26 http://www.eapcct.org/publicfile.php?folder=congress&file=PS_UrineAlkalinization.pdf Also see: Vormann J, Worlitschek M, Goedecke T, Silver B. Supplementation with alkaline minerals reduces symptoms in patients with chronic low back pain. *J Trace Elem Med Biol*. 2001;15(2-3):179-83 Also see: Maurer M, Riesen W, Muser J, Hulter HN, Krapf R. Neutralization of Western diet inhibits bone resorption independently of K intake and reduces cortisol secretion in humans. *Am J Physiol Renal Physiol*. 2003 Jan;284(1):F32-40. Epub 2002 Sep 24. http://ajprenal.physiology.org/cgi/content/full/284/1/F32

[115] "The results show that a disturbed acid-base balance may contribute to the symptoms of low back pain. The simple and safe addition of an alkaline multimineral preparate was able to reduce the pain symptoms in these patients with chronic low back pain." Vormann J, Worlitschek M, Goedecke T, Silver B. Supplementation with alkaline minerals reduces symptoms in patients with chronic low back pain. *J Trace Elem Med Biol*. 2001;15(2-3):179-83

[116] "In postmenopausal women, the oral administration of potassium bicarbonate at a dose sufficient to neutralize endogenous acid improves calcium and phosphorus balance, reduces bone resorption, and increases the rate of bone formation." Sebastian A, Harris ST, Ottaway JH, Todd KM, Morris RC Jr. Improved mineral balance and skeletal metabolism in postmenopausal women treated with potassium bicarbonate. *N Engl J Med*. 1994 Jun 23;330(25):1776-81 http://content.nejm.org/cgi/content/abstract/330/25/1776

[117] "Urine alkalinization is a treatment regimen that increases poison elimination by the administration of intravenous sodium bicarbonate to produce urine with a pH > or = 7.5." Proudfoot AT, Krenzelok EP, Vale JA. Position Paper on urine alkalinization. *J Toxicol Clin Toxicol*. 2004;42:1-26 http://www.eapcct.org/publicfile.php?folder=congress&file=PS_UrineAlkalinization.pdf

Re-educate, rehabilitate, resourcefulness, return to active life, reassure, referral:

- Educate patient on ways to avoid re-injury and to decrease likelihood of recurrence.
- Pre-rehabilitation assessment has three main goals: 1) identification of the type of injury, 2) quantification of the severity of the injury, and 3) determining the appropriate interventions.[118] Rehabilitative exercises **emphasizing strength, coordination, proprioception, range of motion, and functional utility** (appropriate per occupation and hobbies) should be employed.
- **Isometric exercises** can be used to maintain/increase muscle strength in patients for whom range-of-motion exercises are painful or contraindicated.
- **Work hardening** has been defined by the American Physical Therapy Association as "a highly structured goal-oriented, individualized treatment program designed to return a person to work. Work Hardening programs…use real or simulated work activities designed to restore physical, behavioral, and vocational functions."[119] Teperman[120] defined the specific goals of work hardening as:
  1. Improved lifting strength (loading and unloading) to/from different heights, including overhead,
  2. Improved carrying capacity (various objects, different distances, unilateral and bilateral),
  3. Improved functional tolerance (coordination and manipulation) at different levels,
  4. Improved cardiovascular endurance,
  5. Improved dexterity tasks (counting, weighing, sorting, packaging/unpacking)
  6. Improved biomechanics in any setting (work/leisure).
- **Work conditioning** has been defined as "a work-related, intensive, and goal-oriented treatment program specifically designed to restore an individual's systemic, neuromuscular (strength, endurance, flexibility, etc.) and cardiopulmonary function."[121] While overlaps exist between work hardening and work conditioning, and both are generally designed to "return the patient to work", work hardening is focused more on the performance of work-related tasks (task-oriented) while work conditioning tends to focus more on the cardiopulmonary and neuromuscular fitness of the patient (fitness-oriented).
- **Rehabilitation can become more than _restorative_; if the plan is comprehensive and it effects long-term improvements in overall health, then such a program can become _transformative_.** For example, while the oversimplified medical model as commonly practiced in HMO and PPO systems might describe a patient's problem as "low-back pain, refer for physiotherapy and begin Vioxx 25 mg b.i.d.", a more comprehensive assessment and treatment of the same patient's problem might be described as "low-back pain secondary to sedentary lifestyle, obesity, mild systemic inflammation, hypovitaminosis D, and proprioceptive deficits. Begin program of daily general exercise along with specific exercises for low-back region, low-carbohydrate diet to promote weight loss, balance training twice daily, begin supplementation with cholecalciferol 4,000 IU/d and fish oil 3 g/d." Notice that the typical allopathic plan _requires_ and _thus ensures_ patient passivity and does nothing to promote overall health, whereas the comprehensive natural/integrative plan is more in accord with current biomedical literature, requires active patient participation, offers the probability of improved overall health, and will reduce the severity and risk of present and future diseases, respectively.
- Patients should be supported in the tolerance of minor discomfort to avoid overuse of analgesics, to avoid an excessive reduction in activities, and to avoid playing the "sick role." While validating the patient's concerns, physicians should not encourage dysfunctional behavior or contribute to "iatrogenic neurosis."
- **Symptomatic treatment that provides no lasting benefit can foster therapeutic dependency and therapeutic passivity.** "Therapeutic dependency" describes the situation wherein the patient becomes dependent on treatment sessions for secondary gain of attention, physical contact, and time off from work (etc.) rather than focusing on the goal of getting as healthy as possible as quickly as possible. Therapeutic dependency is fostered by doctors who fail to educate patients to take an active role in their own care and by doctors who take on the role of "savior" rather than empowering patients to

[118] Geffen SJ. 3: Rehabilitation principles for treating chronic musculoskeletal injuries. _Med J Aust._ 2003 Mar 3;178(5):238-42
[119] American Physical Therapy Association, "Guidelines for Programs for Injured Workers" 1995. Quoted by Washington State Department of Labor and Industries. http://www.lni.wa.gov/Main/MostAskedQuestions/ClaimsIns/WorkHardFaq.asp. Accessed July 23, 2006
[120] Teperman LJ. Active functional restoration and work hardening program returns patient with 2½-year-old elbow fracture-dislocation to work after 6 months: a case report. _J Can Chiropr Assoc_ 2002; 46(1): 22-30 http://www.jcca-online.org/client/cca/JCCA.nsf/objects/Active+functional+restoration+elbow+fracture-dislocation/$file/5-Teperman.pdf
[121] Howar JM. Keys to Effective Work Hardening and Limited Duty Programs. http://www.eh.doe.gov/feosh/contacts/LimitedDutyPrograms.pdf Accessed July 23, 2006. Ironically, even though the third page of this presentation clearly shows the use of spinal manipulation, chiropractic doctors are notably absent from the list of "Industrial Rehab Specialists" having been usurped even by Occupational Nurses.

take effective action in improving their health. **Therapeutic passivity** is related to **therapeutic dependency** since patients who fail to take responsible action tend to become dependent on healthcare providers to "cure me" and "rescue me."

- While detailed individual descriptions of therapeutic exercise and rehabilitative programs are not the subject of this book, we can readily appreciate the many options that are available to us for the rehabilitation of injuries:
    - <u>Therapeutic exercise</u>: Includes strength training, stretching, improving endurance, and functional training specific to the patient's occupational or athletic activities. These can be tailored to great detail to the patient's condition and goals.[122]
    - <u>Proprioceptive retraining/rehabilitation</u>: As discussed later in this chapter, restoration and optimization of proprioceptive function and balance control is especially important for the long-term functional improvement of patients with proprioceptive deficits, commonly seen in patients with chronic low-back pain[123], neck pain[124], knee arthritis[125], and ankle instability.[126]
    - <u>Weight optimization</u>: For the majority of patients living in our society where obesity is pandemic, weight reduction is important not only to improve overall health and to reduce mechanical stresses on joints, but perhaps even more importantly to reduce the production of proinflammatory chemicals made in adipose tissue (adipokines) which promote an overall internal climate of pain and inflammation. Some patients may need to gain muscle strength to promote healing and avoid re-injury; this can generally be achieved with resistance training and increased protein consumption.
    - <u>Eicosanoid modulation</u>: Historically, the balance of omega-3 to omega-6 fatty acids in the human diet has been approximately 1:1 or 1:2.[127] Since omega-3 fatty acids are generally *anti-inflammatory* while omega-6 fatty acids are generally proinflammatory (with the exception of GLA/DGLA), the former *quantitative* dietary balance translated to a *qualitative* balance with regard to the body's inherent inflammatory tendency. Modern diets today, however, provide a ratio of 1:30, with anti-inflammatory omega-3 fatty acids greatly outnumbered by the proinflammatory omega-6 fatty acids. Thus, human physiology has been altered by the widespread consumption of a ***pro-inflammatory diet***.[128] Correction of this problem at the level of dietary intake rather than by the use of anti-inflammatory medications is essential for the attainment of health and the long-term relief of pain and inflammation.[129,130]
    - <u>Alkalinization</u>: The American/Western style of eating results in subclinical diet-induced pathogenic chronic metabolic acidosis[131] which can be corrected with a Paleo-Mediterranean diet[132] or alkalinizing supplements[133] for the alleviation of musculoskeletal pain in general and low-back pain in particular.[134]
    - <u>Analgesia</u>: Safe and effective natural means for achieving a timely reduction in pain include topical capsaicin, *Harpagophytum*, *Uncaria*, acupuncture, willow, and spinal manipulation.
    - <u>Anti-inflammatory botanicals and nutraceuticals</u>: Fish oil, GLA, vitamin E, *Boswellia*, willow bark, *Harpagophytum*, and *Zingiber* are just a few of the effective natural anti-inflammatory treatments available.

[122] Basmajian JV (ed). Therapeutic Exercise. Fourth Edition. Baltimore: Williams and Wilkins. 1984
[123] Newcomer KL, Jacobson TD, Gabriel DA, Larson DR, Brey RH, An KN. Muscle activation patterns in subjects with and without low back pain. *Arch Phys Med Rehabil*. 2002;83(6):816-21
[124] McPartland JM, Brodeur RR, Hallgren RC. Chronic neck pain, standing balance, and suboccipital muscle atrophy--a pilot study. *J Manipulative Physiol Ther*. 1997 Jan;20(1):24-9
[125] Callaghan MJ, Selfe J, Bagley PJ, Oldham JA. The Effects of Patellar Taping on Knee Joint Proprioception. *J Athl Train*. 2002 Mar;37(1):19-24
[126] Olmsted LC, Carcia CR, Hertel J, Shultz SJ. Efficacy of the Star Excursion Balance Tests in Detecting Reach Deficits in Subjects With Chronic Ankle Instability. *J Athl Train*. 2002 Dec;37(4):501-506
[127] Simopoulos AP. Essential fatty acids in health and chronic disease. *Am J Clin Nutr*. 1999 Sep;70(3 Suppl):560S-569S
[128] Seaman DR. The diet-induced proinflammatory state: a cause of chronic pain and other degenerative diseases? *J Manipulative Physiol Ther*. 2002;25(3):168-79
[129] Vasquez A. A Five-Part Nutritional Protocol that Produces Consistently Positive Results. *Nutritional Wellness* 2005 September Available in the printed version and on-line at http://www.nutritionalwellness.com/archives/2005/sep/09_vasquez.php and http://optimalhealthresearch.com/protocol
[130] Vasquez A. Dietary, Nutritional and Botanical Interventions to Reduce Pain and Inflammation. *Naturopathy Digest* 2006, March *Nutritional Wellness* 2006, March http://optimalhealthresearch.com/archives/anti-inflammation-nutrition
[131] "As a result, healthy adults consuming the standard US diet sustain a chronic, low-grade pathogenic metabolic acidosis that worsens with age as kidney function declines." Cordain L, Eaton SB, Sebastian A, Mann N, Lindeberg S, Watkins BA, O'Keefe JH, Brand-Miller J. Origins and evolution of the Western diet: health implications for the 21st century. *Am J Clin Nutr*. 2005 Feb;81(2):341-54 http://www.ajcn.org/cgi/content/full/81/2/341
[132] Cordain L. The Paleo Diet: Lose Weight and Get Healthy by Eating the Food You Were Designed to Eat. Indianapolis; John Wiley and Sons, 2002
[133] "An acidogenic Western diet results in mild metabolic acidosis in association with a state of cortisol excess, altered divalent ion metabolism, and increased bone resorptive indices." Maurer M, Riesen W, Muser J, Hulter HN, Krapf R. Neutralization of Western diet inhibits bone resorption independently of K intake and reduces cortisol secretion in humans. *Am J Physiol Renal Physiol*. 2003 Jan;284(1):F32-40. Epub 2002 Sep 24. http://ajprenal.physiology.org/cgi/content/full/284/1/F32
[134] "The results show that a disturbed acid-base balance may contribute to the symptoms of low back pain. The simple and safe addition of an alkaline multimineral preparate was able to reduce the pain symptoms in these patients with chronic low back pain." Vormann J, Worlitschek M, Goedecke T, Silver B. Supplementation with alkaline minerals reduces symptoms in patients with chronic low back pain. *J Trace Elem Med Biol*. 2001;15(2-3):179-83

o <u>Treatment of myofascial trigger points</u>: Since joint injuries and chronic pain—*especially in the neck, back and shoulder*—are commonly associated with trigger points[135], addressing this secondary and occult cause of pain is important to maximize pain relief and functional restoration.

o <u>Manipulation, mobilization, and massage</u>: Joint manipulation has numerous physiologic and anatomic effects, most of which are relevant for the alleviation of pain and improvement of joint function. These mechanisms include:

1. Releasing entrapped intraarticular menisci and synovial folds,
2. Acutely reducing intradiscal pressure, thus promoting replacement of decentralized disc material,
3. Stretching of deep periarticular muscles to break the cycle of chronic autonomous muscle contraction by lengthening the muscles and thereby releasing excessive actin-myosin binding,
4. Promoting restoration of proper kinesthesia and proprioception,
5. Promoting relaxation of paraspinal muscles by stretching facet joint capsules,
6. Promoting relaxation of paraspinal muscles via "postactivation depression", which is the temporary depletion of contractile neurotransmitters,
7. Temporarily elevating plasma beta-endorphin,
8. Temporarily enhancing phagocytic ability of neutrophils and monocytes,
9. Activating the diffuse descending pain inhibitory system located in the periaqueductal gray matter—this is an important aspect of nociceptive inhibition by intense sensory/mechanoreceptor stimulation, and
10. Improving neurotransmitter balance and reducing pain (soft-tissue manipulation).[136]

Additional details are provided in numerous published reviews and primary research[137,138,139,140,141,142,143] and by Leach[144], whose extensive description of the mechanisms of action of spinal manipulative therapy is unsurpassed. Given such a wide base of experimental and clinical support published in peer-reviewed journals and widely-available textbooks, denigrations directed toward spinal manipulation on the grounds that it is "unscientific" or "unsupported by research" are unfounded and are indicative of selective ignorance.[145]

o <u>Reassurance</u>: Education, explanation, reassurance, and support help to address the mental and emotional aspects of injury.

o **<u>Referral</u>: Patients with severe pain, serious conditions/complications, or documented noncompliance are excellent candidates for co-management or unidirectional referral.**

- Modify home and occupational workstations to minimize strain and stress on injured tissues. Educate patients to use tools, machines, props, and stepstools to work efficiently and to reduce unnecessary lifting and straining motions.

- Physical activities can be fully resumed when symptoms have decreased and when physical examination findings (e.g., reflexes, strength, range of motion, spinal segmental function, and trigger points) are within normal limits. Note that in many situations returning the patient to their previous duration, frequency, and intensity of activity may predispose to re-injury since the patient is re-entering the situation wherein the original injury occurred; therefore at least one of these lifestyle/occupational/recreational variables must change in order to reduce the likeliness of re-injury.

- Books, websites, and national/local support groups and organizations may be available for emotional, physical, psychological-emotional, and legal assistance.

[135] "The mean number of TrPs present on each neck pain patient was 4.3, of which 2.5 were latent and 1.8 were active TrPs. Control subjects also exhibited TrPs (mean: 2; SD: 0.8). All were latent TrPs." Fernandez-de-Las-Penas C, Alonso-Blanco C, Miangolarra JC. Myofascial trigger points in subjects presenting with mechanical neck pain: A blinded, controlled study. *Man Ther.* 2006 Jun 10
[136] "RESULTS: By the end of the study, the massage therapy group, as compared to the relaxation group, reported experiencing less pain, depression, anxiety and improved sleep. They also showed improved trunk and pain flexion performance, and their serotonin and dopamine levels were higher." Hernandez-Reif M, Field T, Krasnegor J, Theakston H. Lower back pain is reduced and range of motion increased after massage therapy. *Int J Neurosci* 2001;106(3-4):131-45
[137] Maigne JY, Vautravers P. Mechanism of action of spinal manipulative therapy. *Joint Bone Spine.* 2003;70(5):336-41
[138] Brennan PC, Triano JJ, McGregor M, Kokjohn K, Hondras MA, Brennan DC. Enhanced neutrophil respiratory burst as a biological marker for manipulation forces: duration of the effect and association with substance P and tumor necrosis factor. *J Manipulative Physiol Ther.* 1992 Feb;15(2):83-9
[139] Brennan PC, Kokjohn K, Kaltinger CJ, Lohr GE, Glendening C, Hondras MA, McGregor M, Triano JJ. Enhanced phagocytic cell respiratory burst induced by spinal manipulation: potential role of substance P. *J Manipulative Physiol Ther.* 1991 Sep;14(7):399-408
[140] Heikkila H, Johansson M, Wenngren BI. Effects of acupuncture, cervical manipulation and NSAID therapy on dizziness and impaired head repositioning of suspected cervical origin: a pilot study. *Man Ther.* 2000 Aug;5(3):151-7
[141] Rogers RG. The effects of spinal manipulation on cervical kinesthesia in patients with chronic neck pain: a pilot study. *J Manipulative Physiol Ther.* 1997;20(2):80-5
[142] Bergman, Peterson, Lawrence. Chiropractic Technique. New York: Churchill Livingstone 1993. An updated edition is now availabe published by Mosby.
[143] Herzog WH. Mechanical and physiological responses to spinal manipulative treatments. *JNMS: J Neuromusculoskeltal System* 1995; 3: 1-9
[144] Leach RA. (ed). The Chiropractic Theories: A Textbook of Scientific Research, Fourth Edition. Baltimore: Lippincott, Williams & Wilkins, 2004
[145] Vasquez A. The Science of Chiropractic and Spinal Manipulation, Part 2. http://www.mercola.com/2005/mar/12/chiropractic_spine.htm

Nutrition:

- **Protein**: In otherwise healthy patients with no liver, renal, or other metabolic disorders, ensure adequate intake of 0.5-0.9 gram of protein per pound of body weight.[146] Vegetarians may heal more slowly after injury than do omnivores; vegetarians and lacto-vegetarians undergoing cosmetic surgery reportedly have more complications and slower healing than do people eating a diet containing meat.[147] Additionally, low-protein diets have shown to reduce muscle mass and suppress immune function.[148] See the table below for protein intake recommendations:

Recommended <u>Grams of Protein</u> Per <u>Pound</u> of Body Weight Per Day[149]	
Infants and children ages 1-6 years[150]	0.68-0.45
RDA for sedentary adult and children ages 6-18 years[151]	0.4
Adult recreational exerciser	**0.5-0.75**
Adult competitive athlete	0.6-0.9
Adult building muscle mass	0.7-0.9
Dieting athlete	0.7-1.0
Growing teenage athlete	0.9-1.0
Pregnant women need additional protein	Add 15-30 grams/day[152]

- **Water**: Adequate intake of water is important to flush out wastes, toxins, and to prevent constipation. Eight glasses per day is the classic recommendation; however increased fluid intake is appropriate during exercise, heat exposure, stress, and to promote clearance of nitrogenous wastes and xenobiotics. Fluid restriction may be appropriate for persons with adrenal insufficiency to avoid hyponatremia and those with cardiovascular failure, fluid overload, or edema.

- **Vegetables, fruit, and fiber**: Whole foods provide micronutrients, natural anti-inflammatory components, and immune modulators; the fiber/phytonutrient content provides positive effects on gut flora while maintaining proper waste elimination and reducing straining (e.g., reduced need for the Valsalva maneuver).

- **Carbohydrates**: Carbohydrate intake should be adequate to supply energy-expenditure needs and to support healing but should not be excessive such as to unfavorably increase body weight during times of decreased physical activity. Preferred sources of carbohydrates are fruits and vegetables.

- **Identification and elimination of adverse food reactions**: Adverse food reactions—regardless of the underlying mechanism(s) or classification of allergy, intolerance, or sensitivity—can precipitate joint pain and inflammation[153,154,155,156,157,158,159] and a wide range of other health problems.

- **Supplementation with a high-potency broad-spectrum multivitamin and multimineral product**: This will help correct common nutritional deficiencies and support optimal healing. Certain nutrients such as vitamin C, zinc, and copper are commonly considered "specific" for promoting optimal repair of connective tissue.

- **Specific supplements/botanicals**: Supplementation is tailored to the type of tissue that has been injured, such as calcium, magnesium, and vitamins D and K for bone fractures, glucosamine sulfate and niacinamide for cartilage injuries, and proteolytic enzymes for muscle strains.
    - **Niacinamide**: The niacinamide form of vitamin B3 was proven effective against osteoarthritis by Kaufman more than 50 years ago.[160] Furthermore, Kaufman's documentation of an "anti-

[146] Nancy Clark, MS, RD. The Power of Protein. *The Physician and Sportsmedicine* 1996, volume 24, number 4. http://www.physsportsmed.com/issues/1996/04_96/protein.htm

[147] Vegetarians and healing. *JAMA* 1995; 273: 910

[148] Castaneda C, Charnley JM, Evans WJ, Crim MC. Elderly women accommodate to a low-protein diet with losses of body cell mass, muscle function, and immune response. *Am J Clin Nutr* 1995 Jul;62(1):30-9

[149] Slightly modified from Nancy Clark, MS, RD. The Power of Protein. *The Physician and Sportsmedicine* 1996, volume 24, number 4

[150] 1.5-1 g/kg/d (0.68-0.45 grams per pound of body weight. Younger people need proportionately more protein.) Brown ML (ed). Present Knowledge in Nutrition. Sixth Edition. Washington DC: International Life Sciences Institute Nutrition Foundation; 1990 page 68

[151] 0.83 g.kg-1.d-1 (equivalent to 0.37 grams per pound of body weight) "By use of an age-specific scoring system and the mean amino acid composition and digestibility of the US diet, this allowance became 0.83 g.kg-1.d-1 of mixed US dietary protein--a value similar to the previous RDA but derived in a different manner." Pellet PL. Protein requirements in humans. *Am J Clin Nutr.* 1990 May;51(5):723-37

[152] Weinsier RL, Morgan SL (eds). Fundamentals of Clinical Nutrition. St. Louis: Mosby, 1993 page 50

[153] Golding DN. Is there an allergic synovitis? *J R Soc Med.* 1990 May;83(5):312-4

[154] Panush RS. Food induced ("allergic") arthritis: clinical and serologic studies. *J Rheumatol.* 1990 Mar;17(3):291-4

[155] Pacor ML, Lunardi C, Di Lorenzo G, Biasi D, Corrocher R. Food allergy and seronegative arthritis: report of two cases. *Clin Rheumatol.* 2001;20(4):279-81

[156] Schrander JJ, Marcelis C, de Vries MP, van Santen-Hoeufft HM. Does food intolerance play a role in juvenile chronic arthritis? *Br J Rheumatol.* 1997 Aug;36(8):905-8

[157] van de Laar MA, van der Korst JK. Food intolerance in rheumatoid arthritis. I. A double blind, controlled trial of the clinical effects of elimination of milk allergens and azo dyes. *Ann Rheum Dis.* 1992 Mar;51(3):298-302

[158] Haugen MA, Kjeldsen-Kragh J, Forre O. A pilot study of the effect of an elemental diet in the management of rheumatoid arthritis. *Clin Exp Rheumatol.* 1994 May-Jun;12(3):275-9

[159] van de Laar MA, Aalbers M, Bruins FG, van Dinther-Janssen AC, van der Korst JK, Meijer CJ. Food intolerance in rheumatoid arthritis. II. *Ann Rheum Dis.* 1992 Mar;51(3):303-6

[160] Kaufman W. Niacinamide therapy for joint mobility. Therapeutic reversal of a common clinical manifestation of the "normal" aging process. *Conn State Med J* 1953;17:584-591

aging" effect of vitamin supplementation in general and niacinamide therapy in particular[161] is consistent with recent experimental data demonstrating rapid reversion of aging phenotypes by niacinamide through modulation of histone acetylation.[162] A recent double-blind placebo-controlled repeat study found that niacinamide therapy improved joint mobility, reduced objective inflammation as assessed by ESR, reduced the impact of the arthritis on the activities of daily living, and allowed a reduction in analgesic/anti-inflammatory medication use.[163] While the mechanism of action is probably multifaceted, inhibition of joint-destroying nitric oxide appears to be an important benefit.[164] The standard dose of 500 mg given orally 6 times per day is more effective than 1,000 mg 3 times per day. Hepatic dysfunction is rare when daily doses are kept below 3,000 mg per day, yet Gaby[165] suggests measurement of liver enzymes after 3 months of treatment and yearly thereafter. Antirheumatic benefit is generally significant following 2-6 weeks of treatment, and patients may also notice an anxiolytic benefit, possibly mediated by the binding of niacinamide to GABA/benzodiazepine receptors.[166]

- o **Glucosamine sulfate and chondroitin sulfate:** Glucosamine and chondroitin are the "building blocks" from which cartilage is built and oral supplementation is intended to enhance cartilage anabolism and to thus counteract the enhanced cartilage catabolism seen in destructive arthritic processes.[167] Clinical trials with glucosamine and chondroitin sulfates have shown consistently positive results in clinical trials involving patients with osteoarthritis of the hands, hips, knees, temporomandibular joint, and low-back.[168,169,170,171,172,173,174] For example, glucosamine sulfate was superior to placebo for pain reduction and preservation of joint space in a 3-year clinical trial in patients with knee osteoarthritis.[175] Arguments against the use of glucosamine due to inflated concern about inefficacy or exacerbation of diabetes[176] are without scientific merit[177,178] as evidenced by a 90-day trial of diabetic patients consuming 1500 mg of glucosamine hydrochloride with 1200 mg of chondroitin sulfate which showed no significant alterations in serum glucose or hemoglobin A1c[179] and by the previously cited 3-year study which found significant clinical benefit and no adverse effects on glucose homeostasis.[180] The adult dose of glucosamine sulfate is generally 1500-2000 mg per day in divided doses, and the dose of chondroitin sulfate is approximately 1000 mg daily; these treatments can be used singly, in combination, and with other treatments. Both treatments are safe for multiyear use, and rare adverse effects include allergy and nonpathologic gastrointestinal upset. Clinical benefit is generally significant following 4-6 weeks of treatment and is maintained for the duration of treatment. In contrast to coxib and other mislabeled "anti-inflammatory" drugs that consistently elevate the incidence of cardiovascular disease, death, and other adverse effects[181,182,183,184,185], supplementation with

[161] Kaufman W. The use of vitamin therapy to reverse certain concomitants of aging. *J Am Geriatr Soc* 1955;3:927-936
[162] Matuoka K, Chen KY, Takenawa T. Rapid reversion of aging phenotypes by nicotinamide through possible modulation of histone acetylation. *Cell Mol Life Sci.* 2001;58(14):2108-16
[163] Jonas WB, Rapoza CP, Blair WF. The effect of niacinamide on osteoarthritis: a pilot study. *Inflamm Res* 1996 Jul;45(7):330-4
[164] McCarty MF, Russell AL. Niacinamide therapy for osteoarthritis--does it inhibit nitric oxide synthase induction by interleukin 1 in chondrocytes? *Med Hypotheses.* 1999;53(4):350-60
[165] Gaby AR. Literature review and commentary: Niacinamide for osteoarthritis. *Townsend Letter for Doctors and Patients.* 2002: May; 32
[166] Mohler H, Polc P, Cumin R, Pieri L, Kettler R. Nicotinamide is a brain constituent with benzodiazepine-like actions. *Nature.* 1979; 278(5704): 563-5
[167] Vidal y Plana RR, Bizzarri D, Rovati AL. Articular cartilage pharmacology: I. In vitro studies on glucosamine and non steroidal antiinflammatory drugs. *Pharmacol Res Commun.* 1978 Jun;10(6):557-69
[168] "...patients taking GS had a significantly greater decrease in TMJ pain with function, effect of pain, and acetaminophen used between Day 90 and 120 compared with patients taking ibuprofen." Thie NM, Prasad NG, Major PW. Evaluation of glucosamine sulfate compared to ibuprofen for the treatment of temporomandibular joint osteoarthritis: a randomized double blind controlled 3 month clinical trial. *J Rheumatol.* 2001;28(6):1347-55
[169] Braham R, Dawson B, Goodman C. The effect of glucosamine supplementation on people experiencing regular knee pain. *Br J Sports Med.* 2003;37(1):45-9
[170] "...oral glucosamine therapy achieved a significantly greater improvement in articular pain score than ibuprofen, and the investigators rated treatment efficacy as 'good' in a significantly greater proportion of glucosamine than ibuprofen recipients. In comparison with piroxicam, glucosamine significantly improved arthritic symptoms after 12 weeks of therapy..." Matheson AJ, Perry CM. Glucosamine: a review of its use in the management of osteoarthritis. *Drugs Aging.* 2003; 20(14): 1041-60
[171] Uebelhart D, Malaise M, Marcolongo R, DeVathaire F, Piperno M, Mailleux E, Fioravanti A, Matoso L, Vignon E. Intermittent treatment of knee osteoarthritis with oral chondroitin sulfate: a one-year, randomized, double-blind, multicenter study versus placebo. *Osteoarthritis Cartilage.* 2004;12:269-76
[172] van Blitterswijk WJ, van de Nes JC, Wuisman PI. Glucosamine and chondroitin sulfate supplementation to treat symptomatic disc degeneration: biochemical rationale and case report. *BMC Complement Altern Med.* 2003;3(1):2
[173] Morreale P, Manopulo R, Galati M, Boccanera L, Saponati G, Bocchi L. Comparison of the antiinflammatory efficacy of chondroitin sulfate and diclofenac sodium in patients with knee osteoarthritis. *J Rheumatol.* 1996;23(8):1385-91
[174] Mazieres B, Combe B, Phan Van A, Tondut J, Grynfeltt M. Chondroitin sulfate in osteoarthritis of the knee: a prospective, double blind, placebo controlled multicenter clinical study. *J Rheumatol.* 2001;28(1):173-81
[175] Reginster JY, Deroisy R, Rovati LC, Lee RL, Lejeune E, Bruyere O, Giacovelli G, Henrotin Y, Dacre JE, Gossett C. Long-term effects of glucosamine sulphate on osteoarthritis progression: a randomised, placebo-controlled clinical trial. *Lancet.* 2001;357(9252):251-6
[176] Adams ME. Hype about glucosamine. *Lancet.* 1999;354(9176):353-4
[177] Cumming A. Glucosamine in osteoarthritis. *Lancet.* 1999;354(9190):1640-1
[178] Rovati LC, Annefeld M, Giacovelli G, Schmid K, Setnikar I. *Glucosamine in osteoarthritis.* Lancet. 1999;354(9190):1640
[179] Scroggie DA, Albright A, Harris MD. The effect of glucosamine-chondroitin supplementation on glycosylated hemoglobin levels in patients with type 2 diabetes mellitus: a placebo-controlled, double-blinded, randomized clinical trial. *Arch Intern Med.* 2003;163(13):1587-9
[180] Reginster JY, Deroisy R, Rovati LC, Lee RL, Lejeune E, Bruyere O, Giacovelli G, Henrotin Y, Dacre JE, Gossett C. Long-term effects of glucosamine sulphate on osteoarthritis progression: a randomised, placebo-controlled clinical trial. *Lancet.* 2001;357(9252):251-6
[181] Topol EJ. Failing the public health--rofecoxib, Merck, and the FDA. *N Engl J Med.* 2004 Oct 21;351(17):1707-9
[182] Mukherjee D, Nissen SE, Topol EJ. Risk of cardiovascular events associated with selective cox-2 inhibitors. *JAMA* 2001; 286(8):954-9
[183] Ray WA, Griffin MR, Stein CM. Cardiovascular toxicity of valdecoxib. *N Engl J Med.* 2004;351(26):2767

chondroitin sulfate appears to safely reduce the pain and disability associated with osteoarthritis while simultaneously reducing incidence of cardiovascular morbidity and mortality.[186,187]   In a study with animals that spontaneously develop atherosclerosis[188], administration of chondroitin sulfate induced regression of existing atherosclerosis. In a six-year study with 120 patients with established cardiovascular disease, 60 chondroitin-treated patients suffered 6 coronary events and 4 deaths compared to 42 events and 14 deaths in a comparable group of 60 patients receiving "conventional" therapy; chondroitin-treated patients reported enhancement of well-being while no adverse clinical or laboratory effects were noted during the 6 years of treatment.[189]

o Pancreatic/proteolytic enzymes: Orally-administered pancreatic and proteolytic enzymes are absorbed from the gastrointestinal tract into the systemic circulation[190,191] to exert analgesic, anti-inflammatory, anti-edematous benefits with therapeutic relevance for acute and chronic musculoskeletal disorders.[192,193,194,195]

o Vitamin C: Doses of 1-2 grams per day have been suggested to reduce pain and the need for surgery in patients with low-back pain by improving disc integrity.[196] Vitamin C reduces production of isoprostanes, which promote inflammation and pain. Ascorbate is also necessary for the production of the anti-inflammatory prostaglandin E-1. Supplemental vitamin C may also reduce the severity and progression of osteoarthritis.[197]

o Vitamin E, with an emphasis on gamma-tocopherol: The *gamma* form of vitamin E inhibits cyclooxygenase and thus has anti-inflammatory activity.[198] Clinical trials and case reports have suggested benefit of vitamin E supplementation in patients with rheumatoid arthritis[199,200], spondylosis and back pain[201], osteoarthritis[202,203,204], and autoimmune diseases including scleroderma, discoid lupus erythematosus, porphyria cutanea tarda, vasculitis, and polymyositis.[205,206,207]

---

[184] "Patients in the clinical trial taking 400 mg. of Celebrex twice daily had a 3.4 times greater risk of CV events compared to placebo. For patients in the trial taking 200 mg. of Celebrex twice daily, the risk was 2.5 times greater. The average duration of treatment in the trial was 33 months." FDA Statement on the Halting of a Clinical Trial of the cox-2 Inhibitor Celebrex. http://www.fda.gov/bbs/topics/news/2004/NEW01144.html Available on January 4, 2005

[185] "Preliminary information from the study showed some evidence of increased risk of cardiovascular events, when compared to placebo, to patients taking naproxen." FDA Statement on Naproxen. http://www.fda.gov/bbs/topics/news/2004/NEW01148.html Available on January 4, 2005

[186] Morrison LM. Treatment of coronary arteriosclerotic heart disease with chondroitin sulfate-A: preliminary report. *J Am Geriatr Soc.* 1968;16(7):779-85

[187] Morrison LM, Branwood AW, Ershoff BH, Murata K, Quilligan JJ Jr, Schjeide OA, Patek P, Bernick S, Freeman L, Dunn OJ, Rucker P. The prevention of coronary arteriosclerotic heart disease with chondroitin sulfate A: preliminary report. *Exp Med Surg.* 1969;27(3):278-89

[188] Morrison LM, Bajwa GS. Absence of naturally occurring coronary atherosclerosis in squirrel monkeys (Saimiri sciurea) treated with chondroitin sulfate A. *Experientia.* 1972 Dec 15;28(12):1410-1

[189] Morrison LM, Enrick N. Coronary heart disease: reduction of death rate by chondroitin sulfate A. *Angiology.* 1973 May;24(5):269-87

[190] Gotze H, Rothman SS. Enteropancreatic circulation of digestive enzymes as a conservative mechanism. *Nature* 1975; 257(5527): 607-609

[191] Liebow C, Rothman SS. Enteropancreatic Circulation of Digestive Enzymes. *Science* 1975; 189(4201): 472-474

[192] Trickett P. Proteolytic enzymes in treatment of athletic injuries. *Appl Ther.* 1964;30:647-52

[193] Walker JA, Cerny FJ, Cotter JR, Burton HW. Attenuation of contraction-induced skeletal muscle injury by bromelain. *Med Sci Sports Exerc.* 1992 Jan;24(1):20-5

[194] Walker AF, Bundy R, Hicks SM, Middleton RW. Bromelain reduces mild acute knee pain and improves well-being in a dose-dependent fashion in an open study of otherwise healthy adults. *Phytomedicine.* 2002; 9: 681-6

[195] Brien S, Lewith G, Walker A, Hicks SM, Middleton D. Bromelain as a Treatment for Osteoarthritis: a Review of Clinical Studies. *Evidence-based Complementary and Alternative Medicine.* 2004;1(3):251–257

[196] Greenwood J. Optimum vitamin C intake as a factor in the preservation of disc integrity. *Med Ann Dist Columbia.* 1964 Jun;33:274-6

[197] "A 3-fold reduction in risk of OA progression was found for both the middle tertile and highest tertile of vitamin C intake. This related predominantly to a reduced risk of cartilage loss. Those with high vitamin C intake also had a reduced risk of developing knee pain." McAlindon TE, Jacques P, Zhang Y, Hannan MT, Aliabadi P, Weissman B, Rush D, Levy D, Felson DT. Do antioxidant micronutrients protect against the development and progression of knee osteoarthritis? *Arthritis Rheum.* 1996 Apr;39(4):648-56

[198] Jiang Q, Christen S, Shigenaga MK, Ames BN. gamma-tocopherol, the major form of vitamin E in the US diet, deserves more attention. *Am J Clin Nutr* 2001 Dec;74(6):714-22

[199] Helmy M, Shohayeb M, Helmy MH, el-Bassiouni EA. Antioxidants as adjuvant therapy in rheumatoid disease. A preliminary study. *Arzneimittelforschung.* 2001;51(4):293-8

[200] Edmonds SE, Winyard PG, Guo R, Kidd B, Merry P, Langrish-Smith A, Hansen C, Ramm S, Blake DR. Putative analgesic activity of repeated oral doses of vitamin E in the treatment of rheumatoid arthritis. Results of a prospective placebo controlled double blind trial. *Ann Rheum Dis.* 1997 Nov;56(11):649-55

[201] "Vitamin E administration at a dose of 100 mg daily for three weeks resulted in a significant increase in serum vitamin E level accompanied by complete relief of pain... The results therefore strongly indicate that vitamin E is effective in curing spondylosis and most probably due to its antioxidant activity." Mahmud Z, Ali SM. Role of vitamin A and E in spondylosis. *Bangladesh Med Res Counc Bull.* 1992 Apr;18(1):47-59

[202] "The results of this double-blind controlled clinical trial showed that vitamin E was superior to placebo with respect to the relief of pain (pain at rest, pain during movement, pressure-induced pain) and the necessity of additional analgesic treatment. Improvement of mobility was better in the group treated with vitamin E." Blankenhorn G. [Clinical effectiveness of Spondyvit (vitamin E) in activated arthroses. A multicenter placebo-controlled double-blind study] [Article in German] *Z Orthop Ihre Grenzgeb.* 1986 May-Jun;124(3):340-3

[203] This is a very interesting study because the clinical response to vitamin E was proportional to the increase in plasma levels of vitamin E, thus confirming the dose-response relationship that implies causality as well as indicating that the failure of such treatment in some patients may be due to malabsorption or unquenchable systemic oxidative stress rather than the inefficacy of vitamin E supplementation, per se. "There were no significant differences in the efficacy of the two drugs, although one patient in the V-group refused further treatment after 8 days because of inefficacy. V reduced or abolished the pain at rest in 77% (D in 85%), the pain on pressure in 67% (D in 50%), and the pain on movement in 62% (D in 63%). Both treatments appeared to be equally effective in reducing the circumference of the knee joints (p = 0.001) and the walking time (p less than 0.001) and in increasing the joint mobility (p less than 0.002)." Scherak O, Kolarz G, Schodl A, Blankenhorn G. [High dosage vitamin E therapy in patients with activated arthrosis] [Article in German] *Z Rheumatol.* 1990 Nov-Dec;49(6):369-73

[204] Machtey I, Ouaknine L. Tocopherol in Osteoarthritis: a controlled pilot study. *J Am Geriatr Soc.* 1978 Jul;26(7):328-30

[205] Killeen RN, Ayres S Jr, Mihan R. Polymyositis: response to vitamin E. *South Med J.* 1976 Oct;69(10):1372-4

[206] Ayres S Jr, Mihan R. Lupus erythematosus and vitamin E: an effective and nontoxic therapy. *Cutis.* 1979 Jan;23(1):49-52, 54

[207] Ayres S Jr, Mihan R. Is vitamin E involved in the autoimmune mechanism? *Cutis.* 1978 Mar;21(3):321-5

Myofascial trigger points
MFTP

Description/pathophysiology:

- Many patients suffer from chronic pain that originates from myofascial trigger points—localized areas within muscle tissue that produce chronic pain, promote muscle contraction and tightness, and which mediate autonomous autonomic responses. Physicians who take the time to locate and treat MFTP and educate patients about effective home care can often rapidly and permanently reduce their patients' pain in a safe and highly cost-effective manner.
- MFTP have been defined as "a highly localized and hyperirritable spot in a palpable taut band of skeletal muscle fibers"[208] characterized by the following:
    1. Referred pain with compression: Digital compression of the MFTP causes local pain and most often causes referred pain in a distribution similar or identical to the patient's presenting complaint. The distribution of pain may appear radicular and may thus be described as "pseudoradicular."
    2. Twitch response: When digital pressure is applied perpendicularly to the direction of muscle fibers at the location of the MFTP and the muscle is "plucked" or allowed to "snap" as if one were plucking a taut rubber band or the string of a guitar, the muscle being assessed undergoes a rapid contraction.
    3. Muscle tightness: The muscle involved is tighter than usual, and it is resistant to stretch.
    4. Associated autonomic phenomena: Regions of the body near a localized MFTP may display associated autonomic dysregulation such as vasoconstriction, sweating, pilomotor response, and the patient may experience nausea, dizziness, light-headedness[209] or atrial fibrillation.[210]
    5. MFTP may be "active" or "latent": Active MFTP are those which cause spontaneous pain with joint motion or muscle contraction, whereas latent MFTP cause pain only when provoked by an examiner's deep palpation and physical compression. [211]
    6. Normal muscle strength: Muscle weakness and atrophy are not associated with MFTP unless the weakness or atrophy is secondary to pain.
- The initiation and perpetuation of MFTP is complex and commonly associated with previous injury or chronic static posturing (such as sitting in front of a computer for 8-14 hours per day) and also with emotional stress. Since **intrafusal fibers of muscle spindles receive direct sympathetic innervation**, and since adrenaline/epinephrine directly increases the contractile tone and tension of muscles, it is reasonable to conclude that attention to emotional stress and stress management techniques should be part of the comprehensive treatment plan for MFTP. A significant reduction in emotional tension and work-related repetitive strain injuries may follow a comprehensive and "body-based" approach to healthy living and appropriate career choices.[212]
- The pathogenesis and physiology-based treatment of MFTP follow this route are as follows:
    Pathogenesis[213]
    1. Excess calcium is released from the sarcoplasmic reticulum, leading to local muscle fiber contraction.
    2. Intense and chronic muscle contractions cause relative local ischemia.
    3. The reduction in local blood supply limits energy replacement and leads to the depletion of adenosine triphosphate (ATP).
    4. The muscle cell now has insufficient ATP for the active return of calcium from the contractile elements to the sarcoplasmic reticulum, thus maintaining the muscle fibers in a contracted state.

[208] Hong CZ, Simons DG. Pathophysiologic and electrophysiologic mechanisms of myofascial trigger points. *Arch Phys Med Rehabil*. 1998;79(7):863-72
[209] Hubbard DR, Berkoff GM. Myofascial trigger points show spontaneous needle EMG activity. *Spine*. 1993 Oct 1;18(13):1803-7
[210] Simons DG. Cardiology and myofascial trigger points: Janet G. Travell's contribution. *Tex Heart Inst J*. 2003;30(1):3-7
[211] Hubbard DR, Berkoff GM. Myofascial trigger points show spontaneous needle EMG activity. *Spine*. 1993 Oct 1;18(13):1803-7
[212] Jarrow R. Creating the Work You Love: Courage, Commitment and Career. Inner Traditions Intl Ltd; December 1995) [ISBN: 0892815426]
[213] Simons DG. Cardiology and myofascial trigger points: Janet G. Travell's contribution. *Tex Heart Inst J*. 2003;30(1):3-7

Physiology-based treatment:

5. Stretching the muscle fibers reduces the overlap between actin and myosin, which then leads to a reduction in energy demand of the cell and thus helps to "break the cycle" of **contraction** *leading to* **energy depletion** *leading to* **contraction** *leading to* **energy depletion...**

6. Application of ice (or other benign, intense afferent stimuli such as capsaicin or spinal manipulation) floods the dorsal horn and thus blocks transmission of nociceptive stimuli via the hypothesized "gate control" mechanism of pain reception.

7. Magnesium supplementation is appropriate for many patients with MFTP since many patients do not consume sufficient dietary magnesium and since magnesium inhibits calcium release from the sarcoplasmic reticulum[214] and thereby has a muscle relaxing effect. **Magnesium deficiency is an epidemic** in so-called "developed" nations, with 20-40% of different populations showing objective serologic/cytologic evidence of magnesium deficiency.[215,216,217,218]

Clinical presentations:

- The pain pattern from MFTP is varied and is dependent on the muscle(s) involved. Each muscle has a unique pattern of pain referral; e.g., a MFTP in the deltoid or supraspinatus may cause shoulder pain and arm pain that can mimic cervical radiculitis. MFTP in the sternocleidomastoid commonly causes "headache" and pain over the side of the face and TMJ; MFTP in the psoas can cause low back and leg pain. Patients may also subjectively notice numbness or tingling in addition to pain.[219] Differentiation of MFTP pain from radiculitis and radiculopathy should be pursued clinically and documented in the patient chart.

Major differential diagnoses:

- Arthropathy and arthritis: Passive joint provocation tests are negative with MFTP; no laboratory abnormalities (such as elevated CRP) are seen with MFTP.
- Acute muscle injury, strain: History of *recent* injury is often negative; history of *chronic* strain and *previous* injury are common with MFTP
- Radiculitis: The pain associated with MFTP is not dermatomal and is reproduced with local muscle compression, whereas the pain of radiculitis is dermatomal and reproduced with nerve tension tests.
- Radiculopathy: Radiculopathy is associated with muscle weakness, which is not a characteristic of MFTP.

Clinical assessments:

- History/subjective: Pain is always present (although it may be mild or latent).
- Physical examination/objective: The most reliable physical signs of MFTP are **1) spot tenderness within a taut band of muscle, 2) reproduction of pain and referred pain with palpation and provocation**, and 3) local twitch response with palpation and provocation.
- Imaging & laboratory assessments: Lab tests and imaging assessments are normal. Myofascial trigger points show spontaneous electromyographic activity.[220]

[214] "Mg2+ inhibits Ca2+ release from the sarcoplasmic reticulum." Mathew R, Altura BM. The role of magnesium in lung diseases: asthma, allergy and pulmonary hypertension. *Magnes Trace Elem*. 1991-92;10(2-4):220-8
[215] "The American diet is low in magnesium, and with modern water systems, very little is ingested in the drinking water." Innerarity S. Hypomagnesemia in acute and chronic illness. *Crit Care Nurs Q*. 2000 Aug;23(2):1-19
[216] "Altogether 43% of 113 trauma patients had low magnesium levels compared to 30% of noninjured cohorts." Frankel H, Haskell R, Lee SY, Miller D, Rotondo M, Schwab CW. Hypomagnesemia in trauma patients. *World J Surg*. 1999 Sep;23(9):966-9
[217] "There was a 20% overall prevalence of hypomagnesemia among this predominantly female, African American population." Fox CH, Ramsoomair D, Mahoney MC, Carter C, Young B, Graham R. An investigation of hypomagnesemia among ambulatory urban African Americans. *J Fam Pract*. 1999 Aug;48(8):636-9
[218] "Suboptimal levels were detected in 33.7 per cent of the population under study. These data clearly demonstrate that the Mg supply of the German population needs increased attention." Schimatschek HF, Rempis R. Prevalence of hypomagnesemia in an unselected German population of 16,000 individuals. *Magnes Res*. 2001 Dec;14(4):283-90
[219] Hubbard DR, Berkoff GM. Myofascial trigger points show spontaneous needle EMG activity. *Spine*. 1993 Oct 1;18(13):1803-7
[220] Hubbard DR, Berkoff GM. Myofascial trigger points show spontaneous needle EMG activity. *Spine*. 1993 Oct 1;18(13):1803-7

Establishing the diagnosis:

- Reasonable clinical exclusion of acute strain, radiculopathy and radiculitis combined with characteristic clinical findings mentioned above, including at least **1) spot tenderness within a taut band of muscle, 2) reproduction of pain and referred pain with palpation/provocation.**

Complications:

- Many patients with MFTP suffer from pain for years before being properly diagnosed. Many patients are prescribed hazardous and inappropriate medications to treat the pain and symptoms of MFTP, and surgical interventions are periodically used inappropriately in patents who have not been accurately diagnosed. For example when a patient with low back pain due to MFTP is found to have an incidental disc herniation, the patient may undergo surgery on the intervertebral disc only to have pain continue postoperatively until it is treated with simple techniques directed at the MFTP.[221]

Clinical management:

- Simple nutritional and physical treatments as described below.
- Patients should be advised that deep massage of the area is often necessary and that pain may be temporarily exacerbated.
- A sample of notes for educating patients about natural treatment for cervical MFTP and neck pain is available at http://OptimalHealthResearch.com/neck

Treatments:

- Post-isometric stretching: Lewit and Simons described this simple and highly effective treatment succinctly in a highly recommended article[222], "The post-isometric relaxation technique begins by placing the muscle in a stretched position. Then an isometric contraction is exerted against minimal resistance. Relaxation and then gentle stretch follow as the muscle releases." In a large study involving 244 patients, post-isometric stretching "produced **immediate pain relief in 94%, lasting pain relief in 63%**, as well as lasting relief of point tenderness in 23% of the sites treated. Patients who practiced autotherapy on a home program were more likely to realize lasting relief." Clinically the technique is simultaneously performed, explained, and taught by the clinician: 1) stretch the target muscle, 2) weakly contract the target muscle against resistance for 10 seconds, 3) stretch the target muscle to a greater length than before for at least 20 seconds, 4) repeat this procedure 2-3 times. Pretreatment heating or exercising of the target muscles along with post-treatment application of ice helps to increase treatment efficacy and minimize post-treatment soreness, respectively.
- Cold and stretch: The application of cold and the simultaneous stretching of the muscle is an effective treatment for MFTP.[223] Cold can be applied with ice. The previously popular "spray and stretch" technique that used a vapocoolant spray such as Fluori-Methane is unnecessary and is environmentally irresponsible.
- Topical application: Capsaicin helps to relieve neuromuscular pain, too, and may help break the cycle of pain and spasm by 1) providing afferent stimuli to block nociceptive stimuli, and 2) by depleting local tissues of substance P, which not only serves as a transmitter of pain sensations, but may also perpetuate muscle contraction and spasm. Another mechanism by which capsaicin can alleviate trigger points is by desensitizing the vanilloid receptor (VR-1) to ultimately decrease local neurotransmitter release.[224]
- Dry needling or injection of local anesthetic or saline: While local injection of anesthetic or saline may appear more complex and therefore more effective, dry needling (rapid insertion and withdrawal of a needle) directly into the MFTP is just as effective, safer, and is less complicated than using anesthetic or saline solution. Increased efficacy of this technique is associated with the elicitation of a local twitch response immediately upon insertion and withdrawal of the needle. The accuracy of the needle insertion directly into the "sensitive locus" of the MFTP is essential for the effectiveness of this approach. Common locations for MFTP correlate with commonly used acupuncture points, and the

---

[221] Rubin D. Myofascial trigger point syndromes: an approach to management. *Arch Phys Med Rehabil.* 1981 Mar;62(3):107-10

[222] Lewit K, Simons DG. Myofascial pain: relief by post-isometric relaxation. *Arch Phys Med Rehabil.* 1984 Aug;65(8):452-6

[223] Rubin D. Myofascial trigger point syndromes: an approach to management. *Arch Phys Med Rehabil.* 1981 Mar;62(3):107-10

[224] "Massage with capsaicin cream (0.075%, available over the counter) is useful for treating TrPs located in surgical scars,36 which are particularly refractory to treatment." McPartland JM. Travell trigger points--molecular and osteopathic perspectives. *J Am Osteopath Assoc.* 2004 Jun;104(6):244-9 http://www.jaoa.org/cgi/content/full/104/6/244

technique of acupuncture is analogous to the dry needling technique except that dry needling is performed more quickly and with highly localized precision into the MFTP sensitive locus. [225]
- <u>Adjunctive nutritional support</u>: Supplementation with **magnesium** (600 mg per day or to bowel tolerance[226]) and **calcium** are often helpful, particularly when used with an **alkalinizing Paleo-Mediterranean diet** (as discussed in Chapter 2), which—at the very least—promotes renal retention of calcium and magnesium to thus facilitate mineral retention. Other treatments to reduce intracellular calcium levels (intracellular hypercalcinosis[227]) include supplementation with **physiologic doses of vitamin D3**[228] and **fish oil for EPA**[229] along with avoidance/reduction of factors which promote renal loss of calcium and magnesium such as caffeine, sugar, alcohol/ethanol, and psychoemotional stress.

Hypothesized model for the initiation and promotion of myofascial trigger points with self-perpetuating cycles

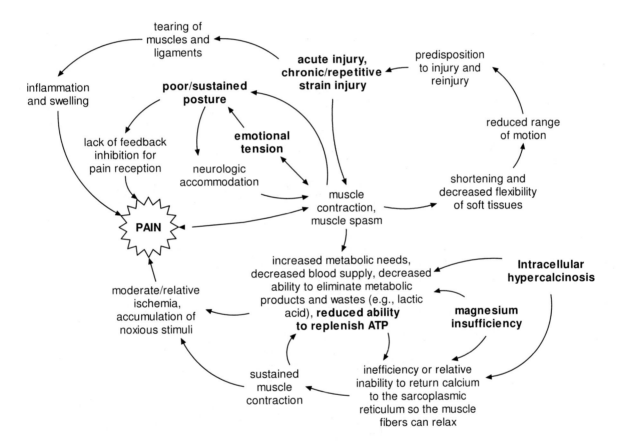

---

[225] Hong CZ, Simons DG. Pathophysiologic and electrophysiologic mechanisms of myofascial trigger points. *Arch Phys Med Rehabil*. 1998 Jul;79(7):863-72

[226] "When the practitioner has been convinced to start Mg on the basis of his diagnosis or through insistence of the patient, the often recommended dose of 300 mg per day is insufficient. Experience of successful therapy indicates that no less than 600 mg per day is required." Liebscher DH, Liebscher DE. About the misdiagnosis of magnesium deficiency. *J Am Coll Nutr*. 2004 Dec;23(6):730S-1S http://www.coldcure.com/html/misdiagnosis-magnesium-deficiency.pdf

[227] See http://optimalhealthresearch.com/archives/intracellular-hypercalcinosis and www.naturopathydigest.com/archives/2006/sep/vasquez.php for additional discussion

[228] Vasquez A, Manso G, Cannell J. The clinical importance of vitamin D (cholecalciferol): a paradigm shift with implications for all healthcare providers. *Altern Ther Health Med*. 2004 Sep-Oct;10(5):28-36 http://optimalhealthresearch.com/monograph04

[229] "This is a consequence of the ability of EPA to release Ca2+ from intracellular stores while inhibiting their refilling via capacitative Ca2+ influx that results in partial emptying of intracellular Ca2+ stores and thereby activation of protein kinase R." Palakurthi SS, Fluckiger R, Aktas H, Changolkar AK, Shahsafaei A, Harneit S, Kilic E, Halperin JA. Inhibition of translation initiation mediates the anticancer effect of the n-3 polyunsaturated fatty acid eicosapentaenoic acid. *Cancer Res*. 2000 Jun 1;60(11):2919-25

Musculoskeletal Manipulation and Manual Medicine: Selection of Commonly Used Chiropractic and Osteopathic Techniques

Manual medicine in general and spinal manipulation in particular are mentioned in nearly every section of **_Integrative Orthopedics_**, and select techniques are described with accompanying text and photographs. Manipulative techniques are included in this textbook to remind practitioners of a few of the more useful and commonly applied maneuvers and to provide descriptions and citations for refinement of their application. However, the level of detail provided here is insufficient unless the reader has received hands-on professionally-supervised training in an accredited institution wherein other important concepts have been taught and implemented under experienced guidance. Competence and proficiency in the art and skill of manipulation cannot be learned from a textbook; these can only be approached with personal mentoring and in-person coursework amply provided in colleges and post-graduate trainings specializing in manipulative technique. **Manipulative medicine** is a _time-space_ objective-subjective-intuitive **kinesthetic phenomenon** which might be described as occurring in four dimensions—_anteroposterior, transverse/horizontal, vertical,_ and _chronological_ due to variations in speed and power; all the while, the doctor is monitoring subjective and objective responses of the what might be considered the fifth dimension—the doctor's dynamic _perception of, influence upon,_ and _interaction with_ the patient's affect, posture, muscle tension, dynamic joint positioning, tissue response, and compressive tension. As the doctor assesses and provides force, the patient's response changes the target, and so the doctor must adapt to a constantly moving target—the lesion being treated.

These sections presume professional training by the reader has already been begun or completed and that the reader is familiar with manipulative concepts, technique, terminology, and commonly used abbreviations. Again, the intention here is to remind clinicians of manipulation in general and these specific techniques in particular; only a few _subjectively chosen_ techniques are included from the several hundred vertebral, myofascial, visceral, and extravertebral/extremity maneuvers that are available.

General Layout and Description of Manipulative Techniques	
Patient position:	• Patient position may be prone, supine, lateral recumbent or "side-posture", standing, or seated
Doctor position:	• Usually standing, either _upright, forward flexed,_ or using an oblique _fencer's stance_; knees are almost always bent in order to bring doctor's torso near treatment area to increase mechanical force from the upper limbs
Assessment:	• <u>Subjective</u>: Patient's experience, sensations, and effect on daily living • <u>Motion palpation</u>: Intersegmental motion analysis generally used for assessing the presence of vertebral motion restrictions or aberrant motion. The patient is relaxed and passive while the doctor takes the joint that is being assessed through its normal range of motion in various directions while palpating near adjacent joint surfaces for nuance of pattern and end-feel. Motion lesions are generally described as **restrictions** and/or **hypermobility** • <u>Static palpation</u>: Boney and other landmarks are compared symmetrically and to the practitioner's experience for the detection of abnormality consistent with subjective, motion, and soft tissue findings; static palpations are usually described in terms of prominence or relative superiority/inferiority when compared symmetrically • <u>Soft tissue palpation</u>: Subcutaneous tissues, tendons, ligaments, muscles, and joint spaces can be palpated to assess myofascial status and function. Soft tissue findings commonly include edema, joint swelling, bogginess, "ropiness" of muscles, tenderness, restricted motion of soft tissues, hypertonicity, spasm, and adhesions
Treatment contact, directive hand:	• Generally the doctor provides therapeutic contact with one of the contact surfaces of the hands—digital, hypothenar, pisiform, index, thumb, thenar, or "calcaneal" when using the heel of the hand[230]; other contacts such as the elbow or chest might be used for deep myofascial or compressive manipulative procedures, respectively. The _treatment contact_ is provided by the _directive hand_—the hand that is delivering the therapeutic _thrust_ or _direction_;

---

[230] Kirk CR, Lawrence DJ, Valvo NL. <u>States Manual of Spinal, Pelvic, and Extravertebral Technics. Second Edition</u>. Lombard, Illinois: National College of Chiropractic; 1985, page 20

	the treatment contact of the directive hand works in cooperation with the *supporting contact* of the *supporting hand*
Supporting contact:	This generally refers to the supportive hand, the one that is either holding or stabilizing the patient in contrast to the hand that is delivering the manipulative force. The indirect hand can provide at least three different types of support • <u>Neutral/stabilizing support</u>: The supportive hand plays a relatively neutral role with regard to the manipulative force • <u>Synergistic/cooperative/assistive support</u>: In this situation, the supportive hand moves with the therapeutic force in the same direction. An example of this would be the head-holding hand moving in the same direction as the directive/treatment hand when performing manipulation of the upper cervical spine • <u>Counterthrust/resistive support</u>: In this situation, the supportive hand moves counter/against the direction of the directive force. A common example is the force applied to the upper torso when performing a side-posture manipulation of the lumbar spine or pelvis. Another important example is the counterthrust by the supportive hand when performing a more forceful manipulation of the cervical spine; in this case the supportive hand is serving to limit the motion that would otherwise be imposed by forceful motion by the directive hand; more forceful manipulations such as used to increase afferent input to joint proprioceptors should *not* result in more motion; rather the increased speed and force of the directive hand is countered rather than assisted by the supportive hand
Pretreatment positioning:	• Joints are generally—but not always—taken to the end range of motion before the manipulative thrust is applied because the general purpose of high-velocity low-amplitude manipulation is to break myofascial restrictions and/or forcefully activate joint proprioceptors. In chiropractic terms, this is described as taking the joint into the **paraphysiologic space** because the physiologic range of motion is temporarily though safely exceeded[231]; in osteopathic terms, this part of the range of motion is described as being within the range of **passive motion** but still within the **anatomic barrier**[232]
Therapeutic action:	• For joint manipulation, this is usually the **chiropractic adjustment** or the **osteopathic HVLA** (high-velocity low-amplitude thrust); <u>**thrust vectors**</u> can be *straight, curvilinear,* or *rotary* into **segmental directions** of *rotation, extension, flexion, side-bending, traction,* and combinations of those directions • Other common manual techniques include stretching, post-isometric stretching, massage, compression, percussion, joint springing, mobilization, articulation, traction
Image:	• Photographs will be provided when relevant and available
Resources:	Textbook and article citations for additional information will be provided in this last row when relevant and available; the most commonly cited works include: • <u>States Manual, Second Edition</u>[233] by Constance Kirk DC, Dana Lawrence DC, Nila Valvo DC • <u>Kimberly Manual, 2006 Edition</u>[234] by Paul Kimberly DO • <u>Chiropractic Technique</u>[235] by Thomas Bergmann DC, David Peterson DC, Dana Lawrence DC • <u>Chiropractic Management of Spine-Related Disorders</u>[236] edited by Meridel Gatterman DC

> The following samples are an obvious underrepresentation of the diversity of manipulative techniques available, which easily numbers into the hundreds. Various techniques are—of course—described with greater range and depth in textbooks wholly dedicated to the topic of manipulation, which by itself is not the subject of this text. Rather, **use these samples as reminders to include or at least consider manipulative therapy** when composing your treatment plan; oftentimes, the manipulative therapy is the fastest and shortest route between *pain* and *relief from pain.*

[231] Leach RA. (ed). <u>The Chiropractic Theories: A Textbook of Scientific Research, Fourth Edition</u>. Baltimore: Lippincott, Williams & Wilkins, 2004, page 32-33
[232] Kimberly PE. <u>Outline of Osteopathic Manipulative Procedures. The Kimberly Manual 2006</u>. Kirksville College of Osteopathic Medicine. Walsworth Publishing , Marceline, Mo, page 7
[233] Kirk CR, Lawrence DJ, Valvo NL. <u>States Manual of Spinal, Pelvic, and Extravertebral Technics. Second Edition</u>. Lombard, Illinois: National College of Chiropractic; 1985
[234] Kimberly PE. <u>Outline of Osteopathic Manipulative Procedures. The Kimberly Manual 2006</u>. Kirksville College of Osteopathic Medicine. Walsworth Publishing , Marceline, Mo
[235] Bergmann TF, Peterson DH, Lawrence DJ. <u>Chiropractic Technique</u>. New York; Churchill Livingstone: 1993
[236] Gatterman MI. <u>Chiropractic Management of Spine Related Disorders</u>. Baltimore; Williams and Wilkins: 1990

Cervical Spine: Rotation Emphasis

Patient position:	• Supine, neck slightly flexed
Doctor position:	• At 45° angle from head of table; may also be in a more lateral position aside the patient's head and neck; while it is acceptable to assess and set-up with straight legs, at the time of impulse, doctor's legs should be bent to provide the doctor with greater power, stability, and biomechanical safety
Assessment:	• <u>Subjective</u>: neck pain, headaches
	• <u>Motion palpation</u>: rotation restriction; primary or compensatory hypermobile segments may be detected above or below the restricted segment
	• <u>Static palpation</u>: vertebra may feel relatively posterior on the side opposite the rotational restriction, e.g., a right rotational restriction may present with a relative left rotational malposition that brings the vertebral lamina and articular pillars posterior on the left
	• <u>Soft tissue</u>: tenderness, may also have muscle spasm
Treatment contact:	• Doctor uses either an index or proximal phalange contact on the posterior aspect of the transverse process and/or articular pillar
	• The doctor's vector and hence the positioning of the forearm of the contact hand must change depending on the level of the cervical spine that is being treated
	• Notice in this photograph that the thumb of the doctor's contact hand is placed on the angle of the mandible, this is more to help anchor the contact and stabilize the doctor's wrist than to assist with the manipulation; very little pressure and zero thrust are applied to the mandible
Supporting contact:	• Head is held into rotation and slight flexion; as with all techniques, nuanced adjustments in flexion-extension, rotation, and side-bending are made until the premanipulative tension is localized to the specific direction/tissue of restriction
Pretreatment positioning:	• Slight flexion and extension may be used below and above the treatment contact to create motion restriction at the adjacent motion segments; this helps to focus the motion and therapeutic force at the specific; importantly the support hand is largely responsible for proper positioning with the correct amount of nuanced flexion-extension and side-bending so that the rotational force is accurately delivered
Therapeutic action:	• Rotational thrust with contact hand; support hand keeps head off table so that rotational motion can occur
Image:	

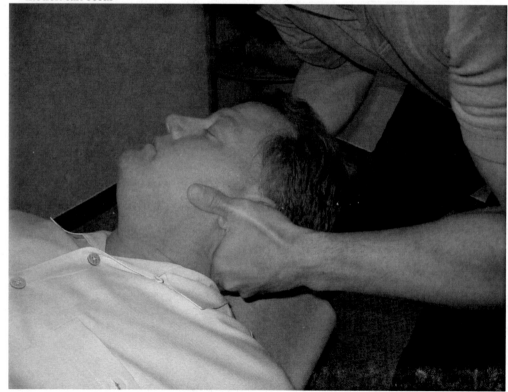

Resources:	• <u>States Manual, Second Edition</u>[237] page 47

[237] Kirk CR, Lawrence DJ, Valvo NL. <u>States Manual of Spinal, Pelvic, and Extravertebral Technics. Second Edition.</u> Lombard, Illinois: National College of Chiropractic; 1985

| **Cervical Spine: Lateral Flexion (Side-Bending) Emphasis; Treatment of Lateral Malposition** |

Patient position:
- Supine, head is neutrally placed—neither flexed nor extended; slight flexion is allowed; this technique can also be adapted for use in a seated position

Doctor position:
- At 45° angle from head of table; may also be in a more lateral position aside the patient's head and neck

Assessment:
- Subjective: neck pain, headaches
- Motion palpation: lateral flexion restriction
- Static palpation: vertebra may feel laterally displaced
- Soft tissue: tenderness, may also have muscle spasm

Treatment contact:
- Using an index (metacarpal-phalangeal) contact at the tip of the transverse process or slightly posterior to the transverse process; an index phalangeal contact can also be used on the articular pillars as long as doctor is careful not to thrust in a rotational direction; notice in this picture how Dr Harris has the forearm of his contact hand perfectly aligned in the treatment vector, which is almost purely in the patient's transverse/horizontal plane; notice also that Dr Harris has his knees bent and is forward flexed to bring his torso closer to his contact and thereby minimize stress and strain on his own shoulders; with slight modifications in vector direction, this technique can be applied throughout the cervical spine from C0-C7

Supporting contact:
- Lateral aspect of head, opposite contact; generally the supporting hand is neutral, however it can supply some traction and can help induce lateral flexion at impulse; with more aggressive adjustments, the supporting hand can supply a counterforce to minimize motion following the application of a faster and more powerful thrust

Pretreatment positioning:
- Lateral flexion at the targeted segment; the slightest amount of contralateral rotation is applied

Therapeutic action:
- Establish minimal premanipulative tension once the end range of motion has been reached, then use quick and very shallow trust to induce lateral flexion

Image:

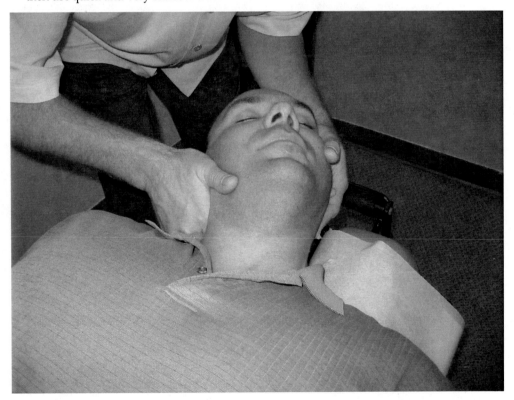

Resources:
- States Manual, Second Edition[238] page 39
- Kimberly Manual, 2006 Edition[239] page 79
- Chiropractic Technique[240] pages 268, 271, 285

[238] Kirk CR, Lawrence DJ, Valvo NL. States Manual of Spinal, Pelvic, and Extravertebral Technics. Second Edition. Lombard, Illinois: National College of Chiropractic; 1985
[239] Kimberly PE. Outline of Osteopathic Manipulative Procedures. The Kimberly Manual 2006. Kirksville College of Osteopathic Medicine. Walsworth Publishing, Marceline, Mo
[240] Bergmann TF, Peterson DH, Lawrence DJ. Chiropractic Technique. New York; Churchill Livingstone: 1993

Thoracic Spine: Supine Thoracic Flexion, "Anterior Thoracic"

Patient position:	• Supine on table; to facilitate positioning, patient's leg opposite doctor may be flexed at hip and knee with foot flat on table
	• Patient is instructed to place right hand on right trapezius and left hand on left trapezius; the patient is instructed, "Do not place your hands behind your neck and do not interlace your fingers."
Doctor position:	• Facing table at 45° angle in fencer stance with feet apart and knees bent
	• Doctor must be midline and balanced at time of impulse in order to provide symmetric force
Assessment:	• <u>Subjective</u>: mechanical midback pain
	• <u>Motion palpation</u>: flexion restriction
	• <u>Static palpation</u>: extension malposition; focal loss of thoracic kyphosis; focal approximation of spinous processes consistent with extension malposition; vertebra may feel anteriorly displaced
	• <u>Soft tissue</u>: local paravertebral myohypertonicity is common; local paresthesia is very common, and patients are often exquisitely sensitive to the lightest touch
Treatment contact:	• Closed fist contact with spinous processes between doctor's distal interphalangeal joints and thenar eminence; the trust is delivered from the doctor's chest through the patient's arms which compress the patient's chest; Dr Harris (pictured as patient) prefers to use a forearm contact to reduce wear-and-tear on his hands and wrists
Supporting contact:	• The supporting contact is the hand-arm that supports the patient's upper torso; the supporting contact pulls toward the doctor and superiorly at time of impulse
Pretreatment positioning:	• Patient lifts head from table; doctor uses supporting hand and arm to lift patient off table to allow placement of contact hand and to facilitate spinal flexion
Therapeutic action:	• Doctor uses **body drop thrust** technique at 45° toward ground and toward the head of the table; the trust should simultaneously generate compression and long-axis traction; the contact hand remains tense to provide solid leverage *inferior* to the targeted motion segment; the supporting hand and arm pull toward doctor at time of impulse to accentuate traction and spinal flexion; patient is instructed to breath deeply then relax and exhale; upon exhalation, the doctor establishes and maintains premanipulative tension to achieve joint flexion, then applies HVLA thrust; the thrust must be fast and shallow; slow and deep impulses can sprain the interspinous ligaments
Image:	

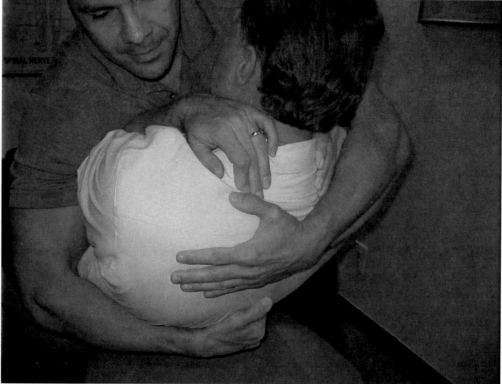

Resources:	• <u>States Manual, Second Edition</u>[241] page 67
	• <u>Kimberly Manual, 2006 Edition</u>[242] page 93-94
	• <u>Chiropractic Technique</u>[243] page 349

[241] Kirk CR, Lawrence DJ, Valvo NL. <u>States Manual of Spinal, Pelvic, and Extravertebral Technics. Second Edition</u>. Lombard, Illinois: National College of Chiropractic; 1985
[242] Kimberly PE. <u>Outline of Osteopathic Manipulative Procedures. The Kimberly Manual 2006</u>. Kirksville College of Osteopathic Medicine. Walsworth Publishing , Marceline, Mo
[243] Bergmann TF, Peterson DH, Lawrence DJ. <u>Chiropractic Technique</u>. New York; Churchill Livingstone: 1993

Lumbar Side-Posture Rotational Manipulation/Mobilization, "Lumbar Roll"	
Patient position:	• Side-posture, lateral recumbent; lower leg is straight; upper leg is flexed at hip and knee with foot behind calf of the leg that is straight on the table
Doctor position:	• Facing table at 45° angle in fencer stance with feet apart and knees bent
	• Notice in the photograph how Dr Harris approximates his center of gravity and biomechanical leverage directly over his therapeutic contact
Assessment:	• <u>Subjective</u>: asymptomatic or with lumbar pain; lumbar disc herniation[244], use a cautious and gentle technique if the patient has radicular symptoms, and as a rule of thumb the patient should be positioned with the symptomatic leg down on the table (e.g., "good leg *up*, bad leg *down*")
	• <u>Motion palpation</u>: focal restrictions with focal pain are perhaps better treated with a lesion-specific technique such as the "push-pull" maneuver; this is an excellent technique if the patient has general discomfort without localization, or has pain and will benefit from rotational manipulation for its muscle stretching and afferent-stimulating analgesic benefits
	• <u>Static palpation</u>: minor displacements and malpositions may be noted; if specific biomechanical lesions are found, use a more specific technique such as the "push-pull" maneuver
	• <u>Soft tissue</u>: palpate for hypertonicity/spasm with or without relative muscle atrophy; patients with chronic low-back pain tend to have weaker extensor muscles than the general population; however, during an acutely painful episode, their otherwise weakened muscles will be hypertonic thus leading to a paradoxical **atrophic hypertonicity**
Treatment contact:	• Doctor uses a palmar/calcaneal ("heel of the hand") contact over the lumbar facet joints
	• Rotation and traction are provided at the time of impulse with the doctor's thigh which is compressed and providing long-axis traction against the patient's upper leg, which is flexed at the hip and knee
Support:	• Doctor's cephalad hand applies rotational resistance to patient's shoulder as shown
Pretreatment positioning:	• Premanipulative tension is attained and maintained prior to **body drop impulse**
	• The premanipulative tension and the therapeutic impulse are established and delivered through the contact hand and the doctor's caudad leg which has compressive contact with the patient's flexed leg
Therapeutic action:	• Body drop thrust impulse with rotational emphasis
	• Notice how Dr Harris has the forearm of his contact hand perpendicular to the patient's coronal plane to direct his impulse in a posterior-to-anterior direction
Image:	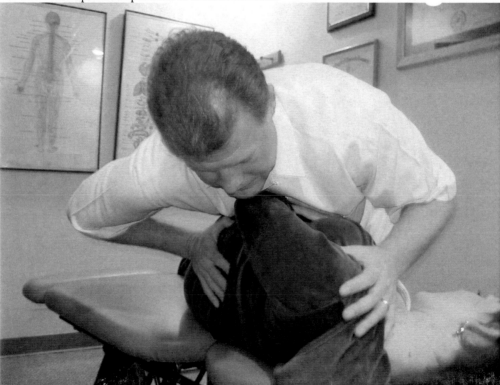
Resources:	• <u>States Manual, Second Edition</u>[245] pages 95, 105, 106

[244] Quon JA, Cassidy JD, O'Connor SM, Kirkaldy-Willis WH. Lumbar intervertebral disc herniation: treatment by rotational manipulation. *J Manipulative Physiol Ther.* 1989 Jun;12(3):220-7
[245] Kirk CR, Lawrence DJ, Valvo NL. <u>States Manual of Spinal, Pelvic, and Extravertebral Technics. Second Edition</u>. Lombard, Illinois: National College of Chiropractic; 1985

Lumbar Spine: Side-Posture Segmental Rotation (Lumbar "Push-Pull")

Patient position:	• Lateral recumbent (side-posture) with no/minimal lateral flexion and minimal thoracic rotation; upper leg is flexed at hip and knee, with foot placed/locked behind the calf that is on the table; the patient grasps his/her own forearms and maintains modest tension to provide anchoring for the doctor's caudad arm, which is placed under the patient's superior arm; the patient's lower leg is straight
Doctor position:	• Doctor is facing the table standing on the cephalad leg while the caudad leg is flexed at the hip and knee and placed atop the patient's flexed upper leg to provide additional leverage at the time of manipulative thrust
	• Regarding the doctor's cephalad arm, the humerus is directed toward the patient's shoulder, and the elbow is bent allowing the forearm to push into the sulcus formed by the pectoralis major and deltoid; doctors forearm emerges under patient's elbow, so that fingertips are on the superior/lateral aspect of the lumbar spinous process of the superior vertebra of the targeted motion segment
	• Regarding the doctor's caudad arm, the elbow is flexed and the forearm is placed along the posterior aspect of the patient's superior ilium; fingers hook the inferior/lateral aspect of the lumbar spinous process of the inferior vertebra of the targeted motion segment
Assessment:	• <u>Subjective</u>: asymptomatic or lumbar pain, which may not be at the affected segment
	• <u>Motion palpation</u>: rotational restriction
	• <u>Static palpation</u>: may have rotational malposition
	• <u>Soft tissue</u>: may have muscle spasm at nearby area of hypermobility
Treatment contact:	• The doctor's cephalad contacts are at the patient's deltopectoral sulcus and directly on the superior/lateral aspect of the lumbar spinous process of the superior vertebra of the targeted motion segment
	• This maneuver has three caudad contacts: 1) doctor's fingertips pull directly on the inferior/lateral aspect of the lumbar spinous process of the inferior vertebra of the targeted motion segment; 2) doctor's forearm on patient's ilium; 3) doctors caudad lower leg is atop patient's flexed leg
Support:	• All contacts are active
Pretreatment positioning:	• Rotational tension is applied and focused at the lumbar spinal segment being treated
	• Thoracic rotation and lateral flexion are minimized to the extent possible
	• Modest lumbar lateral flexion toward the table helps to gap the inferior articular process of the superior segment from the superior articular process of the inferior segment
Therapeutic action:	• 1) Doctor's cephalad elbow thrusts toward patient's shoulder to create simultaneous rotation and long-axis traction; 2) cephalad fingertips push toward the ground while atop the superior/lateral aspect of the lumbar spinous process of the superior vertebra of the targeted motion segment; 3) doctor's caudad fingertips hook and pull the inferior vertebra; 4) forearm pushes patient's ilium into rotation; 5) extension "kick" of doctor's knee quickly creates rotational force. All five actions must occur simultaneously
Image:	

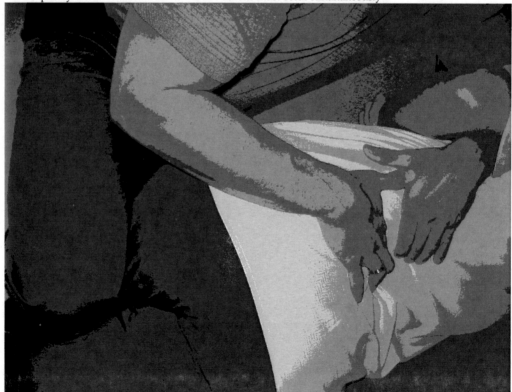

Resources:	• <u>Chiropractic Technique</u>[246] page 428

---

[246] Bergmann TF, Peterson DH, Lawrence DJ. <u>Chiropractic Technique</u>. New York; Churchill Livingstone: 1993

Proprioceptive Rehabilitation and Retraining: An Essential Component in the Comprehensive Management of Chronic Neck and Back Pain as Well as Recurrent Knee and Ankle Injuries

The central nervous system plays a silent and often underappreciated role in the maintenance of joint integrity and the prevention of joint injuries. Finely coordinated, minute alterations in muscle tension and joint position are essential for proper musculoskeletal biomechanics. Impaired coordination of this delicate neuromuscular system—either by injury or more commonly by disuse—predisposes to subtle and gross injuries and the perpetuation of chronic pain. **Muscle spasm, myofascial trigger points, and neuromuscular uncoupling must be viewed within a context that appreciates how the Western diet and lifestyle contribute to the genesis and perpetuation of painful musculoskeletal problems.**

Proprioceptive deficits are common in patients with chronic low-back pain[247], neck pain[248], knee pain and arthritis[249], and ankle instability.[250] Not only does poor proprioception leave joints vulnerable to recurrent microtrauma, but also lack of proprioceptive inhibition of nociceptors negates the proposed "gate-control" mechanism of pain inhibition and thus opens the door to the perception of chronic pain.[251] Thus, **proprioceptive deficits both increase joint injury and increase pain perception.** Chronic pain may lead to functional reorganization in the central nervous system and self-perpetuate pain as "pain memories."[252]

An important component to injury rehabilitation and prevention is proprioceptive retraining.[253] Proprioceptive retraining programs have been shown to reduce the severity of pain and the occurrence and recurrence of injuries. With the simple investment of a few minutes per day, patients and athletes

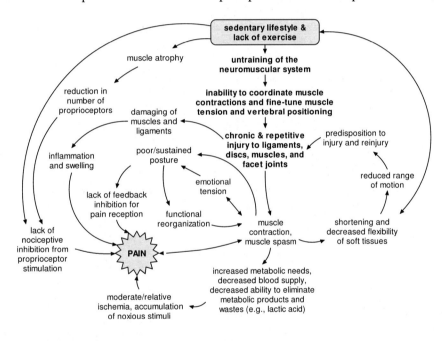

can retrain their nervous systems to respond more quickly and to increase the accuracy of proprioception. Muscle-strengthening rehabilitative programs that fail to address proprioceptive retraining do not result in improved neuromuscular coordination as evaluated by electromyography.[254] Furthermore, muscle-strengthening programs may actually lead to a reduction in postural stability when compared to balance training.[255]

---

[247] Newcomer KL, Jacobson TD, Gabriel DA, Larson DR, Brey RH, An KN. Muscle activation patterns in subjects with and without low back pain. *Arch Phys Med Rehabil.* 2002;83(6):816-21

[248] McPartland JM, Brodeur RR, Hallgren RC. Chronic neck pain, standing balance, and suboccipital muscle atrophy--a pilot study. *J Manipulative Physiol Ther.* 1997 Jan;20(1):24-9

[249] Callaghan MJ, Selfe J, Bagley PJ, Oldham JA. The Effects of Patellar Taping on Knee Joint Proprioception. *J Athl Train.* 2002 Mar;37(1):19-24

[250] Olmsted LC, Carcia CR, Hertel J, Shultz SJ. Efficacy of the Star Excursion Balance Tests in Detecting Reach Deficits in Subjects With Chronic Ankle Instability. *J Athl Train.* 2002 Dec;37(4):501-506 http://www.pubmedcentral.nih.gov/articlerender.fcgi?tool=pubmed&pubmedid=12937574

[251] "The lack of proprioceptive inhibition of nociceptors at the dorsal horn of the spinal cord would result in chronic pain and a loss of standing balance." McPartland JM, Brodeur RR, Hallgren RC. Chronic neck pain, standing balance, and suboccipital muscle atrophy--a pilot study. *J Manipulative Physiol Ther.* 1997 Jan;20(1):24-9

[252] "Functional reorganisation in both the somatosensory and motor system... In patients with chronic low back pain and fibromyalgia... reorganisational change increases with chronicity; ...cortical reorganisation is correlated with the amount of pain... central alterations may be viewed as pain memories ... influence the processing of both painful and nonpainful input..." Flor H. Cortical reorganisation and chronic pain: implications for rehabilitation. *J Rehabil Med.* 2003 May;(41 Suppl):66-72

[253] Murphy DR. Chiropractic rehabilitation of the cervical spine. *J Manipulative Physiol Ther.* 2000 Jul-Aug; 23(6): 404-8

[254] "Unbalanced electromyographic patterns found in patients with LBP given symmetrical tasks were not affected by rehabilitation treatment." Lu WW, Luk KD, Cheung KM, Wong YW, Leong JC. Back muscle contraction patterns of patients with low back pain before and after rehabilitation treatment: an electromyographic evaluation. *J Spinal Disord.* 2001 Aug;14(4):277-82

[255] "RESULTS: After 1 month, back extensor strengthening led to decreased postural stability on hard surface... Balance skill training, however, increased postural stability as indicated by a decreased low-frequency component." Kollmitzer J, Ebenbichler GR, Sabo A, Kerschan K, Bochdansky T. Effects of back extensor strength versus balance training on postural stability. *Med Sci Sports Exerc.* 2000 Oct;32(10):1770-6

The **physical medicine portion** of musculoskeletal rehabilitative programs should generally include:

- Correction of faulty movement patterns: Addressing each of the three major components: 1) initial posture, 2) quality of somatosensory input, and 3) CNS motor programs,
- Promotion of spinal stability: Addressing both the *active* and the *passive* components,
- Proprioceptive/sensorimotor training: Target the neck, torso, lumbar spine, pelvis, and lower extremity,
- Strengthening exercises: Strengthen the neck, shoulders, back, legs, and abdominal and oblique muscles,
- Myofascial and spinal manipulative therapy: Use manual medicine to alleviate pain, facilitate and effect proprioceptive/sensorimotor restoration, and promote optimal joint biomechanics.

A very comprehensive and dense review of this topic was published by Murphy[256] in 2000, and this article is highly recommended for practitioners specializing in rehabilitation.

Clinical techniques for proprioceptive/sensorimotor retraining and rehabilitation:

- Wobble board, balance shoes, foam, exercise ball, or other labile support surface: At the very least, patients should be advised to use a wobble board, balance board, balance shoes or exercise sandals for *at least* 5 minutes 2 times per day every day of the week. Exercise sandals appear to be highly efficient for increasing muscular activity in the lower leg and ankle.[257] Sedentary patients can easily integrate proprioceptive training into their lives—they can use the wobble board or balance shoes while they are watching television. This easy treatment has been shown to facilitate rapid subconscious neuromuscular coordination of the gluteal muscles, thus enhancing pelvic and low-back stability.[258] Other techniques include standing on thick foam or walking in thick sand, which are labile surfaces that require increased neuromuscular control. Standing on one leg and performing gentle motions while blindfolded or with closed eyes further challenges *and therefore improves* the coordination of proprioceptive input with neuromuscular responsiveness.[259,260,261]
- Spinal manipulation: Spinal manipulation appears to improve proprioceptive function.[262]
- Skin taping to increase afferent stimuli: Applying tape to the skin can increase sensory input from cutaneous mechanoreceptors and can improve sensorimotor coordination.[263,264,265,266]
- Vigorous full-body exercise of any and all types, especially those that are relatively fast and require high-frequency complex neuromuscular responses, such as:
  - Swimming: Excellent for promoting fitness in a way that is generally easy on joints and muscles and is without impact; requires and thus promotes coordination and timing
  - Indoor aerobics: Excellent for cardiovascular fitness and weight loss, requires and thus promotes coordination and timing
  - Outdoor cycling (road): Excellent for cardiovascular fitness and weight loss, easy on the joints; requires and promotes coordination and balance
  - Outdoor cycling (mountain and trail): Same as above; requires more balance and coordination than road cycling due to unpredictability of surface; rough surfaces provide flood of afferent stimuli through feet and hands
  - Yoga, Pilates, Calisthenics: Inexpensive, can be done alone or in groups; does not require expensive equipment, can be tailored for low-back rehabilitation[267,268,269]
  - Hiking: Excellent combination of lower extremity strengthening and aerobics; random and uneven trails provide proprioceptive challenge; helps people get in touch with nature.

[256] **Murphy DR. Chiropractic rehabilitation of the cervical spine. *J Manipulative Physiol Ther*. 2000 Jul-Aug;23(6):404-8**
[257] Troy Blackburn J, Hirth CJ, Guskiewicz KM. Exercise Sandals Increase Lower Extremity Electromyographic Activity During Functional Activities. *J Athl Train*. 2003 Sep;38(3):198-203
[258] Bullock-Saxton JE, **Janda V**, Bullock MI.Reflex activation of gluteal muscles in walking. An approach to restoration of muscle function for patients with low-back pain. *Spine* 1993 May;18(6):704-8
[259] Olmsted LC, Carcia CR, Hertel J, Shultz SJ. Efficacy of the Star Excursion Balance Tests in Detecting Reach Deficits in Subjects with Chronic Ankle Instability. *J Athl Train*. 2002 Dec;37(4):501-506
[260] Troy Blackburn J, Hirth CJ, Guskiewicz KM. Exercise Sandals Increase Lower Extremity Electromyographic Activity During Functional Activities. *J Athl Train*. 2003 Sep;38(3):198-203
[261] Willems T, Witvrouw E, Verstuyft J, Vaes P, De Clercq D. Proprioception and Muscle Strength in Subjects With a History of Ankle Sprains and Chronic Instability. *J Athl Train*. 2002 Dec;37(4):487-493
[262] "RESULTS: Subjects receiving manipulation demonstrated a mean reduction in visual analogue scores of 44%, along with a 41% improvement in mean scores for the head repositioning skill." Rogers RG. The effects of spinal manipulation on cervical kinesthesia in patients with chronic neck pain: a pilot study. *J Manipulative Physiol Ther* 1997 Feb;20(2):80-5
[263] "This suggests that ankle taping partly corrects impaired proprioception caused by modern athletic footwear and exercise." Robbins S, Waked E, Rappel R. Ankle taping improves proprioception before and after exercise in young men. *Br J Sports Med*. 1995 Dec;29(4):242-7
[264] "We concluded that increased cutaneous sensory feedback provided by strips of athletic tape applied across the ankle joint of healthy individuals can help improve ankle joint position perception in nonweightbearing, especially for a midrange plantar-flexed ankle position." Simoneau GG, Degner RM, Kramper CA, Kittleson KH. Changes in Ankle Joint Proprioception Resulting From Strips of Athletic Tape Applied Over the Skin. *J Athl Train*. 1997 Apr;32(2):141-147 http://www.pubmedcentral.nih.gov/picrender.fcgi?artid=1319817&blobtype=pdf
[265] Callaghan MJ, Selfe J, Bagley PJ, Oldham JA. The Effects of Patellar Taping on Knee Joint Proprioception. *J Athl Train*. 2002 Mar;37(1):19-24 http://www.pubmedcentral.nih.gov/articlerender.fcgi?tool=pubmed&pubmedid=12937439
[266] "Application of stretch to the skin over VMO via the tape can increase VMO activity, suggesting that cutaneous stimulation may be one mechanism by which patella taping produces a clinical effect." Macgregor K, Gerlach S, Mellor R, Hodges PW. Cutaneous stimulation from patella tape causes a differential increase in vasti muscle activity in people with patellofemoral pain. *J Orthop Res*. 2005 Mar;23(2):351-8
[267] Shiple B. Relieving Low-Back Pain With Exercise. *Physician and Sportsmedicine* 1997; 25: http://www.physsportsmed.com/issues/1997/08aug/shiplepa.htm
[268] Drezner JA. Exercises in the Treatment of Low- Back Pain. *Physician and Sportsmedicine* 2001; 29: http://www.physsportsmed.com/issues/2001/08_01/pa_drezner.htm
[269] Kuritzky L, White J. Extend Yourself for Low-Back Pain Relief. *Physician and Sportsmedicine* 1997; 25: http://www.physsportsmed.com/issues/1997/01jan/back_pa.htm

Reasons to Avoid the Use of Pharmaceutical Nonsteroidal Anti-inflammatory Drugs (NSAIDs) and Selective Cyclooxygenase-2 Inhibitors (coxibs)

Introduction: Nonsteroidal anti-inflammatory drugs (NSAIDs) have many common and serious adverse effects, including the promotion of joint destruction. Paradoxically, these drugs *cause* or *exacerbate* the very symptoms and disease they are supposed to treat: joint pain and destruction. In a tragic exemplification of Orwellian newspeak[270], the habitual utilization and long-term prescription of NSAIDs for joint pain and inflammation as advocated by the pharmaceutical industry[271] and medical textbooks[272] is not described as *malpractice*; rather it is described as the *"standard of care"* and *"first-line therapy."* Adverse effects include:

The Vicious Cycle of NSAID Use: Pain prompts doctors and patients to use NSAIDS, which then promote joint destruction and increased intestinal permeability that promotes systemic inflammation which then contribute to the perpetuation of joint pain.

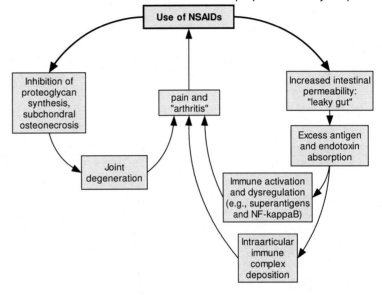

- <u>Gastric ulceration and gastrointestinal bleeding</u>: Nearly all NSAIDs promote gastric ulceration and gastrointestinal bleeding. Among patients who chronically use NSAIDs 65% will develop intestinal inflammation[273] and up to 30% will develop gastroduodenal ulceration.[274] Drugs differ greatly in their propensity to damage the gastrointestinal mucosa and cause bleeding, and aspirin appears to be the most problematic.[275] NSAIDs can also promote and exacerbate colitis and inflammation of the large intestine.[276]

- <u>Increased intestinal permeability</u>: NSAIDs damage the mucosa of the small intestine and promote macromolecular absorption and paracellular permeability—"leaky gut." As described in greater detail later in this text, increased intestinal permeability most certainly contributes to the exacerbation and perpetuation of many rheumatic and musculoskeletal disorders by inducing inflammation via immune activation and by promoting the formation of immune complexes that are then deposited into synovial tissues for the induction of a local inflammatory response inside the joint.[277]

- <u>Promotion of bone necrosis and cartilage destruction</u>: Several NSAIDs cause osteonecrosis[278] and many of these drugs interfere with chondrocyte function and cartilage formation and thus promote the destruction of joints.[279] As noted by Newman and Ling[280], **"...femoral head collapse and acceleration**

[270] Orwell G. <u>1984</u>. New York; Harcourt Brace Jovanovich: 1949. The term "newspeak" is defined by the Merriam-Webster Dictionary (http://www.m-w.com) as "propagandistic language marked by euphemism, circumlocution, and the inversion of customary meanings" and as "a language designed to diminish the range of thought," in the novel *1984* (1949) by George Orwell.
[271] "Congratulations—you've joined the 20 million people who have taken CELEBREX, the #1 doctor-prescribed brand of arthritis medication." http://www.celebrex.com January 24, 2004
[272] "The first drug to treat rheumatoid arthritis is an NSAID." Tierney ML. McPhee SJ, Papadakis MA (eds). <u>Current Medical Diagnosis and Treatment 2002, 41st Edition</u>. New York: Lange Medical Books; 2002. Page 856
[273] "NSAIDs cause small intestinal inflammation in 65% of patients receiving the drugs long-term." Bjarnason I, Macpherson AJ. Intestinal toxicity of non-steroidal anti-inflammatory drugs. *Pharmacol Ther*. 1994 Apr-May;62(1-2):145-57
[274] "Endoscopic studies indicate that up to 30% of chronic NSAID users will develop gastroduodenal ulceration." Blower AL. Considerations for nonsteroidal anti-inflammatory drug therapy: safety. *Scand J Rheumatol Suppl*. 1996;105:13-24
[275] "ASA (1,500 mg/day for 5 days) caused about a 6-fold increase in blood loss. Four days after withdrawal of ASA, faecal blood was still about twice as high as in faeces of subjects given ibuprofen and indoprofen." Porro GB, Corvi G, Fuccella LM, Goldaniga GC, Valzelli G. Gastro-intestinal blood loss during administration of indoprofen, aspirin and ibuprofen. *J Int Med Res* 1977;5(3):155-60
[276] "Non-steroidal anti-inflammatory drugs (NSAIDs) may adversely affect the colon, either by causing a non-specific colitis or by exacerbating a preexisting colonic disease. ... Local and/or systemic effects of NSAIDs on mucosal cells might lead to an increased intestinal permeability, which is a prerequisite for colitis." Faucheron JL, Parc R. Non-steroidal anti-inflammatory drug-induced colitis. *Int J Colorectal Dis*. 1996;11(2):99-101
[277] Inman RD. Antigens, the gastrointestinal tract, and arthritis. *Rheum Dis Clin North Am*. 1991 May; 17(2): 309-21
[278] "The case of a young healthy man, who developed avascular necrosis of head of femur after prolonged administration of indomethacin, is reported here." Prathapkumar KR, Smith I, Attara GA. Indomethacin induced avascular necrosis of head of femur. *Postgrad Med J*. 2000 Sep; 76(899): 574-5
[279] "At...concentrations comparable to those... in the synovial fluid of patients treated with the drug, several NSAIDs suppress proteoglycan synthesis... These NSAID-related effects on chondrocyte metabolism ... are much more profound in osteoarthritic cartilage than in normal cartilage, due to enhanced uptake of NSAIDs by the osteoarthritic cartilage." Brandt KD. Effects of nonsteroidal anti-inflammatory drugs on chondrocyte metabolism in vitro and in vivo. *Am J Med*. 1987 Nov 20; 83(5A): 29-34
[280] Newman NM, Ling RS. Acetabular bone destruction related to non-steroidal anti-inflammatory drugs. *Lancet*. 1985 Jul 6; 2(8445): 11-4

of osteoarthritis have been well documented in association with the NSAIDs..." The subchondral osteonecrosis induced by many NSAIDs may both necessitate and complicate arthroplasty (joint replacement with prosthesis) because of extensive joint damage and because the underlying bone that must hold the new implant is too weak to provide a stable foundation.[281] *In vivo* studies have shown that salicylate, acetylsalicylic acid, fenoprofen, isoxicam, tolmetin, and ibuprofen reduce glycosaminoglycan synthesis.[282] COX-2 inhibition impairs anabolic bone activity that is necessary for the preservation of bone strength.[283,284]

- Promotion of hepatic and renal injury and failure: Chronic use of NSAIDs is an important risk factor for the development of renal failure.[285] Hepatic injury is less common than NSAID-induced renal failure but can be achieved with higher drug doses (especially with the non-NSAID analgesic acetaminophen), coadministration of drugs, and concomitant consumption of alcohol.

- Death: NSAIDs are an impressively significant cause of death in America. According to the review by Singh[286], "**Conservative calculations estimate that approximately 107,000 patients are hospitalized annually for nonsteroidal anti-inflammatory drug (NSAID)-related gastrointestinal (GI) complications and at least 16,500 NSAID-related deaths occur each year among arthritis patients alone. The figures for all NSAID users would be overwhelming, yet the scope of this problem is generally under-appreciated.**"

- Adverse effects specific to Coxibs: Drugs specifically designed to inhibit the isoform of cyclooxygenase known as cyclooxygenase-2 (coxibs) carry their own list of adverse effects, namely membranous glomerulopathy and acute interstitial nephritis[287], acute cholestatic hepatitis[288], toxic epidermal necrolysis[289,290], and—perhaps most importantly—increased risk for cardiovascular disease (e.g., stroke, hypertension, myocardial infarction) and cardiovascular death. Immediately following the withdrawal of the arthritis drug rofecoxib (Vioxx) in late September 2004, Topol[291] extrapolated that as many as 160,000 adverse cardiovascular events (including stroke, myocardial infarction, and death) may have resulted from the overuse of Vioxx/rofecoxib due to the collusion of Merck's intentional failure to withdraw what was known for years to be a dangerous drug, the FDA's failure to enforce regulatory standards to protect the public, and the overutilization of Vioxx by the medical profession, which was well informed of the lethality of Vioxx for several years[292] before Merck's confessionary and belated withdrawal of the drug. Soon thereafter, several other so-called "anti-inflammatory drugs" such as valdecoxib (Bextra)[293], celecoxib (Celebrex)[294], and naproxen (Aleve)[295] were likewise associated with excess cardiovascular injury and death. Although the advertising-induced feeding frenzy on Celebrex made it the most "successful" drug launch in US history with more than 7.4 million prescriptions written within its first 6 months[296], major adverse effects due to the drug were noted within 2 years of its release onto the medical market[297]; current guidelines hold that patients must be informed of the excess cardiovascular risk associated with this drug and that its use should be limited to the lowest dose for the shortest time possible (weeks).[298] When compared with placebo in cardiac surgery patients, Bextra/valdecoxib is associated with a 3-fold to 4-fold increased risk of heart attack,

[281] "This highly significant association between NSAID use and acetabular destruction gives cause for concern, not least because of the difficulty in achieving satisfactory hip replacements in patients with severely damaged acetabula." Newman NM, Ling RS. Acetabular bone destruction related to non-steroidal anti-inflammatory drugs. *Lancet.* 1985 Jul 6; 2(8445): 11-4

[282] Brandt KD. Effects of nonsteroidal anti-inflammatory drugs on chondrocyte metabolism in vitro and in vivo. *Am J Med.* 1987 Nov 20; 83(5A): 29-34

[283] "Histological observations suggest that cox-2 is required for normal endochondral ossification during fracture healing. Because mice lacking Cox2 form normal skeletons, our observations indicate that fetal bone development and fracture healing are different and that cox-2 function is specifically essential for fracture healing." Simon AM, Manigrasso MB, O'Connor JP. Cyclo-oxygenase 2 function is essential for bone fracture healing. *J Bone Miner Res.* 2002 Jun;17(6):963-76

[284] "The results indicate that cox-2 and constitutive NOS are important signaling molecules in the anabolic responses of neonatal tibial bone to the micromechanical load in vitro." Kunnel JG, Igarashi K, Gilbert JL, Stern PH. Bone anabolic responses to mechanical load in vitro involve cox-2 and constitutive NOS. *Connect Tissue Res.* 2004;45(1):40-9

[285] "Patients with chronic arthritis who consume excessive amount of NSAIDs are at risk of developing renal papillary necrosis and chronic renal impairment." Segasothy M, Chin GL, Sia KK, Zulfiqar A, Samad SA. Chronic nephrotoxicity of anti-inflammatory drugs used in the treatment of arthritis. *Br J Rheumatol.* 1995 Feb; 34(2): 162-5

[286] Singh G. Recent considerations in nonsteroidal anti-inflammatory drug gastropathy. *Am J Med.* 1998 Jul 27; 105(1B): 31S-38S

[287] Markowitz GS, Falkowitz DC, Isom R, Zaki M, Imaizumi S, Appel GB, D'Agati VD. Membranous glomerulopathy and acute interstitial nephritis following treatment with celecoxib. *Clin Nephrol.* 2003;59(2):137-42

[288] Grieco A, Miele L, Giorgi A, Civello IM, Gasbarrini G. Acute cholestatic hepatitis associated with celecoxib. *Ann Pharmacother.* 2002;36(12):1887-9

[289] Berger P, Dwyer D, Corallo CE. Toxic epidermal necrolysis after celecoxib therapy. *Pharmacotherapy.* 2002 Sep;22(9):1193-5.

[290] Friedman B, Orlet HK, Still JM, Law E. Toxic epidermal necrolysis due to administration of celecoxib (Celebrex). *South Med J.* 2002;95(10):1213-4

[291] Topol EJ. Failing the public health--rofecoxib, Merck, and the FDA. *N Engl J Med.* 2004 Oct 21;351(17):1707-9

[292] Mukherjee D, Nissen SE, Topol EJ. Risk of cardiovascular events associated with selective cox-2 inhibitors. *JAMA* 2001; 286(8):954-9

[293] Ray WA, Griffin MR, Stein CM. Cardiovascular toxicity of valdecoxib. *N Engl J Med.* 2004;351(26):2767

[294] "Patients in the clinical trial taking 400 mg. of Celebrex twice daily had a 3.4 times greater risk of CV events compared to placebo. For patients in the trial taking 200 mg. of Celebrex twice daily, the risk was 2.5 times greater. The average duration of treatment in the trial was 33 months." FDA Statement on the Halting of a Clinical Trial of the cox-2 Inhibitor Celecoxib. http://www.fda.gov/bbs/topics/news/2004/NEW01144.html Available on January 4, 2005

[295] "Preliminary information from the study showed some evidence of increased risk of cardiovascular events, when compared to placebo, to patients taking naproxen." FDA Statement on Naproxen. http://www.fda.gov/bbs/topics/news/2004/NEW01148.html Available on January 4, 2005

[296] Monsanto, Pfizer celebrate Celebrex. *St. Louis Business Journal.* July 20, 1999 http://www.bizjournals.com/stlouis/stories/1999/07/19/daily5.html Accessed on January 5, 2005

[297] Mukherjee D, Nissen SE, Topol EJ. Risk of cardiovascular events associated with selective cox-2 inhibitors. *JAMA.* 2001 Aug 22-29;286(8):954-9

[298] "Celecoxib should be used in the lowest effective doses for short periods (weeks) only. A risk–benefit discussion is necessary for those requiring the drug for a longer period." Cotter J, Wooltorton E. New restrictions on celecoxib (Celebrex) use and the withdrawal of valdecoxib (Bextra). *CMAJ.* 2005 May 10;172(10):1299. Epub 2005 Apr 15 http://www.cmaj.ca/cgi/content/full/172/10/1299 Accessed September 28, 2005

stroke, and death[299], and recently 7 million arthritis patients, many of whom were already at high risk for cardiovascular disease, were being treated with this drug.[300] Use of Bextra was also strongly associated with toxic epidermal necrolysis, a potentially fatal condition.[301] Due primarily to the adverse cardiovascular effects[302], in the interest of protecting the public from additional adverse effects and unnecessary deaths, in April 2005 the FDA ordered that Bextra/valdecoxib be taken off the market in the US[303], and Health Canada followed suit by removing the drug from Canadian markets.[304] **It is inexcusable that these drugs were so highly utilized despite evidence of relative analgesic inefficacy (not better than earlier NSAIDs like aspirin), exorbitant costs (US $90-180 per month[305]) and clear evidence of danger (e.g., cardiovascular death) by two well-identified biochemical/physiologic mechanisms, namely: 1) inhibiting the formation of vasodilating and anti-aggregatory prostacyclin, which is formed by COX-2, and 2) shunting arachidonate toward formation of pro-atherosclerotic leukotrienes[306] by blocking cyclooxygenase.** Inhibition of prostacyclin formation promotes thrombosis and hypertension.

Perspective: If we summarize that at least 17,000 people die each year from NSAIDs, that other "medication errors" kill over 7,000 people in America[307] and that an additional 180,000 Americans die due to hospital errors[308], then we have a situation where at least 200,000 Americans die each year due to drug effects and hospital/physician errors. Furthermore, according to estimates by David Graham, MD, MPH, (Associate Director for Science, Office of Drug Safety, US FDA), more than 139,000 Americans who took Vioxx suffered serious side effects and between 26,000 and 55,000 people died from using the drug.[309] This aggregate is significantly more than the annual deaths due to diabetes (71,000), suicide (30,000), homicide (20,000) [310], and the September 11, 2001 terrorist attack (up to 3,000) *combined*.[311] Preliminary data indicates that natural treatments such as spinal manipulation[312], glucosamine sulfate[313], and *Harpagophytum*[314] are safer and/or more effective than NSAIDs for the relief of many types of pain. The increased utilization of these nonpharmacologic treatments will result in reductions in morbidity, mortality, and overall healthcare expenses when compared to our current overutilization of NSAIDs and other medical/allopathic pharmacosurgical treatments.[315]

"Only that day dawns to which we are awake."   *Henry David Thoreau*[316]

---

[299] Lenzer J. Pfizer criticised over delay in admitting drug's problems. *BMJ*. 2004;329(7472):935

[300] Ray WA, Griffin MR, Stein CM. Cardiovascular toxicity of valdecoxib. *N Engl J Med*. 2004;351(26):2767

[301] "There is a strong association between Stevens-Johnson syndrome/toxic epidermal necrolysis and the use of the sulfonamide cox-2 inhibitors, particularly valdecoxib." La Grenade L, Lee L, Weaver J, Bonnel R, Karwoski C, Governale L, Brinker A. Comparison of Reporting of Stevens-Johnson Syndrome and Toxic Epidermal Necrolysis in Association with Selective cox-2 Inhibitors. *Drug Saf*. 2005;28(10):917-24

[302] Nussmeier NA, Whelton AA, Brown MT, Langford RM, Hoeft A, Parlow JL, Boyce SW, Verburg KM. Complications of the cox-2 inhibitors parecoxib and valdecoxib after cardiac surgery. *N Engl J Med*. 2005 Mar 17;352(11):1081-91. Epub 2005 Feb 15

[303] "On April 7, the Food and Drug Administration requested that Pfizer suspend sales of BEXTRA in the United States. As a result, BEXTRA will no longer be available to patients in the United States... In light of the FDA's position that there is an increased cardiovascular risk for all prescription non-steroidal anti-inflammatory arthritis medicines, as well as the increased rate of rare, serious skin reactions with BEXTRA, the FDA has requested that sales of BEXTRA be suspended." http://www.bextra.com/ Accessed September 28, 2005

[304] Sibbald B. Pfizer withdraw valdecoxib (Bextra) at Health Canada's request. *CMAJ*. 2005 May 10;172(10):e1298. Epub 2005 Apr 7 http://www.cmaj.ca/cgi/reprint/172/10/e1298 Accessed September 28, 2005

[305] http://www.walgreens.com/library/finddrug/druginfo1.jsp?particularDrug=Celebrex&id=15102 Accessed September 29, 2005

[306] "CONCLUSIONS: Variant 5-lipoxygenase genotypes identify a subpopulation with increased atherosclerosis. The observed diet-gene interactions further suggest that dietary n-6 polyunsaturated fatty acids promote, whereas marine n-3 fatty acids inhibit, leukotriene-mediated inflammation that leads to atherosclerosis in this subpopulation." Dwyer JH, Allayee H, Dwyer KM, Fan J, Wu H, Mar R, Lusis AJ, Mehrabian M. Arachidonate 5-lipoxygenase promoter genotype, dietary arachidonic acid, and atherosclerosis. *N Engl J Med*. 2004 Jan 1;350(1):29-37

[307] "In 1983, 2876 people died from medication errors. ... By 1993, this number had risen to 7,391 - a 2.57-fold increase." Phillips DP, Christenfeld N, Glynn LM. Increase in US medication-error deaths between 1983 and 1993. *Lancet*. 1998 Feb 28;351(9103):643-4

[308] "Recent estimates suggest that each year more than 1 million patients are injured while in the hospital and approximately 180,000 die because of these injuries. Furthermore, drug-related morbidity and mortality are common and are estimated to cost more than $136 billion a year." Holland EG, Degruy FV. Drug-induced disorders. *Am Fam Physician*. 1997;56(7):1781-8, 1791-2

[309] http://www.commondreams.org/views05/0223-35.htm and http://www.fda.gov/cder/drug/infopage/vioxx/vioxxgraham.pdf Accessed July 26, 2006

[310] Centers for Disease Control and Prevention (CDC), National Center for Health Statistics. Deaths: Final Data for 2001. 116 pp. (PHS) 2003-1120. Available at http://www.cdc.gov/nchs/releases/03facts/mortalitytrends.htm on January 18, 2004

[311] "On September 11, 2001, four U.S. planes hijacked by terrorists crashed into the World Trade Center, the Pentagon and a field in Pennsylvania killing nearly 3,000 people in a matter of hours." From http://www.cnn.com/SPECIALS/2001/memorial/ on January 26, 2004

[312] "CONCLUSION: The best evidence indicates that cervical manipulation for neck pain is much safer than the use of NSAIDs, by as much as a factor of several hundred times. There is no evidence that indicates NSAID use is any more effective than cervical manipulation for neck pain." Dabbs V, Lauretti WJ. A risk assessment of cervical manipulation vs. NSAIDs for the treatment of neck pain. *J Manipulative Physiol Ther*. 1995 Oct;18(8):530-6

[313] Muller-Fassbender H, Bach GL, Haase W, Rovati LC, Setnikar I. Glucosamine sulfate compared to ibuprofen in osteoarthritis of the knee. *Osteoarthritis Cartilage*. 1994 Mar;2(1):61-9

[314] Chrubasik S, Model A, Black A, Pollak S. A randomized double-blind pilot study comparing Doloteffin and Vioxx in the treatment of low back pain. *Rheumatology* (Oxford). 2003 Jan;42(1):141-8

[315] Orme-Johnson DW, Herron RE. An innovative approach to reducing medical care utilization and expenditures. *Am J Manag Care*. 1997 Jan;3:135-44 http://www.ajmc.com/Article.cfm?Menu=1&ID=2154

[316] Thoreau HD. (Owen Thomas, Ed). Walden and Civil Disobedience. New York; WW Norton and Company: 1966, page 221

Another Clinically Useful Mnemonic Acronym: "B.e.n.d. S.t.e.m.s."

As an alternative to the "p.r.i.c.e. a. t.u.r.n." acronym previously described, clinicians may use the following alternate, either additively or substitutionally. "B.e.n.d. s.t.e.m.s." is aesthetically more appealing, though it is less complete than *price a turn*. The goal, of course, is to have a useful memory key available when the clinician is formulating the treatment plan. Just as all doctors are familiar with the *s.o.a.p.* format for writing chart notes to ensure their inclusion of *subjective, objective, assessment,* and *plan* for each visit, when arriving to the "p" portion of the note, integrative clinicians can use *price a turn* and/or *bend stems* to help remember key components to integrative and holistic care.

B   **Botanical**: Numerous botanical medicines are available for a wide range of indications. Among the botanical medicines with the best research support for the treatment of musculoskeletal pain and inflammation are willow bark, *Boswellia, Harpagophytum, Uncaria,* ginger, and *Capsicum.*

E   **Ergonomics/posture and Exercise**: Patients can improve their ergonomics at home, at work, and (occasionally) in the car. Likewise, attention to posture—the "style" with which one holds one's body—is important in the prevention of repetitive strain injuries, particularly to the shoulders and neck region. Most patients are overweight, out of shape, weak, and neuromuscularly uncoordinated; problems correctible with exercise.

N   **Nutrition**: Nutritional supplements are extremely valuable in the treatment and prevention of a wide range of mild and serious health problems. Use of high-dose "supranutritional" levels of vitamins can be used to help patients overcome their enzyme and receptor defects to facilitate improved physiological function and improved overall health.[317]

D   **Diet**: In order to remain consistent with the time-proven wisdom of the *Hierarchy of Therapeutics* (discussed in Chapter 2) and to avoid becoming an aimless horde of drug-pushing symptom-suppressors, holistic integrative clinicians must always attend to the basics—the foundational influences which powerfully affect metabolism and thus overall health. Clearly, diet is one of those basics, along with emotions and lifestyle—exercise, work, stress management, outlook, and relationships.

S   **Stretching, strengthening, and stabilization**: Tight muscles can be stretched in the office, where the doctor is able to teach the patient proper methods and is able to refine the diagnosis and specificity of the stretch to ensure that targeted muscles are effectively addressed. Thereafter, the patient *must* continue these stretches at home—both physically and mentally. *Physical stretching* involves the therapeutic lengthening of muscles and fascia to maintain or restore ease of myofascial motion and to alleviate adhesions or restrictions that impair function. *Mental stretching* involves the patient's active use of reframing and discipline in order to attain a higher level of functioning and effectiveness in his/her relationships, lifestyle, work situation, mental outlook, habits and other phenomena in order to overcome the external or internal *adhesions* or *restrictions* that are impairing and preventing optimal function *of the patient as a whole.* Exercise and proproceptive rehabilitation for spinal and peripheral joint stabilization are essential requirements for neuromusculoskeletal health.

T   **Trigger points**: Always remember to address the trigger point component (discussed previously in this chapter) when working with musculoskeletal pain. Seek and ye shall find; treat and the patient will improve. Think outside the region. A trigger point in the low-back or gluteal region may cause the patient to assume an antalgic posture that results in altered biomechanics and leads to a clinical presentation of shoulder or neck pain with chronic tension headaches; direct treatment of the painful shoulders or neck will provide improvement, but cure will not be effected until the cause—often distant from the region of complaint—is effectively addressed.[318]

E   **Educate and Ensure return**: Educate the patient about the condition, its cause and solutions. Educate about PAR-B—procedures, risks, alternatives, and benefits of treatment. Also, educate the patient *in writing* about the importance of follow-up visits and time limitations on treatments; failure to ensure that the patient was educated to return for follow-up visits is grounds for malpractice if the patient's condition changes or deteriorates due to complications associated with the presenting complaint at the last office visit.

M   **Manual medicine—mobilization, manipulation, massage**: Treat the problem effectively and directly with the skilled use of your hands. Practice produces proficiency.

S   **Spirituality (emotions, psychology)**: Perceptions create our emotional and mental realities, and from these subjective realities do we engage the world. Inaccurate perceptions skew and misshape one's interactions with the world. Creating more accurate perceptions—a process that requires intentionality and hard work—enhances *effectiveness* and ultimately *enjoyment* of one's life experience.

---

[317] Ames BN, Elson-Schwab I, Silver EA. High-dose vitamin therapy stimulates variant enzymes with decreased coenzyme binding affinity (increased K(m)): relevance to genetic disease and polymorphisms. *Am J Clin Nutr.* 2002 Apr;75(4):616-58 http://www.ajcn.org/cgi/content/full/75/4/616
[318] "This patient seemed to respond favorably to conservative care that included regions of spine not traditionally associated with headache pain." Stude DE, Sweere JJ. A holistic approach to severe headache symptoms in a patient unresponsive to regional manual therapy. *J Manipulative Physiol Ther.* 1996 Mar-Apr;19(3):202-7

<u>Topics:</u>

- **Food allergy and adverse food reactions**
  - o Allergy, sensitivity, intolerance
  - o Role of food allergy in the induction and perpetuation of autoimmunity and chronic inflammation
  - o Clinical and laboratory diagnosis
  - o Orthomolecular immunomodulation: a four-tiered approach
- **Multifocal dysbiosis**
  - o Overview and mechanisms of disease induction
  - o Gastrointestinal dysbiosis
  - o Genitourinary dysbiosis
  - o Orodental dysbiosis
  - o Parenchymal dysbiosis
  - o Sinorespiratory dysbiosis
  - o Cutaneous dysbiosis
  - o Environmental dysbiosis
- **Xenobiotic Immunotoxicity**
  - o Overview
  - o Chemical xenobiotics
  - o Toxic metals
  - o Therapeutic considerations
- **Orthoendocrinology**
  - o Overview and implications
  - o Assessments and therapeutics
- **Immunonutrigenomics**

<u>Major Modifiable Contributors to Autoimmunity and Immune Dysfunction</u>

Autoimmune phenomena do not occur without *cause*, nor without *multiple causes*. Autoimmunity is a reflection of immune dysfunction. From an allopathic perspective, since nearly all autoimmune diseases are labeled as "idiopathic", the focus is on attaining a diagnosis and then prescribing the "appropriate" drug which interferes with the *expression* of the underlying immune dysfunction but which generally does not address the *causes* of the underlying immune dysfunction. In naturopathic medicine, we seek to restore health by correcting the underlying contributors to illness.

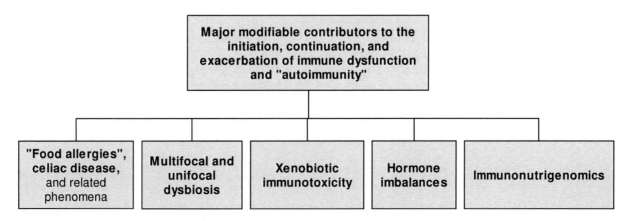

Food Allergy and Adverse Food Reactions

"Adverse food reactions" is a broad and general category that includes food allergy, food sensitivity, and food intolerance. The term "food" here means anything that is ingested other than drugs and medications and includes food, drink, food additives, preservatives, and food dyes. Many studies in the medical literature underestimate the high prevalence and clinical importance of food allergies because of inconsistent terminology, imperfect laboratory assessments[1], and the assumption that an "apparently healthy" person would only be allergic/sensitive to one or two foods—this is an erroneous assumption considering that many patients with food allergy/sensitivity/intolerance must avoid several (common range 3-10) commonly eaten foods to obtain clinical response and maximal improvement.[2,3] Clinical practice differs from basic research in that we as clinicians must often do what is effective while having neither the need nor the luxury for determining the molecular and physiologic basis for the effectiveness of each treatment in each patient. Clinical research has scientifically proven that adverse food reactions, regardless of the underlying mechanism(s) or classification of allergy, intolerance, or sensitivity, can exacerbate a wide range of human illnesses, including thyroid disease[4], mental depression[5,6], asthma, rhinitis,[7] recurrent otitis media[8], migraine[9,10,11], attention deficit and hyperactivity disorders[12], epilepsy[13,14,15], gastrointestinal inflammation[16], hypertension[17], joint pain[18,19,20,21,22,23,24,] and other health problems. **The common view of allergic phenomena it is incomplete and therefore inaccurate because it fails to include the prerequisite immune dysfunction and complex physiologic interconnections.**

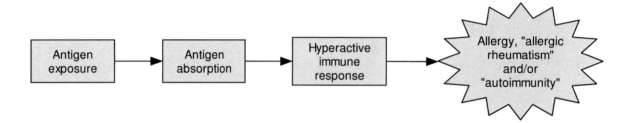

"Food allergy" generally refers to adverse food reactions that are specifically immunoglobulin-mediated. Classically, food allergy is seen with immediate-onset allergy mediated via IgE antibodies which initiate mast cell degranulation and histamine release. The classic symptoms of immediate-onset allergies are skin rash, abdominal pain, angioedema, and bronchoconstriction. However, many doctors recognize the possibility of IgG-mediated allergies and suggest that these might be responsible for the delayed-onset or "hidden" food allergies which are clinically significant but more subtle and difficult to diagnose than the classic IgE-mediated allergies. The binding of antigens with immunoglobulins forms immune complexes

[1] Bindslev-Jensen C, Skov PS, Madsen F, Poulsen LK. Food allergy and food intolerance--what is the difference? *Ann Allergy.* 1994 Apr;72(4):317-20

[2] Grant EC. Food allergies and migraine. *Lancet.* 1979 May 5;1(8123):966-9

[3] Speer F. Multiple food allergy. *Ann Allergy.* 1975 Feb;34(2):71-6

[4] Sategna-Guidetti C, Volta U, Ciacci C, Usai P, Carlino A, De Franceschi L, Camera A, Pelli A, Brossa C. Prevalence of thyroid disorders in untreated adult celiac disease patients and effect of gluten withdrawal: an Italian multicenter study. *Am J Gastroenterol.* 2001 Mar;96(3):751-7

[5] Mills N. Depression and food intolerance: a single case study. *Hum Nutr Appl Nutr.* 1986 Apr;40(2):141-5

[6] Parker G, Watkins T. Treatment-resistant depression: when antidepressant drug intolerance may indicate food intolerance. *Aust N Z J Psychiatry.* 2002 Apr;36(2):263-5

[7] Speer F. The allergic child. *Am Fam Physician.* 1975 Feb;11(2):88-94

[8] Juntti H, Tikkanen S, Kokkonen J, Alho OP, Niinimaki A. Cow's milk allergy is associated with recurrent otitis media during childhood. *Acta Otolaryngol.* 1999;119(8):867-73

[9] Monro J, Carini C, Brostoff J. Migraine is a food-allergic disease. *Lancet.* 1984 Sep 29;2(8405):719-21

[10] Egger J, Carter CM, Wilson J, Turner MW, Soothill JF. Is migraine food allergy? A double-blind controlled trial of oligoantigenic diet treatment. *Lancet.* 1983 Oct 15;2(8355):865-9

[11] Monro J, Brostoff J, Carini C, Zilkha K. Food allergy in migraine. Study of dietary exclusion and RAST. *Lancet.* 1980 Jul 5;2(8184):1-4

[12] Boris M, Mandel FS. Foods and additives are common causes of the attention deficit hyperactive disorder in children. *Ann Allergy.* 1994 May;72(5):462-8

[13] Egger J, Carter CM, Soothill JF, Wilson J. Oligoantigenic diet treatment of children with epilepsy and migraine. *J Pediatr.* 1989;114(1):51-8

[14] Pelliccia A, Lucarelli S, Frediani T, D'Ambrini G, Cerminara C, Barbato M, Vagnucci B, Cardi E. Partial cryptogenetic epilepsy and food allergy/intolerance. A causal or a chance relationship? Reflections on three clinical cases. *Minerva Pediatr.* 1999 May;51(5):153-7

[15] Frediani T, Lucarelli S, Pelliccia A, Vagnucci B, Cerminara C, Barbato M, Cardi E. Allergy and childhood epilepsy: a close relationship? *Acta Neurol Scand.* 2001 Dec;104(6):349-52

[16] Marr HY, Chen WC, Lin LH. Food protein-induced enterocolitis syndrome: report of one case. *Acta Paediatr Taiwan.* 2001;42(1):49-52

[17] Grant EC. Food allergies and migraine. *Lancet.* 1979 May 5;1(8123):966-9

[18] Golding DN. Is there an allergic synovitis? *J R Soc Med.* 1990 May;83(5):312-4

[19] Panush RS. Food induced ("allergic") arthritis: clinical and serologic studies. *J Rheumatol.* 1990 Mar;17(3):291-4

[20] Pacor ML, Lunardi C, Di Lorenzo G, Biasi D, Corrocher R. Food allergy and seronegative arthritis: report of two cases. *Clin Rheumatol.* 2001;20(4):279-81

[21] Schrander JJ, Marcelis C, de Vries MP, van Santen-Hoeufft HM. Does food intolerance play a role in juvenile chronic arthritis? *Br J Rheumatol.* 1997;36(8):905-8

[22] van de Laar MA, van der Korst JK. Food intolerance in rheumatoid arthritis. I. A double blind, controlled trial of the clinical effects of elimination of milk allergens and azo dyes. *Ann Rheum Dis.* 1992 Mar;51(3):298-302

[23] Haugen MA, Kjeldsen-Kragh J, Forre O. A pilot study of the effect of an elemental diet in the management of rheumatoid arthritis. *Clin Exp Rheumatol.* 1994 May-Jun;12(3):275-9

[24] van de Laar MA, Aalbers M, Bruins FG, van Dinther-Janssen AC, van der Korst JK, Meijer CJ. Food intolerance in rheumatoid arthritis. II. Clinical and histological aspects. *Ann Rheum Dis.* 1992 Mar;51(3):303-6

that can deposit in parenchymal and synovial tissues where a localized immune response causes inflammation and organ dysfunction. **"Food sensitivity"** refers to immune-mediated adverse food reactions that are not antibody-mediated but are mediated by some other aspect of the immune/inflammatory system. An example of this is the increased production of specific prostaglandins in food-induced irritable bowel syndrome.[25] **"Food intolerance"** refers to adverse food reactions which are associated with poor nutritional status and/or impaired hepatic detoxification and which are *not* immune-mediated. Classic and well-known examples of this category of adverse food reaction include MSG sensitivity (associated with deficiency of vitamin B-6 and subsequent defects in hepatic transamination), tyramine intolerance that can result in hypertension and headaches, and histamine intolerance that can result in bronchoconstriction.[26] Surely, there is some overlap between allergy, sensitivity, and intolerance in some patients, and regardless of the specific mechanism(s) involved, from a practical clinical standpoint, the following facts are self-evident for any doctor working in the field of nutrition:

1. Some people have adverse food reactions from the foods that they eat.
2. Food-induced reactions may be either immediate-onset (i.e., within minutes) or delayed-onset (within days) of eating the triggering food.
3. The same patient might have immediate-onset reactions to food X with symptoms A and B and simultaneously have a delayed-onset reaction to food Y with symptom C.
4. Food X might cause symptoms D and E in one patient and symptoms F and G in another patient.
5. By avoiding allergens and/or improving immune function, many "diseases" go away with out direct treatment and the patient experiences an improved state of health.
6. Failure to identify and avoid problematic foods combined with failure to correct the underlying immune dysfunction often makes the "disease" recalcitrant to remediation even with "generally effective" treatment. This has been demonstrated in migraine, hypertension[27], and drug-resistant mental depression.[28]

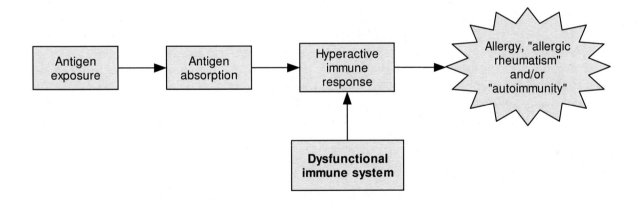

---

[25] "Food intolerance associated with prostaglandin production is an important factor in the pathogenesis of IBS." Jones VA, McLaughlan P, Shorthouse M, Workman E, Hunter JO. Food intolerance: a major factor in the pathogenesis of irritable bowel syndrome. *Lancet.* 1982 Nov 20;2(8308):1115-7

[26] Wantke F, Hemmer W, Haglmuller T, Gotz M, Jarisch R. Histamine in wine. Bronchoconstriction after a double-blind placebo-controlled red wine provocation test. *Int Arch Allergy Immunol.* 1996 Aug;110(4):397-400

[27] "When an average of ten common foods were avoided there was a dramatic fall in the number of headaches per month, 85% of patients becoming headache-free. The 25% of patients with hypertension became normotensive." Grant EC. Food allergies and migraine. *Lancet.* 1979 May 5;1(8123):966-9

[28] "The prevalence of food intolerance as a contributing factor to depressive disorders requires clarification. Clinicians should be aware of the possible syndrome and that it may be worsened by psychotropic medication." Parker G, Watkins T.Treatment-resistant depression: when antidepressant drug intolerance may indicate food intolerance. *Aust N Z J Psychiatry.* 2002 Apr;36(2):263-5

Potential roles of "food allergy" in the induction and perpetuation of autoimmunity and chronic inflammation

Food allergy both *results from* and *contributes to* immune dysfunction and a systemic proinflammatory state. Food allergy contributes to "autoimmunity" and musculoskeletal inflammation via several mechanisms, including but not limited to the following:

1. <u>Stimulation of cytokine release</u>: As will be discussed later, the term "superantigen" classically refers to microbial—viral, bacterial, or fungal—antigens which have the ability to induce production of excessive levels of cytokines and other inflammatory effectors[29], and superantigens appear to be involved in the pathogenesis of inflammatory musculoskeletal disorders such as rheumatoid arthritis.[30,31] **In this section I propose that since food allergens appear capable of inducing cytokine production, they should in certain circumstances be considered "dietary superantigens"** since they invoke cytokine release similarly as do microbial superantigens. An important distinction here, however, is that microbial superantigens generally stimulate cytokine release as an inherent property in *all* patients, whereas **the production of cytokines by dietary (super)antigens is dependent on previous sensitization**; thus cytokine production by allergens is patient-dependent and not an inherent property of the allergen itself. **Mononuclear cells from egg-allergic patients produce much more proinflammatory cytokine (interferon) than do those from nonallergic patients.**[32] Similarly, **in children with autism, who commonly demonstrate immune dysfunction and neuroautoimmunity**[33], **exposure to food allergens greatly increases cytokine release compared to controls.**[34] Food allergy, NFkB activation, cytokine release, and increased intestinal permeability form a self-perpetuating vicious cycle because consumption of dietary allergens causes damage to the intestinal mucosa and stimulates NFkB activation and cytokine release which then increases intestinal permeability, thus allowing for increased absorption of dietary and microbial immunogens for the perpetuation and exacerbation of allergy and immune dysfunction.[35] Generally speaking, cytokines are proinflammatory and would be expected to contribute to autoimmune disease induction via mechanisms such as bystander activation and increased autoantigen processing regardless of their original stimuli.

2. <u>Immune complex formation and deposition</u>: **Dietary antigen-antibody immune complexes are formed following the consumption of allergenic foods by patients with allergy to those foods**[36,37] and these anti-food and anti-IgE immune complexes contribute to allergic symptomatology by a mechanism that has been described as "chronic serum sickness."[38] These immune complexes are then deposited in the joints to localize the resultant proinflammatory response. In the study by Carini et al[39], the authors found that **patients with food-induced joint pain and inflammation had anti-IgE IgG antibodies which formed large immune complexes that were detectable in synovial fluid and which probably contributed to the arthritis.** Anti-IgE IgG antibodies are commonly elevated in patients with allergic/inflammatory diseases such as

---

[29] "The basis of autoimmune disorders due to superantigen is due to greater stimulation of T-lymphocytes and elaborate cytokine production." Hemalatha V, Srikanth P, Mallika M. Superantigens - Concepts, clinical disease and therapy. *Indian J Med Microbiol* 2004;22:204-211

[30] "They also suggest that the etiology of RA may involve initial activation of V beta 14+ T cells by a V beta 14-specific superantigen with subsequent recruitment of a few activated autoreactive v beta 14+ T cell clones to the joints while the majority of other V beta 14+ T cells disappear." Paliard X, West SG, Lafferty JA, Clements JR, Kappler JW, Marrack P, Kotzin BL. Evidence for the effects of a superantigen in rheumatoid arthritis. *Science*. 1991 Jul 19;253(5017):325-9

[31] "Given that binding sites for superantigens have been mapped to the CDR4s of TCR beta chains, the synovial localization of T cells bearing V beta s with significant CDR4 homology indicates that V beta-specific T-cell activation by superantigen may play a role in RA." Howell MD, Diveley JP, Lundeen KA, Esty A, Winters ST, Carlo DJ, Brostoff SW. Limited T-cell receptor beta-chain heterogeneity among interleukin 2 receptor-positive synovial T cells suggests a role for superantigen in rheumatoid arthritis. *Proc Natl Acad Sci U S A*. 1991 Dec 1;88(23):10921-5

[32] "The levels of IFN-gamma production of only IL-2-stimulated or both ovalbumin-stimulated and IL-2-stimulated peripheral blood mononuclear cells from egg-sensitive patients with atopic dermatitis was significantly higher than that of healthy children and that of egg-sensitive children with immediate allergic symptoms." Shinbara M, Kondo N, Agata H, Fukutomi O, Kuwabara N, Kobayashi Y, Miura M, Orii T. Interferon-gamma and interleukin-4 production of ovalbumin-stimulated lymphocytes in egg-sensitive children. *Ann Allergy Asthma Immunol*. 1996;77(1):60-6

[33] "Autistic children, but not normal children, had antibodies to caudate nucleus (49% positive sera), cerebral cortex (18% positive sera) and cerebellum (9% positive sera)." Singh VK, Rivas WH. Prevalence of serum antibodies to caudate nucleus in autistic children. *Neurosci Lett*. 2004 Jan 23;355(1-2):53-6

[34] Jyonouchi H, Sun S, Itokazu N. Innate immunity associated with inflammatory responses and cytokine production against common dietary proteins in patients with autism spectrum disorder. *Neuropsychobiology*. 2002;46(2):76-84

[35] Ma TY, Iwamoto GK, Hoa NT, Akotia V, Pedram A, Boivin MA, Said HM. TNF-alpha-induced increase in intestinal epithelial tight junction permeability requires NF-kappa B activation. *Am J Physiol Gastrointest Liver Physiol*. 2004 Mar;286(3):G367-76 http://ajpgi.physiology.org/cgi/content/full/286/3/G367

[36] "Antigen entry and the formation of immune complexes occur in atopic subjects after food ingestion. ...Food allergic subjects showed, after food challenge, the presence of IgE and IgG immune complexes, which correlates with the subsequent occurrence of symptoms." Carini C, Brostoff J. Evidence for circulating IgE complexes in food allergy. *Ric Clin Lab*. 1987 Oct-Dec;17(4):309-22

[37] "Following challenge, immune complexes containing IgE, IgG, and antigen are detectable in the circulation. Their appearance correlates with the production of symptoms." Carini C, Brostoff J, Wraith DG. IgE complexes in food allergy. *Ann Allergy*. 1987 Aug;59(2):110-7

[38] Marinkovich V. "Immunology and Food Allergy" in "Applying Functional Medicine in Clinical Practice" hosted by the Institute for Functional Medicine. Seattle, Washington: March 2005

[39] "In three food-allergic patients IgG anti-IgE was detectable in a complexed form in the serum samples examined before and after food challenge. The finding of IgG anti-IgE autoantibody in a group of patients with allergic arthralgia is quite exciting." Carini C, Fratazzi C, Aiuti F. Immune complexes in food-induced arthralgia. *Ann Allergy*. 1987 Dec;59(6):422-8

eczema[40], asthma[41], and Crohn's disease[42] and thus tissue damage in these conditions appears mediated at least in part by anti-immunoglobulin immune complexes (i.e., anti-IgE IgG complexed with IgE) rather than the classic antigen-antibody immune complexes. In this way, food allergies cause joint pain and inflammation by the deposition of immune complexes into the synovium and joint cartilage.[43] Conversely, the consumption of a relatively hypoallergenic diet reduces intake of food antigens and helps reduce IgE levels. This explains, in part, the success of hypoallergenic diets in the treatment of immune-complex-mediated diseases such as mixed cryoglobulinemia[44,45], hypersensitivity vasculitis[46], and leukocystoclastic vasculitis with arthritis.[47] In patients with rheumatoid arthritis, the symptomatic and clinical improvement induced by hypoallergenic diets correlates with reductions in antibodies to food antigens.[48]

3. <u>Damage to the intestinal mucosa with resultant increased absorption of dietary and microbial antigens</u>: Consumption of food allergens increases intestinal permeability[49] and thus amplifies the absorption of intestinal contents—dietary and microbial antigens. Patients with food allergy have "leaky gut" that is exacerbated by consumption of allergenic foods; thus lactulose-mannitol assays can be used to assist the diagnosis of food allergy.[50,51] By increasing intestinal permeability, consumption of dietary antigens serves to exacerbate the adverse effects of gastrointestinal dysbiosis by increasing antigen and (anti)metabolite absorption. Since both dietary allergens and bacterial endotoxin stimulate production of cytokines[52], **concomitant exposure to both allergens and intra-intestinal endotoxin leads to an additive increase in proinflammatory cytokine production.**[53] Thus, **consumption of allergenic foods in the presence of gastrointestinal dysbiosis would be expected to lead to more severe and more diverse adverse physiologic and clinical consequences than would be experienced following exposure to either allergens or dysbiosis alone.**

4. <u>Dietary haptenization</u>: **Dietary antigens can complex with human tissues to form** *neoantigens* **that are immunostimulatory**. The best example of this appears to be the induction of autoimmunity by wheat-derived gliadin which haptenizes with intestinal tissue transglutaminase and other extracellular matrix proteins and results in the allergic-autoimmune disease celiac disease.[54,55] **The finding that gliadin proteins haptenize with collagen and can induce the**

[40] "An IgG type of antibody directed against IgE has been studied in serum from healthy and allergic individuals. ... Significantly raised levels of anti-IgE autoantibody were found in patients suffering from atopic disorders in comparison to the controls." Carini C, Fratazzi C, Barbato M. IgG autoantibody to IgE in atopic patients. *Ann Allergy.* 1988 Jan;60(1):48-52

[41] "Significantly enhanced levels of IgE/anti-IgE IC were detected in children with asthma." Ritter C, Battig M, Kraemer R, Stadler BM. IgE hidden in immune complexes with anti-IgE autoantibodies in children with asthma. *J Allergy Clin Immunol.* 1991 Nov;88(5):793-801

[42] "In CD sera no food-specific IgE could be detected, but levels of immune complexes of IgE and IgG anti-IgE autoantibodies were statistically significantly increased compared to healthy controls." Huber A, Genser D, Spitzauer S, Scheiner O, Jensen-Jarolim E. IgE/anti-IgE immune complexes in sera from patients with Crohn's disease do not contain food-specific IgE. *Int Arch Allergy Immunol.* 1998 Jan;115(1):67-72

[43] Inman RD. Antigens, the gastrointestinal tract, and arthritis. *Rheum Dis Clin North Am.* 1991 May;17(2):309-21

[44] "CONCLUSION: These data show that an LAC diet decreases the amount of circulating immune complexes in MC and can modify certain signs and symptoms of the disease." Ferri C, Pietrogrande M, Cecchetti R, et al. Low-antigen-content diet in the treatment of patients with mixed cryoglobulinemia. *Am J Med.* 1989 Nov;87(5):519-24

[45] Pietrogrande M, Cefalo A, Nicora F, Marchesini D. Dietetic treatment of essential mixed cryoglobulinemia. *Ric Clin Lab.* 1986 Apr-Jun;16(2):413-6

[46] "In three cases the vasculitis relapsed following the introduction of food additives; in one case with the addition of potatoes and green vegetables (i.e., beans and green peas) and in the last case with the addition of eggs to the diet." Lunardi C, Bambara LM, Biasi D, Zagni P, Caramaschi P, Pacor ML. Elimination diet in the treatment of selected patients with hypersensitivity vasculitis. *Clin Exp Rheumatol.* 1992 Mar-Apr;10(2):131-5

[47] "Described in this report are two children with severe vasculitis caused by specific foods." Businco L, Falconieri P, Bellioni-Businco B, Bahna SL. Severe food-induced vasculitis in two children. *Pediatr Allergy Immunol.* 2002 Feb;13(1):68-71

[48] Hafstrom I, Ringertz B, Spangberg A, von Zweigbergk L, Brannemark S, Nylander I, Ronnelid J, Laasonen L, Klareskog L. A vegan diet free of gluten improves the signs and symptoms of rheumatoid arthritis: the effects on arthritis correlate with a reduction in antibodies to food antigens. *Rheumatology* (Oxford). 2001 Oct;40(10):1175-9 http://rheumatology.oxfordjournals.org/cgi/content/full/40/10/1175

[49] "When compared to the control group, the 11 patients of the allergic group presented a normal mannitol urinary excretion (16.5 +/- 13.4%, p = NS, Student's t-test) and an increase in the lactulose excretion (1.36 +/- 0.92%, p < 0.001). Moreover, the allergic group showed a lactulose/mannitol ratio that was significantly different (0.105 +/- 0.071, p < 0.001)." Laudat A, Arnaud P, Napoly A, Brion F. The intestinal permeability test applied to the diagnosis of food allergy in paediatrics. *West Indian Med J.* 1994 Sep;43(3):87-8

[50] "After ingestion of food allergens by the patients, mean mannitol recovery fell to 11.57% and mean recovery of lactulose rose to 1.04%, both values being significantly different from those obtained in the fasting patients." Andre C, Andre F, Colin L, Cavagna S. Measurement of intestinal permeability to mannitol and lactulose as a means of diagnosing food allergy and evaluating therapeutic effectiveness of disodium cromoglycate. *Ann Allergy.* 1987 Nov;59(5 Pt 2):127-30

[51] "A provocation IPT with food induced significant L/M ratio changes only in the group in which the food was proved to be responsible for the exacerbation of skin lesions." Dupont C, Barau E, Molkhou P, Raynaud F, Barbet JP, Dehennin L. Food-induced alterations of intestinal permeability in children with cow's milk-sensitive enteropathy and atopic dermatitis. *J Pediatr Gastroenterol Nutr.* 1989 May;8(4):459-65

[52] Jyonouchi H, Sun S, Itokazu N. Innate immunity associated with inflammatory responses and cytokine production against common dietary proteins in patients with autism spectrum disorder. *Neuropsychobiology.* 2002;46(2):76-84

[53] "Thus, endotoxin and allergen acting together could play a role in up-regulating the response of the human asthmatic airway to adenosine. However, our data suggest that the interaction would be additive rather than synergistic." Karmouty Quintana H, Mazzoni L, Fozard JR. Effects of endotoxin and allergen alone and in combination on the sensitivity of the rat airways to adenosine. *Auton Autacoid Pharmacol.* 2005 Oct;25(4):167-70

[54] "Our findings firstly demonstrated that gliadin was directly bound to tTG in duodenal mucosa of coeliacs and controls, and the ability of circulating tTG-autoantibodies to recognize and immunoprecipitate the tTG-gliadin complexes." Ciccocioppo R, Di Sabatino A, Ara C, Biagi F, Perilli M, Amicosante G, Cifone MG, Corazza GR. Gliadin and tissue transglutaminase complexes in normal and coeliac duodenal mucosa. *Clin Exp Immunol.* 2003 Dec;134(3):516-24

[55] "Thus, modification of gluten peptides by tTG, especially deamidation of certain glutamine residues, can enhance their binding to HLA-DQ2 or -DQ8 and potentiate T cell stimulation. Furthermore, tTG-catalyzed cross-linking and consequent haptenization of gluten with extracellular matrix proteins allows for storage and extended availability of gluten in the mucosa." Dieterich W, Esslinger B, Schuppan D. Pathomechanisms in celiac disease. *Int Arch Allergy Immunol.* 2003 Oct;132(2):98-108

formation of anti-collagen antibodies in humans[56] makes clear the pathomechanism by which "wheat allergy" can directly precipitate systemic musculoskeletal autoimmunity. Once initiated and perpetuated by dietary gliadin from wheat, additional autoimmunity ensues (perhaps mediated directly by epitope spreading and/or indirectly by deposition of immune complexes) which is directed against various tissues, most notably the thyroid gland[57], brain[58], and musculoskeletal system.[59] Given the association between lupus and celiac disease[60,61,62], we may speculate that allergy becomes systemic autoimmunity in certain circumstances and in susceptible patients.

5. Dietary molecular mimicry: Just as microbes produce structures similar to human molecules which then incite a cross-reacting immune response—**molecular mimicry** (discussed elsewhere in this chapter in the section on dysbiosis)—certain dietary antigens appear capable of inducing cross reactions. For example, Vojdani et al[63] recently demonstrated **cross-reactivity between anti-gliadin antibodies and anti-cerebellar antibodies in an experimental model that may partly explain the anti-brain autoimmunity seen in autism.** Further expanding this concept of dietary molecular mimicry is the finding that "the virulence factor of C albicans-hyphal wall protein 1 (HWP1)-contains amino acid sequences that are identical or highly homologous to known coeliac disease-related alpha-gliadin and gamma-gliadin T-cell epitopes."[64] This raises three interrelated possibilities: 1) that gastrointestinal overgrowth of *Candida albicans* and the resultant elaboration of HWP1 and immunostimulation may result in sensitivity to gluten, particularly as HWP1 and gliadin are both substrates for transglutaminase, 2) that consumption of wheat gluten may trigger sensitivity to *Candida albicans*, and 3) that wheat gluten and *Candida albicans* must both be present for the development of celiac disease and the ensuant autoimmunity. Additional details on the ability of *C. albicans* to contribute to autoimmunity are discussed in the section on dysbiosis.

6. Enhanced processing of autoantigens: Food-allergic patients may produce autoimmunity-stimulating autoantigens following exposure to foods to which they are sensitized. This has been demonstrated in autistic children, **exposure of lymphocytes from autistic patients to dietary antigens (gliadin and casein peptides) stimulates production of autoantigens that presumably incite and perpetuate autoimmunity.**[65] Thus, at least in autistic patients, we have evidence that food allergy can segue into autoimmunity. This phenomenon is probably not restricted only to autistic patients, as suggested by the association between celiac disease and the systemic autoimmune disease lupus.[66,67,68]

7. Diet-derived xenobiotic immunotoxicity: Foods commonly contain trace amounts of xenobiotics such as pesticides, fungicides, fumigants, fertilizers, preservatives, military propellants such as perchlorate[69], and toxic metals such as mercury. Some of these xenobiotics have been insufficiently studied in humans, while others such as mercury are well-known immunotoxins

[56] "Gliadins alpha1-alpha11, gamma1- gamma6, omega1-omega3, and omega5 were substrates for tTG. tTG catalyzed the crosslinking of gliadin peptides with interstitial collagens type I, III and VI. Coeliac patients showed increased antibody titers against the collagens I, III, V and VI." Dieterich W, Esslinger B, Trapp D, Hahn E, Huff T, Seilmeier W, Wieser H, Schuppan D. Crosslinking to tissue transglutaminase and collagen favours gliadin toxicity in coeliac disease. *Gut*. 2005 Sep 27; [Epub ahead of print]

[57] "Elevated titres of antithyroid antibodies observed in children with coeliac disease (41.1%) in comparison to control group (3.56%) indicate the need for performing the screening tests for antithyroid antibodies in children with CD." Kowalska E, Wasowska-Krolikowska K, Toporowska-Kowalska E. Estimation of antithyroid antibodies occurrence in children with coeliac disease. *Med Sci Monit*. 2000 Jul-Aug;6(4):719-2 http://www.medscimonit.com/pub/vol_6/no_4/1240.pdf

[58] Kieslich M, Errazuriz G, Posselt HG, Moeller-Hartmann W, Zanella F, Boehles H. Brain white-matter lesions in celiac disease: a prospective study of 75 diet-treated patients. *Pediatrics*. 2001 Aug;108(2):E21 http://pediatrics.aappublications.org/cgi/content/full/108/2/e21

[59] "JIA children have an increased prevalence of autoimmune thyroiditis, subclinical hypothyroidism and coeliac disease." Stagi S, Giani T, Simonini G, Falcini F. Thyroid function, autoimmune thyroiditis and coeliac disease in juvenile idiopathic arthritis. *Rheumatology* (Oxford). 2005 Apr;44(4):517-2

[60] Zitouni M, Daoud W, Kallel M, Makni S. Systemic lupus erythematosus with celiac disease: a report of five cases. *Joint Bone Spine*. 2004 Jul;71(4):344-6

[61] Komatireddy GR, Marshall JB, Aqel R, Spollen LE, Sharp GC. Association of systemic lupus erythematosus and gluten enteropathy. *South Med J*. 1995 Jun;88(6):673-6

[62] Rustgi AK, Peppercorn MA. Gluten-sensitive enteropathy and systemic lupus erythematosus. *Arch Intern Med*. 1988 Jul;148(7):1583-4

[63] "This cross-reaction was further confirmed by DOT-immunoblot and inhibition studies. We conclude that a subgroup of patients with autism produce antibodies against Purkinje cells and gliadin peptides, which may be responsible for some of the neurological symptoms in autism." Vojdani A, O'Bryan T, Green JA, Mccandless J, Woeller KN, Vojdani E, Nourian AA, Cooper EL. Immune response to dietary proteins, gliadin and cerebellar peptides in children with autism. *Nutr Neurosci*. 2004 Jun;7(3):151-61

[64] "Subsequently, C albicans might function as an adjuvant that stimulates antibody formation against HWP1 and gluten, and formation of autoreactive antibodies against tissue transglutaminase and endomysium." Nieuwenhuizen WF, Pieters RH, Knippels LM, Jansen MC, Koppelman SJ. Is Candida albicans a trigger in the onset of coeliac disease? *Lancet*. 2003;361(9375):2152-4

[65] Vojdani A, Pangborn JB, Vojdani E, Cooper EL. Infections, toxic chemicals and dietary peptides binding to lymphocyte receptors and tissue enzymes are major instigators of autoimmunity in autism. *Int J Immunopathol Pharmacol*. 2003 Sep-Dec;16(3):189-99

[66] Zitouni M, Daoud W, Kallel M, Makni S. Systemic lupus erythematosus with celiac disease: a report of five cases. *Joint Bone Spine*. 2004 Jul;71(4):344-6

[67] Komatireddy GR, Marshall JB, Aqel R, Spollen LE, Sharp GC. Association of systemic lupus erythematosus and gluten enteropathy. *South Med J*. 1995 Jun;88(6):673-6

[68] Rustgi AK, Peppercorn MA. Gluten-sensitive enteropathy and systemic lupus erythematosus. *Arch Intern Med*. 1988 Jul;148(7):1583-4

[69] "The Bush administration has imposed a gag order on the U.S. Environmental Protection Agency from publicly discussing perchlorate pollution, even as two new studies reveal high levels of the rocket-fuel component may be contaminating the nation's lettuce supply." Peter Waldman. Rocket Fuel Residues Found in Lettuce: Bush administration issues gag order on EPA discussions of possible rocket fuel tainted lettuce. *THE WALL STREET JOURNAL*. See http://www.organicconsumers.org/toxic/lettuce042903.cfm http://www.rhinoed.com/epa's_gag_order.htm http://www.peer.org/press/508.html http://yubanet.com/artman/publish/article_13637.shtml

capable of inducing immune dysfunction which may contribute to autoimmunity. **Mercury poisoning/accumulation can occur in humans as a result of consumption of contaminated foods—especially seafood such as shark, swordfish, king mackerel, tilefish, and albacore ("white") tuna**[70], and the immunologic effects of organic and/or inorganic mercury include immunosuppression, immunostimulation, formation of antinucleolar antibodies targeting fibrillarin, and formation and deposition of immune-complexes, resulting in a syndrome called "mercury-induced autoimmunity" which can be induced by exposure of susceptible animals to mercury.[71] Mercury/"silver" amalgam dental fillings rank highly among the most significant source of mercury exposure in humans, and **implantation of mercury-silver dental amalgams in susceptible animals causes chronic stimulation of the immune system with induction of systemic autoimmunity**.[72] Besides being **a neurotoxin with no safe exposure limit**[73], mercury is **known to modify/antigenize endogenous proteins to promote autoimmunity**[74], and **mercury may also promote autoimmunity by contributing to a pro-inflammatory environment that awakens quiescent autoreactive immunocytes via bystander activation**[75] (detailed later). For example, administration of mercury to "susceptible" mice induces autoimmunity via modification of the nucleolar protein *fibrillarin*[76]; noteworthy in this regard is the fact that antifibrillarin antibodies are characteristic of the autoimmune disease **scleroderma**.[77] Mercury toxicity is commonly encountered in clinical practice (diagnosis and treatment are discussed later), and a recent study published in *JAMA* showed that 8% of American women of childbearing age have sufficient levels of mercury in their bodies to produce neurologic damage in their children.[78] **The mercury-based preservative thimerosol is a type-IV (delayed hypersensitivity) sensitizing agent**[79], and **recent research implicates mercury as an important contributor to the clinical manifestations of autism**[80,81] **and eczema.**[82] Preliminary clinical evidence shows that removal of mercury amalgams, particularly along with implementation of antioxidant therapy and/or mercury chelation, benefits the biochemical status and/or clinical course of autoimmune disease.[83,84]

8. <u>Diet-derived dysbiosis</u>: Induction and exacerbation of dysbiosis following chronic consumption of allergenic foods has been reported to occur in humans. Raw vegetables and salad greens are

---

[70] See http://www.cfsan.fda.gov/~dms/admehg3.html for the white-washed version; see http://www.ewg.org/issues/mercury/20040319/index.php for a more accurate and complete perspective.
[71] Havarinasab S, Hultman P. Organic mercury compounds and autoimmunity. *Autoimmun Rev.* 2005;4(5):270-5 www.generationrescue.org/pdf/havarinasab.pdf Accessed December 27, 2005
[72] "We hypothesize that under appropriate conditions of genetic susceptibility and adequate body burden, heavy metal exposure from dental amalgam may contribute to immunological aberrations, which could lead to overt autoimmunity." Hultman P, Johansson U, Turley SJ, Lindh U, Enestrom S, Pollard KM. Adverse immunological effects and autoimmunity induced by dental amalgam and alloy in mice. *FASEB J.* 1994 Nov;8(14):1183-90 http://www.fasebj.org/cgi/reprint/8/14/1183
[73] University of Calgary Faculty of Medicine. **How Mercury Causes Brain Neuron Degeneration http://commons.ucalgary.ca/mercury/**
[74] Havarinasab S, Hultman P. Organic mercury compounds and autoimmunity. *Autoimmun Rev.* 2005 Jun;4(5):270-5. Full-text available at www.generationrescue.org/pdf/havarinasab.pdf on December 27, 2005
[75] "It is therefore theoretically possible that compounds present in vaccines such as thiomersal or aluminium hydroxyde can trigger autoimmune reactions through bystander effects." Fournie GJ, Mas M, Cautain B, Savignac M, Subra JF, Pelletier L, Saoudi A, Lagrange D, Calise M, Druet P. Induction of autoimmunity through bystander effects. Lessons from immunological disorders induced by heavy metals. *J Autoimmun.* 2001 May;16(3):319-26
[76] Nielsen JB, Hultman P. Mercury-induced autoimmunity in mice. *Environ Health Perspect.* 2002 Oct;110 Suppl 5:877-81 http://ehp.niehs.nih.gov/docs/2002/suppl-5/877-881nielsen/abstract.html
[77] "Since anti-fibrillarin antibodies are specific markers of scleroderma, the present animal model may be valuable for studies of the immunological aberrations which are likely to induce this autoimmune response." Hultman P, Enestrom S, Pollard KM, Tan EM. Anti-fibrillarin autoantibodies in mercury-treated mice. *Clin Exp Immunol.* 1989 Dec;78(3):470-7
[78] "However, approximately 8% of women had concentrations higher than the US Environmental Protection Agency's recommended reference dose (5.8 microg/L), below which exposures are considered to be without adverse effects. Women who are pregnant or who intend to become pregnant should follow federal and state advisories on consumption of fish." Schober SE, Sinks TH, Jones RL, Bolger PM, McDowell M, Osterloh J, Garrett ES, Canady RA, Dillon CF, Sun Y, Joseph CB, Mahaffey KR. Blood mercury levels in US children and women of childbearing age, 1999-2000. *JAMA.* 2003 Apr 2;289(13):1667-74
[79] "Thimerosal is an important preservative in vaccines and ophthalmologic preparations. The substance is known to be a type IV sensitizing agent. High sensitization rates were observed in contact-allergic patients and in health care workers who had been exposed to thimerosal-preserved vaccines." Westphal GA, Schnuch A, Schulz TG, Reich K, Aberer W, Brasch J, Koch P, Wessbecher R, Szliska C, Bauer A, Hallier E. Homozygous gene deletions of the glutathione S-transferases M1 and T1 are associated with thimerosal sensitization. *Int Arch Occup Environ Health.* 2000 Aug;73(6):384-8
[80] Vojdani A, Pangborn JB, Vojdani E, Cooper EL. Infections, toxic chemicals and dietary peptides binding to lymphocyte receptors and tissue enzymes are major instigators of autoimmunity in autism. *Int J Immunopathol Pharmacol.* 2003 Sep-Dec;16(3):189-99
[81] Geier DA, Geier MR. A comparative evaluation of the effects of MMR immunization and mercury doses from thimerosal-containing childhood vaccines on the population prevalence of autism. *Med sci Monit.* 2004 Mar;10(3):PI33-9. Epub 2004 Mar 1. http://www.medscimonit.com/pub/vol_10/no_3/3986.pdf
[82] Weidinger S, Kramer U, Dunemann L, Mohrenschlager M, Ring J, Behrendt H. Body burden of mercury is associated with acute atopic eczema and total IgE in children from southern Germany. *J Allergy Clin Immunol.* 2004 Aug;114(2):457-9
[83] Prochazkova J, Sterzl I, Kucerova H, Bartova J, Stejskal VD. The beneficial effect of amalgam replacement on health in patients with autoimmunity. *Neuro Endocrinol Lett.* 2004 Jun;25(3):211-8. See also: "The MELISA Test is reproducible, sensitive, specific, and reliable for detecting metal sensitivity in metal-sensitive patients." Valentine-Thon E, Schiwara HW. Validity of MELISA for metal sensitivity testing. *Neuro Endocrinol Lett.* 2003 Feb-Apr;24(1-2):57-64. See also: "The hypothesis that metal exposure from dental amalgam can cause ill health in a susceptible part of the exposed population was supported." Lindh U, Hudecek R, Danersund A, Eriksson S, Lindvall A. Removal of dental amalgam and other metal alloys supported by antioxidant therapy alleviates symptoms and improves quality of life in patients with amalgam-associated ill health. *Neuro Endocrinol Lett.* 2002 Oct-Dec;23(5-6):459-82 http://www.nel.edu/23_56/NEL235602A12_Lindh.htm and http://www.nel.edu/pdf_w/23_56/NEL235602A12_Lindh_wr.pdf
[84] "This study documents objective biochemical changes following the removal of these fillings along with other dental materials, utilizing a new health care model of multidisciplinary planning and treatment." Huggins HA, Levy TE. Cerebrospinal fluid protein changes in multiple sclerosis after dental amalgam removal. *Altern Med Rev.* 1998 Aug;3(4):295-300 http://www.thorne.com/altmedrev/.fulltext/3/4/295.pdf

thoroughly contaminated with bacteria and occasionally other microbes. Food can be contaminated with pathogenic microbes via improper preparation, storage, or handling by chefs with contagious diseases and poor hygiene. An inflammatory "reactive" arthritis can result from consumption of food that is contaminated by microorganisms, most commonly *Salmonella*[85,86,87] and *Campylobacter* species.[88] Long-term autoimmune/inflammatory complications of gastrointestinal infections/colonization sourced from food include Reiter's syndrome, Guillain-Barre syndrome (peripheral nerve autoimmunity), uveitis, sacroiliitis, and ankylosing spondylitis.

9. <u>Diet-derived immunodysregulation</u>: Certain foods contain constituents that cause immune dysfunction and the induction or exacerbation of autoimmunity. L-Canavanine sulfate is a non-protein amino acid found in alfalfa sprouts which triggers a condition similar to systemic lupus erythematosus in monkeys[89,90] and which may exacerbate SLE in humans.

10. <u>Dietary xenobiotics</u>: Artificial sweeteners, thickeners, flavor enhancers, emulsifiers, and plasticizers can be found in foods, particularly those which are manufactured and processed. Some of these chemicals have the potential to alter immune mechanisms in favor of autoimmunity. These dietary xenobiotics may be particularly relevant for initiating and promoting Crohn's disease.[91]

11. <u>Immunogenicity induced by cooking—the Maillard reaction (non-enzymatic glycosylation)</u>: Heated exposure of lysine, arginine, and tryptophan to reducing sugars such as fructose and lactose results in the non-enzymatic binding (glycosylation) of the sugar with the amino acid. If the amino acid is a component of a protein, then the structure and antigenicity of the protein is altered as it is now a glycoprotein, which may either serve as a neoantigen or may increase the allergenicity of a protein that was previously hypoallergenic, as seen with the roasting of peanuts.[92,93] Glycoproteins formed from the baking and browning of foods are also called **glycotoxins** and are capable of exacerbating inflammation in patients with diabetes.[94] Similar to the formation of **glycotoxins** is the formation of **acrylamide**, a possible carcinogen, in fried and baked foods.

Common allergy treatments advocated by the pharmaceutical industry create an overly simplistic and inaccurate view of the allergic process which obfuscates the identification and correction of the underlying processes, only two of which are antigen exposure and histamine release. Nutritionally oriented doctors, too, often emphasize the identification and elimination of allergen exposure as the sole means of addressing allergic diathesis with the presumption that allergen avoidance cures the allergy. These simplistic models and the incomplete treatments based upon them fail to address the underlying cause of the allergic phenomenon: immune dysfunction. Allergic manifestations always require at least two factors: 1) exposure of the antigen to the immune system (antigen absorption) and 2) a dysfunctional immune system that "overreacts" to the otherwise benign antigen. Allergy treatment that fails to address

[85] "We describe the case of a patient who became ill with Salmonella Blockley food poisoning while working in Cyprus in August 1994. As his diarrhoea resolved he began to suffer from lower limb joint pains which were diagnosed as acute salmonella reactive arthritis." Wilson IG, Whitehead E. Long-term post-Salmonella reactive arthritis due to Salmonella Blockley. *Jpn J Infect Dis.* 2004 Oct;57(5):210-1

[86] "Reactive joint symptoms after food-borne Salmonella infection may be more frequent than previously thought. The duration of diarrhea is strongly correlated with the occurrence of joint symptoms." Locht H, Molbak K, Krogfelt KA. High frequency of reactive joint symptoms after an outbreak of Salmonella enteritidis. *J Rheumatol.* 2002 Apr;29(4):767-71

[87] Leirisalo-Repo M, Helenius P, Hannu T, Lehtinen A, Kreula J, Taavitsainen M, Koskimies S. Long-term prognosis of reactive salmonella arthritis. *Ann Rheum Dis.* 1997 Sep;56(9):516-20 http://ard.bmjjournals.com/cgi/content/full/56/9/516

[88] "Campylobacter jejuni is the most commonly reported bacterial cause of foodborne infection in the United States. Adding to the human and economic costs are chronic sequelae associated with C. jejuni infection--Guillian-Barre syndrome and reactive arthritis." Altekruse SF, Stern NJ, Fields PI, Swerdlow DL. Campylobacter jejuni--an emerging foodborne pathogen. *Emerg Infect Dis.* 1999 Jan-Feb;5(1):28-35

[89] "L-Canavanine sulfate, a constituent of alfalfa sprouts, was incorporated into the diet and reactivated the syndrome in monkeys in which an SLE-like syndrome had previously been induced by the ingestion of alfalfa seeds or sprouts." Malinow MR, Bardana EJ Jr, Pirofsky B, Craig S, McLaughlin P. Systemic lupus erythematosus-like syndrome in monkeys fed alfalfa sprouts: role of a nonprotein amino acid. *Science.* 1982 Apr 23;216(4544):415-7

[90] "Occurrence of autoimmune hemolytic anemia and exacerbation of SLE have been linked to ingestion of alfalfa tablets containing L-canavanine." Alcocer-Varela J, Iglesias A, Llorente L, Alarcon-Segovia D. Effects of L-canavanine on T cells may explain the induction of systemic lupus erythematosus by alfalfa. *Arthritis Rheum.* 1985 Jan;28(1):52-7

[91] "Various food additives, especially emulsifiants, thickeners, surface-active agents and contaminants like plasticizers share structural domains with mycobacterial lipids. It is therefore hypothesized, that these compounds are able to stimulate by molecular mimicry the CD1 system in the gastrointestinal mucosa and to trigger the pro-inflammatory cytokine cascade." Traunmuller F. Etiology of Crohn's disease: Do certain food additives cause intestinal inflammation by molecular mimicry of mycobacterial lipids? *Med Hypotheses.* 2005;65(5):859-64

[92] "Roasted peanuts exhibited a higher level of IgE binding, which was correlated with a higher level of AGE adducts. We concluded that there is an association between AGE adducts and increased IgE binding (i.e., allergenicity) of roasted peanuts." Chung SY, Champagne ET. Association of end-product adducts with increased IgE binding of roasted peanuts. *J Agric Food Chem.* 2001 Aug;49(8):3911-6

[93] "The data presented here indicate that thermal processing may play an important role in enhancing the allergenic properties of peanuts and that the protein modifications made by the Maillard reaction contribute to this effect." Maleki SJ, Chung SY, Champagne ET, Raufman JP. The effects of roasting on the allergenic properties of peanut proteins. *J Allergy Clin Immunol.* 2000 Oct;106(4):763-8

[94] "A study now reveals that the consumption of foods rich in browned and oxidized products (so-called glycotoxins) induces a chronic inflammatory state in diabetic individuals." Monnier VM, Obrenovich ME. Wake up and smell the maillard reaction. *Sci Aging Knowledge Environ.* 2002 Dec 18;2002(50):pe21

the underlying immune dysfunction is incomplete. Allergy treatment that addresses the underlying immune dysfunction has the opportunity to correct the *total problem*, rather than merely reducing the manifestations of the problem. Therefore, treatment of the allergic diathesis must always address issues of antigen exposure, antigen absorption, *and the dysfunctional immune system* that results in the hyperactive immune response that we call "allergy." Elimination of either antigen exposure or antigen absorption eliminates allergic manifestations, but does not necessarily correct the underlying immune defect(s). Complete correction of the underlying immune defect obviates the need for the identification and avoidance of the allergen. In clinical practice, a combination of both approaches—allergen avoidance and immune modulation—is the most effective approach, affording relatively high effectiveness in symptom reduction even with only modest compliance.

Approaching a More Comprehensive Understanding of "Food Allergy" and Its Contribution to Immune Dysfunction and Musculoskeletal Inflammation

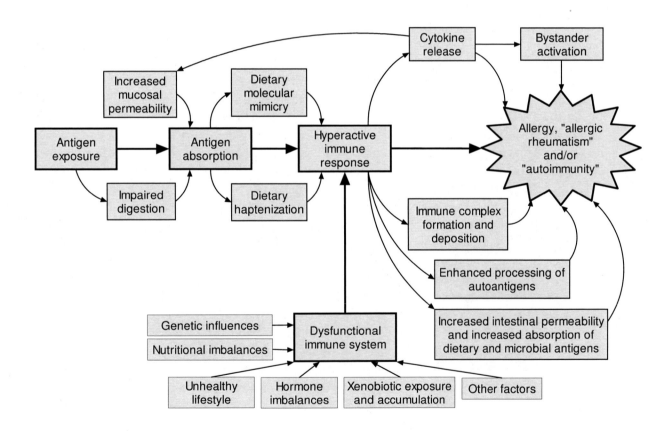

Orthomolecular Immunomodulation: The Author's Approach to Alleviating Allergy

My clinical approach to improving immune function in patients with allergy begins with supplementation of vitamin E, CoQ-10, vitamin B-12, vitamin C, bioflavonoids, honey, and fish oil. Thereafter, I look at hormones, particularly DHEA, estrogen (quantitative and qualitative), testosterone, and cortisol. I also look at diet and bowel health with respect to putrefaction and intestinal permeability. Although rarely powerful when used in isolation, these treatments when used in combinations tailored to the individual patient often result in an impressive reduction in allergic manifestations even when allergen avoidance is either not pursued or not feasible. The process of alleviating allergic disorders is, however, arduous and time-consuming unless the doctor uses a group of protocols such as those described herein which address the most common contributing factors to allergic problems. Here I extend my previous three-step process[95] into a four-tiered approach, with the fourth step including selected pharmaceutical drugs.

Step 1: From initial patient assessment to the first phase of treatment

In a patient with presumed "allergy" who is in otherwise good health, following a basic health assessment and exclusion of significant disease, I begin by correcting problems that are common to patients with allergy. Minor improvements in allergy symptoms as a result of a low-cost low-risk interventions can be multiplied with a specified group of interventions; we aim for a modest improvement with several treatments rather than a "silver bullet" miracle cure with a single intervention. For example, 10% improvement in symptoms may be insignificant in itself; however a 10% improvement from six interventions results in a 60% improvement and enhances patient confidence long enough for other interventions and assessments to be implemented, if necessary. The goal with the first step of treatment is to correct the most common and most likely problems, namely fatty acid imbalances, micronutrient deficiencies, phytonutrient insufficiencies, and dysbiosis.

- Avoidance of suspected food allergens: The most common allergens are wheat, cow's milk, and eggs; however any patient can be allergic to any food. It is not uncommon for patients to have to avoid up to 10 foods before attaining maximal improvement, and up to 85% of migraine patients can be cured of their headaches by the use of allergy avoidance alone.[96] Food allergy avoidance for 1 month helps achieve symptomatic relief and allows the gut to heal and the immune system to recalibrate. The diet should emphasize consumption of lean meats, fruits, vegetables, nuts, seeds, and berries to ensure a systemic anti-inflammatory effect and increased consumption of anti-inflammatory phytonutrients, especially flavonoids. High-glycemic foods are avoided as are "food additives" such as tartrazine, which is known to exacerbate allergic asthma. Some foods like tuna, certain cheeses and wines are high in histamine; frequent consumption of these foods by an allergic individual is analogous to adding fuel to a fire that the patient is simultaneously trying to extinguish. Recall that in breast-feeding infants, the mother will have to consume a hypoallergenic diet to prevent passage of allergens[97] and allergen-antibody immune complexes[98] in breast milk.
- Rotation diet: While select foods should be completely avoided, the remaining foods that are consumed should be rotated in and out of the diet with a periodicity of 3-5 days. Patients should avoid "dietary monotony"[99] by consuming a variety of foods. By rotating different foods in and out of the diet, patients are more likely to consume a nutritious diet and are less likely to develop or perpetuate food allergies.

---

[95] Vasquez A. Improving neuromusculoskeletal health by optimizing immune function and reducing allergic reactions: a review of 16 treatments and a 3-step clinical approach. *Nutritional Perspectives* 2005; October: 27-35, 40 http://optimalhealthresearch.com/part5
[96] Grant EC. Food allergies and migraine. *Lancet.* 1979 May 5;1(8123):966-9
[97] "In all, clinical disappearance of symptoms was observed after removal of milk from the mother's diet and/or elimination from the child's diet of any cow's-milk-based hypoallergenic formula." Barau E, Dupont C. Allergy to cow's milk proteins in mother's milk or in hydrolyzed cow's milk infant formulas as assessed by intestinal permeability measurements. *Allergy.* 1994 Apr;49(4):295-8
[98] The finding of egg-allergen immune complex in breast milk inplies 1) egg protein escapes complete digestion/degradation in the gastrointestinal tract, 2) egg protein is absorbed intact through the mucosa, 3) egg protein escapes filtration by the liver, 4) egg protein stimulates formation IgA immune complexes, and 5) egg-IgA immune complexes are secreted in milk which would then expose the infant to both allergen and immune complex, possibly resulting in clinical disease. Hirose J, Ito S, Hirata N, Kido S, Kitabatake N, Narita H. Occurrence of the major food allergen, ovomucoid, in human breast milk as an immune complex. *Biosci Biotechnol Biochem.* 2001 Jun;65(6):1438-40 http://www.jstage.jst.go.jp/article/bbb/65/6/1438/_pdf
[99] Pelchat ML, Schaefer S. Dietary monotony and food cravings in young and elderly adults. *Physiol Behav.* 2000 Jan;68(3):353-9

- <u>CoQ-10</u>: CoQ-10 levels are low in approximately 40% of patients with allergies, according to a small study conducted by Folkers and Pfeiffer.[100] Asthmatics also have lower levels of CoQ-10 compared to healthy people.[101] In my experience, clinical improvement is commonly seen in allergic patients after supplementation with CoQ-10. I generally prescribe 200 mg per day of CoQ-10 for adults.

- <u>Probiotics</u>: Supplementation with probiotics (beneficial strains of bacteria and yeast) appears to improve intestinal barrier function, promote microecological balance in the gastrointestinal tract, modulate immune function, and thus reduce manifestations of allergic disease.[102,103,104]

- <u>Vitamin E</u>: Vitamin E has been shown to reduce IgE levels in humans and to reduce the manifestations of allergy-related disease.[105] I commonly prescribe 800-2,000 IU per day of mixed tocopherols with approximately 40% gamma tocopherol for patients with allergy.

- <u>Vitamin C</u>: A recent clinical trial showed that 2 grams per day of ascorbic acid reduced blood histamine levels by 38%.[106] Cathcart hypothesized that high doses of vitamin C (i.e., bowel tolerance) may impair the adsorption of IgE with allergens and thus retard the allergic cascade from being initiated.[107] Either of these two mechanisms, perhaps in addition to other mechanisms, may explain the anti-allergy effects of ascorbic acid.[108]

- <u>Bioflavonoids</u>: Bioflavonoids stabilize mast cell membranes and thus reduce the liberation of histamine. Additionally, quercetin and catechin inhibit the action of histidine decarboxylase, which converts histidine into histamine. Many fruits, vegetables, and herbal teas are excellent sources of flavonoids, which can also be consumed in the form of tablets and capsules.

- <u>Vitamin B-12</u>: Vitamin B-12 has been shown to reduce physiologic manifestations of allergy in ovalbumin-sensitized mice.[109] Since vitamin B-12 is safe, non-toxic, and bioavailable when administered orally in large doses to humans, I commonly prescribe 2,500-5,000 mcg per day for allergic patients for a one-month trial. Although the benefit of vitamin B-12 in patients with sulfite-sensitive asthma is biochemically mediated rather than immunologically mediated[110], this research adds tangential support to the use of high-dose vitamin B-12 in selected patients with allergy (particularly asthma), at least for a short-term clinical trial. Hydroxocobalamin and methylcobalamin are preferred over cyanocobalamin due to the content of cyanide in the latter.[111]

Step 2: Additional interventions for moderate or unresponsive allergies.

For patients who do not respond sufficiently to the first phase of treatment, the following interventions can be considered.

- <u>Pancreatic and proteolytic enzymes</u>: Pancreatic enzymes have been shown to alleviate symptoms of food allergy in a controlled clinical trial.[112] Administration of enzyme preparations can alleviate intestinal and extra-intestinal manifestations of food allergy.[113] Proteolytic enzymes are safe and

---

[100] Ye CQ, Folkers K, Tamagawa H, Pfeiffer C. A modified determination of coenzyme Q10 in human blood and CoQ10 blood levels in diverse patients with allergies. *Biofactors*. 1988 Dec;1(4):303-6

[101] Gazdik F, Gvozdjakova A, Nadvornikova R, Repicka L, Jahnova E, Kucharska J, Pijak MR, Gazdikova K. Decreased levels of coenzyme Q(10) in patients with bronchial asthma. *Allergy*. 2002 Sep;57(9):811-4

[102] Majamaa H, Isolauri E. Probiotics: a novel approach in the management of food allergy. *J Allergy Clin Immunol* 1997 Feb;99(2):179-85

[103] von der Weid T, Ibnou-Zekri N, Pfeifer A. Novel probiotics for the management of allergic inflammation. *Dig Liver Dis*. 2002 Sep;34 Suppl 2:S25-8

[104] "The administration of probiotics, strains of bacteria from the healthy human gut microbiota, have been shown to stimulate antiinflammatory, tolerogenic immune responses, the lack of which has been implied in the development of atopic disorders. Thus probiotics may prove beneficial in the prevention and alleviation of allergic disease." Rautava S, Isolauri E. The development of gut immune responses and gut microbiota: effects of probiotics in prevention and treatment of allergic disease. *Curr Issues Intest Microbiol*. 2002 Mar;3(1):15-22

[105] Tsoureli-Nikita E, Hercogova J, Lotti T, Menchini G. Evaluation of dietary intake of vitamin E in the treatment of atopic dermatitis: a study of the clinical course and evaluation of the immunoglobulin E serum levels. *Int J Dermatol*. 2002 Mar;41(3):146-50

[106] "Chemotaxis was inversely correlated to blood histamine (r = -0.32, p = 0.045), and, compared to baseline and withdrawal values, histamine levels were depressed 38% following VC supplementation. ... These data indicate that VC may indirectly enhance chemotaxis by detoxifying histamine in vivo." Johnston CS, Martin LJ, Cai X. Antihistamine effect of supplemental ascorbic acid and neutrophil chemotaxis. *J Am Coll Nutr*. 1992 Apr;11(2):172-6

[107] "Allergic and sensitivity reactions are frequently ameliorated and sometimes completely blocked by massive doses of ascorbate. I now hypothesize that one mechanism in blocking of allergic symptoms is the reducing of the disulfide bonds between the chains in antibody molecules making their bonding antigen impossible." Cathcart RF 3rd. The vitamin C treatment of allergy and the normally unprimed state of antibodies. *Med Hypotheses*. 1986 Nov;21(3):307-21

[108] Bucca C, Rolla G, Oliva A, Farina JC. Effect of vitamin C on histamine bronchial responsiveness of patients with allergic rhinitis. *Ann Allergy*. 1990 Oct;65(4):311-4

[109] "We infer that Cbl administration significantly reduced the IL-2 concentration, and secondarily the IL-4, IgE and histamine concentrations." Funada U, Wada M, Kawata T, Tanaka N, Tadokoro T, Maekawa A. Effect of cobalamin on the allergic response in mice. *Biosci Biotechnol Biochem* 2000 Oct;64(10):2053-8

[110] Anibarro B, Caballero T, Garcia-Ara C, Diaz-Pena JM, Ojeda JA. Asthma with sulfite intolerance in children: a blocking study with cyanocobalamin. *J Allergy Clin Immunol*. 1992 Jul;90(1):103-9

[111] Freeman AG. Cyanocobalamin--a case for withdrawal: discussion paper. *J R Soc Med*. 1992 Nov;85(11):686-7

[112] Raithel M, Weidenhiller M, Schwab D, Winterkamp S, Hahn EG. Pancreatic enzymes: a new group of antiallergic drugs? *Inflamm Res*. 2002 Apr;51 Suppl 1:S13-4

[113] Gaby AR. Pancreatic enzymes block food allergy reactions. *Townsend Letter for Doctors and Patients* 2002; Nov. http://www.townsendletter.com/Nov_2002/gabyliteraturereview1102.htm

effective for the relief of musculoskeletal pain, as reviewed later in this text and elsewhere.[114] When taken with food, pancreatic/proteolytic enzymes facilitate hydrolysis of proteins, fats, and carbohydrates and are then absorbed into the systemic circulation for an anti-inflammatory effect. Although individual enzymes may be used in isolation, enzyme therapy is generally delivered in the form of polyenzyme preparations containing pancreatin, bromelain, papain, amylase, lipase, trypsin and alpha-chymotrypsin.

- NFkB inhibitors: The clinical significance of NFkB and its phytonutritional modulation is detailed later in this book and elsewhere.[115] Nutrients that can be used to downregulate inflammatory responses are vitamin D, curcumin (requires piperine for absorption), lipoic acid, green tea, rosemary, grape seed extract, propolis, resveratrol, selenium, zinc, and N-acetyl-cysteine.

- Eradication of harmful intestinal yeast, bacteria, and other "parasites": I have seen several patients become cured of their "allergies" once we eradicated the dysbiotic bacteria, yeast, amoebas, or other microorganisms from their gastrointestinal tract. Intestinal colonization with harmful bacteria/yeast/protozoa/amebas can cause mucosal injury and result in macromolecular absorption and thus promotes immune sensitization to dietary antigens; in these situations, correction of dysbiosis via eradication of harmful microorganisms can lead to an impressive reduction in food-associated allergic phenomena. Although many indirect mechanisms will be discussed later, the most direct means by which dysbiosis may contribute to "allergy" is via endogenous formation of histamine via bacterial histidine decarboxylase. Galland and Lee[116] reported that eradication of *Giardia lamblia* in patients with chronic digestive complaints lessened the severity of food intolerance/allergy in 54% of patients. The supremely important topic of gastrointestinal dysbiosis is detailed later in this chapter.

Step 3: Treatment for severe allergies

For some patients with severe allergies, we start with selected treatments from Step 2 or Step 3 on the first visit *in addition to* the treatments included in Step 1. Implementation is customized based on history, examination, laboratory findings, and the doctor's experience and good judgment.

- Calcium and magnesium butyrate: Butyrate is a short-chain fatty acid which can be obtained from 1) a limited number of foods, namely butter, 2) intestinal fermentation of carbohydrates by probiotic bacteria, and 3) use of nutritional supplements. It is increasingly well-established that probiotic bacteria have immune-normalizing and "anti-allergy" effects, and this benefit is probably mediated at least in part by probiotic production of butyrate. The mechanisms of the anti-allergy effect of butyrate are manifold, and as a fatty acid butyrate activates peroxisome-proliferator activated receptor-alpha (PPAR-alpha) and thereby results in an immunomodulatory action and a suppressive effect on NFkB.[117,118] Butyrate is also a primary fuel for enterocytes and may improve enterocyte metabolism for the normalization of intestinal permeability. In the treatment of patients with inflammatory bowel disease, 4 grams per day of orally administered butyrate salts safely improves the action of mesalamine[119] as does topical application of butyrate in distal ulcerative colitis.[120] As a normal dietary component and product of the gastrointestinal tract, supplemental calcium and magnesium salts of butyrate are safe and effective for human consumption at doses of 1,000 – 4,500 mg butyrate per day for the alleviation of allergic diseases.[121,122]

[114] Vasquez A. Reducing pain and inflammation naturally - Part 3: Improving overall health while safely and effectively treating musculoskeletal pain. *Nutritional Perspectives* 2005; 28: 34-38, 40-42 www.optimalhealthresearch.com/part3

[115] Vasquez A. Reducing pain and inflammation naturally - part 4: nutritional and botanical inhibition of NF-kappaB, the major intracellular amplifier of the inflammatory cascade. A practical clinical strategy exemplifying anti-inflammatory nutrigenomics. *Nutritional Perspectives*, July 2005:5-12. www.OptimalHealthResearch.com/part4

[116] Galland L, Lee M. Abstract #170 High frequency of giardiasis in patients with chronic digestive complaints. *Am J Gastroenterol* 1989;84:1181

[117] Zapolska-Downar D, Siennicka A, Kaczmarczyk M, Kolodziej B, Naruszewicz M. Butyrate inhibits cytokine-induced VCAM-1 and ICAM-1 expression in cultured endothelial cells: the role of NF-kappaB and PPARalpha. *J Nutr Biochem*. 2004 Apr;15(4):220-8

[118] Luhrs H, Gerke T, Muller JG, Melcher R, Schauber J, Boxberge F, Scheppach W, Menzel T. Butyrate inhibits NF-kappaB activation in lamina propria macrophages of patients with ulcerative colitis. *Scand J Gastroenterol*. 2002 Apr;37(4):458-66

[119] Vernia P, Monteleone G, Grandinetti G, Villotti G, Di Giulio E, Frieri G, Marcheggiano A, Pallone F, Caprilli R, Torsoli A. Combined oral sodium butyrate and mesalazine treatment compared to oral mesalazine alone in ulcerative colitis: randomized, double-blind, placebo-controlled pilot study. *Dig Dis Sci*. 2000 May;45(5):976-81

[120] Vernia P, Annese V, Bresci G, d'Albasio G, D'Inca R, Giaccari S, Ingrosso M, Mansi C, Riegler G, Valpiani D, Caprilli R; Gruppo Italiano per lo Studio del Colon e del Retto. Topical butyrate improves efficacy of 5-ASA in refractory distal ulcerative colitis: results of a multicentre trial. *Eur J Clin Invest*. 2003 Mar;33(3):244-8

[121] Neesby TE. Method for desensitizing the gastrointestinal tract from food allergies. United States Patent 4,721,716. January 26, 1988

[122] Neesby TE. Method for desensitizing the gastrointestinal tract from food allergies. United States Patent 4,735,967. April 5, 1988

- <u>Purified chondroitin sulfate and glucosamine sulfate</u>: Doctors and patients everywhere should already know that chondroitin sulfate and glucosamine sulfate are safe and effective for the treatment of osteoarthritis. Furthermore, purified chondroitin sulfate is cardioprotective and that it helps to reduce the vessel occlusion characteristic of atherosclerosis.[123] Additionally, new experimental evidence shows that chondroitin sulfate and glucosamine sulfate can inhibit allergic reactions.[124] With this in mind, it is reasonable to speculate that many arthritic patients who respond to glucosamine and chondroitin may actually be responding to the anti-allergy benefits of chondroitin and glucosamine *rather than* or *in addition to* the "cartilage building" properties of these supplements. Furthermore, there is evidence that purified chondroitin sulfate can act as a "decoy" and reduce adhesion of harmful bacteria; the role of harmful gastrointestinal bacteria in the genesis and perpetuation of joint pain and inflammation will be discussed in the next article in this series. For now, it will suffice to say that occult gastrointestinal infections (i.e., gastrointestinal dysbiosis) are a major contributor to the systemic pain and inflammation seen in conditions such as rheumatoid arthritis and ankylosing spondylitis.

- <u>Hormones</u>: DHEA, progesterone, testosterone, and cortisol tend to be lower in allergic/autoimmune individuals than in healthy controls. I use either serum testing and/or 24-hour urine samples before prescribing hormones, though I will empirically use progesterone in a woman or a 3-month trial of DHEA in a man with allergies if I find sufficient indications and no contraindications. Treatment is customized per patient. I discuss the hormonal contributions to autoimmunity later in this chapter under the heading of "orthoendocrinology." Much of what applies to "allergy" also applies to "autoimmunity" and visa versa; they are both manifestations of immune dysfunction.[125]

Step 4: Drug treatments

We must acknowledge a place for drug therapy in patients with recalcitrant or severe allergies.

- <u>Prednisone</u>: For patients with allergies that are inconsolable, prednisone becomes a reasonable consideration. The lowest effective dose should be used for the shortest possible period of time. Discontinuation of treatment that has lasted longer than 4 days must be gradual in order to avoid adrenal insufficiency. Topical rather than systemic therapy should be used when appropriate.

- <u>Sodium cromoglycate</u>: Cromoglycate is a mast cell stabilizer which can be applied nasally for allergic rhinitis (Nasalcrom) or taken orally (Gastrocrom) by patients with food allergy to inhibit the local response to type-1 allergies.[126] The drug is poorly absorbed; therefore its anti-allergy effect is mediated at the gastrointestinal mucosa even though the benefits are systemic. Although not officially "approved" in the US for the treatment of food allergy, numerous studies support its use for this purpose.[127] Cromoglycate has been shown to reduce allergy-induced migraine[128] and eczema[129] and prevent the formation of immune complexes following the consumption of allergenic foods. In addition to preventing the allergic phenomena related directly to the consumption of allergenic foods, an additional mechanism of action of sodium cromoglycate is probably that it reduces the allergy-induced increase in intestinal permeability[130] and thereby prohibits absorption of bacterial and other microbial antigens and metabolites; stated differently, some of the manifestations attributed to "food allergy" are probably not mediated by the

---

[123] Morrison LM, Enrick N. Coronary heart disease: reduction of death rate by chondroitin sulfate A. *Angiology*. 1973 May;24(5):269-87

[124] Theoharides TC, Bielory L. Mast cells and mast cell mediators as targets of dietary supplements. *Ann Allergy Asthma Immunol*. 2004 Aug;93(2 Suppl 1):S24-34

[125] Vasquez A. In <u>Textbook of Functional Medicine</u>. In press—see www.functionalmedicine.org for details and purchasing.

[126] http://www.drugs.com/MMX/Cromolyn_Sodium.html Accessed November 24, 2005

[127] "Both the clinician's and patient's preferences and the clinician's evaluation of the specific response to challenge showed a significant benefit from SCG." Dannaeus A, Foucard T, Johansson SG. The effect of orally administered sodium cromoglycate on symptoms of food allergy. *Clin Allergy*. 1977 Mar;7(2):109-15

[128] "Immune complexes were not produced in those patients who were protected by sodium cromoglycate. These observations confirm that a food-allergic reaction is the cause of migraine in this group of patients." Monro J, Carini C, Brostoff J. Migraine is a food-allergic disease. *Lancet*. 1984 Sep 29;2(8405):719-21

[129] "The same atopic patients pretreated with oral sodium cromoglycate had less antigen entry, diminished immune-complex formation, and no atopic symptoms." Paganelli R, Levinsky RJ, Brostoff J, Wraith DG. Immune complexes containing food proteins in normal and atopic subjects after oral challenge and effect of sodium cromoglycate on antigen absorption. *Lancet*. 1979 Jun 16;1(8129):1270-2

[130] "It is suggested that a local IgE-mediated mechanism acts as a "trigger" for the entry of antigen and the formation of immune complexes by altering the permeability of the gut mucosa. The resulting delayed onset symptoms could be viewed as a form of serum sickness with few or many target organs affected." Carini C, Brostoff J, Wraith DG. IgE complexes in food allergy. *Ann Allergy*. 1987 Aug;59(2):110-7

response to food allergens directly but result from the adverse immunologic and metabolic responses toward gut-derived microbial antigens and metabolites which are absorbed in increased amounts following the consumption of allergenic foods which increase intestinal permeability and absorption of "foreign" and "toxic" intraluminal contents which would have otherwise been excluded. Common doses for children are 100 mg 30 minutes before food (up to 400 mg per day) and 100-200 mg qid for adults 30 minutes before meals. Capsules or ampules should be mixed in plain water before consumption.

- Leukotriene antagonists: Montelukast (Singulair®, Merck) is an orally active leukotriene receptor antagonist that blocks leukotriene D4 from the cysteinyl leukotriene CysLT-1 receptor and thereby reduces vasodilation, eosinophilic inflammation, and vascular hyperpermeability. Montelukast is used in the medical treatment of asthma, rhinitis, and eczema.

Objective means for the identification of allergens: skin-prick testing, serum IgE and IgG assays, double-blind placebo-controlled food challenges, and the elimination and challenge technique

- Skin prick testing: IgE-dependent immediate-onset allergies as assessed with a **skin-prick test** are indicative of immediate-onset allergy to the particular allergen, and provide the identity of the allergen, quantification of the severity of the allergic response, *and evidence of underlying immune dysfunction*. Skin-prick testing does not assess for delayed-onset allergies, thus leaving at least one class of adverse food reactions literally unassessed.

- Allergen-specific serum levels of IgE and IgG: Elevated serum levels of IgE and IgG, which are identified as specific for certain foods, also provide the identity of the allergen *and evidence of underlying immune dysfunction*. These "objective" tools are part of the clinician's repertoire for identifying food allergens, while keeping in mind that both skin-prick testing and serum testing are prone to both false positives and false negatives. Serum IgE testing does not assess IgG-mediated allergies, nor does it assess for sensitivity (immune but not immunoglobulin-mediated responses) or intolerance, which tends to be biochemical rather than immunologic. IgG assays and the subclasses of IgG-4 assays have not gained acceptance for their sensitivity or specificity, even though clinicians order them and patients pay for them.

- Double-blind placebo-controlled food challenge: Another commonly mentioned objective means for identifying food allergens is the "double-blind placebo-controlled food challenge" (DBPCFC) wherein food is administered a double-blind fashion with placebo control generally via either capsules or nasogastric tube. Unfortunately, DBPCFC is commonly considered the gold standard for the identification of particular allergens and the establishment of an allergic diathesis. This is unfortunate because the hospital admission and associated costs are expensive, cumbersome and therefore inaccessible for most patients. Some patients will have a false-negative response when challenged with isolated foods because of the lack of "accessory antigens", "accomplice antigens", or "bystander antigens."[131] Some patients will have adverse food reactions only when foods are eaten either with *high frequency* or in *specific combinations* or when *gastrointestinal problems* (e.g., dysbiosis or increased intestinal permeability) are present at the same time as the food challenge. For example, while the patient may tolerate eggs alone and wheat alone without the manifestation of allergic symptoms, the additive insult of the combination of both eggs and wheat may cause sufficient intestinal damage and/or immune activation that clinical manifestations become apparent. With single food challenges given with **DBPCFC**, "real life" situations are not reproduced, and false negative results may erroneously suggest that either the patient has no allergies or that a particular food is not offensive.

- Elimination and challenge: The "**elimination and challenge**" technique (more accurately described as "avoidance and challenge") requires that the patient first clear the diet of all possible

---

[131] "The mechanisms of enhanced permeability to specific and bystander antigens have been delineated as well as the molecular events involved in the sequential phases of allergic reactions." Heyman M. Gut barrier dysfunction in food allergy. *Eur J Gastroenterol Hepatol*. 2005 Dec;17(12):1279-1285

offending foods, either by **fasting** or by **consuming a simple diet of unlikely-to-be-allergenic foods**, such as the classic triad of rice, lamb, and pears or a relatively hypoallergenic hydrolyzed formula such as Vivonex. After 7-14 days of elimination (i.e., avoidance) *and the clearing of symptoms thought to be allergy-mediated*, an offending food is reintroduced by intense consumption (i.e., eaten with every meal) for a period of up to two days. Every two to four days, a new food is added back into the diet, and a correlation is searched for between consumption of a given food and the exacerbation of symptoms. If the symptoms do not abate or disappear with the fasting/elimination phase, then confirming the nature of the disorder as allergic is more difficult and determining the identity of the allergen is additionally unlikely. However, in some cases, clinical signs and symptoms that are indeed allergy-mediated will fail to regress significantly during the brief washout period. This is because the underlying tissue damage is too great to be healed in such a short time. A good example is the thyroid disease induced by gluten-containing grains in people with the severe gluten allergy called celiac disease; simply avoiding gluten for 1-2 weeks does not restore endocrine function because the body needs more time to reacquire homeostasis and to heal injured tissues. A common scenario is one in which symptoms remit during fasting/elimination and then return *gradually* rather than *immediately* when the offending food is eaten. In these situations, the most likely explanations are either 1) a threshold of time was necessary for physiologic abnormalities (e.g., immune complex deposition, increased intestinal permeability, dysbiosis, accumulative immune stimulation) to culminate in the reproduction of symptoms, or 2) synergistic factors may have to be combined in order to produce the symptoms of allergy, such as the induction of IgE-mediated increased intestinal permeability by food R which then leads to the increased absorption of food S, to which the peripheral immune system then responds with an IgG-mediated reaction with resultant clinical manifestations. In the latter case, food R or food S *when eaten alone or on a rotation basis* may be insufficient to produce allergic manifestations, but the combination of R+S, which would not be identified with skin-prick testing, serum tests, or one-at-a-time DBPCFC, may produce allergic manifestations. Since, in real life, foods are eaten in combination when they cause allergic disease (e.g. a headache or joint pain after eating a hamburger with wheat/gluten, cheese/milk, mayonnaise/egg, and pickle/tartrazine/yeast), a reasonable conclusion is that foods will have to be avoided in specific combinations to attain maximal improvement in allergic symptoms since complex foods probably work synergistically to produce allergic manifestations in affected people. Creating chronological distance between the consumption of allergenic foods explains the success of the **rotation diets** in alleviating allergic manifestations, but it does little to address the underlying immune dysfunction other than to reduce the total allergenic load to which the immune system is exposed. **Intestinal dysbiosis** can also increase intestinal permeability and result in increased absorption of food antigens and depletion of detoxification co-factors, which can mimic or perpetuate immune-mediated food allergies. Correction of this problem can begin to normalize immune function and eliminate symptoms attributed to the consumption of specific foods.

Objective Assessments for Adverse Food Reactions—A Quick Clinical Guide

	Advantages	Disadvantages
Skin-prick testing	<ul><li>Proves presence of allergic diathesis.</li><li>Identifies allergen that is being responded to by IgE-mediated reaction.</li><li>Can be used for both food and inhalant allergies.</li></ul>	<ul><li>Numerically impossible to test for all probable allergens due to method of testing, which can be quite painful</li><li>Allergen preparations may not contain full spectrum of immunogenic epitopes that are present in "real food" thus patient may not respond to offensive food, resulting in clinically relevant false negative results.</li><li>Subcutaneous injection is not the natural or physiologic route of allergen exposure.</li><li>Does not assess for IgG or other delayed-onset allergies, thus resulting in clinically relevant false negative results.</li><li>Does not assess for reactions that are mediated by immune complexes, thus resulting in clinically relevant false negative results.</li><li>Procedure is moderately expensive.</li><li>Does not assess for intolerances or biochemical perturbations, thus resulting in clinically relevant false negative results.</li></ul>
Serum IgE assay	<ul><li>Identifies allergen that is being responded to by IgE-mediated reaction.</li><li>Can be used for both food and inhalant allergies.</li><li>Procedure is relatively painless and provides "objective evidence" of food allergies.</li></ul>	<ul><li>Numerically impossible to test for all probable allergens due to method of testing.</li><li>Allergen preparations may not contain full spectrum of immunogenic epitopes that are present in "real food" thus patient may not respond to offensive food, resulting in clinically relevant false negative results.</li><li>Does not assess for IgG or other delayed-onset allergies, thus resulting in clinically relevant false negative results.</li><li>Does not assess for reactions that are mediated by IgG, IgM, or IgA immune complexes, thus resulting in clinically relevant false-negative results.</li><li>Does not assess for intolerances or biochemical perturbations, thus resulting in clinically relevant false negative results.</li></ul>
Serum IgG4 assay	<ul><li>Identifies allergen that is being responded to by IgG-mediated reaction.</li><li>Mostly used in an attempt to identify delayed-onset food allergies.</li><li>Procedure is relatively painless.</li><li>Procedure provides "objective evidence" of food allergies.</li></ul>	<ul><li>Numerically impossible to test for all probable allergens due to method of testing.</li><li>Allergen preparations may not contain full spectrum of immunogenic epitopes that are present in "real food" thus patient may not respond to offensive food, resulting in clinically relevant false negative results.</li><li>Does not assess for IgE or other immediate-onset allergies, thus resulting in clinically relevant false negative results.</li><li>Does not assess for reactions that are mediated by immune complexes, thus resulting in clinically relevant false negative results.</li><li>Procedure is moderately expensive.</li><li>Does not assess for intolerances or biochemical perturbations, thus resulting in clinically relevant false negative results.</li><li>The clinical relevance of IgG4 antibodies to food is controversial.[132]</li></ul>

---

[132] "...it seems unlikely that increased IgG4 antibody levels against egg white is a cause of egg hypersensitivity, and one should pay much attention to IgG1 antibodies, …it is possible that increased IgG4 may reduce the effect of complement-fixing antibodies like IgG1 and/or interfere the action of IgE antibodies." Nakagawa T. Egg white-specific IgE and IgG subclass antibodies and their associations with clinical egg hypersensitivity. *N Engl Reg Allergy Proc.* 1988 Jan-Feb;9(1):67-73

Objective Assessments for Adverse Food Reactions—A Quick Clinical Guide *continued*

	Advantages	Disadvantages
Double-blind placebo-controlled food challenges	<ul><li>Allows for control of interfering factors.</li><li>Removes psychological cues and triggers that can be mistakenly interpreted as adverse food reactions.</li><li>Procedure provides "objective evidence" of food allergies.</li></ul>	<ul><li>Setting and experiment are artificial and not representative of the real environment in which the patient lives and is exposed to allergen(s).</li><li>Testing of single antigens alone is not reflective of real life wherein antigens are consumed in combination.</li><li>Numerically impossible to test for all probable allergens due to method of testing.</li><li>Allergen preparations may not contain full spectrum of immunogenic epitopes that are present in "real food" thus patient may not respond to offensive food, resulting in clinically relevant false negative results.</li><li>Procedure is time-consuming and cumbersome and requires the preparation of both food challenge and placebo, which are administered either by capsules or by nasogastric tube.</li><li>Due to small quantity of allergen and limited time of observation, does not assess for reactions that are quantity-dependent, delayed-onset, or mediated by immune complexes, thus resulting in clinically relevant false negative results.</li><li>Procedure is moderately expensive.</li><li>Does not assess for intolerances or biochemical perturbations, thus resulting in clinically relevant false negative results.</li></ul>
Elimination and challenge	<ul><li>Represents "real life" situations with psychological influences, daily stress, and combinations of foods.</li><li>No financial cost.</li><li>Easy to implement for motivated patients.</li><li>Trains patients to be active in their healthcare and to learn how to diagnose and treat themselves—the true goals of wellness promotion.</li></ul>	<ul><li>Compliance is a challenge for unmotivated or undisciplined patients.</li><li>Identification of offending allergen may take time and repeated cycles of elimination and challenge before the allergen is conclusively identified.</li></ul>

Multifocal Dysbiosis: A Major Promoter of Chronic Inflammation and "Autoimmunity"

Introduction: Microbes contribute to noninfectious human diseases—including chronic inflammation and autoimmunity—by mechanisms which are *numerous, complex, direct* and *indirect*. For the purposes of this discussion, I will use a broad definition of dysbiosis that implies "a relationship of non-acute host-microorganism interaction that adversely affects the human host"; the subtype of dysbiosis can be distinguished based on location: gastrointestinal, orodental, sinorespiratory, genitourinary, dermal, or environmental. Patients may have more than one dysbiotic loci at a time with microbes from more than one kingdom. One of the best clinical examples of autoimmunity/inflammation perpetuated by multifocal dysbiosis is Behcet's syndrome, characterized by subclinical pulmonary infection (sinorespiratory dysbiosis) with *Chlamydia pneumonia*[133], cutaneous colonization (dermal dysbiosis) with *Staphylococcus aureus*[134], and orodental dysbiosis with *Streptococcus sanguis*.[135] Combine with multifocal dysbiosis a few pro-rheumatic genetic traits

> **Dysbiosis**: A relationship of non-acute non-infectious host-microorganism interaction that adversely affects the human host.
>
> **Dysbiosis subtypes** (based on location):
> 1. Orodental
> 2. Sinorespiratory
> 3. Gastrointestinal
> 4. Parenchymal
> 5. Genitourinary
> 6. Cutaneous
> 7. Environmental
>
> **Multifocal dysbiosis**: A clinical condition characterized by a patient's having more than one foci/location of dysbiosis; generally the adverse physiologic and clinical consequences are additive and synergistic.
>
> **Polydysbiosis**: Concurrent dysbiosis with microbes of different species.

(especially HLA-B27) and subclinical proinflammatory nutritional imbalances[136], and it becomes easy to see why rheumatic diseases are generally still considered "idiopathic" when reviewed from a reductionistic medical paradigm that fails to appreciate the interconnected and "holistic" web of influences that synergize to produce systemic inflammation. For the majority of patients in outpatient clinical practice, the location of their dysbiosis is the gut, which is easily assessed with specialized stool testing and parasitology examinations, and which is easily treated with oral botanical antimicrobials and dietary modification. In my own clinical practice, I consider stool testing extremely valuable and estimate that 80% of parasitology examinations return with at least one clinically-relevant abnormality. **Testing for and treating dysbiosis is absolutely essential in patients with chronic fatigue, fibromyalgia, autoimmunity, and any type of "inflammatory arthritis."**[137,138]

At least 70% of patients with chronic arthritis are carriers of "silent infections", according to a 1992 article published in the peer-reviewed medical journal *Annals of the Rheumatic Diseases*.[139] A 2001 article in this same journal which focused exclusively on five bacteria showed that **56% of patients with idiopathic inflammatory arthritis had gastrointestinal or genitourinary dysbiosis**.[140] Indeed, published research strongly and consistently indicates that bacteria, yeast/fungi, amebas, protozoa, and other "parasites" (rarely including helminths/worms) are underappreciated causes of neuromusculoskeletal inflammation. This section will explain the mechanisms by which **silent infections**, **noninfectious microbial colonization**, and **dysbiosis** can cause and perpetuate numerous health problems, and I will also discuss

---

[133] "These finding provide serological evidence of chronic C. pneumoniae infection in association with Behcet's disease." Ayaslioglu E, Duzgun N, Erkek E, Inal A. Evidence of chronic Chlamydia pneumoniae infection in patients with Behcet's disease. *Scand J Infect Dis.* 2004;36(6-7):428-30

[134] "Staphylococcus aureus (41/70, 58.6%, p = 0.008) and Prevotella spp (17/70, 24.3%, p = 0.002) were significantly more common in pustules from BS patients..." Hatemi G, Bahar H, Uysal S, Mat C, Gogus F, Masatlioglu S, Altas K, Yazici H. The pustular skin lesions in Behcet's syndrome are not sterile. *Ann Rheum Dis.* 2004 Nov;63(11):1450-2

[135] "These data indicate that the BD patients are infected with IgA protease-producing S. sanguis strains, which cause an increase of IgA titer against these organisms and IgA protease antigen." Yokota K, Oguma K. IgA protease produced by Streptococcus sanguis and antibody production against IgA protease in patients with Behcet's disease. *Microbiol Immunol.* 1997;41(12):925-31

[136] Seaman DR. The diet-induced proinflammatory state: a cause of chronic pain and other degenerative diseases? *J Manipulative Physiol Ther.* 2002 Mar-Apr;25(3):168-79

[137] **Vasquez A. Reducing Pain and Inflammation Naturally. Part 6: Nutritional and Botanical Treatments Against "Silent Infections" and Gastrointestinal Dysbiosis, Commonly Overlooked Causes of Neuromusculoskeletal Inflammation and Chronic Health Problems.** Nutritional Perspectives 2006; January http://optimalhealthresearch.com/part6

[138] **Vasquez A. Multifocal Dysbiosis: Pathophysiology, Relevance for Inflammatory and Autoimmune Diseases, and Treatment with Nutritional and Botanical Interventions.** *Naturopathy Digest* 2006 June http://www.naturopathydigest.com/archives/2006/jun/vasquez.php

[139] "At the time of initial evaluation, 57 (69%) of the patients with oligoarthritis and 4/20 (20%) of the control subjects were carriers of clinically silent infections." Weyand CM, Goronzy JJ. Clinically silent infections in patients with oligoarthritis: results of a prospective study. *Ann Rheum Dis.* 1992 Feb;51(2):253-8

[140] Fendler C, Laitko S, Sorensen H, Gripenberg-Lerche C, Groh A, Uksila J, Granfors K, Braun J, Sieper J. Frequency of triggering bacteria in patients with reactive arthritis and undifferentiated oligoarthritis and the relative importance of the tests used for diagnosis. *Ann Rheum Dis.* 2001 Apr;60(4):337-43 http://ard.bmjjournals.com/cgi/content/full/60/4/337

basic assessment and treatment measures that can be used clinically to help patients with microbe-induced musculoskeletal inflammation.

A problem that plagues many healthcare providers of all professions is that most doctors are still under the spell of the "Pasteurian paradigm of infectious disease", namely that pathogenic microorganisms cause *disease* by causing "*infection.*" Relatedly, Koch's Postulates first published in 1884 held that "the organism must be found in all animals suffering from the disease, but not in healthy animals" and "the cultured organism should cause disease when introduced into a healthy animal."[141] Such contributions by Pasteur, Koch, and other researchers were essential in providing a preliminary understanding of the role of microorganisms in the genesis of human disease; however, we must appreciate that these simplistic, linear, and rather primitive models do not suffice for explaining all microbe-induced disorders. The major problems with the paradigms proposed by Pasteur and Koch are that both of these models fail to appreciate 1) adverse microbe-host interactions which may not *result in* nor *result from* a true "infection" (thus refuting the Pasteurian paradigm), and 2) the importance of the patient's biochemical individuality and genetic uniqueness which influence the clinical manifestations of dysbiosis-induced disease such that a) not all patients exposed to a pathogenic microbe will express the stereotypic disease, and b) some patients exposed to microorganisms that are generally considered benign commensals will produce a dramatic inflammatory response which results in clinical disease (thus refuting Koch's postulates). Supported amply by the research reviewed herein, **healthcare providers have an obligation to move beyond these simplistic "pathogenic" "infection-based" models of microorganism-induced disease to apprehend the more common "functional" disorders that can result from exposure to microbes**. Readers will note that these new concepts and ideas are amply supported by the references to the biomedical research that are included in the footnotes.[142,143]

One of the common rhetorical positions espoused by undertrained skeptics is, "If infections caused autoimmunity, then antibiotics would cure autoimmune disease." This rhetoric is biophysiologically illogical for several reasons:

1. First, autoimmunity may be incited by microbes and then persist in the absence of those same microbes; when a hammer breaks a window, removing the hammer does not repair the window. Autoimmunity—whether induced by xenobiotics or microorganisms—may have a tendency to persist due to the immune sensitization toward autoantigens that have been haptenized, exposed, or otherwise immunogenized, and due to the secondary endocrinologic changes and xenobiotic accumulation that have been induced by the disease process and which perpetuate the dysregulated proinflammatory state. The autoimmune "reactive arthritis" that follows microbial infection responds only partially to early antibiotic treatment[144], thus indicating that microbe-induced musculoskeletal inflammation—once induced—may persist despite [supposedly] effective antimicrobial treatment. **Pro-inflammatory antigens can persist in synovial immunocytes for years following a bacterial infection that results in chronic inflammatory arthritis.**[145] Conversely, the observation that antimicrobial intervention, particularly with more powerful treatments, can significantly reduce (not eliminate) the development of "autoimmune" phenomena in patients following bacterial infection[146] appears to indicate that 1) microorganisms,

---

[141] Koch's Postulates. http://encyclopedia.thefreedictionary.com/Koch%27s+postulates Accessed October 4, 2005
[142] **Noah PW. The role of microorganisms in psoriasis. Semin Dermatol. 1990 Dec;9(4):269-76**
[143] Samarkos M, Vaiopoulos G. The role of infections in the pathogenesis of autoimmune diseases. Curr Drug Targets Inflamm Allergy. 2005 Feb;4(1):99-10 http://www.bentham.org/cdtia/sample/cdtia4-1/0016L.pdf
[144] Laasila K, Laasonen L, Leirisalo-Repo M. Antibiotic treatment and long term prognosis of reactive arthritis. Ann Rheum Dis. 2003 Jul;62(7):655-8 http://ard.bmjjournals.com/cgi/content/full/62/7/655
[145] "Extensive bacterial cultures of the synovial fluid were negative... We conclude that in patients with reactive arthritis after yersinia infection, microbial antigens can be found in synovial-fluid cells from the affected joints." Granfors K, Jalkanen S, von Essen R, Lahesmaa-Rantala R, Isomaki O, Pekkola-Heino K, Merilahti-Palo R, Saario R, Isomaki H, Toivanen A. Yersinia antigens in synovial-fluid cells from patients with reactive arthritis. N Engl J Med. 1989 Jan 26;320(4):216-2
[146] Yli-Kerttula T, Luukkainen R, Yli-Kerttula U, Mottonen T, Hakola M, Korpela M, Sanila M, Uksila J, Toivanen A. Effect of a three month course of ciprofloxacin on the late prognosis of reactive arthritis. Ann Rheum Dis. 2003 Sep;62(9):880-4 http://ard.bmjjournals.com/cgi/content/full/62/9/880

particularly bacteria, contribute directly to the genesis of specific inflammatory/autoimmune disorders, and that 2) antimicrobial treatment of autoimmune disorders is warranted.

2. Second, all clinicians are aware that no antimicrobial treatment eradicates *all* microbes from *all* surfaces; for example, an orally administered broad-spectrum antibiotic is not appropriate for eradicating a fungal infection located in the sinuses. **Microbial drug resistance is an increasingly large problem in outpatient and hospital-based medicine**[147] where antimicrobial drug therapies are the mainstay treatment of bacterial infections and no consideration is given to effective botanical antimicrobials (reviewed later) and to strengthening host defenses (described throughout this text and particularly in sections on diet and immunonutrition).

3. Third, the administration of antimicrobial therapeutics of a limited scope for a limited time may allow the dysbiosis to return when the antimicrobials are discontinued. The autoimmune condition problem may continue or recur despite even "appropriate" antimicrobial treatment if the duration of antimicrobial treatment is too brief.

4. Fourth, even when the microbe is eradicated, its antigens may persist. **Microbial antigens can persist within the human body for years following clearance of the primary infection.**[148,149,150]

5. Fifth, the microbe-autoimmunity model of autoimmune disease induction does not state that microbes are the *sole cause* of autoimmunity. What I have documented here with an abundance of research is that **microbes are a major contributor to autoimmunity** and that **dysbiosis works in concert with hormonal abnormalities, xenobiotic immunotoxicity, food intolerances, and a proinflammatory lifestyle which synergize to create proinflammatory immune dysfunction that happens to destroy body tissues in a phenomenon that gets labeled "autoimmunity."**

Despite the ability of autoimmunity/inflammation to persist despite the eradication of causative microorganisms, clinicians (and patients) will be pleased to learn that effective oligomicrobial eradication can result in dramatic clinical improvements in patients with autoimmunity. This observation is not merely anecdote from practicing clinicians; **published research and relatively large clinical trials are increasingly documenting that comprehensive antimicrobial treatments do indeed** *promote regression* **and** *initiate cure* **in a growing list of previously "untreatable" autoimmune diseases.**

Mechanisms of Autoimmune Disease Induction by Microorganisms

I have identified at least seventeen mechanisms by which microorganisms can cause immune dysfunction that promotes musculoskeletal inflammation. Each of the following exemplifies a mechanism by which microbes can cause "disease" without causing an "infection." Mechanisms by which microorganisms can contribute to musculoskeletal inflammation without causing "infection" include but are not limited to the following:

1. *Molecular mimicry*: Several microbes have peptides and other structures that resemble or "mimic" the peptides and cell structures found in human tissues. Thus, when the immune system fights against the microbe, the antibodies and T-cells can "cross-react" with the tissues of the human host. In this way, the immune system begins attacking the human body, which is otherwise an innocent bystander—the victim of "friendly fire."[151] As reviewed by Ringrose[152], evidence clearly indicates that specific microbial proteins have amino acid homology with human proteins and/or that homologous bacterial peptides appear to stimulate (auto)immunity toward similar

[147] Sharma R, Sharma CL, Kapoor B. Antibacterial resistance: Current problems and possible solutions. *Indian J Med Sci* [serial online] 2005 [cited 2005 Dec 27];59:120-129. Available from: http://www.indianjmedsci.org/article.asp?issn=0019-5359;year=2005;volume=59;issue=3;spage=120;epage=129;aulast=Sharma

[148] Inman RD. Antigens, the gastrointestinal tract, and arthritis. *Rheum Dis Clin North Am.* 1991 May;17(2):309-21

[149] "These samples were studied by immunochemical techniques for the presence of Yersinia antigens at the beginning of infection and up to 4 years thereafter... This study has, for the first time, directly demonstrated that bacterial antigens persist for a long time in patients who develop ReA after Y. enterocolitica O:3 infection." Granfors K, Merilahti-Palo R, Luukkainen R, Mottonen T, Lahesmaa R, Probst P, Marker-Hermann E, Toivanen P. Persistence of Yersinia antigens in peripheral blood cells from patients with Yersinia enterocolitica O:3 infection with or without reactive arthritis. *Arthritis Rheum.* 1998 May;41(5):855-62

[150] "Extensive bacterial cultures of the synovial fluid were negative... We conclude that in patients with reactive arthritis after yersinia infection, microbial antigens can be found in synovial-fluid cells from the affected joints." Granfors K, Jalkanen S, von Essen R, Lahesmaa-Rantala R, Isomaki O, Pekkola-Heino K, Merilahti-Palo R, Saario R, Isomaki H, Toivanen A. Yersinia antigens in synovial-fluid cells from patients with reactive arthritis. *N Engl J Med.* 1989 Jan 26;320(4):216-2

[151] Wucherpfennig KW. Mechanisms for the induction of autoimmunity by infectious agents. *J Clin Invest.* 2001 Oct;108(8):1097-104 http://www.jci.org/cgi/reprint/108/8/1097

[152] Ringrose JH. HLA-B27 associated spondyloarthropathy, an autoimmune disease based on crossreactivity between bacteria and HLA-B27? *Ann Rheum Dis.* 1999 Oct;58(10):598-610 http://ard.bmjjournals.com/cgi/content/full/58/10/598

neighboring human peptides. Therefore the two underlying bases for autoimmune induction by molecular mimicry—namely 1) homology between human and microbial amino acid sequences, and 2) stimulation of immunity against human peptides—do indeed occur *in vivo*. **Molecular mimicry is strongly implicated in the pathogenesis of reactive arthritis and ankylosing spondylitis.**[153,154]

2. *Superantigens*: Many viral, bacterial, and fungal microbes produce "superantigens", molecules which are capable of causing widespread, nonspecific, and unregulated proinflammatory immune activation. One of the hallmarks of superantigens is their ability to induce polyclonal T- and B-lymphocyte activation and the production of excessive levels of cytokines and other inflammatory effectors.[155] Obviously, when the body is in such a state of unregulated hyper-inflammation, inevitably some of this inflammation will affect the structures of the musculoskeletal system, especially since articular tissues are predisposed to immune attack, if for no other reasons than their proclivity to retain antigens and immune complexes[156,157] to which an exaggerated inflammatory response is promoted by superantigen stimulation. **Several research groups have found evidence of superantigen involvement in the pathogenesis of rheumatoid arthritis.**[158,159]

3. *Enhanced processing of autoantigens*: When the immune system perceives the presence of microbial molecules, mechanisms are enhanced which facilitate the processing and presentation of preexistent antigens to the immune system, which then targets these antigens for destruction. Of course, this is beneficial when fighting a true infection; but there is mounting evidence that chronic silent infections can facilitate the processing and presentation of the body's own antigens (autoantigens) which are then attacked. Clinically, we see the immune system attacking the body, and we call this an "autoimmune disease" even though the original cause of the problem may have been an occult infection or exposure to specific microbial molecules. Ringrose et al[160] showed that infecting HLA-B27-positive human cells with *Salmonella typhimurium* and *Shigella flexneri* caused these cells to express autoantigens, namely human histone H3, human ribosomal protein S17 (two separate amino acid sequences) and the heavy chain of HLA-B27. A similar phenomenon has been demonstrated in autistic children wherein patients exposed to bacterial antigens (streptokinase), toxic chemicals (Thimerosal, ethyl mercury), and dietary antigens (gliadin and casein peptides) produce autoantigens that appear capable of inciting and perpetuating autoimmunity.[161] **Therefore, we have experimental evidence with human cells *in vitro* which demonstrates that *enhanced processing of autoantigens* occurs following exposure to bacterial antigens, dietary allergens, and xenobiotics.**

---

[153] "HLA-B27 and proteins from enteric bacteria are structurally related, in a manner that may affect T cell response to enteric pathogens." Inman RD, Scofield RH. Etiopathogenesis of ankylosing spondylitis and reactive arthritis. *Curr Opin Rheumatol.* 1994 Jul;6(4):360-70

[154] "With respect to bacterial infection, recent findings in bacterial antigenicity, host response through interactions of antigen-presenting cells, T cells, and cytokines are providing new understanding of host-pathogen interactions and the pathogenesis of arthritis." Kim TH, Uhm WS, Inman RD. Pathogenesis of ankylosing spondylitis and reactive arthritis. *Curr Opin Rheumatol.* 2005 Jul;17(4):400-5

[155] "The basis of autoimmune disorders due to superantigen is due to greater stimulation of T-lymphocytes and elaborate cytokine production." Hemalatha V, Srikanth P, Mallika M. Superantigens - Concepts, clinical disease and therapy. *Indian J Med Microbiol* 2004;22:204-211

[156] Inman RD. Antigens, the gastrointestinal tract, and arthritis. *Rheum Dis Clin North Am.* 1991 May;17(2):309-21

[157] "Other factors, like the specific properties of synovial vessels and the adhesion molecules responsible for synovium-specific homing, will contribute to the guiding of the monocytes from the mucosal areas into the joints." Wuorela M, Tohka S, Granfors K, Jalkanen S. Monocytes that have ingested Yersinia enterocolitica serotype O:3 acquire enhanced capacity to bind to nonstimulated vascular endothelial cells via P-selectin. *Infect Immun.* 1999 Feb;67(2):726-32 http://iai.asm.org/cgi/content/full/67/2/726

[158] "They also suggest that the etiology of RA may involve initial activation of V beta 14+ T cells by a V beta 14-specific superantigen with subsequent recruitment of a few activated autoreactive v beta 14+ T cell clones to the joints while the majority of other V beta 14+ T cells disappear." Paliard X, West SG, Lafferty JA, Clements JR, Kappler JW, Marrack P, Kotzin BL. Evidence for the effects of a superantigen in rheumatoid arthritis. *Science.* 1991 Jul 19;253(5017):325-9

[159] "Given that binding sites for superantigens have been mapped to the CDR4s of TCR beta chains, the synovial localization of T cells bearing V beta s with significant CDR4 homology indicates that V beta-specific T-cell activation by superantigen may play a role in RA." Howell MD, Diveley JP, Lundeen KA, Esty A, Winters ST, Carlo DJ, Brostoff SW. Limited T-cell receptor beta-chain heterogeneity among interleukin 2 receptor-positive synovial T cells suggests a role for superantigen in rheumatoid arthritis. *Proc Natl Acad Sci* U S A. 1991 Dec 1;88(23):10921-5

[160] Ringrose JH, Muijsers AO, Pannekoek Y, Yard BA, Boog CJ, van Alphen L, Dankert J, Feltkamp TE. Influence of infection of cells with bacteria associated with reactive arthritis on the peptide repertoire presented by HLA-B27. *J Med Microbiol.* 2001 Apr;50(4):385-9 http://jmm.sgmjournals.org/cgi/reprint/50/4/385

[161] Vojdani A, Pangborn JB, Vojdani E, Cooper EL. Infections, toxic chemicals and dietary peptides binding to lymphocyte receptors and tissue enzymes are major instigators of autoimmunity in autism. *Int J Immunopathol Pharmacol.* 2003 Sep-Dec;16(3):189-99

Schematic Representation of the Interconnected Physiologic Pathways Involved in Dysbiosis-Induced musculoskeletal Inflammation and "Autoimmunity"

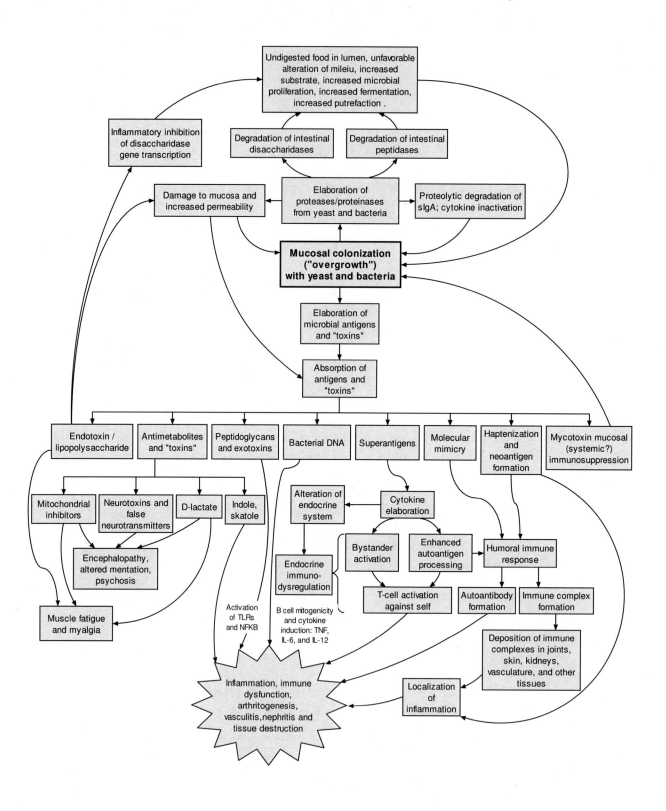

4. *Bystander activation*: Evidence suggests that we all have immunocytes capable of attacking our body tissues, and thus we all have the potential to develop autoimmune disease. Normally, these autoreactive cells are kept anergic, dormant, quiescent, and otherwise inactive through various mechanisms that regulate the immune system; in this way, such autoreactive cells can be considered "bystanders" because they are not really doing anything and are basically "standing by." Bystander activation

> **"Infectious agents can cause autoimmune disease by different mechanisms**, which fall into two categories: *antigen specific* in which pathogen products or elements have a central role e.g. superantigens or epitope (molecular) mimicry, and *antigen non-specific* in which the pathogen provides the appropriate inflammatory setting for **bystander activation**."
>
> Samarkos, Vaiopoulos. The role of infections in the pathogenesis of autoimmune diseases. *Curr Drug Targets Inflamm Allergy*. 2005 Feb

occurs when these cells are awakened by the cascade of inflammatory processes that occur as a result of superantigen exposure, molecular mimicry, immune complex deposition, or xenobiotic immunotoxicity. **Bystander activation appears to contribute to the development of certain autoimmune conditions, such as drug-induced lupus[162], and it may be a contributing pathogenic mechanism in heavy metal-induced autoimmunity.**[163]

5. *Peptidoglycans, teichoic acid, and exotoxins from gram-positive bacteria*: Peptidoglycans from gram-positive bacteria such as group-A streptococci can cause malaise, fever, dermatosis, tenosynovitis, cryoglobulinemia (immune complex disease), and arthritis.[164] Experimental arthritis can be induced in animals by exposing them to group-B streptococci isolated from the nasopharynx of human patients with rheumatoid arthritis.[165] *Staphylococcus aureus* is a gram-positive bacterium, certain strains of which produce the toxic shock syndrome toxin-1 (TSST-1) that causes scalded skin syndrome, toxic shock syndrome, and food poisoning; other strains of *Staphylococcus aureus* that do not produce TSST-1 are also capable of causing toxic shock syndrome from colonization of bone, vagina, wounds, or rectum.[166] Experimental evidence has shown that peptidoglycan-polysaccharide complexes from "good" and "normal" bacteria such as Bifidobacteria and *Lactobacillus casei* can also induce an inflammatory arthritis; this speaks against the "more is better" approach to probiotic supplementation and also demonstrates how **bacterial overgrowth of the small bowel (detailed later) can induce joint pain and inflammation even in the absence of so-called "pathogens."**[167,168]

6. *Endotoxins (lipopolysaccharide) from gram-negative bacteria*: Many different species of gram-negative bacteria produce endotoxin, also known as bacterial lipopolysaccharide (LPS). Even in the absence of viable bacteria, the exposure of humans to endotoxin, say for example by intravenous administration for the purpose of experimentation, produces a wide range of adverse physiologic consequences, including 1) triggering an acute proinflammatory response resembling febrile illness or sepsis, 2) increasing intestinal permeability, causing "leaky gut"[169], 3) inhibiting hepatic detoxification[170], 4) disrupting the blood-brain barrier and promoting neurodegeneration via neuroinflammation.[171,172,173] The pathophysiologic effects of endotoxin/LPS are often *similar to* and *synergistic with* those of

---

[162] "Several mechanisms for induction of autoimmunity will be discussed, including bystander activation of autoreactive lymphocytes due to drug-specific immunity or to non-specific activation of lymphocytes, direct cytotoxicity with release of autoantigens and disruption of central T-cell tolerance." Rubin RL. Drug-induced lupus. *Toxicology*. 2005 Apr 15;209(2):135-47

[163] "It is therefore theoretically possible that compounds present in vaccines such as thiomersal or aluminium hydroxyde can trigger autoimmune reactions through bystander effects." Fournie GJ, Mas M, Cautain B, Savignac M, Subra JF, Pelletier L, Saoudi A, Lagrange D, Calise M, Druet P. Induction of autoimmunity through bystander effects. Lessons from immunological disorders induced by heavy metals. *J Autoimmun*. 2001 May;16(3):319-26

[164] "A characteristic intermittent neutrophilic dermatosis, associated with polyarthritis, tenosynovitis, malaise, fever, and cryoglobulinemia, occurs in 20% of patients who undergo ileojejunal bypass surgery for the treatment of morbid obesity... Peptidoglycans from numerous intestinal bacteria...are suggested as causative of the toxic and immunologic features of this syndrome." Ely PH. The bowel bypass syndrome: a response to bacterial peptidoglycans. *J Am Acad Dermatol*. 1980 Jun;2(6):473-87

[165] "The origin of rheumatoid arthritis (RA) is in our opinion a bacterial infection." Svartz N. The origin of rheumatoid arthritis. *Rheumatology*. 1975;6:322-8

[166] Shandera WX, Moran A. "Infectious diseases: viral and rickettsial." In Tierney LM, McPhee SJ Papadakis MA (eds). Current Medical Diagnosis and Treatment. 44th edition. New York: Lange; 2005, page 1356-8

[167] Simelyte E, Rimpilainen M, Lehtonen L, Zhang X, Toivanen P. Bacterial cell wall-induced arthritis: chemical composition and tissue distribution of four Lactobacillus strains. *Infect Immun*. 2000 Jun;68(6):3535-40 http://iai.asm.org/cgi/reprint/68/6/3535

[168] Toivanen P. Normal intestinal microbiota in the aetiopathogenesis of rheumatoid arthritis. *Ann Rheum Dis*. 2003 Sep;62(9):807-11 http://ard.bmjjournals.com/cgi/reprint/62/9/807

[169] "After endotoxin administration systemic absorption and excretion of lactulose increased almost two-fold... These data suggest that a brief exposure to circulating endotoxin increases the permeability of the normal gut." O'Dwyer ST, Michie HR, Ziegler TR, Revhaug A, Smith RJ, Wilmore DW. A single dose of endotoxin increases intestinal permeability in healthy humans. *Arch Surg*. 1988 Dec;123(12):1459-64

[170] Shedlofsky SI, Israel BC, Tosheva R, Blouin RA. Endotoxin depresses hepatic cytochrome P450-mediated drug metabolism in women. *Br J Clin Pharmacol*. 1997 Jun;43(6):627-32

[171] "Following administration of lipopolysaccharide (LPS) to immunized mice, antibodies gain access to the brain. They bind preferentially to hippocampal neurons and cause neuronal death with resulting cognitive dysfunction and altered hippocampal metabolism..." Kowal C, DeGiorgio LA, Nakaoka T, Hetherington H, Huerta PT, Diamond B, Volpe BT. Cognition and immunity; antibody impairs memory. *Immunity*. 2004 Aug;21(2):179-88 http://www.immunity.com/content/article/abstract?uid=PIIS1074761304001980

[172] Fassbender K, Walter S, Kuhl S, et al. The LPS receptor (CD14) links innate immunity with Alzheimer's disease. *FASEB J*. 2004 Jan;18(1):203-5. Epub 2003 Nov 3 http://www.fasebj.org/cgi/reprint/03-0364fjev1

[173] Laflamme N, Rivest S. Toll-like receptor 4: the missing link of the cerebral innate immune response triggered by circulating gram-negative bacterial cell wall components. *FASEB J*. 2001 Jan;15(1):155-163 http://www.fasebj.org/cgi/reprint/15/1/155.pdf

superantigens to effect altered tissue function and widespread inflammation. **LPS and antigens from gram-negative bacteria (in the absence of viable bacteria) exacerbate arthritis in experimental models[174] and trigger inflammatory arthropathy (reactive arthritis) in humans.[175]**

7. *Immunostimulation by bacterial DNA*: **Bacterial DNA stimulates a proinflammatory response that is comparable to that induced by endotoxin/LPS.** Exposure to single-stranded *bacterial* DNA induces formation of antibodies against single-stranded *mammalian* DNA. These findings may be particularly relevant to patients with systemic lupus erythematosus—a disorder for which the pathogenic hallmark is the formation of anti-DNA antibodies—since these patients have an impaired ability to clear bacterial DNA from the serum and therefore experienced prolonged pro-inflammatory stimulation when exposed to bacterial DNA.[176] Chronic exposure to immunostimulating antigens is a recognized means for the induction of autoimmunity in animal models.

8. *Activation of Toll-like receptors and NF-kappaB*: Microbial products such as peptidoglycans and endotoxins (as well as others) promote inflammation and arthritogenesis by activating receptors and nuclear transcription factors with the resultant non-specific upregulation of proinflammatory genetic expression. Nuclear transcription factor kappaB (NFkB) is considered one of the most important nuclear transcription factors for stimulating genetic expression of proinflammatory genes, and NFkB is activated by microbes and their structures including viruses and endotoxins.[177] Similar to NFkB are the Toll-like receptors (TLRs), which promote an inflammatory response by NFKB-dependent and NFKB-independent pathways following exposure to microbial structures including but not limited to peptidoglycans and lipopolysaccharides.[178] About a dozen different TLRs have been identified, and these play an important role in the joint destruction seen in the classic example of dysbiotic arthropathy—rheumatoid arthritis.[179] From a nutritional perspective, we see that Toll-like receptor activity is stimulated by saturated fatty acids and inhibited by polyunsaturated fatty acids, especially the omega-3 fatty acid docosahexaenoic acid.[180] Likewise, NFkB activity can be modulated by numerous nutrients as I have reviewed later in this text and elsewhere.[181] Of course, nutritional, botanical, or pharmacologic modulation of inflammation should not supersede investigation and correction of the underlying cause(s) of inflammation.

9. *Immune complex formation and deposition due to the activation of B-lymphocytes/plasma cells*: Chronic infection generally results in the increased production of immune complexes, which are polymeric antigen-antibody combinations. Antigen-antibody combinations are formed almost anytime the humoral immune system is fighting against a virus, bacteria, yeast, or food allergen. Although essential for the destruction and clearance of pathogenic antigens, immune complexes pose a problem for the body due to 1) the difficulty in clearing them from the systemic circulation, and 2) their proclivity for deposition in the skin and joints.[182] Indeed, **immune complexes are significant contributors to most "autoimmune" diseases; immune complex deposition is responsible for triggering joint inflammation in rheumatoid arthritis[183] and for the facial rash and many of the other clinical manifestations which characterize systemic lupus erythematosus (SLE, lupus).** Immune complex deposition directly contributes to the renal disease and vasculitis common in patients with autoimmune disease. Patients with autoimmune disease commonly have circulating IgM and IgA antibodies against bacteria from the gastrointestinal and genitourinary tracts[184] clearly

---

[174] "The results showed that administration of LPS was followed by reactivation of AIA in a dose-related fashion." Yoshino S, Yamaki K, Taneda S, Yanagisawa R, Takano H. Reactivation of antigen-induced arthritis in mice by oral administration of lipopolysaccharide. *Scand J Immunol*. 2005 Aug;62(2):117-22

[175] "Extensive bacterial cultures of the synovial fluid were negative... We conclude that in patients with reactive arthritis after yersinia infection, microbial antigens can be found in synovial-fluid cells from the affected joints." Granfors K, Jalkanen S, von Essen R, Lahesmaa-Rantala R, Isomaki O, Pekkola-Heino K, Merilahti-Palo R, Saario R, Isomaki H, Toivanen A. Yersinia antigens in synovial-fluid cells from patients with reactive arthritis. *N Engl J Med*. 1989 Jan 26;320(4):216-2

[176] "The immunostimulatory activities of bacterial DNA are varied and encompass the mitogenicity of B cells and the induction of cytokines including IFN-α/β, IFN-γ, tumor necrosis factor alpha, interleukin 6 (IL-6), and IL-12 (17, 21, 23). Together, these activities resemble those of endotoxin…" Pisetsky DS. Antibody responses to DNA in normal immunity and aberrant immunity. *Clin Diagn Lab Immunol*. 1998 Jan;5(1):1-6 http://cvi.asm.org/cgi/reprint/5/1/1

[177] Tak PP, Firestein GS. NF-kappaB: a key role in inflammatory diseases. *J Clin Invest*. 2001;107(1):7-11 http://www.jci.org/cgi/content/full/107/1/7

[178] Armant MA, Fenton MJ. Toll-like receptors: a family of pattern-recognition receptors in mammals. Genome Biol. 2002 Jul 29;3(8):REVIEWS3011. Epub 2002 Jul 29 http://genomebiology.com/2002/3/8/REVIEWS/3011

[179] Ospelt C, Kyburz D, Pierer M, Seibl R, Kurowska M, Distler O, Neidhart M, Muller-Ladner U, Pap T, Gay RE, Gay S. Toll-like receptors in rheumatoid arthritis joint destruction mediated by two distinct pathways. *Ann Rheum Dis*. 2004 Nov;63 Suppl 2:ii90-ii91 http://ard.bmjjournals.com/cgi/content/full/63/suppl_2/ii90

[180] Lee JY, Sohn KH, Rhee SH, Hwang D. Saturated fatty acids, but not unsaturated fatty acids, induce the _expression of cyclooxygenase-2 mediated through Toll-like receptor 4. J Biol Chem. 2001 May 18;276(20):16683-9. Epub 2001 Mar 2 http://www.jbc.org/cgi/content/full/276/20/16683

[181] Vasquez A. Reducing pain and inflammation naturally - part 4: nutritional and botanical inhibition of NF-kappaB, the major intracellular amplifier of the inflammatory cascade. A practical clinical strategy exemplifying anti-inflammatory nutrigenomics. *Nutritional Perspectives*, July 2005:5-12. www.OptimalHealthResearch.com/part4

[182] Inman RD. Antigens, the gastrointestinal tract, and arthritis. *Rheum Dis Clin North Am*. 1991 May;17(2):309-21

[183] Abramson SB. Mediators of inflammation, tissue destruction, and repair: cellular constituents." In Klippel JH. Primer on the rheumatic diseases. 11th edition. Atlanta: Arthritis Foundation; 1997, page 39

[184] "IgM and IgA anti-Proteus antibodies were significantly higher in patients with RF-positive RA compared with all other patient groups." Newkirk MM, Goldbach-Mansky R, Senior BW, Klippel J, Schumacher HR Jr, El-Gabalawy HS. Elevated levels of IgM and IgA antibodies to Proteus mirabilis and IgM antibodies to Escherichia coli are associated with early rheumatoid factor (RF)-positive rheumatoid arthritis. *Rheumatology* (Oxford). 2005 Aug 9; [Epub ahead of print]

INTEGRATIVE RHEUMATOLOGY *OptimalHealthResearch.com*

indicating an active immune response against these bacteria and suggesting breaches in mucosal integrity. Since IgA-containing immune complexes are cleared from the serum by hepatocytes and are secreted intact into the bile[185,186,187], hepatobiliary phytostimulation may thereby produce an anti-rheumatic benefit; however, this hypothesis requires serologic and outcomes-based validation in a clinical trial.[188]

10. *Haptenization*: **A nonantigenic microbial molecule may bind to a nonantigenic human molecule and result in the formation of a new hybridized or "haptenized" molecule—neoantigen—which stimulates immunologic attack.** Haptenization may be the underlying mechanism by which viruses induce autoimmunity[189] and appears to be a primary mechanism by which *Staphylococcus aureus* contributes to autoimmune vasculitis in Wegener's granulomatosis, namely by producing an antigenic acid phosphatase enzyme which binds with human endothelial cells by a charge interaction—the resultant **hybrid/hapten/neoantigen** formed by the antigen-endothelium complex becomes the target of immune attack, thus creating the phenomenon of "autoimmunity" and the clinical consequences of vasculitis.[190] Similarly, Hwp1 (Hyphal wall protein-1) of *Candida albicans* is a substrate for the tissue transglutaminase enzyme and cross-links with proteins in the mammalian mucosa[191]; the resultant neoantigen that results from this microbe-human haptenization would be a prime candidate to incite autoimmunity, as has been demonstrated by the transglutaminase-mediated haptenization of gliadin with human collagen *in vivo*.[192,193] In fact, since both Hwp1 and gliadin are substrates for tissue transglutaminase, *Candida albicans* may be synergistic with gluten/gliadin in the production of the systemic inflammatory/autoimmune/allergic condition known as **celiac disease**[194]; this may exemplify the interrelated nature of dysbiosis, food allergy, and autoimmunity. Lastly, since many toxic metals, xenobiotics, and drugs appear to trigger autoimmunity via haptenization[195,196,197], the adverse effects of these toxicants will be enhanced by microbe-induced alterations in xenobiotic detoxification and/or the proinflammatory effects of peptidoglycans, exotoxins, endotoxins, lipoteichoic acid, and other antigens and superantigens. In a recent animal study, exposure to bacterial endotoxin exacerbated metal-induced autoimmunity.[198] Endotoxin from gram-negative bacteria impairs detoxification by inhibiting the first cytochrome-p450-mediated step of detoxification[199]; this inhibition of detoxification increases the risk for drug toxicity and chemical accumulation. Bacteria can also adversely affect detoxification by elaborating beta-glucuronidase in the lumen of the intestine which cleaves bile-secreted toxins from their water-soluble conjugation moieties, resulting in increased "enterohepatic

[185] "Clearance of IgA immune complexes was delayed after bile duct ligation." Harmatz PR, Kleinman RE, Bunnell BW, McClenathan DT, Walker WA, Bloch KJ. The effect of bile duct obstruction on the clearance of circulating IgA immune complexes. *Hepatology*. 1984 Jan-Feb;4(1):96-100

[186] Lemaitre-Coelho I, Jackson GD, Vaerman JP. High levels of secretory IgA and free secretory component in the serum of rats with bile duct obstruction. *J Exp Med*. 1978 Mar 1;147(3):934-9 http://www.jem.org/cgi/reprint/147/3/934

[187] "CONCLUSIONS: Biliary obstruction secondary to both calculus or malignancy of the hepatobiliary system causes suppression of bile IgA secretion and elevated serum level of secretory IgA. Bile secretory IgA secretion recovers with endoscopic drainage of the obstructed system." Sung JJ, Leung JC, Tsui CP, Chung SS, Lai KN. Biliary IgA secretion in obstructive jaundice: the effects of endoscopic drainage. *Gastrointest Endosc*. 1995 Nov;42(5):439-44

[188] Vasquez A. Do the Benefits of Botanical and Physiotherapeutic Hepatobiliary Stimulation Result From Enhanced Excretion of IgA Immune Complexes? *Naturopathy Digest* 2006; January: http://www.naturopathydigest.com/archives/2006/jan/vasquez_immune.php

[189] Van Ghelue M, Moens U, Bendiksen S, Rekvig OP. Autoimmunity to nucleosomes related to viral infection: a focus on hapten-carrier complex formation. *J Autoimmun*. 2003;20(2):171-82

[190] Brons RH, Bakker HI, Van Wijk RT, et al. Staphylococcal acid phosphatase binds to endothelial cells via charge interaction; a pathogenic role in Wegener's granulomatosis? *Clin Exp Immunol*. 2000 Mar;119(3):566-73 http://www.blackwell-synergy.com/doi/abs/10.1046/j.1365-2249.2000.01172.x PDF available from this link on November 27, 2005.

[191] "By serving as a microbial substrate for epithelial cell transglutaminase, Hwp1 (Hyphal wall protein 1) of Candida albicans participates in cross-links with proteins on the mammalian mucosa." Staab JF, Bahn YS, Tai CH, Cook PF, Sundstrom P. Expression of transglutaminase substrate activity on Candida albicans germ tubes through a coiled, disulfide-bonded N-terminal domain of Hwp1 requires C-terminal glycosylphosphatidylinositol modification. *J Biol Chem*. 2004 Sep 24;279(39):40737-47 http://www.jbc.org/cgi/content/full/279/39/40737

[192] "Our findings firstly demonstrated that gliadin was directly bound to tTG in duodenal mucosa of coeliacs and controls, and the ability of circulating tTG-autoantibodies to recognize and immunoprecipitate the tTG-gliadin complexes." Ciccocioppo R, Di Sabatino A, Ara C, Biagi F, Perilli M, Amicosante G, Cifone MG, Corazza GR. Gliadin and tissue transglutaminase complexes in normal and coeliac duodenal mucosa. *Clin Exp Immunol*. 2003 Dec;134(3):516-24

[193] "Thus, modification of gluten peptides by tTG, especially deamidation of certain glutamine residues, can enhance their binding to HLA-DQ2 or -DQ8 and potentiate T cell stimulation. Furthermore, tTG-catalyzed cross-linking and consequent haptenization of gluten with extracellular matrix proteins allows for storage and extended availability of gluten in the mucosa." Dieterich W, Esslinger B, Schuppan D. Pathomechanisms in celiac disease. *Int Arch Allergy Immunol*. 2003 Oct;132(2):98-108

[194] "Subsequently, C albicans might function as an adjuvant that stimulates antibody formation against HWP1 and gluten, and formation of autoreactive antibodies against tissue transglutaminase and endomysium." Nieuwenhuizen WF, Pieters RH, Knippels LM, Jansen MC, Koppelman SJ. Is Candida albicans a trigger in the onset of coeliac disease? *Lancet*. 2003;361(9375):2152-4

[195] Rao T, Richardson B. Environmentally induced autoimmune diseases: potential mechanisms. *Environ Health Perspect*. 1999 Oct;107 Suppl 5:737-42 http://ehp.niehs.nih.gov/members/1999/suppl-5/737-742rao/rao-full.html

[196] "Here, Peter Griem and colleagues focus on several aspects of neoantigen formation by xenobiotics: metabolism of xenobiotics into reactive, haptenic metabolites; polymorphisms of metabolizing enzymes; induction of costimulatory signals; and sensitization of T cells." Griem P, Wulferink M, Sachs B, Gonzalez JB, Gleichmann E. Allergic and autoimmune reactions to xenobiotics: how do they arise? *Immunol Today*. 1998 Mar;19(3):133-4

[197] "It appears that the patients' antibodies recognize epitopes consisting of the TFA group plus associated structural features of the protein carriers (100 kDa, 76 kDa, 59 kDa, 57 kDa and 54 kDa), not the TFA hapten alone." Kenna JG, Satoh H, Christ DD, Pohl LR. Metabolic basis for a drug hypersensitivity: antibodies in sera from patients with halothane hepatitis recognize liver neoantigens that contain the trifluoroacetyl group derived from halothane. *J Pharmacol Exp Ther*. 1988 Jun;245(3):1103-9 As an extension of this work, also see: "These investigations have further revealed that the antibodies are directed against distinct polypeptide fractions (100 kDa, 76 kDa, 59 kDa, 57 kDa, 54 kDa) that have been covalently modified by the reactive trifluoroacetyl halide metabolite of halothane." Satoh H, Martin BM, Schulick AH, Christ DD, Kenna JG, Pohl LR. Human anti-endoplasmic reticulum antibodies in sera of patients with halothane-induced hepatitis are directed against a trifluoroacetylated carboxylesterase. *Proc Natl Acad Sci U S A*. 1989 Jan;86(1):322-6 http://www.pnas.org/cgi/reprint/86/1/322

[198] Abedi-Valugerdi M, Nilsson C, Zargari A, Gharibdoost F, DePierre JW, Hassan M. Bacterial lipopolysaccharide both renders resistant mice susceptible to mercury-induced autoimmunity and exacerbates such autoimmunity in susceptible mice. *Clin Exp Immunol*. 2005 Aug;141(2):238-47

[199] Shedlofsky SI, Israel BC, McClain CJ, Hill DB, Blouin RA. Endotoxin administration to humans inhibits hepatic cytochrome P450-mediated drug metabolism. *J Clin Invest*. 1994 Dec;94(6):2209-14

recycling"[200] or "enterohepatic recirculation"[201] as discussed below; increased re-exposure to previously detoxified endogenous and exogenous toxins can result in an upregulation of Phase 1 (cytochrome-p450-mediated biotransformation) leading to the formation of reactive intermediates and a condition commonly described by clinicians as "imbalanced detoxification" or "pathological detoxification."

11. _Damage to the intestinal mucosa_: One of the indirect ways by which gastrointestinal microbes can cause non-infectious disease is by damaging the intestinal mucosa, a situation which results in "leaky gut." The increased absorption of molecular debris from the gut—"antigen overload" from otherwise benign yeast, bacteria, and foods—results in systemic inflammation[202] and immune activation[203], which contribute to enhanced autoantigen processing and bystander activation as discussed above. Exacerbations and relapse of the autoimmune diseases ulcerative colitis and Crohn's disease are preceded by increases in intestinal permeability; this is direct evidence of "leaky gut" preceding clinical disease.[204] Evidence of "leaky gut" is seen in several systemic inflammatory disorders, including asthma[205], eczema[206], psoriasis[207], Behcet's disease[208], seronegative spondyloarthritis[209] and ankylosing spondylitis[210] and nearly all of the so-called "idiopathic" juvenile arthropathies such as enteropathic spondyloarthropathy and oligoarticular juvenile idiopathic arthritis.[211] A "leaky gut" type of intestinal disease (protein-losing enteropathy) has also been documented in some patients with lupus.[212]

12. _Inhibition of detoxification_: **All clinicians must appreciate that bioaccumulation of toxic chemicals can cause autoimmunity.**[213,214,215] Examples of this include the increased autoimmunity seen in humans exposed to pesticides[216,217], the scleroderma-like disease that results from exposure to vinyl chloride[218], the association of mercury and pesticide exposure with lupus[219], and the well-recognized connection between drug and chemical exposure and various autoimmune syndromes such as drug-induced lupus.[220] Indeed, more than 40 pharmaceutical drugs are known to cause

> "Autoimmunity due to chemical exposure was evidenced by elevation of TA1 phenotype frequencies and presence of rheumatoid factor, immune complexes, ANA, and antimyelin basic protein antibodies. We conclude that chemical exposure may induce immune abnormalities including immune suppression and autoimmunity."
>
> Vojdani A, Ghoneum M, Brautbar N. _Toxicology and Industrial Health_ 1992

[200] "Enterohepatic recycling occurs by biliary excretion and intestinal reabsorption of a solute, sometimes with hepatic conjugation and intestinal deconjugation. ... Of particular importance is the potential amplifying effect of enterohepatic variability in defining differences in the bioavailability, apparent volume of distribution and clearance of a given compound." Roberts MS, Magnusson BM, Burczynski FJ, Weiss M. Enterohepatic circulation: physiological, pharmacokinetic and clinical implications. _Clin Pharmacokinet_. 2002;41(10):751-90

[201] Liska DJ. The detoxification enzyme systems. _Altern Med Rev_. 1998 Jun;3(3):187-98 http://www.thorne.com/altmedrev/.fulltext/3/3/187.pdf

[202] Campbell DI, Elia M, Lunn PG. Growth faltering in rural Gambian infants is associated with impaired small intestinal barrier function, leading to endotoxemia and systemic inflammation. _J Nutr_. 2003 May;133(5):1332-8

[203] "Altered gastrointestinal motility and sensation, changed activity of the central nervous system, and increased sympathetic drive and immune activation may be understood as consequences of the host response to SIBO." Lin HC. Small intestinal bacterial overgrowth: a framework for understanding irritable bowel syndrome. _JAMA_. 2004 Aug 18;292(7):852-8

[204] Wyatt J, Vogelsang H, Hubl W, Waldhoer T, Lochs H. Intestinal permeability and the prediction of relapse in Crohn's disease. _Lancet_. 1993 Jun 5;341(8858):1437-9

[205] Hijazi Z, Molla AM, Al-Habashi H, Muawad WM, Molla AM, Sharma PN. Intestinal permeability is increased in bronchial asthma. _Arch Dis Child_. 2004 Mar;89(3):227-9

[206] Ukabam SO, Mann RJ, Cooper BT. Small intestinal permeability to sugars in patients with atopic eczema. _Br J Dermatol_. 1984 Jun;110(6):649-52

[207] "The 24-h urine excretion of 51Cr-EDTA from psoriatic patients was 2.46 +/- 0.81%. These results differed significantly from controls (1.95 +/- 0.36%; P less than 0.05)." Humbert P, Bidet A, Treffel P, Drobacheff C, Agache P. Intestinal permeability in patients with psoriasis. _J Dermatol Sci_. 1991 Jul;2(4):324-6

[208] Fresko I, Hamuryudan V, Demir M, Hizli N, Sayman H, Melikoglu M, Tunc R, Yurdakul S, Yazici H. Intestinal permeability in Behcet's syndrome. _Ann Rheum Dis_. 2001 Jan;60(1):65-6

[209] Di Leo V, D'Inca R, Bettini MB, Podswiadek M, Punzi L, Mastropaolo G, Sturniolo GC. Effect of Helicobacter pylori and eradication therapy on gastrointestinal permeability. Implications for patients with seronegative spondyloarthritis. _J Rheumatol_. 2005 Feb;32(2):295-300

[210] "Patients with AS have altered small intestinal, but not gastric, permeability. NSAID use cannot explain all the abnormality. Bowel permeability abnormalities, possibly genetically determined, may antedate development of bowel or joint symptoms." Vaile JH, Meddings JB, Yacyshyn BR, Russell AS, Maksymowych WP. Bowel permeability and CD45RO expression on circulating CD20+ B cells in patients with ankylosing spondylitis and their relatives. _J Rheumatol_. 1999 Jan;26(1):128-35

[211] Picco P, Gattorno M, Marchese N, Vignola S, Sormani MP, Barabino A, Buoncompagni A. Increased gut permeability in juvenile chronic arthritides. A multivariate analysis of the diagnostic parameters. _Clin Exp Rheumatol_. 2000 Nov-Dec;18(6):773-8

[212] "Fourteen cases of primary lupus-associated protein-losing enteropathy have now been reported in the English-language literature." Perednia DA, Curosh NA. Lupus-associated protein-losing enteropathy. _Arch Intern Med_. 1990 Sep;150(9):1806-10

[213] "Autoimmunity due to chemical exposure was evidenced by elevation of TA1 phenotype frequencies and presence of rheumatoid factor, immune complexes, ANA, and anti myelin basic protein antibodies. We conclude that chemical exposure may induce immune abnormalities including immune suppression and autoimmunity." Vojdani A, Ghoneum M, Brautbar N. Immune alteration associated with exposure to toxic chemicals. _Toxicol Ind Health_ 1992;8:239-253

[214] Crinnion WJ. Results of a decade of naturopathic treatment for environmental illnesses. _J Naturopathic Med_ 1994;17:21-27

[215] Crinnion WJ. Environmental medicine, part one: the human burden of environmental toxins and their common health effects. _Altern Med Rev_. 2000 Feb;5(1):52-63 http://www.thorne.com/altmedrev/.fulltext/5/1/52.pdf See also: Crinnion WJ. Environmental medicine, part 2 - health effects of and protection from ubiquitous airborne solvent exposure. _Altern Med Rev_. 2000 Apr;5(2):133-43 http://www.thorne.com/altmedrev/.fulltext/5/2/133.pdf

[216] "IgG levels decreased with increasing p,p'-DDE levels, with a statistically significant decrease of approximately 50% in the highest two categories of exposure. Sixteen (12%) were positive for antinuclear antibodies... These analyses provide evidence that p,p'-DDE modulates immune responses in humans." Cooper GS, Martin SA, Longnecker MP, Sandler DP, Germolec DR. Associations between plasma DDE levels and immunologic measures in African-American farmers in North Carolina. _Environ Health Perspect_. 2004 Jul;112(10):1080-4

[217] "Twelve individuals who were exposed to chlorpyrifos were studied 1-4.5 y following exposure to determine changes in the peripheral immune system. The subjects were found to have a high rate of atopy and antibiotic sensitivities, elevated CD26 cells (p < .01), and a higher rate of autoimmunity, compared with two control groups." Thrasher JO, Madison R, Broughton A. Immunologic abnormalities in humans exposed to chlorpyrifos: preliminary observations. _Arch Environ Health_ 1993;48:89-93

[218] "Vinyl chloride (VC) monomer can induce a scleroderma-like syndrome in a proportion of workers exposed to it during production of polyvinyl chloride." Black CM, Welsh KI, Walker AE, Bernstein RM, Catoggio LJ, McGregor AR, Jones JK. Genetic susceptibility to scleroderma-like syndrome induced by vinyl chloride. _Lancet_. 1983 Jan 1;1(8314-5):53-5

[219] "...reported occupational exposure to mercury (OR 3.6), mixing pesticides for agricultural work (OR 7.4), and among dental workers (OR 7.1, 95% CI 2.2, 23.4). ...these associations were fairly strong and statistically significant..." Cooper GS, Parks CG, Treadwell EL, St Clair EW, Gilkeson GS, Dooley MA. Occupational risk factors for the development of systemic lupus erythematosus. _J Rheumatol_. 2004 Oct;31(10):1928-33

[220] Hess EV. Environmental chemicals and autoimmune disease: cause and effect. _Toxicology_. 2002 Dec 27;181-182:65-70

drug-induced lupus, and bystander activation appears to be one of the primary mechanisms involved.[221] Thus having established the general premise that *chemical exposure can cause autoimmune disease*, it seems logical and probable that anything which would inhibit the body's ability to detoxify these chemicals would likewise increase the risk for autoimmunity. Stated differently, factors that inhibit detoxification and which therefore increase the body-burden of immunotoxic xenobiotics would serve to indirectly contribute to immunodysfunction and the resultant autoimmunity. Indeed, **patients with lupus and systemic sclerosis show defects in detoxification[222], and different detoxification defects have been documented in patients with ankylosing spondylitis.**[223] Surmounting detoxification defects and xenobiotic exposure by the use of comprehensive detoxification programs (discussed later) is clinically beneficial.[224,225,226,227] Dysbiotic bacterial overgrowth of the gastrointestinal tract directly impairs detoxification via the following four mechanisms:

❶ cP450/phase-1 inhibition: Bacterial lipopolysaccharide (endotoxin) has been shown to significantly impair Phase 1 of chemical detoxification.[228] Obviously when major cytochrome p450 pathways are inhibited by endotoxin, then detoxification/biotransformation of xenobiotics and drugs is greatly impaired.[229]

❷ Deconjugation and enterohepatic recirculation: Several species of bacteria produce deconjugating enzymes (such as beta-glucuronidase) that cleave previously "detoxified" toxins from their water-soluble moieties thus allowing the toxin to be reabsorbed in a mechanism termed "enterohepatic recycling"[230] or "enterohepatic recirculation."[231]

❸ Increased intestinal permeability: Damage to the intestinal mucosa increases absorption of intraluminal contents and thus increase the toxic load placed on the detoxification mechanisms, which are mostly located in the liver; eventually these pathways become depleted, rendering the host susceptible to the consequences of nutritional depletion and impaired detoxification.[232]

❹ Constipation: Bacterial overgrowth can lead to excess production of methane which causes constipation[233] and thus increases the "toxic load" in the colon which then increases the load on the liver via the portal circulation.

Taken together, these enterometabolic mechanisms are consistent with the observance of increased risk for xenobiotic-associated diseases such as breast cancer[234,235] and Parkinson's disease[236,237] in

---

[221] "Drug-induced lupus has been reported as a side-effect of long-term therapy with over 40 medications… Several mechanisms for induction of autoimmunity will be discussed, including bystander activation of autoreactive lymphocytes due to drug-specific immunity or to non-specific activation of lymphocytes, direct cytotoxicity with release of autoantigens ..." Rubin RL. Drug-induced lupus. *Toxicology.* 2005;209(2):135-47

[222] "The observed increased frequencies of the CYP1A1 mutant Val-allele and the slow acytalator phenotype in idiopathic autoimmune disease support our concept that in slow acetylators non-acetylated xenobiotics may accumulate and are subsequently metabolized by other enzymes into reactive intermediates. Thus, enhanced formation of reactive metabolites could alter self-proteins..." von Schmiedeberg S, Fritsche E, Ronnau AC, Specker C, Golka K, Richter-Hintz D, Schuppe HC, Lehmann P, Ruzicka T, Esser C, Abel J, Gleichmann E. Polymorphisms of the xenobiotic-metabolizing enzymes CYP1A1 and NAT-2 in systemic sclerosis and lupus erythematosus. *Adv Exp Med Biol.* 1999;455:147-52

[223] "Homozygosity for poor metabolizer alleles was found to be associated with AS... Significant within-family association of CYP2D6*4 alleles and AS was demonstrated. Weak linkage was also demonstrated between CYP2D6 and AS. We postulate that altered metabolism of a natural toxin or antigen by the CYP2D6 gene may increase susceptibility to AS." Brown MA, Edwards S, Hoyle E, Campbell S, Laval S, Daly AK, Pile KD, Calin A, Ebringer A, Weeks DE, Wordsworth BP. Polymorphisms of the CYP2D6 gene increase susceptibility to ankylosing spondylitis. *Hum Mol Genet.* 2000 Jul 1;9(11):1563-6 http://hmg.oxfordjournals.org/cgi/content/full/9/11/1563

[224] Crinnion WJ. Results of a decade of naturopathic treatment for environmental illnesses. *J Naturopathic Med* 1994;17:21-27

[225] Crinnion WJ. Environmental medicine, part one: the human burden of environmental toxins and their common health effects. *Altern Med Rev.* 2000 Feb;5(1):52-63 http://www.thorne.com/altmedrev/.fulltext/5/1/52.pdf See also: Crinnion WJ. Environmental medicine, part 2 - health effects of and protection from ubiquitous airborne solvent exposure. *Altern Med Rev.* 2000 Apr;5(2):133-43 http://www.thorne.com/altmedrev/.fulltext/5/2/133.pdf

[226] Krop J. Chemical sensitivity after intoxication at work with solvents: response to sauna therapy. *J Altern Complement Med.* 1998 Spring;4(1):77-86

[227] "Retesting following the detoxification program showed significantly improved scores on: three memory tests, block design, trails B, and embedded figures. Thus, there was significant reversibility of impairment after the detoxification interval." Kilburn KH, Warsaw RH, Shields MG. Neurobehavioral dysfunction in firemen exposed to polychlorinated biphenyls (PCBs): possible improvement after detoxification. *Arch Environ Health.* 1989 Nov-Dec;44(6):345-50

[228] Shedlofsky SI, Israel BC, McClain CJ, Hill DB, Blouin RA. **Endotoxin administration to humans inhibits hepatic cytochrome P450-mediated drug metabolism.** *J Clin Invest.* 1994 Dec;94(6):2209-14 http://www.pubmedcentral.nih.gov.proxy.hsc.unt.edu/articlerender.fcgi?tool=pubmed&pubmedid=7989576

[229] "CONCLUSIONS: These data show that endotoxin-induced inflammation decreases hepatic cytochrome P450-mediated metabolism of selected probe drugs in women as it does in men." Shedlofsky SI, Israel BC, Tosheva R, Blouin RA. Endotoxin depresses hepatic cytochrome P450-mediated drug metabolism in women. *Br J Clin Pharmacol.* 1997 Jun;43(6):627-32

[230] "Enterohepatic recycling occurs by biliary excretion and intestinal reabsorption of a solute, sometimes with hepatic conjugation and intestinal deconjugation. ... Of particular importance is the potential amplifying effect of enterohepatic variability in defining differences in the bioavailability, apparent volume of distribution and clearance of a given compound." Roberts MS, Magnusson BM, Burczynski FJ, Weiss M. Enterohepatic circulation: physiological, pharmacokinetic and clinical implications. *Clin Pharmacokinet.* 2002;41(10):751-90

[231] Liska DJ. The detoxification enzyme systems. *Altern Med Rev.* 1998 Jun;3(3):187-98

[232] Lunn PG, Northrop-Clewes CA, Downes RM. Intestinal permeability, mucosal injury, and growth faltering in Gambian infants. *Lancet.* 1991 Oct 12;338(8772):907-1

[233] Lin HC. Small intestinal bacterial overgrowth: a framework for understanding irritable bowel syndrome. *JAMA.* 2004 Aug 18;292(7):852-8

[234] "These observations are consistent with an hypothesized association between constipation and increased risk of breast cancer." Micozzi MS, Carter CL, Albanes D, Taylor PR, Licitra LM. Bowel function and breast cancer in US women. *Am J Public Health.* 1989 Jan;79(1):73-5

[235] Petrakis NL, King EB. Cytological abnormalities in nipple aspirates of breast fluid from women with severe constipation. *Lancet.* 1981 Nov 28;2(8257):1203-4

[236] "…lower frequency bowel movements predict the future risk of PD. …They also hypothesize that some yet undefined toxins break through the mucosal barrier of the intestine and are incorporated into the axon terminal of the vagus nerve and transported in a retrograde manner to the vagus nucleus." Ueki A, Otsuka M. Life style risks of Parkinson's disease: association between decreased water intake and constipation. *J Neurol.* 2004 Oct;251 Suppl 7:vII18-23

[237] "CONCLUSIONS: Findings indicate that infrequent bowel movements are associated with an elevated risk of future PD." Abbott RD, Petrovitch H, White LR, Masaki KH, Tanner CM, Curb JD, Grandinetti A, Blanchette PL, Popper JS, Ross GW. Frequency of bowel movements and the future risk of Parkinson's disease. *Neurology.* 2001 Aug 14;57(3):456-62

patients with chronic constipation. Furthermore, we would expect that patients with endotoxin-producing bacterial overgrowth of the small intestine would be more susceptible to the chemical accumulation that leads to multiple chemical sensitivity syndrome (MCS) and the xenobiotic-induced immune dysfunction that may result. In my own clinical practice, I have seen many patients with **multiple chemical sensitivity** respond very favorably to the eradication of their intestinal bacterial overgrowth, and I consider this treatment essential for all patients with autoimmune disease.

13. *Antimetabolites*: Yeast and bacteria can produce certain molecules which *jam up, monkey wrench*, or otherwise interfere with normal human cellular metabolism. The best example is **D-lactic acid**, which impairs human metabolic pathways that are designed to work with the "human" form of this metabolite: L-lactic acid. Commonly resulting in headache, fatigue, depression, and sometimes death, D-lactic acidosis is extensively well documented in the medical research literature and commonly occurs in association with bacterial overgrowth of the intestine, particularly following intestinal bypass surgery.[238] Other antimetabolites produced from (intestinal) microbes which are associated with human disease and dysfunction include **ammonia, tryptamine, tyramine, octopamine, mercaptates, aldehydes, alcohol, tartaric acid, indolepropionic acid, indoleacetic acid, skatole, indole, putrescine, and cadaverine**. Many of these metabolites are seen in higher amounts in patients with migraine, depression, weakness, confusion, schizophrenia, agitation, hepatic encephalopathy, chronic arthritis and rheumatoid arthritis. **Gut-derived neurotoxins** from bacteria and yeast may contribute to autistic symptomatology[239,240], and case reports have consistently demonstrated that excess absorption of bacterial metabolites can alter behavior in humans and result in acute neurocognitive decline and behavioral abnormalities in children.[241] **Hydrogen sulfide**, produced by intestinal bacteria such as *Citrobacter freundii*[242], is a mitochondrial poison[243] and is strongly associated with disease activity in ulcerative colitis.[244] Degradation of tryptophan by bacterial tryptophanase predisposes to a "functional tryptophan deficiency" and may result in insufficiency of serotonin which would contribute to hyperalgesia, depression, impaired adrenal responsiveness[245] ("hypoadrenalism"), and insomnia; **indole** and **skatole**, which are gut-derived bacterial degradation products of tryptophan, produce an inflammatory arthritis that is identical to rheumatoid arthritis in animal models.[246,247]

14. *"Autointoxication", "hepatic encephalopathy" and "intestinal arthritis-dermatitis syndrome"*: The term "autointoxication" fell out of favor among American allopaths in the 1940s despite the recognition and objective documentation that systemically absorbed microbial metabolites/toxins from the colon could adversely affect systemic health, particularly neurocognitive function.[248] "Hepatic encephalopathy" seems to be one of the currently acceptable terms for this phenomenon, and it is probable that the condition exists among some outpatients to a milder degree than that which is classically seen in patients with fulminant liver failure. Recognition that excess or abnormal microbes in the gut could cause neuropsychiatric symptoms contributed to the rationale for the use of colonic irrigation in clinical practice which was fully endorsed by the American Medical Association in a position paper published in 1932.[249] Concurrently, an article published in the *New England Journal of Medicine*[250] in this same year documented the clinical benefits of colonic irrigation in patients with mental disease; the treatment was deemed effective against most cases of dementia, depression, neurosis and many cases

---

[238] "D-Lactic acidosis is a potentially fatal clinical condition seen in patients with a short small intestine and an intact colon. Excessive production of D-lactate by abnormal bowel flora overwhelms normal metabolism of D-lactate and leads to an accumulation of this enantiomer in the blood." Vella A, Farrugia G. D-lactic acidosis: pathologic consequence of saprophytism. *Mayo Clin Proc*. 1998 May;73(5):451-6

[239] Sandler RH, Finegold SM, Bolte ER, et al. Short-term benefit from oral vancomycin treatment of regressive-onset autism. *J Child Neurol*. 2000 Jul;15(7):429-35

[240] Shaw W, Kassen E, Chaves E. Increased urinary excretion of analogs of Krebs cycle metabolites and arabinose in two brothers with autistic features. *Clin Chem*. 1995;41(8 Pt 1):1094-104

[241] "The neurological features consisted of a depressed conscious state, confusion, aggressive behaviour, slurred speech and ataxia. The organic acid profile of urine demonstrated increased amounts of lactic, 3-hydroxypropionic, 3-hydroxyisobutyric, 2-hydroxyisocaproic, phenyllactic, 4-hydroxyphenylacetic and 4-hydroxyphenyllactic acids. Of the lactic acid 99% was D-lactic acid." Haan E, Brown G, Bankier A, et al. Severe illness caused by the products of bacterial metabolism in a child with a short gut. *Eur J Pediatr*. 1985 May;144(1):63-5

[242] Lennette EH (editor in chief). Manual of Clinical Microbiology. Fourth Edition. Washington DC; American Society for Microbiology: 1985, page 269. See also http://web.indstate.edu/thcme/micro/GI/general/sld038.htm Accessed 10/27/2005

[243] "Treatment of H2S poisoning may benefit from interventions aimed at minimizing ROS-induced damage and reducing mitochondrial damage." Eghbal MA, Pennefather PS, O'Brien PJ. H2S cytotoxicity mechanism involves reactive oxygen species formation and mitochondrial depolarisation. *Toxicology*. 2004 Oct 15;203(1-3):69-76

[244] "CONCLUSIONS: Metabolic effects of sodium hydrogen sulfide on butyrate oxidation along the length of the colon closely mirror metabolic abnormalities observed in active ulcerative colitis, and the increased production of sulfide in ulcerative colitis suggests that the action of mercaptides may be involved in the genesis of ulcerative colitis." Roediger WE, Duncan A, Kapaniris O, Millard S. Reducing sulfur compounds of the colon impair colonocyte nutrition: implications for ulcerative colitis. *Gastroenterology*. 1993 Mar;104(3):802-9

[245] "This hypothesis is supported by the findings in chronic MS patients of a significantly diminished adrenal cortisol reactivity to insulin-induced hypoglycemia which is considered a stress response mediated through the 5-HT system. Consequently, since patients with MS exhibit an abnormal response to stress it follows that increased tryptophan availability through dietary supplementation would diminish their vulnerability to psychological stress." Sandyk R. Tryptophan availability and the susceptibility to stress in multiple sclerosis: a hypothesis. *Int J Neurosci*. 1996 Jul;86(1-2):47-53

[246] Nakoneczna I, Forbes JC, Rogers KS. The arthritogenic effect of indole, skatole and other tryptophan metabolites in rabbits. *Am J Pathol*. 1969 Dec;57(3):523-38

[247] Rogers KS, Forbes JC, Nakoneczna I. Arthritogenic properties of lipophilic, aryl molecules. *Proc Soc Exp Biol Med*. 1969 Jun;131(2):670-2

[248] Person JR, Bernhard JD. Autointoxication revisited. *J Am Acad Dermatol*. 1986;15(3):559-63

[249] Bastedo WA. Colon irrigations: their administration, therapeutic applications, and dangers. *Journal of the American Medical Association* 1932; 98(9): 734-6

[250] Marshall HK, Thomson CR. Colon irrigation in the treatment of mental disease. N Engl J Med 1932; 207 (Sept 8): 454-7

of irritability, headaches, and hypertension. Enemas and colonics, which promote hepatobiliary detoxification[251,252] and cleanse the bowel of harmful microbes, were valued by clinicians as a cure or adjunctive treatment for numerous systemic diseases.[253] Although the term "autointoxication" is eschewed as "unscientific", all medical professionals recognize that gastrointestinal dysbiosis can cause clinical conditions characterized by inflammatory vasculitis, dermatitis, and arthritis; current terms for this condition include "bowel-associated dermatosis-arthritis syndrome"[254], "intestinal arthritis-dermatitis syndrome"[255], and "bypass disease"[256]—all of which are largely mediated by the gut-derived formation and systemic deposition of immune complexes in skin, joints, kidneys, and vascular endothelium. Bacterial overgrowth of the small bowel is also a cause of gastroesophageal reflux disease (GERD) because products of bacterial fermentation relax the *lower esophageal sphincter*[257] and retard intestinal transit[258]; reducing the phenomenon of intestinal bacterial overgrowth by simply "starving" the bacteria of carbohydrate by implementation of a **low-carbohydrate diet** alleviates GERD symptoms and substantiates the cause-and-effect relationship.[259,260]

15. *Impairment of mucosal and systemic defenses*: Microbial colonization of mucosal surfaces can result in impaired local immunity by causing loss of protective secretory IgA or by causing direct tissue damage that results in increased absorption of microbial, dietary, or environmental antigens. Several microorganisms such as *Entamoeba histolytica*[261], *Streptococcus sanguis*[262], and *Candida albicans*[263] externalize a protein-digesting enzyme (proteinase) that "digests" defensive immunoglobulins, including secretory IgA and humoral immunoglobulins. The proteinases produced by *Candida* are capable of lysing not only sIgA but also keratin and collagen[264], obviously providing for a breach of protection from other infections and antigens. In this way, mucosal microbial colonization with yeast/bacteria that secrete proteases/proteinases can "open the door" to previously excluded microbes or antigens to promote the resultant "infection" or "allergy", respectively. Furthermore, because IgA is destroyed by the protease, the infection is allowed to fester, resulting in on-going immune stimulation and its consequences such as bystander activation. This may explain why women with chronic vaginal candidiasis, which always implies chronic yeast overgrowth of the intestine[265], have nearly double the incidence of allergic rhinitis compared to patients without chronic yeast overgrowth.[266] Further supporting the link between yeast and allergy is another recent study showing that allergy/atopy is more common in patients with chronic yeast infections.[267] *Candida* produces an immunotoxin called "gliotoxin", which suppresses human immune function.[268] The combination of mucosal damage, destruction of sIgA, immunosuppression, and microbial overgrowth synergize to sensitize the systemic immune system toward allergic and proinflammatory disease.[269] Lastly, bacterial proteases work synergistically with biofilm formation to nullify immunologic attack (via

[251] Garbat, AL, Jacobi, HG: Secretion of Bile in Response to Rectal Installations. *Arch Intern Med* 1929; 44: 455-462

[252] "Caffeine enemas cause dilation of bile ducts, which facilitates excretion of toxic cancer breakdown products by the liver and dialysis of toxic products from blood across the colonic wall. The therapy must be used as an integrated whole." Gerson M. The cure of advanced cancer by diet therapy: a summary of 30 years of clinical experimentation. *Physiol Chem Phys.* 1978;10(5):449-64

[253] Snyder RG. The value of colonic irrigations in countering auto-intoxication of intestinal origin. *Medical Clinics of North America* 1939; May: 781-788

[254] Jorizzo JL, Apisarnthanarax P, Subrt P, et al. Bowel-bypass syndrome without bowel bypass. Bowel-associated dermatosis-arthritis syndrome. *Arch Intern Med.* 1983 Mar;143(3):457-61

[255] Stein HB, Schlappner OL, Boyko W, Gourlay RH, Reeve CE. The intestinal bypass: arthritis-dermatitis syndrome. *Arthritis Rheum.* 1981 May;24(5):684-90

[256] Utsinger PD. Systemic immune complex disease following intestinal bypass surgery: bypass disease. *J Am Acad Dermatol.* 1980 Jun;2(6):488-95

[257] "In summary, we have shown that colonic fermentation, through the production of SCFAs, exerts a controlled feedback on LES motor function." Piche T, Zerbib F, Varannes SB, Cherbut C, Anini Y, Roze C, le Quellec A, Galmiche JP. Modulation by colonic fermentation of LES function in humans. *Am J Physiol Gastrointest Liver Physiol.* 2000 Apr;278(4):G578-84 http://ajpgi.physiology.org/cgi/content/full/278/4/G578

[258] "Altered gastrointestinal motility and sensation, changed activity of the central nervous system, and increased sympathetic drive and immune activation may be understood as consequences of the host response to SIBO." Lin HC. Small intestinal bacterial overgrowth: a framework for understanding irritable bowel syndrome. *JAMA.* 2004 Aug 18;292(7):852-8

[259] "These data suggest that a very low-carbohydrate diet in obese individuals with GERD significantly reduces distal esophageal acid exposure and improves symptoms." Austin GL, Thiny MT, Westman EC, Yancy WS Jr, Shaheen NJ. A very low-carbohydrate diet improves gastroesophageal reflux and its symptoms. *Dig Dis Sci.* 2006 Aug;51(8):1307-12

[260] "The 5 individuals described in these case reports experienced resolution of GERD symptoms after self-initiation of a low-carbohydrate diet." Yancy WS Jr, Provenzale D, Westman EC. Improvement of gastroesophageal reflux disease after initiation of a low-carbohydrate diet: five brief case reports. *Altern Ther Health Med.* 2001 Nov-Dec;7(6):120, 116-9

[261] Kelsall BL, Ravdin JI. Degradation of human IgA by Entamoeba histolytica. *J Infect Dis.* 1993 Nov;168(5):1319-22

[262] "These data indicate that the BD patients are infected with IgA protease-producing S. sanguis strains, which cause an increase of IgA titer against these organisms and IgA protease antigen." Yokota K, Oguma K. IgA protease produced by Streptococcus sanguis and antibody production against IgA protease in patients with Behcet's disease. *Microbiol Immunol.* 1997;41(12):925-31

[263] Kaminishi H, Miyaguchi H, Tamaki T, et al. Degradation of humoral host defense by Candida albicans proteinase. *Infect Immun.* 1995 Mar;63(3):984-8

[264] "The enzymes produced by these yeasts are all carboxyl proteinases capable of degrading secretory IgA, the major immunoglobulin of mucous membranes. Some have keratino- or collagenolytic activity." Douglas LJ. Candida proteinases and candidosis. *Crit Rev Biotechnol.* 1988;8(2):121-9

[265] "The results showed that if C albicans was cultured from the vagina, it was always found in the stool... The gut-reservoir concept may well apply to other forms of candidiasis." Miles MR, Olsen L, Rogers A. Recurrent vaginal candidiasis. Importance of an intestinal reservoir. *JAMA.* 1977 Oct 24;238(17):1836-7

[266] Moraes PS. Recurrent vaginal candidiasis and allergic rhinitis: a common association. *Ann Allergy Asthma Immunol.* 1998 Aug;81(2):165-9

[267] Neves NA, Carvalho LP, De Oliveira MA, et al. Association between atopy and recurrent vaginal candidiasis. *Clin Exp Immunol.* 2005 Oct;142(1):167-71

[268] "This study suggests a previously unrecognized potential virulence factor of C. albicans that could contribute to persistence of yeast colonization or recurrence of symptomatic infection through diminished host resistance." Shah DT, Jackman S, Engle J, Larsen B. Effect of gliotoxin on human polymorphonuclear neutrophils. *Infect Dis Obstet Gynecol* 1998;6(4):168-75

[269] "Studies performed in humans show that selective IgA deficiency, preterm delivery, intestinal helminth infection and type of feeding during the neonatal period may influence antigen uptake by the intestinal epithelium. These conditions...may cause increased absorption of intraluminal antigens and result in the synergy of allergic type responses." Reinhardt MC. Macromolecular absorption of food antigens in health and disease. *Ann Allergy.* 1984 Dec;53(6 Pt 2):597-601

immunosuppression and cytokine inactivation) and are important for the establishment of chronic mucosal colonization.[270]

16. _Impairment of mucosal digestion by microbial proteases and inflammation_: Similar to the degradation of human IgA by microbial proteases/proteinases is the degradation of mucosal digestive enzymes such as the disaccharidases (sucrase, maltase, lactase, and isomaltase) and dipeptidases. First, impaired digestion of carbohydrates skews the intestinal milieu toward one favorable to bacterial/yeast overgrowth by increasing the levels of carbohydrate substrate upon which microbes feed. Impaired peptide breakdown promotes immune sensitization, protein malnutrition, and putrefaction. Second, inflammation resultant from intestinal dysbiosis further impairs carbohydrate digestion via downregulation of sucrase-isomaltase gene expression by inflammatory cytokines.[271] Third, destruction of microvilli exacerbates loss of mucosal enzymes and leads to additional malabsorption, maldigestion, and increased macromolecular absorption, such as seen in patients with intestinal giardiasis.[272] Impairment/reduction of disaccharidases and dipeptidases is also seen in patients with inflammatory bowel disease.[273]

17. _Inflammation-induced endocrine dysfunction_: Although research in this area is less conclusive, the pattern of emerging research indicates that the multifaceted phenomenon of inflammation, particularly the elaboration of cytokines, alters endocrine function, and these inflammation-induced endocrine alterations further promote additional musculoskeletal inflammation. Endocrine changes induced by chronic inflammation include increased production of proinflammatory **prolactin**, reduced production of anti-inflammatory and immunoregulatory **cortisol** and **androgens**. The effects of altered endocrine function is discussed in the following section detailing orthoendocrinology. The link between dysbiosis and inflammation-induced changes in endocrine status has only recently begun to be documented, and some of these conclusions are logical though somewhat speculative. However, the nature of holistic healthcare requires us to consider _all_ potentially significant contributions and interconnections, and thus microbe-endocrine links are briefly outlined here based on _highly suggestive_—yet not _wholly conclusive_—data. What is very clear is that autoimmune patients have alterations in hypothalamic-pituitary-adrenal/gonadal function. What is not yet clear is whether or not these are primary initiators of disease or secondary results of the disease process. Here I propose that both of these statements are true, namely that 1) endocrine dysfunction predisposes to the immune dysfunction that results in autoimmunity, and that 2) systemic inflammation further exacerbates endocrine dysfunction. Further, I speculate and add that 3) in some patients, chronic dysbiosis and subclinical inflammation and bacterial endotoxinemia/exotoxinemia can initiate the endocrine dysfunction and pro-inflammatory state that can eventually cross a diagnostic threshold to become overt clinical autoimmunity. Research support is provided here:

- Altered hypothalamic responsiveness and circadian rhythm: The region of the basal hypothalamus is not protected by the blood-brain barrier and is sensitive and vulnerable to substances in the blood.[274] Because of this, hypothalamic and thus pituitary responses can be tuned to or altered by circulating prostaglandins, cytokines, and bacterial endotoxins and exotoxins. Patients with rheumatoid arthritis show hypothalamic/endocrine disturbances including blunted responsiveness to ACTH, abnormal circadian rhythm of prolactin and cortisol, and abnormalities in growth hormone secretion.[275] Furthermore, arginine vasopressin (AVP) is secreted from the hypothalamus in response to stress, is inherently pro-inflammatory, and is capable of augmenting prolactin secretion to further increase inflammation.[276]

- Increased production of prolactin: Prolactin is a highly proinflammatory hormone produced by the anterior pituitary gland as well as by peripheral lymphocytes. As a model of infection-

[270] "The two proteases, alkaline protease and elastase, inhibit the function of the cells of the immune system (phagocytes, NK cells, T cells), inactivate several cytokines (IL-1, IL-2, IFN-r, TNF), cleave immunoglobulins and inactivate complement. Inhibition of the local immune response by bacterial proteases provides an environment for the colonization and establishment of chronic infection." Kharazmi A. Mechanisms involved in the evasion of the host defence by Pseudomonas aeruginosa. _Immunol Lett._ 1991 Oct;30(2):201-5

[271] Ziambaras T, Rubin DC, Perlmutter DH. Regulation of sucrase-isomaltase gene expression in human intestinal epithelial cells by inflammatory cytokines. _J Biol Chem._ 1996 Jan 12;271(2):1237-42 http://www.jbc.org/cgi/content/full/271/2/1237

[272] Buret AG. Immunopathology of giardiasis. _Mem Inst Oswaldo Cruz._ 2005 Mar;100 Suppl 1:185-90 http://www.scielo.br/pdf/mioc/v100s1/v100ns1a31.pdf

[273] "A significant reduction of the specific activity of disaccharidases (lactase, sucrase and trehalase) in jejunal mucosal homogenate occurred in patients with inflammatory bowel disease. ... Several dipeptidases such as glycyl-leucine, leucyl-glycine, glycyl-glycine and valyl-proline hydrolase activities were lower in patients with inflammatory bowel disease than in controls." Arvanitakis C. Abnormalities of jejunal mucosal enzymes in ulcerative colitis and Crohn's disease. _Digestion._ 1979;19(4):259-66

[274] Waxman SG. Clinical Neuroanatomy 25th Edition. McGraw Hill Medical, New York, 2003, p 160

[275] Anisman H, Baines MG, Berczi I, Bernstein CN, Blennerhassett MG, Gorczynski RM, Greenberg AH, Kisil FT, Mathison RD, Nagy E, Nance DM, Perdue MH, Pomerantz DK, Sabbadini ER, Stanisz A, Warrington RJ. Neuroimmune mechanisms in health and disease: 2. Disease. _CMAJ._ 1996 Oct 15;155(8):1075-82 http://www.pubmedcentral.nih.gov/articlerender.fcgi?tool=pubmed&pubmedid=8873636

[276] Chikanza IC, Grossman AS. Hypothalamic-pituitary-mediated immunomodulation: arginine vasopressin is a neuroendocrine immune mediator. _Br J Rheumatol._ 1998 Feb;37(2):131-6 http://rheumatology.oxfordjournals.org/cgi/reprint/37/2/131

induced inflammation, **sepsis is generally associated with increased prolactin production in humans.**[277] Prolactin levels increase due to chronic psychoemotional stress. **The classic exemplification of dysbiosis-induced musculoskeletal inflammation—reactive arthritis—is frequently associated with hyperprolactinemia.**[278]

- Reduced production of cortisol: Cortisol is an immunoregulatory hormone which tends to suppress excess immune activity, and relative reductions in cortisol production are commonly seen in patients with autoimmunity and allergic disorders.[279,280] **Cortisol production is reduced by chronic psychoemotional stress**[281], and the stress of chronic inflammation due to dysbiosis may impair normal endocrine function.

- Reduced production and bioavailability of androgens: High-intensity stress associated with military training leads to 60-80% reductions in androgens[282]; the chronic stress and pain associated with musculoskeletal inflammation may contribute to a similar profile on a subacute and chronic basis. Hyperprolactinemia further complicates this problem by simulating hepatic production of sex hormone binding globulin (SHBG) which adsorbs androgens and reduces their bioavailability. Indeed, **the clinical manifestations of hypogonadism may exist despite adequate production of androgens when prolactin stimulates increased SHBG production and results in reduced bioavailability of androgens.**[283]

In conclusion, **this survey of the literature has supported the concept that intestinal dysbiosis can contribute to systemic pain, inflammation, and immune activation by numerous mechanisms, and that many of these "silent infections" are self-perpetuating by inducing alterations in local milieu and systemic immunity.** Clinical experience has demonstrated again and again that eradicating dysbiosis helps normalize immune function, alleviate autoimmunity and allergy, reduce inflammation, improve detoxification, and to help "cure" people of their previously "incurable" multiple chemical sensitivity, environmental illness, and autoimmunity.

---

[277] "Prolactin levels are regularly elevated in sepsis although to variable degrees." Dennhardt R, Gramm HJ, Meinhold K, Voigt K. Patterns of endocrine secretion during sepsis. *Prog Clin Biol Res.* 1989;308:751-6

[278] "Hyperprolactinemia (PRL > 20 ng/ml) was found in 9 of 25 (36%) patients with RS." Jara LJ, Silveira LH, Cuellar ML, Pineda CJ, Scopelitis E, Espinoza LR. Hyperprolactinemia in Reiter's syndrome. *J Rheumatol.* 1994 Jul;21(7):1292-7

[279] "Yet evidence that patients with rheumatoid arthritis improved with small, physiologic dosages of cortisol or cortisone acetate was reported over 25 years ago, and that patients with chronic allergic disorders or unexplained chronic fatigue also improved with administration of such small dosages was reported over 15 years ago..." Jefferies WM. Mild adrenocortical deficiency, chronic allergies, autoimmune disorders and the chronic fatigue syndrome: a continuation of the cortisone story. *Med Hypotheses.* 1994 Mar;42(3):183-9 http://www.thebuteykocentre.com/Irish_%20Buteykocenter_files/further_studies/med_hyp2.pdf and http://members.westnet.com.au/pkolb/med_hyp2.pdf

[280] "The etiology of rheumatoid arthritis ...explained by a combination of three factors: (i) a relatively mild deficiency of cortisol, ..., (ii) a deficiency of DHEA, ...and (iii) infection by organisms such as mycoplasma,..." Jefferies WM. The etiology of rheumatoid arthritis. *Med Hypotheses.* 1998 Aug;51(2):111-4

[281] "Prolonged psychological stress is associated with a transient suppression of the HPA axis, manifested by low morning cortisol and reduced cortisol response to ACTH. The reduction of cortisol response is sufficient to cause false diagnosis of HPA insufficiency." Zarkovic M, Stefanova E, Ciric J, Penezic Z, Kostic V, Sumarac-Dumanovic M, Macut D, Ivovic MS, Gligorovic PV. Prolonged psychological stress suppresses cortisol secretion. *Clin Endocrinol* (Oxf). 2003 Dec;59(6):811-6

[282] "Plasma levels of testosterone, free testosterone, dehydroepiandrosterone, 17 alpha-hydroxyprogesterone, and androstenedione decreased by 60-80% during the course." Opstad PK. Androgenic hormones during prolonged physical stress, sleep, and energy deficiency. *J Clin Endocrinol Metab.* 1992 May;74(5):1176-83

[283] "The pitfalls of measuring only total serum testosterone are illustrated by a 52 year old man whose hyperprolactinaemia was associated with normal total serum testosterone but a raised sex-hormone-binding globulin, giving a low free testosterone. Prolactin suppression with bromocriptine normalized sex-hormone-binding globulin and free testosterone..." Hardy KJ, Seckl JR. Endocrine assessment of impotence--pitfalls of measuring serum testosterone without sex-hormone-binding globulin. *Postgrad Med J.* 1994 Nov;70(829):836-7

The Seven Main Loci of Dysbiosis

For a microorganism to induce a systemic proinflammatory immunodysregulatory response in a human, the microbe or its metabolic products must be exposed to a susceptible host. Non-infectious microbial overgrowth can occur inside the body (gastrointestinal, sinus, respiratory tract and lungs, genitourinary, or orodental), on the surface of the body (dermal), or outside of the body (environmental). The adverse physiologic and clinical effects can be similar regardless of the location of the microorganism. The term "dysbiosis" is classically applied to harmful, non-infectious relationships between the human host and yeast, bacteria, protozoans, amoebas, or other "parasites" located specifically in the gastrointestinal tract, and "dysbiosis" is now an accepted term in the medical literature.[284] However, we must also appreciate that harmful, noninfectious microbe-host interactions can also occur when microbes are localized in the sinuses, oral cavity, genitourinary tract, skin, and in the external environment. I prefer to use a broad definition of dysbiosis that implies "a relationship of non-infectious host-microorganism interaction that adversely affects the human host" and then to specify the subtype based on the location: gastrointestinal, oral, sinus, genitourinary, dermatologic, or environmental. Gastrointestinal dysbiosis is clearly the prototype for understanding other types of dysbiosis; this is because it seems to be the most common form of dysbiosis, perhaps due to the large numbers and types of microbes in the gut and the extensive surface area of the gastrointestinal tract. Clinicians must appreciate the anatomical interconnections that can segue one type of loci of dysbiosis into another. Orodental dysbiosis may result in gastrointestinal dysbiosis if the microbes can survive in the gastrointestinal tract. Sinus dysbiosis could likewise drain into the lungs and gastrointestinal tract. In women, close relationships between gastrointestinal dysbiosis and vaginal dysbiosis are well documented.[285] Bacterial and fungal superantigens from the surrounding environment can contribute to a proinflammatory response in the lungs and on the skin and which becomes systemic, leading to autoimmunity.[286,287]

Correlation of Dysbiosis with Autoimmune and Rheumatic Diseases

Disease & dysbiosis	Gastrointestinal dysbiosis	Orodental dysbiosis	Sinorespiratory dysbiosis	Genitourinary dysbiosis	Parenchymal dysbiosis	Cutaneous dysbiosis	Environmental dysbiosis
SLE	+		+				
RA	✓			✓	+ osteomyel		
ReA	✓		✓	✓	✓ pneumonia		
Psor	✓	✓	✓	✓		✓	✓
PM-DM	+	+	+				
Spond-AS	✓			✓			
Sclerod	+						
Weg	+	✓	✓				
Vasc	✓				✓ viral hep		
Sarc			✓				
Behc		✓	✓			✓	
Neuro	✓			✓			✓

✓ = **Positive research and clinical evidence in humans;** + = **Weak research in humans, substantive research in animal models, biologic plausibility**; N = Negative findings; No correlation; SLE = lupus; RA = rheumatoid arthritis; ReA = reactive arthritis; Psor = Psoriasis or psoriatic arthritis; PM-DM = polymyositis/dermatomyositis; PMR = polymyalgia rheumatica; Sjo = Sjogren's syndrome; Spond-AS = spondyloarthropathy and ankylosing spondylitis; Sclerod = scleroderma; Weg = Wegener's granulomatosis; Vasc = vasculitis; Sarc = sarcoidosis; Behc = Behcet's syndrome; Neuro = neurologic autoimmunity, which is not detailed in this text

---

[284] Tamboli CP, Neut C, Desreumaux P, Colombel JF. Dysbiosis in inflammatory bowel disease. *Gut*. 2004 Jan;53(1):1-4

[285] "The results showed that if C albicans was cultured from the vagina, it was always found in the stool... The gut-reservoir concept may well apply to other forms of candidiasis." Miles MR, Olsen L, Rogers A. Recurrent vaginal candidiasis. Importance of an intestinal reservoir. *JAMA*. 1977 Oct 24;238(17):1836-7

[286] Campbell AW, Thrasher JD, Madison RA, Vojdani A, Gray MR, Johnson A. Neural autoantibodies and neurophysiologic abnormalities in patients exposed to molds in water-damaged buildings. *Arch Environ Health*. 2003 Aug;58(8):464-74

[287] Gray MR, Thrasher JD, Crago R, Madison RA, Arnold L, Campbell AW, Vojdani A. Mixed mold mycotoxicosis: immunological changes in humans following exposure in water-damaged buildings. *Arch Environ Health*. 2003 Jul;58(7):410-20

Gastrointestinal Dysbiosis: *Overview of the Prototype of All Forms of Dysbiosis*

We all have bacteria and occasionally small quantities of yeast in our intestines, and this is normal and generally healthy. However, problems arise when these yeast/bacteria become imbalanced or when *harmful* yeast, bacteria, parasites take up residence within the gut. Particularly in the European research literature, this condition has been more widely researched and described as "dysbacteriosis" or "dysbacterosis."[288] These latter terms are somewhat unfortunate because they imply that the problem has a *bacterial* origin, which is partially (and therefore significantly) misleading since dysbiosis commonly involves bacteria *and yeast* (including but not limited to *Candida albicans*) and commonly other harmful non-bacterial microbes such as *Giardia lamblia, Blastocystis hominis, Endolimax nana, Entamoeba histolytica* and a cast of other malcontents that adversely affect the overall health of their human host.[289] "Candidiasis" and yeast-related problems have been described in the research literature and general press.[290] Dysbiosis is probably a major aspect of the phenomenon that was previously referred to in the medical literature as "autointoxication" and which was effectively treated with dietary modifications, nutritional supplementation, and colonic irrigation.[291] **Given that endotoxin/lipopolysaccharide is one of the major activators of nuclear factor kappa-B (NFkB)[292], and that NFkB activation is a major rate-limiting step in the production of proinflammatory cytokines and in the induction of proinflammatory enzymes such as cyclooxygenase, lipoxygenase, and inducible nitric oxide synthase,[293] then the link between dysbiosis and systemic inflammation becomes clear: gastrointestinal bacterial overgrowth leads to excess production and absorption of endotoxin, which then initiates immune dysfunction and a systemic proinflammatory response.** Intestinal overgrowth of gram-negative bacteria is, in this author's opinion, highly problematic since endotoxin/lipopolysaccharide, of which there are varying degrees of toxicity, can cause intestinal inflammation, leaky gut, inhibition of hepatic detoxification, hyperalgesia[294], brain dysfunction[295] and immune dysfunction by acting as superantigens.[296] **Indeed, many of the systemic manifestations associated with dysbiosis are clearly not mediated by the infecting organism but are mediated by the host response to microbial toxins and to the systemic dysfunction induced by increased intestinal permeability and subsequent alterations in hepatic and immune function. Thus, the sequelae of dysbiosis are mediated by alterations in human physiology rather than being directly caused by the microbe.** Current research has linked several microbes with human autoimmune/inflammatory diseases, for example *Entamoeba histolytica* has been linked with Henoch Schonlein purpura[297], *Klebsiella pneumoniae* with ankylosing spondylitis[298], *Proteus mirabilis* with rheumatoid arthritis[299,300] and ankylosing spondylitis[301], *Pseudomonas aeruginosa* with multiple sclerosis[302], and *Helicobacter pylori* with reactive arthritis.[303]

[288] Lizko NN. Problems of microbial ecology in man space mission. *Acta Astronaut.* 1991;23:163-9

[289] Galland L. Intestinal protozoan infection is a common unsuspected cause of chronic illness. *J Advancement Med.* 1989;2: 539-552

[290] Crook W. The Yeast Connection. Professional Books. Jackson. Tennessee. 1983

[291] "The writer has observed numerous cases suffering from such conditions as chronic arthritis, hypertension, coronary disease, chronic abdominal distention, constipation, and colitis, in which the element of constipation, auto-intoxication and possible colon infection seemed to play a prominent part, which responded very satisfactorily to colonic irrigations after failure to improve following the usual forms of medical treatment." Snyder RG. The value of colonic irrigations in countering auto-intoxication of intestinal origin. *Medl Clin North America* 1939; May: 781-788

[292] D'Acquisto F, May MJ, Ghosh S. Inhibition of Nuclear Factor Kappa B (NF-B):: An Emerging Theme in Anti-Inflammatory Therapies. *Mol Interv.* 2002 Feb;2(1):22-35 http://molinterv.aspetjournals.org/cgi/content/full/2/1/22

[293] Tak PP, Firestein GS. NF-kappaB: a key role in inflammatory diseases. *J Clin Invest.* 2001 Jan;107(1):7-1 http://www.jci.org/cgi/content/full/107/1/7

[294] "We have recently shown that 'illness'-inducing agents, such as intraperitoneally administered lipopolysaccharide (LPS; bacterial endotoxin), can produce prolonged hyperalgesia." Watkins LR, Wiertelak EP, Furness LE, Maier SF. Illness-induced hyperalgesia is mediated by spinal neuropeptides and excitatory amino acids. *Brain Res.* 1994 Nov 21;664(1-2):17-24

[295] "The immunogen E. coli lipopolysaccharide (LPS, endotoxin) has been widely used to stimulate immune/inflammatory responses both systemically and in the CNS… LPS appears to release glutamate, which then acts at non-NMDA receptors to remove the voltage-sensitive Mg2+ block of NMDA receptors, thus permitting NMDA receptors to be activated…" Wang YS, White TD. The bacterial endotoxin lipopolysaccharide causes rapid inappropriate excitation in rat cortex. *J Neurochem.* 1999 Feb;72(2):652-60

[296] "Superantigens are potent activators of CD4+ T cells, causing rapid and massive proliferation of cells and cytokine production… Superantigens have also been implicated in acute diseases such as food poisoning and TSS, and in chronic diseases such as psoriasis and rheumatoid arthritis." Torres BA, Kominsky S, Perrin GQ, Hobeika AC, Johnson HM. Superantigens: the good, the bad, and the ugly. *Exp Biol Med* (Maywood). 2001 Mar;226(3):164-76

[297] Demircin G, Oner A, Erdogan O, Bulbul M, Memis L. Henoch Schonlein purpura and amebiasis. *Acta Paediatr Jpn.* 1998 Oct; 40(5): 489-91

[298] Ahmadi K, Wilson C, Tiwana H, Binder A, Ebringer A. Antibodies to Klebsiella pneumoniae lipopolysaccharide in patients with ankylosing spondylitis. *Br J Rheumatol.* 1998 Dec;37(12):1330-3

[299] Ebringer A, Rashid T, Wilson C. Rheumatoid arthritis: proposal for the use of anti-microbial therapy in early cases. *Scand J Rheumatol* 2003;32(1):2-11

[300] Rashid T, Darlington G, Kjeldsen-Kragh J, Forre O, Collado A, Ebringer A. Proteus IgG antibodies and C-reactive protein in English, Norwegian and Spanish patients with rheumatoid arthritis. *Clin Rheumatol* 1999;18(3):190-5

[301] Wilson C, Rashid T, Tiwana H, Beyan H, Hughes L, Bansal S, Ebringer A, Binder A. Cytotoxicity responses to Peptide antigens in rheumatoid arthritis and ankylosing spondylitis. *J Rheumatol* 2003 May;30(5):972-8

[302] Hughes LE, Bonell S, Natt RS, Wilson C, Tiwana H, Ebringer A, Cunningham P, Chamoun V, Thompson EJ, Croker J, Vowles J. Antibody responses to Acinetobacter spp. and Pseudomonas aeruginosa in multiple sclerosis: prospects for diagnosis using the myelin-acinetobacter-neurofilament antibody index. *Clin Diagn Lab Immunol.* 2001 Nov;8(6):1181-8

[303] "Our findings suggest that HP may be included in the list of possible arthritis triggering microbes." Melby KK, Kvien TK, Glennas A. Helicobacter pylori--a trigger of reactive arthritis? *Infection.* 1999;27:252-5

Building upon a previous four-subtype categorization proposed by Galland[304], here I describe six different types of gastrointestinal dysbiosis:

1. <u>Insufficiency dysbiosis</u>: This results when there is an insufficient quantity of the "good bacteria." Absence of "good bacteria" such as *Bifidobacteria* and *Lactobacillus* leaves the gastrointestinal tract vulnerable to colonization with pathogens and is associated with increased risk for bacterial overgrowth and other intestinal diseases. Furthermore, **beneficial bacteria in the intestines helps to normalize systemic immune response and promote proper digestion, elimination and nutrient absorption**. Numerous scientific studies have documented the powerful benefits of supplementing with good bacteria (probiotics), supporting their growth with fermentable carbohydrates such as inulin and fructooligosaccharides (prebiotics), and by co-administering probiotics with prebiotics (synbiotics).

2. <u>Bacterial overgrowth</u>: This is a quantitative excess of yeast and bacteria in the gut. Bacterial overgrowth of the small bowel is a well-established medical problem that is particularly common in patients who are diabetic, elderly, immunosuppressed (such as with corticosteroids/prednisone[305,306]), naturally hypochlorhydric or iatrogenically hypochlorhydric due to "antacid" drugs.[307] This commonly results in gas, bloating, malabsorption, constipation and/or diarrhea, "irritable bowel syndrome", as well as myalgias and systemic immune activation.[308] **Animal studies have proven that it is possible to reactivate peripheral arthritis by inducing bacterial overgrowth of the small bowel; endotoxins and other microbial products stimulate a systemic proinflammatory state which re-activates inflammation of joints and periarticular structures.**[309] Bacterial overgrowth of the small intestine is seen in 84% of patients with irritable bowel syndrome[310] and in **100% of patients with fibromyalgia**.[311] Researchers recently demonstrated that endotoxins can lead to impairment of muscle function and a lowered lactate threshold[312], thereby explaining the link between intestinal dysbiosis and chronic musculoskeletal pain that is not responsive to drugs or manual therapies. Drs. Over and Bucknall[313] describe a patient with **systemic sclerosis** who achieved **long-term remission** of her disease following **antibiotic treatment for intestinal bacterial overgrowth**. Bacterial overgrowth generally leads to pathologically synergistic clinical effects mediated by fermentation, putrefaction, constipation, increased enterohepatic recycling, bile acid deconjugation, malabsorption (particularly fat-soluble nutrients and vitamin B-12), nutritional deficiencies, sugar cravings, increased intestinal permeability, immune complex formation, and induction of a systemic proinflammatory response with immune complexes that is particularly prone to manifest as vasculitis and arthritis.[314,315,316]

3. <u>Immunosuppressive dysbiosis</u>: Some microbes, particularly yeast, produce toxins that suppress immune function. The immunosuppressive mycotoxin produced by *Candia albicans* is called gliotoxin[317], and it is produced at the site of yeast overgrowth, thus suppressing local—and possibly, systemic—immune function.[318] Since secretory IgA is the first line of defense against allergens and

---

[304] Attributed to Galland L. "Fire in the belly: update on gut fermentation." Presented to Great Lakes Association of Clinical Medicine, circa 1996. Also, personal email from Leo Galland dated October 28, 2005: "I have used the concept of 4 types of dysbiosis (putrefaction, fermentation, depletion and immune activation forms) in several presentations and in one written document."

[305] "A 63-year-old man with systemic lupus erythematosus and selective IgA deficiency developed intractable diarrhoea the day after treatment with prednisone, 50 mg daily, was started. The diarrhoea was considered to be caused by bacterial overgrowth and was later successfully treated with doxycycline." Denison H, Wallerstedt S. Bacterial overgrowth after high-dose corticosteroid treatment. *Scand J Gastroenterol.* 1989 Jun;24(5):561-4

[306] "These bacteria also translocated to the mesenteric lymph nodes in mice injected with cyclophosphamide or prednisone." Berg RD, Wommack E, Deitch EA. Immunosuppression and intestinal bacterial overgrowth synergistically promote bacterial translocation. *Arch Surg.* 1988 Nov;123(11):1359-64

[307] Saltzman JR, Russell RM. Nutritional consequences of intestinal bacterial overgrowth. *Compr Ther.* 1994;20(9):523-30

[308] Lin HC. Small intestinal bacterial overgrowth: a framework for understanding irritable bowel syndrome. *JAMA.* 2004 Aug 18;292(7):852-8

[309] Lichtman SN, Wang J, Sartor RB, Zhang C, Bender D, Dalldorf FG, Schwab JH. Reactivation of arthritis induced by small bowel bacterial overgrowth in rats: role of cytokines, bacteria, and bacterial polymers. *Infect Immun.* 1995 Jun;63(6):2295-301

[310] Lin HC. Small intestinal bacterial overgrowth: a framework for understanding irritable bowel syndrome. *JAMA.* 2004 Aug 18;292(7):852-8

[311] Pimentel M, et al. A link between irritable bowel syndrome and fibromyalgia may be related to findings on lactulose breath testing. *Ann Rheum Dis.* 2004 Apr;63(4):450-2

[312] Bundgaard H, Kjeldsen K, Suarez Krabbe K, et al. Endotoxemia stimulates skeletal muscle Na+-K+-ATPase and raises blood lactate under aerobic conditions in humans. *Am J Physiol Heart Circ Physiol.* 2003 Mar;284(3):H1028-34. http://ajpheart.physiology.org/cgi/reprint/284/3/H1028

[313] Over KE, Bucknall RC. Regression of skin changes in a patient with systemic sclerosis following treatment for bacterial overgrowth with ciprofloxacin. *Br J Rheumatol.* 1998 Jun;37(6):696

[314] Lin HC. Small intestinal bacterial overgrowth: a framework for understanding irritable bowel syndrome. *JAMA.* 2004 Aug 18;292(7):852-8

[315] Zaidel O, Lin HC. Uninvited guests: the impact of small intestinal bacterial overgrowth on nutrition. *Practical Gastroenterology* 2003; 27(7):27-34 http://www.healthsystem.virginia.edu/internet/digestive-health/zaidelarticle.pdf

[316] "The initial skin changes were frankly vasculitic with 'target' lesions, whilst older lesions showed a psoriasiform scale and a tendency to central clearing. The illness was associated with raised levels of IgM and IgG containing circulating immune complexes and deposition of IgM and IgG in the dermis." Fairris GM, Ashworth J, Cotterill JA. A dermatosis associated with bacterial overgrowth in jejunal diverticula. *Br J Dermatol.* 1985 Jun;112(6):709-13

[317] "Candida albicans is known to produce gliotoxin, which has several prominent biological effects, including immunosuppression." Shah DT, Jackman S, Engle J, Larsen B. Effect of gliotoxin on human polymorphonuclear neutrophils. *Infect Dis Obstet Gynecol.* 1998;6(4):168-75

[318] "Based on the recent finding that C. albicans is able to produce an immunosuppressive mycotoxin, gliotoxin, we analyzed vaginal samples of 3 women severely symptomatic for vaginal candidiasis and found that they contained significant levels of gliotoxin." Shah DT, Glover DD, Larsen B. In situ mycotoxin production by Candida albicans in women with vaginitis. *Gynecol Obstet Invest.* 1995;39(1):67-9

infections in the gastrointestinal tract, its destruction by microbes such as *Candida albicans* and *Entamoeba histolytica* retards this immune barrier, and this can be considered a form of local immunosuppression.

4. Hypersensitivity/allergic dysbiosis: **Some people have an exaggerated immune response to otherwise "normal" yeast and bacteria. In this situation, we have to eradicate their "normal" yeast or bacteria in order to alleviate their hypersensitivity reaction.** The best example of this is the **severe intestinal inflammation that some patients develop in response to intestinal colonization with *Candida albicans***, which is generally considered "nonpathogenic" in small amounts. In susceptible patients, *Candida* can induce a severe local inflammatory reaction, such as colitis, that only remits with antifungal treatment.[319] **Gastrointestinal overgrowth of *Candida albicans* and *C. glabrata* caused near-fatal hypersensitivity alveolitis that remitted with eradication of gastrointestinal candidiasis.**[320] Some women become "allergic" to their own vaginal *Candida albicans*[321]; undoubtedly there are also men who are likewise allergic to their own intestinal yeast. In patients with lupus, gastrointestinal bacteria are abnormal (decreased colonization resistance[322]), and it is possible that gastrointestinal bacteria in these patients may translocate into the systemic circulation to induce formation of antibodies that cross-react with double-stranded DNA to produce the clinical manifestations of the disease.[323,324] With regard to dermal dysbiosis, **most (57%) of patients with atopic dermatitis show evidence of IgE-mediated histamine release (i.e., "allergy") to exotoxins secreted from *Staphylococcus aureus***, which commonly colonizes eczematous skin[325]; in other words: most eczema patients are allergic to their own dermal bacteria and can thus be said to have *hypersensitivity dermal dysbiosis*.

5. Inflammatory dysbiosis and reactive arthritis: People with specific genotypes and HLA markers are susceptible to a proinflammatory "autoimmune" syndrome that occurs following exposure to specific microbial molecules that are structurally similar to human body tissues—a phenomenon previously described as molecular mimicry. The best-known example of systemic musculoskeletal inflammation caused by microbial exposure is "reactive arthritis" such as Reiter's syndrome, which is classically seen in patients with the genotype HLA-B27 following urogenital exposure to *Chlamydia trachomatis*.

6. Amoebas, cysts, protozoas, and other parasites: In this case when we use the term "parasites'" we are not talking about worms/helminths, *per se*, although these are occasionally found with parasitology examinations. Certain microorganisms are not consistent with optimal health and should be eliminated even though the microbe is not classically identified as a "pathogen." Interestingly, 97% of patients severely infected with the gastrointestinal "parasite" *Entamoeba histolytica* develop self-destructive ANCA[326], suggesting the possibility that this microbe can induce or sustain autoimmunity.

---

[319] Doby T. Monilial esophagitis and colitis. *J Maine Med Assoc.* 1971 May;62(5):109-14

[320] "We conclude that the disease was induced by C.a.-antigen reaching the lungs from the intestinal tract via the bloodstream." Schreiber J, Struben C, Rosahl W, Amthor M. Hypersensitivity alveolitis induced by endogenous candida species. *Eur J Med Res.* 2000 Mar 27;5(3):126

[321] Ramirez De Knott HM, McCormick TS, Do SO, Goodman W, Ghannoum MA, Cooper KD, Nedorost ST. Cutaneous hypersensitivity to Candida albicans in idiopathic vulvodynia. *Contact Dermatitis.* 2005 Oct;53(4):214-8

[322] "Colonization Resistance (CR)...tended to be lower in active SLE patients than in healthy individuals. This could indicate that in SLE more and different bacteria translocate across the gut wall due to a lower CR. Some of these may serve as polyclonal B cell activators or as antigens cross-reacting with DNA." Apperloo-Renkema HZ, Bootsma H, Mulder BI, Kallenberg CG, van der Waaij D. Host-microflora interaction in systemic lupus erythematosus (SLE): colonization resistance of the indigenous bacteria of the intestinal tract. *Epidemiol Infect.* 1994;112(2):367-73

[323] "The lower IgG antibacterial antibody titres in active SLE might possibly result from sequestration of these IgG antibodies in immune complexes, indicating a possible role for antibacterial antibodies in exacerbations of SLE." Apperloo-Renkema HZ, Bootsma H, Mulder BI, Kallenberg CG, van der Waaij D. Host-microflora interaction in systemic lupus erythematosus (SLE): circulating antibodies to the indigenous bacteria of the intestinal tract. *Epidemiol Infect.* 1995 Feb;114(1):133-41

[324] Pisetsky DS. Antibody responses to DNA in normal immunity and aberrant immunity. *Clin Diagn Lab Immunol* 1998;5:1-6 http://cdli.asm.org/cgi/content/full/5/1/1?view=long&pmid=9455870

[325] "These data indicate that a subset of patients with AD mount an IgE response to SEs that can be grown from their skin." Leung DY, Harbeck R, Bina P, Reiser RF, Yang E, Norris DA, Hanifin JM, Sampson HA. Presence of IgE antibodies to staphylococcal exotoxins on the skin of patients with atopic dermatitis. Evidence for a new group of allergens. *J Clin Invest.* 1993 Sep;92(3):1374-80 http://www.pubmedcentral.gov/articlerender.fcgi?tool=pubmed&pubmedid=7690780

[326] George J, Levy Y, Kallenberg CG, Shoenfeld Y. Infections and Wegener's granulomatosis--a cause and effect relationship? *QJM.* 1997 May;90(5):367-73 http://qjmed.oxfordjournals.org/cgi/reprint/90/5/367

- *History*: Clinicians should suspect gastrointestinal dysbiosis in their patients with gas, bloating, alternating constipation/diarrhea, irritable bowel syndrome, fibromyalgia, chronic fatigue syndrome, multiple chemical sensitivity, severe allergies, and autoimmunity, especially Crohn's disease, ulcerative colitis, rheumatoid arthritis, and ankylosing spondylitis. Frequent gas and bloating indicates excess gastrointestinal fermentation by yeast and/or overgrowth of aerobic bacteria. Abdominal pain, chronic constipation, and/or diarrhea are clear indications for stool testing; however, clinicians must remember that **many of the most heavily colonized patients will have no gastrointestinal symptoms**. Thus, **assessment and treatment for gastrointestinal dysbiosis is not unnecessary simply because the patient lacks gastrointestinal symptoms**.

- *Breath testing*: Bacterial overgrowth of the small bowel can be objectively documented with measurement of a **post-carbohydrate hydrogen/methane breath test**, but I consider a history of postprandial gas and bloating to be sufficiently diagnostic.

- *Lactulose-mannitol assay for "leaky gut"*: The intestinal wall should function as a tightly regulated barrier that accomplishes two tasks: 1) **efficient absorption** of nutrients, and 2) **selective exclusion** of antigens, foreign debris, microbes and microbial antigens, and indigestible food residues. Compromise of the intestinal barrier results in impairments in nutrient absorption and/or toxin exclusion. Impaired nutrient absorption predisposes to and commonly results in micro- or macro-nutrient deficiencies. Impaired exclusion results in increased absorption of microbes, antigens, waste products, and debris into the systemic circulation. This phenomenon of altered intestinal permeability is referred to in the lay public and increasingly in the medical literature as "leaky gut" or "leaky gut syndrome."[327,328] In many patients this injury is occult, and **they have no gastrointestinal symptoms at all**; other patients may have a spectrum of signs and symptoms including diarrhea, constipation, abdominal pain, fatigue, general malaise, dyscognition, and an increase in the number and severity of food allergies, food sensitivities, and food intolerances. The **lactulose and mannitol assay** evaluates paracellular (pathologic) and transcellular (physiologic) absorption, respectively; and an increased lactulose:mannitol ratio is a non-specific finding that indicates gastrointestinal damage, generally due to 1) enterotoxin consumption such as with alcohol or NSAIDs, 2) malnutrition, 3) food allergy including celiac disease, 4) inflammatory bowel disease, and/or 5) dysbiosis—excess/harmful yeast, bacteria, or parasites. **Recall that "leaky gut" is only a symptom or manifestation of another, larger problem**.

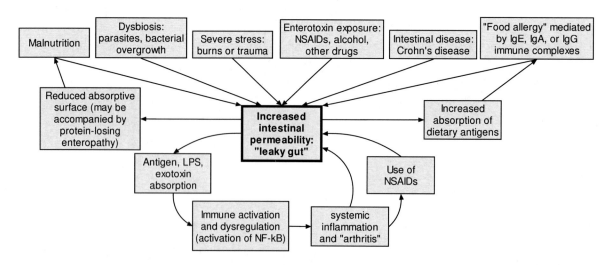

- **Comprehensive stool analysis and comprehensive parasitology**: The single best test for the assessment of gastrointestinal dysbiosis is a comprehensive stool analysis and comprehensive parasitology examination performed by a specialty laboratory that provides bacterial culture, yeast culture, microscopic exam, and measurement of sIgA to assess mucosal immune response, along with markers of inflammation such as

---

[327] Hollander D. Intestinal permeability, leaky gut, and intestinal disorders. *Curr Gastroenterol Rep*. 1999 Oct;1(5):410-6
[328] Keshavarzian A, Holmes EW, Patel M, Iber F, Fields JZ, Pethkar S. Leaky gut in alcoholic cirrhosis: a possible mechanism for alcohol-induced liver damage. *Am J Gastroenterol*. 1999 Jan;94(1):200-7

lactoferrin, calprotectin, and/or lysozyme. Comprehensive parasitology examinations (x3) to assess for bacteria, yeast, and parasites should be followed by culture and sensitivity to fine-tune the identification of the microbes and to guide treatment. These tests should be performed by a specialty laboratory rather than a regular medical or hospital laboratory. Additional markers can help put microbiological findings into the proper context; for example, in a patient with no "pathogens" other than normal *Candida albicans*, the finding of an exaggerated inflammatory response suggests a hypersensitivity/allergic dysbiosis that should be eradicated.

- **Stool testing must be performed by a specialty laboratory** because the quality of testing provided by most standard "medical labs" and hospitals is completely inadequate. Initial samples should be collected on three separate occasions by the patient and each sample should be analyzed separately by the laboratory.
- Important qualitative and quantitative markers include the following:
  - Beneficial bacteria (" probiotics"): Microbiological testing should quantify and identify various beneficial bacteria, which should be present at "+4" levels on a 0-4 scale.
  - Harmful and potentially harmful bacteria, protozoans, amebas, etc.: Questionable or harmful microbes should be eradicated even if they are not identified as true pathogens in the paleo-classic Pasteurian/Kochian sense.[329]
  - Yeast and mycology: At least two tests must be performed for a complete assessment: 1) yeast culture, and 2) microscopic examination for yeast elements. (See Chapter 1 for additional discussion.)
  - Microbial sensitivity testing: An important component to parasitology testing is the determination of which anti-microbial agents (natural and synthetic) the microbe is sensitive to. This helps to guide and enhance the effectiveness of anti-microbial therapy.
  - Secretory IgA: SIgA levels are elevated in patients who are having an immune response to either food or microbial antigens.[330] Thus, in a patient with minimal dysbiosis, say for example with *Candida albicans*, an elevated sIgA can indicate that the patient is having a hypersensitivity reaction to an otherwise benign microbe—in this case, eradication of the microbe is warranted and may result in a positive clinical response. Low sIgA suggests either primary or secondary immune defect such as selective sIgA deficiency[331] or malnutrition, stress, prednisone/corticosteroids, or possibly mycotoxicosis (immunosuppression due to fungal immunotoxins).
  - Short-chain fatty acids: These are produced by intestinal bacteria. Quantitative excess indicates bacterial overgrowth of the intestines, while insufficiency indicates a lack of probiotics or an insufficiency of dietary substrate, i.e., soluble fiber. Abnormal patterns of individual short-chain fatty acids indicate qualitative/quantitative abnormalities in gastrointestinal microflora, particularly anaerobic bacteria that cannot be identified with routine bacterial cultures.
  - Beta-glucuronidase: This is an enzyme produced by several different intestinal bacteria. High levels of beta-glucuronidase in the intestinal lumen serve to nullify the benefits of detoxification (specifically glucuronidation) by cleaving the toxicant from its glucuronide conjugate. This can result in re-absorption of the toxicant through the intestinal mucosa which then re-exposes the patient to the toxin that was previously detoxified ("enterohepatic recirculation" or "enterohepatic recycling"[332]). This is an exemplary aspect of "auto-intoxication" that results in chronic fatigue and upregulation of Phase 1 detoxification systems (chapter 4 of *Integrative Rheumatology*).
  - Lactoferrin: The iron-binding glycoprotein lactoferrin is an inflammatory marker that helps distinguish functional disorders (i.e., IBS) from more serious diseases (i.e., IBD).
  - Lysozyme: Elevated in proportion to intestinal inflammation in dysbiosis and IBD.
  - Other markers: Other markers of digestion, inflammation, and absorption are reported with the more comprehensive panels performed on stool samples. These tests are not always necessary, but such additional information is always helpful when working with complex patients. These markers are relatively self-explanatory and/or are described on the results of the test by the laboratory.

---

[329] **Vasquez A. Reducing Pain and Inflammation Naturally. Part 6: Nutritional and Botanical Treatments Against "Silent Infections" and Gastrointestinal Dysbiosis, Commonly Overlooked Causes of Neuromusculoskeletal Inflammation and Chronic Health Problems.** *Nutr Perspect* **2006; Jan** http://optimalhealthresearch.com/part6
[330] Quig DW, Higley M. Noninvasive assessment of intestinal inflammation: inflammatory bowel disease vs. irritable bowel syndrome. *Townsend Letter for Doctors and Patients* 2006;Jan:74-5
[331] "Selective IgA deficiency is the most common form of immunodeficiency. Certain select populations, including allergic individuals, patients with autoimmune and gastrointestinal tract disease and patients with recurrent upper respiratory tract illnesses, have an increased incidence of this disorder." Burks AW Jr, Steele RW. Selective IgA deficiency. *Ann Allergy.* 1986;57:3-13
[332] Parker RJ, Hirom PC, Millburn P.Enterohepatic recycling of phenolphthalein, morphine, lysergic acid diethylamide (LSD) and diphenylacetic acid in the rat. Hydrolysis of glucuronic acid conjugates in the gut lumen. *Xenobiotica.* 1980 Sep;10(9):689-70

Gastrointestinal Dysbiosis, "Leaky Gut" and Impaired Detoxification: a Hypothetical Model of Interconnected Scenarios and Clinical Remediation[333]

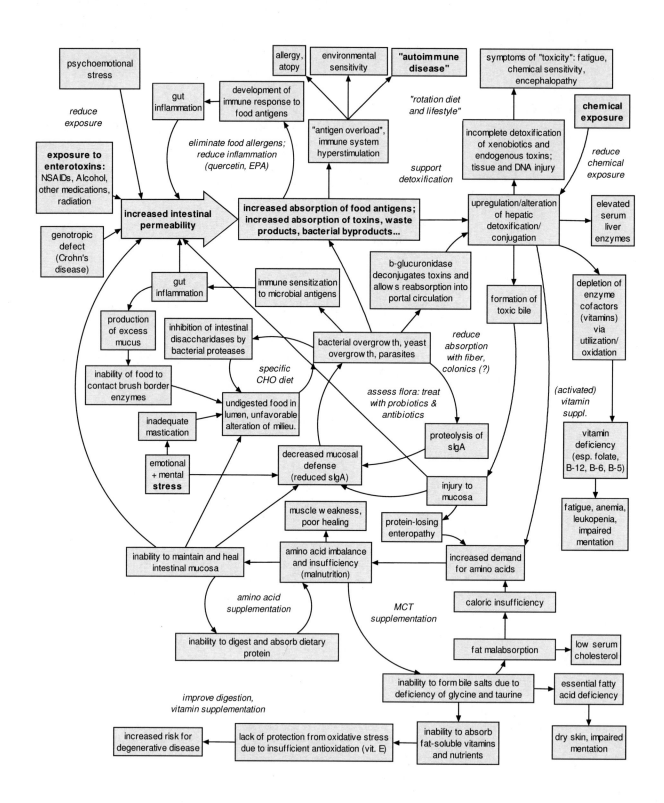

[333] Originally published in *Integrative Orthopedics* in 2004. An earlier, color version of this diagram is available at the website: www.OptimalHealthResearch.com/gastro

Orodental Dysbiosis

- *Introduction*: The human oral cavity is heavily populated by microbes, and these microbes and their products such as endotoxin can enter the bloodstream to induce a proinflammatory response via "metastatic infection" and "**metastatic inflammation**", respectively.[334] The systemic inflammatory response triggered by mild oral/dental "infections" is now believed to exacerbate conditions associated with inflammation, such as cardiovascular disease and diabetes.[335]

- *Assessments*: Obviously, any major microbial infestations of the mouth, such as gingivitis or thrush, need to be treated regardless of the presence or absence of systemic inflammatory disease. **Culture of mouth, throat, dentures for yeast and bacteria can be performed** (see Noah[336]). Palpation/provocation of the gums and teeth should not cause pain; the presence of pain suggests underlying inflammation, which in turn indicates underlying infection. If flossing causes bleeding and pain, this is indicative of unhealthy gums due to an overgrowth of bacteria below the gum line. Mild gum regression and the development of deep dental pockets is an indication for intervention with fastidious oral hygiene and professional dental care. Patients with systemic disease including chronic unwellness may have asymptomatic infections of the mandible that can only be detected with non-standard imaging techniques such as computer-enhanced mandibular ultrasound (Cavitat).[337]

- *Specific treatment considerations*: A professional cleaning by a dentist or oral hygienist is a reasonable start. Thereafter, twice-daily brushing, flossing, and the use of an antiseptic mouthwash and a plaque-removing solution should be employed. Toothbrushes should be periodically disinfected and replaced. Electric toothbrushes are more efficient than manual toothbrushes, and three-dimensional and ultrasound toothbrushes can cleanse below the gum line. Avoiding sucrose and refined carbohydrates is essential. Sugar-free chewing gums help to reduce bacterial loads at least in part by stimulating saliva production, and chewing gums with xylitol significantly reduce bacterial colonization of the oral cavity.[338,339] Immunonutrition as described later should be used to improve overall systemic defenses; particular attention should be given to glutamine, bovine colostrum and IgG, and thymus extract. In an animal study of experimental dental disease, administration of thymus extract was shown to normalize immune function and reduce orodental dysbiosis.[340]

Sinorespiratory Dysbiosis

- *Introduction*: **Sinorespiratory dysbiosis refers to adverse health consequences resultant from noninfectious colonization of the respiratory tract.** Patients with acute and chronic rhinosinusitis commonly display a rich mixture of bacteria and fungi in their sinuses. Regarding bacteria, both anaerobic and aerobic bacteria are seen, as are gram-positives such as *Staphylococcus aureus*, *Streptococcus* sp, Peptococcus/Peptostreptococcus, and gram-negative (endotoxin-producing) species including *Klebsiella pneumoniae*, *Proteus mirabilis*, *Bacteroides*, *Haemophilus parainfluenzae*, and *Haemophilus influenzae*.[341,342] Regarding fungi, **almost all patients with chronic sinus congestion have occult fungal sinus infections**, as shown in a landmark article wherein the authors concluded, "*Fungal cultures of nasal secretions were positive in 202 (96%) of 210 consecutive chronic rhinosinusitis patients.*"[343] **Reactive arthritis** and **cutaneous**

---

[334] Li X, Kolltveit KM, Tronstad L, Olsen I. Systemic diseases caused by oral infection. *Clin Microbiol Rev*. 2000 Oct;13(4):547-58 http://cmr.asm.org/cgi/content/full/13/4/547

[335] Amar S, Han X. The impact of periodontal infection on systemic diseases. *Med Sci Monit*. 2003 Dec;9(12):RA291-9 http://www.medscimonit.com/pub/vol_9/no_12/3776.pdf

[336] **Noah PW. The role of microorganisms in psoriasis. *Semin Dermatol*. 1990 Dec;9(4):269-76**

[337] "...the first commercially available TAU device, the Cavitat CAV 4000 (Cavitat Medical Technologies, Inc., Alba, TX)." Imbeau J. Introduction to through-transmission alveolar ultrasonography (TAU) in dental medicine. *Cranio*. 2005 Apr;23(2):100-12

[338] "Chewing 100% xylitol gum caused significant reductions on salivary MS scores (p < 0.025) which was little different from the 55% xylitol group. The results suggest that the use of xylitol chewing gum can reduce the levels of MS in plaque and saliva." Thaweboon S, Thaweboon B, Soo-Ampon S. The effect of xylitol chewing gum on mutans streptococci in saliva and dental plaque. *Southeast Asian J Trop Med Public Health*. 2004 Dec;35(4):1024-7

[339] "Especially xylitol-containing chewing gum may significantly reduce the growth of mutans streptococci and dental plaque which may be associated with dental caries." Makinen KK, Isotupa KP, Makinen PL, Soderling E, Song KB, Nam SH, Jeong SH. Six-month polyol chewing-gum programme in kindergarten-age children: a feasibility study focusing on mutans streptococci and dental plaque. *Int Dent J*. 2005 Apr;55(2):81-8

[340] Manti F, Kornman K, Goldschneider I. Effects of an immunomodulating agent on peripheral blood lymphocytes and subgingival microflora in ligature-induced periodontitis. *Infect Immun*. 1984 Jul;45(1):172-9 http://www.pubmedcentral.gov/articlerender.fcgi?tool=pubmed&pubmedid=6234232

[341] "Aspirates of 72 chronically inflamed maxillary sinuses were processed for aerobic and anaerobic bacteria. Bacterial growth was present in 66 of the 72 specimens (92%).... The predominant anaerobic organisms were anaerobic cocci and Bacteroides sp, and the predominant aerobes or facultatives were Streptococcus sp and Staphylococcus aureus." Brook I. Bacteriology of chronic maxillary sinusitis in adults. *Ann Otol Rhinol Laryngol*. 1989 Jun;98(6):426-8

[342] "The most frequently isolated bacteria were Streptococcus viridans, Klebsiella pneumoniae, Proteus mirabilis, and Hemophilus parainfluenzae." Jiang RS, Hsu CY, Leu JF. Bacteriology of ethmoid sinus in chronic rhinosinusitis. *Am J Rhinol*. 1997 Mar-Apr;11(2):133-7

[343] Ponikau JU, Sherris DA, Kern EB, Homburger HA, Frigas E, Gaffey TA, Roberts GD. The diagnosis and incidence of allergic fungal sinusitis. *Mayo Clin Proc*. 1999 Sep;74(9):877-84 http://www.aspergillus.man.ac.uk/secure/laboratory_protocols/Ponikau.pdf

vasculitis have been reported in an HLA-B27-negative patient with *Chlamydia pneumoniae* pneumonia.[344] Perhaps the best current exemplification of the link between sinus infections and chronic inflammatory disease is seen in patients with **Wegener's granulomatosis**, who have a high incidence of sinus colonization with *Staphylococcus aureus*. In these patients, *Staphylococcus aureus* produces a superantigen as well as an antigenic acid phosphatase which induces autoimmune vasculitis, nephritis, the production of antineutrophil anticytoplasmic antibody (ANCA), and the formation of immune complexes. **Antimicrobial treatment to eradicate *Staphylococcus aureus* results in clinical remission of the "autoimmune" disease[345], thus proving the microbe-autoimmune link.** Increased nasal colonization with *Staphylococcus aureus* has also been documented in other inflammatory/autoimmune diseases, including **systemic lupus erythematosus**[346] and **psoriasis.**[347]

- *Assessments*: Several studies documenting fungal and bacterial colonization of the sinuses have used diagnostic/surgical techniques that are not routinely available to clinicians working in outpatient settings. **Nasal swab and culture, throat culture for bacteria and yeasts should be performed** (see Noah[348]). Accessing the sinuses is generally not feasible on a clinical/nonsurgical basis. Response to antimicrobial treatment implies cure of the occult infection. In severe cases, MRI or CT can be used to assess for occult infectious sinusitis.

- *Specific treatment considerations*: Systemic antibiotics are commonly used by allopaths when treating sinus infections. Nasal lavage with saline is highly efficacious for relieving sinus congestion.[349] The basic solution is approximately one cup of warm water with one-half teaspoon of salt (sodium chloride) and one-half teaspoon baking soda (sodium bicarbonate). Distilled, bottled, or otherwise filtered and purified water may be preferred to avoid the microbial contaminants that are found in municipal tap water. To this can be added antimicrobial botanicals such as berberine, hyperforin (highly effective against *Staphylococcus aureus*[350]), artemisinin, and others (discussed later) as well as diluted iodine[351] and powdered Nystatin (sugar-free only.) Irrigation with a bulb syringe (such as used to clear an infant's nostrils) or Neti lota pot (aka: Neti pot, or Jala neti pot) can be performed by the patient while leaning over the sink. In the author's experience, 10-15 drops of povidone iodine 10% solution can be added to one cup of nasal lavage; higher amounts of iodine cause a burning sensation. Irrigating while kneeling with the head on the floor is the most effective technique for irrigating the maxillary sinuses and frontal recess; however most techniques are inefficient for accessing the sphenoid and frontal sinuses.[352] Nasal sprays and nebulizers with saline and/or antimicrobial herbs and medications can also be utilized.[353] However, clinicians and patients must remember that the creation of microbial imbalance is possible in the sinuses just as it is in the gastrointestinal tract, namely that the use of an antibacterial agent may result in fungal overgrowth or proliferation of resistant pathogens. Patients with sinus dysbiosis should integrate antimicrobial sinus lavage into their daily hygiene routine, such as at the same time they brush their teeth in the morning and evening. I suspect that as we gain additional experience in the treatment of sinorespiratory dysbiosis, we will find that many cases of recalcitrant gastrointestinal dysbiosis have been difficult to treat because of the continual gastrointestinal "seeding" of dysbiotic microbes from the sinorespiratory tract.

---

[344] "Here we present the case history of a patient with C. pneumoniae community acquired pneumonia (CAP) who subsequently developed a ReA and a cutaneous vasculitis." Cascina A, Marone Bianco A, Mangiarotti P, Montecucco CM, Meloni F. Cutaneous vasculitis and reactive arthritis following respiratory infection due to Chlamydia pneumoniae: report of a case. *Clin Exp Rheumatol*. 2002 Nov-Dec;20(6):845-7

[345] Popa ER, Stegeman CA, Kallenberg CG, Tervaert JW. Staphylococcus aureus and Wegener's granulomatosis. *Arthritis Res*. 2002;4(2):77-9 http://arthritis-research.com/content/4/2/077

[346] Medline abstract from Polish research: "In 9 from 14 patients with (64.3%) a.b. very massive growth of Staphylococcus aureus in culture from vestibulae of the nose swab was, in other cultures very massive growth of physiological flora was seen. ...clinical significance of asymptomatic bacteriuria and pathogenic bacteria colonisation of nostrils as a precedence to symptomatic infections needs further investigations." Koseda-Dragan M, Hebanowski M, Galinski J, Krzywinska E, Bakowska A. [Asymptomatic bacteriuria in women diagnosed with systemic lupus erythematosus (SLE)] *Pol Arch Med Wewn*. 1998 Oct;100(4):321-30.

[347] "The nasal carriage rate of Staphylococcus aureus in psoriatics was higher than the control groups." Singh G, Rao DJ. Bacteriology of psoriatic plaques. *Dermatologica*. 1978;157(1):21-7

[348] **Noah PW. The role of microorganisms in psoriasis. *Semin Dermatol*. 1990 Dec;9(4):269-76**

[349] "Endonasal irrigations with salt solutions are effective in the treatment of chronic sinusitis..." Bachmann G, Hommel G, Michel O. Effect of irrigation of the nose with isotonic salt solution on adult patients with chronic paranasal sinus disease. *Eur Arch Otorhinolaryngol*. 2000 Dec;257(10):537-41

[350] Schempp CM, Pelz K, Wittmer A, Schopf E, Simon JC. Antibacterial activity of hyperforin from St John's wort, against multiresistant Staphylococcus aureus and gram-positive bacteria. *Lancet*. 1999 Jun 19;353(9170):2129

[351] "Gargling with povidone-iodine before oral intubation reduces the transport of bacteria into the trachea." Ogata J, Minami K, Miyamoto H, Horishita T, Ogawa M, Sata T, Taniguchi H. Gargling with povidone-iodine reduces the transport of bacteria during oral intubation. *Can J Anaesth*. 2004 Nov;51(9):932-6 http://www.cja-jca.org/cgi/content/full/51/9/932 See also: "...a technique with facial, nasal vestibule and nasal cavity disinfection with a povidone-iodine solution followed by a cleansing of the nasal cavity (N = 87 patients and 166 samples)." Rombaux P, Collet S, Hamoir M, Eloy P, Bertrand B, Jamart F, Gigi J. The role of nasal cavity disinfection in the bacteriology of chronic sinusitis. *Rhinology*. 2005 Jun;43(2):125-9

[352] "...nasal douching while kneeling with the head on the floor. ...Nasal douches are more effective in distributing irrigation solution to the maxillary sinus and frontal recess. This should be the method of choice for irrigating these areas." Wormald PJ, Cain T, Oates L, Hawke L, Wong I. A comparative study of three methods of nasal irrigation. *Laryngoscope*. 2004 Dec;114(12):2224-7

[353] "Therapy with a 4-week course of large-particle nebulized aerosol therapy improves symptomatology and objective parameters of rhinosinusitis in patients refractory to surgical and medical therapies. Addition of tobramycin appears of minimal benefit." Desrosiers MY, Salas-Prato M. Treatment of chronic rhinosinusitis refractory to other treatments with topical antibiotic therapy delivered by means of a large-particle nebulizer: results of a controlled trial. *Otolaryngol Head Neck Surg*. 2001 Sep;125(3):265-9

Parenchymal Dysbiosis

- *Introduction*: Infections and microbial colonization of internal organs is generally incompatible with life and unlikely to be a silent/asymptomatic locus of inflammatory stimuli due to the appropriate febrile response that typically characterizes such infections. However, exceptions to these rules do exist, and infections of parenchymal tissue—especially of liver or bone—have been reported as initiators/mimickers of systemic rheumatic/inflammatory disease. **Viral hepatitis may present with polyarthropathy while the hepatitis is asymptomatic and serum levels of liver enzymes are within normal limits**; in these cases, the underlying dysbiosis/infection is identified with the use of specific serologic testing.[354] **Polyarteritis nodosa** is an autoimmune/inflammatory vasculitic syndrome strongly associated with hepatitis B infection, and 90% of patients with the immune complex vasculitis cryoglobulinemia have hepatitis C.[355] Robertson and Hickling[356] describe the case of a young girl who was **tentatively diagnosed with juvenile rheumatoid arthritis before being more accurately diagnosed with "recurrent multifocal osteomyelitis."** Dysbiosis (characterized by the acute nature of the microbial colonization) can segue into a true "infection." An advantage to the term *dysbiosis* in this situation is that it encourages clinicians to search for inflammation-generating microbial foci that may exist despite the absence of organ failure or classic/standard characteristics associated with parenchymal infection.

- *Assessments*: Given the increasing prevalence of viral hepatitis and its protean manifestations, specific serologic testing for viral hepatitis is warranted in patients with constitutional symptoms and inflammatory/idiopathic arthralgia. Likewise, occult osteomyelitis—particularly of the mandible—is increasingly appreciated, particularly as newer imaging techniques are facilitating detection. Bone scans can be helpful for detecting occult bone infections; otherwise, assessment for internal bacterial/viral/fungal infections can be used as and when clinically indicated.

- *Specific treatment considerations*: Treatment is determined by the underlying identity, nature, and location of the infection.

Genitourinary dysbiosis

- *Introduction*: All doctors know that genitourinary infection with *Chlamydia trachomatis* can produce inflammatory arthropathy—**"reactive arthritis"**—and result in the condition previously known as Reiter's syndrome.[357] Often fatal, **toxic shock syndrome results from the absorption of toxins and superantigens from *Staphylococcus aureus* directly through the genitourinary mucosa. In a study of 234 patients with inflammatory arthritis, 44% of patients had a silent genitourinary infection, mostly due to *Chlamydia*, *Mycoplasma*, or *Ureaplasma*.**[358] Men with chronic prostatitis have elevated endotoxin levels in their expressed prostatic secretions[359], and plasma endotoxin levels are elevated in all types of chronic urinary tract infections[360], thus clearly demonstrating the *systemic* inflammatory nature of these *localized* infections. **Microbial contamination of the genitourinary tract can cause a systemic pro-inflammatory arthritogenic response in susceptible individuals.**[361]

> **"Urogenital swab culture is a sensitive diagnostic method to identify the triggering infection in reactive arthritis."**
>
> Erlacher et al. *Br J Rheumatol* 1995

---

[354] "HCV arthritis should be considered in the differential diagnosis of seronegative arthritis of undetermined etiology even in the setting of normal liver chemistries." Akhtar AJ, Funnye AS. Hepatitis C virus associated arthritis in absence of clinical, biochemical and histological evidence of liver disease--responding to interferon therapy. *Med Sci Monit.* 2005 Jul;11(7):CS37-9 http://www.medscimonit.com/pub/vol_11/no_7/6300.pdf

[355] Tierney ML. McPhee SJ, Papadakis MA (eds). Current Medical Diagnosis and Treatment 2006. 45th edition. New York; Lange Medical Books: 2006, pages 844-850

[356] Robertson LP, Hickling P. Chronic recurrent multifocal osteomyelitis is a differential diagnosis of juvenile idiopathic arthritis. *Ann Rheum Dis.* 2001 Sep;60(9):828-31 http://ard.bmjjournals.com/cgi/reprint/60/9/828

[357] Kobayashi S, Kida I. Reactive arthritis: recent advances and clinical manifestations. *Intern Med.* 2005 May;44(5):408-12 http://www.jstage.jst.go.jp/article/internalmedicine/44/5/408/_pdf

[358] "Urogenital swab cultures showed a microbial infection in 44% of the patients with oligoarthritis (15% Chlamydia, 14% Mycoplasma, 28% Ureaplasma), whereas in the control group only 26% had a positive result (4% Chlamydia, 7% Mycoplasma, 21% Ureaplasma)." Erlacher L, Wintersberger W, Menschik M, Benke-Studnicka A, Machold K, Stanek G, Soltz-Szots J, Smolen J, Graninger W. Reactive arthritis: urogenital swab culture is the only useful diagnostic method for the detection of the arthritogenic infection in extra-articularly asymptomatic patients with undifferentiated oligoarthritis. *Br J Rheumatol.* 1995 Sep;34(9):838-42 http://rheumatology.oxfordjournals.org/cgi/content/abstract/34/9/838

[359] Dai YP, Sun XZ, Zheng KL. Endotoxins in the prostatic secretions of chronic prostatitis patients. *Asian J Androl.* 2005 Mar;7(1):45-7 http://www.blackwell-synergy.com/toc/ajan/7/1

[360] "RESULTS: The mean plasma endotoxin concentrations in patients with sterile pyuria, chronic complicated cystitis, acute uncomplicated pyelonephritis or acute exacerbation of chronic complicated pyelonephritis, chronic complicated pyelonephritis, and acute bacterial prostatitis or epididymitis were significantly higher than those in healthy individuals and in patients with acute uncomplicated cystitis." Goto T, Makinose S, Ohi Y. Plasma endotoxin concentrations in patients with urinary tract infections. *Int J Urol.* 1995 Sep;2(4):238-42

[361] "Urogenital swab cultures showed a microbial infection in 44% of the patients with oligoarthritis (15% Chlamydia, 14% Mycoplasma, 28% Ureaplasma), whereas in the control group only 26% had a positive result (4% Chlamydia, 7% Mycoplasma, 21% Ureaplasma)." Erlacher L, Wintersberger W, Menschik M, Benke-Studnicka A, Machold K, Stanek G, Soltz-Szots J, Smolen J, Graninger W. Reactive arthritis: urogenital swab culture is the only useful diagnostic method for the detection of the arthritogenic infection in extra-articularly asymptomatic patients with undifferentiated oligoarthritis. *Br J Rheumatol.* 1995 Sep;34(9):838-42 http://rheumatology.oxfordjournals.org/cgi/content/abstract/34/9/838

- *Assessments*: Basic assessment begins with a serum chemistry/metabolic panel to assess basic renal function, CBC to screen for any signs of classic infection, and urinalysis to assess for WBC, mucus, leukocyte esterase, bacteria and other basic markers. Serum tests for STDs can be performed. Urethral/vaginal swab for culture and DNA polymerase chain reaction is generally sufficient for the detection of the majority of urogenital infections. **Culture and sensitivity testing should be performed for all organisms from clean-catch urine specimens; assessment of sexual partners is advised** (see excellent review by Noah[362]). Women should undergo complete pelvic examinations, and men should undergo assessment of expressed prostatic secretions. Similar to the protocol evaluation of men with elevated PSA, a clinical trial of antibiotics/antimicrobials may reduce systemic inflammation and thereby implicate a dysbiotic stimulus to the inflammation.

- *Specific treatment considerations*: In women, particular attention must be given to correcting gastrointestinal dysbiosis due to the close anatomical proximity and therefore microbiologic communication between the anus and vagina.[363] Sexual partners should also be tested; barrier methods (e.g., condoms) should be used to prevent transmission/cross-contamination. Products containing Uva Ursi[364], buchu[365] and cranberry[366] are commonly used as urinary antiseptics. Pharmaceutical antibiotics can be used as indicated.

Cutaneous Dysbiosis, Dermal Dysbiosis

- *Introduction*: Microorganisms from dermal infections such as acne can incite systemic inflammation either by dermal absorption of bacterial[367] and fungal[368] (super)antigens and by serving as loci for metastatic infections which produce septic arthritis.[369] **Patients with the autoimmune vasculitic syndrome known as Behcet's disease are more likely to develop arthritis if their skin lesions are infected, thus implicating absorption of an inflammatory immunogen.**[370] Most (57%) of patients with atopic dermatitis show evidence of IgE-mediated histamine release (i.e., "allergy") to exotoxins secreted from *Staphylococcus aureus*, which commonly colonizes eczematous skin[371]; in other words: most eczema patients are allergic to their own dermal bacteria and can thus be said to have *hypersensitivity dermal dysbiosis*.

- *Assessments*: Routine physical examination of the skin and scalp is generally sufficient to screen for obvious infections and any lesions that may be presumed to be colonized. Dermal scrapings and swabs are taken for bacterial, viral, and fungal cultures and microscopic examination. Skin/nail culture, Giemsa staining, culture of lesioned skin on blood agar, MacConkey agar, Sabouraud plates can be performed; see the review by Noah[372] for additional details.

- *Specific treatment considerations*: Topical and/or systemic antimicrobial treatment along with immunonutrition (detailed later) may be necessary for complete treatment of patients with inflammation perpetuated by dermal dysbiosis. Topical *Mahonia/Berberis aquifolium* is effective for dermal psoriasis[373] via its combined anti-inflammatory and antimicrobial benefits. Other botanical antimicrobials available in topical creams, gels, and soaps include grape seed extract, artemesinin from *Artemisia annua*, and tea tree oil. Clothes, bedding, and the environments in the car, home, and work should be disinfected and/or routinely washed; see section on *environmental dysbiosis*.

[362] Noah PW. **The role of microorganisms in psoriasis.** *Semin Dermatol.* 1990 Dec;9(4):269-76
[363] "The results showed that if C albicans was cultured from the vagina, it was always found in the stool... The gut-reservoir concept may well apply to other forms of candidiasis." Miles MR, Olsen L, Rogers A. Recurrent vaginal candidiasis. Importance of an intestinal reservoir. *JAMA.* 1977 Oct 24;238(17):1836-7
[364] Yarnell E. Botanical medicines for the urinary tract. *World J Urol.* 2002 Nov;20(5):285-93
[365] "Buchu preparations are now used as a diuretic and for a wide range of conditions including stomach aches, rheumatism, bladder and kidney infections and coughs and colds." Simpson D. Buchu--South Africa's amazing herbal remedy. *Scott Med J* 1998 Dec;43(6):189-91
[366] Lynch DM. Cranberry for prevention of urinary tract infections. *Am Fam Physician.* 2004 Dec 1;70(11):2175-7 http://www.aafp.org/afp/20041201/2175.pdf
[367] Delyle LG, Vittecoq O, Bourdel A, Duparc F, Michot C, Le Loet X. Chronic destructive oligoarthritis associated with Propionibacterium acnes in a female patient with acne vulgaris: septic-reactive arthritis? *Arthritis Rheum.* 2000 Dec;43(12):2843-7
[368] Hemalatha V, Srikanth P, Mallika M. Superantigens - Concepts, clinical disease and therapy. *Indian J Med Microbiol* 2004;22:204-211
[369] Schaeverbeke T, Lequen L, de Barbeyrac B, Labbe L, Bebear CM, Morrier Y, Bannwarth B, Bebear C, Dehais J. Propionibacterium acnes isolated from synovial tissue and fluid in a patient with oligoarthritis associated with acne and pustulosis. *Arthritis Rheum.* 1998 Oct;41(10):1889-93
[370] Diri E, Mat C, Hamuryudan V, Yurdakul S, Hizli N, Yazici H. Papulopustular skin lesions are seen more frequently in patients with Behcet's syndrome who have arthritis: a controlled and masked study. *Ann Rheum Dis.* 2001 Nov;60(11):1074-6
[371] "These data indicate that a subset of patients with AD mount an IgE response to SEs that can be grown from their skin." Leung DY, Harbeck R, Bina P, Reiser RF, Yang E, Norris DA, Hanifin JM, Sampson HA. Presence of IgE antibodies to staphylococcal exotoxins on the skin of patients with atopic dermatitis. Evidence for a new group of allergens. *J Clin Invest.* 1993 Sep;92(3):1374-80 http://www.pubmedcentral.gov/articlerender.fcgi?tool=pubmed&pubmedid=7690780
[372] Noah PW. **The role of microorganisms in psoriasis.** *Semin Dermatol.* 1990 Dec;9(4):269-76
[373] "Taken together, these clinical studies conducted by several investigators in several countries indicate that Mahonia aquifolium is a safe and effective treatment of patients with mild to moderate psoriasis." Gulliver WP, Donsky HJ. A report on three recent clinical trials using Mahonia aquifolium 10% topical cream and a review of the worldwide clinical experience with Mahonia aquifolium for the treatment of plaque psoriasis. *Am J Ther.* 2005 Sep-Oct;12(5):398-406

Environmental dysbiosis

- *Introduction*: Patients may develop inflammation/autoimmunity from exposures to microbial toxins from their home, work, or recreational environments. Many microorganisms, particularly yeasts/molds, defend themselves via elaboration of toxins to fend off other microbes that might otherwise invade their territory. Environmental and occupational researchers appreciate that **yeast/mold commonly elaborate immunomodulating bioaerosols, while gram-negative bacteria exude endotoxin, which is a common contaminant of "house dust."**[374] We may reasonably speculate that a susceptible person might have a systemic inflammatory response from the inhalation of bioaerosols and/or endotoxin in the air of their home and/or work environments. **Airborne immunogens include fungi, bacteria, actinomycetes, endotoxin, ß(1,3)-glucans, peptidoglycans, microbial volatile organic compounds (MVOC), and mycotoxins.**[375] "Toxic mold syndrome" and more recently "mixed mold mycotoxicosis"[376] describes patients with systemic health problems resultant from exposure to fungal bioaerosols, classically associated with mold-contaminated buildings following water damage. Such individuals develop systemic autoimmunity that resembles **multiple sclerosis** and **chronic inflammatory polyneuropathy** mediated in part by antibodies against endogenous neuronal structures.[377] Additional evidence proves that **mold exposure can lead to proinflammatory immune activation and resultant multisystem (especially neurologic) autoimmunity.**[378] This is yet another example of how microorganisms can cause human disease without causing "infection." Obviously, patients with inflammatory lung disorders such as asthma, idiopathic pulmonary fibrosis, and especially **acute pulmonary hemorrhage in infants**[379] are candidates for environmental evaluation and intervention. Patients with **Crohn's disease** are well-known to have exquisite sensitivity to the yeast *Saccharomyces cerevisiae*, and a few doctors have reported improvement in Crohn's patients following environmental disinfection. Of related interest is the finding that intraperitoneal exposure of autoimmune-prone mice to fungal components stimulates **autoimmune arthritis resembling rheumatoid arthritis.**[380]

- *Assessments*: Location-specific exacerbation of symptoms is an important historical indicator. Home, work, and recreational environments can be surveyed for microbial contamination, particularly mold. Pier-and-beam homes should be inspected for mold and water in the crawlspace; likewise, attics should be inspected for occult leaks and mold. Mold plates, Petri dishes, and filter cartridges can be used to identify airborne microbes. *Fusarium*, *Trichoderma*, and *Stachybotrys* produce mycotoxins.[381] Thorough cleaning/sanitization of wigs, shoes, furniture, whirlpool/pool water should be implemented; again, see the review by Noah.[382]

- *Specific treatment considerations*: Walls, windows, utility closets, bathrooms, and under-sink cabinets should be assessed for mold and thoroughly cleaned. High-efficiency air filters can be used in the HVAC system; stand-alone air purifiers and dehumidifiers can be used. Bedding, sheets, blankets, pillows, carpets, furniture and drapes should be inspected for contamination and thoroughly cleaned. Eucalyptus oil can be added to washing detergent to kill dust mites[383], as described in the following section.

---

[374] Douwes J, Thorne P, Pearce N, Heederik D. Bioaerosol health effects and exposure assessment: progress and prospects. *Ann Occup Hyg*. 2003 Apr;47(3):187-200 http://annhyg.oxfordjournals.org/cgi/content/full/47/3/187

[375] Douwes J, Thorne P, Pearce N, Heederik D. Bioaerosol health effects and exposure assessment: progress and prospects. *Ann Occup Hyg*. 2003 Apr;47(3):187-200

[376] Gray MR, Thrasher JD, Crago R, Madison RA, Arnold L, Campbell AW, Vojdani A. Mixed mold mycotoxicosis: immunological changes in humans following exposure in water-damaged buildings. *Arch Environ Health*. 2003 Jul;58(7):410-20

[377] "The authors concluded that exposure to molds in water-damaged buildings increased the risk for development of neural autoantibodies, peripheral neuropathy, and neurophysiologic abnormalities in exposed individuals." Campbell AW, Thrasher JD, Madison RA, Vojdani A, Gray MR, Johnson A. Neural autoantibodies and neurophysiologic abnormalities in patients exposed to molds in water-damaged buildings. *Arch Environ Health*. 2003 Aug;58(8):464-74

[378] "Abnormally high levels of ANA, ASM, and CNS myelin (immunoglobulins [Ig]G, IgM, IgA) and PNS myelin (IgG, IgM, IgA)... showing an increased risk for autoimmunity. ...exposure to mixed molds and their associated mycotoxins in water-damaged buildings leads to multiple health problems involving the CNS and the immune system... Mold exposure also initiates inflammatory processes." Gray MR, Thrasher JD, Crago R, Madison RA, Arnold L, Campbell AW, Vojdani A. Mixed mold mycotoxicosis: immunological changes in humans following exposure in water-damaged buildings. *Arch Environ Health*. 2003 Jul;58(7):410-20

[379] "Mean colony counts for all fungi averaged 29227 colony-forming units (CFU)/m3 in homes of patients and 707 CFU/m3 in homes of controls... Conclusion Infants with pulmonary hemorrhage and hemosiderosis were more likely than controls to live in homes with toxigenic S atra and other fungi in the indoor air." Etzel RA, Montana E, Sorenson WG, et al. Acute pulmonary hemorrhage in infants associated with exposure to Stachybotrys atra and other fungi. *Arch Pediatr Adolesc Med*. 1998 Aug;152(8):757-62

[380] Yoshitomi H, Sakaguchi N, Kobayashi K, et al. A role for fungal {beta}-glucans and their receptor Dectin-1 in the induction of autoimmune arthritis in genetically susceptible mice. *J Exp Med*. 2005 Mar 21;201(6):949-60 http://www.jem.org/cgi/content/full/201/6/949

[381] Am Acad Pediatrics.Toxic effects of indoor molds. Committee on Environ Health.*Pediatrics* 1998;101(4 Pt1):712-4 http://aappolicy.aappublications.org/cgi/content/full/pediatrics;101/4/712

[382] **Noah PW. The role of microorganisms in psoriasis. *Semin Dermatol*. 1990 Dec;9(4):269-76**

[383] Tovey ER, McDonald LG. A simple washing procedure with eucalyptus oil for controlling house dust mites and their allergens in clothing and bedding. *J Allergy Clin Immunol*. 1997 Oct;100(4):464-6

Cleaning the home/work/recreational environment of microbial contaminants

Household "dust" is actually a complex mixture of microscopic particles such as fabric fragments (from bedding, carpet, clothing, etc.), pollen (from outdoor plants), dirt (which has settled from the air), dead skin cells (from humans and pets), bacteria and mold, and the feces of dust mites and other insects. Since dust, especially the feces from dust mites, is very allergenic, particularly for patients with eczema, we are wise to take effective steps to reduce the amount of dust/contaminants to which we are exposed. Reducing the amount of "dust" in a home environment involves 3 general steps:

1. **Dust, mold, and chemical removal**
   - Cleaning: Periodically, use a damp cloth on furniture to remove dust that accumulates.
   - Vacuuming: Vacuum the floors/carpet and ensure that the vacuum is equipped with an *allergy filter* or HEPA filter to ensure that the dust is not simply transposed from the floor back into the air and onto furniture, bedding, and clothes. In severe cases, patients with inflammatory disorders, allergies/eczema, and environmental sensitivity may choose to have carpets removed and replaced either with a low-offgassing/outgassing flooring such as bamboo hardwoods or ceramic tile.
   - Exclude pollen/mold: Close doors and windows on days the pollen/mold count is high.
   - Pet control: If you have pets, it is often helpful to 1) wash them regularly, 2) keep them off the bedding, and/or 3) allow them to stay outdoors as much as is possible and practical.
   - Using air filters for the central cooling/heating unit: Consider the "Filterete Allergen Reducing Filter" from 3M (comes with a purple label). Other, more expensive and effective options are available for complicated cases.
   - Vinyl/hypoallergenic mattress cover: Buy and use a simple hypoallergenic or vinyl mattress cover to eliminate exposure to years of accumulated dust inside the mattress which is slept on for 8 hours each night. The goal is create an airtight seal around the mattress to contain the dust and antigens. Vinyl mattress covers are inexpensive and widely available.
2. **Reducing the amount of moisture in the air**. Ideally, the steam from bathing and cooking areas should be vented outdoors so that moisture does not accumulate inside the living area. Moisture is necessary for dust mites and mold to live and to create allergens; if the air is very moist then the inflammation-producing activities of the dust mites and mold are stimulated. Conversely, by reducing the humidity in the air, we are able to impair the microbes and thus reduce the amount of antigens. Reducing the amount of moisture in the air by use of an electric dehumidifier may be necessary to help reduce the amount of both dust allergen and mold in a home.
3. **Wash clothes/linens with eucalyptus oil to eliminate dust mites:** The combination of 1) hot water, 2) detergent, and 3) eucalyptus oil is an effective and natural way to get rid of dust mites and dust allergens. As validated by research published in *Journal of Allergy and Clinical Immunology*[384], this is an effective technique for killing and eliminating dust mites from clothing and bed sheets. "Bi-O-Klean Hand Dishwashing Liquid" available at Whole Foods Market or "Kit liquid dishwashing detergent concentrate" meet the criteria for the selection of a detergent for this purpose. Eucalyptus oil must never be applied to the skin or taken internally.

Metric measurements from the original study	"American" unit translation	One-half recipe
1. **Eucalyptus oil**: 100 mL	6 tablespoons or 3.4 oz.	3 tablespoons or 1½ oz.
2. **Detergent**: 25 mL liquid concentrated dishwashing detergent	1 ½ tablespoons or 0.8 oz.	¾ tablespoons or 0.4 oz.
3. **Warm water** (30°C): 50 L	86°F water: 13 gallons	86°F water: 6 gallons
4. **Soak in hot detergent-eucalyptus solution for 15-30 minutes, then wash in machine as usual.**		

---

[384] 1) When mixed, the oil-detergent mixture should dissolve to form a clear homogenous solution, and 2) five mL (1 teaspoon) of the mixture stirred with 200 mL (6 oz.) of water should form a "milky, opaque solution that is stable (does not "break oil") for at least 10 minutes." Tovey ER, McDonald LG. A simple washing procedure with eucalyptus oil for controlling house dust mites and their allergens in clothing and bedding. *J Allergy Clin Immunol*. 1997 Oct;100(4):464-6

Problematic Bacteria, Yeast, and Parasites: A Listing of Commonly Encountered Dysbiotic Microorganisms

All of the following yeast, bacteria, and "parasites" have been observed in various patients in my private practice of chiropractic and naturopathic medicine. Even though several of these microbes are considered nonpathogenic by outdated medical paradigms[385,386,387] that are still hypnotized by Pasteur and Koch, their presence is generally inconsistent with optimal health and their eradication is rewarding for both doctor and patient. In other words, **even if a microbe is not a true pathogen and is thus not a therapeutic target from a** *disease-oriented paradigm*, **we as clinicians are still justified in eradicating it from our chronically ill patient from a** *wellness-oriented paradigm* **because we know that 1) eradicating potentially harmful bacteria will do no harm to the patient, and 2) in many cases—indeed** *the majority of cases*—**patients experience a significant and sustained clinical improvement regardless of their presenting complaint, thus implying a causal relationship between the microbe and the non-infectious illness.**

The following microbes are commonly detected with stool testing performed by a specialty laboratory. **One of the benefits of specialized stool testing is that it allows the presence of microbes to be determined within a context that evaluates the patient's individualized response.** For example, the finding of a mild degree of *Candida albicans* ("+1" on a 0-4 scale) might be considered insignificant; however if no other pathogens are identified, and the secretory IgA, lactoferrin, and lysozyme levels are elevated, then the clinician is justified in determining that the patient is having a hypersensitivity reaction to an otherwise "benign" yeast. **Remember, we are not looking for classic "infection" here; we are looking to determine which underlying disruptions may be exacerbating inflammation and the patient's symptomatology.** We have to look beyond the *disease-associated characteristics of the microbe* to see *the patient's individualized response to the microbe*. **Often what we find when working with autoimmune/inflammatory patients is that they are having a** *pathogenic inflammatory response* **to a** *nonpathogenic* **microbe.**

Commonly Encountered Dysbiotic Microorganisms

Dysbiotic microbe	*Pathophysiology and clinical manifestations*
Aeromonas hydrophila	• *Aeromonas hydrophila* can cause colitis and should therefore be eradicated immediately upon detection.[388]
Blastocystis hominis	• Many infections are asymptomatic • Can cause abdominal pain, nausea, vomiting, diarrhea, weight loss[389,390] as well as fever, chills, malaise, anorexia, flatus, and eosinophilia[391] • Fecal leukocytes are occasionally seen[392] • Can cause colitis[393]

[385] "…standard of care in developed countries is to maintain schizophrenia patients on neuroleptics, this practice is not supported by the 50-year research record for the drugs. …**this paradigm of care worsens long-term outcomes**, … 40% of all schizophrenia patients would fare better if they were not so medicated." Whitaker R. The case against antipsychotic drugs: a 50-year record of doing more harm than good. *Med Hypotheses.* 2004;62(1):5-1   Available at http://psychrights.org/Research/Digest/Chronicity/50yearecord.pdf on January 1, 2006
[386] Hyman M. **Paradigm shift**: the end of "normal science" in medicine understanding function in nutrition, health, and disease. *Altern Ther Health Med.* 2004 Sep-Oct;10(5):10-5, 90-4
[387] Heaney RP. Vitamin D, nutritional deficiency, and the **medical paradigm**. *J Clin Endocrinol Metab.* 2003 Nov;88(11):5107-8 http://jcem.endojournals.org/cgi/content/full/88/11/5107
[388] Farraye FA, Peppercorn MA, Ciano PS, Kavesh WN. Charles A. Segmental colitis associated with Aeromonas hydrophila. *Am J Gastroenterol.* 1989 Apr;84(4):436-8
[389] O'Gorman MA, Orenstein SR, Proujansky R, Wadowsky RM, Putnam PE, Kocoshis SA. Prevalence and characteristics of Blastocystis hominis infection in children. *Clin Pediatr* (Phila) 1993 Feb;32(2):91-6
[390] Telalbasic S, Pikula ZP, Kapidzic M. Blastocystis hominis may be a potential cause of intestinal disease. *Scand J Infect Dis* 1991;23(3):389-90
[391] Sheehan DJ, Raucher BG, McKitrick JC. Association of Blastocystis hominis with signs and symptoms of human disease. *J Clin Microbiol.* 1986;24(4):548-50
[392] Diaczok BJ, Rival J. Diarrhea due to Blastocystis hominis: an old organism revisited. *South Med J* 1987 Jul;80(7):931-2
[393] Russo AR, Stone SL, Taplin ME, Snapper HJ, Doern GV. Presumptive evidence for Blastocystis hominis as a cause of colitis. *Arch Intern Med.* 1988 May;148(5):1064

Commonly Encountered Dysbiotic Microorganisms—*continued*

Microbe	*Pathophysiology and clinical manifestations*
Candida albicans and *other yeasts*	• Although normal in small amounts ("+1"), excess *Candida* in the intestines is never a sign of optimal health. Patients may have mild general symptoms such as fatigue and dyscognition ("brain fog"); gas and intestinal bloating following consumption of carbohydrates are common. • *Candida* produces an immunosuppressive myotoxin called gliotoxin as well as an IgA-destroying protease and can cause watery diarrhea, particularly in elderly, ill, and immunosuppressed patients.[394] • *Candida* is always present in the gastrointestinal tract of women with recurrent yeast vaginitis.[395] • Some people have an inflammatory hypersensitivity to *Candida*, as it can cause **local allergic dermatitis/mucositis**[396], **colitis**[397], and **pulmonary inflammation** (**hypersensitivity alveolitis** from gastrointestinal colonization).[398] • Other yeasts such as *Candida parapsilosis* and *Geotrichum capitatum* are occasionally seen and should be eradicated.
Citrobacter rodentium *Citrobacter freundii*	• *Citrobacter freundii* is a gram-negative anaerobe; it produces pro-inflammatory endotoxin • *Citrobacter* species may cause **gastroenteritis** in humans[399] • Most strains of *Citrobacter freundii* produce hydrogen sulfide[400] which interferes with mitochondrial function and energy production and may be a major causative molecule in **ulcerative colitis**.[401] • Animal studies have shown that this bacterium can induce an intense inflammatory response in the gastrointestinal tract that resembles **inflammatory bowel disease**.[402] • Gastrointestinal dysbiosis with *Citrobacter freundii* may be causative in so-called "rheumatoid arthritis" in some patients.[author's experience]
Dientamoeba fragilis	• *Dientamoeba fragilis* is a flagellate protozoan that can cause **diarrhea, abdominal pain, nausea, vomiting, fatigue, malaise, eosinophilia, urticaria, pruritus and/or weight loss**. It is commonly associated with pinworm infection and may produce a clinical picture that mimics **food allergy, colitis, or eosinophilic enteritis**.[403]

[394] Gupta TP, Ehrinpreis MN. Candida-associated diarrhea in hospitalized patients. *Gastroenterology* 1990 Mar;98(3):780-5
[395] Miles MR, Olsen L, Rogers A. Recurrent vaginal candidiasis. Importance of an intestinal reservoir. *JAMA*. 1977 Oct 24;238(17):1836-7
[396] Ramirez De Knott HM, McCormick TS, et al. Cutaneous hypersensitivity to Candida albicans in idiopathic vulvodynia. *Contact Dermatitis*. 2005 Oct;53(4):214-8
[397] Doby T. Monilial esophagitis and colitis. *J Maine Med Assoc*. 1971 May;62(5):109-14
[398] "We conclude that the disease was induced by C.a.-antigen reaching the lungs from the intestinal tract via the bloodstream." Schreiber J, Struben C, Rosahl W, Amthor M. Hypersensitivity alveolitis induced by endogenous candida species. *Eur J Med Res*. 2000 Mar 27;5(3):126
[399] "Members of this genus can cause neonatal meningitis and, perhaps, gastroenteritis in both children and adults." Lipsky BA, Hook EW 3rd, Smith AA, Plorde JJ. Citrobacter infections in humans: experience at the Seattle Veterans Administration Medical Center and a review of the literature. *Rev Infect Dis*. 1980 Sep-Oct;2(5):746-60
[400] Lennette EH (editor in chief). Manual of Clinical Microbiology. Fourth Edition. Washington DC; American Society for Microbiology: 1985, page 269. See also http://web.indstate.edu/thcme/micro/GI/general/sld038.htm Accessed 10/27/2005
[401] "CONCLUSIONS: Metabolic effects of sodium hydrogen sulfide on butyrate oxidation along the length of the colon closely mirror metabolic abnormalities observed in active ulcerative colitis, and the increased production of sulfide in ulcerative colitis suggests that the action of mercaptides may be involved in the genesis of ulcerative colitis." Roediger WE, Duncan A, Kapaniris O, Millard S. Reducing sulfur compounds of the colon impair colonocyte nutrition: implications for ulcerative colitis. Gastroenterology. 1993 Mar;104(3):802-9
[402] Higgins LM, Frankel G, Douce G, Dougan G, MacDonald TT. Citrobacter rodentium infection in mice elicits a mucosal Th1 cytokine response and lesions similar to those in murine inflammatory bowel disease. *Infect Immun*. 1999 Jun;67(6):3031-9 This article is available on-line at http://iai.asm.org/cgi/reprint/67/6/3031.pdf as of December 26, 2003
[403] Cuffari C, Oligny L, Seidman EG. Dientamoeba fragilis masquerading as allergic colitis. *J Pediatr Gastroenterol Nutr*. 1998 Jan;26(1):16-20

Commonly Encountered Dysbiotic Microorganisms—*continued*

Dysbiotic microbe	Pathophysiology and clinical manifestations
Endolimax nana	• *Endolimax nana*, a protozoa, has a world-wide distribution and is commonly considered an harmless commensal of the intestine.[404] • Intestinal infection with *Endolimax nana* can cause a **peripheral arthropathy** that is clinically similar to **rheumatoid arthritis** and which remits with effective parasite eradication.[405] • In my own clinical practice, I have seen several cases of intestinal colonization with *Endolimax nana* in patients who presented with **chronic fatigue, myalgia, eczema**, and especially refractory **chronic vaginitis.**
Entamoeba histolytica	• Induces tissue damage, **amebic colitis**, and **liver abscess.**[406] • Associated with **Henoch Schonlein purpura** in a single case report[407] • **Amebic colitis** may be misdiagnosed as **ulcerative colitis.**[408] • May contribute to **irritable bowel syndrome, rheumatoid arthritis, fibromyalgia, food allergy**, or **multiple chemical sensitivity** and can **exacerbate HIV infection.**[409] • Hepatic infection is associated with induction of antineutrophil cytoplasmic antibodies (ANCA) such as seen with the vasculitic disease Wegener's granulomatosis.[410]
Gamma strep *Enterococcus*	• "Gamma strep", *Enterococcus faecalis*, and *Streptococcus faecalis* are somewhat interchangeable terms.[411,412,413] These terms refer to gram-positive *Enterococcus* species such as *Enterococcus faecalis*, which cause **urinary tract infections, bacteremia, intra-abdominal infections, and endocarditis.** • Enterococci produce **lipoteichoic acid** which is proinflammatory in a manner similar to endotoxin from gram-negative bacteria, and these gram-positive bacteria also appear to produce a superantigen.[414] • "Gamma strep" is commonly identified in stool tests of patients with **chronic unwellness and fatigue.**
Giardia lamblia *"Beaver fever"*	• Causatively associated with **abdominal pain, diarrhea, constipation, bloating, chronic fatigue, and food allergy/intolerance.**[415] • May contribute to **irritable bowel syndrome, rheumatoid arthritis, food allergy, or multiple chemical sensitivity.**[416] • Extraintestinal symptoms of gastrointestinal *Giardia* infection can include **fever, maculopapular rashes, geographic tongue, pulmonary infiltrates, lymphadenopathy, polyarthritis, aphthous ulcers, and urticaria.**[417]

[404] Information available at http://www2.provlab.ab.ca/bugs/webbug/parasite/artifact/enana.htm as of December 26, 2003
[405] "Endolimax nana grew on stool sample. Both the patient's diarrhea and arthritis responded effectively to therapy with metronidazole. The diagnosis of parasitic rheumatism was made in retrospect." Burnstein SL, Liakos S. Parasitic rheumatism presenting as rheumatoid arthritis. *J Rheumatol.* 1983 Jun;10(3):514-5
[406] Huston CD. Parasite and host contributions to the pathogenesis of amebic colitis. *Trends Parasitol.* 2004 Jan; 20(1): 23-6
[407] Demircin G, Oner A, Erdogan O, Bulbul M, Memis L. Henoch Schonlein purpura and amebiasis. *Acta Paediatr Jpn.* 1998 Oct; 40(5): 489-91
[408] Galland L. Intestinal protozoan infection is a common unsuspected cause of chronic illness. *J Advancement Med.* 1989;2: 539-552
[409] Galland L. Intestinal protozoan infection is a common unsuspected cause of chronic illness. *J Advancement Med.* 1989;2: 539-552
[410] George J, Levy Y, Kallenberg CG, Shoenfeld Y. Infections and Wegener's granulomatosis--a cause and effect relationship? QJM. 1997 May;90(5):367-73 http://qjmed.oxfordjournals.org/cgi/reprint/90/5/367
[411] "Figure 38: "Gamma *Streptococcus*" : *Enterococcus faecalis*" and "The genus *Enterococcus* was once a part of the *Streptococcus* genus, was considered a "gamma *Streptococcus* species." http://www.microbelibrary.org/asmonly/details_print.asp?id=1986&lang
[412] "Enterococcus faecalis. Synonyms: group D strep, Streptococcus faecalis. Classification: facultative anaerobic, gram+ bacteria, cocci." http://medinfo.ufl.edu/year2/mmid/bms5300/bugs/strfaeca.html
[413] "Microscopically, Gram-positive cocci occurring in chains or pairs with individual cells being somewhat elongated can be presumed to be streptococci or enterococci." http://members.tripod.com/piece_de_resistance/SAARS/bugs/menteroc.htm
[414] Lynn E. Hancock and Michael S. Gilmore. Department of Microbiology and Immunology, University of Oklahoma Health Sciences Center. Pathogenicity of Enterococci published in "Gram-Positive Pathogens" edited by Fischetti V et al. http://w3.ouhsc.edu/enterococcus/lynn_revirew.asp
[415] Galland L, Lee M. #170 High frequency of giardiasis in patients with chronic digestive complaints. *Am J Gastroenterol* 1989;84:1181
[416] Galland L. Intestinal protozoan infection is a common unsuspected cause of chronic illness. *J Advancement Med.* 1989;2: 539-552
[417] Corsi A, Nucci C, Knafelz D, Bulgarini D, Di Iorio L, Polito A, De Risi F, Ardenti Morini F, Paone FM. Ocular changes associated with Giardia lamblia infection in children. *Br J Ophthalmol.* 1998 Jan;82(1):59-62 http://bjo.bmjjournals.com/cgi/content/full/82/1/59

Microbe	Pathophysiology and clinical manifestations
Giardia lamblia [continued from previous page]	• **Ocular complications** from gastrointestinal infection include iridocyclitis, choroiditis, retinal hemorrhages, anterior and posterior uveitis, retinal vasculitis, and "salt and pepper" retinal degeneration. These complications are most likely due to deposition of **immune complexes** in the retinal epithelium.[418] • Reported to have caused numerous cases of **reactive arthritis (peripheral arthritis and/or sacroiliitis)** in patients who are either positive or negative for HLA-B27[419]; "beaver fever" is a cause of reactive arthritis.[420] • Antigen detection appears superior to microscopic examination for detection.[421]
Hafnia alvei	• *Hafnia alvei* is a gram-negative bacterium capable of causing **reactive arthritis** from gastrointestinal infection; the reactive arthritis associated with *Hafnia alvei* occurs without association with HLA-B27.[422]
Helicobacter pylori	• *H. pylori* is a gram-negative endotoxin-producing rod that causes stomach ulcers and appears to cause **reactive arthritis** in some patients.[423] • *H. pylori* colonization is increased in patients with **scleroderma.**[424] • *H. pylori* is commonly found in the middle ear of patients with acute otitis media.[425]
Klebsiella pneumoniae	• Many cases of gastrointestinal colonization with this microorganism produce no acute gastrointestinal symptoms such as nausea, vomiting, constipation, or diarrhea. Patients may have mild general symptoms such as fatigue and dyscognition ("brain fog"). • Can cause **diarrhea**[426] and **acute gastroenteritis.**[427] • Associated with **reactive arthritis** such as **ankylosing spondylitis.**[428] • Gram-negative bacteria, produces endotoxin/lipopolysaccharide that is capable of impairing cytochrome p-450 and **reducing hepatic clearance and urinary/biliary excretion of drugs.**[429]
Proteus mirabilis	• Gram-negative bacteria, produces endotoxin/lipopolysaccharide.[430] • Gastrointestinal and urinary tract colonization is associated with **rheumatoid arthritis**[431,432] and **ankylosing spondylitis.**[433] • In one of my patients, gastrointestinal dysbiosis with *Proteus* incited "**idiopathic inflammatory polyneuropathy**" that disappeared within one month of parasite eradication and which coincided with normalization of hsCRP.

[418] "The retinal changes associated with giardiasis are more than likely caused by immune mechanisms. Wania reported that circulating immune complexes were found in all of the patients with ocular complications he examined." Corsi A, Nucci C, Knafelz D, Bulgarini D, Di Iorio L, Polito A, De Risi F, Ardenti Morini F, Paone FM. Ocular changes associated with Giardia lamblia infection in children. *Br J Ophthalmol.* 1998 Jan;82(1):59-62 http://bjo.bmjjournals.com/cgi/content/full/82/1/59

[419] Layton MA, Dziedzic K, Dawes PT. Sacroiliitis in an HLA B27-negative patient following giardiasis. *Br J Rheumatol.* 1998 May;37(5):581-3 http://rheumatology.oxfordjournals.org/cgi/reprint/37/5/581

[420] "Giardia lamblia infection is rarely associated with adult reactive arthritis. We report the first North American case and review the pediatric and adult literature to date. Antimicrobial treatment is essential to eradicate the parasite and control the arthritis." Tupchong M, Simor A, Dewar C. Beaver fever--a rare cause of reactive arthritis. *J Rheumatol.* 1999 Dec;26(12):2701-2

[421] "For all patients, microscopy was uniformly negative, but 6 of 13 patients were antigen positive... Giardiasis, an increasing problem in family practice, should be considered early in patients with GI disturbances. New, sensitive immunodiagnostic tests that usually require a single specimen are more useful than microscopy." Chappell CL, Matson CC. Giardia antigen detection in patients with chronic gastrointestinal disturbances. *J Fam Pract.* 1992 Jul;35(1):49-53

[422] Toivanen P, Toivanen A. Two forms of reactive arthritis? *Ann Rheum Dis.* 1999 Dec;58(12):737-41 http://ard.bmjjournals.com/cgi/content/full/58/12/737 See also: Newmark JJ, Hobbs WN, Wilson BE. Reactive arthritis associated with Hafnia alvei enteritis. *Arthritis Rheum.* 1994 Jun;37(6):960

[423] "Our findings suggest that HP may be included in the list of possible arthritis triggering microbes." Melby KK, Kvien TK, Glennas A. Helicobacter pylori--a trigger of reactive arthritis? *Infection.* 1999;27(4-5):252-5

[424] "Patients with SSc have H. pylori infection at a higher prevalence than the general population." Yazawa N, Fujimoto M, Kikuchi K, Kubo M, Ihn H, Sato S, Tamaki T, Tamaki K. High seroprevalence of Helicobacter pylori infection in patients with systemic sclerosis: association with esophageal involvement. *J Rheumatol.* 1998 Apr;25(4):650-3

[425] "Twelve of 15 smears for MEE were positive for HP by immunohistochemistry and 14 by Giemsa that were Gram-negative." Morinaka S, Tominaga M, Nakamura H. Detection of Helicobacter pylori in the middle ear fluid of patients with otitis media with effusion. *Otolaryngol Head Neck Surg.* 2005 Nov;133(5):791-4

[426] Niyogi SK, Pal A, Mitra U, Dutta P. Enteroaggregative Klebsiella pneumoniae in association with childhood diarrhoea. *Indian J Med Res* 2000 Oct;112:133-4

[427] Ananthan, Raju S, Alavandi S. Enterotoxigenicity of Klebsiella pneumoniae associated with childhood gastroenteritis in Madras, India. *Jpn J Infect Dis* 1999 Feb;52(1):16-7

[428] Ahmadi K, Wilson C, Tiwana H, Binder A, Ebringer A. Antibodies to Klebsiella pneumoniae lipopolysaccharide in patients with ankylosing spondylitis. *Br J Rheumatol.* 1998 Dec;37(12):1330-3

[429] Hasegawa T, Takagi K, Kitaichi K. Effects of bacterial endotoxin on drug pharmacokinetics. *Nagoya J Med Sci* 1999 May;62(1-2):11-28

[430] Kondakova AN, Fudala R, Senchenkova SN, Shashkov AS, Knirel YA, Kaca W. Structural and serological studies of the O-antigen of Proteus mirabilis O-9. *Carbohydr Res* 2003 May 23;338(11):1191-6

[431] Ebringer A, Rashid T, Wilson C. Rheumatoid arthritis: proposal for the use of anti-microbial therapy in early cases. *Scand J Rheumatol* 2003;32(1):2-11

[432] Rashid T, Darlington G, Kjeldsen-Kragh J, Forre O, Collado A, Ebringer A. Proteus IgG antibodies and C-reactive protein in English, Norwegian and Spanish patients with rheumatoid arthritis. *Clin Rheumatol* 1999;18(3):190-5

[433] Wilson C, Rashid T, Tiwana H, Beyan H, Hughes L, Bansal S, Ebringer A, Binder A. Cytotoxicity responses to Peptide antigens in rheumatoid arthritis and ankylosing spondylitis. *J Rheumatol* 2003 May;30(5):972-8

Commonly Encountered Dysbiotic Microorganisms—*continued*

Microbe	*Pathophysiology and clinical manifestations*
Pseudomonas aeruginosa	• Many cases of gastrointestinal colonization with this microorganism produce no acute gastrointestinal symptoms such as nausea, vomiting, constipation, or diarrhea. Patients may have mild general symptoms such as fatigue and dyscognition ("brain fog"). • *Pseudomonas aeruginosa* is a gram-negative bacterium, produces endotoxin[434] and can cause antibiotic-associated diarrhea.[435,436] • Patients with **multiple sclerosis** show evidence of a heightened immune response against *Pseudomonas aeruginosa*, suggesting the possibility of immune cross-reactivity.[437]
Staphylococcus aureus *Staphylococcus epidermidis*	• **Any and all *Staphylococcus aureus* should be eradicated immediately due to the well-known inflammatory consequences of the toxins and superantigens this bacterium produces.** *Staphylococcus aureus* is a gram-positive bacterium, certain strains of which produce the toxic shock syndrome toxin-1 (TSST-1) that produces scalded skin syndrome, toxic shock syndrome, and food poisoning; other strains of *Staphylococcus aureus* that do not produce TSST-1 are also capable of causing toxic shock syndrome from colonization of bone, vagina, wounds, or rectum.[438] • Gastrointestinal colonization with *Staphylococcus aureus* is a known cause of **acute colitis**[439], and nasal carriage of this bacterium is documented in patients with several autoimmune disorders, including **Wegener's granulomatosis**[440], **systemic lupus erythematosus**[441] and **psoriasis**.[442, 443] • *Staphylococcus aureus* can trigger **reactive arthritis**.[444] • *Staphylococcus epidermidis* can trigger **reactive arthritis and sacroiliitis**.[445] • Patients with **Behcet's syndrome** commonly have skin lesions that are colonized by *Staphylococcus aureus*.[446] • Most (57%) of patients with **atopic dermatitis** show evidence of IgE-mediated histamine release (i.e., "allergy") to exotoxins secreted from *Staphylococcus aureus*, which commonly colonizes eczematous skin[447]; in other words: most eczema patients are allergic to their own dermal bacteria and can thus be said to have *hypersensitivity dermal dysbiosis*.

[434] Bergan T. Pathogenetic factors of Pseudomonas aeruginosa. *Scand J Infect Dis Suppl.* 1981;29:7-12

[435] Kim SW, Peck KR, Jung SI, Kim YS, Kim S, Lee NY, Song JH. Pseudomonas aeruginosa as a potential cause of antibiotic-associated diarrhea. *J Korean Med Sci.* 2001 Dec;16(6):742-4

[436] Porco FV, Visconte EB. Pseudomonas aeruginosa as a cause of infectious diarrhea successfully treated with oral ciprofloxacin. *Ann Pharmacother.* 1995 Nov;29(11):1122-3

[437] Hughes LE, Bonell S, Natt RS, Wilson C, Tiwana H, Ebringer A, Cunningham P, Chamoun V, Thompson EJ, Croker J, Vowles J. Antibody responses to Acinetobacter spp. and Pseudomonas aeruginosa in multiple sclerosis: prospects for diagnosis using the myelin-acinetobacter-neurofilament antibody index. *Clin Diagn Lab Immunol.* 2001 Nov;8(6):1181-8

[438] Shandera WX, Moran A. "Infectious diseases: viral and rickettsial." In Tierney LM, McPhee SJ Papadakis MA (eds). Current Medical Diagnosis and Treatment. 44th edition. New York: Lange; 2005, page 1356-8

[439] Watanabe H, Masaki H, Asoh N, Watanabe K, Oishi K, Kobayashi S, Sato A, Nagatake T. Enterocolitis caused by methicillin-resistant Staphylococcus aureus: molecular characterization of respiratory and digestive tract isolates. *Microbiol Immunol.* 2001;45(9):629-34 http://www.jstage.jst.go.jp/article/mandi/45/9/629/_pdf

[440] Popa ER, Stegeman CA, Kallenberg CG, Tervaert JW. Staphylococcus aureus and Wegener's granulomatosis. *Arthritis Res.* 2002;4(2):77-9 http://arthritis-research.com/content/4/2/077

[441] Medline abstract from Polish research: "In 9 from 14 patients with (64.3%) a.b. very massive growth of Staphylococcus aureus in culture from vestibulae of the nose swab was, in other cultures very massive growth of physiological flora was seen. ...clinical significance of asymptomatic bacteriuria and pathogenic bacteria colonisation of nostrils as a precedence to symptomatic infections needs further investigations." Koseda-Dragan M, Hebanowski M, Galinski J, Krzywinska E, Bakowska A. [Asymptomatic bacteriuria in women diagnosed with systemic lupus erythematosus (SLE)] *Pol Arch Med Wewn.* 1998 Oct;100(4):321-30.

[442] "The nasal carriage rate of Staphylococcus aureus in psoriatics was higher than the control groups." Singh G, Rao DJ. Bacteriology of psoriatic plaques. *Dermatologica.* 1978;157(1):21-7

[443] "In this study, S aureus was present in more than 50% of patients with AD and PS. We found that the severity of AD and PS significantly correlated to enterotoxin production of the isolated S aureus strains." Tomi NS, Kranke B, Aberer E. Staphylococcal toxins in patients with psoriasis, atopic dermatitis, and erythroderma, and in healthy control subjects. *J Am Acad Dermatol.* 2005 Jul;53(1):67-72

[444] "CONCLUSION--Reactive arthritis may rarely follow Staph aureus infection. HLA-B27 negativity may be associated with a self limited arthritis in these cases." Siam AR, Hammoudeh M. Staphylococcus aureus triggered reactive arthritis. *Ann Rheum Dis.* 1995 Feb;54(2):131-3

[445] "We report an unusual case of a patient with SE bacteriaemia, who developed elbow arthritis, asymmetrical sacroiliitis, keratoderma and restrictive cardiomyopathy." Giordano N, Senesi M, Battisti E, Palumbo F, Mondillo S, Bargagli G, Palazzuoli V, Nardi P, Gennari C. Reactive arthritis by staphylococcus epidermidis: report of an unusual case. *Clin Rheumatol.* 1996;15(1):59-61

[446] "At least one type of microorganism was grown from each pustule. Staphylococcus aureus (41/70, 58.6%, p = 0.008) and Prevotella spp (17/70, 24.3%, p = 0.002) were significantly more common in pustules from BS patients, and coagulase negative staphylococci (17/37, 45.9%, p = 0.007) in pustules from acne patients. CONCLUSIONS: The pustular lesions of BS are not usually sterile." Hatemi G, Bahar H, Uysal S, Mat C, Gogus F, Masatlioglu S, Altas K, Yazici H. The pustular skin lesions in Behcet's syndrome are not sterile. *Ann Rheum Dis.* 2004 Nov;63(11):1450-2

[447] "These data indicate that a subset of patients with AD mount an IgE response to SEs that can be grown from their skin." Leung DY, Harbeck R, Bina P, Reiser RF, Yang E, Norris DA, Hanifin JM, Sampson HA. Presence of IgE antibodies to staphylococcal exotoxins on the skin of patients with atopic dermatitis. Evidence for a new group of allergens. *J Clin Invest.* 1993 Sep;92(3):1374-80 http://www.pubmedcentral.gov/articlerender.fcgi?tool=pubmed&pubmedid=7690780

Commonly encountered dysbiotic microorganisms—*continued*

Dysbiotic microbe	Pathophysiology and clinical manifestations
Streptococcus pyogenes *Group A streptococci*	• Intestinal overgrowth of this bacterium, which produces peptidoglycans, can cause **dermatosis, <u>inflammatory polyarthritis</u>, tenosynovitis, malaise, fever, and cryoglobulinemia**.[448] • Non-infectious manifestations precipitated by infection with *S. pyogenes* include **autoimmune neuropsychiatric disorders** (including obsessive-compulsive disorder and Sydenham's chorea), **dystonia, glomerulonephritis, and reactive arthritis**.[449] • Group A streptococci can cause **reactive arthritis** in humans.[450] • *Streptococcus pyogenes* is a very likely trigger of **psoriasis**[451]; chronic penicillin treatment leads to clinical improvement of recalcitrant psoriasis.[452] • Certain strains of *S. pyogenes* produce an exotoxin that can cause toxic shock syndrome.[453]

Clinical Benefits of Identifying and Eradicating Dysbiosis

In the previous section, I described the biochemical/physiologic mechanisms by which microorganisms can contribute to disease *without causing a classic "infection"* and promote systemic inflammation and human disease. Thus having developed the precept that **microorganisms can cause inflammatory disease by noninfectious means**, I will (re)state here that the cure of human disease by eradication of harmful microbes is not a requirement to prove the validity of this thesis. Inflammation and autoimmunity are self-perpetuating phenomena that can persist despite the effective eradication of the principle cause, and research has demonstrated that microbial antigens can remain present in synovial fluid for several years after the eradication of the primary infection.[454] With that said, we are fortunate to observe that **many patients with autoimmunity are indeed benefited and occasionally "cured" by removal of instigating microbes**. I have seen this on numerous occasions in my clinical practice, and this phenomenon has also been documented in the research literature. Examples published in the research include the amelioration of one patient's scleroderma with the eradication of intestinal bacterial overgrowth[455], the amelioration of Wegener's granulomatosis with antimicrobial therapy against *Staphylococcus aureus*[456,457], and the alleviation of inflammatory arthritis following the use of antibiotics against genitourinary *Chlamydia trachomatis* and gastrointestinal *Salmonella enteritidis*, *Yersinia enterocolitica*, *Shigella flexneri* or *Campylobacter jejuni*.[458] Treatments for addressing dysbiosis and its numerous sequelae are described in the pages that follow.

> "We have repeatedly observed psoriatic flares associated with microbial infection, sequestered antigen, and colonization.
>
> **Removal of these microbial foci results in clearing of the disease.**"
>
> Patricia Noah PhD from University of Tennessee College of Medicine. *Semin Dermatol.* 1990;9:269

---

[448] Ely PH. The bowel bypass syndrome: a response to bacterial peptidoglycans. *J Am Acad Dermatol.* 1980 Jun;2(6):473-87

[449] Hahn RG, Knox LM, Forman TA. Evaluation of poststreptococcal illness. *Am Fam Physician.* 2005 May 15;71(10):1949-54 http://www.aafp.org/afp/20050515/1949.pdf

[450] "We present a patient whose clinical features are more consistent with post-streptococcal reactive arthritis than acute rheumatic fever." Howell EE, Bathon J. A case of post-streptococcal reactive arthritis. *Md Med J.* 1999 Nov-Dec;48(6):292-4

[451] "These findings justify the hypothesis that S pyogenes infections are more important in the pathogenesis of chronic plaque psoriasis than has previously been recognized, and indicate the need for further controlled therapeutic trials of antibacterial measures in this common skin disease." El-Rachkidy RG, Hales JM, Freestone PP, Young HS, Griffiths CE, Camp RD. Increased Blood Levels of IgG Reactive with Secreted Streptococcus pyogenes Proteins in Chronic Plaque Psoriasis. *J Invest Dermatol.* 2007 Mar 8; [Epub ahead of print]

[452] "Total duration of the study was two years. Initially benzathine penicillin 1.2 million units, was given I.M. AST fortnightly. After 24 weeks benzathine penicillin was reduced to 1.2 million units once a month... Significant improvement in the PASI score was noted from 12 weeks onwards. All patients showed excellent improvement at 2 years." Saxena VN, Dogra J. Long-term use of penicillin for the treatment of chronic plaque psoriasis. *Eur J Dermatol.* 2005 Sep-Oct;15(5):359-62 http://www.john-libbey-eurotext.fr/en/revues/medecine/ejd/e-docs/00/04/10/A4/article.md?type=text.html

[453] Chikkamuniyappa S. Streptococcal toxic shock syndrome and sepsis manifesting in a patient with chronic rheumatoid arthritis. *Dermatol Online J.* 2004 Jul 15;10(1):7

[454] "Extensive bacterial cultures of the synovial fluid were negative... We conclude that in patients with reactive arthritis after yersinia infection, microbial antigens can be found in synovial-fluid cells from the affected joints." Granfors K, Jalkanen S, von Essen R, Lahesmaa-Rantala R, Isomaki O, Pekkola-Heino K, Merilahti-Palo R, Saario R, Isomaki H, Toivanen A. Yersinia antigens in synovial-fluid cells from patients with reactive arthritis. *N Engl J Med.* 1989 Jan 26;320(4):216-2

[455] Over KE, Bucknall RC. Regression of skin changes in a patient with systemic sclerosis following treatment for bacterial overgrowth with ciprofloxacin. *Br J Rheumatol.* 1998 Jun;37(6):696

[456] Popa ER, Stegeman CA, Kallenberg CG, Tervaert JW. Staphylococcus aureus and Wegener's granulomatosis. *Arthritis Res.* 2002;4(2):77-9 http://arthritis-research.com/content/4/2/077

[457] George J, Levy Y, Kallenberg CG, Shoenfeld Y. Infections and Wegener's granulomatosis--a cause and effect relationship? *QJM.* 1997 May;90(5):367-73 http://qjmed.oxfordjournals.org/cgi/reprint/90/5/367

[458] Kobayashi S, Kida I. Reactive arthritis: recent advances and clinical manifestations. *Intern Med.* 2005 May;44(5):408-12 http://www.jstage.jst.go.jp/article/internalmedicine/44/5/408/_pdf

Natural Treatments for the Eradication of Dysbiosis and Related Immune-complex Diseases

Although antimicrobial drugs may be used, these are not universally curative and are not necessarily "more powerful" or "more effective" than natural treatments. Treatments for gastrointestinal dysbiosis may be somewhat summarized as follows: "*Starve, Poison, Crowd, Purge, and Support Immunity*." The following concepts and therapeutics are particularly—though not exclusively—relevant for the treatment of *gastrointestinal* dysbiosis.

1. **Diet modifications ("*starve the microbes*")**: The diet plan should ensure **avoidance of sugar**, grains, soluble fiber, gums, prebiotics, and dairy products since these contain **fermentable carbohydrates that promote overgrowth of bacteria and other microorganisms in the gut**. Short-term **fasting** starves intestinal microbes, temporarily eliminates dietary antigens, alleviates "autointoxication", and stimulates the humoral immune system in the gut to more effectively destroy local microbes.[459,460] Thus, implementation of the "**specific carbohydrate diet**" popularized by Gottschall[461] along with periodic fasting, which has obvious anti-inflammatory benefits[462], can be used therapeutically in patients with conditions associated with dysbiosis-induced inflammation. Plant-based low-carbohydrate diets can lead to favorable changes in the quality and quantity of intestinal microflora. Hypoallergenic diets are proven beneficial for the treatment of the **immune complex disease** called mixed cryoglobulinemia.[463,464]

2. **Antimicrobial treatments ("*poison the microbes, not the patient*")**: Anti-microbial herbs can be used which directly kill or strongly inhibit the intestinal microbes. The most commonly used and well-documented botanicals in this regard are listed in the section below. Antimicrobial treatment is frequently continued for 1-3 months, and co-administration of drugs can be utilized when appropriate. Sometimes antimicrobial drugs are necessary, especially for acute and severe infections; often nutritional and botanical interventions are safer and more effective. Although these herbs are generally taken orally, some of them can also be applied topically (in a cream or lotion), and nasally (in a saline water lavage, as detailed previously). Botanical medicines are generally used in combination, and lower doses of each can be used when used in combination compared to the doses that are necessary when the herbs are used in isolation.

   - **Oregano oil in an emulsified and time-released tablet**: Botanical oils that are not emulsified do not attain maximal dispersion in the gastrointestinal tract; products that are not time-released may be absorbed before reaching the colon in sufficient concentrations. Emulsified oil of oregano in a time-released tablet is proven effective in the eradication of harmful gastrointestinal microbes, including *Blastocystis hominis*, *Entamoeba hartmanni*, and *Endolimax nana*.[465] An in vitro study[466] and clinical experience support the use of emulsified oregano against *Candida albicans*. The common dose is 600 mg per day in divided doses for at least 6 weeks.[467]

   - **Berberine**: Berberine is an alkaloid extracted from plant such as *Berberis vulgaris*, and *Hydrastis canadensis*, and it shows effectiveness against *Giardia*, *Candida*, and *Streptococcus* in addition to its direct anti-inflammatory and antidiarrheal actions. Oral dose of 400 mg per day is common for adults.[468] Topical *Mahonia/Berberis aquifolium* is effective for dermal psoriasis[469] via its combined anti-inflammatory and antimicrobial benefits.

[459] Trollmo C, Verdrengh M, Tarkowski A. Fasting enhances mucosal antigen specific B cell responses in rheumatoid arthritis. *Ann Rheum Dis*. 1997 Feb;56(2):130-4

[460] Ramakrishnan T, Stokes P. Beneficial effects of fasting and low carbohydrate diet in D-lactic acidosis associated with short-bowel syndrome. *JPEN J Parenter Enteral Nutr*. 1985 May-Jun;9(3):361-3

[461] Gottschall E. Breaking the Vicious Cycle: Intestinal Health Through Diet. Kirkton Press; Rev edition (August 1, 1994)

[462] "The pooling of these studies showed a statistically and clinically significant beneficial long-term effect." Muller H, de Toledo FW, Resch KL. Fasting followed by vegetarian diet in patients with rheumatoid arthritis: a systematic review. *Scand J Rheumatol*. 2001;30(1):1-10

[463] "CONCLUSION: These data show that an LAC diet decreases the amount of circulating immune complexes in MC and can modify certain signs and symptoms of the disease." Ferri C, Pietrogrande M, Cecchetti R, et al. Low-antigen-content diet in the treatment of patients with mixed cryoglobulinemia. *Am J Med*. 1989 Nov;87(5):519-24

[464] Pietrogrande M, Cefalo A, Nicora F, Marchesini D. Dietetic treatment of essential mixed cryoglobulinemia. *Ric Clin Lab*. 1986 Apr-Jun;16(2):413-6

[465] Force M, Sparks WS, Ronzio RA. Inhibition of enteric parasites by emulsified oil of oregano in vivo. *Phytother Res*. 2000 May;14(3):213-4

[466] Stiles JC, Sparks W, Ronzio RA. The inhibition of Candida albicans by oregano. *J Applied Nutr* 1995;47:96–102

[467] Force M, Sparks WS, Ronzio RA. Inhibition of enteric parasites by emulsified oil of oregano in vivo. *Phytother Res*. 2000 May;14(3):213-4

[468] Berberine. Altern Med Rev. 2000 Apr;5(2):175-7 http://www.thorne.com/altmedrev/.fulltext/5/2/175.pdf

[469] "Taken together, these clinical studies conducted by several investigators in several countries indicate that Mahonia aquifolium is a safe and effective treatment of patients with mild to moderate psoriasis." Gulliver WP, Donsky HJ. A report on three recent clinical trials using Mahonia aquifolium 10% topical cream and a review of the worldwide clinical experience with Mahonia aquifolium for the treatment of plaque psoriasis. *Am J Ther*. 2005 Sep-Oct;12(5):398-406

- *Artemisia annua*: Artemisinin has been safely used for centuries in Asia for the treatment of malaria[470,471], and it also has **effectiveness against anaerobic bacteria** due to the pro-oxidative sesquiterpene endoperoxide. In a recent study treating patients with malaria, "the adult artemisinin dose was 500 mg; children aged < 15 years received 10 mg/kg per dose" and thus the dose for an 80-lb child would be 363 mg per day by these criteria.[472] I commonly use **artemisinin at 100 mg twice per day (with other antimicrobial botanicals such as berberine) in divided doses for adults with dysbiosis.** One of the additional benefits of artemisinin is its systemic bioavailability.

- St. John's Wort (*Hypericum perforatum*): Best known for its antidepressant action, **hyperforin from *Hypericum perforatum* also shows impressive antibacterial action, particularly against gram-positive bacteria such as *Staphylococcus aureus*, *Streptococcus pyogenes* and *Streptococcus agalactiae*.** According to in vitro studies, the lowest effective hyperforin concentration is 0.1 mcg/mL against *Corynebacterium diphtheriae* with increasing effectiveness against multiresistant *Staphylococcus aureus* at higher concentrations of 100 mcg/mL.[473] Since oral dosing with hyperforin can result in serum levels of 500 nanogram /mL (equivalent to 0.5 microgram/mL) then it is possible that high-dose hyperforin will have systemic antibacterial action. Regardless of its possible systemic antibacterial effectiveness, **hyperforin should clearly have antibacterial action when applied "topically" such as when it is taken orally against gastric and upper intestinal colonization.** Extracts from St. John's Wort hold particular promise against multidrug-resistant *Staphylococcus aureus*[474] and perhaps *Helicobacter pylori*.[475]

- **Myrrh (*Commiphora molmol*)**: Myrrh is remarkably effective against parasitic infections.[476] A recent clinical trial against **schistosomiasis**[477] showed "The parasitological cure rate after three months was 97.4% and 96.2% for *S. haematobium* and *S. mansoni* cases with the marvelous clinical cure without any side-effects."[478]

- **Bismuth**: Bismuth is commonly used in the empiric treatment of diarrhea (e.g., "Pepto-<u>Bismol</u>") and is commonly combined with other antimicrobial agents to reduce drug resistance and increase antibiotic effectiveness.[479]

- **Peppermint (*Mentha piperita*)**: Peppermint shows antimicrobial and antispasmodic actions and has demonstrated clinical effectiveness in patients with bacterial overgrowth of the small bowel.

- **Uva Ursi**: Uva ursi can be used against gastrointestinal pathogens on a limited basis per culture and sensitivity findings; its primary historical and modern use is as a urinary antiseptic which is effective only when the urine pH is alkaline.[480] Components of uva ursi potentiate antibiotics.[481] **This herb has some ocular and neurologic toxicity and should be used with professional supervision for low-dose and/or short-term administration only.**[482]

- **Garlic**: Garlic shows *in vitro* antimicrobial action against numerous microorganisms, including *H. pylori*, *Pseudomonas aeruginosa*, and *Candida albicans*, and this effect is mediated *directly* via microbicidal actions as well as *indirectly* via dissolution of microbial biofilms[483] and inhibition of quorum sensing.[484] However, since the antimicrobial components of garlic are likely absorbed in the upper gastrointestinal tract, I propose that it is unlikely that garlic can exert a clinically significant anti-

[470] Dien TK, de Vries PJ, Khanh NX, Koopmans R, Binh LN, Duc DD, Kager PA, van Boxtel CJ. Effect of food intake on pharmacokinetics of oral artemisinin in healthy Vietnamese subjects. *Antimicrob Agents Chemother.* 1997 May;41(5):1069-72

[471] Giao PT, Binh TQ, Kager PA, Long HP, Van Thang N, Van Nam N, de Vries PJ. Artemisinin for treatment of uncomplicated falciparum malaria: is there a place for monotherapy? *Am J Trop Med Hyg.* 2001 Dec;65(6):690-5

[472] Giao PT, Binh TQ, Kager PA, Long HP, Van Thang N, Van Nam N, de Vries PJ. Artemisinin for treatment of uncomplicated falciparum malaria: is there a place for monotherapy? *Am J Trop Med Hyg.* 2001 Dec;65(6):690-5 http://www.ajtmh.org/cgi/reprint/65/6/690

[473] Schempp CM, Pelz K, Wittmer A, Schopf E, Simon JC. Antibacterial activity of hyperforin from St John's wort, against multiresistant Staphylococcus aureus and gram-positive bacteria. *Lancet.* 1999 Jun 19;353(9170):2129

[474] Gibbons S, Ohlendorf B, Johnsen I. The genus Hypericum--a valuable resource of anti-Staphylococcal leads. *Fitoterapia.* 2002 Jul;73(4):300-4

[475] "A butanol fraction of St. John's Wort revealed anti-Helicobacter pylori activity with MIC values ranging between 15.6 and 31.2 microg/ml." Reichling J, Weseler A, Saller R. A current review of the antimicrobial activity of Hypericum perforatum L. *Pharmacopsychiatry.* 2001 Jul;34 Suppl 1:S116-8

[476] El Baz MA, Morsy TA, El Bandary MM, Motawea SM. Clinical and parasitological studies on the efficacy of Mirazid in treatment of schistosomiasis haematobium in Tatoon, Etsa Center, El Fayoum Governorate. *J Egypt Soc Parasitol.* 2003 Dec;33(3):761-76

[477] Schistosomiasis. http://www.dpd.cdc.gov/dpdx/HTML/Schistosomiasis.htm

[478] Abo-Madyan AA, Morsy TA, Motawea SM. Efficacy of Myrrh in the treatment of schistosomiasis (haematobium and mansoni) in Ezbet El-Bakly, Tamyia Center, El-Fayoum Governorate, Egypt. *J Egypt Soc Parasitol.* 2004 Aug;34(2):423-46

[479] Veldhuyzen van Zanten SJ, Sherman PM, Hunt RH. Helicobacter pylori: new developments and treatments. *CMAJ.* 1997;156(11):1565-74 http://www.cmaj.ca/cgi/reprint/156/11/1565.pdf

[480] Yarnell E. Botanical medicines for the urinary tract. *World J Urol.* 2002 Nov;20(5):285-93

[481] Shimizu M, Shiota S, Mizushima T, Ito H, Hatano T, Yoshida T, Tsuchiya T. Marked potentiation of activity of beta-lactams against methicillin-resistant Staphylococcus aureus by corilagin. *Antimicrob Agents Chemother.* 2001 Nov;45(11):3198-201 http://aac.asm.org/cgi/reprint/45/11/3198

[482] "A 56-year-old woman who ingested uva ursi for 3 years noted a decrease in visual acuity within the past year. Ocular examination including fluorescein angiography revealed a typical bull's-eye maculopathy bilaterally." Wang L, Del Priore LV. Bull's-eye maculopathy secondary to herbal toxicity from uva ursi. *Am J Ophthalmol.* 2004 Jun;137(6):1135-7

[483] "Sub-MICs of allicin also diminished the biofilm formations by S. epidermidis." Perez-Giraldo C, Cruz-Villalon G, Sanchez-Silos R, Martinez-Rubio R, Blanco MT, Gomez-Garcia AC. In vitro activity of allicin against Staphylococcus epidermidis and influence of subinhibitory concentrations on biofilm formation. *J Appl Microbiol.* 2003;95(4):709-11

[484] "The results indicate that a QS-inhibitory extract of garlic renders P. aeruginosa sensitive to tobramycin, respiratory burst and phagocytosis by PMNs, as well as leading to an improved outcome of pulmonary infections." Bjarnsholt T, Jensen PO, Rasmussen TB, Christophersen L, Calum H, Hentzer M, Hougen HP, Rygaard J, Moser C, Eberl L, Hoiby N, Givskov M. Garlic blocks quorum sensing and promotes rapid clearing of pulmonary Pseudomonas aeruginosa infections. *Microbiology.* 2005 Dec;151(Pt 12):3873-80. The in vivo portion of this study was performed in animals, not humans.

dysbiotic effect in the lower small intestine and colon. In fact, two studies in humans have shown that—despite its *in vitro* effectiveness against *H. pylori*—garlic is ineffective in the treatment of gastric *H. pylori* colonization.[485,486] While these studies argue against the use of garlic as antimicrobial monotherapy, the possibility remains that garlic may enhance the clinical effectiveness of other antimicrobial therapeutics via its aforementioned ability to weaken microbial biofilms and to impair quorum sensing, which otherwise serve to protect yeast/bacteria from immune attack and from antibacterial/antifungal therapeutics.

- **Cranberry**: Particularly effective for the prevention and adjunctive treatment of urinary tract infections, mostly by inhibiting adherence of *E. coli* to epithelial cells.[487]

- **Thyme (*Thymus vulgaris*)**: Thyme extracts have direct antimicrobial actions and also potentiate the effectiveness of tetracycline against drug-resistant *Staphylococcus aureus*.[488] Thyme also appears effective against *Aeromonas hydrophila*.[489]

- **Clove (*Syzygium* species)**: Clove's eugenol has been shown in animal studies to have a potent antifungal effect.[490]

- **Anise**: Although it has weak antibacterial action when used alone, anise does show in vitro activity against molds.[491]

- **Buchu/betulina**: Buchu has a long history of use against urinary tract infections and systemic infections.[492]

- **Caprylic acid and undecylenic acid**: Caprylic acid is a medium chain fatty acid that is commonly used in patients with dysbiosis, particularly that which has a fungal/yeast component. Beside empiric use, caprylic acid may be indicated by culture-sensitivity results provided with comprehensive parasitology. When bacterial/fungal sensitivity tests indicate caprylic acid, many clinicians prefer to use undecylenic acid which is reportedly up to six times more powerful than caprylic acid.[493] Commercial preparations delivering 50 mg undecylenic acid per gelcap can be taken orally in doses of 3-5 gelcaps three times per day. Anti-candidal action has been reported[494], and my impression is that undecylenic acid is among the more valuable therapeutics in the treatment of gastrointestinal dysbiosis.

- **Dill (*Anethum graveolens*)**: Dill shows activity against several types of mold and yeast.[495]

- ***Brucea javanica***: Extract from *Brucea javanica* fruit shows *in vitro* activity against *Babesia gibsoni*, *Plasmodium falciparum*[496], *Entamoeba histolytica*[497] and *Blastocystis hominis*.[498,499]

- ***Acacia catechu***: Acacia catechu shows moderate *in vitro* activity against *Salmonella typhi*.[500]

[485] "This study did not support a role for either garlic or jalapenos in the treatment of H. pylori infection. Caution must be used when attempting to extrapolate data from in vitro studies to the in vivo condition." Graham DY, Anderson SY, Lang T. Garlic or jalapeno peppers for treatment of Helicobacter pylori infection. *Am J Gastroenterol*. 1999 May;94(5):1200-2

[486] "Five patients completed the study. There was no evidence of either eradication or suppression of H. pylori or symptom improvement whilst taking garlic oil." McNulty CA, Wilson MP, Havinga W, Johnston B, O'Gara EA, Maslin DJ. A pilot study to determine the effectiveness of garlic oil capsules in the treatment of dyspeptic patients with Helicobacter pylori. *Helicobacter*. 2001 Sep;6(3):249-53

[487] Lynch DM. Cranberry for prevention of urinary tract infections. *Am Fam Physician*. 2004 Dec 1;70(11):2175-7 http://www.aafp.org/afp/20041201/2175.pdf

[488] Fujita M, Shiota S, Kuroda T, Hatano T, Yoshida T, Mizushima T, Tsuchiya T. Remarkable synergies between baicalein and tetracycline, and baicalein and beta-lactams against methicillin-resistant Staphylococcus aureus. *Microbiol Immunol*. 2005;49(4):391-6

[489] "...thyme essential oil showed the greatest inhibition against A. hydrophila." Fabio A, Corona A, Forte E, Quaglio P. Inhibitory activity of spices and essential oils on psychrotrophic bacteria. *New Microbiol*. 2003 Jan;26(1):115-20

[490] Chami N, Chami F, Bennis S, Trouillas J, Remmal A. Antifungal treatment with carvacrol and eugenol of oral candidiasis in immunosuppressed rats. *Braz J Infect Dis*. 2004 Jun;8(3):217-26 http://www.scielo.br/pdf/bjid/v8n3/21619.pdf

[491] "Anise oil was not particularly inhibitory to bacteria (inhibition zone, approximately 25 mm); however, anise oil was highly inhibitory to molds." Elgayyar M, Draughon FA, Golden DA, Mount JR. Antimicrobial activity of essential oils from plants against selected pathogenic and saprophytic microorganisms. *J Food Prot*. 2001 Jul;64(7):1019-24

[492] "Buchu preparations are now used as a diuretic and for a wide range of conditions including stomach aches, rheumatism, bladder and kidney infections and coughs and colds." Simpson D. Buchu--South Africa's amazing herbal remedy. *Scott Med J* 1998 Dec;43(6):189-91

[493] Undecylenic acid. Monograph. *Altern Med Rev*. 2002 Feb;7(1):68-70 http://www.thorne.com/altmedrev/.fulltext/7/1/68.pdf

[494] McLain N, Ascanio R, Baker C, Strohaver RA, Dolan JW. Undecylenic acid inhibits morphogenesis of Candida albicans. *Antimicrob Agents Chemother*. 2000 Oct;44(10):2873-5 http://aac.asm.org/cgi/content/full/44/10/2873?view=long&pmid=10991877

[495] "Antimicrobial testings showed high activity of the essential A. graveolens oil against the mold Aspergillus niger and the yeasts Saccharomyces cerevisiae and Candida albicans." Jirovetz L, Buchbauer G, Stoyanova AS, Georgiev EV, Damianova ST. Composition, quality control, and antimicrobial activity of the essential oil of long-time stored dill (Anethum graveolens L.) seeds from Bulgaria. *J Agric Food Chem*. 2003 Jun 18;51(13):3854-7

[496] Murnigsih T, Subeki, Matsuura H, et al. Evaluation of the inhibitory activities of the extracts of Indonesian traditional medicinal plants against Plasmodium falciparum and Babesia gibsoni. *J Vet Med Sci*. 2005 Aug;67(8):829-31 http://www.jstage.jst.go.jp/article/jvms/67/8/829/_pdf

[497] Wright CW, O'Neill MJ, Phillipson JD, Warhurst DC. Use of microdilution to assess in vitro antiamoebic activities of Brucea javanica fruits, Simarouba amara stem, and a number of quassinoids. *Antimicrob Agents Chemother*. 1988 Nov;32(11):1725-9 http://www.pubmedcentral.gov/articlerender.fcgi?tool=pubmed&pubmedid=2908094

[498] "Dichloromethane and methanol extracts from the Brucea javanica seed and a methanol extract from Quercus infectoria nut gall showed the highest activity." Sawangjaroen N, Sawangjaroen K. The effects of extracts from anti-diarrheic Thai medicinal plants on the in vitro growth of the intestinal protozoa parasite: Blastocystis hominis. *J Ethnopharmacol*. 2005 Apr 8;98(1-2):67-72

[499] "The crude extracts of Coptis chinensis (CC) and Brucea javanica (BJ) were found to be most active against B. hominis." Yang LQ, Singh M, Yap EH, Ng GC, Xu HX, Sim KY. In vitro response of Blastocystis hominis against traditional Chinese medicine. *J Ethnopharmacol*. 1996 Dec;55(1):35-42

[500] "Moderate antimicrobial activity was shown by Picorhiza kurroa, Acacia catechu, ..." Rani P, Khullar N. Antimicrobial evaluation of some medicinal plants for their anti-enteric potential against multi-drug resistant Salmonella typhi. *Phytother Res*. 2004 Aug;18(8):670-3

3. _Oral administration of proteolytic enzymes_: The use of polyenzyme therapy in patients with dysbiotic inflammation is justified for at least four reasons. First, orally administered proteolytic enzymes are efficiently absorbed by the gastrointestinal tract into the systemic circulation[501] to then provide a **clinically significant anti-inflammatory benefit** as I reviewed recently.[502] Second and more specifically, oral administration of proteolytic enzymes is generally believed to effect a **reduction in immune complexes and their clinical consequences**[503], and immune complexes are probably a major mechanism of dysbiosis-induced disease and are pathogenic in rheumatoid arthritis[504] and many other autoimmune diseases such as systemic lupus erythematosus, dermatomyositis, Sjogren's syndrome, and polyarteritis nodosa.[505] Third, proteolytic enzymes have been shown to **stimulate immune function**[506] and may thereby promote clearance of occult infections. Fourth, **proteolytic enzymes inhibit formation of microbial biofilms** and increase immune penetration and the effectiveness of antimicrobial therapeutics.[507] Although individual enzymes may be used in isolation, enzyme therapy is generally delivered in the form of polyenzyme preparations containing pancreatin, bromelain, papain, amylase, lipase, trypsin and alpha-chymotrypsin.[508]

4. **Probiotic supplementation ("_crowd out the bad with the good_")**: Given that "healthy" intestinal bacteria can alleviate disease and promote normal immune function[509], then it is conversely true that a condition of harmful or suboptimal intestinal bacteria could promote disease and lead to immune dysfunction. For patients with gastrointestinal and genitourinary dysbiosis, supplementation with _Bifidobacteria, Lactobacillus_, and perhaps _Saccharomyces_ and other beneficial strains is mandatory. The wide-ranging and well-documented benefits seen with probiotic supplementation provide direct support for the importance of microbial balance in health and disease. Supplementation with probiotics (live bacteria) is the best option, however prebiotics (such as fructooligosaccarides), and synbiotics (probiotics + prebiotics) may also be used. Synbiotic supplementation has been shown to reduce endotoxinemia and clinical symptoms in 50% of patients with minimal hepatic encephalopathy[510], and probiotic supplementation safely ameliorated the adverse effects of bacterial overgrowth in a clinical study of patients with renal failure.[511]

5. **Immunonutrition**: Obviously, the diet should be nutritious and free of sugars and other "junk foods" that promote inflammation and suppress immune function.[512] Especially in patients with gastrointestinal dysbiosis, vitamin and mineral supplementation should be used to counteract the effects of malabsorption, maldigestion, and hypermetabolism that accompany immune activation. Additionally, oral glutamine in doses of six grams three times daily can help normalize intestinal permeability, enhance immune function, and improve clinical outcomes in severely ill patients.[513] Zinc and vitamin A supplementation are each well known to support immune function against infection. Selenium has anti-inflammatory and antiviral actions.[514] Vitamin D supplementation reduces inflammation, protects against autoimmunity, and promotes immunity against viral and bacterial infections.[515] Supplementation with IgG from bovine colostrum can also provide benefit

[501] Liebow C, Rothman SS. Enteropancreatic Circulation of Digestive Enzymes. _Science_ 1975; 189(4201): 472-474

[502] Vasquez A. Reducing pain and inflammation naturally - Part 3: Improving overall health while safely and effectively treating musculoskeletal pain. _Nutritional Perspectives_ 2005; 28: 34-38, 40-42 http://optimalhealthresearch.com/part3

[503] Galebskaya LV, Ryumina EV, Niemerovsky VS, Matyukov AA. Human complement system state after wobenzyme intake. _VESTNIK MOSKOVSKOGO UNIVERSITETA. KHIMIYA._ 2000. Vol. 41, No. 6. Supplement. Pages 148-149

[504] Edwards JC, Cambridge G. Rheumatoid arthritis: the predictable effect of small immune complexes in which antibody is also antigen. _Br J Rheumatol._ 1998 Feb;37(2):126-30 http://rheumatology.oxfordjournals.org/cgi/reprint/37/2/126

[505] Jancar S, Sanchez Crespo M. Immune complex-mediated tissue injury: a multistep paradigm. _Trends Immunol._ 2005 Jan;26(1):48-55 http://www.i3u.org/i3u-papers/MSC-2005-TIMM.pdf

[506] Zavadova E, Desser L, Mohr T. Stimulation of reactive oxygen species production and cytotoxicity in human neutrophils in vitro and after oral administration of a polyenzyme preparation. _Cancer Biother._ 1995 Summer;10(2):147-52

[507] "The enzymes were shown to inhibit the biofilm formation. When appliilied to the formed associations, the enzymes potentiated the effect of antibiotics on the bacteria located in them." Tets VV, Knorring GIu, Artemenko NK, Zaslavskaia NV, Artemenko KL. [Impact of exogenic proteolytic enzymes on bacteria][Article in Russian] _Antibiot Khimioter._ 2004;49(12):9-13

[508] Vasquez A. Reducing pain and inflammation naturally - Part 3: Improving overall health while safely and effectively treating musculoskeletal pain. _Nutritional Perspectives_ 2005; 28: 34-38, 40-42 http://optimalhealthresearch.com/part3

[509] Isolauri E, Sutas Y, Kankaanpaa P, Arvilommi H, Salminen S. Probiotics: effects on immunity. _Am J Clin Nutr._ 2001 Feb;73(2 Suppl):444S-450S http://www.ajcn.org/cgi/reprint/73/2/444S

[510] Liu Q, Duan ZP, Ha da K, et al. Synbiotic modulation of gut flora: effect on minimal hepatic encephalopathy in patients with cirrhosis. _Hepatology._ 2004 May;39(5):1441-9

[511] Simenhoff ML, Dunn SR, Zollner GP, Fitzpatrick ME, Emery SM, Sandine WE, Ayres JW. Biomodulation of the toxic and nutritional effects of small bowel bacterial overgrowth in end-stage kidney disease using freeze-dried Lactobacillus acidophilus. _Miner Electrolyte Metab._ 1996;22(1-3):92-6

[512] Seaman DR. The diet-induced proinflammatory state: a cause of chronic pain and other degenerative diseases? _J Manipulative Physiol Ther._ 2002 Mar-Apr;25(3):168-79. See also Vasquez A. Chiropractic and Naturopathic Medicine for the Promotion of Wellness and Alleviation of Pain and Inflammation. http://optimalhealthresearch.com/monograph05

[513] Miller AL. Therapeutic considerations of L-glutamine: a review of the literature. _Altern Med Rev._ 1999 Aug;4(4):239-48 http://www.thorne.com/altmedrev/.fulltext/4/4/239.pdf

[514] Beck MA. Nutritionally induced oxidative stress: effect on viral disease. _Am J Clin Nutr._ 2000 Jun;71(6 Suppl):1676S-81S http://www.ajcn.org/cgi/content/full/71/6/1676S

[515] Vasquez A, Manso G, Cannell J. The clinical importance of vitamin D (cholecalciferol): a paradigm shift with implications for all healthcare providers. _Altern Ther Health Med._ 2004 Sep-Oct;10(5):28-36 http://optimalhealthresearch.com/monograph04

against chronic and acute infections.[516,517]   Extracts from bovine thymus are safe for clinical use in humans and have shown anti-infective and anti-inflammatory benefits in elderly patients[518] as well as antirheumatic/anti-inflammatory benefits in patients with autoimmune diseases[519,520,521]; in an animal study of experimental dental disease, administration of thymus extract was shown to normalize immune function and reduce orodental dysbiosis.[522]

6. **Hepatobiliary stimulation for IgA-complex removal**: The binding of immunoglobuin A (IgA) with antigen creates IgA immune complexes that contribute to tissue destruction by complement activation (alternate pathway) and other pathomechanisms in IgA nephropathy[523], Henoch-Schonlein purpura[524], rheumatoid vasculitis[525], lupus[526], and Sjogren's syndrome.[527]   Autoreactive IgA antibodies are a characteristic of lupus and Sjogren's syndrome[528] and correlate strongly with disease activity in rheumatoid arthritis.[529]   **Immune complexes containing secretory IgA that has been reabsorbed from mucosal surfaces mediate many of the clinical phenomenon of dysbiosis-related musculoskeletal disease[530], and these same IgA-containing immune complexes are eliminated from the systemic circulation via the liver and biliary system[531,532], thus providing the rationale for the use of botanicals and physiotherapeutics that promote liver function and bile flow in the treatment of IgA-mediated inflammatory disorders.**   Numerous experimental studies in animals have shown that circulating IgA immune complexes are taken up by hepatocytes and then secreted into the bile for elimination.[533,534]   The fact that bile duct obstruction retards systemic clearance of IgA immune complexes and that **normalization/optimization of bile flow reduces serum IgA levels by enhancing biliary excretion in animals[535,536] and humans[537]** proves the importance of ensuring optimal hepatobiliary function and supports the use of botanical and physiological therapeutics that facilitate bile flow.   A 1929 clinical study with human patients published in *Archives of Internal Medicine* provided irrefutable radiographic documentation that **therapeutic enemas safely and effectively stimulate bile flow for 45-60 minutes following administration[538]**, and this finding, along with the obvious quantitative reduction in intestinal microbes induced by such "cleansing", helps explain the reported benefits of colonics/enemas in patients with systemic illness[539,540,541,542] and

[516] Mero A, Kahkonen J, Nykanen T, Parviainen T, Jokinen I, Takala T, Nikula T, Rasi S, Leppaluoto J. IGF-I, IgA, and IgG responses to bovine colostrum supplementation during training. *J Appl Physiol*. 2002 Aug;93(2):732-9 http://jap.physiology.org/cgi/content/full/93/2/732

[517] "The preparation has high antibacterial antibody titres, and a high capacity for the neutralization of bacterial toxins. It is well tolerated and highly effective in the treatment of severe diarrhoea, e.g. in AIDS patients." Stephan W, Dichtelmuller H, Lissner R. Antibodies from colostrum in oral immunotherapy. *J Clin Chem Clin Biochem*. 1990 Jan;28(1):19-23

[518] Pandolfi F, Quinti I, Montella F, Voci MC, Schipani A, Urasia G, Aiuti F. T-dependent immunity in aged humans. II. Clinical and immunological evaluation after three months of administering a thymic extract. *Thymus*. 1983 Apr;5(3-4):235-40

[519] Lavastida MT, Goldstein AL, Daniels JC. Thymosin administration in autoimmune disorders. *Thymus*. 1981 Feb;2(4-5):287-95

[520] Thrower PA, Doyle DV, Scott J, Huskisson EC. Thymopoietin in rheumatoid arthritis. *Rheumatol Rehabil*. 1982 May;21(2):72-7

[521] Malaise MG, Hauwaert C, Franchimont P, et al. Treatment of active rheumatoid arthritis with slow intravenous injections of thymopentin. A double-blind placebo-controlled randomised study. *Lancet*. 1985 Apr 13;1(8433):832-6

[522] Manti F, Kornman K, Goldschneider I. Effects of an immunomodulating agent on peripheral blood lymphocytes and subgingival microflora in ligature-induced periodontitis. *Infect Immun*. 1984 Jul;45(1):172-9 http://www.pubmedcentral.gov/articlerender.fcgi?tool=pubmed&pubmedid=6234232

[523] "...it is likely that the usual instance of IgA-associated glomerulonephritis is due to deposition of circulating immune complexes containing IgA." McPhaul JJ Jr. IgA-associated glomerulonephritis. *Annu Rev Med*. 1977;28:37-42

[524] "... it is generally considered to be an immune complex-mediated disease characterized by the presence of polymeric IgA1 (pIgA1)-containing immune complexes predominantly in dermal, gastrointestinal, and glomerular capillaries. ...also been observed in the kidneys of patients with liver cirrhosis, dermatitis herpetiformis, celiac disease, and chronic inflammatory disease of the lung. " Rai A, Nast C, Adler S. Henoch-Schonlein purpura nephritis. *J Am Soc Nephrol*. 1999 Dec;10(12):2637-44 http://jasn.asnjournals.org/cgi/content/full/10/12/2637

[525] Voskuyl AE, Hazes JM, Zwinderman AH, van der Meer FJ, Daha MR, Breedveld FC. Diagnostic strategy for the assessment of rheumatoid vasculitis. *Ann Rheum Dis*. 2003 May;62(5):407-13 http://ard.bmjjournals.com/cgi/reprint/62/5/407

[526] Sikander FF, Salgaonkar DS, Joshi VR. Cryoglobulin studies in systemic lupus erythematosus. *J Postgrad Med* 1989;35:139-43

[527] Pourmand N, Wahren-Herlenius M, Gunnarsson I, et al. Ro/SSA and La/SSB specific IgA autoantibodies in serum of patients with Sjogren's syndrome and systemic lupus erythematosus. *Ann Rheum Dis*. 1999 Oct;58(10):623-9 http://ard.bmjjournals.com/cgi/content/full/58/10/623

[528] Pourmand N, Wahren-Herlenius M, Gunnarsson I, et al. Ro/SSA and La/SSB specific IgA autoantibodies in serum of patients with Sjogren's syndrome and systemic lupus erythematosus. *Ann Rheum Dis*. 1999 Oct;58(10):623-9 http://ard.bmjjournals.com/cgi/content/full/58/10/623

[529] Jonsson T, Valdimarsson H. What about IgA rheumatoid factor in rheumatoid arthritis? *Ann Rheum Dis*. 1998 Jan;57(1):63-4 http://ard.bmjjournals.com/cgi/content/full/57/1/63

[530] Inman RD. Antigens, the gastrointestinal tract, and arthritis. *Rheum Dis Clin North Am*. 1991 May;17(2):309-21

[531] Russell MW, Brown TA, Claflin JL, Schroer K, Mestecky J. Immunoglobulin A-mediated hepatobiliary transport constitutes a natural pathway for disposing of bacterial antigens. *Infect Immun*. 1983 Dec;42(3):1041-8 http://www.pubmedcentral.gov/articlerender.fcgi?tool=pubmed&pubmedid=6642659

[532] "The liver therefore appears to be singularly capable of transporting both free and complexed IgA into its secretion, the bile." Russell MW, Brown TA, Mestecky J. Preferential transport of IgA and IgA-immune complexes to bile compared with other external secretions. *Mol Immunol*. 1982 May;19(5):677-82

[533] "These results indicate that mouse hepatocytes are involved in the uptake and hepatobiliary transport of pIgA and pIgA-IC of low mol. wt." Phillips JO, Komiyama K, Epps JM, Russell MW, Mestecky J. Role of hepatocytes in the uptake of IgA and IgA-containing immune complexes in mice. *Mol Immunol*. 1988 Sep;25(9):873-9

[534] "Thus hepatobiliary transport appears to be the major pathway for the clearance of both IgA IC and free IgA from the circulation." Brown TA, Russell MW, Kulhavy R, Mestecky J. IgA-mediated elimination of antigens by the hepatobiliary route. *Fed Proc*. 1983 Dec;42(15):3218-21

[535] "Clearance of IgA immune complexes was delayed after bile duct ligation." Harmatz PR, Kleinman RE, Bunnell BW, McClenathan DT, Walker WA, Bloch KJ. The effect of bile duct obstruction on the clearance of circulating IgA immune complexes. *Hepatology*. 1984 Jan-Feb;4(1):96-100

[536] Lemaitre-Coelho I, Jackson GD, Vaerman JP. High levels of secretory IgA and free secretory component in the serum of rats with bile duct obstruction. *J Exp Med*. 1978 Mar 1;147(3):934-9 http://www.jem.org/cgi/reprint/147/3/934

[537] "CONCLUSIONS: Biliary obstruction secondary to both calculus or malignancy of the hepatobiliary system causes suppression of bile IgA secretion and elevated serum level of secretory IgA. Bile secretory IgA secretion recovers with endoscopic drainage of the obstructed system." Sung JJ, Leung JC, Tsui CP, Chung SS, Lai KN. Biliary IgA secretion in obstructive jaundice: the effects of endoscopic drainage. *Gastrointest Endosc*. 1995 Nov;42(5):439-44

[538] Garbat AL, Jacobi HG. Secretion of Bile in Response to Rectal Installations. *Arch Intern Med* 1929; 44: 455-462

[539] Crinnion WJ. Results of a decade of naturopathic treatment for environmental illnesses. *J Naturopathic Med* 1994;17:21-27

other immune-complex associated diseases such as cancer.[543]   Validation of this concept is demonstrated by the significant efficacy of immunoadsorption[544] and plasmapheresis[545,546] (techniques for removing immune complexes) in patients with lupus. Furthermore, this directly supports the naturopathic concept of "treating the liver" in patients with systemic disease by the use of dietary and botanical therapeutics that stimulate bile flow, such as beets, ginger[547], curcumin/turmeric[548], *Picrorhiza*[549], milk thistle[550], *Andrographis paniculata*[551], and *Boerhaavia diffusa*.[552]   Investigation of an antirheumatic benefit from phytophysiotherapeutic hepatobiliary stimulation is worthy of clinical trials with pre- and post-intervention measurement of serum immune complexes and other clinical indexes.[553]

7. **Ensure generous bowel movements and consider therapeutic purgatives** (*purge: to free from impurities*): Dysbiotic patients should consume a low-fermentation fiber-rich diet that allows for 1-2 very generous bowel movements per day. Constipation must absolutely be eliminated; **there is no place for constipation in patients being treated for dysbiosis of any type**. Patients with severe or recalcitrant dysbiosis can start the day with a laxative dose of ascorbic acid (e.g., 20 grams with 4 cups of water) and should expect liquid diarrhea within 30-60 minutes. The goal here is purgative physical removal of enteric microbes; in high concentrations, ascorbic acid has a direct antibacterial effect. Magnesium in elemental doses of 500-1,500 mg also helps soften stool and promote laxation.

The clinical implementation of an anti-dysbiosis program must be tailored to the patient's overall condition and his/her willingness to implement the above-mentioned treatment options. Some patients are only willing to take a few treatments, while empowered autonomous nonmasochistic patients are more willing to do **whatever is necessary** in order to regain their health, even if it means taking numerous supplements, improving diet, starting/ending the day with enemas, and making appropriate changes in lifestyle and relationships to improve immune function. To the extent that we *first, do no harm*, all of the above-mentioned therapeutic interventions are reasonable "alternatives" to life-long medicalization, surgery, and immune-system destroying high-dose chemotherapy, which is astoundingly expensive, highly hazardous, and incompletely effective. **Patients with autoimmune diseases have numerous, largely untapped options for the treatment of their autoimmune diseases**; therefore, (pseudo)justifying lethal and expensive and devastating medical interventions on the basis of a "lack of other treatment alternatives"[554] when reasonable, safe, and effective options have not been implemented is scientifically inaccurate, ethically untenable, and medicolegally questionable.

[540] Snyder RG. The value of colonic irrigations in countering auto-intoxication of intestinal origin. *Medical Clinics of North America* 1939; May: 781-788
[541] Marshall HK, Thomson CR. Colon irrigation in the treatment of mental disease. *N Engl J Med* 1932; 207 (Sept 8): 454-7
[542] Bastedo WA. Colon irrigations: their administration, therapeutic applications, and dangers. *Journal of the American Medical Association* 1932; 98(9): 734-6
[543] Gonzalez NJ, Isaacs LL. Evaluation of pancreatic proteolytic enzyme treatment of adenocarcinoma of the pancreas, with nutrition and detoxification support. Nutr Cancer. 1999;33(2):117-24
[544] Braun N, Erley C, Klein R, Kotter I, Saal J, Risler T. Immunoadsorption onto protein A induces remission in severe systemic lupus erythematosus. *Nephrol Dial Transplant*. 2000 Sep;15(9):1367-72 http://ndt.oxfordjournals.org/cgi/reprint/15/9/1367
[545] Santos-Ocampo AS, Mandell BF, Fessler BJ. Alveolar hemorrhage in systemic lupus erythematosus: presentation and management. *Chest*. 2000 Oct;118(4):1083-90 http://www.chestjournal.org/cgi/content/full/118/4/1083
[546] Choi BG, Yoo WH. Successful treatment of pure red cell aplasia with plasmapheresis in a patient with systemic lupus erythematosus. *Yonsei Med J*. 2002 Apr;43(2):274-8 http://www.eymj.org/2002/pdf/04274.pdf
[547] "Further analyses for the active constituents of the acetone extracts through column chromatography indicated that [6]-gingerol and [10]-gingerol, which are the pungent principles, are mainly responsible for the cholagogic effect of ginger." Yamahara J, Miki K, Chisaka T, Sawada T, Fujimura H, Tomimatsu T, Nakano K, Nohara T. Cholagogic effect of ginger and its active constituents. *J Ethnopharmacol*. 1985;13(2):217-25
[548] "On the basis of the present findings, it appears that curcumin induces contraction of the human gall-bladder." Rasyid A, Lelo A. The effect of curcumin and placebo on human gall-bladder function: an ultrasound study. *Aliment Pharmacol Ther*. 1999 Feb;13(2):245-9
[549] "Significant anticholestatic activity was also observed against carbon tetrachloride induced cholestasis in conscious rat, anaesthetized guinea pig and cat. Picroliv was more active than the known hepatoprotective drug silymarin." Saraswat B, Visen PK, Patnaik GK, Dhawan BN. Anticholestatic effect of picroliv, active hepatoprotective principle of Picrorhiza kurrooa, against carbon tetrachloride induced cholestasis. *Indian J Exp Biol*. 1993 Apr;31(4):316-8
[550] "We conclude that SIL counteracts TLC-induced cholestasis by preventing the impairment in both the BS-dependent and -independent fractions of the bile flow." Crocenzi FA, Sanchez Pozzi EJ, Pellegrino JM, Rodriguez Garay EA, Mottino AD, Roma MG. Preventive effect of silymarin against taurolithocholate-induced cholestasis in the rat. *Biochem Pharmacol*. 2003 Jul 15;66(2):355-64
[551] "Andrographolide from the herb Andrographis paniculata (whole plant) per se produces a significant dose (1.5-12 mg/kg) dependent choleretic effect (4.8-73%) as evidenced by increase in bile flow, bile salt, and bile acids in conscious rats and anaesthetized guinea pigs." Shukla B, Visen PK, Patnaik GK, Dhawan BN. Choleretic effect of andrographolide in rats and guinea pigs. *Planta Med*. 1992 Apr;58(2):146-9
[552] "The extract also produced an increase in normal bile flow in rats suggesting a strong choleretic activity." Chandan BK, Sharma AK, Anand KK. Boerhaavia diffusa: a study of its hepatoprotective activity. *J Ethnopharmacol*. 1991 Mar;31(3):299-307
[553] Vasquez A. Do the Benefits of Botanical and Physiotherapeutic Hepatobiliary Stimulation Result From Enhanced Excretion of IgA Immune Complexes? *Naturopathy Digest* 2006; January: http://www.naturopathydigest.com/archives/2006/jan/vasquez_immune.php
[554] Binks M, Passweg JR, Furst D, McSweeney P, Sullivan K, Besenthal C, Finke J, Peter HH, van Laar J, Breedveld FC, Fibbe WE, Farge D, Gluckman E, Locatelli F, Martini A, van den Hoogen F, van de Putte L, Schattenberg AV, Arnold R, Bacon PA, Emery P, Espigado I, Hertenstein B, Hiepe F, Kashyap A, Kotter I, Marmont A, Martinez A, Pascual MJ, Gratwohl A, Prentice HG, Black C, Tyndall A. Phase I/II trial of autologous stem cell transplantation in systemic sclerosis: procedure related mortality and impact on skin disease. Ann Rheum Dis. 2001 Jun;60(6):577-84 http://ard.bmjjournals.com/cgi/content/full/60/6/577

Xenobiotic Immunotoxicity and its Treatment by Therapeutic Detoxification: An Ultracondensed Clinical Review

Chemicals such as pesticides, synthetic fertilizers, herbicides, fungicides, industrial pollution, car exhaust, solvents, and innumerable others are bioaccumulative and can alter immune function. The classic manifestation of xenobiotic immunotoxicity is the combination of reduced resistance to infections and increased allergic and autoimmune disorders. The subject of environmental medicine and detoxification is much to broad and complex to review completely in this textbook, and while naturopathic physicians are trained in these topics, other healthcare professionals are not unless they attend post-graduate training and take the time to read articles and textbooks on these topics. Readers for whom these topics are new are encouraged to access the following citations for additional information.[555,556,557,558,559] What follows here will be an ultracondensed clinical review focusing on major concepts and problem-specific solutions.

For the sake of simplicity and with recognition of the various nuances of different xenobiotics, I generalize toxicity into two categories, either *chemicals* or *heavy metals*. Most patients have an overlay of these two problems, so that the clinical manifestations and treatments have several commonalities.

- Chemical toxicity: Accumulation of xenobiotics can cause immune dysfunction and can contribute to the development of "autoimmunity." Examples of xenobiotic-induced autoimmunity include 1) the increased autoimmunity seen in farmers exposed to pesticides[560], 2) the scleroderma-like disease that results from exposure to vinyl chloride[561], 3) the association of mercury and pesticide exposure with lupus[562], and 4) the well-recognized connection between drug and chemical exposure and various autoimmune syndromes such as drug-induced lupus.[563] More than 40 pharmaceutical drugs are known to cause drug-induced lupus.[564] Every one of us is exposed to toxic chemicals every day, and every one of us has chemical accumulation and the potential for xenobiotic-induced disease. Except for denial (shown to be clinically ineffective), we cannot escape from the chemical consequences of living in a world with tens of thousands of synthetic chemicals. According to limited analyses, the average American has accumulated at least 18 different chemicals[565], and analyses that are more detailed show that even more chemicals and metals have been accumulated.[566] Common sources of these chemicals include pesticides, synthetic fertilizers, herbicides, fungicides, industrial pollution, car exhaust, solvents, paints, perfumes, plastic food/drink containers, non-stick cookware, Styrofoam, trichloroethylene from dry cleaning, rubber, carpet, plastics, glues, propellants, petroleum fuels such as gasoline, detergents, and other "cleaners." Clinical consequences of chemical toxicity are diverse, can

[555] "Caffeine enemas cause dilation of bile ducts, which facilitates excretion of toxic cancer breakdown products by the liver and dialysis of toxic products from blood across the colonic wall. The therapy must be used as an integrated whole." Gerson M. The cure of advanced cancer by diet therapy: a summary of 30 years of clinical experimentation. *Physiol Chem Phys.* 1978;10(5):449-64

[556] "The writer has observed numerous cases suffering from such conditions as chronic arthritis, hypertension, coronary disease, chronic abdominal distention, constipation, and colitis, in which the element of constipation, auto-intoxication and possible colon infection seemed to play a prominent part, which responded very satisfactorily to colonic irrigations after failure to improve following the usual forms of medical treatment." Snyder RG. The value of colonic irrigations in countering auto-intoxication of intestinal origin. *Medical Clinics of North America* 1939; May: 781-788

[557] Gonzalez NJ, Isaacs LL. Evaluation of pancreatic proteolytic enzyme treatment of adenocarcinoma of the pancreas, with nutrition and detoxification support. *Nutr Cancer.* 1999;33(2):117-24

[558] Crinnion WJ. Results of a decade of naturopathic treatment for environmental illness: a review of clinical records. *J Naturopathic Med* 1997;7:21-27

[559] Sherman JD. Chemical exposure and disease. Diagnostic and investigative techniques. Princeton Scientific Publishing; 1994

[560] "IgG levels decreased with increasing p,p'-DDE levels, with a statistically significant decrease of approximately 50% in the highest two categories of exposure. Sixteen (12%) were positive for antinuclear antibodies... These analyses provide evidence that p,p'-DDE modulates immune responses in humans." Cooper GS, Martin SA, Longnecker MP, Sandler DP, Germolec DR. Associations between plasma DDE levels and immunologic measures in African-American farmers in North Carolina. *Environ Health Perspect.* 2004 Jul;112(10):1080-4

[561] "Vinyl chloride (VC) monomer can induce a scleroderma-like syndrome in a proportion of workers exposed to it during production of polyvinyl chloride." Black CM, Welsh KI, Walker AE, Bernstein RM, Catoggio LJ, McGregor AR, Jones JK. Genetic susceptibility to scleroderma-like syndrome induced by vinyl chloride. *Lancet.* 1983 Jan 1;1(8314-5):53-5

[562] "...reported occupational exposure to mercury (OR 3.6), mixing pesticides for agricultural work (OR 7.4), and among dental workers (OR 7.1, 95% CI 2.2, 23.4). ...these associations were fairly strong and statistically significant..." Cooper GS, Parks CG, Treadwell EL, St Clair EW, Gilkeson GS, Dooley MA. Occupational risk factors for the development of systemic lupus erythematosus. *J Rheumatol.* 2004 Oct;31(10):1928-33

[563] Hess EV. Environmental chemicals and autoimmune disease: cause and effect. *Toxicology.* 2002 Dec 27;181-182:65-70

[564] "Drug-induced lupus has been reported as a side-effect of long-term therapy with over 40 medications... Several mechanisms for induction of autoimmunity will be discussed, including bystander activation of autoreactive lymphocytes due to drug-specific immunity or to non-specific activation of lymphocytes, direct cytotoxicity with release of autoantigens ..." Rubin RL. Drug-induced lupus. *Toxicology.* 2005;209(2):135-47

[565] Kristin S. Schafer, Margaret Reeves, Skip Spitzer, Susan E. Kegley. Chemical Trespass: Pesticides in Our Bodies and Corporate Accountability. Pesticide Action Network North America. May 2004 Available at http://www.panna.org/campaigns/docsTrespass/chemicalTrespass2004.dv.html on August 1, 2004

[566] Body Burden: The Pollution in People. http://ewg.org/issues/siteindex/issues.php?issueid=5004 Accessed February 6, 2006

affect nearly every organ system, and may be predicted to some extent by the pattern of chemical exposure since some chemicals have characteristic sequelae. Most chemicals, especially those which are fat-soluble, can readily enter the body via respiratory, gastrointestinal, and transdermal routes. Once in the bloodstream, chemicals are either detoxified (inactivated and/or solubilized) by the liver and then excreted via urine or bile, or to a lesser extent exhaled from the lungs or excreted via sweat. Chemicals which are not excreted from the body are stored in the tissues, particularly lipid-rich organs such as the liver, adipose, and brain. Molecular turnover and recycling (particularly lipolysis) liberates fat-stored xenobiotics for another opportunity for either detoxification or additional toxicity. The main route for detoxification is the liver, which hydrosolublizes xenobiotics via oxidation ("phase one") and conjugation ("phase two"). Generally speaking, oxidation reactions are dependent on the cytochrome P-450 system, which can be inhibited by various drugs (e.g., ketoconazole, erythromycin, ritonavir, cimetidine, omeprazole, ethanol), foods such as ethanol and grapefruit juice, bacterial endotoxin from bacterial overgrowth of the intestines, and/or by genetic defects known as single nucleotide polymorphisms ("SNiPs") which reduce xenobiotic clearance. Similarly, conjugation reactions can be inhibited by a low-vegetable diet, SNiPs, and insufficiencies of conjugation moieties such as glutathione, glycine, glutamine, taurine, ornithine, sulfur, and methyl groups. If oxidation is too slow, then xenobiotics are insufficiently detoxicated and insufficiently processed for conjugation, leading to xenobiotic accumulation. If oxidation is too fast relative to conjugation, then reactive intermediates are formed which are commonly more toxic than the original xenobiotic, and insufficient conjugation results in accumulation of reactive xenobiotics which are inherently prone to tissue haptenization (which can incite autoimmunity) and DNA intercalation (which promotes damage to DNA and the resultant mutation and oncogenesis). Optimally oxidized and conjugated xenobiotics are excreted in the urine (smaller molecules with molecular weight less than 400-600) or expelled in the bile (larger molecules with molecular weight greater than 400-600). Supranormal hydration and urinary alkalinization enhance renal clearance of weakly acidic xenobiotics and drugs, whereas dehydration and urinary acidity impair toxin excretion, generally speaking. Conjugated toxins expelled in the bile can be deconjugated by bacteria so that the toxin is reabsorbed, a phenomenon commonly referred to as "enterohepatic recycling"[567] or "enterohepatic recirculation."[568] Such recirculation is obviously less likely if gastrointestinal status and diet have been optimized to minimize the presence of deconjugating bacteria and to maximize fiber intake and laxation for the adsorption and expulsion of intraluminal toxins. Therapeutic colonics and enemas can be employed to stimulate bile flow from the liver[569,570] and to remove bile-secreted toxins from the gut before deconjugation and re-absorption occur. Bile formation and expulsion are further stimulated by botanical medicines such as beets, ginger[571], curcumin/turmeric[572], *Picrorhiza*[573], milk thistle[574], *Andrographis paniculata*[575] and *Boerhaavia diffusa*.[576] Respiratory exhalation of toxins is enhanced by deep breathing and exercise, and hyperventilation promotes respiratory alkalosis which elevates urine

---

[567] "Enterohepatic recycling occurs by biliary excretion and intestinal reabsorption of a solute, sometimes with hepatic conjugation and intestinal deconjugation. ... Of particular importance is the potential amplifying effect of enterohepatic variability in defining differences in the bioavailability, apparent volume of distribution and clearance of a given compound." Roberts MS, Magnusson BM, Burczynski FJ, Weiss M. Enterohepatic circulation: physiological, pharmacokinetic and clinical implications. *Clin Pharmacokinet*. 2002;41(10):751-90

[568] Liska DJ. The detoxification enzyme systems. *Altern Med Rev*. 1998 Jun;3(3):187-98

[569] Garbat, AL, Jacobi, HG: Secretion of Bile in Response to Rectal Installations. *Arch Intern Med* 1929; 44: 455-462

[570] "Caffeine enemas cause dilation of bile ducts, which facilitates excretion of toxic cancer breakdown products by the liver and dialysis of toxic products from blood across the colonic wall. The therapy must be used as an integrated whole." Gerson M. The cure of advanced cancer by diet therapy: a summary of 30 years of clinical experimentation. *Physiol Chem Phys*. 1978;10(5):449-64

[571] "Further analyses for the active constituents of the acetone extracts through column chromatography indicated that [6]-gingerol and [10]-gingerol, which are the pungent principles, are mainly responsible for the cholagogic effect of ginger." Yamahara J, Miki K, Chisaka T, Sawada T, Fujimura H, Tomimatsu T, Nakano K, Nohara T. Cholagogic effect of ginger and its active constituents. *J Ethnopharmacol*. 1985;13(2):217-25

[572] "On the basis of the present findings, it appears that curcumin induces contraction of the human gall-bladder." Rasyid A, Lelo A. The effect of curcumin and placebo on human gall-bladder function: an ultrasound study. *Aliment Pharmacol Ther*. 1999 Feb;13(2):245-9

[573] "Significant anticholestatic activity was also observed against carbon tetrachloride induced cholestasis in conscious rat, anaesthetized guinea pig and cat. Picroliv was more active than the known hepatoprotective drug silymarin." Saraswat B, Visen PK, Patnaik GK, Dhawan BN. Anticholestatic effect of picroliv, active hepatoprotective principle of Picrorhiza kurrooa, against carbon tetrachloride induced cholestasis. *Indian J Exp Biol*. 1993 Apr;31(4):316-8

[574] "We conclude that SIL counteracts TLC-induced cholestasis by preventing the impairment in both the BS-dependent and -independent fractions of the bile flow." Crocenzi FA, Sanchez Pozzi EJ, Pellegrino JM, Rodriguez Garay EA, Mottino AD, Roma MG. Preventive effect of silymarin against taurolithocholate-induced cholestasis in the rat. *Biochem Pharmacol*. 2003 Jul 15;66(2):355-64

[575] "Andrographolide from the herb Andrographis paniculata (whole plant) per se produces a significant dose (1.5-12 mg/kg) dependent choleretic effect (4.8-73%) as evidenced by increase in bile flow, bile salt, and bile acids in conscious rats and anaesthetized guinea pigs." Shukla B, Visen PK, Patnaik GK, Dhawan BN. Choleretic effect of andrographolide in rats and guinea pigs. *Planta Med*. 1992 Apr;58(2):146-9

[576] "The extract also produced an increase in normal bile flow in rats suggesting a strong choleretic activity." Chandan BK, Sharma AK, Anand KK. Boerhaavia diffusa: a study of its hepatoprotective activity. *J Ethnopharmacol*. 1991 Mar;31(3):299-307

pH and promotes excretion of weakly acidic drugs and xenobiotics as previously mentioned. Dermal excretion of toxins via sweat and expedited lipolysis are stimulated via low-temperature saunas and regular aerobic exercise. Xenobiotic oxidation can be promoted (cautiously) by reducing endotoxins from the gut and by the use of botanicals such as *Hypericum perforatum* which induce several isoforms of cytochrome P-450 via activation of the pregane X receptor. Xenobiotic conjugation is likewise promoted via nutrigenomic induction stimulated by cruciferous vegetables and their derivatives such as indole-3-carbinol (I3C) and dimethylindolylemethane (DIM). The plant-based diet is employed to provide fiber for bowel cleansing and the urinary alkalinization that is necessary for optimal urinary excretion of toxins, the majority of which are weak acids and are thus excreted more efficiently in alkaline urine. Sodium bicarbonate can also be used to induce urinary alkalinization. The diet must contain high-quality protein and can be supplemented with amino acids to support amino acid and glutathione conjugation. Serum, urine, and adipose samples can be analyzed to determine the intensity and diversity of chemical accumulation; I tend reserve such testing for patients who have been exposed to a specific chemical, particularly in occupational settings. For most patients, their chemical accumulation is so diverse that they may not display abnormally high levels of a specific chemical; their clinical manifestations are rather a manifestation of a wide plethora of different chemicals, which individually may be only modestly increased. Detoxification genotype can be determined by genomic testing for SNPs in oxidation and conjugation enzymes. Phenotype can be assessed by serum and urine measurements of post-challenge detoxification of benzoate, caffeine, acetylsalicylic acid, and acetaminophen. Amino acid status can be quantified and qualified via serum or urine amino acid analysis. Stool testing assesses digestion, absorption, and microflora status. Clinical implementation follows a screening physical examination and basic laboratory assessment (minimally including CBC, metabolic panel, and urinalysis). Stool testing is always reasonable when working with patients with fatigue and/or autoimmunity; however, this and the other detoxification-related tests can often be deferred and/or used selectively. The Paleo-Mediterranean diet provides ample high-quality protein, alkalinization, fiber, and phytonutrients to which may be added supplements of protein, amino acids (especially NAC, glycine, and glutamine), and vitamins and minerals. Antioxidant teas and fresh fruit and vegetable juices are consumed to increase frequency of urination and promote urinary alkalinization, due primarily to the content of potassium citrate. Exercise and low-temperature saunas promote sweating and xenobiotic-mobilizing lipolysis. Colonics and enemas cleanse the bowel and stimulate bile flow.[577,578] Bile flow is further stimulated by consumption of beets, ginger, curcumin/turmeric, *Picrorhiza*, milk thistle, *Andrographis paniculata* and *Boerhaavia diffusa*. These interventions work in concert to enhance xenobiotic depuration ("The act or process of depurating or freeing from foreign or impure matter "[579]) and cleanse the tissues of accumulated toxins. Intervention can be acute or periodic, but must be maintained for the long-term in order to resist the re-accumulation that is destined to result from the chemical onslaught that is inescapable in our polluted world.

- Heavy metal toxicity: In contrast to chemical toxicity for which a generalized non-specific cleansing protocol is appropriate, toxic metals more commonly require specific interventions; treatment is determined by the identity of the metal. Metals which are considered toxic or which are linked to the induction of human diseases include aluminum, arsenic, cadmium, lead, and mercury. Other metals and minerals such as manganese, lithium, copper, and iron can be toxic when present in high amounts. In this section I will limit the discussion to mercury since this

---

[577] Garbat, AL, Jacobi, HG: Secretion of Bile in Response to Rectal Installations. *Arch Intern Med* 1929; 44: 455-462

[578] "Caffeine enemas cause dilation of bile ducts, which facilitates excretion of toxic cancer breakdown products by the liver and dialysis of toxic products from blood across the colonic wall. The therapy must be used as an integrated whole." Gerson M. The cure of advanced cancer by diet therapy: a summary of 30 years of clinical experimentation. *Physiol Chem Phys.* 1978;10(5):449-64

[579] "The act or process of depurating or freeing from foreign or impure matter." http://www.thefreedictionary.com/Depuration Verified March 11, 2007

metal is 1) commonly elevated in chronically toxic patients, and 2) because this metal can contribute to autoimmunity.

- o Mercury: Chronic mercury toxicity is commonly discovered in clinical practice in patients with chronic unwellness, and a recent study published in *JAMA* showed that 8% of American women of childbearing age have sufficient levels of mercury in their bodies to produce neurologic damage in their children.[580] Accumulating evidence implicates mercury in the induction of immune dysfunction and the exacerbation of autoimmunity and allergy, and clinical trials indicate the benefit of mercury removal.

  - Mercury induces autoimmunity, immune complex formation and deposition, and the formation of antinuclear antibodies and antinucleolar antibodies in animal experiments.[581,582,583]

  - In a case-control study of 265 recently diagnosed lupus patients, occupational exposure to mercury increased the risk of developing lupus by 360%, while working in a dental office increased the risk by 710%.[584]

  - Patients with eczema have an increase body burden of mercury[585], suggesting the probability that mercury accumulation induces immune dysfunction and contributes to the clinical picture of immune-induced skin inflammation, to which is affixed the label of "eczema."

  - Leukocytes from autistic patients produce autoantigens when exposed to ethyl mercury (Thimerosal), thus clearly implicating mercury in the incitement and perpetuation of autoimmunity.[586]

  - A slight increase in risk for multiple sclerosis was noted among patients with many long-term mercury amalgam fillings.[587]

  - It is highly probable that chronic mercury exposure, whether from diet or dental amalgams, alters gastrointestinal flora in favor of dysbiosis in general and antibiotic resistance in particular.[588] Thus, mercury may indirectly contribute to autoimmunity by promoting treatment-resistant dysbiosis, which then directly effects pro-inflammatory immune dysfunction.

  - In a clinical trial with 35 patients, 71% experienced improvement in overall health following removal of mercury amalgams; the patients with the most improvement were patients with multiple sclerosis.[589] Whether this was due to reducing autoimmunity or to reducing neurotoxicity is not clear; certainly both

---

[580] "However, approximately 8% of women had concentrations higher than the US Environmental Protection Agency's recommended reference dose (5.8 microg/L), below which exposures are considered to be without adverse effects. Women who are pregnant or who intend to become pregnant should follow federal and state advisories on consumption of fish." Schober SE, Sinks TH, Jones RL, Bolger PM, McDowell M, Osterloh J, Garrett ES, Canady RA, Dillon CF, Sun Y, Joseph CB, Mahaffey KR. Blood mercury levels in US children and women of childbearing age, 1999-2000. *JAMA.* 2003 Apr 2;289(13):1667-74

[581] "It is well established that in susceptible mouse strains, chronic treatment with subtoxic doses of mercuric chloride (HgCl2) induces a systemic autoimmune disease, which is characterized by increased serum levels of IgG1 and IgE antibodies, by the production of anti-nucleolar antibodies and by the development of immune complex-mediated glomerulonephritis." al-Balaghi S, Moller E, Moller G, Abedi-Valugerdi M. Mercury induces polyclonal B cell activation, autoantibody production and renal immune complex deposits in young (NZB x NZW)F1 hybrids. *Eur J Immunol.* 1996 Jul;26(7):1519-26

[582] "It is well demonstrated that mercury induces a systemic autoimmune disease in susceptible mouse strains... The dominant antibody in the kidney eluate of mercury-injected mice was of IgG1 isotype and found to be directed against double-stranded DNA, collagen, cardiolipin, phosphatidylethanolamine, and the hapten trinitrophenol, but not against nucleolar antigens." Abedi-Valugerdi M, Hu H, Moller G. Mercury-induced renal immune complex deposits in young (NZB x NZW)F1 mice: characterization of antibodies/autoantibodies. *Clin Exp Immunol.* 1997 Oct;110(1):86-91

[583] Abedi-Valugerdi M, Hu H, Moller G. Mercury-induced anti-nucleolar autoantibodies can transgress the membrane of living cells in vivo and in vitro. *Int Immunol.* 1999 Apr;11(4):605-15 http://intimm.oxfordjournals.org/cgi/content/full/11/4/605

[584] "...reported occupational exposure to mercury (OR 3.6), mixing pesticides for agricultural work (OR 7.4), and among dental workers (OR 7.1, 95% CI 2.2, 23.4). ...these associations were fairly strong and statistically significant..." Cooper GS, Parks CG, Treadwell EL, St Clair EW, Gilkeson GS, Dooley MA. Occupational risk factors for the development of systemic lupus erythematosus. *J Rheumatol.* 2004 Oct;31(10):1928-33

[585] Weidinger S, Kramer U, Dunemann L, Mohrenschlager M, Ring J, Behrendt H. Body burden of mercury is associated with acute atopic eczema and total IgE in children from southern Germany. *J Allergy Clin Immunol.* 2004 Aug;114(2):457-9

[586] Vojdani A, Pangborn JB, Vojdani E, Cooper EL. Infections, toxic chemicals and dietary peptides binding to lymphocyte receptors and tissue enzymes are major instigators of autoimmunity in autism. *Int J Immunopathol Pharmacol.* 2003 Sep-Dec;16(3):189-99

[587] "Although a suggestive elevated risk was found for those individuals with a large number of dental amalgams, and for a long period of time, the difference between cases and controls was not statistically significant." Bangsi D, Ghadirian P, Ducic S, Morisset R, Ciccocioppo S, McMullen E, Krewski D. Dental amalgam and multiple sclerosis: a case-control study in Montreal, Canada. *Int J Epidemiol.* 1998 Aug;27(4):667-71 http://ije.oxfordjournals.org/cgi/reprint/27/4/667

[588] Pike R, Lucas V, Stapleton P, Gilthorpe MS, Roberts G, Rowbury R, Richards H, Mullany P, Wilson M. Prevalence and antibiotic resistance profile of mercury-resistant oral bacteria from children with and without mercury amalgam fillings. *J Antimicrob Chemother.* 2002 May;49(5):777-83 http://jac.oxfordjournals.org/cgi/content/full/49/5/777 This seems to be a rather tragic article insofar as the researchers' conclusions are inconsistent with their findings; they state that mercury does not contribute to increased prevalence or numbers of antibiotic resistant bacteria, yet their data in Table 4 clearly demonstrate that patients with dental amalgams have more drug-resistant isolates than do patients without such toxic implantations. Note also that the bacteria studied here were from the oral cavity, not the gastrointestinal tract. A much better article on this topic is the following: "Our findings indicate that mercury released from amalgam fillings can cause an enrichment of mercury resistance plasmids in the normal bacterial floras of primates. Many of these plasmids also carry antibiotic resistance, implicating the exposure to mercury from dental amalgams in an increased incidence of multiple antibiotic resistance plasmids in the normal floras of nonmedicated subjects." Summers AO, Wireman J, Vimy MJ, Lorscheider FL, Marshall B, Levy SB, Bennett S, Billard L. Mercury released from dental "silver" fillings provokes an increase in mercury- and antibiotic-resistant bacteria in oral and intestinal floras of primates. *Antimicrob Agents Chemother.* 1993 Apr;37(4):825-34 http://www.pubmedcentral.gov/articlerender.fcgi?tool=pubmed&pubmedid=8280208

[589] " Out of 35 patients, 25 patients (71%) showed improvement of health... The highest rate of improvement was observed in patients with multiple sclerosis... Mercury-containing amalgam may be an important risk factor for patients with autoimmune diseases." Prochazkova J, Sterzl I, Kucerova H, Bartova J, Stejskal VD. The beneficial effect of amalgam replacement on health in patients with autoimmunity. *Neuro Endocrinol Lett.* 2004 Jun;25(3):211-8

mechanisms may explain the improvement. Mercury is directly neurotoxic independently from its almost certain ability to contribute to neuroautoimmunity; this is visually demonstrated in a video of brain neuron degeneration following exposure to mercury, available on-line from the University of Calgary at http://commons.ucalgary.ca/mercury/.[590]

Very interestingly, the patients most sensitive to mercury compounds appear to be those with a genotypic defect in phase-2 xenobiotic conjugation, specifically glutathione-S-transferase (GST).[591] What makes this even more interesting is the finding that mercury compounds can inhibit GST and produce a GST-deficient phenotype even when the original genotype was GST-normal.[592] Even though this latter finding was documented in *ex vivo* research with human erythrocytes, it correlates with the clinical experience of doctors who specialize in environmental medicine, namely that mercury accumulation appears to inhibit chemical xenobiotic detoxification. Thus mercury and chemical xenobiotics may work synergistically for the induction of immune dysfunction, with the former inhibiting the detoxification/conjugation of the latter. Regardless of the mechanisms involved, which are clearly numerous and synergistic, given that no safe level of mercury has been established, clinicians are justified in treating patients with evidence of mercury accumulation, chronic mercury toxicity. Based on numerous case reports documenting safety and efficacy of dimercaptosuccinic acid (DMSA), when used in children and adults[593,594,595,596,597], it is my chelating agent of choice for most patients with lead and mercury toxicity as I review in the DMSA monograph in the pages that follow. Clinical implementation of metal detoxification can be performed simultaneously with the chemical detoxification program described previously and outlined in the pages that follow. The difference is the addition of DMSA first thing in the morning on an empty stomach at a dose of 10-30 mg per kg. Screening examination for overall health and kidney function should be performed before full-dose administration of DMSA, and sensitivity testing with <100 mg of DMSA is also reasonable to exclude allergy or idiosyncratic reactions to DMSA, which may indeed occur. DMSA is given in an "on and off" schedule, such as four days "on" and 3 days "off." Bile flow stimulation with botanicals and colonics for expulsion of mercury is the same as for xenobiotic detoxification. Two to four hours after consumption of DMSA, metal adsorbents such as phytochelatins and alginate can be used to bind metals in the gut and reduce enterohepatic recirculation. Antioxidants, especially selenium, are supplemented, and the diet is fresh, hypoallergenic, and Paleo-Mediterranean.

[590] University of Calgary. How Mercury Causes Brain Neuron Degeneration. http://commons.ucalgary.ca/mercury/ Accessed November 24, 2005
[591] "The combined deletion (GSTT1-/GSTM1-) was markedly more frequent among thimerosal-sensitized patients than in healthy controls (17.6% vs. 6.5%, P = 0.0093) and in the "para-compound" group (17.6% vs. 6.1%, P =0.014), revealing a synergistic effect of these enzyme deficiencies." Westphal GA, Schnuch A, Schulz TG, Reich K, Aberer W, Brasch J, Koch P, Wessbecher R, Szliska C, Bauer A, Hallier E. Homozygous gene deletions of the glutathione S-transferases M1 and T1 are associated with thimerosal sensitization. *Int Arch Occup Environ Health*. 2000 Aug;73(6):384-8
[592] "Thus, sufficiently high doses of thimerosal may be able to change the phenotypic status of an individual--at least in vitro--by inhibition of the GST T1 enzyme." Muller M, Westphal G, Vesper A, Bunger J, Hallier E. Inhibition of the human erythrocytic glutathione-S-transferase T1 (GST T1) by thimerosal. Int J Hyg Environ Health. 2001 Jul;203(5-6):479-81
[593] Bradstreet J, Geier DA, Kartzinel JJ, Adams JB, Geier MR. A case-control study of mercury burden in children with autistic spectrum disorders. *Journal of American Physicians and Surgeons* 2003; 8: 76-79 http://www.jpands.org/vol8no3/geier.pdf
[594] Crinnion WJ. Environmental medicine, part three: long-term effects of chronic low-dose mercury exposure. *Altern Med Rev*. 2000 Jun;5(3):209-23 http://www.thorne.com/altmedrev/.fulltext/5/3/209.pdf
[595] Forman J, Moline J, Cernichiari E, Sayegh S, Torres JC, Landrigan MM, Hudson J, Adel HN, Landrigan PJ. A cluster of pediatric metallic mercury exposure cases treated with meso-2,3-dimercaptosuccinic acid (DMSA). *Environ Health Perspect*. 2000 Jun;108(6):575-7 http://ehp.niehs.nih.gov/docs/2000/108p575-577forman/abstract.html
[596] Miller AL. Dimercaptosuccinic acid (DMSA), a non-toxic, water-soluble treatment for heavy metal toxicity. *Altern Med Rev*. 1998 Jun;3(3):199-207 http://www.thorne.com/altmedrev/.fulltext/3/3/199.pdf
[597] DMSA. *Altern Med Rev*. 2000 Jun;5(3):264-7 http://thorne.com/altmedrev/.fulltext/5/3/264.pdf

Problems and Solutions in Clinical Detoxification

Effects	Cause	Solutions
1) Toxicant exposure and accumulation	• Excess exposure in relation to genotypic/phenotypic detoxification capabilities	• Total load of all xenobiotics must be reduced because of the similar/identical pathways used for the elimination of chemicals. Avoid the following: paint fumes, perfume, varnish, new carpet, formaldehyde, food colors, food additives, artificial sweeteners, pesticides, herbicides, and industrial waste.[598] • Since the vast majority of toxicants originate from irresponsible corporations, social/political action is necessary to effect fundamental change.[599]
2) Phase 1 Oxidation inhibited, too slow	• SNiPs and genotypic variations • Certain drugs • Certain food components: arachidonate and flavonoids such as bergapten (67%), quercetin (55%), naringenin (39%) naringin (6%) • Viral infections • Heavy metals • Nutritional deficiencies • Gut-derived LPS/endotoxin	• Reduce drug need by restoring health and addressing underlying problems • Address viral infections and promote glutathione production, e.g., NAC[600] and lipoic acid[601] • Vitamin/mineral supplements to correct common deficiencies in American diet[602] and to induce activity of detoxifying enzymes[603] • Paleo[604]/Mediterranean diet[605] to provide foundational nutrition and improve health • Avoidance of excess arachidonate and grapefruit • Eliminate unfavorable microflora and reflorestate to reduce LPS/endotoxin load[606] • Chelate metals with chelating agent such as DMSA[607]

[598] Ross GH. Treatment options in multiple chemical sensitivity. *Toxicol Ind Health.* 1992 Jul-Aug;8(4):87-94

[599] Kristin S. Schafer, Margaret Reeves, Skip Spitzer, Susan E. Kegley. Chemical Trespass: Pesticides in Our Bodies and Corporate Accountability. Pesticide Action Network North America. May 2004 Available at http://www.panna.org/campaigns/docsTrespass/chemicalTrespass2004.dv.html on August 1, 2004

[600] "NAC treatment was well tolerated and resulted in a significant decrease in the frequency of influenza-like episodes, severity, and length of time confined to bed. Both local and systemic symptoms were sharply and significantly reduced in the NAC group." De Flora S, Grassi C, Carati L. Attenuation of influenza-like symptomatology and improvement of cell-mediated immunity with long-term N-acetylcysteine treatment. *Eur Respir J.* 1997 Jul;10(7):1535-41 Available on-line at http://erj.ersjournals.com/cgi/reprint/10/7/1535 on October 18, 2004

[601] "These findings confirm the involvement of ROI in NF-kappaB-mediated HIV gene expression as well as the efficacy of LA as a therapeutic regimen for HIV infection and acquired immunodeficiency syndrome (AIDS)." Merin JP, Matsuyama M, Kira T, Baba M, Okamoto T. Alpha-lipoic acid blocks HIV-1 LTR-dependent expression of hygromycin resistance in THP-1 stable transformants. *FEBS Lett.* 1996 Sep 23;394(1):9-13

[602] Fletcher RH, Fairfield KM. Vitamins for chronic disease prevention in adults: clinical applications. *JAMA.* 2002 Jun 19;287(23):3127-9

[603] Ames BN, Elson-Schwab I, Silver EA. High-dose vitamin therapy stimulates variant enzymes with decreased coenzyme binding affinity (increased K(m)): relevance to genetic disease and polymorphisms. *Am J Clin Nutr.* 2002 Apr;75(4):616-58

[604] O'Keefe JH Jr, Cordain L. Cardiovascular disease resulting from a diet and lifestyle at odds with our Paleolithic genome: how to become a 21st-century hunter-gatherer. *Mayo Clin Proc.* 2004 Jan;79(1):101-8

[605] Knoops KT, de Groot LC, Kromhout D, Perrin AE, Moreiras-Varela O, Menotti A, van Staveren WA. Mediterranean diet, lifestyle factors, and 10-year mortality in elderly European men and women: the HALE project. *JAMA.* 2004 Sep 22;292(12):1433-9

[606] Shedlofsky SI, Israel BC, Tosheva R, Blouin RA. Endotoxin depresses hepatic cytochrome P450-mediated drug metabolism in women. *Br J Clin Pharmacol.* 1997 Jun;43(6):627-32

[607] Miller AL. Dimercaptosuccinic Acid (DMSA), A Non-Toxic, Water-Soluble Treatment For Heavy Metal Toxicity. *Altern Med Rev* 1998;3(3):199-207

Schematic Overview of Toxicant Exposure and Detoxification/Depuration

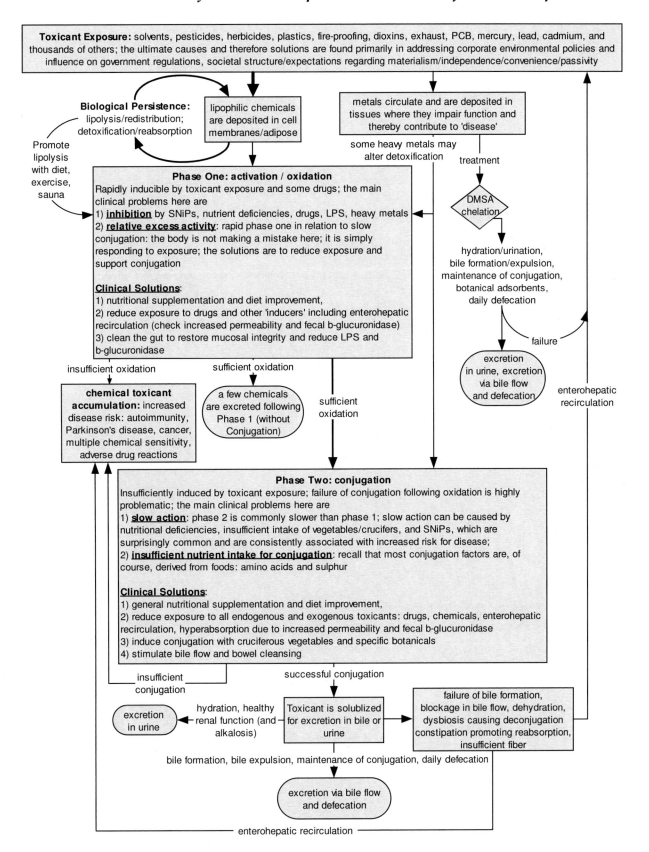

Toxicant Exposure: solvents, pesticides, herbicides, plastics, fire-proofing, dioxins, exhaust, PCB, mercury, lead, cadmium, and thousands of others; the ultimate causes and therefore solutions are found primarily in addressing corporate environmental policies and influence on government regulations, societal structure/expectations regarding materialism/independence/convenience/passivity

Biological Persistence: lipolysis/redistribution; detoxification/reabsorption

lipophilic chemicals are deposited in cell membranes/adipose

metals circulate and are deposited in tissues where they impair function and thereby contribute to 'disease'

Promote lipolysis with diet, exercise, sauna

some heavy metals may alter detoxification

treatment

DMSA chelation

Phase One: activation / oxidation
Rapidly inducible by toxicant exposure and some drugs; the main clinical problems here are
1) **inhibition** by SNiPs, nutrient deficiencies, drugs, LPS, heavy metals
2) **relative excess activity**: rapid phase one in relation to slow conjugation: the body is not making a mistake here; it is simply responding to exposure; the solutions are to reduce exposure and support conjugation

Clinical Solutions:
1) nutritional supplementation and diet improvement,
2) reduce exposure to drugs and other 'inducers' including enterohepatic recirculation (check increased permeability and fecal b-glucuronidase)
3) clean the gut to restore mucosal integrity and reduce LPS and b-glucuronidase

hydration/urination, bile formation/expulsion, maintenance of conjugation, botanical adsorbents, daily defecation

failure

insufficient oxidation

sufficient oxidation

excretion in urine, excretion via bile flow and defecation

enterohepatic recirculation

chemical toxicant accumulation: increased disease risk: autoimmunity, Parkinson's disease, cancer, multiple chemical sensitivity, adverse drug reactions

a few chemicals are excreted following Phase 1 (without Conjugation)

sufficient oxidation

Phase Two: conjugation
Insufficiently induced by toxicant exposure; failure of conjugation following oxidation is highly problematic; the main clinical problems here are
1) **slow action**: phase 2 is commonly slower than phase 1; slow action can be caused by nutritional deficiencies, insufficient intake of vegetables/crucifers, and SNiPs, which are surprisingly common and are consistently associated with increased risk for disease;
2) **insufficient nutrient intake for conjugation**: recall that most conjugation factors are, of course, derived from foods: amino acids and sulphur

Clinical Solutions:
1) general nutritional supplementation and diet improvement,
2) reduce exposure to all endogenous and exogenous toxicants: drugs, chemicals, enterohepatic recirculation, hyperabsorption due to increased permeability and fecal b-glucuronidase
3) induce conjugation with cruciferous vegetables and specific botanicals
4) stimulate bile flow and bowel cleansing

insufficient conjugation

successful conjugation

excretion in urine

hydration, healthy renal function (and alkalosis)

Toxicant is solubilized for excretion in bile or urine

failure of bile formation, blockage in bile flow, dehydration, dysbiosis causing deconjugation constipation promoting reabsorption, insufficient fiber

bile formation, bile expulsion, maintenance of conjugation, daily defecation

excretion via bile flow and defecation

enterohepatic recirculation

Problems and Solutions in Clinical Detoxification—*continued*

Effects	*Cause*	*Solutions*
3) Phase 1 Oxidation imbalanced, too fast relative to Phase 2	▪ Certain drugs or other toxicant exposure from endogenous or exogenous sources leads to upregulation of Phase 1	▪ Reduce drug need by restoring health and addressing underlying problems ▪ Suspect excess enterohepatic recirculation (via excess fecal β-glucuronidase): assess and optimize gastrointestinal flora by eliminating harmful bacteria and using probiotics[608] ▪ Upregulate phase 2 with diet and botanicals, such as cruciferous vegetables[609,610]
4) Phase 2 Conjugation too slow	▪ SNiPs: single nucleotide polymorphism defects in detoxification enzymes ▪ Fluoridated water: inhibits glucuronidation in some patients with Gilbert's syndrome[611] ▪ Lack of stimulation with diet and botanicals (i.e., insufficient intake of cruciferous vegetables)	▪ Avoid fluoridated water ▪ Upregulate phase 2 with diet and botanicals (citations above) ▪ Create balance by addressing the toxicant exposure that is upregulating phase 1
5) Phase 2 Conjugation Unsupported	▪ Insufficient protein for amino acids and sulfur; insufficient vitamins/minerals ▪ Poor digestion	▪ Paleo-Mediterranean diet with plenty of protein (this is not the time to be a *junkitarian* or *breaditarian*)[612] ▪ Cofactor supplementation: NAC, glutamine, glycine, taurine, sulfur, whey[613,614] ▪ Custom amino acid blend for recalcitrant cases[615]

---

[608] "Also they inhibited the harmful enzymes (beta-glucosidase, beta-glucuronidase, tryptophanase and urease) and ammonia production of intestinal microflora, and lowered pH of the culture media by increasing lactic acid bacteria of intestinal microflora." Park HY, Bae EA, Han MJ, Choi EC, Kim DH. Inhibitory effects of Bifidobacterium spp. isolated from a healthy Korean on harmful enzymes of human intestinal microflora. *Arch Pharm Res*. 1998 Feb;21(1):54-61

[609] "In conclusion, consumption of glucosinolate-containing Brussels sprouts for 1 week results in increased rectal GST-alpha and -pi isozyme levels. We hypothesize that these enhanced detoxification enzyme levels may partly explain the epidemiological association between a high intake of glucosinolates (cruciferous vegetables) and a decreased risk of colorectal cancer." Nijhoff WA, Grubben MJ, Nagengast FM, Jansen JB, Verhagen H, van Poppel G, Peters WH. Effects of consumption of Brussels sprouts on intestinal and lymphocytic glutathione S-transferases in humans. *Carcinogenesis*. 1995 Sep;16(9):2125-8

[610] "...human CYP1A2 and other CYP enzymes involved in oestrone 2-hydroxylation are induced by dietary broccoli." Kall MA, Vang O, Clausen J. Effects of dietary broccoli on human in vivo drug metabolizing enzymes: evaluation of caffeine, oestrone and chlorzoxazone metabolism. *Carcinogenesis*. 1996 Apr;17(4):793-9

[611] Lee J. Gilbert's disease and fluoride intake. *Fluoride* 1983; 16: 139-45

[612] O'Keefe JH Jr, Cordain L. Cardiovascular disease resulting from a diet and lifestyle at odds with our Paleolithic genome: how to become a 21st-century hunter-gatherer. *Mayo Clin Proc*. 2004 Jan;79(1):101-8 http://www.thepaleodiet.com/articles/Hunter-Gatherer%20Mayo.pdf

[613] "CONCLUSION: Supplementation with whey proteins persistently increased plasma glutathione levels in patients with advanced HIV-infection. The treatment was well tolerated." Micke P, Beeh KM, Buhl R. Effects of long-term supplementation with whey proteins on plasma glutathione levels of HIV-infected patients. *Eur J Nutr*. 2002 Feb;41(1):12-8

[614] "A significant increase in mononuclear cell glutathione was also observed in subjects receiving the WPI supplement following the 40 km simulated cycling trial." Middleton N, Jelen P, Bell G. Whole blood and mononuclear cell glutathione response to dietary whey protein supplementation in sedentary and trained male human subjects. *Int J Food Sci Nutr*. 2004 Mar;55(2):131-41

[615] Bralley JA. Lord RS. Treatment of chronic fatigue syndrome with specific amino acid supplementation. *Journal of Applied Nutrition* 1994; 46(3): 74-78

Problems and Solutions in Clinical Detoxification—*continued*

Effects	*Cause*	*Solutions*
6) Insufficient bile flow	▪ "Normal" bile flow appears too slow to keep pace with supraphysiologic toxicant exposure	▪ Stimulate bile flow with rectal instillations[616,617] and botanical medicines such as *Picrorhiza kurroa*[618] and *Andrographis paniculata*[619]
7) Urinary excretion insufficient due to insufficient hydration	▪ Subclinical dehydration is common and is exacerbated by diuretics such as ethanol and caffeine	▪ Drink water and antioxidant-rich teas and juices
8) Renal pH too acidic for optimal toxicant excretion	▪ Western/American diet promotes an acidic renal pH[620] which is known to reduce toxicant excretion[621]	▪ Vegetarian or Paleo-Mediterranean diet to alkalinize renal pH ▪ Fruit/vegetable juices provide potassium and citrate for effective alkalinization of urine[622] ▪ Use sodium bicarbonate[623] and/or potassium citrate as needed
9) Enterohepatic recirculation	▪ Constipation ▪ Excess microflora (quantitative or qualitative) producing β-glucuronidase ▪ Leaky gut	▪ Promote generous laxation: magnesium, fiber, vegetables, fruit, nuts, seeds ▪ Optimize gastrointestinal microflora ▪ Assess and normalize mucosal integrity ▪ Rectal instillations may be used to cleanse the bowel and to increase bile flow as previously documented radiographically[624]; this appears to improve detoxification clinical results[625,626] presumably due to expedition of toxicant removal[627]

[616] Garbat, AL, Jacobi, HG: Secretion of Bile in Response to Rectal Installations. *Arch Intern Med* 1929; 44: 455-462

[617] "Caffeine enemas cause dilation of bile ducts, which facilitates excretion of toxic cancer breakdown products by the liver and dialysis of toxic products from blood across the colonic wall. The therapy must be used as an integrated whole." Gerson M. The cure of advanced cancer by diet therapy: a summary of 30 years of clinical experimentation. *Physiol Chem Phys.* 1978;10(5):449-64

[618] Vaidya AB, Antarkar DS, Doshi JC, Bhatt AD, Ramesh VV, Vora PV, Perissond DD, Baxi AJ, Kale PM. Picrorhiza kurroa (Kutaki) Royle ex Benth as a hepatoprotective agent--experimental & clinical studies. *J Postgrad Med* 1996;42:105-8 Available on October 18, 2004 at http://www.jpgmonline.com/article.asp?issn=0022-3859;year=1996;volume=42;issue=4;spage=105;epage=8;aulast=Vaidya

[619] "Andrographolide from the herb Andrographis paniculata (whole plant) per se produces a significant dose (1.5-12 mg/kg) dependent choleretic effect (4.8-73%) as evidenced by increase in bile flow, bile salt, and bile acids in conscious rats and anaesthetized guinea pigs." Shukla B, Visen PK, Patnaik GK, Dhawan BN. Choleretic effect of andrographolide in rats and guinea pigs. *Planta Med* 1992 Apr;58(2):146-9

[620] Cordain L: *The Paleo Diet: Lose weight and get healthy by eating the food you were designed to eat.* John Wiley & Sons Inc., New York 2002

[621] Proudfoot AT, Krenzelok EP, Vale JA. Position Paper on urine alkalinization. *J Toxicol Clin Toxicol.* 2004;42(1):1-26

[622] "New Guinean hunter-gatherer tribal group living in "the primitive feral condition" ...urine pH of adults was usually between 7.5 and 9.0." Sebastian A, Frassetto LA, Sellmeyer DE, Merriam RL, Morris RC Jr. Estimation of the net acid load of the diet of ancestral preagricultural Homo sapiens and their hominid ancestors. *Am J Clin Nutr.* 2002 Dec;76(6):1308-16

[623] "Urine alkalinization is a treatment regimen that increases poison elimination by the administration of intravenous sodium bicarbonate to produce urine with a pH > or = 7.5." Proudfoot AT, Krenzelok EP, Vale JA. Position Paper on urine alkalinization. *J Toxicol Clin Toxicol.* 2004;42(1):1-26

[624] "Caffeine enemas cause dilation of bile ducts, which facilitates excretion of toxic cancer breakdown products by the liver and dialysis of toxic products from blood across the colonic wall. The therapy must be used as an integrated whole." Gerson M. The cure of advanced cancer by diet therapy: a summary of 30 years of clinical experimentation. *Physiol Chem Phys.* 1978;10(5):449-64

[625] Snyder RG. The value of colonic irrigations in countering auto-intoxication of intestinal origin. *Medical Clinics of North America* 1939; May: 781-788

[626] Gonzalez NJ, Isaacs LL. Evaluation of pancreatic proteolytic enzyme treatment of adenocarcinoma of the pancreas, with nutrition and detoxification support. *Nutr Cancer.* 1999;33(2):117-24

[627] Crinnion WJ. Results of a decade of naturopathic treatment for environmental illness: a review of clinical records. *J Naturopathic Med* 1997;7:21-27

Effects	Cause	Solutions
10) Deconjugation by microflora	▪ Excess microflora (quantitative or qualitative) producing β-glucuronidase ▪ Constipation must be eliminated[628]	▪ Botanical and/or pharmaceutical antimicrobials/antifungals to reduce bacterial load in the intestines, similar to the use of antibiotics in the treatment of hepatic encephalopathy ▪ Prebiotics and probiotics to optimize gut flora ▪ Dietary fiber may be used to promote laxation and excretion of toxicants before enterohepatic recirculation; cholestyramine may be used in selected cases to augment fecal elimination of toxicants such as pesticides[629]
11) Heavy metal toxicity 12) Metal-induced alteration of detoxification (upregulation or downregulation of specific processes)	▪ Heavy metal exposure appears to inhibit Phase 1 oxidation (*in vitro*[630])	▪ Reduce exposure to toxicants ▪ Chelation, such as with DMSA which appears effective for mercury[631] and lead[632] ▪ Promote generous laxation: magnesium, fiber, vegetables, fruit, nuts, seeds ▪ Optimize gastrointestinal microflora ▪ Fruit/vegetable juices provide potassium and citrate for effective urinary alkalinization
13) Disease promotion via toxicants stored in body tissues, particularly adipose and brain	▪ Chemical toxicants are inherently biologically persistent ▪ Defective detoxification	▪ Sauna, hyperthermia, exercise to promote sweating and lipolysis[633,634] ▪ "Fat exchange" via low-fat diet to effect weight loss followed by supplementation of health-promoting uncontaminated fatty acids[635] ▪ Weight loss for obese patients only after detoxification program is well established

[628] "Enemas and suppositories stimulate colonic contractions and soften stools. Water, saline, soap suds, hypertonic sodium phosphate, and mineral oil are used as enemas. Acute water intoxication can occur with water enemas, especially in infants, children, and the elderly, if they have difficulty evacuating the water." Dosh SA. Evaluation and treatment of constipation. *J Fam Pract.* 2002 Jun;51(6):555-9 Available at http://www.jfponline.com/content/2002/06/jfp_0602_00541.asp on October 18, 2004

[629] "Output of chlordecone in bile was 10 to 20 times greater than in stool, suggesting that chlordecone is reabsorbed in the intestine. Cholestyramine, an anion-exchange resin that binds chlordecone, increased its fecal excretion by seven times." Cohn WJ, Boylan JJ, Blanke RV, Fariss MW, Howell JR, Guzelian PS. Treatment of chlordecone (Kepone) toxicity with cholestyramine. Results of a controlled clinical trial. *N Engl J Med.* 1978 Feb 2;298(5):243-8

[630] "All four of the metals investigated decreased the extent of CYP1A1 induction in HepG2 cells by at least one of the five PAHs, in some cases decreases were marked. The same order of effectiveness of metal-mediated decreases in CYP1A1 were cadmium > arsenic > lead > mercury for all the PAHs." Vakharia DD, Liu N, Pause R, Fasco M, Bessette E, Zhang QY, Kaminsky LS. Polycyclic aromatic hydrocarbon/metal mixtures: effect on PAH induction of CYP1A1 in human HEPG2 cells. Drug Metab Dispos. 2001 Jul;29(7):999-1006 Available at http://dmd.aspetjournals.org/cgi/content/full/29/7/999 on October 18, 2004

[631] "Thus, oral chelation with DMSA produced a significant mercury diuresis in these children. We observed no adverse side effects of treatment. DMSA appears to be an effective and safe chelating agent for treatment of pediatric overexposure to metallic mercury." Forman J, Moline J, Cernichiari E, Sayegh S, Torres JC, Landrigan MM, Hudson J, Adel HN, Landrigan PJ. A cluster of pediatric metallic mercury exposure cases treated with meso-2,3-dimercaptosuccinic acid (DMSA). *Environ Health Perspect.* 2000 Jun;108(6):575-7 Available at http://ehp.niehs.nih.gov/members/2000/108p575-577forman/108p575.pdf on October 18, 2004

[632] "To conclude, awareness and early diagnosis of lead toxicity is important. Succimer is an effective chelator in patients for lead toxicity. It can be administered orally and hospitalization eliminated. However, chelation therapy should never be used as a substitute for environmental assessment and lead abatement for lead poisoned children." Kalra V, Dua T, Kumar V, Kaul B. Succimer in symptomatic lead poisoning. *Indian Pediatr.* 2002 Jun;39(6):580-5 Available at http://www.indianpediatrics.net/june2002/june-580-585.htm on October 18, 2004

[633] Schnare DW, Ben M, Shields MG. Body Burden Reductions of PCBs, PBBs and Chlorinated Pesticide Residues in Human Subjects. Ambio 1984; 13 (5-6): 378-380

[634] Krop J. Chemical sensitivity after intoxication at work with solvents: response to sauna therapy. *J Altern Complement Med* 1998 Spring;4(1):77-86

[635] "Repeated fasting and refeeding with fish oil facilitated plasma exchange of n-3 for n-6 PUFA, improved BP, clinical metabolic parameters and lowered platelet reactivity in the vessel wall (primary hemostasis)." Yosefy C, Viskoper JR, Varon D, Ilan Z, Pilpel D, Lugassy G, Schneider R, Savyon N, Adan Y, Raz A. Repeated fasting and refeeding with 20:5, n-3 eicosapentaenoic acid (EPA): a novel approach for rapid fatty acid exchange and its effect on blood pressure, plasma lipids and hemostasis. *J Hum Hypertens* 1996 Sep;10 Suppl 3:S135-9

Therapeutic: ## Dimercaptosuccinic acid

Common name: # DMSA

Applications and mechanisms of action:

- DMSA is a well documented chelating agent that is FDA-approved for the treatment of lead poisoning.[636] It has been used safely and successfully in children and adults with lead and/or mercury toxicity, whether acute or chronic. The sulfur-containing moiety of the molecule binds to heavy metals, rendering them soluble, and then the metal-DMSA complex is excreted in urine or bile.

A few of the better articles on this topic are listed here:

- **DMSA-mercury testing in autistic children**: Two-hundred-twenty-one children with autism were challenged with 30 mg/kg of DMSA and showed significantly higher urinary mercury excretion compared to control subjects. The specific protocol is described as follows: "The Arizona State University Institutional Review Board approved our retrospective examination of cases and controls in this study. ... Informed consent was obtained from both cases and controls for DMSA chelation treatment. Controls and cases were both challenged with a three-day oral treatment of **DMSA (10 mg/kg per dose given three times daily).** After the ninth dose, the first voided morning urine was collected (when possible), or an overnight urine collection bag was worn. All laboratory analyses were performed by the Doctors Data, Inc., in Chicago, Ill."[637] No adverse effects were reported.

- **Mercury review by Dr. Walter Crinnion**: As one of the most experienced environmental medicine doctors in the US, Dr. Crinnion provides his perspective on the treatment of mercury toxicity, and states, "DMSA can be given to an adult at a dose of 500 mg tid... DMSA (30 mg/kg)... It is generally recommended that these agents be given in several day courses repeatedly, with rest periods in between."[638]

- **Nine cases of pediatric mercury poisoning safely treated with DMSA**: Nine mercury-poisoned children were treated with DMSA 30 mg/kg for 5 days followed by 20 mg/kg for 2 weeks; mercury levels declined in all children, and no adverse effects occurred.[639]

- **DMSA monographs**: monographs on the basic science and clinical applications of DMSA.[640,641]

- **Acute poisoning review**: A "nutshell" review of the management of acute poisoning.[642]

---

[636] "The Food and Drug Administration has recently licensed the drug DMSA (succimer) for reduction of blood lead levels >/= 45 micrograms/dl. This decision was based on the demonstrated ability of DMSA to reduce blood lead levels. An advantage of this drug is that it can be given orally." Goyer RA, Cherian MG, Jones MM, Reigart JR. Role of chelating agents for prevention, intervention, and treatment of exposures to toxic metals. *Environ Health Perspect.* 1995 Nov;103(11):1048-52 Http://ehp.niehs.nih.gov/docs/1995/103-11/meetingreport.html
[637] Bradstreet J, Geier DA, Kartzinel JJ, Adams JB, Geier MR. A case-control study of mercury burden in children with autistic spectrum disorders. *Journal of American Physicians and Surgeons* 2003; 8: 76-79   http://www.jpands.org/vol8no3/geier.pdf
[638] Crinnion WJ. Environmental medicine, part three: long-term effects of chronic low-dose mercury exposure. *Altern Med Rev.* 2000 Jun;5(3):209-23 http://www.thorne.com/altmedrev/.fulltext/5/3/209.pdf
[639] Forman J, Moline J, Cernichiari E, Sayegh S, Torres JC, Landrigan MM, Hudson J, Adel HN, Landrigan PJ. A cluster of pediatric metallic mercury exposure cases treated with meso-2,3-dimercaptosuccinic acid (DMSA). *Environ Health Perspect.* 2000 Jun;108(6):575-7 http://ehp.niehs.nih.gov/docs/2000/108p575-577forman/abstract.html
[640] Miller AL. Dimercaptosuccinic acid (DMSA), a non-toxic, water-soluble treatment for heavy metal toxicity. *Altern Med Rev.* 1998 Jun;3(3):199-207 http://www.thorne.com/altmedrev/.fulltext/3/3/199.pdf
[641] DMSA. *Altern Med Rev.* 2000 Jun;5(3):264-7 http://thorne.com/altmedrev/.fulltext/5/3/264.pdf
[642] Greene SL, Dargan PI, Jones AL. Acute poisoning: understanding 90% of cases in a nutshell. *Postgrad Med J.* 2005 Apr;81(954):204-16 http://pmj.bmjjournals.com/cgi/content/full/81/954/204

Toxicity:	▪ DMSA has a very favorable risk:benefit ratio when used in patients without renal/hepatic impairment and who are at average or greater-than-average risk for heavy metal accumulation/toxicity. Toxicity is very rare. Some articles make fleeting mention of bone marrow suppression, but this is almost never precipitated clinically and is practically never documented in the case reports and clinical studies using DMSA for the treatment of heavy metal toxicity. Patients should be tested for hematologic and metabolic status prior to DMSA administration; a CBC and metabolic/chemistry panel is sufficient.
	▪ Allergic-type reactions to DMSA and/or the mobilization of heavy metals, especially mercury, are infrequent but not rare. To reduce the risk of precipitating such reactions, a trial dose of 100 mg (or less for children) should be used on a single occasion to ensure that IgE-mediated allergy or anaphylaxis does not occur with the higher doses used therapeutically. Like any drug, DMSA may precipitate idiosyncratic reactions, but these are by definition nearly impossible to predict. However, since idiosyncratic drug reactions appear to reflect imbalanced Phase 1 / Phase 2 detoxification, the likelihood of such a reaction can probably be reduced by ensuring that the patient is supplemented with antioxidants, fortified with sufficient protein for supporting Phase 2 conjugation reactions, and abstinent from other drugs which induce Phase 1 upregulation. Patients with adverse reactions to DMSA should either not use DMSA or should do so carefully, such as with a lower dose or after the underlying cause of the sensitivity has been addressed.
Dosage and administration:	▪ <u>Screening laboratory tests</u>: Urinalysis, CBC and chemistry panel with BUN, creatinine, and hepatic markers are sufficient for assessing renal, hepatic, and marrow status.
	▪ <u>Empty stomach</u>: DMSA should be taken on an empty stomach, preferably 1-2 hours away from food. In particular, mineral supplements containing zinc and copper (etc) should be avoided for 4 hours before and after DMSA supplementation. Generally, first morning supplementation with a delayed or skipped breakfast is ideal.
	▪ <u>The lowest therapeutic dose is generally 10 mg/kg per day, and the highest therapeutic dose is generally 30 mg/kg per day</u>. The 30 mg/kg dose is generally delivered in three divided doses (i.e., 10 mg/kg TID); however, a single-dose 30 mg/kg dose may be used provocatively for diagnostic purposes. Lower dosage schemes are appropriate for children or those with severe sensitivities. The highest scheme may also be appropriate for children but might otherwise be reserved for adult patients who are in otherwise good health.

Body weight in lbs (kg)	10 mg/kg dose	30 mg/kg dose (bolus or divided)
40 lbs (18 kg)	180 mg	540 mg
80 lbs (36 kg)	360 mg	1080 mg
120 lbs (54 kg)	540 mg	1620 mg
160 lbs (72 kg)	720 mg	2,160 mg (limit to 2,000) mg
200 lbs (90 kg)	900 mg	2,700 (limit to 2,000) mg
240 lbs (108 kg)	1080 mg	3,240 (limit to 2,000) mg
280 lbs (126 kg)	1260 mg	3,780 (limit to 2,000) mg

Dosage and administration (continued):	▪ <u>Cyclical dosing</u>: DMSA is generally "cycled" which means that it is taken for a few days, the discontinued for a few days, then resumed, etc. This can be customized per patient for ease of compliance and variations in scheduling. For example, the patient might use DMSA for 5 days of the week, taking the weekends "off", or might use DMSA for 4 days on and 3 days off, etc. Every-other-day dosing is also reasonable. Treatment is generally continued for 1-2 months.
	▪ <u>Plenty of water</u>: DMSA should be taken with 16 ounces of water. An additional 1-2 liters should be consumed over the next 2-4 hours.
Additional information:	▪ DMSA increases urinary excretion of copper in humans[643]; if treatment were excessively prolonged then theoretically this might lead to copper deficiency. Additionally, DMSA might be useful for people with excess copper. These areas require more research.
	▪ Co-supplementation with the following can increase urinary metal excretion and/or reduce enterohepatic recycling of toxic metals. These can be used during DMSA treatment but should not be taken within 2-4 hours of DMSA supplementation so as not to bind with or otherwise interfere with DMSA absorption and utilization.

- *Fruit and vegetable juices*: Potassium citrate has been shown to significantly increase mercury excretion in humans when used alone and/or with DMSA.[644,645] Fruit and vegetable juices are rich sources of potassium citrate and should be consumed liberally by patients undergoing detoxification. Furthermore, since urinary alkalinization greatly increases the urinary excretion of chemical/xenobiotics toxicants[646], essentially all patients undergoing detoxification programs should increase consumption of fruit and vegetable juices as well as fruits and vegetables.
- *Phytochelatins*: Phytochelatins are metal-binding moieties from plants and algae.[647] Clinically, doctors use phytochelatin supplementation to bind metals in the gut for enhanced excretion, i.e., to prevent re-absorption of metals that have been detoxified into the gut lumen via the bile. High-fiber plant-based diets are beneficial for the same purpose.
- *Selenium*: Selenium has many important actions in the body, one of which is that of an antioxidant. It is generally dosed at 200 mcg per day, but doses up to 1,000 mcg per day are generally safe for most adults. Clinical studies evaluating the effect of selenium on mercury kinetics are rare, and the study by Seppanen et al[648] appears of limited clinical relevance.

---

[643] "The Food and Drug Administration has recently licensed the drug DMSA (succimer) for reduction of blood lead levels >/= 45 micrograms/dl. This decision was based on the demonstrated ability of DMSA to reduce blood lead levels. An advantage of this drug is that it can be given orally." Goyer RA, Cherian MG, Jones MM, Reigart JR. Role of chelating agents for prevention, intervention, and treatment of exposures to toxic metals. *Environ Health Perspect*. 1995 Nov;103(11):1048-52 Http://ehp.niehs.nih.gov/docs/1995/103-11/meetingreport.html

[644] "Based on the increase in urinary Hg concentrations after single doses, compared with controls, the order of efficacy was: DMPS plus K Cit., NAC plus K Cit. and DMSA (each producing an increase of 163%), then in descending order, DMSA plus K Cit., DMPS, NAC and K Cit." Hibberd AR, Howard MA, Hunnisett AG. Mercury from dental amalgam fillings studies on oral chelating agents for assessing and reducing mercury burdens in humans. *J Nutr Environ Med* 1998;8:219-231

[645] Crinnion WJ. Environmental medicine, part three: long-term effects of chronic low-dose mercury exposure. *Altern Med Rev*. 2000 Jun;5(3):209-23 http://www.thorne.com/altmedrev/.fulltext/5/3/209.pdf

[646] Proudfoot AT, Krenzelok EP, Vale JA. Position Paper on urine alkalinization. *J Toxicol Clin Toxicol*. 2004;42(1):1-26. This is a very important paper. Posted by the European Association of Poisons Centres and Clinical Toxicologists at http://www.eapcct.org/publicfile.php?folder=congress&file=PS_UrineAlkalinization.pdf accessed October 28, 2005

[647] Cobbett CS. Phytochelatins and their roles in heavy metal detoxification. *Plant Physiol*. 2000 Jul;123(3):825-32 http://www.plantphysiol.org/cgi/content/full/123/3/825 This is a basic science review with relevance for plant biology that discusses the use of phytochelatins to bind metals in the plant's environment. It does not discuss relevance of phytochelatins for the treatment of heavy metal exposure in humans.

[648] "The selenium supplementation group received daily 100 micrograms of selenomethionine. Selenium supplementation reduced pubic hair mercury level by 34% (p = 0.005) and elevated serum selenium by 73% and blood selenium by 59% in the supplemented group (p < 0.001 for both). The study indicates that mercury accumulation in pubic hair can be reduced by dietary supplementation with small daily amounts of organic selenium in a short range of time." Seppanen K, Kantola M, Laatikainen R, Nyyssonen K, Valkonen VP, Kaarlopp V, Salonen JT. Effect of supplementation with organic selenium on mercury status as measured by mercury in pubic hair. *J Trace Elem Med Biol*. 2000 Jun;14(2):84-7

Information about DMSA and lead/mercury toxicity

- *About lead and mercury*: Lead and mercury are toxic metals that accumulate in some people and cause serious health problems. Diagnosis and treatment of heavy metal accumulation is important for alleviating current symptoms and preventing future illness.
- *About DMSA*: DMSA is an over-the-counter nutritional supplement that provides succinate, a substance found in every cell of the body.
- *What it DMSA does*: DMSA helps the body rid itself of harmful minerals and metals, and it has been used in many studies in adults and children.
- *Potential risks and benefits*: The vast majority of studies have shown DMSA to be safe and highly effective. In healthcare, we always look at treatments in terms of the "risk-to-benefit ratio" and in the case of DMSA the risks appear small and the potential benefit is large when we are talking about removing toxic heavy metals. Side-effects are very rare, but have been reported to include temporary liver damage and mild gastrointestinal upset. Some doctors and companies mention that bone marrow suppression can also be a temporary side effect, but I have never seen this described in the research.
- *How DMSA has been used*: DMSA has been safely and effectively used in the treatment of people who have been either acutely or chronically poisoned with toxic metals such as lead and mercury. It has been used in children and adults. DMSA has been approved by the FDA for the treatment of lead poisoning in children. DMSA is also used by doctors to assist in the diagnosis of heavy metal toxicity—in this case, a "provocation" dose of DMSA is administered by mouth to increase the excretion of mercury in the urine; a urine sample is then sent to the laboratory for analysis.
- *How DMSA is dosed*: **For testing**, most experts recommend doses range from 10 mg/kg up to 30mg/kg with a limit of 2,000 mg per day. These doses are generally safe and effective and are well supported by the research. **For treatment**, a reasonable plan would be DMSA 10 mg/kg per day for 4 days "on" followed by 3 days "off." Some experts might consider this to be under-treatment, and your doctor may choose to use a higher dose.
- *Supportive treatments*: Patients must drink plenty of water, such as 3 liters per day for adults. The diet must be high in fiber to ensure generous bowel movements. DMSA treatment is not allowed in patients with constipation. High intake of fruit and vegetable juices to provide potassium citrate will significantly assist in the excretion of mercury in the urine. Binding agents such as fiber, phytochelatins, and alginate can be used to help reduce re-absorption of mercury in the gut. Supplementation with selenium and other antioxidants is advised.

Additional articles and sources of information so you can be informed of the risks and benefits:
- http://www.thorne.com/pdf/journal/5-3/environmental_3_mercury.pdf
- http://www.thorne.com/altmedrev/.fulltext/3/3/199.pdf
- http://www.jpands.org/vol8no3/geier.pdf
- http://ehp.niehs.nih.gov/docs/2000/108p575-577forman/abstract.html
- http://www.thorne.com/altmedrev/.fulltext/5/3/264.pdf

Sample schedule for "on" days:
- *First thing in the morning*: Take your dose of DMSA on an empty stomach with plenty of liquid, either tea, coffee, or fruit vegetable juice.
- *At least 1 hour later and preferably 2 hours after the DMSA dose*: OK to eat solid foods: emphasize fruits, vegetables, nuts and seeds (i.e., natural plant foods). Protein foods are also recommended, particularly soy and whey proteins; fish and poultry are also acceptable. This would also be an appropriate time to begin taking additional treatments such as "liver herbs" to simulate bile flow as well as plant fibers and phytochelatins to bind the mercury that will be released into the intestine from the liver.
- *Rest of the day*: Consume a healthy natural diet such as the one described by Dr. Loren Cordain in The Paleo Diet.
- Discontinue treatment and consult your healthcare provider if you experience any significant adverse effects. If symptoms are severe, call 911 or go to the nearest hospital.

Orthoendocrinology

<u>**Introduction**</u>: Steroidal hormones have significant immunomodulating properties, and a characteristic pattern of disruption is commonly seen in patients with autoimmunity. Relatively simple natural and/or pharmacologic interventions can be used to safely and effectively correct hormonal disturbances with the dual benefits of improved overall health and the amelioration of autoimmunity. I have coined the term "orthoendocrinology"[649] to describe this technique of addressing numerous disturbances in endocrine function by using the "right hormones" based on a similar conceptual model to Linus Pauling's suggestion that health might be optimized by the use of the "right molecules" (orthomolecular medicine, orthomolecular nutrition) rather than endless reliance on the cyclical prescriptions of what he called "toximolecular" substances. I will keep this overview and application straightforward, simple, and clinically relevant.

> **"The altered hormonal status could result in relative immunological hyperactivity contributing to enhance tissue damage and disease severity."**
>
> Mirone, Barini, Barini. Androgen and prolactin levels in systemic sclerosis: relationship to disease severity. *Ann N Y Acad Sci* 2006

The typical hormonal pattern that is seen in patients with systemic autoimmunity is:
- High prolactin
- High estrogen
- Low testosterone
- Low cortisol
- Low DHEA
- Hypothyroidism and/or thyroid autoimmunity
- Progesterone status is variable, apparently less important, and can be assessed per patient

<u>***Testing and treatment hormonal status in patients with autoimmunity***</u>: Patients with autoimmune disorders commonly have deficiencies and imbalances in their hormones, particularly steroid and "sex" hormones, which are potent immunomodulators. The classic pattern which may be expressed incompletely in an individual patient, is that of excess prolactin and estrogen, and insufficient cortisol, testosterone, and DHEA. The role of progesterone seems less clear, with some patients showing normal, excess, or insufficient amounts; obviously, this can be tested in an individual patient (random serum test in men or 21st-day/midluteal serum sample from a premenopausal woman). All testing methods—via serum, saliva, or urine—have their individual advantages and disadvantages. Generally however, serum is considered the standard; following this I prefer polyhormonal assessment with 24-hour urine collections, and the last resort is saliva testing, which is the most controversial and least reliable. Thyroid autoimmunity and hypothyroidism are both common in autoimmune/inflammatory patients; comprehensive thyroid assessment with TSH, T4, and anti-TPO antibodies can be justified in nearly any rheumatic patient.

> "Multiple lines of evidence support the concept that **the anterior pituitary hormone prolactin has a pathogenic role in rheumatic and autoimmune diseases** including, but not limited to, rheumatoid arthritis (RA), systemic lupus erythematosus (SLE), Reiter's syndrome, psoriatic arthritis, and uveitis."
>
> McMurray RW. *Semin Arthritis Rheum.* 2001

- **<u>Hyperprolactinemia and latent hyperprolactinemia</u>**: Besides its obvious role in lactation, prolactin is a polyfunctional hormone that, at the very least, stimulates the liver to produce excess sex-hormone-binding globulin (SHBG) which adsorbs sex hormones, rendering them less effective due to reduced bioavailability; the resultant *functional hypogonadism* deprives the immune system of the modulation/suppression normally effected by

---

[649] As of November 15, 2005 the word "orthoendocrinology" cannot be found either on Pubmed, Medline or an Internet search using Google, Yahoo, or MSN search engines.

these hormones. Beyond these well-known physiologic roles, **prolactin is now known to be powerfully proinflammatory.**[650] **Patients with RA and SLE have higher basal and stress-induced levels of prolactin compared with normal controls.**[651,652] **Patients with scleroderma have relatively high prolactin**[653] **and low DHEA.**[654] **Patients with polymyalgia rheumatica have elevated prolactin that correlates with increased symptomatology.**[655] Elevated prolactin levels may further exacerbate immune dysfunction by increasing hepatic production of sex-hormone binding globulin and reducing bioavailability of testosterone, thus depriving cells and tissues of testosterone's potent anti-inflammatory and immunoregulatory properties. Prolactin is routinely measured in serum; high values should be reduced with effective treatment, whether nutritional, botanical, or pharmacologic.

- o <u>Thyroid hormone</u>: **Hypothyroidism frequently causes hyperprolactinemia** that is reversible upon effective treatment of hypothyroidism. Conversely, due to its immunodysregulating effects, elevated prolactin appears capable of inducing hypothyroidism and autoimmune thyroiditis.[656] Assessing hyperprolactinemic patients for thyroid disturbances with TSH, T4, T3, and anti-TPO antibodies is strongly advised. Thyroid status should be evaluated in all patients with hyperprolactinemia.

- o <u>High-dose pyridoxine</u>: B6 (250 mg qd-bid with food) is used by some doctors to lower prolactin despite the lack of consistently demonstrated benefit in the research literature.

- o *<u>Vitex astus-cagnus</u> and other supporting botanicals and nutrients*: **Vitex lowers serum prolactin in humans**[657,658] **via a dopaminergic effect.**[659] Vitex is considered safe for clinical use; mild and reversible adverse effects possibly associated with Vitex include nausea, headache, gastrointestinal disturbances, menstrual disorders, acne, pruritus and erythematous rash. No drug interactions are known, but given the herb's dopaminergic effect it should probably be used with some caution in patients treated with dopamine antagonists such as the so-called antipsychotic drugs (most of which do not work very well and/or carry intolerable adverse effects[660,661]). In a recent review, Bone[662] stated that daily doses can range from 500 mg to 2,000 mg DHE (dry herb equivalent) and can be tailored to the suppression of prolactin. Due at least in part to its content of L-dopa, *Mucuna pruriens* **shows clinical dopaminergic activity** as evidenced by its effectiveness in Parkinson's disease[663]; up to 15-30 gm/d of mucuna has been used clinically but doses will be dependent on preparation and phytoconcentration. Triptolide and other **extracts from** *Tripterygium wilfordii* **Hook F** exert clinically significant anti-inflammatory action in patients

[650] "Multiple lines of evidence support the concept that the anterior pituitary hormone prolactin has a pathogenic role in rheumatic and autoimmune diseases including, but not limited to, rheumatoid arthritis (RA), systemic lupus erythematosus (SLE), Reiter's syndrome, psoriatic arthritis, and uveitis." McMurray RW. Bromocriptine in rheumatic and autoimmune diseases. *Semin Arthritis Rheum.* 2001 Aug;31(1):21-32

[651] Dostal C, Moszkorzova L, Musilova L, Lacinova Z, Marek J, Zvarova J. Serum prolactin stress values in patients with systemic lupus erythematosus. *Ann Rheum Dis.* 2003 May;62(5):487-8 http://ard.bmjjournals.com/cgi/content/full/62/5/487

[652] "RESULTS: A significantly higher rate of elevated PRL levels was found in SLE patients (40.0%) compared with the healthy controls (14.8%). No proof was found of association with the presence of anti-ds-DNA or with specific organ involvement. Similarly, elevated PRL levels were found in RA patients (39.3%)." Moszkorzova L, Lacinova Z, Marek J, Musilova L, Dohnalova A, Dostal C. Hyperprolactinaemia in patients with systemic lupus erythematosus. *Clin Exp Rheumatol.* 2002 Nov-Dec;20(6):807-12

[653] Straub RH, Zeuner M, Lock G, Scholmerich J, Lang B. High prolactin and low dehydroepiandrosterone sulphate serum levels in patients with severe systemic sclerosis. *Br J Rheumatol.* 1997 Apr;36(4):426-32 http://rheumatology.oxfordjournals.org/cgi/reprint/36/4/426

[654] "CONCLUSION: Our data show that, as in other autoimmune diseases, low serum DHEAS is a feature of premenopausal SSc patients. More extensive prospective studies are needed to define the exact role of DHEAS dysregulation in SSc." La Montagna G, Baruffo A, Buono G, Valentini G. Dehydroepiandrosterone sulphate serum levels in systemic sclerosis. *Clin Exp Rheumatol.* 2001 Jan-Feb;19(1):21-6

[655] Straub RH, Georgi J, Helmke K, Vaith P, Lang B. In polymyalgia rheumatica serum prolactin is positively correlated with the number of typical symptoms but not with typical inflammatory markers. *Rheumatology* (Oxford). 2002 Apr;41(4):423-9 http://rheumatology.oxfordjournals.org/cgi/content/full/41/4/423

[656] "...PRL level is higher in SLE patients and that in the presence of hyperPRL there is increased prevalence of antithyroid antibodies, evidencing the association of PRL and autoimmunity and pointing to the appropriateness of assessing and monitoring the progress of these markers in patients affected by these disorders." Kramer CK, Tourinho TF, de Castro WP, da Costa Oliveira M. Association between systemic lupus erythematosus, rheumatoid arthritis, hyperprolactinemia and thyroid autoantibodies. *Arch Med Res.* 2005 Jan-Feb;36(1):54-8

[657] "Since AC extracts were shown to have beneficial effects on premenstrual mastodynia serum prolactin levels in such patients were also studied in one double-blind, placebo-controlled clinical study. Serum prolactin levels were indeed reduced in the patients treated with the extract." Wuttke W, Jarry H, Christoffel V, Spengler B, Seidlova-Wuttke D. Chaste tree (Vitex agnus-castus)--pharmacology and clinical indications. *Phytomedicine.* 2003 May;10(4):348-57

[658] German abstract from Medline: "The prolactin release was reduced after 3 months, shortened luteal phases were normalised and deficits in the luteal progesterone synthesis were eliminated." Milewicz A, Gejdel E, Sworen H, Sienkiewicz K, Jedrzejak J, Teucher T, Schmitz H. [Vitex agnus castus extract in the treatment of luteal phase defects due to latent hyperprolactinemia. Results of a randomized placebo-controlled double-blind study] *Arzneimittelforschung.* 1993 Jul;43(7):752-6

[659] "Our results indicate a dopaminergic effect of Vitex agnus-castus extracts and suggest additional pharmacological actions via opioid receptors." Meier B, Berger D, Hoberg E, Sticher O, Schaffner W. Pharmacological activities of Vitex agnus-castus extracts in vitro. *Phytomedicine.* 2000 Oct;7(5):373-81

[660] "The majority of patients in each group discontinued their assigned treatment owing to inefficacy or intolerable side effects or for other reasons." Lieberman JA, Stroup TS, McEvoy JP, Swartz MS, Rosenheck RA, Perkins DO, Keefe RS, Davis SM, Davis CE, Lebowitz BD, Severe J, Hsiao JK; Clinical Antipsychotic Trials of Intervention Effectiveness (CATIE) Investigators. Effectiveness of antipsychotic drugs in patients with chronic schizophrenia. *N Engl J Med.* 2005 Sep 22;353(12):1209-23

[661] Whitaker R. The case against antipsychotic drugs: a 50-year record of doing more harm than good. *Med Hypotheses.* 2004;62(1):5-13

[662] "In conditions such as endometriosis and fibroids, for which a significant estrogen antagonist effect is needed, doses of at least 2 g/day DHE may be required and typically are used by professional herbalists." Bone K. New Insights Into Chaste Tree. *Nutritional Wellness* 2005 November http://www.nutritionalwellness.com/archives/2005/nov/11_bone.php

[663] "CONCLUSIONS: The rapid onset of action and longer on time without concomitant increase in dyskinesias on mucuna seed powder formulation suggest that this natural source of L-dopa might possess advantages over conventional L-dopa preparations in the long term management of PD." Katzenschlager R, Evans A, Manson A, Patsalos PN, Ratnaraj N, Watt H, Timmermann L, Van der Giessen R, Lees AJ. Mucuna pruriens in Parkinson's disease: a double blind and pharmacological study. *J Neurol Neurosurg Psychiatry.* 2004 Dec;75(12):1672-7

with rheumatoid arthritis[664,665] and also offer protection to dopaminergic neurons.[666,667] Ironically, even though tyrosine is the nutritional precursor to dopamine with evidence of clinical effectiveness (e.g., narcolepsy[668], enhancement of memory[669] and cognition[670]), **supplementation with tyrosine appears to actually increase rather than decrease prolactin levels[671]; therefore tyrosine should be used cautiously if at all in patients with systemic inflammation.** Furthermore, the finding that **high-protein meals stimulate prolactin release[672]** may partly explain the benefits of vegetarian diets in the treatment of systemic inflammation; since vegetarian diets are comparatively low in protein compared to omnivorous diets, they may lead to a relative reduction in prolactin production due to lack of stimulation.

o Bromocriptine: Bromocriptine has long been considered the pharmacologic treatment of choice for elevated prolactin.[673] Typical dose is 2.5 mg per day (effective against lupus[674]); gastrointestinal upset and sedation are common.[675] **Clinical intervention with bromocriptine appears warranted in patients with RA, SLE, Reiter's syndrome, psoriatic arthritis, and probably multiple sclerosis and uveitis.[676]**

o Cabergoline/Dostinex: Cabergoline/Dostinex is a newer dopamine agonist with few adverse effects; typical dose starts at 0.5 mg per week (0.25 mg twice per week).[677] Several studies have indicated that cabergoline is safer and more effective than bromocriptine for reducing prolactin levels[678] and the dose can often be reduced after successful prolactin reduction, allowing for reductions in cost and adverse effects.[679] Although fewer studies have been published supporting the antirheumatic benefits of cabergoline than bromocriptine, the scientific rationale for its use is derived from the success of bromocriptine in various rheumatic/autoimmune diseases. Erb et al[680] published a case report of a woman with unremitting rheumatoid arthritis who achieved remarkable clinical improvement and who was able to reduce her need for other antirheumatic drugs with the use of cabergoline 0.5 mg per day.

[664] "The ethanol/ethyl acetate extract of TWHF shows therapeutic benefit in patients with treatment-refractory RA. At therapeutic dosages, the TWHF extract was well tolerated by most patients in this study." Tao X, Younger J, Fan FZ, Wang B, Lipsky PE. Benefit of an extract of Tripterygium Wilfordii Hook F in patients with rheumatoid arthritis: a double-blind, placebo-controlled study. *Arthritis Rheum.* 2002 Jul;46(7):1735-43

[665] "CONCLUSION: The EA extract of TWHF at dosages up to 570 mg/day appeared to be safe, and doses > 360 mg/day were associated with clinical benefit in patients with RA." Tao X, Cush JJ, Garret M, Lipsky PE. A phase I study of ethyl acetate extract of the chinese antirheumatic herb Tripterygium wilfordii hook F in rheumatoid arthritis. *J Rheumatol.* 2001 Oct;28(10):2160-7

[666] "Our data suggests that triptolide may protect dopaminergic neurons from LPS-induced injury and its efficiency in inhibiting microglia activation may underlie the mechanism." Li FQ, Lu XZ, Liang XB, Zhou HF, Xue B, Liu XY, Niu DB, Han JS, Wang XM. Triptolide, a Chinese herbal extract, protects dopaminergic neurons from inflammation-mediated damage through inhibition of microglial activation. *J Neuroimmunol.* 2004 Mar;148(1-2):24-31

[667] "Moreover, tripchlorolide markedly prevented the decrease in amount of dopamine in the striatum of model rats. Taken together, our data provide the first evidence that tripchlorolide acts as a neuroprotective molecule that rescues MPP+ or axotomy-induced degeneration of dopaminergic neurons, which may imply its therapeutic potential for Parkinson's disease." Li FQ, Cheng XX, Liang XB, Wang XH, Xue B, He QH, Wang XM, Han JS. Neurotrophic and neuroprotective effects of tripchlorolide, an extract of Chinese herb Tripterygium wilfordii Hook F, on dopaminergic neurons. *Exp Neurol.* 2003 Jan;179(1):28-37

[668] "Of twenty-eight visual analogue scales rating mood and arousal, the subjects' ratings in the tyrosine treatment (9 g daily) and placebo periods differed significantly for only three (less tired, less drowsy, more alert)." Elwes RD, Crewes H, Chesterman LP, Summers B, Jenner P, Binnie CD, Parkes JD. Treatment of narcolepsy with L-tyrosine: double-blind placebo-controlled trial. *Lancet.* 1989 Nov 4;2(8671):1067-9

[669] "Ten men and 10 women subjects underwent these batteries 1 h after ingesting 150 mg/kg of l-tyrosine or placebo. Administration of tyrosine significantly enhanced accuracy and decreased frequency of list retrieval on the working memory task during the multiple task battery compared with placebo." Thomas JR, Lockwood PA, Singh A, Deuster PA. Tyrosine improves working memory in a multitasking environment. *Pharmacol Biochem Behav.* 1999 Nov;64(3):495-500

[670] "Ten subjects received five daily doses of a protein-rich drink containing 2 g tyrosine, and 11 subjects received a carbohydrate rich drink with the same amount of calories (255 kcal)." Deijen JB, Wientjes CJ, Vullinghs HF, Cloin PA, Langefeld JJ. Tyrosine improves cognitive performance and reduces blood pressure in cadets after one week of a combat training course. *Brain Res Bull.* 1999 Jan 15;48(2):203-9

[671] "Tyrosine (when compared to placebo) had no effect on any sleep related measure, but it did stimulate prolactin release." Waters WF, Magill RA, Bray GA, Volaufova J, Smith SR, Lieberman HR, Rood J, Hurry M, Anderson T, Ryan DH. A comparison of tyrosine against placebo, phentermine, caffeine, and D-amphetamine during sleep deprivation. *Nutr Neurosci.* 2003;6(4):221-35

[672] "Whereas carbohydrate meals had no discernible effects, high protein meals induced a large increase in both PRL and cortisol; high fat meals caused selective release of PRL." Ishizuka B, Quigley ME, Yen SS. Pituitary hormone release in response to food ingestion: evidence for neuroendocrine signals from gut to brain. *J Clin Endocrinol Metab.* 1983 Dec;57(6):1111-6

[673] Beers MH, Berkow R (eds). The Merck Manual. Seventeenth Edition. Whitehouse Station; Merck Research Laboratories 1999 Page 77-78

[674] "A prospective, double-blind, randomized, placebo-controlled study compared BRC at a fixed daily dosage of 2.5 mg with placebo... Long term treatment with a low dose of BRC appears to be a safe and effective means of decreasing SLE flares in SLE patients." Alvarez-Nemegyei J, Cobarrubias-Cobos A, Escalante-Triay F, Sosa-Munoz J, Miranda JM, Jara LJ. Bromocriptine in systemic lupus erythematosus: a double-blind, randomized, placebo-controlled study. *Lupus.* 1998;7(6):414-9

[675] Serri O, Chik CL, Ur E, Ezzat S. Diagnosis and management of hyperprolactinemia. *CMAJ.* 2003 Sep 16;169(6):575-81 http://www.cmaj.ca/cgi/content/full/169/6/575

[676] "...clinical observations and trials support the use of bromocriptine as a nonstandard primary or adjunctive therapy in the treatment of recalcitrant RA, SLE, Reiter's syndrome, and psoriatic arthritis and associated conditions unresponsive to traditional approaches." McMurray RW. Bromocriptine in rheumatic and autoimmune diseases. *Semin Arthritis Rheum.* 2001 Aug;31(1):21-32

[677] Serri O, Chik CL, Ur E, Ezzat S. Diagnosis and management of hyperprolactinemia. *CMAJ.* 2003 Sep 16;169(6):575-81 http://www.cmaj.ca/cgi/content/full/169/6/575

[678] "CONCLUSION: These data indicate that cabergoline is a very effective agent for lowering the prolactin levels in hyperprolactinemic patients and that it appears to offer considerable advantage over bromocriptine in terms of efficacy and tolerability." Sabuncu T, Arikan E, Tasan E, Hatemi H. Comparison of the effects of cabergoline and bromocriptine on prolactin levels in hyperprolactinemic patients. *Intern Med.* 2001 Sep;40(9):857-61

[679] "Cabergoline also normalized PRL in the majority of patients with known bromocriptine intolerance or -resistance. Once PRL secretion was adequately controlled, the dose of cabergoline could often be significantly decreased, which further reduced costs of therapy." Verhelst J, Abs R, Maiter D, van den Bruel A, Vandeweghe M, Velkeniers B, Mockel J, Lamberigts G, Petrossians P, Coremans P, Mahler C, Stevenaert A, Verlooy J, Raftopoulos C, Beckers A. Cabergoline in the treatment of hyperprolactinemia: a study in 455 patients. *J Clin Endocrinol Metab.* 1999 Jul;84(7):2518-22 http://jcem.endojournals.org/cgi/content/full/84/7/2518

[680] Erb N, Pace AV, Delamere JP, Kitas GD. Control of unremitting rheumatoid arthritis by the prolactin antagonist cabergoline. *Rheumatology* (Oxford). 2001 Feb;40(2):237-9 http://rheumatology.oxfordjournals.org/cgi/content/full/40/2/237

- **Estrogen (excess):** Nearly all autoimmune disorders are more common in females than males, suggesting a possible immunodysregulation by estrogen. Despite the complex and multifaceted nature of the endocrine system, we may safely generalize that the estrogens are immunostimulatory and immunodysregulatory while androgens are immunosuppressive and immunoregulatory[681]; thus, elevated estrogen:androgen ratios promote/exacerbate autoimmunity. Furthermore, many chemical/pollutant xenobiotics have estrogen-like effects ("xenoestrogens") and are consistently associated with induction or exacerbation of autoimmunity. So-called **"estrogen-replacement therapy" used in postmenopausal women increases the risk for lupus and scleroderma.**[682] **Men with rheumatoid arthritis show an excess of estradiol** and a decrease in DHEA, and the **excess estrogen is proportional to the degree of inflammation.**[683] Estrogen(s) can be measured in serum and/or 24-hour urine samples. Beyond looking at estrogens from a *quantitative* standpoint, they can also be *qualitatively* analyzed with respect to the ratio of estrone:estradiol:estriol as well as the balance between the "good" 2-hydroxyestrone relative to the purportedly carcinogenic and proinflammatory 16-alpha-hydroxyestrone. Interventions to lower estrogen levels can include the following:
  - Weight loss and weight optimization: Excess adiposity and obesity raise estrogen levels due to high levels of aromatase (the hormone that makes estrogens from androgens) in adipose tissue; weight optimization and loss of excess fat helps normalize hormone levels and reduce inflammation. In overweight patients, *weight loss* is the means to attaining the goal of *weight optimization*; the task is not complete until the body mass index is normalized/optimized.
  - Avoidance of ethanol: Ethanol stimulates estrogen production, particularly in men.
  - Surgical correction of varicocele in affected men: Men with varicocele have higher estrogen levels due to temperature-induced alterations in enzyme function in the testes; surgical correction of the varicocele lowers estrogen levels.
  - "Anti-estrogen diet": Foods and supplements such as green tea, diindolylmethane (DIM), indole-3-carbinol (I3C), licorice, and a high-fiber crucifer-based "anti-estrogenic diet" can also be used; monitoring clinical status and serum estradiol will prove or disprove efficacy. Whereas **16-alpha-hydroxyestrone is pro-inflammatory and immunodysregulatory, 2-hydroxyestrone has anti-inflammatory action**[684] and has been described as "the good estrogen"[685] due to its anticancer and comparatively health-preserving qualities. **In a recent short-term study using I3C in patients with SLE, I3C supplementation at 375 mg per day was well tolerated and resulted in modest treatment-dependent clinical improvement as well as favorable modification of estrogen metabolism away from 16-alpha-hydroxyestrone and toward 2-hydroxyestrone.**[686]

    > "Using **antiestrogen medication** [tamoxifen or anastrozole] in women with dermatomyositis may result in a significant improvement in their rash, possibly via the inhibition of TNF-alpha production by immune or other cells."
    >
    > Sereda D, Werth VP. *Arch Dermatol.* 2006

  - Anastrozole/Arimidex: In our office, we commonly measure serum estradiol in men and administer the aromatase inhibitor anastrozole/arimidex 1 mg (2-3 doses per week) to men whose estradiol level is greater than 32 picogram/mL. The Life Extension Foundation[687] proposes that the optimal serum estradiol level for a man is 10-30 picogram/mL. Clinical studies using anastrozole/Arimidex in men have shown that aromatase blockade lowers

[681] "In general, androgens seem to inhibit immune activity, while oestrogen seems to have a more powerful effect on immune cells and to stimulate immune activity." Tanriverdi F, Silveira LF, MacColl GS, Bouloux PM. The hypothalamic-pituitary-gonadal axis: immune function and autoimmunity. *J Endocrinol.* 2003 Mar;176(3):293-304 http://joe.endocrinology-journals.org/cgi/content/abstract/176/3/293

[682] "These studies indicate that estrogen replacement therapy in postmenopausal women increases the risk of developing lupus, scleroderma, and Raynaud disease..." Mayes MD. Epidemiologic studies of environmental agents and systemic autoimmune diseases. *Environ Health Perspect.* 1999 Oct;107 Suppl 5:743-8

[683] "RESULTS: DHEAS and estrone concentrations were lower and estradiol was higher in patients compared with healthy controls. DHEAS differed between RF positive and RF negative patients. Estrone did not correlate with any disease variable, whereas estradiol correlated strongly and positively with all measured indices of inflammation." Tengstrand B, Carlstrom K, Fellander-Tsai L, Hafstrom I. Abnormal levels of serum dehydroepiandrosterone, estrone, and estradiol in men with rheumatoid arthritis: high correlation between serum estradiol and current degree of inflammation. *J Rheumatol.* 2003 Nov;30(11):2338-43

[684] "Micromolar concentrations of beta-estradiol, estrone, 16-alpha-hydroxyestrone and estriol enhance the oxidative metabolism of activated human PMNL's. The corresponding 2-hydroxylated estrogens 2-OH-estradiol, 2-OH-estrone and 2-OH-estriol act on the contrary as powerful inhibitors of cell activity." Jansson G. Oestrogen-induced enhancement of myeloperoxidase activity in human polymorphonuclear leukocytes--a possible cause of oxidative stress in inflammatory cells. *Free Radic Res Commun.* 1991;14(3):195-208

[685] "Even more dramatically, in the case of laryngeal papillomas induction of 2-hydroxylation with indole-3-carbinol (I3C) has resulted in inhibition of tumor growth during the time that the patients continue to take I3C or vegetables rich in this compound." Bradlow HL, Telang NT, Sepkovic DW, Osborne MP. 2-hydroxyestrone: the 'good' estrogen. *J Endocrinol.* 1996 Sep;150 Suppl:S259-65

[686] "Women with SLE can manifest a metabolic response to I3C and might benefit from its antiestrogenic effects." McAlindon TE, Gulin J, Chen T, Klug T, Lahita R, Nuite M. Indole-3-carbinol in women with SLE: effect on estrogen metabolism and disease activity. *Lupus.* 2001;10(11):779-83

[687] Male Hormone Modulation Therapy, Page 4 Of 7: http://www.lef.org/protocols/prtcl-130c.shtml Accessed October 30, 2005

estradiol and raises testosterone[688]; generally speaking, this is exactly the result that we want in patients with severe systemic autoimmunity. Frequency of dosing is based on serological and clinical responses. Of course, anastrozole/Arimidex can be administered to women in 1 mg doses ranging from once per week to 5-7 times per week depending on clinical and serologic response. **In two recent case reports, administration of anti-estrogen medication—either tamoxifen or anastrozole—resulted in clinical improvements in two women with dermatomyositis.[689]**

The aromatase enzyme converts androgens to estrogens: If estrogens are high and androgens are low, then estrogens can be lowered and androgens raised via inhibition of aromatase. If androgens are low and estrogens are low, then administration of androgens will raise both the androgens and the estrogens, possibly necessitating the coadministration of an aromatase inhibitor.

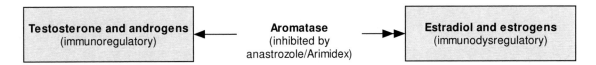

- **Testosterone (insufficiency):** Androgen deficiencies predispose to, are exacerbated by, and contribute to autoimmune/inflammatory disorders. **A large proportion of men with lupus or RA have low testosterone[690]** and suffer the effects of hypogonadism: fatigue, weakness, depression, slow healing, low libido, and difficulties with sexual performance. Particularly in men, blood samples should be drawn for *free* and *total* testosterone along with serum estradiol. Since some labs accept ridiculously low levels of testosterone as "within normal limits" clinicians should not necessarily wait until the patient is pathologically hypogonadal before implementing treatment. Clinicians must appreciate the interrelationship of testosterone with estrogen in order to interpret the patient's status appropriately and implement proper treatment. Since testosterone is converted to estradiol by aromatase, a patient with low testosterone and high estradiol is properly treated with aromatase inhibition (e.g., Arimidex/anastrozole) rather than testosterone; administration of Arimidex/anastrozole to men simultaneously lowers estradiol and raises testosterone.[691] Conversely, low testosterone along with low estrogen indicates the appropriateness of testosterone replacement. The need for co-administration of testosterone and Arimidex/anastrozole is not uncommon in order to raise testosterone without leading to an iatrogenic increase in estrogen due to shunting by aromatase. Follow-up testing of testosterone and estradiol 4-8 weeks after the implementation of testosterone replacement is advised to ensure optimal hormone status and that the additional *immunoregulatory* testosterone is not being shunted into *immunodysregulatory* estradiol. Doses of Arimidex/anastrozole typically range from 1 mg administered 1-4 times per week; the drug appears to have a wide margin of safety, and doses of 10 mg per day are used in women with estrogen-responsive breast cancer. As with any modulation/administration of testosterone and estrogen, follow-up testing of hormones and serum lipids is recommended to ensure the attainment of optimal status and the avoidance of

[688] "These data demonstrate that aromatase inhibition increases serum bioavailable and total testosterone levels to the youthful normal range in older men with mild hypogonadism." Leder BZ, Rohrer JL, Rubin SD, Gallo J, Longcope C. Effects of aromatase inhibition in elderly men with low or borderline-low serum testosterone levels. *J Clin Endocrinol Metab*. 2004 Mar;89(3):1174-80 http://jcem.endojournals.org/cgi/reprint/89/3/1174
[689] "Using antiestrogen medication in women with DM may result in a significant improvement in their rash, possibly via the inhibition of TNF-alpha production by immune or other cells." Sereda D, Werth VP. Improvement in dermatomyositis rash associated with the use of antiestrogen medication. *Arch Dermatol*. 2006 Jan;142(1):70-2
[690] Karagiannis A, Harsoulis F. Gonadal dysfunction in systemic diseases. *Eur J Endocrinol*. 2005 Apr;152(4):501-13 http://www.eje-online.org/cgi/content/full/152/4/501
[691] "These data demonstrate that aromatase inhibition increases serum bioavailable and total testosterone levels to the youthful normal range in older men with mild hypogonadism. Serum estradiol levels decrease modestly but remain within the normal male range." Leder BZ, Rohrer JL, Rubin SD, Gallo J, Longcope C. Effects of aromatase inhibition in elderly men with low or borderline-low serum testosterone levels. *J Clin Endocrinol Metab*. 2004 Mar;89(3):1174-80 http://jcem.endojournals.org/cgi/content/full/89/3/1174

complications, such as suppression of HDL synthesis which would be expected to have adverse cardiovascular consequences. Assessing serum PSA is a prerequisite to testosterone administration in men. **Testosterone therapy improves clinical status and wellbeing in women with rheumatoid arthritis.**[692] Transdermal testosterone creams can be used with dose tailored to serum and clinical response.

- **Cortisol (insufficiency):** In physiologic doses cortisol is immunoregulatory and mildly yet significantly immunosuppressive ("*physiologic immunosuppression*"), while at higher doses the hormone becomes immunosuppressive ("*pharmacologic immunosuppression*") and brings additional adverse effects such as weight gain, truncal obesity, hypertension, glucose intolerance and increased susceptibility to infections—the classic manifestations of hypercortisolemia seen in Cushing's disease.[693] Insufficiencies of cortisol production contribute to the development and perpetuation of allergies, fatigue, inflammation, and autoimmunity.[694] The works of Drs. John Tintera and William Jefferies have remained important despite being ignored by most endocrinologists; Jefferies' books[695] and articles[696] are still widely available and provide concepts and clinically relevant applications. In a 1998 summary by Jefferies[697] on the etiology of rheumatoid arthritis, he reviewed evidence suggesting that subacute hypoadrenalism results in insufficiencies of cortisol and DHEA, both of which are necessary for immunomodulation and

> ## Criteria for the diagnosis of adrenal insufficiency in children and adults
>
> - **First-morning cortisol less than 8-10 mcg/dL**: An 8:00 am serum cortisol concentration less than 8-10 mcg/dL suggests adrenal insufficiency.
> - **Serum cortisol less than 18 mcg/dL during illness or stress or with elevated ACTH**: Serum cortisol concentration less than 18 mcg/dL in a sick and stressed patient, or associated with an elevated ACTH, is highly suggestive of adrenal insufficiency.
> - **Post-ACTH serum cortisol less than 18 mcg/dL**: Serum cortisol less than 18 mcg/dL obtained 30-60 minutes following ACTH injection is diagnostic of adrenal insufficiency.
> - **Serum cortisol that fails to double within 30-60 minutes after ACTH injection**: This test involves three steps: 1) blood sample is taken for serum cortisol, 2) ACTH is injected, 3) blood sample for serum cortisol is taken again at 30-60 minutes. Cortisol production should double following injection of ACTH; this is a demonstration of adrenal reserve and the ability of the adrenal glands to respond to stress.
> - **Low output of adrenal hormones measured in 24-hour urine samples**: This provides sufficient objective data to justify a clinical trial of cortisol replacement in patients with a suggestive clinical picture and lack of contraindications.
> - **Proper dosing of cosyntropin/ACTH**: Injections of "ACTH" are generally performed with the intravenous or intramuscular injection of "Cosyntropin" which is a synthetic peptide fragment of ACTH used for adrenal stimulation. According to the review by Wilson, the **standard dose for adults is 250 mcg**. "For infants, the author suggests 50 mcg of cosyntropin (approximately 250 mg/m2)."
>
> References:
> - Jefferies WMcK. Safe Uses of Cortisol. Second Edition. Springfield, CC Thomas, 1996 page 39
> - http://www.medicinenet.com/cosyntropin-injectable/article.htm Accessed December 7, 2006
> - Wilson TA. Adrenal Hypoplasia. eMedicine Last Updated: July 10, 2003 http://www.emedicine.com/PED/topic45.htm Accessed November 18, 2005

immunocompetence; insufficiencies of these hormones leaves the body vulnerable to chronic infections (i.e., multifocal dysbiosis, as detailed previously) and the systemic proinflammatory

---

[692] "An improvement in ESR, Dutch health assessment questionnaire, and pain was noted. …Testosterone may improve the general wellbeing of postmenopausal women with active rheumatoid arthritis." Booji A, Biewenga-Booji CM, Huber-Bruning O, Cornelis C, Jacobs JW, Bijlsma JW. Androgens as adjuvant treatment in postmenopausal female patients with rheumatoid arthritis. *Ann Rheum Dis.* 1996 Nov;55(11):811-5

[693] Kirk LF Jr, Hash RB, Katner HP, Jones T. Cushing's disease: clinical manifestations and diagnostic evaluation. *Am Fam Physician.* 2000 Sep 1;62(5):1119-27, 1133-4 http://www.aafp.org/afp/20000901/1119.html

[694] "Yet evidence that patients with rheumatoid arthritis improved with small, physiologic dosages of cortisol or cortisone acetate was reported over 25 years ago, and that patients with chronic allergic disorders or unexplained chronic fatigue also improved with administration of such small dosages was reported over 15 years ago..." Jefferies WM. Mild adrenocortical deficiency, chronic allergies, autoimmune disorders and the chronic fatigue syndrome: a continuation of the cortisone story. *Med Hypotheses.* 1994 Mar;42(3):183-9 http://www.thebuteykocentre.com/Irish_%20Buteykocenter_files/further_studies/med_hyp2.pdf and http://members.westnet.com.au/pkolb/med_hyp2.pdf

[695] Jefferies WMcK. Safe Uses of Cortisol. Second Edition. Springfield, CC Thomas, 1996

[696] "Yet evidence that patients with rheumatoid arthritis improved with small, physiologic dosages of cortisol or cortisone acetate was reported over 25 years ago, and that patients with chronic allergic disorders or unexplained chronic fatigue also improved with administration of such small dosages was reported over 15 years ago..." Jefferies WM. Mild adrenocortical deficiency, chronic allergies, autoimmune disorders and the chronic fatigue syndrome: a continuation of the cortisone story. *Med Hypotheses.* 1994 Mar;42(3):183-9 http://www.thebuteykocentre.com/Irish_%20Buteykocentre_files/further_studies/med_hyp2.pdf and http://members.westnet.com.au/pkolb/med_hyp2.pdf

[697] "The etiology of rheumatoid arthritis …explained by a combination of three factors: (i) a relatively mild deficiency of cortisol, …, (ii) a deficiency of DHEA, …and (iii) infection by organisms such as mycoplasma,..." Jefferies WM. The etiology of rheumatoid arthritis. *Med Hypotheses.* 1998 Aug;51(2):111-4

sequelae that result in so-called "autoimmunity." Differential diagnoses in patients with low adrenal function include congenital adrenal hypoplasia, adrenoleukodystrophy, autoimmune Addison disease, and chronic hypopituarism. A small short-term randomized crossover clinical trial published in *The Lancet* showed benefit of 5-10 mg/day of cortisol in patients with chronic fatigue syndrome.[698] Supplementation with up to 20 mg per day of cortisol/Cortef is physiologic; higher doses in the range of 40 mg per day may benefit patients, especially during times of stress, but are adrenosuppressive. My preference is to dose 10 mg first thing in the morning, then 5 mg in late morning and 5 mg in midafternoon in an attempt to replicate the diurnal variation and normal morning peak of cortisol levels. In patients with hypoadrenalism, administration of pregnenolone in doses of 10-60 mg in the morning may also be beneficial; DHEA supplementation is beneficial for patients with adrenal insufficiency.

- **DHEA (insufficiency and supraphysiologic supplementation):** Patients with autoimmunity should be tested for DHEA insufficiency by measurement of serum DHEA-sulfate; insufficiencies should generally be corrected except in cases of concomitant hormone-responsive cancer such as breast cancer or prostate cancer. Physiologic doses are approximately 15-25 mg for women and 25-50 mg for men. However, many patients with autoimmunity will respond favorably to supraphysiologic doses in the range of 200 mg per day. The rationale for using high-dose DHEA in patients with autoimmune diseases is supported by the following:
  1. DHEA is a natural metabolite/hormone of the human body made in the adrenal glands.
  2. Patients with autoimmune diseases are commonly treated with prednisone and other corticosteroids for months or years at a time. Use of prednisone causes adrenal suppression with resultant suppression of DHEA levels.[699]
  3. As a consequence of prednisone treatment, many patients lose bone mass and develop osteoporosis. DHEA has been shown to reverse the osteoporosis and loss of bone mass induced by corticosteroid treatment.[700]
  4. DHEA shows no acute or subacute toxicity even when used in supraphysiologic doses, even when used in sick patients. For example, in a study of 32 patients with HIV, DHEA doses of 750 mg – 2,250 mg per day were well tolerated and produced no dose-limiting adverse effects.[701] This lack of toxicity compares favorably with any and all so-called "antirheumatic" drugs, nearly all of which show alarming comparable toxicity.
  5. DHEA is inexpensive. Even at the relatively high dose of 200 mg per day, the cost is less than $40 per month.
  6. When used at doses of 200 mg per day, DHEA safely provides clinical benefit for patients with various autoimmune diseases, including ulcerative colitis, Crohn's disease[702], and SLE.[703]
  7. 200 mg per day of DHEA allows SLE patients to reduce their dose of prednisone (thus avoiding its adverse effects) while achieving symptomatic improvement. In other words, it allows for improved health and reduced medication use and therefore fewer side effects.[704]

---

[698] "In some patients with chronic fatigue syndrome, low-dose hydrocortisone reduces fatigue levels in the short term." Cleare AJ, Heap E, Malhi GS, Wessely S, O'Keane V, Miell J. Low-dose hydrocortisone in chronic fatigue syndrome: a randomised crossover trial. *Lancet*. 1999 Feb 6;353(9151):455-8
[699] "Basal serum DHEA and DHEAS concentrations were suppressed to a greater degree than was cortisol during both daily and alternate day prednisone treatments. ...Thus, adrenal androgen secretion was more easily suppressed than was cortisol secretion by this low dose of glucocorticoid, but there was no advantage to alternate day therapy." Rittmaster RS, Givner ML. Effect of daily and alternate day low dose prednisone on serum cortisol and adrenal androgens in hirsute women. *J Clin Endocrinol Metab*. 1988 Aug;67(2):400-3
[700] "CONCLUSION: Prasterone treatment prevented BMD loss and significantly increased BMD at both the lumbar spine and total hip in female patients with SLE receiving exogenous glucocorticoids." Mease PJ, Ginzler EM, Gluck OS, Schiff M, Goldman A, Greenwald M, Cohen S, Egan R, Quarles BJ, Schwartz KE. Effects of prasterone on bone mineral density in women with systemic lupus erythematosus receiving chronic glucocorticoid therapy. *J Rheumatol*. 2005 Apr;32(4):616-21
[701] "Thirty-one subjects were evaluated and monitored for safety and tolerance. The oral drug was administered three times daily in doses ranging from 750 mg/day to 2,250 mg/day for 16 weeks. ... The drug was well tolerated and no dose-limiting side effects were noted." Dyner TS, Lang W, Geaga J, Golub A, Stites D, Winger E, Galmarini M, Masterson J, Jacobson MA. An open-label dose-escalation trial of oral dehydroepiandrosterone tolerance and pharmacokinetics in patients with HIV disease. *J Acquir Immune Defic Syndr*. 1993 May;6(5):459-65
[702] "CONCLUSIONS: In a pilot study, dehydroepiandrosterone was effective and safe in patients with refractory Crohn's disease or ulcerative colitis." Andus T, Klebl F, Rogler G, Bregenzer N, Scholmerich J, Straub RH. Patients with refractory Crohn's disease or ulcerative colitis respond to dehydroepiandrosterone: a pilot study. *Aliment Pharmacol Ther*. 2003 Feb;17(3):409-14
[703] "CONCLUSION: The overall results confirm that DHEA treatment was well-tolerated, significantly reduced the number of SLE flares, and improved patient's global assessment of disease activity." Chang DM, Lan JL, Lin HY, Luo SF. Dehydroepiandrosterone treatment of women with mild-to-moderate systemic lupus erythematosus: a multicenter randomized, double-blind, placebo-controlled trial. *Arthritis Rheum*. 2002 Nov;46(11):2924-7
[704] "CONCLUSION: Among women with lupus disease activity, reducing the dosage of prednisone to < or = 7.5 mg/day for a sustained period of time while maintaining stabilization or a reduction of disease activity was possible in a significantly greater proportion of patients treated with oral prasterone, 200 mg once daily, compared with patients treated with placebo." Petri MA, Lahita RG, Van Vollenhoven RF, Merrill JT, Schiff M, Ginzler EM, Strand V, Kunz A, Gorelick KJ, Schwartz KE; GL601 Study Group. Effects of prasterone on corticosteroid requirements of women with systemic lupus erythematosus: a double-blind, randomized, placebo-controlled trial. *Arthritis Rheum*. 2002 Jul;46(7):1820-9

Thus, based on these financial, safety, and effectiveness considerations, the administration of DHEA is reasonable for patients with moderate or severe autoimmune disease. Furthermore, since optimal clinical response appears to correlate with serum levels that are supraphysiologic[705], treatment may be implemented with little regard for initial DHEA levels, particularly when 1) the dose of DHEA is kept as low as possible, 2) duration is kept as short as possible, 3) other interventions are used to address the underlying cause of the disease, 4) the patient is deriving benefit and the risk-to-benefit ratio is favorable.

- **Thyroid (insufficiency or autoimmunity):** Hypothyroidism is a common concomitant to many of the autoimmune diseases. Overt or imminent hypothyroidism is suggested by TSH greater than 2 mU/L[706] or 3 mU/L[707], low T4 or T3, and/or the presence of anti-thyroid peroxidase antibodies.[708] Specific treatment considerations include the following:
    - Selenium: Supplementation with either selenomethionine[709] or sodium selenite[710,711] can reduce thyroid autoimmunity and improve peripheral conversion of T4 to T3. Selenium may be started at 500-800 mcg per day (for 1-3 months) and tapered to 200-400 mcg per day for maintenance.[712]
    - L-thyroxine/levothyroxine/Synthroid—prescription synthetic T4: 25-50 mcg per day is a common starting dose which can be adjusted based on clinical and laboratory response. Thyroid hormone supplements must be consumed separately from soy products (by at least 1-2 hours) and preferably on an empty stomach to avoid absorption interference by food, fiber, and minerals, especially calcium. Doses are generally started at one-half of the daily dose for the first 10 days after which the full dose is used. Caution must be applied in patients with adrenal insufficiency and/or those with cardiovascular disease.
    - Liothyronine, Cytomel®: Cytomel is prescription synthetic T3. Except in patients with myxedema for whom the appropriate starting dose is 5 mcg per day, treatment generally starts with 25 mcg per day and can be increased to 75 mcg per day; dose is adjusted based on clinical and laboratory response.[713] As stated previously, thyroid hormone supplements must be consumed separately from soy products (by at least 1-2 hours) and preferably on an empty stomach to avoid absorption interference by food, fiber, and minerals, especially calcium. Time-released T3 can be obtained from a compounding pharmacy.
    - Armour thyroid—prescription natural T4 and T3 from cow/pig thyroid gland: 60 mg (one grain) is a common starting and maintenance dose. Since administration of Armour thyroid frequently increases serum levels of anti-thyroid antibodies in patients with preexisting thyroid autoimmunity, **many doctors choose to not use Armour thyroid in patients with thyroid autoimmunity**. Some patients prefer to divide their daily dose to maintain constant serum levels of T3.
    - Thyrolar/Liotrix—prescription synthetic T4 with T3: Dosed incrementally as "1", "2", or "3." This product has been difficult to obtain for the past few years due to manufacturing problems (http://thyrolar.com/); previously it was my treatment of choice

[705] "CONCLUSION: The clinical response to DHEA was not clearly dose dependent. Serum levels of DHEA and DHEAS correlated only weakly with lupus outcomes, but suggested an optimum serum DHEAS of 1000 microg/dl." Barry NN, McGuire JL, van Vollenhoven RF. Dehydroepiandrosterone in systemic lupus erythematosus: relationship between dosage, serum levels, and clinical response. J Rheumatol. 1998 Dec;25(12):2352-6
[706] Weetman AP. Hypothyroidism: screening and subclinical disease. BMJ. 1997 Apr 19;314(7088):1175-8 http://bmj.bmjjournals.com/cgi/content/full/314/7088/1175
[707] "Now AACE encourages doctors to consider treatment for patients who test outside the boundaries of a narrower margin based on a target TSH level of 0.3 to 3.0. AACE believes the new range will result in proper diagnosis for millions of Americans who suffer from a mild thyroid disorder, but have gone untreated until now." American Association of Clinical Endocrinologists (AACE). 2003 Campaign Encourages Awareness of Mild Thyroid Failure, Importance of Routine Testing http://www.aace.com/pub/tam2003/press.php November 26, 2005
[708] Beers MH, Berkow R (eds). The Merck Manual. Seventeenth Edition. Whitehouse Station; Merck Research Laboratories 1999 Page 96
[709] Duntas LH, Mantzou E, Koutras DA. Effects of a six month treatment with selenomethionine in patients with autoimmune thyroiditis. Eur J Endocrinol. 2003 Apr;148(4):389-93 http://eje-online.org/cgi/reprint/148/4/389
[710] Gartner R, Gasnier BC, Dietrich JW, Krebs B, Angstwurm MW. Selenium supplementation in patients with autoimmune thyroiditis decreases thyroid peroxidase antibodies concentrations. J Clin Endocrinol Metab. 2002 Apr;87(4):1687-91 http://jcem.endojournals.org/cgi/content/full/87/4/1687
[711] "We recently conducted a prospective, placebo-controlled clinical study, where we could demonstrate, that a substitution of 200 wg sodium selenite for three months in patients with autoimmune thyroiditis reduced thyroid peroxidase antibody (TPO-Ab) concentrations significantly." Gartner R, Gasnier BC. Selenium in the treatment of autoimmune thyroiditis. Biofactors. 2003;19(3-4):165-70
[712] Bruns F, Micke O, Bremer M. Current status of selenium and other treatments for secondary lymphedema. J Support Oncol. 2003 Jul-Aug;1(2):121-30 http://www.supportiveoncology.net/journal/articles/0102121.pdf
[713] http://www.kingpharm.com/uploads/pdf_inserts/Cytomel_Web_PI.pdf

due to the combination of T4 and T3 and the lack of antigenicity compared to gland-derived products.

- o Thyroid glandular—nonprescription T3: Producers of nutritional products are able to distribute T3 because it is not listed by the FDA as a prescription item. Nutritional supplement companies may start with Armour thyroid, remove the T4, and sell the thyroid glandular with active T3 thereby providing a nonprescription source of active thyroid hormone. For many patients, one tablet per day is at least as effective as a prescription source of thyroid hormone. Since it is derived from a glandular and therefore potentially antigenic source, thyroid glandular is not used in patients with thyroid autoimmunity due to its ability to induce increased production of anti-thyroid antibodies.

- o L-tyrosine and iodine: Some patients with mild hypothyroidism respond to supplementation with L-tyrosine and iodine. Tyrosine is commonly used in doses of 4-9 grams per day in divided doses. According to Abraham and Wright[714], doses of iodine may be as high as 12.5 milligrams (12,500 micrograms), which is slightly less than the average daily intake in Japan at 13.8 mg per day.

- **Pregnenolone:** Several reviews and clinical trials from the early 1950s showed moderate clinical effectiveness and absence of adverse effects from oral administration of pregnenolone in doses as high as 500-1,000 mg/d in patients with rheumatoid arthritis and other rheumatic conditions.[715,716,717,718] Following oral administration of pregnenolone in doses of approximately 500 mg/d, beneficial results are noted in approximately 50-80% of patients. Responders will show reduced pain, swelling, and objective reductions in inflammation measured by ESR and will have increased strength and mobility. No important adverse effects have been reported, particularly with regard to pulse rate, blood pressure, or glucose homeostasis. In contrast to the adverse withdrawal effects noted with prednisone/prednisolone, discontinuance of pregnenolone does not immediately result in exacerbation of inflammation and has never been reported to incite adrenal insufficiency. Oral administration of pregnenolone produces better clinical response than does intramuscular administration, apparently due to the relative insolubility of parenteral pregnenolone. The low cost and absence of adverse effects makes pregnenolone a reasonable therapeutic intervention in patients with rheumatic disease because the treatment may provide benefit and/or mitigate the need for treatments with greater toxicity and cost. However, this treatment should not be relied upon as monotherapy and/or in patients with important inflammatory complications such as iritis, scleritis, or temporal arteritis. In contrast to the much higher doses of 500-1,000 mg/d reported in the studies cited above in this paragraph, I generally limit pregnenolone doses to 10-50 mg/d taken in the morning in patients who may derive benefit; some patients—generally those with hypoadrenalism—notice a marked improvement in energy (to the point of causing insomnia) with doses as low as 5-10 mg/d.

[714] Wright JV. Why you need 83 times more of this essential, cancer-fighting nutrient than the "experts" say you do. *Nutrition and Healing* 2005; volume 12, issue 4.
[715] Freeman H, Pincus G, Johnson CW, Bachrach S, McCabe GE, MacGilpin H. Therapeutic efficacy of delta-5-pregnenolone in rheumatoid arthritis. *JAMA: Journal of the American Medical Association* 1950; April 15: 1124-8
[716] Stock JP, McClure EC. Pregnenolone in the treatment of rheumatoid arthritis. *Lancet* 1950 Jul 22;2(4):125-8
[717] Dordick JR, Ehrlich ME, Alexander S, Kissin M. Pregnenolone in rheumatoid arthritis. *N Engl J Med.* 1951 Mar 1;244(9):324-6
[718] Freeman H, Pincus G, Bachrach S, Johnson CW, McCabe GE, MacGilpin HH Jr. Oral steroid medication in rheumatoid arthritis. *J Clin Endocrinol Metab.* 1950 Dec;10(12):1523-32

Immunonutrigenomics and Nutritional Immunomodulation

We must look beyond the nutritional properties of foods to appreciate that dietary patterns and the consumption of specific foods can influence genetic expression and either promote or retard the development of inflammation and related clinical disorders. The purpose of this section is to help clinicians attain a more profound understanding of the value of nutrition and its critical role as a foundational component in the treatment plan of patients with inflammatory disorders. The "correct" diet for the vast majority of patients with inflammatory disorders is the "supplemented Paleo-Mediterranean diet" which I have detailed previously in this text and elsewhere.[719,720] The diet is modified for the specific exclusion of allergenic foods; it is implemented on a rotation basis, and it allows for periodic fasting and vegetarianism/veganism. The implementation of health-promoting dietary modifications is an *absolutely mandatory* component of the treatment plan, upon which other treatments depend for their success.

The study of how dietary components and nutritional supplements influence genetic expression is referred to as *nutrigenomics* or *nutritional genomics* and has been described as "the next frontier in the postgenomic era."[721] Various nutrients have been shown to modulate genetic expression and thus alter phenotypic manifestations of disease by upregulating or downregulating specific genes, interacting with nuclear receptors, altering hormone receptors, and modifying the influence of transcription factors, such as pro-inflammatory NF-kappaB (NFkB) and the anti-inflammatory peroxisome-proliferator activated receptors (PPARs).[722,723,724,725] **The previous view that nutrients only interact with human physiology at the metabolic/post-transcriptional level must be updated in light of current research showing that nutrients can, in fact, modify human physiology and phenotype at the genetic/pre-transcriptional level.**

Fatty acids and their *eicosanoid, leukotriene,* and *isoprostane* intermediates and end-products modulate genetic expression in several ways. In general, n-3 fatty acids decrease inflammation and promote health while n-6 fatty acids (except for GLA, which is generally health-promoting) increase inflammation, oxidative stress, and the manifestation of disease. Corn oil, probably as a result of its high n-6 LA (linoleic acid) content, rapidly activates NFkB and thus promotes tumor development, atherosclerosis, and elaboration of proinflammatory mediators such as TNFa.[726,727,728] Similarly n-6 arachidonic acid increases production of the free radical *superoxide* approximately 4-fold when added to isolated Kupffer cells *in vitro*. Prostaglandin-E2 is produced from arachidonic acid by cyclooxygenase and increases genetic expression of cyclooxygenase and IL-6; thus, an increase in PG-E2 leads to

Health-promoting polyunsaturated fatty acids (PUFA): names, abbreviations, and sources
1. <u>alpha-linolenic acid (ALA)</u>: n-3 PUFA primarily from flaxseed oil
2. <u>gamma-linolenic acid (GLA)</u>: n-6 PUFA from borage oil, evening primrose oil, hemp oil, and black currant seed oil
3. <u>Eicosapentaenoic acid (EPA)</u>: n-3 PUFA from fish oil
4. <u>Docosahexaenoic acid (DHA)</u>: n-3 PUFA from fish oil and marine algae
5. <u>Oleic acid</u>: n-9 monounsaturated fatty acid primarily from olive oil; also found in flaxseed oil and borage oil

[719] Vasquez A. A Five-Part Nutritional Protocol that Produces Consistently Positive Results. *Nutritional Wellness* 2005 September Available in the printed version and on-line at http://www.nutritionalwellness.com/archives/2005/sep/09_vasquez.php

[720] Vasquez A. Implementing the Five-Part Nutritional Wellness Protocol for the Treatment of Various Health Problems. *Nutritional Wellness* 2005 November Available in the printed version and on-line at http://www.nutritionalwellness.com/archives/2005/nov/11_vasquez.php

[721] Kaput J, Rodriguez RL. Nutritional genomics: the next frontier in the postgenomic era. *Physiol Genomics*. 2004 Jan 15;16(2):166-77 http://physiolgenomics.physiology.org/cgi/content/full/16/2/166

[722] Vamecq J, Latruffe N. Medical significance of peroxisome proliferator-activated receptors. *Lancet*. 1999;354:141-8

[723] Ehrmann J Jr, Vavrusova N, Collan Y, Kolar Z. Peroxisome proliferator-activated receptors (PPARs) in health and disease. *Biomed Pap Med Fac Univ Palacky Olomouc Czech Repub*. 2002 Dec;146(2):11-4 http://publib.upol.cz/~obd/fulltext/Biomed/2002/2/11.pdf

[724] Kliewer SA, Xu HE, Lambert MH, Willson TM. Peroxisome proliferator-activated receptors: from genes to physiology. *Recent Prog Horm Res*. 2001;56:239-63

[725] Delerive P, Fruchart JC, Staels B. Peroxisome proliferator-activated receptors in inflammation control. *J Endocrinol*. 2001;169(3):453-9

[726] Rusyn I, Bradham CA, Cohn L, Schoonhoven R, Swenberg JA, Brenner DA, Thurman RG. Corn oil rapidly activates nuclear factor-kappaB in hepatic Kupffer cells by oxidant-dependent mechanisms. *Carcinogenesis*. 1999 Nov;20(11):2095-100

[727] Rose DP, Hatala MA, Connolly JM, Rayburn J. Effect of diets containing different levels of linoleic acid on human breast cancer growth and lung metastasis in nude mice. *Cancer Res*. 1993 Oct 1;53(19):4686-90

[728] Dichtl W, Ares MP, Jonson AN, Jovinge S, Pachinger O, Giachelli CM, Hamsten A, Eriksson P, Nilsson J. Linoleic acid-stimulated vascular adhesion molecule-1 expression in endothelial cells depends on nuclear factor-kappaB activation. *Metabolism*. 2002 Mar;51(3):327-33

additive expression of cyclooxygenase, which further increases inflammation and elevates C-reactive protein.[729] Some of the unique health-promoting effects of GLA are nutrigenomically mediated via activation of PPAR-gamma, resultant inhibition of NFkB, and impairment of estrogen receptor function.[730,731] Supplementation with ALA leads to a dramatic reduction of prostaglandin formation in humans[732], and this effect is probably mediated by downregulation of proinflammatory gene transcription, as evidenced by reductions in CRP, IL-6, and serum amyloid A.[733] EPA appears to exert much of its anti-inflammatory benefit by suppressing NFkB activation and thus reducing elaboration of proinflammatory mediators.[734,735] EPA also indirectly modifies gene expression and cell growth by reducing intracellular calcium levels and thus activating protein kinase R which impairs eukaryotic initiation factor-2alpha and inhibits protein synthesis at the level of translation initiation, thereby mediating an anti-cancer benefit.[736] DHA is the precursor to docosatrienes and resolvins which downregulate gene expression for proinflammatory IL-1, inhibit of TNFa, and reduce neutrophil entry to sites of inflammation.[737] Oxidized EPA activates PPAR-alpha and thereby suppresses NFkB and the activation of proinflammatory genes.[738,739] Other nutrients that inhibit the activation of NFkB include vitamin D[740,741], lipoic acid[742], green tea[743], rosemary[744], grape seed extract[745], resveratrol[746,747], caffeic acid phenethyl ester (CAPE) from bee propolis[748], indole-3-carbinol[749], N-acetyl-L-cysteine[750], selenium[751], and zinc.[752] **Therefore, we see that fatty acids and nutrients directly affect gene expression by complex and multiple mechanisms, as graphically illustrated in the accompanying diagram, and the synergism and potency of these anti-inflammatory nutraceuticals supports the rationale for the use of nutrition and select botanicals for the safe and effective treatment of inflammatory disorders.**

[729] Bagga D, Wang L, Farias-Eisner R, Glaspy JA, Reddy ST. Differential effects of prostaglandin derived from omega-6 and omega-3 polyunsaturated fatty acids on COX-2 expression and IL-6 secretion. *Proc Natl Acad Sci U S A.* 2003 Feb 18;100(4):1751-6. http://www.pnas.org/cgi/reprint/100/4/1751.pdf
[730] Menendez JA, Colomer R, Lupu R. Omega-6 polyunsaturated fatty acid gamma-linolenic acid (18:3n-6) is a selective estrogen-response modulator in human breast cancer cells: gamma-linolenic acid antagonizes estrogen receptor-dependent transcriptional activity, transcriptionally represses estrogen receptor expression and synergistically enhances tamoxifen and ICI 182,780 (Faslodex) efficacy in human breast cancer cells. *Int J Cancer.* 2004 May 10;109(6):949-54
[731] Jiang WG, Redfern A, Bryce RP, Mansel RE. Peroxisome proliferator activated receptor-gamma (PPAR-gamma) mediates the action of gamma linolenic acid in breast cancer cells. *Prostaglandins Leukot Essent Fatty Acids.* 2000 Feb;62(2):119-27
[732] Adam O, Wolfram G, Zollner N. Effect of alpha-linolenic acid in the human diet on linoleic acid metabolism and prostaglandin biosynthesis. *J Lipid Res.* 1986 Apr;27(4):421-6
[733] Rallidis LS, Paschos G, Liakos GK, Velissaridou AH, Anastasiadis G, Zampelas A. Dietary alpha-linolenic acid decreases C-reactive protein, serum amyloid A and interleukin-6 in dyslipidaemic patients. *Atherosclerosis.* 2003 Apr;167(2):237-42
[734] Zhao Y, Joshi-Barve S, Barve S, Chen LH. Eicosapentaenoic acid prevents LPS-induced TNF-alpha expression by preventing NF-kappaB activation. *J Am Coll Nutr.* 2004 Feb;23(1):71-8
[735] Mishra A, Chaudhary A, Sethi S. Oxidized omega-3 fatty acids inhibit NF-kappaB activation via a PPARalpha-dependent pathway. *Arterioscler Thromb Vasc Biol.* 2004 Sep;24(9):1621-7
[736] Palakurthi SS, Fluckiger R, Aktas H, Changolkar AK, Shahsafaei A, Harneit S, Kilic E, Halperin JA. Inhibition of translation initiation mediates the anti-cancer effect of the n-3 polyunsaturated fatty acid eicosapentaenoic acid. *Cancer Res.* 2000 Jun 1;60(11):2919-25
[737] "These results indicate that DHA is the precursor to potent protective mediators generated via enzymatic oxygenations to novel docosatrienes and 17S series resolvins that each regulate events of interest in inflammation and resolution." Hong S, Gronert K, Devchand PR, Moussignac RL, Serhan CN. Novel docosatrienes and 17S-resolvins generated from docosahexaenoic acid in murine brain, human blood, and glial cells. Autacoids in anti-inflammation. *J Biol Chem.* 2003 Apr 25;278(17):14677-87
[738] Mishra A, Chaudhary A, Sethi S. Oxidized omega-3 fatty acids inhibit NF-kappaB activation via a PPARalpha-dependent pathway. *Arterioscler Thromb Vasc Biol.* 2004 Sep;24(9):1621-7
[739] Delerive P, Fruchart JC, Staels B. Peroxisome proliferator-activated receptors in inflammation control. *J Endocrinol.* 2001;169(3):453-9
[740] "1 Alpha,25-dihydroxyvitamin D3 (1,25-(OH)2-D3), the active metabolite of vitamin D, can inhibit NF-kappaB activity in human MRC-5 fibroblasts, targeting DNA binding of NF-kappaB but not translocation of its subunits p50 and p65." Harant H, Wolff B, Lindley IJ. 1Alpha,25-dihydroxyvitamin D3 decreases DNA binding of nuclear factor-kappaB in human fibroblasts. *FEBS Lett.* 1998 Oct 9;436(3):329-34
[741] "Thus, 1,25(OH)2D3 may negatively regulate IL-12 production by downregulation of NF-kB activation and binding to the p40-kB sequence." D'Ambrosio D, Cippitelli M, Cocciolo MG, Mazzeo D, Di Lucia P, Lang R, Sinigaglia F, Panina-Bordignon P. Inhibition of IL-12 production by 1,25-dihydroxyvitamin D3. Involvement of NF-kappaB downregulation in transcriptional repression of the p40 gene. *J Clin Invest.* 1998 Jan 1;101(1):252-62
[742] "ALA reduced the TNF-alpha-stimulated ICAM-1 expression in a dose-dependent manner, to levels observed in unstimulated cells. Alpha-lipoic acid also reduced NF-kappaB activity in these cells in a dose-dependent manner." Lee HA, Hughes DA.Alpha-lipoic acid modulates NF-kappaB activity in human monocytic cells by direct interaction with DNA. *Exp Gerontol.* 2002 Jan-Mar;37(2-3):401-10
[743] "In conclusion, EGCG is an effective inhibitor of IKK activity. This may explain, at least in part, some of the reported anti-inflammatory and anti-cancer effects of green tea." Yang F, Oz HS, Barve S, de Villiers WJ, McClain CJ, Varilek GW. The green tea polyphenol (-)-epigallocatechin-3-gallate blocks nuclear factor-kappa B activation by inhibiting I kappa B kinase activity in the intestinal epithelial cell line IEC-6. *Mol Pharmacol.* 2001 Sep;60(3):528-33
[744] "These results suggest that carnosol suppresses the NO production and iNOS gene expression by inhibiting NF-kappaB activation, and provide possible mechanisms for its anti-inflammatory and chemopreventive action." Lo AH, Liang YC, Lin-Shiau SY, Ho CT, Lin JK. Carnosol, an antioxidant in rosemary, suppresses inducible nitric oxide synthase through down-regulating nuclear factor-kappaB in mouse macrophages. *Carcinogenesis.* 2002 Jun;23(6):983-91
[745] "Constitutive and TNFalpha-induced NF-kappaB DNA binding activity was inhibited by GSE at doses > or =50 microg/ml and treatments for > or =12 h." Dhanalakshmi S, Agarwal R, Agarwal C. Inhibition of NF-kappaB pathway in grape seed extract-induced apoptotic death of human prostate carcinoma DU145 cells. *Int J Oncol.* 2003 Sep;23(3):721-7
[746] "Resveratrol's anticarcinogenic, anti-inflammatory, and growth-modulatory effects may thus be partially ascribed to the inhibition of activation of NF-kappaB and AP-1 and the associated kinases." Manna SK, Mukhopadhyay A, Aggarwal BB. Resveratrol suppresses TNF-induced activation of nuclear transcription factors NF-kappa B, activator protein-1, and apoptosis: potential role of reactive oxygen intermediates and lipid peroxidation. *J Immunol.* 2000 Jun 15;164(12):6509-19
[747] "Both resveratrol and quercetin inhibited NF-kappaB-, AP-1- and CREB-dependent transcription to a greater extent than the glucocorticosteroid, dexamethasone." Donnelly LE, Newton R, Kennedy GE, Fenwick PS, Leung RH, Ito K, Russell RE, Barnes PJ. Anti-inflammatory Effects of Resveratrol in Lung Epithelial Cells: Molecular Mechanisms. *Am J Physiol Lung Cell Mol Physiol.* 2004 Jun 4 [Epub ahead of print]
[748] "Caffeic acid phenethyl ester (CAPE) is an anti-inflammatory component of propolis (honeybee resin). CAPE is reportedly a specific inhibitor of nuclear factor-kappaB (NF-kappaB)." Fitzpatrick LR, Wang J, Le T. Caffeic acid phenethyl ester, an inhibitor of nuclear factor-kappaB, attenuates bacterial peptidoglycan polysaccharide-induced colitis in rats. *J Pharmacol Exp Ther.* 2001 Dec;299(3):915-20
[749] Takada Y, Andreeff M, Aggarwal BB. Indole-3-carbinol suppresses NF-{kappa}B and I{kappa}B{alpha} kinase activation causing inhibition of expression of NF-{kappa}B-regulated antiapoptotic and metastatic gene products and enhancement of apoptosis in myeloid and leukemia cells. Blood. 2005 Apr 5; [Epub ahead of print]
[750] Paterson RL, Galley HF, Webster NR. The effect of N-acetylcysteine on nuclear factor-kappa B activation, interleukin-6, interleukin-8, and intercellular adhesion molecule-1 expression in patients with sepsis. Crit Care Med. 2003 Nov;31(11):2574-8
[751] Faure P, Ramon O, Favier A, Halimi S. Selenium supplementation decreases nuclear factor-kappa B activity in peripheral blood mononuclear cells from type 2 diabetic patients. *Eur J Clin Invest.* 2004;34(7):475-81
[752] Uzzo RG, Leavis P, Hatch W, Gabai VL, Dulin N, Zvartau N, Kolenko VM. Zinc inhibits nuclear factor-kappa B activation and sensitizes prostate cancer cells to cytotoxic agents. *Clin Cancer Res.* 2002;8(11):3579-83

Schematic Representation of Nutrigenomics and Fatty Acid Modulation of Eicosanoid Production and Genetic Expression[753]

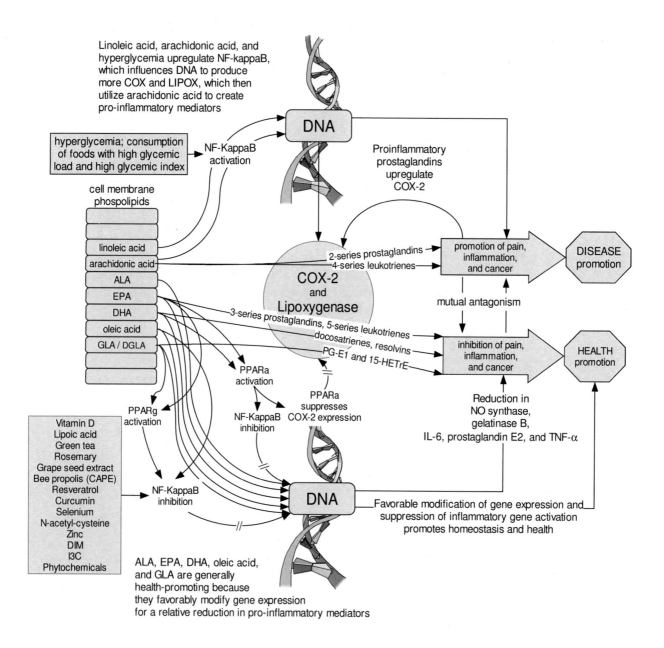

[753] See also: Vasquez A. Reducing Pain and Inflammation Naturally. Part 2: New Insights into Fatty Acid Supplementation and Its Effect on Eicosanoid Production and Genetic Expression. *Nutritional Perspectives* 2005; January: 5-16 www.optimalhealthresearch.com/part2

Clinical Management of Patients with Systemic Autoimmune Diseases

In this textbook, I provide what—to the best of my knowledge—is an original conceptualization of rheumatic diseases. In Chapter 4 and the disease-specific chapters that follow, I will provide additional scientific rationale for *theses* that I originally presented elsewhere[1,2,3]:
1) Autoimmunity is a manifestation of immune dysfunction.
2) "Different" autoimmune diseases have much in common despite the different labels applied and manifestations observed. The commonalities in their etiologies and pathogenesis provides the rationale for the similarities in their treatments and a focus on identifying and ameliorating the underlying causes of autoimmunity as detailed in Chapter 4: 1) food allergies/incompatibilities, 2) multifocal dysbiosis, 3) hormonal imbalances, 4) xenobiotic immunotoxicity, and 5) a pro-inflammatory diet and lifestyle.
3) Autoimmunity can be *ameliorated* (not always eliminated) in the majority of patients with combined and coordinated effort on the part of the physician and the patient to address the most common cause**s** of immune dysfunction, which rarely operate in isolation and are generally found in synergistic combination.
4) Since the etiopathogenesis is generally complex and multifaceted, treatment must be assertive and likewise multifaceted. Only rarely will a simple "silver bullet" cure be possible and sustainable.

Of the four major healthcare paradigms in Western medicine—i.e., osteopathic, chiropractic, naturopathic, and allopathic—the naturopathic paradigm is uniquely—and perhaps *solitarily*—well-suited for the successful assessment of and intervention for most autoimmune diseases. For it is only in naturopathic medicine that we find the specific admonishment to *Treat the Cause*, and this is a critical differentiation from the allopathic model which codifies and compels the use of symptom-suppressing and immune-suppressing medications. The original chiropractic model acknowledges the multifaceted nature of health and disease but is too vague in this context to direct assessment and treatment. The original osteopathic model did not include an appreciation of biochemical/nutritional considerations and environmental contributions which are essential for the treatment of autoimmunity. It will be obvious to any student of rheumatology that the allopathic paradigm which turns to symptom-suppressing drugs as "first line treatment" for rheumatic disease is an abysmal failure except that it reduces symptomatology and protracts the disease while imposing an impressive array of medication side-effects and nearly unbearable financial burdens. The failure of the modern allopathic medical paradigm is evidenced in the increased utilization of high-dose chemotherapy and stem-cell transplantation for the treatment of autoimmune diseases[4], an action which seems to confess, "Since we were unsuccessful with our first use of a hammer, instead of trying a different approach, we will just use a bigger hammer." It is thus with the firmly established scaffolding of the naturopathic paradigm that we begin our ascent to a vantage point high enough to allow a blurring of the rhetorical boundaries between diseases and from which we can ascertain the best path by which to traverse these complex and intricate labyrinths.

[1] Vasquez A. "Inflammation and Autoimmunity: A Functional Medicine Approach." David S. Jones, MD (Editor-in-Chief). Textbook of Functional Medicine. Gig Harbor, WA; Institute for Functional Medicine (www.FunctionalMedicine.org): 2006, pages 409-417
[2] Vasquez A. Web-like Interconnections of Physiological Factors. *Integrative Medicine: A Clinician's Journal* 2006, April/May, 32-37
[3] Vasquez A. Reducing Pain and Inflammation Naturally. Part 6: Nutritional and Botanical Treatments Against "Silent Infections" and Gastrointestinal Dysbiosis, Commonly Overlooked Causes of Neuromusculoskeletal Inflammation and Chronic Health Problems. *Nutritional Perspectives* 2006; January http://www.optimalhealthresearch.com/part6
[4] "Hematopoietic stem cell transplantation is an increasingly used therapy for treatment of autoimmune diseases and severe immune-mediated disorders." Burt RK, Verda L, Statkute L, Quigley K, Yaung K, Brush M, Oyama Y. Stem cell transplantation for autoimmune diseases. *Clin Adv Hematol Oncol*. 2004 May;2(5):313-9

Rules of Engagement: A Note Especially to Students and Recent Licensees

Even if you are a board-certified rheumatologist and an assertive and astute clinician with years of experience, the consideration of these guidelines may help protect **you** from malpractice liability and **your patient** from harm. Practicing "good medicine" is inherently defensive and in the best interests of the patient and the doctor.

1. **Document the specifics of your treatment plan and the rationale behind it.**
2. **Do not tell your patient to discontinue their anti-rheumatic drugs unless these drugs are in your scope of practice *and* discontinuing such drugs is therapeutically appropriate.**
3. **Give your patient written instructions, and specifically delineate time parameters for the next visit to monitor for therapeutic effectiveness, adverse effects, and disease progression/regression.**
4. **Always have an internist or rheumatologist (or appropriate specialist) on-board as part of the clinical team in case the patient experiences an exacerbation and needs to be hospitalized or acutely immunosuppressed.**
5. **When working with patients that have potentially serious diseases such as most of the autoimmune diseases, you should have a back-up plan integrated into your treatment plan from day one.** You might consider having patients sign a consent form that includes language consistent with the following:

   - *"Due to the uniqueness of each disease and each individual, including his or her willingness and ability to implement the treatment plan, no guarantees of successful treatment can be offered."*

   - *"Dr.___ may not be available on a 24-hour basis at all times. If you have a serious health problem that requires immediate attention, you should call your other doctors(s), call 911, or have someone take you to the nearest hospital emergency room. If you notice an adverse effect from one of the components of your health plan, you should discontinue it then call Dr.__ and inform him/her of what occurred."*

   - *"Treatments with other physicians or healthcare providers are not necessarily to be discontinued. Please let Dr.__ know if you are being treated by other healthcare providers (physicians, counselors, therapists, etc.). Consult your prescribing doctor before discontinuing medications."*

6. **Test responsibly.**
7. **Treat responsibly.**
8. **Re-test to document effectiveness of your intervention.**
9. **When in doubt, refer the patient for co-management.** If you are working with a serious life-threatening disease, and *your plan* or *the patient's implementation of it* is unable to produce documentable results, then you should refer the patient for allopathic/osteopathic/specialist co-management for the sake of protecting the patient from harm and for protecting yourself from undue liability.
10. **Practice defensively.** You will thereby safeguard your patient and your livelihood.

Rheumatoid Arthritis
"RA"

<u>Description/pathophysiology</u>:

- From the allopathic perspective, RA is seen as a chronic "idiopathic" inflammatory disorder primarily affecting the peripheral joints but also affecting the axial skeleton and internal organs; it is generally treated with NSAIDs and other "anti-inflammatory" and immunosuppressive drugs, which are palliative and have no chance of providing cure. Conversely, from the perspective of naturopathic medicine and functional medicine, the condition is considered highly amenable to treatment that addresses the allergic, dysbiotic, and endocrinologic components of this multifaceted phenomenon.
- RA is a persistent, symmetric, destructive, inflammatory peripheral arthritis.
- A pathogenic hallmark of the disease is immune complex formation and intra-articular deposition with resultant release of cytokines and other pro-inflammatory mediators. Immune complexes are important instigators of rheumatoid arthritis and vasculitis, and rheumatoid factor (RF) antibodies are important contributors to these immune complexes.[1,2] The chronic inflammation leads to synovial thickening, villous hypertrophy (pannus formation), and intraarticular colonization with activated lymphocytes and plasma cells. The localized immunocytes cause inflammation and tissue destruction via elaboration of matrix metalloproteinases (including collagenases), prostaglandins, and cytokines such as IL-1.
- **Affects 0.8-1% of all populations: considered the second most common rheumatic diagnosis**[3] after "osteoarthritis", many cases of which are actually hemochromatosis, the most common hereditary condition in the human population.[4]
- **Etiological considerations include:**
    - **Genetic predisposition: associated with HLA-DR:** HLA-DR4 is positive in 70% of RA patients, compared to 28% of control patients; Other HLA-D subsets are seen in various populations. "Genetic risk factors do not fully account for the incidence of RA, suggesting that environmental factors also play a role in the etiology of the disease. …[C]limate and urbanization have a major impact on the incidence and severity of RA in groups of similar genetic background."[5]
    - **Female gender / estrogen**: women are affected 2-3x more often than men. Male RA patients tend to have relative reductions in DHEA and testosterone and relative excess of estrogen and prolactin.
    - **Occult viral, bacterial or parasitic infections.**
        - *Viral*: "Cytomegalovirus and rubella viruses have been cultured from the synovium in patients with rheumatoid arthritis…" "Some evidence suggests hepatitis C virus as a possible trigger to rheumatoid arthritis."[6] The implications of this data are unclear; however, possibilities include: 1) virus *directly* provoking joint destruction, 2) virus *indirectly* provoking joint destruction, such as via immune complexes, 3) noncausal, coincidental finding, 4) inability of RA patients to clear this infection due to immunologic deficits which accompany immune dysfunction. Remember, "unhealthy people are unhealthy", and an *associated* abnormality does not imply a *causal* relationship. Sick people tend to get sicker

[1] Beers MH, Berkow R (eds). The Merck Manual. Seventeenth Edition. Whitehouse Station; Merck Research Laboratories: 1999, page 416
[2] Jonsson T, Valdimarsson H. What about IgA rheumatoid factor in rheumatoid arthritis? *Ann Rheum Dis.* 1998 Jan;57(1):63-4 http://ard.bmjjournals.com/cgi/content/full/57/1/63
[3] Hardin JG, Waterman J, Labson LH. Rheumatic disease: Which diagnostic tests are useful? *Patient Care* 1999; March 15: 83-102
[4] Vasquez A. Musculoskeletal disorders and iron overload disease: comment on the American College of Rheumatology guidelines for the initial evaluation of the adult patient with acute musculoskeletal symptoms. *Arthritis Rheum.* 1996 Oct;39(10):1767-8
[5] Fauci AS, Braunwald E, Isselbacher KJ, et al., eds. Harrison's Principles of Internal Medicine. 14th ed. New York, NY: McGraw-Hill; 1998, page 1881
[6] Siegel LB, Gall EP. Viral infection as a cause of arthritis. *Am Fam Physician* 1996 Nov 1;54(6):2009-15

and enter vicious cycles that can amplify the original illness and lead to the genesis of new, additive health problems.

- ▪ *Bacterial (specific species and generalized gut overgrowth)*: RA is associated with gastrointestinal and genitourinary colonization with *Proteus mirabilis.*[7,8] **Approximately 40% of patients with rheumatoid arthritis have bacterial overgrowth of the small bowel, and the severity of bacterial overgrowth correlates positively with the severity of the musculoskeletal inflammation,** suggesting the probability of a causal relationship.[9] Relatedly, clinicians may recall that peptidoglycans, bacterial cell wall debris[10,11], endotoxins, indole, skatole[12,13] and numerous other gut-derived "toxins" can promote joint inflammation and that the gastrointestinal dysbiotic contribution to rheumatoid arthritis is likely to be both *qualitative* (related to specific inciting microbes) and *quantitative* (related to total, nonspecific bacterial overgrowth of the gut).
- ▪ *Parasitic*: Gastrointestinal parasite infections, such as with *Endolimax nana*[14], can induce a systemic inflammatory response that mimics rheumatoid arthritis and is cured with parasite eradication.

Clinical presentations:

- • Variable course with exacerbations and remissions; the general trend is one of progressive joint destruction and systemic inflammation-induced damage.
- • The disease begins slowly in 2/3 of patients and can be slow to reach a diagnostic threshold—generally takes 9 months between initial onset and diagnosis. May affect only one joint initially.
- • 10% have acute onset polyarthritis.
- • **Typical autoimmune systemic manifestations: fatigue, malaise, fever (don't overlook infection), anorexia, and weight loss.**
- • Classic presentation: can affect any age, either gender, and clinical presentations will vary.
  - ○ 2-3x more common in women than men
  - ○ Age of onset is typically 25-50 y
  - ○ Polyarticular: peripheral symmetric polyarthropathy
  - ○ Symmetrical distribution of joint swelling
  - ○ Morning stiffness > 1 hour
- • Musculoskeletal:
  - ○ The joints most commonly affected are the wrists, MCP, PIP, MTP (metatarsophalangeal) joints, and knees (Baker's cyst is common). In severe or advanced disease, essentially any joint in the body—including the TMJ and upper cervical spine—can be involved.
  - ○ Most common at PIP, MCP joints, wrists (i.e., "knuckles and wrists")
  - ○ Upper cervical spine involvement can lead to atlantoaxial instability
  - ○ Muscle atrophy surrounding joints—due to inflammation and disuse
  - ○ Osteoporosis is common due to inflammation, disuse, hypogonadism, and drug effects
  - ○ Advanced complications include radial deviation of the wrists and ulnar deviation of the fingers, PIP hyperextension (swan neck deformity), flexion of DIP (boutonniere deformity)

[7] Ebringer A, Rashid T, Wilson C. Rheumatoid arthritis: proposal for the use of anti-microbial therapy in early cases. *Scand J Rheumatol* 2003;32(1):2-11

[8] Rashid T, Darlington G, Kjeldsen-Kragh J, Forre O, Collado A, Ebringer A. Proteus IgG antibodies and C-reactive protein in English, Norwegian and Spanish patients with rheumatoid arthritis. *Clin Rheumatol* 1999;18(3):190-5

[9] "Eight (32%) of the patients with RA had hypochlorhydria or achlorhydria... A high frequency of small intestinal bacterial overgrowth was found in patients with RA; it was associated with a high disease activity and observed in patients with hypochlorhydria or achlorhydria and in those with normal acid secretion." Henriksson AE, Blomquist L, Nord CE, Midtvedt T, Uribe A. Small intestinal bacterial overgrowth in patients with rheumatoid arthritis. *Ann Rheum Dis*. 1993 Jul;52(7):503-10

[10] Simelyte E, Rimpilainen M, Lehtonen L, Zhang X, Toivanen P. Bacterial cell wall-induced arthritis: chemical composition and tissue distribution of four Lactobacillus strains. *Infect Immun*. 2000 Jun;68(6):3535-40 http://iai.asm.org/cgi/reprint/68/6/3535

[11] Toivanen P. Normal intestinal microbiota in the aetiopathogenesis of rheumatoid arthritis. *Ann Rheum Dis*. 2003 Sep;62(9):807-11 http://ard.bmjjournals.com/cgi/reprint/62/9/807

[12] Nakoneczna I, Forbes JC, Rogers KS. The arthritogenic effect of indole, skatole and other tryptophan metabolites in rabbits. *Am J Pathol*. 1969 Dec;57(3):523-38

[13] Rogers KS, Forbes JC, Nakoneczna I. Arthritogenic properties of lipophilic, aryl molecules. *Proc Soc Exp Biol Med*. 1969 Jun;131(2):670-2

[14] "Endolimax nana grew on stool culture. Both the patient's diarrhea and arthritis responded effectively to therapy with metronidazole. The diagnosis of parasitic rheumatism was made in retrospect." Burnstein SL, Liakos S. Parasitic rheumatism presenting as rheumatoid arthritis. *J Rheumatol*. 1983 Jun;10(3):514-5

- <u>Skin</u>: Rheumatoid nodules (subcutaneous inflammatory granulomas) are seen in up to 30% of patients. Also rarely seen in patients with hemochromatoic arthropathy mimicking RA.[15]
- <u>Arteries and vessels</u>: Rheumatoid vasculitis leads to impaired circulation, causing necrosis of affected tissues/organs: fingers, skin, internal organs, and nerves (peripheral neuropathy).
- <u>Pulmonary manifestations</u> (more common in men): dyspnea, pulmonary nodules, fibrosis
- <u>Eye</u>: complications are seen in 1% of patients but can lead to rapid blindness
- <u>Other autoimmune diseases</u>: up to 20% of patients with RA develop Sjogren's syndrome

Major differential diagnoses:

- <u>Hemochromatosis and iron overload</u>: essential diagnostic consideration.[16,17] Test serum ferritin and transferrin saturation as discussed in Chapter 1 in the section dealing with laboratory assessments
- <u>Osteoarthritis (OA)</u>: OA tends to be monoarticular or oligoarticular rather than Polyarticular; OA is generally only minimally inflammatory (except after the progression of joint destruction) whereas RA is clearly more inflammatory as assessed clinically and serologically (with ESR or CRP). OA is more likely to be asymmetric whereas RA is nearly always symmetric (except in cases of stroke, paralysis, or peripheral nerve lesion due to interference with neurogenic inflammation). Lab tests such as ANA and RF are normal in OA; CRP and ESR may be moderately elevated in severe OA but inflammatory markers are generally much lower than the levels seen in RA.
- <u>SLE</u>:differentiated by nonerosive arthritis, anti-DS-DNA antibodies, low complement
- <u>Septic arthritis</u>: differentiated by monoarthritis, fever, and purulent joint aspiration
  - **Septic arthritis may complicate pre-existing rheumatoid arthritis**, and patients with RA appear to be predisposed to septic arthritis; reasons for this septic predisposition include immune dysfunction, use of prednisone or other immunosuppressant medications, and concomitant obesity and/or diabetes. **Patients may lack the classic systemic manifestations of septic arthritis (fever, chills, leukocytosis) due to age, disease, or pharmaceutical immunosuppression.**[18,19] Patients may have concomitant respiratory or urinary tract infections, which makes the clinical diagnosis particularly difficult. Treatment may require systemic antibiotics (oral or intravenous) and joint lavage with antibiotics.[20] **Failure to diagnose and treat septic arthritis promptly may result in deformity, disability, or death.**
- <u>Reactive arthritis</u>: differentiated by the recent history of infection, greatly increased prevalence of HLA-B27, and the presence of uveitis/iritis, sacroiliac and lumbar involvement, inflammation of the heels, knees, hips[21]
- <u>Gout and other crystal-induced arthropathy</u>: asymmetric arthritis, crystals demonstrated with joint aspiration
- <u>Arthritis related to viral infection</u>: such as parvovirus and hepatitis C[22]
- <u>Psoriatic arthritis</u>: skin lesions, nail pitting, asymmetric arthritis, negative RF and CCP

---

[15] "These manifestations which are common to rheumatoid arthritis may be seen in hemochromatotic arthropathy." Bensen WG, Laskin CA, Little HA, Fam AG. Hemochromatotic arthropathy mimicking rheumatoid arthritis. A case with subcutaneous nodules, tenosynovitis, and bursitis. *Arthritis Rheum.* 1978 Sep-Oct;21(7):844-8

[16] Vasquez A. Musculoskeletal disorders and iron overload disease: comment on the American College of Rheumatology guidelines for the initial evaluation of the adult patient with acute musculoskeletal symptoms. *Arthritis Rheum.* 1996 Oct;39(10):1767-8

[17] "These manifestations which are common to rheumatoid arthritis may be seen in hemochromatotic arthropathy." Bensen WG, Laskin CA, Little HA, Fam AG. Hemochromatotic arthropathy mimicking rheumatoid arthritis. A case with subcutaneous nodules, tenosynovitis, and bursitis. *Arthritis Rheum.* 1978 Sep-Oct;21(7):844-8

[18] "Many patients lacked distinctive features of joint sepsis (fever, chills) and only one half had leukocytosis." Blackburn WD Jr, Dunn TL, Alarcon GS. Infection versus disease activity in rheumatoid arthritis: eight years' experience. *South Med J.* 1986 Oct;79(10):1238-41

[19] "Pain and loss of motion in the affected joint were prominent, but toxic features of pyogenic infections--hectic fever, chills, sweats, local warmth, or erythema--were conspicuously absent. Two patients had moderate fever and three patients had mild leukocytosis." Kraft SM, Panush RS, Longley S. Unrecognized staphylococcal pyarthrosis with rheumatoid arthritis. *Semin Arthritis Rheum.* 1985 Feb;14(3):196-201

[20] Septic arthritis complicating rheumatoid arthritis was due to Staphylococcus aureus (12 cases) and Escherichia coli (1 case). Recommended treatment: "The authors recommend as the treatment of choice: systemic antibiotic therapy and immediate arthrotomy followed by through-and-through irrigation with fluid containing the appropriate antibiotics." Gristina AG, Rovere GD, Shoji H. Spontaneous septic arthritis complicating rheumatoid arthritis. *J Bone Joint Surg Am.* 1974 Sep;56(6):1180-4

[21] Author's note: I think rheumatoid arthritis should be considered a variant of reactive arthritis, with RA being triggered by multifocal dysbiosis (several subclinical infections) whereas the latter is triggered by a single true infection.

[22] Siegel LB, Gall EP. Viral infection as a cause of arthritis. *Am Fam Physician* 1996 Nov 1;54(6):2009-15

- **Adult Still's disease**: Diagnosis relies on *all of the following*: high fevers (>102.2°F), arthralgia/arthritis, RF<80, ANA<1:100, *plus two of the following*: skin rash (generalized and confluent red papules and plaques), pleuritis/pericarditis, WBC count >15,000 cells/mm³, and hepatomegally/spenomegally/lymphadenopathy.
- **Ewing's sarcoma**: an aggressive bone malignancy that typically presents in children and young adults with periarticular bone pain and fever which can mimic inflammatory monoarthritis

Clinical assessment:
- **History/subjective**:
  - Systemic manifestations with symmetric peripheral polyarthropathy
  - Morning stiffness lasting more than 30-60 minutes is common
- **Physical examination/objective**:
  - Assess joints, especially the distal/peripheral joints of the wrists/hands and ankles/feet. Remember that the initial manifestation of RA, like all inflammatory arthropathies, can affect any joint in the body, including the atlantoaxial joint. Flexion contractures and ulnar deviation of the fingers are common, classic findings of developed disease.
  - Clinically assess patient for exclusion of other diseases. Some patients with RA will develop other autoimmune diseases, especially hypothyroidism and Sjogren's syndrome.
- **Laboratory assessments**: Goals of laboratory testing are 1) exclude serious life-threatening conditions (e.g., septic arthritis), 2) quantitatively and qualitatively assess patient's health status, 3) determine identity and nature of underlying diseases and disorders
  - **CCP: Cyclic citrullinated protein antibody; Citrullinated protein antibodies (CPA); anti-CCP antibodies: anti-cyclic citrullinated peptide antibody**: Anti-CCP antibodies have 98% specificity for RA[23] and is likely to become the future laboratory standard in the diagnosis and prognosis of RA.[24] **The best current data indicates that anti-CCP antibodies are sensitive and specific for RA[25], and clinicians should use this test to diagnose and confirm RA.** Anti-CCP antibodies with a positive rheumatoid factor (RF) is termed "composite seropositivity" and appears to be more specific than isolated anti-CCP antibodies or RF.[26]
  - C-reactive protein: CRP can be used to support the diagnosis (as it indicates inflammation) and can be used to monitor the disease and the response to treatment.[27]
  - Erythrocyte sedimentation rate: ESR is elevated in 90% of patients and can be used to support the diagnosis (as it indicates inflammation) and can be used to monitor the disease and the response to treatment.[28]
  - Complete blood count: CBC may reveal anemia or suggest nutritional deficiencies (namely B12 and folic acid as discussed in Chapter 1); elevated WBC suggests infection.
  - Ferritin: Ferritin is elevated by inflammation and concomitant iron overload. However, transferrin saturation and serum iron should be low in RA due to inflammation, whereas they are commonly elevated in patients with iron overload. In order to determine the acute phase contribution to an elevated ferritin level, an independent marker of inflammation such as CRP or ESR should be tested simultaneously. When in doubt, iron overload can be excluded with diagnostic phlebotomy, liver MRI, liver biopsy (especially if liver enzymes are elevated), or the response to therapeutic phlebotomy.[29]

[23] Hill J, Cairns E, Bell DA. The joy of citrulline: new insights into the diagnosis, pathogenesis, and treatment of rheumatoid arthritis. *J Rheumatol.* 2004 Aug;31(8):1471-3
[24] "We conclude that, at present, the antibody response directed to citrullinated antigens has the most valuable diagnostic and prognostic potential for RA." van Boekel MA, Vossenaar ER, van den Hoogen FH, van Venrooij WJ. Autoantibody systems in rheumatoid arthritis: specificity, sensitivity and diagnostic value. *Arthritis Res.* 2002;4(2):87-93 http://arthritis-research.com/content/4/2/87
[25] "Serum antibodies reactive with citrullinated proteins/peptides are a very sensitive and specific marker for rheumatoid arthritis." Migliorini P, Pratesi F, Tommasi C, Anzilotti C. The immune response to citrullinated antigens in autoimmune diseases. *Autoimmun Rev.* 2005 Nov;4(8):561-4
[26] "...our findings suggest that a positive anti-CCP antibody result does not necessarily exclude SLE in African American patients presenting with inflammatory arthritis. In such patients, the additional assessment of IgA-RF or IgM-RF isotypes may be of added value since composite seropositivity appears to be nearly exclusive to patients with RA." Mikuls TR, Holers VM, Parrish L, Kuhn KA, Conn DL, Gilkeson G, Smith EA, Kamen DL, Jonas BL, Callahan LF, Alarcon GS, Howard G, Moreland LW, Bridges SL Jr. Anti-cyclic citrullinated peptide antibody and rheumatoid factor isotypes in African Americans with early rheumatoid arthritis. *Arthritis Rheum.* 2006 Sep;54(9):3057-9
[27] Gabay C, Kushner I. Acute-phase proteins and other systemic responses to inflammation. *N Engl J Med.* 1999 Feb 11;340(6):448-54
[28] Klippel JH (ed). Primer on the Rheumatic Diseases. 11th Edition. Atlanta: Arthritis Foundation. 1997 page 94
[29] "Therapeutic phlebotomy is used to remove excess iron and maintain low normal body iron stores, and it should be initiated in men with serum ferritin levels of 300 microg/L or more and in women with serum ferritin levels of 200 microg/L or more, regardless of the presence or absence of symptoms." Barton JC, McDonnell SM, Adams PC, Brissot P, Powell LW, Edwards CQ, Cook JD, Kowdley KV. Management of hemochromatosis. Hemochromatosis Management Working Group. *Ann Intern Med.* 1998 Dec 1;129(11):932-9

o Rheumatoid factor: RF is positive in 70-80% of patients with RA but is not specific and is not necessary for the diagnosis of RA; provides supportive evidence; high levels indicate more severe disease and worse prognosis. IgA-RF appears to have clinical superiority over other forms of RF.[30] RF is seen in 5% of normal people, and it is present in some patients with iron overload, thus making the distinction between RA and hemochromatoic arthropathy all the more difficult.[31] Diseases (other than RA) associated with RF positivity include iron overload, chronic infections, hepatitis, sarcoidosis, and bacterial endocarditis.

o Thyroid assessment: Hypothyroidism can mimic systemic rheumatic disease by causing an inflammatory oligoarthropathy and myopathy, complete with elevations of CRP and ESR.[32] Overt or imminent hypothyroidism is suggested by TSH greater than 2 mU/L[33] or 3 mU/L[34], low T4 or T3, and/or the presence of anti-thyroid peroxidase antibodies (anti-TPO).[35]

o Complete hormone assessment: Patients with RA commonly show elevations of prolactin and estradiol along with insufficiencies of testosterone, cortisol, and DHEA. These can be tested in serum, and early-morning serum cortisol is more accurate than late-day cortisol. Other options and details are provided in the following section under Treatments and in the previous section in Chapter 4 on Orthoendocrinology.

o Lactulose-mannitol assay for "leaky gut": Increased intestinal permeability is a common contributor to and complication of many inflammatory/rheumatic diseases including psoriasis[36], Behcet's disease[37], ankylosing spondylitis[38] and seronegative spondyloarthritis[39], enteropathic spondyloarthropathy and oligoarticular juvenile idiopathic arthritis[40], and lupus.[41] This test may be used for the evaluation of gastrointestinal mucosal integrity, which serves as a barometer of systemic health. An elevated lactulose:mannitol ratio may indicate the presence of food allergies, NSAID enterotoxicity, and/or gastrointestinal dysbiosis, the latter of which then needs to be characterized with comprehensive stool testing and comprehensive parasitology.

o Comprehensive stool analysis and comprehensive parasitology with bacterial and fungal culture and sensitivity: **All patients with rheumatoid arthritis should be considered to have gastrointestinal dysbiosis until proven otherwise. A three-sample comprehensive parasitology examination performed by a specialty laboratory is strongly recommended as a minimal component of basic care. In lieu of a comprehensive parasitology test, patients can be treated for 4-8 weeks with broad-spectrum antimicrobial treatment that is effective against gram-positive and gram-negative bacteria, aerobes and anaerobes, yeast, protozoa and amebas.** For additional details, see the Section on *multifocal dysbiosis* in Chapter 4.

- **Imaging**:
  o Radiographic changes are not seen in early disease.

[30] Jonsson T, Valdimarsson H. What about IgA rheumatoid factor in rheumatoid arthritis? *Ann Rheum Dis.* 1998 Jan;57(1):63-4 http://ard.bmjjournals.com/cgi/content/full/57/1/63
[31] "These manifestations which are common to rheumatoid arthritis may be seen in hemochromatotic arthropathy." Bensen WG, Laskin CA, Little HA, Fam AG. Hemochromatotic arthropathy mimicking rheumatoid arthritis. A case with subcutaneous nodules, tenosynovitis, and bursitis. *Arthritis Rheum.* 1978 Sep-Oct;21(7):844-8
[32] Bowman CA, Jeffcoate WJ, Pattrick M, Doherty M. Bilateral adhesive capsulitis, oligoarthritis and proximal myopathy as presentation of hypothyroidism. *Br J Rheumatol.* 1988;27(1):62-4
[33] Weetman AP. Hypothyroidism: screening and subclinical disease. *BMJ.* 1997 Apr 19;314(7088):1175-8 http://bmj.bmjjournals.com/cgi/content/full/314/7088/1175
[34] "Now AACE encourages doctors to consider treatment for patients who test outside the boundaries of a narrower margin based on a target TSH level of 0.3 to 3.0. AACE believes the new range will result in proper diagnosis for millions of Americans who suffer from a mild thyroid disorder, but have gone untreated until now." American Association of Clinical Endocrinologists (AACE). 2003 Campaign Encourages Awareness of Mild Thyroid Failure, Importance of Routine Testing http://www.aace.com/pub/tam2003/press.php November 26, 2005
[35] Beers MH, Berkow R (eds). The Merck Manual. Seventeenth Edition. Whitehouse Station; Merck Research Laboratories 1999 Page 96
[36] Humbert P, Bidet A, Treffel P, Drobacheff C, Agache P. Intestinal permeability in patients with psoriasis. *J Dermatol Sci.* 1991 Jul;2(4):324-6
[37] Fresko I, Hamuryudan V, Demir M, Hizli N, Sayman H, Melikoglu M, Tunc R, Yurdakul S, Yazici H. Intestinal permeability in Behcet's syndrome. *Ann Rheum Dis.* 2001 Jan;60(1):65-6
[38] Vaile JH, Meddings JB, Yacyshyn BR, Russell AS, Maksymowych WP. Bowel permeability and CD45RO expression on circulating CD20+ B cells in patients with ankylosing spondylitis and their relatives. *J Rheumatol.* 1999 Jan;26(1):128-35
[39] Di Leo V, D'Inca R, Bettini MB, Podswiadek M, Punzi L, Mastropaolo G, Sturniolo GC. Effect of Helicobacter pylori and eradication therapy on gastrointestinal permeability. Implications for patients with seronegative spondyloarthritis. *J Rheumatol.* 2005 Feb;32(2):295-300
[40] Picco P, Gattorno M, Marchese N, Vignola S, Sormani MP, Barabino A, Buoncompagni A. Increased gut permeability in juvenile chronic arthritides. A multivariate analysis of the diagnostic parameters. *Clin Exp Rheumatol.* 2000 Nov-Dec;18(6):773-8
[41] "Fourteen cases of primary lupus-associated protein-losing enteropathy have now been reported in the English-language literature." Perednia DA, Curosh NA. Lupus-associated protein-losing enteropathy. *Arch Intern Med.* 1990 Sep;150(9):1806-10

- o Radiographic findings when clustered are relatively specific in developed disease: soft tissue swelling, periarticular osteoporosis, joint space narrowing due to loss of cartilage, marginal erosions, ulnar/lateral deviation of the fingers; subluxation and dislocation may occur.
- **Establishing the diagnosis**:
  - o The diagnosis is established by pattern recognition of the typical clinical manifestations and laboratory abnormalities. Criteria are listed below; however, "Failure to meet these criteria does not exclude the diagnosis."[42]

Criteria for diagnosing rheumatoid arthritis[43] (must have 4 of the following 7 manifestations):
Morning stiffness > 1 hour
Idiopathic, non-traumatic arthritis of at least 3 joints for > 6 weeks
Arthritis of the wrists/hands/knuckles/fingers
Symmetric arthritis (not applicable in patients with peripheral neuropathy, stroke, or hemiplegia)
Rheumatoid nodules
Positive RF (note that these criteria were developed before the use of antibodies to cyclic citrullinated proteins)
Radiographic manifestations: must include erosions or periarticular osteoporosis

Complications:

- Decreased life expectancy by 3-7 years, mostly due to infection and gastrointestinal bleeding.
- Mild disease results in mild symptoms and manageable impact on ADL (activities of daily living) and QOL (quality of life). Severe disease is painful, minimally responsive to *medical* treatment, disfiguring and generally devastating.

Clinical management:

Medical treatments:

1. Discouraging nutritional quackery—according to the Merck Manual, "Food and diet quackery is common and should be discouraged."[44]

2. NSAIDs as first-line treatment (despite the exacerbation of increased intestinal permeability and food allergies[45], and destruction of articular structures[46,47,48,49]),

3. Immunosuppression with prednisone, methotrexate, or other DMARD (disease-modifying antirheumatic drugs). **Despite the clinical drawbacks and philosophical inadequacies, pharmacologic immunosuppression has a role in the management of patients with autoimmunity when their disease flares and threatens vital structures, particularly the heart, brain, and kidneys.** Allopathically, immunosuppression is followed by gold compounds, hydroxychloroquine, sulfasalazine, cyclosporine, and other drugs. Immunosuppression with corticosteroids/prednisone promotes bacterial overgrowth of the small bowel in humans[50], and animal studies have demonstrated increased bacterial translocation following prednisone administration[51]; recall that intestinal bacterial

[42] Fauci AS, Braunwald E, Isselbacher KJ, et al., eds. Harrison's Principles of Internal Medicine. 14th ed. New York, NY: McGraw-Hill; 1998, page 1885

[43] Beers MH, Berkow R (eds). The Merck Manual. Seventeenth Edition. Whitehouse Station; Merck Research Laboratories: 1999, page 418

[44] Beers MH, Berkow R (eds). The Merck Manual. Seventeenth Edition. Whitehouse Station; Merck Research Laboratories: 1999, page 419

[45] Abbreviations: cow's milk beta-lactoglobulin absorption (BLG), acetylsalicylic acid (ASA), disodium chromoglycate (DSCG). "ASA administration strongly increased BLG absorption, not prevented by DSCG pretreatment. In normal controls treated with a single dose of ASA we obtained similar results. Our results suggest that prolonged treatment with nonsteroidal anti-inflammatory drugs induces an increase of food antigen absorption, apparently not related to anaphylaxis mediator release, with possible clinical effects." Fagiolo U, Paganelli R, Ossi E, Quinti I, Cancian M, D'Offizi GP, Fiocco U. Intestinal permeability and antigen absorption in rheumatoid arthritis. Effects of acetylsalicylic acid and sodium chromoglycate. Int Arch Allergy Appl Immunol. 1989;89(1):98-102

[46] "At...concentrations comparable to those... in the synovial fluid of patients treated with the drug, several NSAIDs suppress proteoglycan synthesis... These NSAID-related effects on chondrocyte metabolism ... are much more profound in osteoarthritic cartilage than in normal cartilage, due to enhanced uptake of NSAIDs by the osteoarthritic cartilage." Brandt KD. Effects of nonsteroidal anti-inflammatory drugs on chondrocyte metabolism in vitro and in vivo. Am J Med. 1987 Nov 20; 83(5A): 29-34

[47] "The case of a young healthy man, who developed avascular necrosis of head of femur after prolonged administration of indomethacin, is reported here." Prathapkumar KR, Smith I, Attara GA. Indomethacin induced avascular necrosis of head of femur. Postgrad Med J. 2000 Sep; 76(899): 574-5

[48] "This highly significant association between NSAID use and acetabular destruction gives cause for concern, not least because of the difficulty in achieving satisfactory hip replacements in patients with severely damaged acetabula." Newman NM, Ling RS. Acetabular bone destruction related to non-steroidal anti-inflammatory drugs. Lancet. 1985 Jul 6; 2(8445): 11-4

[49] Vidal y Plana RR, Bizzarri D, Rovati AL. Articular cartilage pharmacology: I. In vitro studies on glucosamine and non steroidal anti-inflammatory drugs. Pharmacol Res Commun. 1978 Jun;10(6):557-69

[50] "A 63-year-old man with systemic lupus erythematosus and selective IgA deficiency developed intractable diarrhoea the day after treatment with prednisone, 50 mg daily, was started. The diarrhoea was considered to be caused by bacterial overgrowth and was later successfully treated with doxycycline." Denison H, Wallerstedt S. Bacterial overgrowth after high-dose corticosteroid treatment. Scand J Gastroenterol. 1989 Jun;24(5):561-4

[51] "These bacteria also translocated to the mesenteric lymph nodes in mice injected with cyclophosphamide or prednisone." Berg RD, Wommack E, Deitch EA. Immunosuppression and intestinal bacterial overgrowth synergistically promote bacterial translocation. Arch Surg. 1988 Nov;123(11):1359-64

overgrowth/translocation are both pro-inflammatory and arthritogenic. A common general sequence of medicalization used by rheumatologists is ❶ begin first-visit treatment with daily/PRN low-dose prednisone (5-7.5 mg/day) and weekly methotrexate (7.5-15 mg/week), ❷ eventually add hydroxychloroquine and/or sulfasalazine, ❸ then when the patient becomes "resistant to treatment" add either an oral immunosuppressant or one of the "biologics" such as the parenterally-administered TNF/cytokine blockers: etanercept, infliximab, adalimumab—these drugs generally cost more than $10,000 per year and carry complications such as increased risk and severity of opportunistic infections (especially tuberculosis), exacerbation of heart failure, and increased risk for lymphoma and—less commonly—SLE and CNS demyelination similar to multiple sclerosis.

4. Surgery is used for deformities and other orthopedic complications, including atlantoaxial instability.

- Avoidance of pro-inflammatory foods: Pro-inflammatory foods act *directly* and *indirectly* to promote and exacerbate systemic inflammation. *Direct* mechanisms include the activation of Toll-like receptors and NF-kappaB, while *indirect* mechanisms include depleting the body of anti-inflammatory nutrients and dietary displacement of more nutrient-dense anti-inflammatory foods. Arachidonic acid (found in cow's milk, beef, liver, pork, and lamb) is the direct precursor to pro-inflammatory prostaglandins and leukotrienes[52] and pain-promoting isoprostanes.[53] Saturated fats promote inflammation by activating/enabling pro-inflammatory Toll-like receptors, which are otherwise "specific" for inducing pro-inflammatory responses to microorganisms.[54] Consumption of saturated fat in the form of cream creates marked oxidative stress and lipid peroxidation that lasts for at least 3 hours postprandially.[55] Corn oil rapidly activates NF-kappaB (in hepatic Kupffer cells) for a pro-inflammatory effect[56]; similarly, consumption of PUFA and linoleic acid promotes antioxidant depletion and may thus promote oxidation-mediated inflammation via activation of NF-kappaB. Linoleic acid causes intracellular oxidative stress and calcium influx and results in increased NF-kappaB-stimulated transcription of pro-inflammatory genes.[57] High glycemic foods cause oxidative stress[58,59] and inflammation via activation of NF-kappaB and other mechanisms—e.g., *white bread causes inflammation*[60] as does *a high-fat high-carbohydrate fast-food-style breakfast.*[61] High glycemic foods suppress immune function[62,63] and thus promote the perpetuation of infection/dysbiosis. Delivery of a high carbohydrate load to the gastrointestinal lumen promotes bacterial overgrowth[64,65], which is inherently pro-inflammatory[66,67] and which appears to be myalgenic in humans[68] at least in part

[52] Vasquez A. Reducing Pain and Inflammation Naturally. Part 2: New Insights into Fatty Acid Supplementation and Its Effect on Eicosanoid Production and Genetic Expression. *Nutritional Perspectives* 2005; January: 5-16 www.optimalhealthresearch.com/part2
[53] Evans AR, Junger H, Southall MD, Nicol GD, Sorkin LS, Broome JT, Bailey TW, Vasko MR. Isoprostanes, novel eicosanoids that produce nociception and sensitize rat sensory neurons. *J Pharmacol Exp Ther*. 2000 Jun;293(3):912-20
[54] Lee JY, Sohn KH, Rhee SH, Hwang D. Saturated fatty acids, but not unsaturated fatty acids, induce the expression of cyclooxygenase-2 mediated through Toll-like receptor 4. *J Biol Chem*. 2001 May 18;276(20):16683-9. Epub 2001 Mar 2 http://www.jbc.org/cgi/content/full/276/20/16683
[55] "CONCLUSIONS: Both fat and protein intakes stimulate ROS generation. The increase in ROS generation lasted 3 h after cream intake and 1 h after protein intake. Cream intake also caused a significant and prolonged increase in lipid peroxidation." Mohanty P, Ghanim H, Hamouda W, Aljada A, Garg R, Dandona P. Both lipid and protein intakes stimulate increased generation of reactive oxygen species by polymorphonuclear leukocytes and mononuclear cells. *Am J Clin Nutr*. 2002 Apr;75(4):767-72 http://www.ajcn.org/cgi/content/full/75/4/767
[56] Rusyn I, Bradham CA, Cohn L, Schoonhoven R, Swenberg JA, Brenner DA, Thurman RG. Corn oil rapidly activates nuclear factor-kappaB in hepatic Kupffer cells by oxidant-dependent mechanisms. *Carcinogenesis*. 1999 Nov;20(11):2095-100 http://carcin.oxfordjournals.org/cgi/content/full/20/11/2095
[57] "Exposing endothelial cells to 90 micromol linoleic acid/L for 6 h resulted in a significant increase in lipid hydroperoxides that coincided wih an increase in intracellular calcium concentrations." Hennig B, Toborek M, Joshi-Barve S, Barger SW, Barve S, Mattson MP, McClain CJ. Linoleic acid activates nuclear transcription factor-kappa B (NF-kappa B) and induces NF-kappa B-dependent transcription in cultured endothelial cells. *Am J Clin Nutr*. 1996 Mar;63(3):322-8 http://www.ajcn.org/cgi/reprint/63/3/322
[58] Mohanty P, Hamouda W, Garg R, Aljada A, Ghanim H, Dandona P. Glucose challenge stimulates reactive oxygen species (ROS) generation by leucocytes. *J Clin Endocrinol Metab*. 2000 Aug;85(8):2970-3 http://jcem.endojournals.org/cgi/content/full/85/8/2970 Glucose/carbohydrate and saturated fat consumption appear to be the two biggest offenders in the food-stimulated production of oxidative stress. The effect by protein is much less. "CONCLUSIONS: Both fat and protein intakes stimulate ROS generation. The increase in ROS generation lasted 3 h after cream intake and 1 h after protein intake. Cream intake also caused a significant and prolonged increase in lipid peroxidation." Mohanty P, Ghanim H, Hamouda W, Aljada A, Garg R, Dandona P. Both lipid and protein intakes stimulate increased generation of reactive oxygen species by polymorphonuclear leukocytes and mononuclear cells. *Am J Clin Nutr*. 2002 Apr;75(4):767-72 http://www.ajcn.org/cgi/content/full/75/4/767
[59] Koska J, Blazicek P, Marko M, Grna JD, Kvetnansky R, Vigas M. Insulin, catecholamines, glucose and antioxidant enzymes in oxidative damage during different loads in healthy humans. *Physiol Res*. 2000;49 Suppl 1:S95-100 http://www.biomed.cas.cz/physiolres/pdf/2000/49_S95.pdf
[60] "Conclusion - The present study shows that high GI carbohydrate, but not low GI carbohydrate, mediates an acute proinflammatory process as measured by NF-kappaB activity." Dickinson S, Hancock DP, Petocz P, Brand-Miller JC..High glycemic index carbohydrate mediates an acute proinflammatory process as measured by NF-kappaB activation. *Asia Pac J Clin Nutr*. 2005;14 Suppl:S120
[61] Aljada A, Mohanty P, Ghanim H, Abdo T, Tripathy D, Chaudhuri A, Dandona P. Increase in intranuclear nuclear factor kappaB and decrease in inhibitor kappaB in mononuclear cells after a mixed meal: evidence for a proinflammatory effect. *Am J Clin Nutr*. 2004 Apr;79(4):682-90 http://www.ajcn.org/cgi/content/full/79/4/682
[62] Sanchez A, Reeser JL, Lau HS, et al. Role of sugars in human neutrophilic phagocytosis. *Am J Clin Nutr*. 1973 Nov;26(11):1180-4
[63] "Postoperative infusion of carbohydrate solution leads to moderate fall in the serum concentration of inorganic phosphate. ... The hypophosphatemia was associated with significant reduction of neutrophil phagocytosis, intracellular killing, consumption of oxygen and generation of superoxide during phagocytosis." Rasmussen A, Segel E, Hessov I, Borregaard N. Reduced function of neutrophils during routine postoperative glucose infusion. *Acta Chir Scand*. 1988 Jul-Aug;154(7-8):429-33
[64] Ramakrishnan T, Stokes P. Beneficial effects of fasting and low carbohydrate diet in D-lactic acidosis associated with short-bowel syndrome. *JPEN J Parenter Enteral Nutr*. 1985 May-Jun;9(3):361-3
[65] Gottschall E. Breaking the Vicious Cycle: Intestinal Health Through Diet. Kirkton Press; Rev edition (August 1, 1994)
[66] Lin HC. Small intestinal bacterial overgrowth: a framework for understanding irritable bowel syndrome. *JAMA*. 2004 Aug 18;292(7):852-8

due to the ability of endotoxin to impair muscle function.[69]   Overconsumption of high-carbohydrate low-phytonutrient grains, potatoes, and manufactured foods displaces phytonutrient-dense foods such as fruits, vegetables, nuts, seeds, and berries which contain more than 8,000 phytonutrients, many of which have antioxidant and thus anti-inflammatory actions.[70,71]

- Supplemented Paleo-Mediterranean diet: The health-promoting diet of choice for the majority of people is a diet based on abundant consumption of fruits, vegetables, seeds, nuts, omega-3 and monounsaturated fatty acids, and lean sources of protein such as lean meats, fatty cold-water fish, soy and whey proteins.   This diet obviates overconsumption of chemical preservatives, artificial sweeteners, and carbohydrate-dominant foods such as candies, pastries, breads, potatoes, grains, and other foods with a high glycemic load and high glycemic index.   This "Paleo-Mediterranean Diet" is a combination of the "Paleolithic" or "Paleo diet" and the well-known "Mediterranean diet", both of which are well described in peer-reviewed journals and the lay press. (See Chapter 2 and my other publications[72,73] for details).   This diet is the most nutrient-dense diet available, and its benefits are further enhanced by supplementation with vitamins, minerals, and the health-promoting fatty acids: ALA, GLA, EPA, DHA.

- Avoidance of allergenic foods: **Gluten-free vegetarian diets benefit patients with rheumatoid arthritis.**[74]   Any patient may be allergic to any food, even if the food is generally considered a health-promoting food.   Generally speaking, the most notorious allergens are wheat, citrus (especially juice due to the industrial use of fungal hemicellulases), cow's milk, eggs, peanuts, chocolate, and yeast-containing foods. According to a study in patients with migraine, some patients will have to avoid as many as 10 specific foods in order to become symptom-free.[75] **Celiac disease can present with inflammatory oligoarthritis that resembles rheumatoid arthritis and which remits with avoidance of wheat/gluten.** The inflammatory arthropathy of celiac disease has preceded bowel symptoms and/or an accurate diagnosis by as many as 3-15 years.[76,77] Clinicians must explain to their patients that celiac disease and wheat allergy are two different clinical entities and that exclusion of one does not exclude the other, and in neither case does mutual exclusion obviate the promotion of intestinal bacterial overgrowth (i.e., pro-inflammatory dysbiosis) by indigestible wheat oligosaccharides.

- Gluten-free vegetarian/vegan diet: **Gluten-free vegetarian diets benefit patients with rheumatoid arthritis.**[78] Vegetarian/vegan diets have a place in the treatment plan of all patients with autoimmune/inflammatory disorders[79,80,81]; this is also true for patients for whom long-term

---

[67] Lichtman SN, Wang J, Sartor RB, Zhang C, Bender D, Dalldorf FG, Schwab JH. Reactivation of arthritis induced by small bowel bacterial overgrowth in rats: role of cytokines, bacteria, and bacterial polymers. *Infect Immun.* 1995 Jun;63(6):2295-301

[68] Pimentel M, et al. A link between irritable bowel syndrome and fibromyalgia may be related to findings on lactulose breath testing. *Ann Rheum Dis.* 2004 Apr;63(4):450-2

[69] Bundgaard H, Kjeldsen K, Suarez Krabbe K, van Hall G, Simonsen L, Qvist J, Hansen CM, Moller K, Fonsmark L, Lav Madsen P, Klarlund Pedersen B. Endotoxemia stimulates skeletal muscle Na+-K+-ATPase and raises blood lactate under aerobic conditions in humans. *Am J Physiol Heart Circ Physiol.* 2003 Mar;284(3):H1028-34. Epub 2002 Nov 21
http://ajpheart.physiology.org/cgi/reprint/284/3/H1028

[70] "We propose that the additive and synergistic effects of phytochemicals in fruit and vegetables are responsible for their potent antioxidant and anticancer activities, and that the benefit of a diet rich in fruit and vegetables is attributed to the complex mixture of phytochemicals present in whole foods." Liu RH. Health benefits of fruit and vegetables are from additive and synergistic combinations of phytochemicals. *Am J Clin Nutr.* 2003 Sep;78(3 Suppl):517S-520S

[71] Seaman DR. The diet-induced proinflammatory state: a cause of chronic pain and other degenerative diseases? *J Manipulative Physiol Ther.* 2002;25(3):168-79

[72] Vasquez A. A Five-Part Nutritional Protocol that Produces Consistently Positive Results. *Nutritional Wellness* 2005 September Available in the printed version and on-line at
http://www.nutritionalwellness.com/archives/2005/sep/09_vasquez.php and http://optimalhealthresearch.com/protocol

[73] Vasquez A. Implementing the Five-Part Nutritional Wellness Protocol for the Treatment of Various Health Problems. *Nutritional Wellness* 2005 November. Available on-line at
http://www.nutritionalwellness.com/archives/2005/nov/11_vasquez.php and http://optimalhealthresearch.com/protocol

[74] "The immunoglobulin G (IgG) antibody levels against gliadin and beta-lactoglobulin decreased in the responder subgroup in the vegan diet-treated patients, but not in the other analysed groups." Hafstrom I, Ringertz B, Spangberg A, von Zweigbergk L, Brannemark S, Nylander I, Ronnelid J, Laasonen L, Klareskog L. A vegan diet free of gluten improves the signs and symptoms of rheumatoid arthritis: the effects on arthritis correlate with a reduction in antibodies to food antigens. *Rheumatology* (Oxford). 2001 Oct;40(10):1175-9
http://rheumatology.oxfordjournals.org/cgi/content/abstract/40/10/1175

[75] Grant EC. Food allergies and migraine. *Lancet.* 1979 May 5;1(8123):966-9

[76] "We report six patients with coeliac disease in whom arthritis was prominent at diagnosis and who improved with dietary therapy. Joint pain preceded diagnosis by up to three years in five patients and 15 years in one patient." Bourne JT, Kumar P, Huskisson EC, Mageed R, Unsworth DJ, Wojtulewski JA. Arthritis and coeliac disease. *Ann Rheum Dis.* 1985 Sep;44(9):592-8

[77] "A 15-year-old girl, with synovitis of the knees and ankles for 3 years before a diagnosis of gluten-sensitive enteropathy, is described." Pinals RS. Arthritis associated with gluten-sensitive enteropathy. *J Rheumatol.* 1986 Feb;13(1):201-4

[78] "The immunoglobulin G (IgG) antibody levels against gliadin and beta-lactoglobulin decreased in the responder subgroup in the vegan diet-treated patients, but not in the other analysed groups." Hafstrom I, Ringertz B, Spangberg A, von Zweigbergk L, Brannemark S, Nylander I, Ronnelid J, Laasonen L, Klareskog L. A vegan diet free of gluten improves the signs and symptoms of rheumatoid arthritis: the effects on arthritis correlate with a reduction in antibodies to food antigens. *Rheumatology* (Oxford). 2001 Oct;40(10):1175-9
http://rheumatology.oxfordjournals.org/cgi/content/abstract/40/10/1175

[79] "After four weeks at the health farm the diet group showed a significant improvement in number of tender joints, Ritchie's articular index, number of swollen joints, pain score, duration of morning stiffness, grip strength, erythrocyte sedimentation rate, C-reactive protein, white blood cell count, and a health assessment questionnaire score." Kjeldsen-Kragh J, Haugen M, Borchgrevink CF, Laerum E, Eek M, Mowinkel P, Hovi K, Forre O. Controlled trial of fasting and one-year vegetarian diet in rheumatoid arthritis. *Lancet.* 1991 Oct 12;338(8772):899-902

[80] "During fasting, arthralgia was less intense in many subjects. In some types of skin diseases (pustulosis palmaris et plantaris and atopic eczema) an improvement could be demonstrated during the fast. During the vegan diet, both signs and symptoms returned in most patients, with the exception of some patients with psoriasis who experienced an improvement." Lithell H, Bruce A, Gustafsson IB, Hoglund NJ, Karlstrom B, Ljunghall K, Sjolin K, Venge P, Werner I, Vessby B. A fasting and vegetarian diet treatment trial on chronic inflammatory disorders. *Acta Derm Venereol.* 1983;63(5):397-403

exclusive reliance on a meat-free vegetarian diet is either not appropriate or not appealing. No scientist or clinician familiar with the research literature doubts the antirheumatic power and anti-inflammatory advantages of vegetarian diets, whether used short-term or long term.[82] The benefits of gluten-free vegetarian diets are well documented, and the mechanisms of action are well elucidated, including reduced intake of pro-inflammatory linoleic[83] and arachidonic acids[84], iron[85], common food antigens[86], gluten[87] and gliadin[88,89], pro-inflammatory sugars[90] and increased intake of omega-3 fatty acids, micronutrients[91], and anti-inflammatory and antioxidant phytonutrients.[92] Vegetarian diets also effect subtle yet biologically and clinically important changes—both *qualitative* and *quantitative*—in intestinal flora[93,94] that correlate with clinical improvement.[95] Patients who rely on the Paleo-Mediterranean diet (which is inherently omnivorous) can use vegetarian *meals* on a daily basis or for days at a time—for example, by having a daily vegetarian meal, or one week per month of vegetarianism. Some (not all) patients can use a purely vegetarian diet long-term provided that nutritional needs (especially protein and cobalamin) are consistently met.

- Short-term fasting: Whether the foundational diet is Paleo-Mediterranean, vegetarian, vegan, or a combination of all of these, autoimmune/inflammatory patients will still benefit from periodic fasting, whether on a weekly (e.g., every Saturday), monthly (every first week or weekend of the month, or every other month), or yearly (1-2 weeks of the year) basis. Since consumption of food—particularly unhealthy foods—induces an inflammatory effect[96], abstinence from food provides a relative anti-inflammatory effect. Fasting indeed provides a distinct anti-inflammatory benefit and may help "re-calibrate" metabolic and homeostatic mechanisms by breaking self-perpetuating "vicious cycles"[97] that autonomously promote inflammation independent of pro-inflammatory stimuli. Water-only fasting is completely hypoallergenic (assuming that the patient is not sensitive to chlorine, fluoride, or other contaminants), and subsequent re-introduction of foods provides the ideal opportunity to identify offending foods. Fasting deprives intestinal microbes of substrate[98], stimulates intestinal B-cell immunity[99],

[81] Tanaka T, Kouda K, Kotani M, Takeuchi A, Tabei T, Masamoto Y, Nakamura H, Takigawa M, Suemura M, Takeuchi H, Kouda M. Vegetarian diet ameliorates symptoms of atopic dermatitis through reduction of the number of peripheral eosinophils and of PGE2 synthesis by monocytes. *J Physiol Anthropol Appl Human Sci*. 2001 Nov;20(6):353-61 http://www.jstage.jst.go.jp/article/jpa/20/6/20_353/_article/-char/en

[82] "For the patients who were randomised to the vegetarian diet there was a significant decrease in platelet count, leukocyte count, calprotectin, total IgG, IgM rheumatoid factor (RF), C3-activation products, and the complement components C3 and C4 after one month of treatment." Kjeldsen-Kragh J, Mellbye OJ, Haugen M, Mollnes TE, Hammer HB, Sioud M, Forre O. Changes in laboratory variables in rheumatoid arthritis patients during a trial of fasting and one-year vegetarian diet. *Scand J Rheumatol*. 1995;24(2):85-93

[83] Rusyn I, Bradham CA, Cohn L, Schoonhoven R, Swenberg JA, Brenner DA, Thurman RG. Corn oil rapidly activates nuclear factor-kappaB in hepatic Kupffer cells by oxidant-dependent mechanisms. *Carcinogenesis*. 1999 Nov;20(11):2095-100 http://carcin.oxfordjournals.org/cgi/content/full/20/11/2095

[84] Vasquez A. Reducing Pain and Inflammation Naturally. Part 2: New Insights into Fatty Acid Supplementation and Its Effect on Eicosanoid Production and Genetic Expression. *Nutritional Perspectives* 2005; January: 5-16 http://optimalhealthresearch.com/part2

[85] Dabbagh AJ, Trenam CW, Morris CJ, Blake DR. Iron in joint inflammation. *Ann Rheum Dis*. 1993 Jan;52(1):67-73

[86] Hafstrom I, Ringertz B, Spangberg A, von Zweigbergk L, Brannemark S, Nylander I, Ronnelid J, Laasonen L, Klareskog L. A vegan diet free of gluten improves the signs and symptoms of rheumatoid arthritis: the effects on arthritis correlate with a reduction in antibodies to food antigens. *Rheumatology* (Oxford). 2001 Oct;40(10):1175-9 http://rheumatology.oxfordjournals.org/cgi/reprint/40/10/1175

[87] "The data provide evidence that dietary modification may be of clinical benefit for certain RA patients, and that this benefit may be related to a reduction in immunoreactivity to food antigens eliminated by the change in diet." Hafstrom I, Ringertz B, Spangberg A, von Zweigbergk L, Brannemark S, Nylander I, Ronnelid J, Laasonen L, Klareskog L. A vegan diet free of gluten improves the signs and symptoms of rheumatoid arthritis: the effects on arthritis correlate with a reduction in antibodies to food antigens. *Rheumatology* (Oxford). 2001 Oct;40(10):1175-9

[88] "Despite the increased AGA [antigliadin antibodies] positivity found distinctively in patients with recent-onset RA, none of the RA patients showed clear evidence of coeliac disease." Paimela L, Kurki P, Leirisalo-Repo M, Piirainen H. Gliadin immune reactivity in patients with rheumatoid arthritis. *Clin Exp Rheumatol*. 1995 Sep-Oct;13(5):603-7

[89] "The median IgA antigliadin ELISA index was 7.1 (range 2.1-22.4) for the RA group and 3.1 (range 0.3-34.9) for the controls (p = 0.0001)." Koot VC, Van Straaten M, Hekkens WT, Collee G, Dijkmans BA. Elevated level of IgA gliadin antibodies in patients with rheumatoid arthritis. *Clin Exp Rheumatol*. 1989 Nov-Dec;7(6):623-6

[90] Seaman DR. The diet-induced proinflammatory state: a cause of chronic pain and other degenerative diseases? *J Manipulative Physiol Ther*. 2002 Mar-Apr;25(3):168-79

[91] Hagfors L, Nilsson I, Skoldstam L, Johansson G. Fat intake and composition of fatty acids in serum phospholipids in a randomized, controlled, Mediterranean dietary intervention study on patients with rheumatoid arthritis. *Nutr Metab* (Lond). 2005 Oct 10;2:26 http://www.nutritionandmetabolism.com/content/2/1/26

[92] Liu RH. Health benefits of fruit and vegetables are from additive and synergistic combinations of phytochemicals. *Am J Clin Nutr* 2003;78(3 Suppl):517S-520S http://www.ajcn.org/cgi/content/full/78/3/517S

[93] "Significant alteration in the intestinal flora was observed when the patients changed from omnivorous to vegan diet. ... This finding of an association between intestinal flora and disease activity may have implications for our understanding of how diet can affect RA." Peltonen R, Kjeldsen-Kragh J, Haugen M, Tuominen J, Toivanen P, Forre O, Eerola E. Changes of faecal flora in rheumatoid arthritis during fasting and one-year vegetarian diet. *Br J Rheumatol*. 1994 Jul;33(7):638-43

[94] Toivanen P, Eerola E. A vegan diet changes the intestinal flora. *Rheumatology* (Oxford). 2002 Aug;41(8):950-1 http://rheumatology.oxfordjournals.org/cgi/reprint/41/8/950

[95] "We conclude that a vegan diet changes the faecal microbial flora in RA patients, and changes in the faecal flora are associated with improvement in RA activity." Peltonen R, Nenonen M, Helve T, Hanninen O, Toivanen P, Eerola E. Faecal microbial flora and disease activity in rheumatoid arthritis during a vegan diet. *Br J Rheumatol*. 1997 Jan;36(1):64-8 http://rheumatology.oxfordjournals.org/cgi/reprint/36/1/64

[96] Aljada A, Mohanty P, Ghanim H, Abdo T, Tripathy D, Chaudhuri A, Dandona P. Increase in intranuclear nuclear factor kappaB and decrease in inhibitor kappaB in mononuclear cells after a mixed meal: evidence for a proinflammatory effect. *Am J Clin Nutr*. 2004 Apr;79(4):682-90 http://www.ajcn.org/cgi/content/full/79/4/682

[97] "The ability of therapeutic fasts to break metabolic vicious cycles may also contribute to the efficacy of fasting in the treatment of type 2 diabetes and autoimmune disorders." McCarty MF. A preliminary fast may potentiate response to a subsequent low-salt, low-fat vegan diet in the management of hypertension - fasting as a strategy for breaking metabolic vicious cycles. *Med Hypotheses*. 2003 May;60(5):624-33

[98] Ramakrishnan T, Stokes P. Beneficial effects of fasting and low carbohydrate diet in D-lactic acidosis associated with short-bowel syndrome. *JPEN J Parenter Enteral Nutr*. 1985 May-Jun;9(3):361-3

[99] Trollmo C, Verdrengh M, Tarkowski A. Fasting enhances mucosal antigen specific B cell responses in rheumatoid arthritis. *Ann Rheum Dis*. 1997 Feb;56(2):130-4 http://ard.bmjjournals.com/cgi/content/full/56/2/130

improves the bactericidal action of neutrophils[100], reduces lysozyme release and leukotriene formation[101], and ameliorates intestinal hyperpermeability.[102] In case reports and clinical trials, short-term fasting (or protein-sparing fasting) has been documented as safe and effective treatment for SLE[103], RA[104], and non-rheumatic diseases such as chronic severe hypertension[105], moderate hypertension[106], obesity[107,108], type-2 diabetes[109], and epilepsy.[110]

- <u>Broad-spectrum fatty acid therapy with ALA, EPA, DHA, GLA and oleic acid</u>: Fatty acid supplementation should be delivered in the form of combination therapy with ALA, GLA, DHA, and EPA. Given at doses of 3,000 – 9,000 mg per day, ALA from flaxseed oil has impressive anti-inflammatory benefits demonstrated by its ability to halve prostaglandin production in humans.[111] **Numerous studies have demonstrated the benefit of GLA in the treatment of rheumatoid arthritis when used at doses between 500 mg – 4,000 mg per day.[112,113] Fish oil provides EPA and DHA which have well-proven anti-inflammatory benefits in rheumatoid arthritis[114,115,116] and lupus.[117,118]** ALA, EPA, DHA, and GLA need to be provided in the form of supplements; when using high doses of therapeutic oils, *liquid* supplements that can be mixed in juice or a smoothie are generally more convenient and palatable than are *capsules*. For example, at the upper end of oral fatty acid administration, the patient may be consuming as much as one-quarter cup per day of fatty acid supplementation; this same dose administered in the form of pills would require at least 72 capsules to attain the equivalent doses of ALA, EPA, DHA, and GLA. Therapeutic amounts of oleic acid can be obtained from generous use of olive oil, preferably on fresh vegetables. Supplementation with polyunsaturated fatty acids warrants increased intake of antioxidants from diet, from fruit and vegetable juices, and from properly formulated supplements. Since patients with systemic inflammation are generally in a pro-oxidative state, consideration must be given to the timing and starting dose of fatty acid supplementation and the need for antioxidant protection; some patients should start with a low dose of fatty acid supplementation until inflammation and the hyperoxidative state have been reduced; see the final chapter in this text on Therapeutics for more fatty acid details and biochemical pathways. Clinicians must realize that fatty acids are not clinically or biochemically

[100] "An association was found between improvement in inflammatory activity of the joints and enhancement of neutrophil bactericidal capacity. Fasting appears to improve the clinical status of patients with RA." Uden AM, Trang L, Venizelos N, Palmblad J. Neutrophil functions and clinical performance after total fasting in patients with rheumatoid arthritis. *Ann Rheum Dis*. 1983 Feb;42(1):45-51

[101] "We thus conclude that a reduced ability to generate cytotaxins, reduced release of enzyme, and reduced leukotriene formation from RA neutrophils, together with an altered fatty acid composition of membrane phospholipids, may be mechanisms for the decrease of inflammatory symptoms that results from fasting." Hafstrom I, Ringertz B, Gyllenhammar H, Palmblad J, Harms-Ringdahl M. Effects of fasting on disease activity, neutrophil function, fatty acid composition, and leukotriene biosynthesis in patients with rheumatoid arthritis. *Arthritis Rheum*. 1988 May;31(5):585-92

[102] "The results indicate that, unlike lactovegetarian diet, fasting may ameliorate the disease activity and reduce both the intestinal and the non-intestinal permeability in rheumatoid arthritis." Sundqvist T, Lindstrom F, Magnusson KE, Skoldstam L, Stjernstrom I, Tagesson C. Influence of fasting on intestinal permeability and disease activity in patients with rheumatoid arthritis. *Scand J Rheumatol*. 1982;11(1):33-8

[103] Fuhrman J, Sarter B, Calabro DJ. Brief case reports of medically supervised, water-only fasting associated with remission of autoimmune disease. *Altern Ther Health Med*. 2002 Jul-Aug;8(4):112, 110-1

[104] "An association was found between improvement in inflammatory activity of the joints and enhancement of neutrophil bactericidal capacity. Fasting appears to improve the clinical status of patients with RA." Uden AM, Trang L, Venizelos N, Palmblad J. Neutrophil functions and clinical performance after total fasting in patients with rheumatoid arthritis. *Ann Rheum Dis*. 1983 Feb;42(1):45-51

[105] "The average reduction in blood pressure was 37/13 mm Hg, with the greatest decrease being observed for subjects with the most severe hypertension. Patients with stage 3 hypertension (those with systolic blood pressure greater than 180 mg Hg, diastolic blood pressure greater than 110 mm Hg, or both) had an average reduction of 60/17 mm Hg at the conclusion of treatment." Goldhamer A, Lisle D, Parpia B, Anderson SV, Campbell TC. Medically supervised water-only fasting in the treatment of hypertension. *J Manipulative Physiol Ther*. 2001 Jun;24(5):335-9 http://www.healthpromoting.com/335-339Goldhamer115263.QXD.pdf

[106] "RESULTS: Approximately 82% of the subjects achieved BP at or below 120/80 mm Hg by the end of the treatment program. The mean BP reduction was 20/7 mm Hg, with the greatest decrease being observed for subjects with the highest baseline BP." Goldhamer AC, Lisle DJ, Sultana P, Anderson SV, Parpia B, Hughes B, Campbell TC. Medically supervised water-only fasting in the treatment of borderline hypertension. *J Altern Complement Med*. 2002 Oct;8(5):643-50 http://www.healthpromoting.com/Articles/articles/study%202/acmpaper5.pdf

[107] Vertes V, Genuth SM, Hazelton IM. Supplemented fasting as a large-scale outpatient program. *JAMA*. 1977 Nov 14;238(20):2151-3

[108] Bauman WA, Schwartz E, Rose HG, Eisenstein HN, Johnson DW. Early and long-term effects of acute caloric deprivation in obese diabetic patients. *Am J Med*. 1988 Jul;85(1):38-46

[109] Goldhamer AC. Initial cost of care results in medically supervised water-only fasting for treating high blood pressure and diabetes. *J Altern Complement Med*. 2002 Dec;8(6):696-7 http://www.healthpromoting.com/Articles/pdf/Study%2032.pdf

[110] "The ketogenic diet should be considered as alternative therapy for children with difficult-to-control seizures. It is more effective than many of the new anticonvulsant medications and is well tolerated by children and families when it is effective." Freeman JM, Vining EP, Pillas DJ, Pyzik PL, Casey JC, Kelly LM. The efficacy of the ketogenic diet-1998: a prospective evaluation of intervention in 150 children. *Pediatrics*. 1998 Dec;102(6):1358-63 http://pediatrics.aappublications.org/cgi/reprint/102/6/1358

[111] Adam O, Wolfram G, Zollner N. Effect of alpha-linolenic acid in the human diet on linoleic acid metabolism and prostaglandin biosynthesis. *J Lipid Res*. 1986 Apr;27(4):421-6 http://www.jlr.org/cgi/reprint/27/4/421

[112] "Other results showed a significant reduction in morning stiffness with gamma-linolenic acid at 3 months and reduction in pain and articular index at 6 months with olive oil." Brzeski M, Madhok R, Capell HA. Evening primrose oil in patients with rheumatoid arthritis and side-effects of non-steroidal anti-inflammatory drugs. *Br J Rheumatol*. 1991 Oct;30(5):370-2

[113] Rothman D, DeLuca P, Zurier RB. Botanical lipids: effects on inflammation, immune responses, and rheumatoid arthritis. *Semin Arthritis Rheum*. 1995 Oct;25(2):87-96

[114] Adam O, Beringer C, Kless T, Lemmen C, Adam A, Wiseman M, Adam P, Klimmek R, Forth W. Anti-inflammatory effects of a low arachidonic acid diet and fish oil in patients with rheumatoid arthritis. *Rheumatol Int*. 2003 Jan;23(1):27-36

[115] Lau CS, Morley KD, Belch JJ. Effects of fish oil supplementation on non-steroidal anti-inflammatory drug requirement in patients with mild rheumatoid arthritis--a double-blind placebo controlled study. *Br J Rheumatol*. 1993 Nov;32(11):982-9

[116] Kremer JM, Jubiz W, Michalek A, Rynes RI, Bartholomew LE, Bigaouette J, Timchalk M, Beeler D, Lininger L. Fish-oil fatty acid supplementation in active rheumatoid arthritis. A double-blinded, controlled, crossover study. *Ann Intern Med*. 1987 Apr;106(4):497-503

[117] Walton AJ, Snaith ML, Locniskar M, Cumberland AG, Morrow WJ, Isenberg DA. Dietary fish oil and the severity of symptoms in patients with systemic lupus erythematosus. *Ann Rheum Dis*. 1991 Jul;50(7):463-6

[118] Duffy EM, Meenagh GK, McMillan SA, Strain JJ, Hannigan BM, Bell AL. The clinical effect of dietary supplementation with omega-3 fish oils and/or copper in systemic lupus erythematosus. *J Rheumatol*. 2004 Aug;31(8):1551-6

interchangeable and that one fatty acid does not substitute for another; each of the fatty acids must be supplied in order for its benefits to be obtained.[119]

- <u>Vitamin D3 supplementation with physiologic doses and/or tailored to serum 25(OH)D levels</u>: Vitamin D deficiency is common in the general population and is even more common in patients with chronic illness and chronic musculoskeletal pain.[120] Correction of vitamin D deficiency supports normal immune function against infection and provides a clinically significant anti-inflammatory[121] and analgesic benefit in patients with back pain[122] and limb pain.[123] Reasonable daily doses for children and adults are 1,000-2,000 and 4,000 IU, respectively.[124] Deficiency and response to treatment are monitored with serum 25(OH)vitamin D while safety is monitored with serum calcium; inflammatory granulomatous diseases and certain drugs such as hydrochlorothiazide greatly increase the propensity for hypercalcemia and warrant increment dosing and frequent monitoring of serum calcium. Vitamin D2 (ergocalciferol) is not a human nutrient and should not be used in clinical practice.

- **Assessment for dysbiosis: All patients with rheumatoid arthritis have gastrointestinal dysbiosis until proven otherwise by the combination of 1) three-sample comprehensive parasitology examinations performed by a specialty laboratory and 2) clinical response to at least two 2-4 week courses of broad-spectrum antimicrobial treatment.** Yeast, bacteria, and parasites are treated as indicated based on identification and sensitivity results from comprehensive parasitology assessments. Patients taking immunosuppressant drugs such as corticosteroids/prednisone have increased risk of intestinal bacterial overgrowth and translocation.[125,126] Other dysbiotic loci should be investigated as discussed in Chapter 4 in the section on multifocal dysbiosis.

  - <u>Gastrointestinal dysbiosis</u>: Additionally or empirically, treatment for gastrointestinal dysbiosis may include the following:
    - <u>Oregano oil</u>: Emulsified oil of oregano in a time-released tablet is proven effective in the eradication of harmful gastrointestinal microbes, including *Blastocystis hominis*, *Entamoeba hartmanni*, and *Endolimax nana*.[127] An *in vitro* study[128] and clinical experience support the use of emulsified oregano against *Candida albicans* and various bacteria. The common dose is 600 mg per day in divided doses for 6 weeks.[129]
    - <u>Berberine</u>: Berberine is an alkaloid extracted from plants such as *Berberis vulgaris*, and *Hydrastis canadensis*, and it shows effectiveness against *Giardia*, *Candida*, and *Streptococcus* in addition to its direct anti-inflammatory and antidiarrheal actions. Oral dose of 400 mg per day is common for adults.[130]
    - *Artemisia annua*: Artemisinin has been safely used for centuries in Asia for the treatment of malaria, and it also has effectiveness against anaerobic bacteria due

[119] Vasquez A. Reducing Pain and Inflammation Naturally. Part 2: New Insights into Fatty Acid Supplementation and Its Effect on Eicosanoid Production and Genetic Expression. *Nutritional Perspectives* 2005; January: 5-16 http://optimalhealthresearch.com/part2

[120] Plotnikoff GA, Quigley JM. Prevalence of severe hypovitaminosis D in patients with persistent, nonspecific musculoskeletal pain. *Mayo Clin Proc.* 2003 Dec;78(12):1463-70

[121] Timms PM, Mannan N, Hitman GA, Noonan K, Mills PG, Syndercombe-Court D, Aganna E, Price CP, Boucher BJ. Circulating MMP9, vitamin D and variation in the TIMP-1 response with VDR genotype: mechanisms for inflammatory damage in chronic disorders? *QJM.* 2002 Dec;95(12):787-96 http://qjmed.oxfordjournals.org/cgi/content/full/95/12/787

[122] Al Faraj S, Al Mutairi K. Vitamin D deficiency and chronic low back pain in Saudi Arabia. *Spine.* 2003 Jan 15;28(2):177-9

[123] Masood H, Narang AP, Bhat IA, Shah GN. Persistent limb pain and raised serum alkaline phosphatase the earliest markers of subclinical hypovitaminosis D in Kashmir. *Indian J Physiol Pharmacol.* 1989 Oct-Dec;33(4):259-61

[124] Vasquez A, Manso G, Cannell J. The clinical importance of vitamin D (cholecalciferol): a paradigm shift with implications for all healthcare providers. *Altern Ther Health Med.* 2004 Sep-Oct;10(5):28-36 http://optimalhealthresearch.com/monograph04

[125] "A 63-year-old man with systemic lupus erythematosus and selective IgA deficiency developed intractable diarrhoea the day after treatment with prednisone, 50 mg daily, was started. The diarrhoea was considered to be caused by bacterial overgrowth and was later successfully treated with doxycycline." Denison H, Wallerstedt S. Bacterial overgrowth after high-dose corticosteroid treatment. *Scand J Gastroenterol.* 1989 Jun;24(5):561-4

[126] "These bacteria also translocated to the mesenteric lymph nodes in mice injected with cyclophosphamide or prednisone." Berg RD, Wommack E, Deitch EA. Immunosuppression and intestinal bacterial overgrowth synergistically promote bacterial translocation. *Arch Surg.* 1988 Nov;123(11):1359-64

[127] Force M, Sparks WS, Ronzio RA. Inhibition of enteric parasites by emulsified oil of oregano in vivo. *Phytother Res.* 2000 May;14(3):213-4

[128] Stiles JC, Sparks W, Ronzio RA. The inhibition of Candida albicans by oregano. *J Applied Nutr* 1995;47:96-102

[129] Force M, Sparks WS, Ronzio RA. Inhibition of enteric parasites by emulsified oil of oregano in vivo. *Phytother Res.* 2000 May;14(3):213-4

[130] Berberine. *Altern Med Rev.* 2000 Apr;5(2):175-7 http://www.thorne.com/altmedrev/.fulltext/5/2/175.pdf

to the pro-oxidative sesquiterpene endoperoxide.[131,132] I commonly use artemisinin at 200 mg per day in divided doses for adults with dysbiosis.

- St. John's Wort (*Hypericum perforatum*): Hyperforin from *Hypericum perforatum* also shows impressive antibacterial action, particularly against gram-positive bacteria such as *Staphylococcus aureus*, *Streptococcus pyogenes*, *Streptococcus agalactiae*[133] and perhaps *Helicobacter pylori*.[134] Up to 600 mg three times per day of a 3% hyperforin standardized extract is customary in the treatment of depression.

- Bismuth: Bismuth is commonly used in the empiric treatment of diarrhea (e.g., "Pepto-Bismol") and is commonly combined with other antimicrobial agents to reduce drug resistance and increase antibiotic effectiveness.[135]

- Undecylenic acid: Derived from castor bean oil, undecylenic acid has antifungal properties and is commonly indicated by sensitivity results obtained by stool culture. Common dosages are 150-250 mg tid (up to 750 mg per day).[136]

- Peppermint *(Mentha piperita)*: Peppermint shows antimicrobial and antispasmodic actions and has demonstrated clinical effectiveness in patients with bacterial overgrowth of the small bowel.

- Commonly used antibiotic/antifungal drugs: The most commonly employed drugs for intestinal bacterial overgrowth are described here.[137] Treatment duration is generally at least 2 weeks and up to 8 weeks, depending on clinical response and the severity and diversity of the intestinal overgrowth. With all anti*bacterial* treatments, use empiric anti*fungal* treatment to prevent yeast overgrowth; some patients benefit from antifungal treatment that is continued for *months* and occasionally *years*. Drugs can generally be coadministered with natural antibiotics/antifungals for improved efficacy. Treatment can be guided by identification of the dysbiotic microbes and the results of culture and sensitivity tests.

  ⇒ Metronidazole: 250-500 mg BID-QID (generally limit to 1.5 g/d); metronidazole has systemic bioavailability and effectiveness against a wide range of dysbiotic microbes, including protozoans, amebas/Giardia, *H. pylori*, *Clostridium difficile* and most anaerobic gram-negative bacilli.[138] Adverse effects are generally limited to stomatitis, nausea, diarrhea, and—rarely and/or with long-term use—peripheral neuropathy, dizziness, and metallic taste; the drug must not be consumed with alcohol. Metronidazole resistance by *Blastocystis hominis* and other parasites has been noted.

  ⇒ Erythromycin: 250-500 mg TID-QID; this drug is a widely used antibiotic that also has intestinal promotility benefits (thus making it an ideal treatment for intestinal bacterial overgrowth associated with or caused by intestinal dysmotility/hypomotility such as seen in scleroderma[139,140]). Do not combine erythromycin with the promotility drug **cisapride** due to risk for serious cardiac arrhythmia.

[131] Dien TK, de Vries PJ, Khanh NX, Koopmans R, Binh LN, Duc DD, Kager PA, van Boxtel CJ. Effect of food intake on pharmacokinetics of oral artemisinin in healthy Vietnamese subjects. *Antimicrob Agents Chemother*. 1997 May;41(5):1069-72

[132] Giao PT, Binh TQ, Kager PA, Long HP, Van Thang N, Van Nam N, de Vries PJ. Artemisinin for treatment of uncomplicated falciparum malaria: is there a place for monotherapy? *Am J Trop Med Hyg*. 2001 Dec;65(6):690-5

[133] Schempp CM, Pelz K, Wittmer A, Schopf E, Simon JC. Antibacterial activity of hyperforin from St John's wort, against multiresistant Staphylococcus aureus and gram-positive bacteria. *Lancet*. 1999 Jun 19;353(9170):2129

[134] "A butanol fraction of St. John's Wort revealed anti-Helicobacter pylori activity with MIC values ranging between 15.6 and 31.2 microg/ml." Reichling J, Weseler A, Saller R. A current review of the antimicrobial activity of Hypericum perforatum L. *Pharmacopsychiatry*. 2001 Jul;34 Suppl 1:S116-8

[135] Veldhuyzen van Zanten SJ, Sherman PM, Hunt RH. Helicobacter pylori: new developments and treatments. *CMAJ*. 1997;156(11):1565-74 http://www.cmaj.ca/cgi/reprint/156/11/1565.pdf

[136] "Adult dosage is usually 450-750 mg undecylenic acid daily in three divided doses." Undecylenic acid. Monograph. *Altern Med Rev*. 2002 Feb;7(1):68-70 http://www.thorne.com/altmedrev/.fulltext/7/1/68.pdf

[137] Saltzman JR, Russell RM. Nutritional consequences of intestinal bacterial overgrowth. *Compr Ther*. 1994;20(9):523-30

[138] Tierney ML. McPhee SJ, Papadakis MA. Current Medical Diagnosis and Treatment 2006. 45th edition. New York; Lange Medical Books: 2006, pages 1578-1577

[139] "Prokinetic agents effective in pseudoobstruction include metoclopramide, domperidone, cisapride, octreotide, and erythromycin. ... The combination of octreotide and erythromycin may be particularly effective in systemic sclerosis." Sjogren RW. Gastrointestinal features of scleroderma. *Curr Opin Rheumatol*. 1996 Nov;8(6):569-75

[140] "CONCLUSIONS: Erythromycin accelerates gastric and gallbladder emptying in scleroderma patients and might be helpful in the treatment of gastrointestinal motor abnormalities in these patients." Fiorucci S, Distrutti E, Bassotti G, Gerli R, Chiucchiu S, Betti C, Santucci L, Morelli A. Effect of erythromycin administration on upper gastrointestinal motility in scleroderma patients. *Scand J Gastroenterol*. 1994 Sep;29(9):807-13

⇒ <u>Tetracycline</u>: 250-500 mg QID

⇒ <u>Ciproflaxacin</u>: 500 mg BID

⇒ <u>Cephalexin/kelfex</u>: 250 mg QID

⇒ <u>Minocycline</u>: **Minocycline (200 mg/day)[141] has received the most attention in the treatment of rheumatoid arthritis due to its superior response (65%) over placebo (13%)[142]; in addition to its antibacterial action, the drug is also immunomodulatory and anti-inflammatory.** Ironically, minocycline can cause drug-induced autoimmunity, especially lupus.[143,144]

⇒ <u>Nystatin</u>: Nystatin 500,000 units bid with food; duration of treatment begins with a minimum duration of 2-4 weeks and may continue as long as the patient is deriving benefit.

⇒ <u>Ketoconazole</u>: As a systemically bioavailable antifungal drug, ketoconazole has inherent anti-inflammatory benefits which may be helpful; however the drug inhibits androgen formation and may lead to exacerbation of the hypoandrogenism that is commonly seen in autoimmune patients and which contributes to the immune dysfunction.

- <u>Probiotics</u>: Live cultures in the form of tablets, capsules, yogurt, or kefir can be used per patient preference and tolerance. Obviously, dairy-based products should be avoided by patients with dairy allergy.

- <u>*Saccharomyces boulardii*</u>: A non-colonizing, non-pathogenic yeast that increases sIgA production and can aid in the elimination of pathogenic/dysbiotic yeast, bacteria, and parasites. It is particularly useful during antibiotic treatment to help prevent secondary Candidal infections. Common dose is 250 mg thrice daily.

- <u>Supplemented Paleo-Mediterranean diet / Specific Carbohydrate Diet</u>: The specifications of the *specific carbohydrate diet* (SCD) detailed by Gottschall[145] are met with adherence to the Paleo diet by Cordain.[146] The combination of both approaches and books will give patients an excellent combination of informational understanding and culinary versatility.

- <u>Orthoendocrinology</u>: Assess prolactin, cortisol, DHEA, free and total testosterone, serum estradiol, and thyroid status (e.g., TSH, T4, *and* anti-thyroid peroxidase antibodies).

  o <u>Prolactin (excess)</u>: **Patients with RA and SLE have higher basal and stress-induced levels of prolactin compared with normal controls.[147,148] Men with RA have higher serum levels of prolactin, and these levels correlate with the severity and duration of the disorder.[149,150]** Serum prolactin is the standard assessment of prolactin status. Since elevated prolactin may be a sign of pituitary tumor, assessment for headaches, visual deficits, and other abnormalities of pituitary hormones (e.g., GH and TSH) should be performed; CT or MRI must be considered. Patients with prolactin levels less than 100 ng/mL and normal CT/MRI findings can be managed conservatively with effective prolactin-lowering treatment and annual

---

[141] "...48-week trial of oral minocycline (200 mg/d) or placebo." Tilley BC, Alarcon GS, Heyse SP, Trentham DE, Neuner R, Kaplan DA, Clegg DO, Leisen JC, Buckley L, Cooper SM, Duncan H, Pillemer SR, Tuttleman M, Fowler SE. Minocycline in rheumatoid arthritis. A 48-week, double-blind, placebo-controlled trial. MIRA Trial Group. *Ann Intern Med.* 1995 Jan 15;122(2):81-9

[142] "In patients with early seropositive RA, therapy with minocycline is superior to placebo." O'Dell JR, Haire CE, Palmer W, Drymalski W, Wees S, Blakely K, Churchill M, Eckhoff PJ, Weaver A, Doud D, Erikson N, Dietz F, Olson R, Maloley P, Klassen LW, Moore GF. Treatment of early rheumatoid arthritis with minocycline or placebo: results of a randomized, double-blind, placebo-controlled trial. *Arthritis Rheum.* 1997 May;40(5):842-8

[143] "...many cases of drug-induced lupus related to minocycline have been reported. Some of those reports included pulmonary lupus..." Christodoulou CS, Emmanuel P, Ray RA, Good RA, Schnapf BM, Cawkwell GD. Respiratory distress due to minocycline-induced pulmonary lupus. *Chest.* 1999 May;115(5):1471-3 http://www.chestjournal.org/cgi/content/full/115/5/1471

[144] Lawson TM, Amos N, Bulgen D, Williams BD.Minocycline-induced lupus: clinical features and response to rechallenge. *Rheumatology* (Oxford). 2001 Mar;40(3):329-35 http://rheumatology.oxfordjournals.org/cgi/content/full/40/3/329

[145] Gotschall E. Breaking the Vicious Cycle: Intestinal health though diet. Kirkton Press; Rev edition (August, 1994) http://www.scdiet.com/

[146] Cordain L: The Paleo Diet: Lose weight and get healthy by eating the food you were designed to eat. John Wiley & Sons Inc., New York 2002 http://thepaleodiet.com/

[147] Dostal C, Moszkorzova L, Musilova L, Lacinova Z, Marek J, Zvarova J. Serum prolactin stress values in patients with systemic lupus erythematosus. *Ann Rheum Dis.* 2003 May;62(5):487-8 http://ard.bmjjournals.com/cgi/content/full/62/5/487

[148] "RESULTS: A significantly higher rate of elevated PRL levels was found in SLE patients (40.0%) compared with the healthy controls (14.8%). No proof was found of association with the presence of anti-ds-DNA or with specific organ involvement. Similarly, elevated PRL levels were found in RA patients (39.3%)." Moszkorzova L, Lacinova Z, Marek J, Musilova L, Dohnalova A, Dostal C. Hyperprolactinaemia in patients with systemic lupus erythematosus. *Clin Exp Rheumatol.* 2002 Nov-Dec;20(6):807-12

[149] "CONCLUSION: Men with RA have high serum PRL levels and concentrations increase with longer disease evolution and worse functional stage." Mateo L, Nolla JM, Bonnin MR, Navarro MA, Roig-Escofet D. High serum prolactin levels in men with rheumatoid arthritis. *J Rheumatol.* 1998 Nov;25(11):2077-82

[150] "Male patients affected by RA showed high serum PRL levels. The serum PRL concentration was found to be increased in relation to the duration and the activity of the disease. Serum PRL levels do not seem to have any relationship with the BMD, at least in RA." Seriolo B, Ferretti V, Sulli A, Fasciolo D, Cutolo M. Serum prolactin concentrations in male patients with rheumatoid arthritis. *Ann N Y Acad Sci.* 2002 Jun;966:258-62

radiologic assessment (less necessary with favorable serum response).[151, see review 152]   Specific treatment options include the following:

- **Thyroid hormone**: Hypothyroidism frequently causes hyperprolactinemia which is reversible upon effective treatment of hypothyroidism. Obviously therefore, thyroid status should be evaluated in all patients with hyperprolactinemia. Thyroid assessment and treatment is reviewed later in this section.

- *Vitex astus-cagnus* and other supporting botanicals and nutrients: **Vitex lowers serum prolactin in humans**[153,154] **via a dopaminergic effect.**[155]   Vitex is considered safe for clinical use; mild and reversible adverse effects possibly associated with Vitex include nausea, headache, gastrointestinal disturbances, menstrual disorders, acne, pruritus and erythematous rash. No drug interactions are known, but given the herb's dopaminergic effect it should probably be used with some caution in patients treated with dopamine antagonists such as the so-called antipsychotic drugs (most of which do not work very well and/or carry intolerable adverse effects[156,157]). Bone[158] stated that daily doses can range from 500 mg to 2,000 mg DHE (dry herb equivalent) and can be tailored to the suppression of prolactin. Due at least in part to its content of L-dopa, *Mucuna pruriens* **shows clinical dopaminergic activity** as evidenced by its effectiveness in Parkinson's disease[159]; up to 15-30 gm/d of mucuna has been used clinically but doses will be dependent on preparation and phytoconcentration. **Triptolide and other extracts from *Tripterygium wilfordii* Hook F exert clinically significant anti-inflammatory action in patients with rheumatoid arthritis**[160,161] **and also offer protection to dopaminergic neurons.**[162,163] Ironically, even though tyrosine is the nutritional precursor to dopamine with evidence of clinical effectiveness (e.g., narcolepsy[164], enhancement of memory[165] and cognition[166]), **supplementation with tyrosine appears to actually increase rather than decrease prolactin levels[167]; therefore tyrosine should be used cautiously (if at all) in patients with systemic inflammation and elevated prolactin.**

[151] Beers MH, Berkow R (eds). The Merck Manual. Seventeenth Edition. Whitehouse Station; Merck Research Laboratories 1999 Page 77-78

[152] Serri O, Chik CL, Ur E, Ezzat S. Diagnosis and management of hyperprolactinemia. *CMAJ*. 2003 Sep 16;169(6):575-81 http://www.cmaj.ca/cgi/content/full/169/6/575

[153] "Since AC extracts were shown to have beneficial effects on premenstrual mastodynia serum prolactin levels in such patients were also studied in one double-blind, placebo-controlled clinical study. Serum prolactin levels were indeed reduced in the patients treated with the extract." Wuttke W, Jarry H, Christoffel V, Spengler B, Seidlova-Wuttke D. Chaste tree (Vitex agnus-castus)--pharmacology and clinical indications. *Phytomedicine*. 2003 May;10(4):348-57

[154] German abstract from Medline: "The prolactin release was reduced after 3 months, shortened luteal phases were normalised and deficits in the luteal progesterone synthesis were eliminated." Milewicz A, Gejdel E, Sworen H, Sienkiewicz K, Jedrzejak J, Teucher T, Schmitz H. [Vitex agnus castus extract in the treatment of luteal phase defects due to latent hyperprolactinemia. Results of a randomized placebo-controlled double-blind study] *Arzneimittelforschung*. 1993 Jul;43(7):752-6

[155] "Our results indicate a dopaminergic effect of Vitex agnus-castus extracts and suggest additional pharmacological actions via opioid receptors." Meier B, Berger D, Hoberg E, Sticher O, Schaffner W. Pharmacological activities of Vitex agnus-castus extracts in vitro. *Phytomedicine*. 2000 Oct;7(5):373-81

[156] "The majority of patients in each group discontinued their assigned treatment owing to inefficacy or intolerable side effects or for other reasons." Lieberman JA, Stroup TS, McEvoy JP, Swartz MS, Rosenheck RA, Perkins DO, Keefe RS, Davis SM, Davis CE, Lebowitz BD, Severe J, Hsiao JK; Clinical Antipsychotic Trials of Intervention Effectiveness (CATIE) Investigators. Effectiveness of antipsychotic drugs in patients with chronic schizophrenia. *N Engl J Med*. 2005 Sep 22;353(12):1209-23

[157] Whitaker R. The case against antipsychotic drugs: a 50-year record of doing more harm than good. *Med Hypotheses*. 2004;62(1):5-13

[158] "In conditions such as endometriosis and fibroids, for which a significant estrogen antagonist effect is needed, doses of at least 2 g/day DHE may be required and typically are used by professional herbalists." Bone K. New Insights Into Chaste Tree. *Nutritional Wellness* 2005 November http://www.nutritionalwellness.com/archives/2005/nov/11_bone.php

[159] "CONCLUSIONS: The rapid onset of action and longer on time without concomitant increase in dyskinesias on mucuna seed powder formulation suggest that this natural source of L-dopa might possess advantages over conventional L-dopa preparations in the long term management of PD." Katzenschlager R, Evans A, Manson A, Patsalos PN, Ratnaraj N, Watt H, Timmermann L, Van der Giessen R, Lees AJ. Mucuna pruriens in Parkinson's disease: a double blind clinical and pharmacological study. *J Neurol Neurosurg Psychiatry*. 2004 Dec;75(12):1672-7

[160] "The ethanol/ethyl acetate extract of TWHF shows therapeutic benefit in patients with treatment-refractory RA. At therapeutic dosages, the TWHF extract was well tolerated by most patients in this study." Tao X, Younger J, Fan FZ, Wang B, Lipsky PE. Benefit of an extract of Tripterygium Wilfordii Hook F in patients with rheumatoid arthritis: a double-blind, placebo-controlled study. *Arthritis Rheum*. 2002 Jul;46(7):1735-43

[161] "CONCLUSION: The EA extract of TWHF at dosages up to 570 mg/day appeared to be safe, and doses > 360 mg/day were associated with clinical benefit in patients with RA." Tao X, Cush JJ, Garret M, Lipsky PE. A phase I study of ethyl acetate extract of the chinese antirheumatic herb Tripterygium wilfordii hook F in rheumatoid arthritis. *J Rheumatol*. 2001 Oct;28(10):2160-7

[162] "Our data suggests that triptolide may protect dopaminergic neurons from LPS-induced injury and its efficiency in inhibiting microglia activation may underlie the mechanism." Li FQ, Lu XZ, Liang XB, Zhou HF, Xue B, Liu XY, Niu DB, Han JS, Wang XM. Triptolide, a Chinese herbal extract, protects dopaminergic neurons from inflammation-mediated damage through inhibition of microglial activation. *J Neuroimmunol*. 2004 Mar;148(1-2):24-31

[163] "Moreover, tripchlorolide markedly prevented the decrease in amount of dopamine in the striatum of model rats. Taken together, our data provide the first evidence that tripchlorolide acts as a neuroprotective molecule that rescues MPP+ or axotomy-induced degeneration of dopaminergic neurons, which may imply its therapeutic potential for Parkinson's disease." Li FQ, Cheng XX, Liang XB, Wang XH, Xue B, He QH, Wang XM, Han JS. Neurotrophic and neuroprotective effects of tripchlorolide, an extract of Chinese herb Tripterygium wilfordii Hook F, on dopaminergic neurons. *Exp Neurol*. 2003 Jan;179(1):28-37

[164] "Of twenty-eight visual analogue scales rating mood and arousal, the subjects' ratings in the tyrosine treatment (9 g daily) and placebo periods differed significantly for only three (less tired, less drowsy, more alert)." Elwes RD, Crewes H, Chesterman LP, Summers B, Jenner P, Binnie CD, Parkes JD. Treatment of narcolepsy with L-tyrosine: double-blind placebo-controlled trial. *Lancet*. 1989 Nov 4;2(8671):1067-9

[165] "Ten men and 10 women subjects underwent these batteries 1 h after ingesting 150 mg/kg of l-tyrosine or placebo. Administration of tyrosine significantly enhanced accuracy and decreased frequency of list retrieval on the working memory task during the multiple task battery compared with placebo." Thomas JR, Lockwood PA, Singh A, Deuster PA. Tyrosine improves working memory in a multitasking environment. *Pharmacol Biochem Behav*. 1999 Nov;64(3):495-500

[166] "Ten subjects received five daily doses of a protein-rich drink containing 2 g tyrosine, and 11 subjects received a carbohydrate rich drink with the same amount of calories (255 kcal)." Deijen JB, Wientjes CJ, Vullinghs HF, Cloin PA, Langefeld JJ. Tyrosine improves cognitive performance and reduces blood pressure in cadets after one week of a combat training course. *Brain Res Bull*. 1999 Jan 15;48(2):203-9

[167] "Tyrosine (when compared to placebo) had no effect on any sleep related measure, but it did stimulate prolactin release." Waters WF, Magill RA, Bray GA, Volaufova J, Smith SR, Lieberman HR, Rood J, Hurry M, Anderson T, Ryan DH. A comparison of tyrosine against placebo, phentermine, caffeine, and D-amphetamine during sleep deprivation. *Nutr Neurosci*. 2003;6(4):221-35

Furthermore, the finding that **high-protein meals stimulate prolactin release**[168] may partly explain the benefits of vegetarian diets in the treatment of systemic inflammation; since vegetarian diets are comparatively low in protein compared to omnivorous diets, they may lead to a relative reduction in prolactin production due to lack of stimulation.

- Bromocriptine: Bromocriptine has long been considered the pharmacologic treatment of choice for elevated prolactin.[169] Typical dose is 2.5 mg per day (effective against lupus[170]); gastrointestinal upset and sedation are common.[171] Clinical intervention with bromocriptine appears warranted in patients with RA, SLE, Reiter's syndrome, psoriatic arthritis, and probably multiple sclerosis and uveitis.[172]

- Cabergoline/Dostinex: Cabergoline/Dostinex is a newer dopamine agonist with few adverse effects; typical dose starts at 0.5 mg per week (0.25 mg twice per week).[173] Several studies have indicated that cabergoline is safer and more effective than bromocriptine for reducing prolactin levels[174] and the dose can often be reduced after successful prolactin reduction, allowing for reductions in cost and adverse effects.[175] Although fewer studies have been published supporting the antirheumatic benefits of cabergoline than bromocriptine, its antirheumatic benefits have been documented.[176]

o Estrogen (excess): **Men with rheumatoid arthritis show an excess of estradiol** and a decrease in DHEA, and the **excess estrogen is proportional to the degree of inflammation**.[177] Serum estradiol is commonly used to assess estrogen status; estrogens can also be measured in 24-hour urine samples. Beyond looking at estrogens from a *quantitative* standpoint, they can also be *qualitatively* analyzed with respect to the ratio of estrone:estradiol:estriol as well as the balance between the "good" 2-hydroxyestrone relative to the purportedly carcinogenic and proinflammatory 16-alpha-hydroxyestrone. Interventions to combat high estrogen levels may include any effective combination of the following:

- Weight loss and weight optimization: In overweight patients, *weight loss* is the means to attaining the goal of *weight optimization*; the task is not complete until the body mass index is normalized/optimized. Excess adiposity and obesity raise estrogen levels due to high levels of aromatase (the hormone that makes estrogens from androgens) in adipose tissue; weight optimization and loss of excess fat helps normalize hormone levels and reduce inflammation.

- Avoidance of ethanol: Estrogen production is stimulated by ethanol intake.

---

[168] "Whereas carbohydrate meals had no discernible effects, high protein meals induced a large increase in both PRL and cortisol; high fat meals caused selective release of PRL." Ishizuka B, Quigley ME, Yen SS. Pituitary hormone release in response to food ingestion: evidence for neuroendocrine signals from gut to brain. *J Clin Endocrinol Metab.* 1983 Dec;57(6):1111-6

[169] Beers MH, Berkow R (eds). The Merck Manual. Seventeenth Edition. Whitehouse Station; Merck Research Laboratories 1999 Page 77-78

[170] "A prospective, double-blind, randomized, placebo-controlled study compared BRC at a fixed daily dosage of 2.5 mg with placebo... Long term treatment with a low dose of BRC appears to be a safe and effective means of decreasing SLE flares in SLE patients." Alvarez-Nemegyei J, Cobarrubias-Cobos A, Escalante-Triay F, Sosa-Munoz J, Miranda JM, Jara LJ. Bromocriptine in systemic lupus erythematosus: a double-blind, randomized, placebo-controlled study. *Lupus.* 1998;7(6):414-9

[171] Serri O, Chik CL, Ur E, Ezzat S. Diagnosis and management of hyperprolactinemia. *CMAJ.* 2003 Sep 16;169(6):575-81 http://www.cmaj.ca/cgi/content/full/169/6/575

[172] "...clinical observations and trials support the use of bromocriptine as a nonstandard primary or adjunctive therapy in the treatment of recalcitrant RA, SLE, Reiter's syndrome, and psoriatic arthritis and associated conditions unresponsive to traditional approaches." McMurray RW. Bromocriptine in rheumatic and autoimmune diseases. *Semin Arthritis Rheum.* 2001 Aug;31(1):21-32

[173] Serri O, Chik CL, Ur E, Ezzat S. Diagnosis and management of hyperprolactinemia. *CMAJ.* 2003 Sep 16;169(6):575-81 http://www.cmaj.ca/cgi/content/full/169/6/575

[174] "CONCLUSION: These data indicate that cabergoline is a very effective agent for lowering the prolactin levels in hyperprolactinemic patients and that it appears to offer considerable advantage over bromocriptine in terms of efficacy and tolerability." Sabuncu T, Arikan E, Tasan E, Hatemi H. Comparison of the effects of cabergoline and bromocriptine on prolactin levels in hyperprolactinemic patients. *Intern Med.* 2001 Sep;40(9):857-61

[175] "Cabergoline also normalized PRL in the majority of patients with known bromocriptine intolerance or -resistance. Once PRL secretion was adequately controlled, the dose of cabergoline could often be significantly decreased, which further reduced costs of therapy." Verhelst J, Abs R, Maiter D, van den Bruel A, Vandeweghe M, Velkeniers B, Mockel J, Lamberigts G, Petrossians P, Coremans P, Mahler C, Stevenaert A, Verlooy J, Raftopoulos C, Beckers A. Cabergoline in the treatment of hyperprolactinemia: a study in 455 patients. *J Clin Endocrinol Metab.* 1999 Jul;84(7):2518-22 http://jcem.endojournals.org/cgi/content/full/84/7/2518

[176] Erb N, Pace AV, Delamere JP, Kitas GD. Control of unremitting rheumatoid arthritis by the prolactin antagonist cabergoline. *Rheumatology* (Oxford). 2001 Feb;40(2):237-9 http://rheumatology.oxfordjournals.org/cgi/content/full/40/2/237

[177] "RESULTS: DHEAS and estrone concentrations were lower and estradiol was higher in patients compared with healthy controls. DHEAS differed between RF positive and RF negative patients. Estrone did not correlate with any disease variable, whereas estradiol correlated strongly and positively with all measured indices of inflammation." Tengstrand B, Carlstrom K, Fellander-Tsai L, Hafstrom I. Abnormal levels of serum dehydroepiandrosterone, estrone, and estradiol in men with rheumatoid arthritis: high correlation between serum estradiol and current degree of inflammation. *J Rheumatol.* 2003 Nov;30(11):2338-43

- **Consider surgical correction of varicocele in affected men**: Men with varicocele have higher estrogen levels due to temperature-induced alterations in enzyme function in the testes; surgical correction of the varicocele lowers estrogen levels.
- **"Anti-estrogen diet"**: Foods and supplements such as green tea, diindolylmethane (DIM), indole-3-carbinol (I3C), licorice, and a high-fiber crucifer-based "anti-estrogenic diet" can also be used; monitoring clinical status and serum estradiol will prove or disprove efficacy. Whereas 16-alpha-hydroxyestrone is pro-inflammatory and immunodysregulatory, 2-hydroxyestrone has anti-inflammatory action[178] and been described as "the good estrogen"[179] due to its anticancer and comparatively health-preserving qualities. **In a recent short-term study using I3C in patients with SLE, I3C supplementation at 375 mg per day was well tolerated and resulted in modest treatment-dependent clinical improvement as well as favorable modification of estrogen metabolism away from 16-alpha-hydroxyestrone and toward 2-hydroxyestrone.[180]**
- **Anastrozole/Arimidex**: In our office, we commonly measure serum estradiol in men and administer the aromatase inhibitor anastrozole/arimidex 1 mg (2-3 doses per week) to men whose estradiol level is greater than 32 picogram/mL. The Life Extension Foundation[181] advocates that the optimal serum estradiol level for a man is 10-30 picogram/mL. Clinical studies using anastrozole/arimidex in men have shown that aromatase blockade lowers estradiol and raises testosterone[182]; generally speaking, this is exactly the result that we want in patients with severe systemic autoimmunity. Frequency of dosing is based on serum and clinical response.

- **Cortisol (insufficiency)**: Cortisol has immunoregulatory and "immunosuppressive" actions at physiological concentrations. Low adrenal function is common in patients with chronic inflammation.[183,184,185] Assessment of cortisol production and adrenal function was detailed in Chapter 4 under the section of Orthoendocrinology. Supplementation with 20 mg per day of cortisol/Cortef is physiologic; my preference is to dose 10 mg first thing in the morning, then 5 mg in late morning and 5 mg in midafternoon in an attempt to replicate the diurnal variation and normal morning peak of cortisol levels. In patients with hypoadrenalism, administration of pregnenolone in doses of 10-60 mg in the morning may also be beneficial.

- **Testosterone (insufficiency)**: Androgen deficiencies predispose to, are exacerbated by, and contribute to autoimmune/inflammatory disorders. **A large proportion of men with SLE or RA have low testosterone**[186,187] and suffer the effects of hypogonadism: fatigue, weakness, depression, slow healing, low libido, and difficulties with sexual performance. Testosterone levels may rise following DHEA supplementation (especially in women)

[178] "Micromolar concentrations of beta-estradiol, estrone, 16-alpha-hydroxyestrone and estriol enhance the oxidative metabolism of activated human PMNL's. The corresponding 2-hydroxylated estrogens 2-OH-estradiol, 2-OH-estrone and 2-OH-estriol act on the contrary as powerful inhibitors of cell activity." Jansson G. Oestrogen-induced enhancement of myeloperoxidase activity in human polymorphonuclear leukocytes--a possible cause of oxidative stress in inflammatory cells. *Free Radic Res Commun.* 1991;14(3):195-208

[179] "Even more dramatically, in the case of laryngeal papillomas induction of 2-hydroxylation with indole-3-carbinol (I3C) has resulted in inhibition of tumor growth during the time that the patients continue to take I3C or vegetables rich in this compound." Bradlow HL, Telang NT, Sepkovic DW, Osborne MP. 2-hydroxyestrone: the 'good' estrogen. *J Endocrinol.* 1996 Sep;150 Suppl:S259-65

[180] "Women with SLE can manifest a metabolic response to I3C and might benefit from its antiestrogenic effects." McAlindon TE, Gulin J, Chen T, Klug T, Lahita R, Nuite M. Indole-3-carbinol in women with SLE: effect on estrogen metabolism and disease activity. *Lupus.* 2001;10(11):779-83

[181] Male Hormone Modulation Therapy, Page 4 Of 7: http://www.lef.org/protocols/prtcl-130c.shtml Accessed October 30, 2005

[182] "These data demonstrate that aromatase inhibition increases serum bioavailable and total testosterone levels to the youthful normal range in older men with mild hypogonadism." Leder BZ, Rohrer JL, Rubin SD, Gallo J, Longcope C. Effects of aromatase inhibition in elderly men with low or borderline-low serum testosterone levels. *J Clin Endocrinol Metab.* 2004 Mar;89(3):1174-80 http://jcem.endojournals.org/cgi/reprint/89/3/1174

[183] "Yet evidence that patients with rheumatoid arthritis improved with small, physiologic dosages of cortisol or cortisone acetate was reported over 25 years ago, and that patients with chronic allergic disorders or unexplained chronic fatigue also improved with administration of such small dosages was reported over 15 years ago..." Jefferies WM. Mild adrenocortical deficiency, chronic allergies, autoimmune disorders and the chronic fatigue syndrome: a continuation of the cortisone story. *Med Hypotheses.* 1994 Mar;42(3):183-9 http://www.thebuteykocentre.com/Irish_%20Buteykocenter_files/further_studies/med_hyp2.pdf http://members.westnet.com.au/pkolb/med_hyp2.pdf

[184] "The etiology of rheumatoid arthritis ...explained by a combination of three factors: (i) a relatively mild deficiency of cortisol, ..., (ii) a deficiency of DHEA, ...and (iii) infection by organisms such as mycoplasma,..." Jefferies WM. The etiology of rheumatoid arthritis. *Med Hypotheses.* 1998 Aug;51(2):111-4

[185] Jefferies W McK. Safe Uses of Cortisol. Second Edition. Springfield, CC Thomas, 1996

[186] Karagiannis A, Harsoulis F. Gonadal dysfunction in systemic diseases. *Eur J Endocrinol.* 2005 Apr;152(4):501-13 http://www.eje-online.org/cgi/content/full/152/4/501

[187] "Using analysis of covariance, patients with rheumatoid arthritis showed significantly lower serum testosterone (p less than 0.05) and derived free testosterone (p less than 0.01) concentrations and significantly higher serum LH and FSH concentrations (p less than 0.05) compared with controls." Gordon D, Beastall GH, Thomson JA, Sturrock RD. Androgenic status and sexual function in males with rheumatoid arthritis and ankylosing spondylitis. *Q J Med.* 1986 Jul;60(231):671-9

and can be elevated in men by the use of anastrozole/arimidex. Otherwise, transdermal testosterone such as Androgel or Testim can be applied as indicated.

- o <u>DHEA (insufficiency / supraphysiologic supplementation)</u>: DHEA is an anti-inflammatory and immunoregulatory hormone that is commonly deficient in patients with autoimmunity and inflammatory arthritis.[188] DHEA levels are suppressed by prednisone[189], and DHEA supplementation has been shown to reverse the osteoporosis and loss of bone mass induced by corticosteroid treatment.[190] DHEA shows no acute or subacute toxicity even when used in supraphysiologic doses, even when used in sick patients. For example, in a study of 32 patients with HIV, DHEA doses of 750 mg – 2,250 mg per day were well-tolerated and produced no dose-limiting adverse effects.[191] This lack of toxicity compares favorably with any and all so-called "antirheumatic" drugs, nearly all of which show impressive comparable toxicity. When used at doses of 200 mg per day, DHEA safely provides clinical benefit for patients with various autoimmune diseases, including ulcerative colitis, Crohn's disease[192], and SLE.[193] In patients with SLE, DHEA supplementation allows for reduced dosing of prednisone (thus avoiding its adverse effects) while providing symptomatic improvement.[194] Optimal clinical response appears to correlate with serum levels that are supraphysiologic[195], and therefore treatment may be implemented with little regard for initial/baseline DHEA levels provided that the patient is free of contraindications, particularly high risk for sex-hormone-dependent malignancy. Other than mild adverse effects predictable with any androgen (namely voice deepening, transient acne, and increased facial hair), DHEA supplementation does not cause serious adverse effects[196], and it is appropriate for routine clinical use particularly when 1) the dose of DHEA is kept as low as possible, 2) duration is kept as short as possible, 3) other interventions are used to address the underlying cause of the disease, 4) the patient is deriving benefit, and 5) the risk-to-benefit ratio is favorable.

- o <u>Thyroid (insufficiency or autoimmunity)</u>: Overt or imminent hypothyroidism is suggested by TSH greater than 2 mU/L[197] or 3 mU/L[198], low T4 or T3, and/or the presence of anti-thyroid peroxidase antibodies.[199] Hypothyroidism can cause an inflammatory myopathy that can resemble polymyositis, and hypothyroidism is a frequent complication of any and all autoimmune diseases. Specific treatment considerations include the following:

[188] "DHEAS concentrations were significantly decreased in both women and men with inflammatory arthritis (IA) (P < 0.001)." Dessein PH, Joffe BI, Stanwix AE, Moomal Z. Hyposecretion of the adrenal androgen dehydroepiandrosterone sulfate and its relation to clinical variables in inflammatory arthritis. *Arthritis Res.* 2001;3(3):183-8. Epub 2001 Feb 21. http://arthritis-research.com/content/3/3/183

[189] "Basal serum DHEA and DHEAS concentrations were suppressed to a greater degree than was cortisol during both daily and alternate day prednisone treatments. ...Thus, adrenal androgen secretion was more easily suppressed than was cortisol secretion by this low dose of glucocorticoid, but there was no advantage to alternate day therapy." Rittmaster RS, Givner ML. Effect of daily and alternate day low dose prednisone on serum cortisol and adrenal androgens in hirsute women. *J Clin Endocrinol Metab.* 1988 Aug;67(2):400-3

[190] "CONCLUSION: Prasterone treatment prevented BMD loss and significantly increased BMD at both the lumbar spine and total hip in female patients with SLE receiving exogenous glucocorticoids." Mease PJ, Ginzler EM, Gluck OS, Schiff M, Goldman A, Greenwald M, Cohen S, Egan R, Quarles BJ, Schwartz KE. Effects of prasterone on bone mineral density in women with systemic lupus erythematosus receiving chronic glucocorticoid therapy. *J Rheumatol.* 2005 Apr;32(4):616-21

[191] "Thirty-one subjects were evaluated and monitored for safety and tolerance. The oral drug was administered three times daily in doses ranging from 750 mg/day to 2,250 mg/day for 16 weeks. ... The drug was well tolerated and no dose-limiting side effects were noted." Dyner TS, Lang W, Geaga J, Golub A, Stites D, Winger E, Galmarini M, Masterson J, Jacobson MA. An open-label dose-escalation trial of oral dehydroepiandrosterone tolerance and pharmacokinetics in patients with HIV disease. *J Acquir Immune Defic Syndr.* 1993 May;6(5):459-65

[192] "CONCLUSIONS: In a pilot study, dehydroepiandrosterone was effective and safe in patients with refractory Crohn's disease or ulcerative colitis." Andus T, Klebl F, Rogler G, Bregenzer N, Scholmerich J, Straub RH. Patients with refractory Crohn's disease or ulcerative colitis respond to dehydroepiandrosterone: a pilot study. *Aliment Pharmacol Ther.* 2003 Feb;17(3):409-14

[193] "CONCLUSION: The overall results confirm that DHEA treatment was well-tolerated, significantly reduced the number of SLE flares, and improved patient's global assessment of disease activity." Chang DM, Lan JL, Lin HY, Luo SF. Dehydroepiandrosterone treatment of women with mild-to-moderate systemic lupus erythematosus: a multicenter randomized, double-blind, placebo-controlled trial. *Arthritis Rheum.* 2002 Nov;46(11):2924-7

[194] "CONCLUSION: Among women with lupus disease activity, reducing the dosage of prednisone to < or = 7.5 mg/day for a sustained period of time while maintaining stabilization or a reduction of disease activity was possible in a significantly greater proportion of patients treated with oral prasterone, 200 mg once daily, compared with patients treated with placebo." Petri MA, Lahita RG, Van Vollenhoven RF, Merrill JT, Schiff M, Ginzler EM, Strand V, Kunz A, Gorelick KJ, Schwartz KE; GL601 Study Group. Effects of prasterone on corticosteroid requirements of women with systemic lupus erythematosus: a double-blind, randomized, placebo-controlled trial. *Arthritis Rheum.* 2002 Jul;46(7):1820-9

[195] "CONCLUSION: The clinical response to DHEA was not clearly dose dependent. Serum levels of DHEA and DHEAS correlated only weakly with lupus outcomes, but suggested an optimum serum DHEAS of 1000 microg/dL." Barry NN, McGuire JL, van Vollenhoven RF. Dehydroepiandrosterone in systemic lupus erythematosus: relationship between dosage, serum levels, and clinical response. *J Rheumatol.* 1998 Dec;25(12):2352-6

[196] Tierney ML. McPhee SJ, Papadakis MA. Current Medical Diagnosis and Treatment 2006. 45th edition. New York; Lange Medical Books: 2006, page 1721

[197] Weetman AP. Hypothyroidism: screening and subclinical disease. *BMJ.* 1997 Apr 19;314(7088):1175-8 http://bmj.bmjjournals.com/cgi/content/full/314/7088/1175

[198] "Now AACE encourages doctors to consider treatment for patients who test outside the boundaries of a narrower margin based on a target TSH level of 0.3 to 3.0. AACE believes the new range will result in proper diagnosis for millions of Americans who suffer from a mild thyroid disorder, but have gone untreated until now." American Association of Clinical Endocrinologists (AACE). 2003 Campaign Encourages Awareness of Mild Thyroid Failure, Importance of Routine Testing http://www.aace.com/pub/tam2003/press.php November 26, 2005

[199] Beers MH, Berkow R (eds). The Merck Manual. Seventeenth Edition. Whitehouse Station; Merck Research Laboratories 1999 Page 96

- **Selenium**: Supplementation with either selenomethonine[200] or sodium selenite[201,202] can reduce thyroid autoimmunity and improve peripheral conversion of T4 to T3. Selenium may be started at 500-800 mcg per day and tapered to 200-400 mcg per day for maintenance.[203]
- **L-thyroxine/levothyroxine/Synthroid—prescription synthetic T4**: 25-50 mcg per day is a common starting dose which can be adjusted based on clinical and laboratory response. Thyroid hormone supplements must be consumed separately from soy products (by at least 1-2 hours) and preferably on an empty stomach to avoid absorption interference by food, fiber, and minerals, especially calcium. Doses are generally started at one-half of the daily dose for the first 10 days after which the full dose is used. Caution must be applied in patients with adrenal insufficiency and/or those with cardiovascular disease.
- **Armour thyroid—prescription natural T4 and T3 from cow/pig thyroid gland**: 60 mg (one grain) is a common starting and maintenance dose. Due to the exacerbating effect on thyroid autoimmunity, Armour thyroid is never used in patients with thyroid autoimmunity.
- **Thyrolar/Liotrix—prescription synthetic T4 with T3**: Dosed as "1" (low), "2" (intermediate), or "3" (high). Although this product has been difficult to obtain for the past few years due to manufacturing problems (http://thyrolar.com/), it has been my treatment of choice due to the combination of T4 and T3 and the lack of antigenicity compared to gland-derived products.
- **Thyroid glandular—nonprescription T3**: Producers of nutritional products are able to distribute T3 because it is not listed by the FDA as a prescription item. Nutritional supplement companies may start with Armour thyroid, remove the T4, and sell the thyroid glandular with active T3 thereby providing a nonprescription source of active thyroid hormone. For many patients, one tablet per day is at least as effective as a prescription source of thyroid hormone. Since it is derived from a glandular and therefore potentially antigenic source, thyroid glandular is not used in patients with thyroid autoimmunity due to its ability to induce increased production of anti-thyroid antibodies.
- **L-tyrosine and iodine**: Some patients with mild hypothyroidism respond to supplementation with L-tyrosine and iodine. Tyrosine is commonly used in doses of 4-9 grams per day in divided doses. According to Abraham and Wright[204], doses of iodine may be as high as 12.5 milligrams (12,500 micrograms), which is slightly less than the average daily intake in Japan at 13.8 mg per day.

- Oral enzyme therapy with proteolytic/pancreatic enzymes: Polyenzyme supplementation is used to ameliorate the pathophysiology induced by immune complexes, such as rheumatoid arthritis.[205]
- *Uncaria tomentosa, Uncaria guianensis*: Cat's claw has been safely and successfully used in the treatment of osteoarthritis[206] and **rheumatoid arthritis**.[207] High-quality extractions from reputable manufacturers used according to directions are recommended. Most products contain between

[200] Duntas LH, Mantzou E, Koutras DA. Effects of a six month treatment with selenomethionine in patients with autoimmune thyroiditis. *Eur J Endocrinol*. 2003 Apr;148(4):389-93 http://eje-online.org/cgi/reprint/148/4/389
[201] Gartner R, Gasnier BC, Dietrich JW, Krebs B, Angstwurm MW. Selenium supplementation in patients with autoimmune thyroiditis decreases thyroid peroxidase antibodies concentrations. *J Clin Endocrinol Metab*. 2002 Apr;87(4):1687-91 http://jcem.endojournals.org/cgi/content/full/87/4/1687
[202] "We recently conducted a prospective, placebo-controlled clinical study, where we could demonstrate, that a substitution of 200 wg sodium selenite for three months in patients with autoimmune thyroiditis reduced thyroid peroxidase antibody (TPO-Ab) concentrations significantly." Gartner R, Gasnier BC. Selenium in the treatment of autoimmune thyroiditis. *Biofactors*. 2003;19(3-4):165-70
[203] Bruns F, Micke O, Bremer M. Current status of selenium and other treatments for secondary lymphedema. *J Support Oncol*. 2003 Jul-Aug;1(2):121-30 http://www.supportiveoncology.net/journal/articles/0102121.pdf
[204] Wright JV. Why you need 83 times more of this essential, cancer-fighting nutrient than the "experts" say you do. *Nutrition and Healing* 2005; volume 12, issue 4.
[205] Galebskaya LV, Ryumina EV, Niemerovsky VS, Matyukov AA. Human complement system state after wobenzyme intake. *VESTNIK MOSKOVSKOGO UNIVERSITETA. KHIMIYA*. 2000. Vol. 41, No. 6. Supplement. Pages 148-149
[206] Piscoya J, Rodriguez Z, Bustamante SA, Okuhama NN, Miller MJ, Sandoval M.Efficacy and safety of freeze-dried cat's claw in osteoarthritis of the knee: mechanisms of action of the species Uncaria guianensis. *Inflamm Res*. 2001 Sep;50(9):442-8
[207] "This small preliminary study demonstrates relative safety and modest benefit to the tender joint count of a highly purified extract from the pentacyclic chemotype of UT in patients with active RA taking sulfasalazine or hydroxychloroquine." Mur E, Hartig F, Eibl G, Schirmer M. Randomized double blind trial of an extract from the pentacyclic alkaloid-chemotype of uncaria tomentosa for the treatment of rheumatoid arthritis. *J Rheumatol*. 2002 Apr;29(4):678-81

250-500 mg and are standardized to 3.0% alkaloids and 15% total polyphenols; QD-TID po dosing should be sufficient as *part* of a comprehensive plan.

- *Harpagophytum procumbens*: Harpagophytum is a moderately effective botanical analgesic.[208,209,210,211,212] Products are generally standardized for the content of harpagosides, with a target dose of 60 mg harpagoside per day when used in isolation.[213]

- Willow bark: Extracts from willow bark have proven safe and effective in the alleviation of moderate/severe low-back pain.[214,215] The mechanism of action appears to be inhibition of prostaglandin formation via inhibition of cyclooxygenase-2 gene transcription[216] by salicylates, phytonutrients which are widely present in fruits, vegetables, herbs and spices and which are partly responsible for the anti-cancer, anti-inflammatory, and health-promoting benefits of plant consumption.[217,218] According to a letter by Vasquez and Muanza[219], the only adverse effect that has been documented in association with willow bark was a single case of anaphylaxis in a patient previously sensitized to acetylsalicylic acid.

- *Boswellia serrata*: *Boswellia* shows clear anti-inflammatory and analgesic action via inhibition of 5-lipoxygenase[220] and clinical benefits have been demonstrated in patients with osteoarthritis of the knees[221] as well as asthma[222] and ulcerative colitis.[223] Products are generally standardized to contain 37.5–65% boswellic acids, with a target dose is approximately 150 mg of boswellic acids TID; dose and number of capsules/tablets will vary depending upon the concentration found in differing products. A German study showing that *Boswellia* was ineffective for rheumatoid arthritis[224] was poorly conducted, with inadequate follow-up, inadequate controls, and abnormal dosing of the herb.

- Topical *Capsicum annuum, Capsicum frutescens* (Cayenne pepper, hot chili pepper): Controlled clinical trials have conclusively demonstrated capsaicin's ability to deplete sensory fibers of the neuropeptide **substance P** and to thus reduce pain. Topical capsaicin has been proven effective in relieving the pain associated with diabetic neuropathy[225], chronic low back pain[226], chronic neck pain[227], osteoarthritis[228], and **rheumatoid arthritis.**[229] Given the important role of neurogenic inflammation in chronic arthritis[230,231], **the use of topical *Capsicum* should not be viewed as merely symptomatic; by depleting neurons of substance P it has the ability to help break the vicious cycle of neurogenic-immunogenic inflammation.**

[208] Chrubasik S, Thanner J, Kunzel O, Conradt C, Black A, Pollak S. Comparison of outcome measures during treatment with the proprietary Harpagophytum extract doloteffin in patients with pain in the lower back, knee or hip. *Phytomedicine* 2002 Apr;9(3):181-94

[209] Chantre P, Cappelaere A, Leblan D, Guedon D, Vandermander J, Fournie B. Efficacy and tolerance of Harpagophytum procumbens versus diacerhein in treatment of osteoarthritis. *Phytomedicine* 2000 Jun;7(3):177-83

[210] Leblan D, Chantre P, Fournie B. Harpagophytum procumbens in the treatment of knee and hip osteoarthritis. Four-month results of a prospective, multicenter, double-blind trial versus diacerhein. *Joint Bone Spine* 2000;67(5):462-7

[211] "...subgroup analyses suggested that the effect was confined to patients with more severe and radiating pain accompanied by neurological deficit. ...a slightly different picture, with the benefits seeming, if anything, to be greatest in the H600 group and in patients without more severe pain, radiation or neurological deficit." Chrubasik S, Junck H, Breitschwerdt H, Conradt C, Zappe H. Effectiveness of Harpagophytum extract WS 1531 in the treatment of exacerbation of low back pain: a randomized, placebo-controlled, double-blind study. *Eur J Anaesthesiol* 1999 Feb;16(2):118-29

[212] Chrubasik S, Model A, Black A, Pollak S. A randomized double-blind pilot study comparing Doloteffin and Vioxx in the treatment of low back pain. *Rheumatology* (Oxford). 2003 Jan;42(1):141-8

[213] "They took an 8-week course of Doloteffin at a dose providing 60 mg harpagoside per day.... Doloteffin is well worth considering for osteoarthritic knee and hip pain and nonspecific low back pain." Chrubasik S, Thanner J, Kunzel O, Conradt C, Black A, Pollak S. Comparison of outcome measures during treatment with the proprietary Harpagophytum extract doloteffin in patients with pain in the lower back, knee or hip. *Phytomedicine* 2002 Apr;9(3):181-94

[214] Chrubasik S, Eisenberg E, Balan E, Weinberger T, Luzzati R, Conradt C. Treatment of low-back pain exacerbations with willow bark extract: a randomized double-blind study. *Am J Med*. 2000;109:9-14

[215] Chrubasik S, Kunzel O, Model A, Conradt C, Black A. Treatment of low-back pain with a herbal or synthetic anti-rheumatic: a randomized controlled study. Willow bark extract for low-back pain. *Rheumatology* (Oxford). 2001;40:1388-93

[216] Hare LG, Woodside JV, Young IS. Dietary salicylates. *J Clin Pathol* 2003 Sep;56(9):649-50

[217] Lawrence JR, Peter R, Baxter GJ, Robson J, Graham AB, Paterson JR. Urinary excretion of salicyluric and salicylic acids by non-vegetarians, vegetarians, and patients taking low dose aspirin. *J Clin Pathol*. 2003 Sep;56(9):651-3

[218] Paterson JR, Lawrence JR. Salicylic acid: a link between aspirin, diet and the prevention of colorectal cancer. *QJM*. 2001 Aug;94(8):445-8

[219] Vasquez A, Muanza DN. Evaluation of Presence of Aspirin-Related Warnings with Willow Bark: Comment on the Article by Clauson et al. *Ann Pharmacotherapy* 2005 Oct;39(10):1763

[220] Wildfeuer A, Neu IS, Safayhi H, Metzger G, Wehrmann M, Vogel U, Ammon HP. Effects of boswellic acids extracted from a herbal medicine on the biosynthesis of leukotrienes and the course of experimental autoimmune encephalomyelitis. *Arzneimittelforschung* 1998 Jun;48(6):668-74

[221] Kimmatkar N, Thawani V, Hingorani L, Khiyani R. Efficacy and tolerability of Boswellia serrata extract in treatment of osteoarthritis of knee--a randomized double blind placebo controlled trial. *Phytomedicine*. 2003 Jan;10(1):3-7

[222] Gupta I, Gupta V, Parihar A, Gupta S, Ludtke R, Safayhi H, Ammon HP. Effects of Boswellia serrata gum resin in patients with bronchial asthma: results of a double-blind, placebo-controlled, 6-week clinical study. *Eur J Med Res*. 1998 Nov 17;3(11):511-4

[223] Gupta I, Parihar A, Malhotra P, Singh GB, Ludtke R, Safayhi H, Ammon HP. Effects of Boswellia serrata gum resin in patients with ulcerative colitis. *Eur J Med Res*. 1997 Jan;2(1):37-43

[224] Sander O, Herborn G, Rau R. [Is H15 (resin extract of Boswellia serrata, "incense") a useful supplement to established drug therapy of chronic polyarthritis? Results of a double-blind pilot study] [Article in German] *Z Rheumatol*. 1998 Feb;57(1):11-6

[225] Treatment of painful diabetic neuropathy with topical capsaicin. A multicenter, double-blind, vehicle-controlled study. The Capsaicin Study Group. [No authors listed] *Arch Intern Med*. 1991 Nov;151(11):2225-9

[226] Keitel W, Frerick H, Kuhn U, Schmidt U, Kuhlmann M, Bredehorst A. Capsicum pain plaster in chronic non-specific low back pain. *Arzneimittelforschung*. 2001 Nov;51(11):896-903

[227] Mathias BJ, Dillingham TR, Zeigler DN, Chang AS, Belandres PV. Topical capsaicin for chronic neck pain. A pilot study. *Am J Phys Med Rehabil* 1995 Jan-Feb;74(1):39-44

[228] McCarthy GM, McCarty DJ. Effect of topical capsaicin in the therapy of painful osteoarthritis of the hands. *J Rheumatol*. 1992;19(4):604-7

[229] Deal CL, Schnitzer TJ, Lipstein E, Seibold JR, Stevens RM, Levy MD, Albert D, Renold F. Treatment of arthritis with topical capsaicin: a double-blind trial. *Clin Ther*. 1991 May-Jun;13(3):383-95

[230] Gouze-Decaris E, Philippe L, Minn A, Haouzi P, Gillet P, Netter P, Terlain B. Neurophysiological basis for neurogenic-mediated articular cartilage anabolism alteration. *Am J Physiol Regul Integr Comp Physiol*. 2001;280(1):R115-22 http://ajpregu.physiology.org/cgi/content/full/280/1/R115

[231] Decaris E, Guingamp C, Chat M, Philippe L, Grillasca JP, Abid A, Minn A, Gillet P, Netter P, Terlain B. Evidence for neurogenic transmission inducing degenerative cartilage damage distant from local inflammation. *Arthritis Rheum*. 1999;42(9):1951-60

- Phytonutritional modulation of NF-kappaB: As a stimulator of pro-inflammatory gene transcription, NF-kappaB is almost universally activated in conditions associated with inflammation.[232,233] As we would expect, **NF-kappaB plays a central role in the pathogenesis of synovitis and joint destruction seen in RA.**[234] Nutrients and botanicals which either directly or indirectly inhibit NF-kappaB for an anti-inflammatory benefit include vitamin D[235,236], curcumin[237] (requires piperine for absorption[238]), lipoic acid[239], green tea[240], rosemary[241], grape seed extract[242], propolis[243], zinc[244], high-dose selenium[245], indole-3-carbinol[246,247], N-acetyl-L-cysteine[248], resveratrol[249,250], isohumulones[251], GLA via PPAR-gamma[252] and EPA via PPAR-alpha.[253] I have reviewed the phytonutritional modulation of NF-kappaB later in this text and elsewhere.[254] Several phytonutritional products targeting NF-kappaB are available.
- Glucosamine sulfate and chondroitin sulfate: Glucosamine and chondroitin sulfates are well tolerated and well documented in the treatment of osteoarthritis.[255,256,257,258] Since these serve as substrate for the "rebuilding" and preservation of joint cartilage, they would clearly help shift the balance toward anabolism and away from catabolism within articular tissues.
- Creative self-expression and therapeutic writing: Limited evidence indicates that self-expressive writing can significantly reduce symptomatology in patients with RA.[259]

---

[232] Tak PP, Firestein GS. NF-kappaB: a key role in inflammatory diseases. *J Clin Invest.* 2001 Jan;107(1):7-11 http://www.jci.org/cgi/content/full/107/1/7

[233] D'Acquisto F, May MJ, Ghosh S. Inhibition of Nuclear Factor KappaB (NF-B): An Emerging Theme in Anti-Inflammatory Therapies. *Mol Interv.* 2002 Feb;2(1):22-35 http://molinterv.aspetjournals.org/cgi/content/abstract/2/1/22

[234] "NF-B plays a central role in the pathogenesis of synovitis in RA and PsA." Foell D, Kane D, Bresnihan B, Vogl T, Nacken W, Sorg C, Fitzgerald O, Roth J. Expression of the pro-inflammatory protein S100A12 (EN-RAGE) in rheumatoid and psoriatic arthritis. *Rheumatology* (Oxford). 2003 Nov;42(11):1383-9 http://rheumatology.oxfordjournals.org/cgi/content/full/42/11/1383

[235] "1Alpha,25-dihydroxyvitamin D3 (1,25-(OH)2-D3), the active metabolite of vitamin D, can inhibit NF-kappaB activity in human MRC-5 fibroblasts, targeting DNA binding of NF-kappaB but not translocation of its subunits p50 and p65." Harant H, Wolff B, Lindley IJ. 1Alpha,25-dihydroxyvitamin D3 decreases DNA binding of nuclear factor-kappaB in human fibroblasts. *FEBS Lett.* 1998 Oct 9;436(3):329-34

[236] "Thus, $1,25(OH)_2D_3$ may negatively regulate IL-12 production by downregulation of NF-kB activation and binding to the p40-kB sequence." D'Ambrosio D, Cippitelli M, Cocciolo MG, Mazzeo D, Di Lucia P, Lang R, Sinigaglia F, Panina-Bordignon P. Inhibition of IL-12 production by 1,25-dihydroxyvitamin D3. Involvement of NF-kappaB downregulation in transcriptional repression of the p40 gene. *J Clin Invest.* 1998 Jan 1;101(1):252-62

[237] "Curcumin, EGCG and resveratrol have been shown to suppress activation of NF-kappa B." Surh YJ, Chun KS, Cha HH, Han SS, Keum YS, Park KK, Lee SS. Molecular mechanisms underlying chemopreventive activities of anti-inflammatory phytochemicals: down-regulation of COX-2 and iNOS through suppression of NF-kappa B activation. *Mutat Res.* 2001 Sep 1;480-481:243-68

[238] Shoba G, Joy D, Joseph T, Majeed M, Rajendran R, Srinivas PS. Influence of piperine on the pharmacokinetics of curcumin in animals and human volunteers. *Planta Med.* 1998 May;64(4):353-6

[239] "ALA reduced the TNF-alpha-stimulated ICAM-1 expression in a dose-dependent manner, to levels observed in unstimulated cells. Alpha-lipoic acid also reduced NF-kappaB activity in these cells in a dose-dependent manner." Lee HA, Hughes DA.Alpha-lipoic acid modulates NF-kappaB activity in human monocytic cells by direct interaction with DNA. *Exp Gerontol.* 2002 Jan-Mar;37(2-3):401-10

[240] "In conclusion, EGCG is an effective inhibitor of IKK activity. This may explain, at least in part, some of the reported anti-inflammatory and anticancer effects of green tea." Yang F, Oz HS, Barve S, de Villiers WJ, McClain CJ, Varilek GW. The green tea polyphenol (-)-epigallocatechin-3-gallate blocks nuclear factor-kappa B activation by inhibiting I kappa B kinase activity in the intestinal epithelial cell line IEC-6. *Mol Pharmacol.* 2001 Sep;60(3):528-33

[241] "These results suggest that carnosol suppresses the NO production and iNOS gene expression by inhibiting NF-kappaB activation, and provide possible mechanisms for its anti-inflammatory and chemopreventive action." Lo AH, Liang YC, Lin-Shiau SY, Ho CT, Lin JK. Carnosol, an antioxidant in rosemary, suppresses inducible nitric oxide synthase through down-regulating nuclear factor-kappaB in mouse macrophages. *Carcinogenesis.* 2002 Jun;23(6):983-91

[242] "Constitutive and TNFalpha-induced NF-kappaB DNA binding activity was inhibited by GSE at doses > or =50 microg/ml and treatments for > or =12 h." Dhanalakshmi S, Agarwal R, Agarwal C. Inhibition of NF-kappaB pathway in grape seed extract-induced apoptotic death of human prostate carcinoma DU145 cells. *Int J Oncol.* 2003 Sep;23(3):721-7

[243] "Caffeic acid phenethyl ester (CAPE) is an anti-inflammatory component of propolis (honeybee resin). CAPE is reportedly a specific inhibitor of nuclear factor-kappaB (NF-kappaB)." Fitzpatrick LR, Wang J, Le T. Caffeic acid phenethyl ester, an inhibitor of nuclear factor-kappaB, attenuates bacterial peptidoglycan polysaccharide-induced colitis in rats. *J Pharmacol Exp Ther.* 2001 Dec;299(3):915-20

[244] "Our results suggest that zinc supplementation may lead to downregulation of the inflammatory cytokines through upregulation of the negative feedback loop A20 to inhibit induced NF-kappaB activation." Prasad AS, Bao B, Beck FW, Kucuk O, Sarkar FH. Antioxidant effect of zinc in humans. *Free Radic Biol Med.* 2004 Oct 15;37(8):1182-90

[245] Note that the patients in this study received a very high dose of selenium: 960 micrograms per day. This is at the top—and some would say over the top—of the safe and reasonable dose for long-term supplementation. In this case, the study lasted for three months. "In patients receiving selenium supplementation, selenium NF-kappaB activity was significantly reduced, reaching the same level as the nondiabetic control group. CONCLUSION: In type 2 diabetic patients, activation of NF-kappaB measured in peripheral blood monocytes can be reduced by selenium supplementation, confirming its importance in the prevention of cardiovascular diseases." Faure P, Ramon O, Favier A, Halimi S. Selenium supplementation decreases nuclear factor-kappa B activity in peripheral blood mononuclear cells from type 2 diabetic patients. *Eur J Clin Invest.* 2004 Jul;34(7):475-81

[246] Takada Y, Andreeff M, Aggarwal BB. Indole-3-carbinol suppresses NF-{kappa}B and I{kappa}B{alpha} kinase activation causing inhibition of expression of NF-{kappa}B-regulated antiapoptotic and metastatic gene products and enhancement of apoptosis in myeloid and leukemia cells. *Blood.* 2005 Apr 5; [Epub ahead of print]

[247] "Overall, our results indicated that indole-3-carbinol inhibits NF-kappaB and NF-kappaB-regulated gene expression and that this mechanism may provide the molecular basis for its ability to suppress tumorigenesis." Takada Y, Andreeff M, Aggarwal BB. Indole-3-carbinol suppresses NF-kappaB and IkappaBalpha kinase activation, causing inhibition of expression of NF-kappaB-regulated antiapoptotic and metastatic gene products and enhancement of apoptosis in myeloid and leukemia cells. *Blood.* 2005 Jul 15;106(2):641-9. Epub 2005 Apr 5.

[248] "CONCLUSIONS: Administration of N-acetylcysteine results in decreased nuclear factor-kappa B activation in patients with sepsis, associated with decreases in interleukin-8 but not interleukin-6 or soluble intercellular adhesion molecule-1. These pilot data suggest that antioxidant therapy with N-acetylcysteine may be useful in blunting the inflammatory response to sepsis." Paterson RL, Galley HF, Webster NR. The effect of N-acetylcysteine on nuclear factor-kappa B activation, interleukin-6, interleukin-8, and intercellular adhesion molecule-1 expression in patients with sepsis. *Crit Care Med.* 2003 Nov;31(11):2574-8

[249] "Resveratrol's anticarcinogenic, anti-inflammatory, and growth-modulatory effects may thus be partially ascribed to the inhibition of activation of NF-kappaB and AP-1 and the associated kinases." Manna SK, Mukhopadhyay A, Aggarwal BB. Resveratrol suppresses TNF-induced activation of nuclear transcription factors NF-kappa B, activator protein-1, and apoptosis: potential role of reactive oxygen intermediates and lipid peroxidation. *J Immunol.* 2000 Jun 15;164(12):6509-19

[250] "Both resveratrol and quercetin inhibited NF-kappaB-, AP-1- and CREB-dependent transcription to a greater extent than the glucocorticosteroid, dexamethasone." Donnelly LE, Newton R, Kennedy GE, Fenwick PS, Leung RH, Ito K, Russell RE, Barnes PJ.Anti-inflammatory Effects of Resveratrol in Lung Epithelial Cells: Molecular Mechanisms. *Am J Physiol Lung Cell Mol Physiol.* 2004 Jun 4 [Epub ahead of print]

[251] Yajima H, Ikeshima E, Shiraki M, Kanaya T, Fujiwara D, Odai H, Tsuboyama-Kasaoka N, Ezaki O, Oikawa S, Kondo K. Isohumulones, bitter acids derived from hops, activate both peroxisome proliferator-activated receptor alpha and gamma and reduce insulin resistance. *J Biol Chem.* 2004 Aug 6;279(32):33456-62. Epub 2004 Jun 3. http://www.jbc.org/cgi/content/full/279/32/33456

[252] "Thus, PPAR gamma serves as the receptor for GLA in the regulation of gene expression in breast cancer cells. " Jiang WG, Redfern A, Bryce RP, Mansel RE. Peroxisome proliferator activated receptor-gamma (PPAR-gamma) mediates the action of gamma linolenic acid in breast cancer cells. *Prostaglandins Leukot Essent Fatty Acids.* 2000 Feb;62(2):119-27

[253] "...EPA requires PPARalpha for its inhibitory effects on NF-kappaB." Mishra A, Chaudhary A, Sethi S. Oxidized omega-3 fatty acids inhibit NF-kappaB activation via a PPARalpha-dependent pathway. *Arterioscler Thromb Vasc Biol.* 2004 Sep;24(9):1621-7. Epub 2004 Jul 1. http://atvb.ahajournals.org/cgi/content/full/24/9/1621

[254] "Indeed, the previous view that nutrients only interact with human physiology at the metabolic/post-transcriptional level must be updated in light of current research showing that nutrients can, in fact, modify human physiology and phenotype at the genetic/pre-transcriptional level." Vasquez A. Reducing pain and inflammation naturally - part 4: nutritional and botanical inhibition of NF-kappaB, the major intracellular amplifier of the inflammatory cascade. A practical clinical strategy exemplifying anti-inflammatory nutrigenomics. *Nutritional Perspectives*, July 2005:5-12. www.OptimalHealthResearch.com/part4

[255] Braham R, Dawson B, Goodman C. The effect of glucosamine supplementation on people experiencing regular knee pain. *Br J Sports Med.* 2003;37(1):45-9

[256] Nguyen P, Mohamed SE, Gardiner D, Salinas T. A randomized double-blind clinical trial of the effect of chondroitin sulfate and glucosamine hydrochloride on temporomandibular joint disorders: a pilot study. *Cranio.* 2001 Apr;19(2):130-9

[257] "…oral glucosamine therapy achieved a significantly greater improvement in articular pain score than ibuprofen, and the investigators rated treatment efficacy as 'good' in a significantly greater proportion of glucosamine than ibuprofen recipients. In comparison with piroxicam, glucosamine significantly improved arthritic symptoms after 12 weeks of therapy..." Matheson AJ, Perry CM. Glucosamine: a review of its use in the management of osteoarthritis. *Drugs Aging.* 2003; 20(14): 1041-60

[258] Muller-Fassbender H, Bach GL, Haase W, Rovati LC, Setnikar I. Glucosamine sulfate compared to ibuprofen in osteoarthritis of the knee. *Osteoarthritis Cartilage.* 1994 Mar;2(1):61-9

[259] "Rheumatoid arthritis patients in the experimental group showed improvements in overall disease activity (a mean reduction in disease severity from 1.65 to 1.19 [28%] on a scale of 0 [asymptomatic] to 4 [very severe] at the 4-month follow-up; P=.001), whereas control group patients did not change." Smyth JM, Stone AA, Hurewitz A, Kaell A. Effects of writing about stressful experiences on symptom reduction in patients with asthma or rheumatoid arthritis: a randomized trial. *JAMA.* 1999 Apr 14;281(14):1304-9

Systemic Lupus Erythematosus
"SLE"
"Lupus"

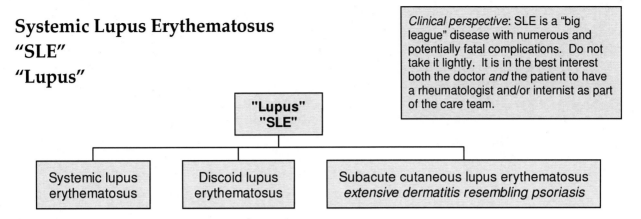

Clinical perspective: SLE is a "big league" disease with numerous and potentially fatal complications. Do not take it lightly. It is in the best interest both the doctor *and* the patient to have a rheumatologist and/or internist as part of the care team.

```
              "Lupus"
               "SLE"

Systemic lupus    Discoid lupus    Subacute cutaneous lupus erythematosus
erythematosus     erythematosus    extensive dermatitis resembling psoriasis
```

Description/pathophysiology:

- This condition is generally considered "idiopathic" in most cases, though in some patients the disease is induced by pharmaceutical drugs and is then generally reversible upon discontinuation of the drug. Most people with complement deficiencies (a group of congenital immune defects) develop SLE. Other precipitating/contributing factors include ultraviolet light, chemical exposure), and consumption of alfalfa sprouts (based on animal data[1] and very little human data). Abnormal hormone metabolism has also been noted and may play a role in the pathogenesis as described in the section on *Orthoendocrinology*.

- Tissue damage is largely mediated by **autoantibodies—particularly anti-DNA antibodies—**and **immune complexes**, cryoglobulins, and the resultant inflammatory cascade.[2,3,4,5] **Patients with SLE have impaired ability to clear immune complexes via hepatic and splenic routes**[6,7]; therapeutic implications are discussed below.

Clinical presentations:

- 85-90% of new patients are young women in their childbearing years; the ratio of women to men is 7:1 except among prepubertal children and older/postmenopausal men and women in which the ratio is 2:1.[8] The much higher prevalence of the disorder among women of childbearing age compared to men of the same age (11:1) implicates sex hormones and hormonal fluctuations as causative factors that predispose young women to this disorder.

- 4x more common in women of African descent (1 per 250) than Caucasian women (1 per 1000).[9]

    - *Comment and hypothesis*: The increased prevalence of SLE in dark-skinned women may be due at least in part to their higher prevalence of vitamin D deficiency, which unquestionably predisposes to inflammation, immune dysfunction, and the clinical manifestation of autoimmunity.[10] Although administration of vitamin D3 to cholecalciferol-deficient adults clearly has anti-inflammatory action[11,12], important windows of opportunity appear to occur *in utero* and within the first few postnatal

[1] "L-Canavanine sulfate, a constituent of alfalfa sprouts, was incorporated into the diet and reactivated the syndrome in monkeys in which an SLE-like syndrome had previously been induced by the ingestion of alfalfa seeds or sprouts." Malinow MR, Bardana EJ Jr, Pirofsky B, Craig S, McLaughlin P. Systemic lupus erythematosus-like syndrome in monkeys fed alfalfa sprouts: role of a nonprotein amino acid. *Science*. 1982 Apr 23;216(4544):415-7

[2] Tierney ML. McPhee SJ, Papadakis MA (eds). Current Medical Diagnosis and Treatment 2006. 45th edition. New York; Lange Medical Books: 2006, pages 833-837

[3] Suzuki N, Mihara S, Sakane T. Development of pathogenic anti-DNA antibodies in patients with systemic lupus erythematosus. *FASEB J*. 1997 Oct;11(12):1033-8 http://www.fasebj.org/cgi/reprint/11/12/1033

[4] "Pisetsky DS. Antibody responses to DNA in normal immunity and aberrant immunity. *Clin Diagn Lab Immunol*. 1998 Jan;5(1):1-6 http://cvi.asm.org/cgi/reprint/5/1/1

[5] Sikander FF, Salgaonkar DS, Joshi VR. Cryoglobulin studies in systemic lupus erythematosus. *J Postgrad Med* [serial online] 1989 [cited 2005 Nov 2];35:139-43

[6] "These observations support the hypothesis that IC handling is abnormal in SLE." Davies KA, Peters AM, Beynon HL, Walport MJ. Immune complex processing in patients with systemic lupus erythematosus. In vivo imaging and clearance studies. *J Clin Invest*. 1992 Nov;90(5):2075-83 http://www.pubmedcentral.gov/articlerender.fcgi?tool=pubmed&pubmedid=1430231

[7] "These results indicate that Fc-mediated clearance of ICs is defective in patients with SLE and suggest that ligation of ICs by Fc receptors is critical for their efficient binding and retention by the fixed MPS in the liver." Davies KA, Robson MG, Peters AM, Norsworthy P, Nash JT, Walport MJ. Defective Fc-dependent processing of immune complexes in patients with systemic lupus erythematosus. *Arthritis Rheum*. 2002 Apr;46(4):1028-38

[8] Manzi S. Epidemiology of systemic lupus erythematosus. *Am J Manag Care*. 2001 Oct;7(16 Suppl):S474-9 http://www.ajmc.com/files/articlefiles/A01_131_2001octManziS474_9.pdf

[9] Tierney ML. McPhee SJ, Papadakis MA. Current Medical Diagnosis and Treatment 2006. 45th edition. New York; Lange Medical Books: 2006, pages 833-837

[10] Cantorna MT. Vitamin D and autoimmunity: is vitamin D status an environmental factor affecting autoimmune disease prevalence? *Proc Soc Exp Biol Med*. 2000;223(3):230-3

[11] Timms PM, Mannan N, Hitman GA, Noonan K, Mills PG, Syndercombe-Court D, Aganna E, Price CP, Boucher BJ. Circulating MMP9, vitamin D and variation in the TIMP-1 response with VDR genotype: mechanisms for inflammatory damage in chronic disorders? *QJM*. 2002;95:787-96 http://qjmed.oxfordjournals.org/cgi/content/full/95/12/787

[12] Van den Berghe G, Van Roosbroeck D, Vanhove P, Wouters PJ, De Pourcq L, Bouillon R. Bone turnover in prolonged critical illness: effect of vitamin D. *J Clin Endocrinol Metab*. 2003;88(10):4623-32

months and years; for example, administration of vitamin D to **infants** reduces the subsequent incidence of type-1 *autoimmune-mediated* diabetes by 78%.[13] Vitamin D sufficiency appears to support immune function and thereby reduce the acquisition of infectious diseases[14]; thus, vitamin D may exert an anti-*rheumatic* benefit by exerting an anti-*infectious* benefit; i.e., by preventing the dysbiotic infections that may serve to trigger autoimmunity. Given the strength of evidence supporting the routine use of vitamin D3 supplementation in infants, children, and adults, healthcare providers should ensure adequate vitamin D status in their patients[15,16,17] for the treatment and prevention of long-latency deficiency diseases[18] and alleviation of systemic inflammation.[19]

- Positive family history of the disease is common: daughters of a mother with SLE have a 1 in 40 prevalence of SLE, whereas sons have a 1 in 250 prevalence
- Clinical course may be slow or acute, involving many organ systems or only one, and is characterized by exacerbations and remissions
- **Classic autoimmune systemic manifestations: fatigue, malaise, low-grade fever, anorexia, weight loss, peripheral polyarthritis**. Septicemia and septic arthritis should always be considered in patients with SLE, especially those taking immunosuppressive drugs and those experiencing what appears to be an exacerbation of the disease.
  - Skin:
    - Malar "butterfly" rash over the cheeks and bridge of the nose: this is a classic manifestation of the disease but is seen in less than half of SLE patients.
    - Photosensitivity: erythematous skin rash develops readily on sun-exposed areas.
    - Hair loss.
    - Nail infarcts, periungual erythema, splinter hemorrhages.
    - Purpura.
  - Musculoskeletal:
    - 90% of patients have polyarthralgia—most commonly affecting the peripheral joints of the hands, wrists, knees, feet.
    - Polymyalgia, myositis, and myopathy; avascular necrosis due to corticosteroids.
  - Renal/kidney:
    - Glomerulonephritis: 50% of patients have clinical nephritis, hematuria, and proteinuria; renal function commonly declines during exacerbation of disease and then improves with disease remission.
    - **Renal failure is a leading cause of death in patients with SLE.**[20]
  - CNS:
    - 70% have EEG abnormalities
    - **Neuropsychiatric lupus is a medical emergency**[21]: characteristics include psychosis, seizures, transient ischemic attacks, severe depression, delirium, confusion. Exclude adverse drug effect (especially corticosteroid psychosis), infection, and hyponatremia.
    - Headaches, migraine, stroke
    - Peripheral and cranial neuropathies, transverse myelitis
    - Increased risk for meningitis when immunosuppressive therapy is used.

[13] "Children who regularly took the recommended dose of vitamin D (2000 IU daily) had a RR of 0.22 (0.05-0.89) compared with those who regularly received less than the recommended amount." Hypponen E, Laara E, Reunanen A, Jarvelin MR, Virtanen SM. Intake of vitamin D and risk of type 1 diabetes: a birth-cohort study. *Lancet.* 2001;358(9292):1500-3
[14] Wayse V, Yousafzai A, Mogale K, Filteau S. Association of subclinical vitamin D deficiency with severe acute lower respiratory infection in Indian children under 5 y. *Eur J Clin Nutr.* 2004;58(4):563-7
[15] Vasquez A, Manso G, Cannell J. The clinical importance of vitamin D (cholecalciferol): a paradigm shift with implications for all healthcare providers. *Altern Ther Health Med.* 2004 Sep-Oct;10(5):28-36 http://optimalhealthresearch.com/monograph04
[16] Heaney RP. Vitamin D, nutritional deficiency, and the medical paradigm. *J Clin Endocrinol Metab.* 2003 Nov;88(11):5107-8 http://jcem.endojournals.org/cgi/content/full/88/11/5107
[17] Hollis BW, Wagner CL. Assessment of dietary vitamin D requirements during pregnancy and lactation. *Am J Clin Nutr.* 2004 May;79(5):717-26 http://www.ajcn.org/cgi/content/full/79/5/717
[18] Heaney RP. Long-latency deficiency disease: insights from calcium and vitamin D. *Am J Clin Nutr.* 2003;78(5):912-9 http://jcem.endojournals.org/cgi/content/full/88/11/5107
[19] Timms PM, Mannan N, Hitman GA, Noonan K, Mills PG, Syndercombe-Court D, Aganna E, Price CP, Boucher BJ. Circulating MMP9, vitamin D and variation in the TIMP-1 response with VDR genotype: mechanisms for inflammatory damage in chronic disorders? *QJM.* 2002;95:787-96 http://qjmed.oxfordjournals.org/cgi/content/full/95/12/787
[20] Suzuki N, Mihara S, Sakane T. Development of pathogenic anti-DNA antibodies in patients with systemic lupus erythematosus. *FASEB J.* 1997 Oct;11(12):1033-8 http://www.fasebj.org/cgi/reprint/11/12/1033
[21] McInnes I, Sturrock R. Rheumatological emergencies. *Practitioner.* 1994 Mar;238(1536):220-4

- o Cardiovascular and circulation:
  - ▪ Vasculitis
  - ▪ Thrombosis and **increased risk for myocardial infarction**
  - ▪ Pericarditis, myocarditis: may result in sudden death, heart failure, arrhythmias
  - ▪ Hypertension due to renal injury
  - ▪ Raynaud's phenomenon—periodic vasospasm affecting the hands and fingers
  - ▪ Antiphospholipid antibody syndrome—a major cause of complications
- o Lungs/pulmonary:
  - ▪ Pneumonitis: presents with fever, cough, dyspnea—important to **assess with radiographs and exclude infection**
  - ▪ Pleurisy, pleural effusion; **alveolar hemorrhage can be life-threatening**
- o Hematologic/CBC abnormalities:
  - ▪ Leukopenia, lymphopenia
  - ▪ Thrombocytopenia
  - ▪ Anemia
  - ▪ Immune complexes: Immune complexes are elevated in patients with active SLE[22]
- o Gastrointestinal:
  - ▪ Nausea
  - ▪ Diarrhea
  - ▪ **Intestinal/mesenteric vasculitis and infarct—surgical emergency**—postprandial abdominal pain, cramps, vomiting, diarrhea
  - ▪ Pancreatitis
  - ▪ Increased intestinal permeability, occasionally of such severity that a protein-losing enteropathy results[23]
- o Eyes:
  - ▪ **Retinal vasculitis** (look for exudates with fundoscopic examination) can cause blindness in days—**treat as an emergency**
  - ▪ Other manifestations include conjunctivitis, photophobia, blurred vision
- o Other:
  - ▪ Edema—may be seen with cardiac or renal damage
  - ▪ Lymphadenopathy
  - ▪ Mucocutaneous ulcerations
  - ▪ Increased risk of miscarriage and congenital heart block

Major differential diagnoses:
- • Infection
- • Cancer, lymphoma
- • RA or other autoimmune disease such as scleroderma, vasculitis, sarcoidosis
- • Iron overload
- • Fibromyalgia
- • Porphyria cutanea tarda
- • Drug hypersensitivity and drug-induced lupus: SLE is differentiated from drug-induced lupus by the following characteristics of drug-induced lupus: 1) temporal association with drug/medication use; remission of disease following drug discontinuation, and 2) lack of fully characteristic pattern of clinical and laboratory manifestations: lack of renal and CNS involvement, lack of hypocomplementemia and anti-native DNA antibodies. Clinicians must exclude drug-induced lupus before making diagnosis of SLE.

---

[22] Suzuki N, Mihara S, Sakane T. Development of pathogenic anti-DNA antibodies in patients with systemic lupus erythematosus. *FASEB J.* 1997 Oct;11(12):1033-8 http://www.fasebj.org/cgi/reprint/11/12/1033
[23] "Fourteen cases of primary lupus-associated protein-losing enteropathy have now been reported in the English-language literature." Perednia DA, Curosh NA. Lupus-associated protein-losing enteropathy. *Arch Intern Med.* 1990 Sep;150(9):1806-10

Clinical assessments:

- **History and physical examination:** consistent with the clinical presentations listed previously
- **Laboratory assessments:** See flow diagram.
    - **ANA: anti-nuclear antibodies: ANA is the best screening test and is now considered positive in 100% of patients.**[24] ANA levels correlate with disease activity. Previous editions of standard medical textbooks reported that this test was less than 100% sensitive for SLE; it may be that improvements in laboratory analysis now account for the 100% sensitivity. A positive ANA test result—even with a high titer—does not necessarily indicate that the patient has SLE, especially if no other signs or symptoms are present.
    - Anti-double stranded (DS, native) DNA antibodies (anti-dsDNA): positive in ~60% of patients; specific (not sensitive) for SLE; when positive, anti-dsDNA levels correlate with disease activity.
    - Anti-Sm (anti-Smith) antibodies: positive in ~30% of patients; specific (not sensitive) for SLE.[25]
    - Anti-histone antibodies: seen in drug-induced lupus.
    - Anti-Ro antibodies (SSA: Sjogren's syndrome antibodies): Seen with cutaneous SLE, Sjogren's syndrome, and neonatal lupus.[26]
    - CRP is a sensitive indicator of inflammation, *except in SLE* where CRP levels can be normal even with severe active disease.[27,28]
    - ESR is not useful in all patients with SLE.[29]
    - Use other tests (metabolic panels, UA, CBC, etc.) to assess for complications and concomitant disease.
    - Complement levels (CH50): Complement levels are lowered in accord with complement activation by immune complexes; levels tend to normalize when disease is in remission.
    - HLA-DR2 and HLA-DR3: These are more common in patients with SLE than in the general population.
    - Serologic testing for syphilis (VDRL): A false-positive test for syphilis is characteristic of SLE and is a reflection of antiphospholipid antibodies.
    - Anticardiolipin antibodies: One of several types of antiphospholipid antibodies; associated with significantly increased risk for venous and arterial thrombosis. Commonly elevated in patients with SLE, particularly those with thrombosis. In SLE patients with antiphospholipid antibodies, treatment with anticoagulants such as warfarin/coumadin are commonly used.
        - INR: International Normalized Ratio is a standardized quantification of Prothrombin Time (PT), which is a measure of clotting/bleeding tendency. INR is used to monitor dosing of warfarin/coumadin; in this case the INR should be kept between 2.0-3.0.[30]
    - Comprehensive testing for celiac disease and wheat allergy: Some patients diagnosed with "systemic lupus erythematosus" actually have autoimmunity and systemic inflammation due to occult celiac disease. These patients achieve clinical remission after avoiding gluten/gliadin-containing grains such as wheat.[31,32] **More than 23% of patients with SLE have anti-gliadin antibodies.**[33] In addition to IgA and IgG anti-gliadin antibodies, serologic testing for celiac disease includes IgA and IgG antiendomysial and anti-transglutaminase antibodies which should be interpreted along with a test for total serum IgA to identify those patients with selective IgA deficiency.

[24] Tierney ML. McPhee SJ, Papadakis MA. Current Medical Diagnosis and Treatment 2006. 45th edition. New York; Lange Medical Books: 2006, pages 833-837

[25] Shojania K. Rheumatology: 2. What laboratory tests are needed? CMAJ. 2000 Apr 18;162(8):1157-63 http://www.cmaj.ca/cgi/content/full/162/8/1157

[26] Shojania K. Rheumatology: 2. What laboratory tests are needed? CMAJ. 2000 Apr 18;162(8):1157-63 http://www.cmaj.ca/cgi/content/full/162/8/1157

[27] Deodhar SD. C-reactive protein: the best laboratory indicator available for monitoring disease activity. Cleve Clin J Med 1989 Mar-Apr;56(2):126-30

[28] Gabay C, Kushner I. Acute-phase proteins and other systemic responses to inflammation. N Engl J Med. 1999 Feb 11;340(6):448-54

[29] Klippel JH (ed). Primer on the Rheumatic Diseases. 11th Edition. Atlanta: Arthritis Foundation. 1997 page 94

[30] Tierney ML. McPhee SJ, Papadakis MA. Current Medical Diagnosis and Treatment 2006. 45th edition. New York; Lange Medical Books: 2006, pages 833-837

[31] "The immunological profile of IgA deficiency and/or raised double stranded DNA in the absence of antinuclear factor together with raised inflammatory markers and symptoms suggestive of an immune diathesis should alert the physician to the possibility of gluten sensitivity." Hadjivassiliou M, Sanders DS, Grunewald RA, Akil M. Gluten sensitivity masquerading as systemic lupus erythematosus. Ann Rheum Dis. 2004 Nov;63(11):1501-3 http://ard.bmjjournals.com/cgi/content/full/63/11/1501

[32] "Villous atrophy on duodenal biopsy specimens with a favorable response to a gluten-free diet was noted in all five patients." Zitouni M, Daoud W, Kallel M, Makni S. Systemic lupus erythematosus with celiac disease: a report of five cases. Joint Bone Spine. 2004 Jul;71(4):344-6

[33] "Twenty-four of 103 (23.3%) systemic lupus erythematosus patients tested positive for either antigliadin antibody, whereas none of the 103 patients tested positive for antiendomysial antibody." Rensch MJ, Szyjkowski R, Shaffer RT, Fink S, Kopecky C, Grissmer L, Enzenhauer R, Kadakia S. The prevalence of celiac disease autoantibodies in patients with systemic lupus erythematosus. Am J Gastroenterol. 2001 Apr;96(4):1113-5 For the authors to state that these patients did not have celiac disease simply because their intestinal biopsies were normal seems to indicate that the authors were ignorant of the modern paradigm of celiac disease which acknowledges that the disease can be present in the absence of gastrointestinal lesions.

- **Imaging**:
  - o Imaging is used to in the assessment of complications and exclusion of concomitant diseases.
  - o The arthritis of SLE is typically mild (compared to rheumatoid arthritis) and is nondeforming.

Establishing the diagnosis: Clinical presentation and lab tests; more positives = more confident DX.

- **Qualification for a diagnosis of SLE requires at least four of the following eleven criteria**:
  1. Malar/cheek rash
  2. Discoid rash
  3. Photosensitivity
  4. Ulcerations of oral mucosa
  5. Joint pain and inflammation not attributable to other disease or trauma
  6. Serositis: Inflammation of the serous tissues, which line the lungs (pleura), heart (pericardium), and the inner lining of the abdomen (peritoneum) and associated organs
  7. Renal disease (any of the following): >3+ proteinuria measured by dipstick; cellular casts; proteinuria >0.5 grams per day
  8. CNS involvement: seizures or psychosis without other cause
  9. Hematologic abnormalities (any of the following): hemolytic anemia, leucopenia (45%), lymphopenia, thrombocytopenia (30%), anemia of chronic disease
  10. **Positive ANA**
  11. Additional serologic tests (any of the following):
      a. Positive LE cell prep
      b. Anti-native DNA antibody (50%)
      c. Anti-Sm antibody (20%)
      d. False-positive test for syphilis (25%)

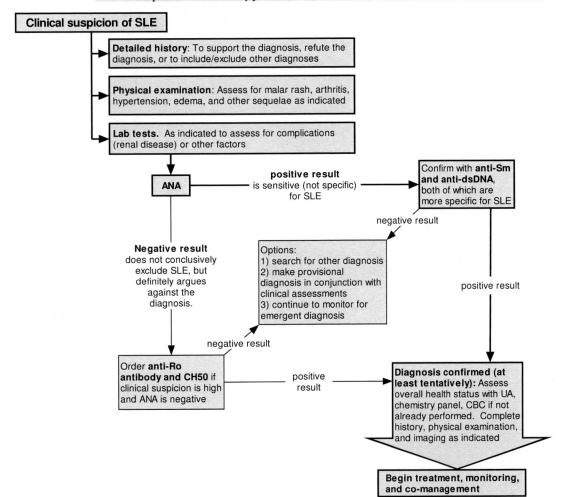

Life-threatening complications and medical emergencies:

- **Infection**—Infections are now the leading cause of death in patients with SLE[34]
- **SLE complications: renal failure and CNS involvement**
- **Stroke, myocardial infarction**—Increased risk with male gender and antiphospholipid antibodies
- Septic arthritis
- Thromboembolism
- 10-year survival is >85%[35]

Overview of clinical management:

- **The clinical course of the disease is variable, marked by exacerbations and remissions. Life-threatening complications can develop rapidly and must be managed effectively to prevent patient morbidity and practitioner liability.**
- Treat patient safely and effectively. If you cannot get good results, refer them to someone who can. Refer if clinical outcome is unsatisfactory or if serious complications are possible. Stable patients are seen every 3-6 months for monitoring of disease activity, re-examination, and treatment recalibration.[36] Patients must understand that acute exacerbations and/or new symptoms—especially fever—must be evaluated promptly.
- Treatment must be customized to the patient and must be flexible to accommodate the natural exacerbations and remissions of the disease.
- To the extent possible, discourage use of NSAIDs since these drugs exacerbate joint destruction, renal impairment, and increased intestinal permeability which increases exposure to dietary and microbial antigens.

Treatments:

Drug treatments:

1. **NSAIDs** are used for joint pain[37] despite adverse effects on the gut[38], joints[39,,40,41], and kidneys.
2. **Antimalarial drug: hydroxychloroquine/Plaquenil):** Adverse effects include retinal damage, neuropathy, myopathy. As with anticonvulsant drugs, hydroxychloroquine/Plaquenil interferes with conversion of 25-hydroxycholecalciferol to the more active 1-25-dihydroxycholecalciferol[42]; this would be expected to exacerbate immune dysfunction, inflammation, hypertension, and depression.
3. **Danazol is an androgenic corticosteroid:** particularly used against thrombocytopenia
4. **Immunosuppression** with <u>prednisone</u> (promotes bacterial overgrowth and osteoporosis), <u>cyclophosphamide</u> (especially for renal involvement), <u>mycophenolate mofetil</u>, <u>azathioprine</u>, or other DMARD (disease-modifying antirheumatic drugs) is commonly used, particularly for the more serious complications of the disease such as those affecting the brain, heart, lungs, and kidneys. **Despite the clinical drawbacks and philosophical inadequacies, pharmacologic immunosuppression has a role in the management of patients with autoimmunity when their disease flares and threatens vital structures, particularly the heart, brain, and kidneys.**
5. **Anticoagulant drugs such as <u>warfarin</u>** are used for patients with antiphospholipid antibodies and resultant thrombotic complications.

- <u>Anti-autoantibody interventions</u>: **Patients with SLE have impaired ability to clear immune complexes via hepatic and splenic routes.**[43,44] Given that anti-DNA and related immune complexes and cryoglobulins are considered the most fundamental abnormalities in the pathogenesis of this disorder, we can explore at least three routes of clinical intervention based on this limited focus. First, therapeutic interventions might be used that inhibit the *de novo* formation of autoantibodies, particularly those that are directed against double-

[34] Tierney ML. McPhee SJ, Papadakis MA. Current Medical Diagnosis and Treatment 2006. 45th edition. New York; Lange Medical Books: 2006, pages 833-837

[35] Tierney ML. McPhee SJ, Papadakis MA. Current Medical Diagnosis and Treatment 2006. 45th edition. New York; Lange Medical Books: 2006, pages 833-837

[36] Manzi S. Epidemiology of systemic lupus erythematosus. Am J Manag Care. 2001 Oct;7(16 Suppl):S474-9 http://www.ajmc.com/files/articlefiles/A01_131_2001octManziS474_9.pdf

[37] Tierney ML. McPhee SJ, Papadakis MA. Current Medical Diagnosis and Treatment 2006. 45th edition. New York; Lange Medical Books: 2006, pages 833-837

[38] Abbreviations: cow's milk beta-lactoglobulin absorption (BLG), acetylsalicylic acid (ASA), disodium chromoglycate (DSCG). "ASA administration strongly increased BLG absorption, not prevented by DSCG pretreatment. In normal controls treated with a single dose of ASA we obtained similar results. Our results suggest that prolonged treatment with nonsteroidal anti-inflammatory drugs induces an increase of food antigen absorption, apparently not related to anaphylaxis mediator release, with possible clinical effects." Fagiolo U, Paganelli R, Ossi E, Quinti I, Cancian M, D'Offizi GP, Fiocco U. Intestinal permeability and antigen absorption in rheumatoid arthritis. Effects of acetylsalicylic acid and sodium chromoglycate. Int Arch Allergy Appl Immunol. 1989;89(1):98-102

[39] "At...concentrations comparable to those... in the synovial fluid of patients treated with the drug, several NSAIDs suppress proteoglycan synthesis...." Brandt KD. Effects of nonsteroidal anti-inflammatory drugs on chondrocyte metabolism in vitro and in vivo. Am J Med. 1987 Nov 20; 83(5A): 29-34

[40] "This highly significant association between NSAID use and acetabular destruction gives cause for concern, not least because of the difficulty in achieving satisfactory hip replacements in patients with severely damaged acetabula." Newman NM, Ling RS. Acetabular bone destruction related to non-steroidal anti-inflammatory drugs. Lancet. 1985 Jul 6; 2(8445): 11-4

[41] Vidal y Plana RR, et al. Articular cartilage pharmacology: I. In vitro studies on glucosamine and non steroidal anti-inflammatory drugs. Pharmacol Res Commun. 1978 Jun;10(6):557-69

[42] "CONCLUSION: Half the SLE and FM patients had 25(OH)-vitamin D levels < 50 nmol/l, a level at which PTH stimulation occurs. Our data suggest that in SLE patients HCQ might inhibit conversion of 25(OH)-vitamin D to 1,25(OH)2-vitamin D." Huisman AM, White KP, Algra A, Harth M, Vieth R, Jacobs JW, Bijlsma JW, Bell DA. Vitamin D levels in women with systemic lupus erythematosus and fibromyalgia. J Rheumatol. 2001 Nov;28(11):2535-9

[43] "These observations support the hypothesis that IC handling is abnormal in SLE." Davies KA, Peters AM, Beynon HL, Walport MJ. Immune complex processing in patients with systemic lupus erythematosus. In vivo imaging and clearance studies. J Clin Invest. 1992 Nov;90(5):2075-83 http://www.pubmedcentral.gov/articlerender.fcgi?tool=pubmed&pubmedid=1430231

[44] "These results indicate that Fc-mediated clearance of ICs is defective in patients with SLE and suggest that ligation of ICs by Fc receptors is critical for their efficient binding and retention by the fixed MPS in the liver." Davies KA, Robson MG, Peters AM, Norsworthy P, Nash JT, Walport MJ. Defective Fc-dependent processing of immune complexes in patients with systemic lupus erythematosus. Arthritis Rheum. 2002 Apr;46(4):1028-38

stranded DNA. This could be accomplished via bio-logical immunomodulation, pharmacologic/anti-biological immunosuppression, or by removing the underlying stimuli ("etiologic/anticausative approach"). Second, treatments might be implemented to nullify or diminish the adverse effects of these antibodies. Third, we might use interventions that remove the autoantibodies that are formed so that they are not significantly available to contribute to disease pathogenesis. As discussed previously in the section on treatments for multifocal dysbiosis, at least two primary mechanisms exist for the removal of autoantibody-containing immune complexes, namely 1) phagocytosis and proteolytic degradation by macrophages embedded in the liver and spleen, and 2) transport via hepatocytes directly into the bile for excretion. IgG double-stranded DNA antibodies are consumed and proteolytically degraded by monocytes/phagocytes[45] while IgA-containing immune complexes are preferentially consumed by hepatocytes and exported intact into the bile for excretion.

Treatments to reduce the adverse effects of autoantibodies and immune complexes: a conceptual overview with interventional considerations					
Reduce *de novo* formation of autoantibodies	→	Biological immunomodulation	→	Orthoendocrinology, particularly supraphysiologic DHEA supplementation	
			→	Anti-inflammatory hypoallergenic diet	
			→	Anti-inflammatory nutrition: ALA, GLA, EPA, DHA, cholecalciferol, antioxidants, NF-kappaB inhibitors, and anti-inflammatory botanicals	
			→	Xenobiotic detoxification	
	→	Pharmacologic immunosuppression	→	Prednisone and other corticosteroids	
			→	Antibiologics such as hydroxychloroquine which exert their clinical benefits via interfering with normal immunologic function, not by improving overall health or addressing underlying etiologic factors	
	→	Removal/correction of primary stimuli for antibody formation *per patient*	→	Orthoendocrinology	
			→	Xenobiotic detoxification	
			→	Antidysbiotic interventions: assessment and correction of multifocal dysbiosis	
Reduce effects of autoantibodies	→	Anti-inflammatory treatments	→	Anti-inflammatory nutrition: ALA, GLA, EPA, DHA, cholecalciferol, antioxidants, NF-kappaB inhibitors, and anti-inflammatory botanicals	
	→	Proteolytic enzymes	→	Proteolytic/pancreatic enzymes appear to reduce *de novo* formation of immune complexes	
Enhance clearance of autoantibodies	→	Allopathic interventions	→	Immunoadsorption[46]	
			→	Plasmapheresis[47,48]	
	→	Naturopathic interventions (theoretical[49])	→	Choleretic and cholagogic botanicals: beets, ginger[50], curcumin[51], *Picrorhiza*[52], milk thistle[53], *Andrographis paniculata*[54] and *Boerhaavia diffusa*.[55]	
			→	Low-volume enemas[56]	

[45] " In the presence of U937 [monocytic] cells, both the AHP-anti-dsDNA and C3b-opsonized ICs were rapidly removed from the erythrocytes; at 37 degrees C, more than half of the complexes were removed in 2 minutes." Craig ML, Bankovich AJ, McElhenny JL, Taylor RP. Clearance of anti-double-stranded DNA antibodies: the natural immune complex clearance mechanism. *Arthritis Rheum*. 2000 Oct;43(10):2265-75

[46] Braun N, Erley C, Klein R, Kotter I, Saal J, Risler T. Immunoadsorption onto protein A induces remission in severe systemic lupus erythematosus. *Nephrol Dial Transplant*. 2000 Sep;15(9):1367-72 http://ndt.oxfordjournals.org/cgi/reprint/15/9/1367

[47] Santos-Ocampo AS, Mandell BF, Fessler BJ. Alveolar hemorrhage in systemic lupus erythematosus: presentation and management. *Chest*. 2000 Oct;118(4):1083-90

[48] Choi BG, Yoo WH. Successful treatment of pure red cell aplasia with plasmapheresis in a patient with systemic lupus erythematosus. *Yonsei Med J*. 2002 Apr;43(2):274-8

[49] Vasquez A. Do the Benefits of Botanical and Physiotherapeutic Hepatobiliary Stimulation Result From Enhanced Excretion of IgA Immune Complexes? *Naturopathy Digest* 2006; January: http://www.naturopathydigest.com/archives/2006/jan/vasquez_immune.php

[50] "Further analyses for the active constituents of the acetone extracts through column chromatography indicated that [6]-gingerol and [10]-gingerol, which are the pungent principles, are mainly responsible for the cholagogic effect of ginger." Yamahara J, Miki K, Chisaka T, Sawada T, Fujimura H, Tomimatsu T, Nakano K, Nohara T. Cholagogic effect of ginger and its active constituents. *J Ethnopharmacol*. 1985;13(2):217-25

[51] "On the basis of the present findings, it appears that curcumin induces contraction of the human gall-bladder." Rasyid A, Lelo A. The effect of curcumin and placebo on human gall-bladder function: an ultrasound study. *Aliment Pharmacol Ther*. 1999 Feb;13(2):245-9

[52] "Significant anticholestatic activity was also observed against carbon tetrachloride induced cholestasis in conscious rat, anaesthetized guinea pig and cat. Picroliv was more active than the known hepatoprotective drug silymarin." Saraswat B, Visen PK, Patnaik GK, Dhawan BN. Anticholestatic effect of picroliv, active hepatoprotective principle of Picrorhiza kurrooa, against carbon tetrachloride induced cholestasis. *Indian J Exp Biol*. 1993 Apr;31(4):316-8

[53] Crocenzi FA, Sanchez Pozzi EJ, Pellegrino JM, Rodriguez Garay EA, Mottino AD, Roma MG. Preventive effect of silymarin against taurolithocholate-induced cholestasis in the rat. *Biochem Pharmacol*. 2003 Jul 15;66(2):355-64

[54] Shukla B, Visen PK, Patnaik GK, Dhawan BN. Choleretic effect of andrographolide in rats and guinea pigs. *Planta Med*. 1992 Apr;58(2):146-9

[55] Chandan BK, Sharma AK, Anand KK. Boerhaavia diffusa: a study of its hepatoprotective activity. *J Ethnopharmacol*. 1991 Mar;31(3):299-307

[56] Garbat AL, Jacobi HG. Secretion of Bile in Response to Rectal Installations. *Arch Intern Med* 1929; 44: 455-462

- <u>Avoidance of proinflammatory foods</u>: Pro-inflammatory foods act *directly* and *indirectly* to promote and exacerbate systemic inflammation. *Direct* mechanisms include the activation of Toll-like receptors and NF-kappaB, while *indirect* mechanisms include depleting the body of anti-inflammatory nutrients and dietary displacement of more nutrient-dense anti-inflammatory foods. Arachidonic acid (found in cow's milk, beef, liver, pork, and lamb) is the direct precursor to pro-inflammatory prostaglandins and leukotrienes[57] and pain-promoting isoprostanes.[58] Saturated fats promote inflammation by activating/enabling pro-inflammatory Toll-like receptors, which are otherwise "specific" for inducing pro-inflammatory responses to microorganisms.[59] Consumption of saturated fat in the form of cream creates marked oxidative stress and lipid peroxidation that lasts for at least 3 hours postprandially.[60] Corn oil rapidly activates NF-kappaB (in hepatic Kupffer cells) for a pro-inflammatory effect[61]; similarly, consumption of PUFA and linoleic acid promotes antioxidant depletion and may thus promote oxidation-mediated inflammation via activation of NF-kappaB. Linoleic acid causes intracellular oxidative stress and calcium influx and results in increased NF-kappaB-stimulated transcription of pro-inflammatory genes.[62] High glycemic foods cause oxidative stress[63,64] and inflammation via activation of NF-kappaB and other mechanisms—e.g., *white bread causes inflammation*[65] as does *a high-fat high-carbohydrate fast-food-style breakfast*.[66] High glycemic foods suppress immune function[67,68] and thus promote the perpetuation of infection/dysbiosis. Delivery of a high carbohydrate load to the gastrointestinal lumen promotes bacterial overgrowth[69,70], which is inherently pro-inflammatory[71,72] and which appears to be myalgenic in humans[73] at least in part due to the ability of endotoxin to impair muscle function.[74] Overconsumption of high-carbohydrate low-phytonutrient grains, potatoes, and manufactured foods displaces phytonutrient-dense foods such as fruits, vegetables, nuts, seeds, and berries which contain more than 8,000 phytonutrients, many of which have antioxidant and thus anti-inflammatory actions.[75,76]

[57] Vasquez A. Reducing Pain and Inflammation Naturally. Part 2: New Insights into Fatty Acid Supplementation and Its Effect on Eicosanoid Production and Genetic Expression. *Nutritional Perspectives* 2005; January: 5-16 www.optimalhealthresearch.com/part2

[58] Evans AR, Junger H, Southall MD, Nicol GD, Sorkin LS, Broome JT, Bailey TW, Vasko MR. Isoprostanes, novel eicosanoids that produce nociception and sensitize rat sensory neurons. *J Pharmacol Exp Ther*. 2000 Jun;293(3):912-20

[59] Lee JY, Sohn KH, Rhee SH, Hwang D. Saturated fatty acids, but not unsaturated fatty acids, induce the expression of cyclooxygenase-2 mediated through Toll-like receptor 4. *J Biol Chem*. 2001 May 18;276(20):16683-9. Epub 2001 Mar 2 http://www.jbc.org/cgi/content/full/276/20/16683

[60] "CONCLUSIONS: Both fat and protein intakes stimulate ROS generation. The increase in ROS generation lasted 3 h after cream intake and 1 h after protein intake. Cream intake also caused a significant and prolonged increase in lipid peroxidation." Mohanty P, Ghanim H, Hamouda W, Aljada A, Garg R, Dandona P. Both lipid and protein intakes stimulate increased generation of reactive oxygen species by polymorphonuclear leukocytes and mononuclear cells. *Am J Clin Nutr*. 2002 Apr;75(4):767-72 http://www.ajcn.org/cgi/content/full/75/4/767

[61] Rusyn I, Bradham CA, Cohn L, Schoonhoven R, Swenberg JA, Brenner DA, Thurman RG. Corn oil rapidly activates nuclear factor-kappaB in hepatic Kupffer cells by oxidant-dependent mechanisms. *Carcinogenesis*. 1999 Nov;20(11):2095-100 http://carcin.oxfordjournals.org/cgi/content/full/20/11/2095

[62] "Exposing endothelial cells to 90 micromol linoleic acid/L for 6 h resulted in a significant increase in lipid hydroperoxides that coincided wih an increase in intracellular calcium concentrations." Hennig B, Toborek M, Joshi-Barve S, Barger SW, Barve S, Mattson MP, McClain CJ. Linoleic acid activates nuclear transcription factor-kappa B (NF-kappa B) and induces NF-kappa B-dependent transcription in cultured endothelial cells. *Am J Clin Nutr*. 1996 Mar;63(3):322-8 http://www.ajcn.org/cgi/reprint/63/3/322

[63] Mohanty P, Hamouda W, Garg R, Aljada A, Ghanim H, Dandona P. Glucose challenge stimulates reactive oxygen species (ROS) generation by leucocytes. *J Clin Endocrinol Metab*. 2000 Aug;85(8):2970-3 http://jcem.endojournals.org/cgi/content/full/85/8/2970 Glucose/carbohydrate and saturated fat consumption appear to be the two biggest offenders in the food-stimulated production of oxidative stress. The effect by protein is much less. "CONCLUSIONS: Both fat and protein intakes stimulate ROS generation. The increase in ROS generation lasted 3 h after cream intake and 1 h after protein intake. Cream intake also caused a significant and prolonged increase in lipid peroxidation." Mohanty P, Ghanim H, Hamouda W, Aljada A, Garg R, Dandona P. Both lipid and protein intakes stimulate increased generation of reactive oxygen species by polymorphonuclear leukocytes and mononuclear cells. *Am J Clin Nutr*. 2002 Apr;75(4):767-72 http://www.ajcn.org/cgi/content/full/75/4/767

[64] Koska J, Blazicek P, Marko M, Grna JD, Kvetnansky R, Vigas M. Insulin, catecholamines, glucose and antioxidant enzymes in oxidative damage during different loads in healthy humans. *Physiol Res*. 2000;49 Suppl 1:S95-100 http://www.biomed.cas.cz/physiolres/pdf/2000/49_S95.pdf

[65] "Conclusion - The present study shows that high GI carbohydrate, but not low GI carbohydrate, mediates an acute proinflammatory process as measured by NF-kappaB activity." Dickinson S, Hancock DP, Petocz P, Brand-Miller JC..High glycemic index carbohydrate mediates an acute proinflammatory process as measured by NF-kappaB activation. *Asia Pac J Clin Nutr*. 2005;14 Suppl:S120

[66] Aljada A, Mohanty P, Ghanim H, Abdo T, Tripathy D, Chaudhuri A, Dandona P. Increase in intranuclear nuclear factor kappaB and decrease in inhibitor kappaB in mononuclear cells after a mixed meal: evidence for a proinflammatory effect. *Am J Clin Nutr*. 2004 Apr;79(4):682-90 http://www.ajcn.org/cgi/content/full/79/4/682

[67] Sanchez A, Reeser JL, Lau HS, et al. Role of sugars in human neutrophilic phagocytosis. *Am J Clin Nutr*. 1973 Nov;26(11):1180-4

[68] "Postoperative infusion of carbohydrate solution leads to moderate fall in the serum concentration of inorganic phosphate. ... The hypophosphatemia was associated with significant reduction of neutrophil phagocytosis, intracellular killing, consumption of oxygen and generation of superoxide during phagocytosis." Rasmussen A, Segel E, Hessov I, Borregaard N. Reduced function of neutrophils during routine postoperative glucose infusion. *Acta Chir Scand*. 1988 Jul-Aug;154(7-8):429-33

[69] Ramakrishnan T, Stokes P. Beneficial effects of fasting and low carbohydrate diet in D-lactic acidosis associated with short-bowel syndrome. *JPEN J Parenter Enteral Nutr*. 1985 May-Jun;9(3):361-3

[70] Gottschall E. <u>Breaking the Vicious Cycle: Intestinal Health Through Diet</u>. Kirkton Press; Rev edition (August 1, 1994)

[71] Lin HC. Small intestinal bacterial overgrowth: a framework for understanding irritable bowel syndrome. *JAMA*. 2004 Aug 18;292(7):852-8

[72] Lichtman SN, Wang J, Sartor RB, Zhang C, Bender D, Dalldorf FG, Schwab JH. Reactivation of arthritis induced by small bowel bacterial overgrowth in rats: role of cytokines, bacteria, and bacterial polymers. *Infect Immun*. 1995 Jun;63(6):2295-301

[73] Pimentel M, et al. A link between irritable bowel syndrome and fibromyalgia may be related to findings on lactulose breath testing. *Ann Rheum Dis*. 2004 Apr;63(4):450-2

[74] Bundgaard H, Kjeldsen K, Suarez Krabbe K, van Hall G, Simonsen L, Qvist J, Hansen CM, Moller K, Fonsmark L, Lav Madsen P, Klarlund Pedersen B. Endotoxemia stimulates skeletal muscle Na+-K+-ATPase and raises blood lactate under aerobic conditions in humans. *Am J Physiol Heart Circ Physiol*. 2003 Mar;284(3):H1028-34. Epub 2002 Nov 21 http://ajpheart.physiology.org/cgi/reprint/284/3/H1028

[75] "We propose that the additive and synergistic effects of phytochemicals in fruit and vegetables are responsible for their potent antioxidant and anticancer activities, and that the benefit of a diet rich in fruit and vegetables is attributed to the complex mixture of phytochemicals present in whole foods." Liu RH. Health benefits of fruit and vegetables are from additive and synergistic combinations of phytochemicals. *Am J Clin Nutr*. 2003 Sep;78(3 Suppl):517S-520S

[76] Seaman DR. The diet-induced proinflammatory state: a cause of chronic pain and other degenerative diseases? *J Manipulative Physiol Ther*. 2002;25(3):168-79

- <u>Avoidance of allergenic foods</u>: Any patient may be allergic to any food, even if the food is generally considered a health-promoting food. Generally speaking, the most notorious allergens are wheat, citrus (especially juice due to the industrial use of fungal hemicellulases), cow's milk, eggs, peanuts, chocolate, and yeast-containing foods; according to a study in patients with migraine, some patients will have to avoid as many as 10 specific foods in order to become symptom-free.[77] Celiac disease can present with inflammatory oligoarthritis that resembles rheumatoid arthritis and which remits with avoidance of wheat/gluten; the inflammatory arthropathy of celiac disease has preceded bowel symptoms and/or an accurate diagnosis by as many as 3-15 years.[78,79] **Some patients diagnosed with "systemic lupus erythematosus" actually have autoimmunity and systemic inflammation due to occult celiac disease, and they achieve remarkable improvement—complete remission of systemic inflammation and the ability to discontinue all anti-inflammatory drugs—after avoiding gluten/gliadin-containing grains—most notoriously, wheat.[80]** In a study of 103 SLE patients, **more than 23% of SLE patients had anti-gliadin antibodies.[81]** Clinicians must explain to their patients that celiac disease and wheat allergy are two different clinical entities and that exclusion of one does not exclude the other, and in neither case does mutual exclusion obviate the promotion of intestinal bacterial overgrowth (i.e., proinflammatory dysbiosis) by indigestible wheat oligosaccharides.
- <u>Cardiovascular disease (CVD) risk reduction</u>: **Patients with SLE have an increased risk of cardiovascular disease due to the synergistic effects of inflammation, oxidative stress, antiphospholipid antibodies, and elevated homocysteine.** Obviously, the risk for CVD will be exacerbated if the SLE patient has other risk factors such as tobacco use, diabetes, obesity, hypertension, or physical inactivity. Therapeutic and interventional considerations specific to the prevention of cardiovascular disease include but are not limited to the following:
  - <u>Cardioprotective diet</u>: Paleo-Mediterranean diet
  - <u>Fatty acid supplementation</u>: Combination fatty acid supplementation with ALA, GLA, EPA, DHA[82,83]
  - <u>Magnesium supplementation</u>: > 200 mg up to bowel tolerance
  - <u>Treatments to lower homocysteine</u>: Doses given here for various treatments are for adults:
    - <u>Folic acid</u>: 5-10 mg, should be used with high-dose vitamin B-12
    - <u>Hydroxocobalamin</u>: 2,000-6,000 mcg/d orally, or 1,000-4,000 mcg/wk by injection
    - <u>Pyridoxine</u>: 250 mg/day with meals, co-administered with magnesium (e.g., >200 mg/d)
    - <u>NAC</u>: 600 mg tid
    - <u>Betaine/ trimethylglycine</u>: 1-2 grams tid (>6 grams daily when used alone)
    - <u>Lecithin</u>: 2.6 g choline/d (as phosphatidylcholine) decreased mean fasting plasma homocysteine by 18%.[84] Attaining this high dose might require as many as 45 capsules of commercially available supplements; an equivalent dose in the form

[77] Grant EC. Food allergies and migraine. *Lancet.* 1979 May 5;1(8123):966-9

[78] "We report six patients with coeliac disease in whom arthritis was prominent at diagnosis and who improved with dietary therapy. Joint pain preceded diagnosis by up to three years in five patients and 15 years in one patient." Bourne JT, Kumar P, Huskisson EC, Mageed R, Unsworth DJ, Wojtulewski JA. Arthritis and coeliac disease. *Ann Rheum Dis.* 1985 Sep;44(9):592-8

[79] "A 15-year-old girl, with synovitis of the knees and ankles for 3 years before a diagnosis of gluten-sensitive enteropathy, is described." Pinals RS. Arthritis associated with gluten-sensitive enteropathy. *J Rheumatol.* 1986 Feb;13(1):201-4

[80] "The immunological profile of IgA deficiency and/or raised double stranded DNA in the absence of antinuclear factor together with raised inflammatory markers and symptoms suggestive of an immune diathesis should alert the physician to the possibility of gluten sensitivity." Hadjivassiliou M, Sanders DS, Grunewald RA, Akil M. Gluten sensitivity masquerading as systemic lupus erythematosus. *Ann Rheum Dis.* 2004 Nov;63(11):1501-3
http://ard.bmjjournals.com/cgi/content/full/63/11/1501

[81] "Twenty-four of 103 (23.3%) systemic lupus erythematosus patients tested positive for either antigliadin antibody, whereas none of the 103 patients tested positive for antiendomysial antibody." Rensch MJ, Szyjkowski R, Shaffer RT, Fink S, Kopecky C, Grissmer L, Enzenhauer R, Kadakia S. The prevalence of celiac disease autoantibodies in patients with systemic lupus erythematosus. *Am J Gastroenterol.* 2001 Apr;96(4):1113-5. For the authors to state that these patients did not have celiac disease simply because their intestinal biopsies were normal seems to indicate that the authors were ignorant of the modern paradigm of celiac disease which acknowledges that the disease can be present in the absence of gastrointestinal lesions.

[82] Vasquez A. Reducing Pain and Inflammation Naturally. Part 2: New Insights into Fatty Acid Supplementation and Its Effect on Eicosanoid Production and Genetic Expression. *Nutritional Perspectives* 2005; January: 5-16 www.optimalhealthresearch.com/part2

[83] Laidlaw M, Holub BJ. Effects of supplementation with fish oil-derived n-3 fatty acids and gamma-linolenic acid on circulating plasma lipids and fatty acid profiles in women. *Am J Clin Nutr.* 2003 Jan;77(1):37-42 http://www.ajcn.org/cgi/content/full/77/1/37

[84] Olthof MR, Brink EJ, Katan MB, Verhoef P. Choline supplemented as phosphatidylcholine decreases fasting and postmethionine-loading plasma homocysteine concentrations in healthy men. *Am J Clin Nutr.* 2005 Jul;82(1):111-7

of powdered lecithin granules delivered in a smoothie may be better tolerated than the capsules.

- ▪ <u>Thyroid hormone</u>: as indicated
  - ○ <u>Policosanol</u>: Policosanol (20 mg per day)[85,86] derived from sugar cane, standardized for content of octacosanol. In addition to its ability to favorably modulate lipid parameters, Policosanol also exerts an anticoagulant effect and therefore exerts cardioprotective benefits independent from its lipid-lowering characteristics. Policosanol may be used with low-dose aspirin in this regard; in some cases, the cardioprotective/antithrombotic benefit of *low-dose* aspirin justifies its use despite its adverse effects, such as increased intestinal permeability.

- <u>Alcohol/ethanol avoidance</u>: Consumption of alcoholic beverages—even in low doses—increases intestinal permeability and can exacerbate inflammatory disorders, particularly those associated with food allergies, gastrointestinal dysbiosis, and/or overproduction of estrogen.

- <u>Supplemented Paleo-Mediterranean diet</u>: The health-promoting diet of choice for the majority of people is a diet based on abundant consumption of fruits, vegetables, seeds, nuts, omega-3 and monounsaturated fatty acids, and lean sources of protein such as lean meats, fatty cold-water fish, soy and whey proteins. This diet obviates overconsumption of chemical preservatives, artificial sweeteners, and carbohydrate-dominant foods such as candies, pastries, breads, potatoes, grains, and other foods with a high glycemic load and high glycemic index. This "Paleo-Mediterranean Diet" is a combination of the "Paleolithic" or "Paleo diet" and the well-known "Mediterranean diet", both of which are well described in peer-reviewed journals and the lay press. (See Chapter 2 and my other publications[87,88] for details). This diet is the most nutrient-dense diet available, and its benefits are further enhanced by supplementation with vitamins, minerals, probiotics, and the health-promoting fatty acids: ALA, GLA, EPA, DHA.

- <u>Gluten-free vegetarian diet</u>: Vegetarian/vegan diets have a place in the treatment plan of all patients with autoimmune/inflammatory disorders[89,90]; this is also true for patients for whom long-term exclusive reliance on a meat-free vegetarian diet is either not appropriate or not appealing. No legitimate scientist or literate clinician doubts the antirheumatic power and anti-inflammatory advantages of vegetarian diets, whether used short-term or long term.[91] The benefits of gluten-free vegetarian diets are well documented, and the mechanisms of action are well elucidated, including reduced intake of proinflammatory linoleic[92] and arachidonic acids[93], iron[94], common food antigens[95], gluten[96] and gliadin[97,98], proinflammatory sugars[99] and increased

[85] "These results show that policosanol-treated CHD patients improved clinical evolution, and exercise-ECG responses, owing to the amelioration of myocardial ischemia, even more when administered with aspirin." Stusser R, Batista J, Padron R, Sosa F, Pereztol O. Long-term therapy with policosanol improves treadmill exercise-ECG testing performance of coronary heart disease patients. *Int J Clin Pharmacol Ther*. 1998 Sep;36(9):469-73
[86] "Policosanol seems to be a very promising phytochemical alternative to classic lipid-lowering agents such as the statins and deserves further evaluation." Gouni-Berthold I, Berthold HK.Policosanol: clinical pharmacology and therapeutic significance of a new lipid-lowering agent. *Am Heart J*. 2002 Feb;143(2):356-65
[87] Vasquez A. A Five-Part Nutritional Protocol that Produces Consistently Positive Results. *Nutritional Wellness* 2005 September Available in the printed version and on-line at http://www.nutritionalwellness.com/archives/2005/sep/09_vasquez.php and http://optimalhealthresearch.com/protocol
[88] Vasquez A. Implementing the Five-Part Nutritional Wellness Protocol for the Treatment of Various Health Problems. *Nutritional Wellness* 2005 November. Available on-line at http://www.nutritionalwellness.com/archives/2005/nov/11_vasquez.php and http://optimalhealthresearch.com/protocol
[89] "After four weeks at the health farm the diet group showed a significant improvement in number of tender joints, Ritchie's articular index, number of swollen joints, pain score, duration of morning stiffness, grip strength, erythrocyte sedimentation rate, C-reactive protein, white blood cell count, and a health assessment questionnaire score." Kjeldsen-Kragh J, Haugen M, Borchgrevink CF, Laerum E, Eek M, Mowinkel P, Hovi K, Forre O. Controlled trial of fasting and one-year vegetarian diet in rheumatoid arthritis. *Lancet*. 1991 Oct 12;338(8772):899-902
[90] "During the vegan diet, both signs and symptoms returned in most patients, with the exception of some patients with psoriasis who experienced an improvement." Lithell H, Bruce A, Gustafsson IB, Hoglund NJ, Karlstrom B, Ljunghall K, Sjolin K, Venge P, Werner I, Vessby B. A fasting and vegetarian diet treatment trial on chronic inflammatory disorders. *Acta Derm Venereol*. 1983;63(5):397-403
[91] "For the patients who were randomised to the vegetarian diet there was a significant decrease in platelet count, leukocyte count, calprotectin, total IgG, IgM rheumatoid factor (RF), C3-activation products, and the complement components C3 and C4 after one month of treatment." Kjeldsen-Kragh J, Mellbye OJ, Haugen M, Mollnes TE, Hammer HB, Sioud M, Forre O. Changes in laboratory variables in rheumatoid arthritis patients during a trial of fasting and one-year vegetarian diet. *Scand J Rheumatol*. 1995;24(2):85-93
[92] Rusyn I, Bradham CA, Cohn L, Schoonhoven R, Swenberg JA, Brenner DA, Thurman RG. Corn oil rapidly activates nuclear factor-kappaB in hepatic Kupffer cells by oxidant-dependent mechanisms. *Carcinogenesis*. 1999 Nov;20(11):2095-100 http://carcin.oxfordjournals.org/cgi/content/full/20/11/2095
[93] Vasquez A. Reducing Pain and Inflammation Naturally. Part 2: New Insights into Fatty Acid Supplementation and Its Effect on Eicosanoid Production and Genetic Expression. *Nutritional Perspectives* 2005; January: 5-16 http://optimalhealthresearch.com/part2
[94] Dabbagh AJ, Trenam CW, Morris CJ, Blake DR. Iron in joint inflammation. *Ann Rheum Dis*. 1993 Jan;52(1):67-73
[95] Hafstrom I, Ringertz B, Spangberg A, von Zweigbergk L, Brannemark S, Nylander I, Ronnelid J, Laasonen L, Klareskog L. A vegan diet free of gluten improves the signs and symptoms of rheumatoid arthritis: the effects on arthritis correlate with a reduction in antibodies to food antigens. *Rheumatology* (Oxford). 2001 Oct;40(10):1175-9 http://rheumatology.oxfordjournals.org/cgi/reprint/40/10/1175
[96] "The data provide evidence that dietary modification may be of clinical benefit for certain RA patients, and that this benefit may be related to a reduction in immunoreactivity to food antigens eliminated by the change in diet." Hafstrom I, Ringertz B, Spangberg A, von Zweigbergk L, Brannemark S, Nylander I, Ronnelid J, Laasonen L, Klareskog L. A vegan diet free of gluten improves the signs and symptoms of rheumatoid arthritis: the effects on arthritis correlate with a reduction in antibodies to food antigens. *Rheumatology* (Oxford). 2001 Oct;40(10):1175-9
[97] "Despite the increased AGA [antigliadin antibodies] positivity found distinctively in patients with recent-onset RA, none of the RA patients showed clear evidence of coeliac disease." Paimela L, Kurki P, Leirisalo-Repo M, Piirainen H. Gliadin immune reactivity in patients with rheumatoid arthritis. Clin Exp Rheumatol. 1995 Sep-Oct;13(5):603-7
[98] "The median IgA antigliadin ELISA index was 7.1 (range 2.1-22.4) for the RA group and 3.1 (range 0.3-34.9) for the controls (p = 0.0001)." Koot VC, Van Straaten M, Hekkens WT, Collee G, Dijkmans BA. Elevated level of IgA gliadin antibodies in patients with rheumatoid arthritis. Clin Exp Rheumatol. 1989 Nov-Dec;7(6):623-6
[99] Seaman DR. The diet-induced proinflammatory state: a cause of chronic pain and other degenerative diseases? *J Manipulative Physiol Ther*. 2002 Mar-Apr;25(3):168-79

intake of omega-3 fatty acids and micronutrients[100], and anti-inflammatory and anti-oxidant phytonutrients[101]; vegetarian diets also effect profound changes—both *qualitative* and *quantitative*—in intestinal flora[102,103] that correlate with clinical improvement.[104] **Some patients diagnosed "systemic lupus erythematosus" have autoimmunity and systemic inflammation due to occult celiac disease, and they achieve complete remission of systemic inflammation and the ability to discontinue all anti-inflammatory drugs after avoiding gluten/gliadin-containing grains.[105]** Patients who rely on the Paleo-Mediterranean Diet can use vegetarian meals, on a daily basis or for days at a time, for example, by having a daily vegetarian meal, or one week per month of vegetarianism. Of course, some (not all) patients can use a purely vegetarian diet long-term provided that nutritional needs (especially protein and cobalamin) are consistently met.

- <u>Short-term fasting</u>: Whether the foundational diet is Paleo-Mediterranean, vegetarian, vegan, or a combination of all of these, autoimmune/inflammatory patients will still benefit from periodic fasting, whether on a weekly (e.g., every Saturday), monthly (every first week or weekend of the month, or every other month), or yearly (1-2 weeks of the year) basis. Since consumption of food—particularly unhealthy foods—induces an inflammatory effect[106], abstinence from food provides a relative anti-oxidative and anti-inflammatory benefit[107] with many of the antioxidant benefits beginning within 24 hours of the initiation of the fast.[108] Fasting indeed provides a distinct anti-inflammatory benefit and may help "re-calibrate" metabolic and homeostatic mechanisms by breaking self-perpetuating "vicious cycles"[109] that autonomously promote inflammation independent from proinflammatory stimuli. Of course, water-only fasting is completely hypoallergenic (assuming that the patient is not sensitive to chlorine, fluoride, or other contaminants), and subsequent re-introduction of foods provides the ideal opportunity to identify offending foods. Fasting deprives intestinal microbes of substrate[110], stimulates intestinal B-cell immunity[111], improves the bactericidal action of neutrophils[112], reduces lysozyme release and leukotriene formation[113], and ameliorates intestinal hyperpermeability.[114] In case reports and clinical trials, short-term fasting (or protein-sparing fasting) has been documented as safe and

---

[100] Hagfors L, Nilsson I, Skoldstam L, Johansson G. Fat intake and composition of fatty acids in serum phospholipids in a randomized, controlled, Mediterranean dietary intervention study on patients with rheumatoid arthritis. *Nutr Metab* (Lond). 2005 Oct 10;2:26 http://www.nutritionandmetabolism.com/content/2/1/26
[101] Liu RH. Health benefits of fruit and vegetables are from additive and synergistic combinations of phytochemicals. *Am J Clin Nutr* 2003;78(3 Suppl):517S-520S http://www.ajcn.org/cgi/content/full/78/3/517S
[102] "Significant alteration in the intestinal flora was observed when the patients changed from omnivorous to vegan diet. ... This finding of an association between intestinal flora and disease activity may have implications for our understanding of how diet can affect RA." Peltonen R, Kjeldsen-Kragh J, Haugen M, Tuominen J, Toivanen P, Forre O, Eerola E. Changes of faecal flora in rheumatoid arthritis during fasting and one-year vegetarian diet. *Br J Rheumatol.* 1994 Jul;33(7):638-43
[103] Toivanen P, Eerola E. A vegan diet changes the intestinal flora. *Rheumatology* (Oxford). 2002 Aug;41(8):950-1 http://rheumatology.oxfordjournals.org/cgi/reprint/41/8/950
[104] "We conclude that a vegan diet changes the faecal microbial flora in RA patients, and changes in the faecal flora are associated with improvement in RA activity." Peltonen R, Nenonen M, Helve T, Hanninen O, Toivanen P, Eerola E. Faecal microbial flora and disease activity in rheumatoid arthritis during a vegan diet. *Br J Rheumatol.* 1997 Jan;36(1):64-8 http://rheumatology.oxfordjournals.org/cgi/reprint/36/1/64
[105] "The immunological profile of IgA deficiency and/or raised double stranded DNA in the absence of antinuclear factor together with raised inflammatory markers and symptoms suggestive of an immune diathesis should alert the physician to the possibility of gluten sensitivity." Hadjivassiliou M, Sanders DS, Grunewald RA, Akil M. Gluten sensitivity masquerading as systemic lupus erythematosus. *Ann Rheum Dis.* 2004 Nov;63(11):1501-3 http://ard.bmjjournals.com/cgi/content/full/63/11/1501
[106] Aljada A, Mohanty P, Ghanim H, Abdo T, Tripathy D, Chaudhuri A, Dandona P. Increase in intranuclear nuclear factor kappaB and decrease in inhibitor kappaB in mononuclear cells after a mixed meal: evidence for a proinflammatory effect. *Am J Clin Nutr.* 2004 Apr;79(4):682-90 http://www.ajcn.org/cgi/content/full/79/4/682
[107] "This is the first demonstration of ...a decrease in reactive oxygen species generation by leukocytes and oxidative damage to lipids, proteins, and amino acids after dietary restriction and weight loss in the obese over a short period." Dandona P, Mohanty P, Ghanim H, Aljada A, Browne R, Hamouda W, Prabhala A, Afzal A, Garg R. The suppressive effect of dietary restriction and weight loss in the obese on the generation of reactive oxygen species by leukocytes, lipid peroxidation, and protein carbonylation. *J Clin Endocrinol Metab.* 2001 Jan;86(1):355-62 http://jcem.endojournals.org/cgi/content/full/86/1/355
[108] "Thus, a 48h fast may reduce ROS generation, total oxidative load and oxidative damage to amino acids." Dandona P, Mohanty P, Hamouda W, Ghanim H, Aljada A, Garg R, Kumar V. Inhibitory effect of a two day fast on reactive oxygen species (ROS) generation by leucocytes and plasma ortho-tyrosine and meta-tyrosine concentrations. *J Clin Endocrinol Metab.* 2001 Jun;86(6):2899-902 http://jcem.endojournals.org/cgi/content/abstract/86/6/2899
[109] "The ability of therapeutic fasts to break metabolic vicious cycles may also contribute to the efficacy of fasting in the treatment of type 2 diabetes and autoimmune disorders." McCarty MF. A preliminary fast may potentiate response to a subsequent low-salt, low-fat vegan diet in the management of hypertension - fasting as a strategy for breaking metabolic vicious cycles. *Med Hypotheses.* 2003 May;60(5):624-33
[110] Ramakrishnan T, Stokes P. Beneficial effects of fasting and low carbohydrate diet in D-lactic acidosis associated with short-bowel syndrome. *JPEN J Parenter Enteral Nutr.* 1985 May-Jun;9(3):361-3
[111] Trollmo C, Verdrengh M, Tarkowski A. Fasting enhances mucosal antigen specific B cell responses in rheumatoid arthritis. *Ann Rheum Dis.* 1997 Feb;56(2):130-4 http://ard.bmjjournals.com/cgi/content/full/56/2/130
[112] "An association was found between improvement in inflammatory activity of the joints and enhancement of neutrophil bactericidal capacity. Fasting appears to improve the clinical status of patients with RA." Uden AM, Trang L, Venizelos N, Palmblad J. Neutrophil functions and clinical performance after total fasting in patients with rheumatoid arthritis. *Ann Rheum Dis.* 1983 Feb;42(1):45-51
[113] "We thus conclude that a reduced ability to generate cytotaxins, reduced release of enzyme, and reduced leukotriene formation from RA neutrophils, together with an altered fatty acid composition of membrane phospholipids, may be mechanisms for the decrease of inflammatory symptoms that results from fasting." Hafstrom I, Ringertz B, Gyllenhammar H, Palmblad J, Harms-Ringdahl M. Effects of fasting on disease activity, neutrophil function, fatty acid composition, and leukotriene biosynthesis in patients with rheumatoid arthritis. *Arthritis Rheum.* 1988 May;31(5):585-92
[114] "The results indicate that, unlike lactovegetarian diet, fasting may ameliorate the disease activity and reduce both the intestinal and the non-intestinal permeability in rheumatoid arthritis." Sundqvist T, Lindstrom F, Magnusson KE, Skoldstam L, Stjernstrom I, Tagesson C. Influence of fasting on intestinal permeability and disease activity in patients with rheumatoid arthritis. *Scand J Rheumatol.* 1982;11(1):33-8

effective treatment for SLE[115], RA[116], and non-rheumatic diseases such as chronic severe hypertension[117], moderate hypertension[118], obesity[119,120], type-2 diabetes[121], and epilepsy.[122] **The combination of energy restriction and fish oil supplementation was shown highly beneficial in an animal model of SLE.[123]**

- Broad-spectrum fatty acid therapy with ALA, EPA, DHA, GLA and oleic acid: **Fish oil provides EPA and DHA which have well-proven anti-inflammatory benefits when used in the treatment of SLE.[124,125,126]** Fatty acid supplementation should be delivered in the form of combination therapy with ALA, GLA, DHA, and EPA. Given at doses of 3,000 – 9,000 mg per day, ALA from flax oil has impressive anti-inflammatory benefits demonstrated by its ability to halve prostaglandin production in humans.[127] Numerous studies have demonstrated the benefit of GLA in the treatment of rheumatoid arthritis when used at doses between 500 mg – 4,000 mg per day.[128,129] Fish oil provides EPA and DHA which have well-proven anti-inflammatory benefits in RA[130,131,132] and SLE.[133,134] ALA, EPA, DHA, and GLA need to be provided in the form of supplements; when using high doses of therapeutic oils, liquid supplements that can be mixed in juice or a smoothie are generally more convenient and palatable than capsules. Therapeutic amounts of oleic acid can be obtained from generous use of olive oil, preferably on fresh vegetables. Supplementation with polyunsaturated fatty acids warrants increased intake of antioxidants from diet, fruit and vegetable juices, and properly formulated supplements; since patients with systemic inflammation are generally in a pro-oxidative state, consideration must be given to the timing and starting dose of fatty acid supplementation and the need for anti-oxidant protection. See chapter on Therapeutics for more details and biochemical pathways. Clinicians must realize that fatty acids are not clinically or biochemically interchangeable and that one fatty acid does not substitute for another; each of the fatty acids must be supplied in order for its benefits to be obtained.[135]

[115] Fuhrman J, Sarter B, Calabro DJ. Brief case reports of medically supervised, water-only fasting associated with remission of autoimmune disease. *Altern Ther Health Med*. 2002 Jul-Aug;8(4):112, 110-1

[116] "An association was found between improvement in inflammatory activity of the joints and enhancement of neutrophil bactericidal capacity. Fasting appears to improve the clinical status of patients with RA." Uden AM, Trang L, Venizelos N, Palmblad J. Neutrophil functions and clinical performance after total fasting in patients with rheumatoid arthritis. *Ann Rheum Dis*. 1983 Feb;42(1):45-51

[117] "The average reduction in blood pressure was 37/13 mm Hg, with the greatest decrease being observed for subjects with the most severe hypertension. Patients with stage 3 hypertension (those with systolic blood pressure greater than 180 mg Hg, diastolic blood pressure greater than 110 mg Hg, or both) had an average reduction of 60/17 mm Hg at the conclusion of treatment." Goldhamer A, Lisle D, Parpia B, Anderson SV, Campbell TC. Medically supervised water-only fasting in the treatment of hypertension. *J Manipulative Physiol Ther*. 2001 Jun;24(5):335-9 http://www.healthpromoting.com/335-339Goldhamer115263.QXD.pdf

[118] "RESULTS: Approximately 82% of the subjects achieved BP at or below 120/80 mm Hg by the end of the treatment program. The mean BP reduction was 20/7 mm Hg, with the greatest decrease being observed for subjects with the highest baseline BP." Goldhamer AC, Lisle DJ, Sultana P, Anderson SV, Parpia B, Hughes B, Campbell TC. Medically supervised water-only fasting in the treatment of borderline hypertension. *J Altern Complement Med*. 2002 Oct;8(5):643-50 http://www.healthpromoting.com/Articles/articles/study%202/acmpaper5.pdf

[119] Vertes V, Genuth SM, Hazelton IM. Supplemented fasting as a large-scale outpatient program. *JAMA*. 1977 Nov 14;238(20):2151-3

[120] Bauman WA, Schwartz E, Rose HG, Eisenstein HN, Johnson DW. Early and long-term effects of acute caloric deprivation in obese diabetic patients. *Am J Med*. 1988 Jul;85(1):38-46

[121] Goldhamer AC. Initial cost of care results in medically supervised water-only fasting for treating high blood pressure and diabetes. *J Altern Complement Med*. 2002 Dec;8(6):696-7 http://www.healthpromoting.com/Articles/pdf/Study%2032.pdf

[122] "The ketogenic diet should be considered as alternative therapy for children with difficult-to-control seizures. It is more effective than many of the new anticonvulsant medications and is well tolerated by children and families when it is effective." Freeman JM, Vining EP, Pillas DJ, Pyzik PL, Casey JC, Kelly LM. The efficacy of the ketogenic diet-1998: a prospective evaluation of intervention in 150 children. *Pediatrics*. 1998 Dec;102(6):1358-63 http://pediatrics.aappublications.org/cgi/reprint/102/6/1358

[123] "In conclusion, our data strongly indicate that ER and FO maintain antioxidant status and GSH:GSSG ratio, thereby protecting against renal deterioration from oxidative insults during ageing." Kelley VE, Ferretti A, Izui S, Strom TB. A fish oil diet rich in eicosapentaenoic acid reduces cyclooxygenase metabolites, and suppresses lupus in MRL-lpr mice. *J Immunol*. 1985 Mar;134(3):1914-9

[124] "No major side effects were noted, and it is suggested that dietary modification with additional marine oil may be a useful way of modifying disease activity in systemic lupus erythematosus." Walton AJ, Snaith ML, Locniskar M, Cumberland AG, Morrow WJ, Isenberg DA. Dietary fish oil and the severity of symptoms in patients with systemic lupus erythematosus. *Ann Rheum Dis*. 1991 Jul;50(7):463-6

[125] "CONCLUSION: In the management of SLE, dietary supplementation with fish oil may be beneficial in modifying symptomatic disease activity." Duffy EM, Meenagh GK, McMillan SA, Strain JJ, Hannigan BM, Bell AL. The clinical effect of dietary supplementation with omega-3 fish oils and/or copper in systemic lupus erythematosus. *J Rheumatol*. 2004 Aug;31(8):1551-6 http://www.jrheum.com/subscribers/04/08/tables/PDF/1551.pdf

[126] "Oral supplementation of EPA and DHA induced prolonged remission of SLE in 10 consecutive patients without any side-effects. These results suggest that n-3 fatty acids, EPA and DHA, are useful in the management of SLE and possibly, other similar collagen vascular diseases." Das UN. Beneficial effect of eicosapentaenoic and docosahexaenoic acids in the management of systemic lupus erythematosus and its relationship to the cytokine network. *Prostaglandins Leukot Essent Fatty Acids*. 1994 Sep;51(3):207-13

[127] Adam O, Wolfram G, Zollner N. Effect of alpha-linolenic acid in the human diet on linoleic acid metabolism and prostaglandin biosynthesis. *J Lipid Res*. 1986 Apr;27(4):421-6 http://www.jlr.org/cgi/reprint/27/4/421

[128] "Other results showed a significant reduction in morning stiffness with gamma-linolenic acid at 3 months and reduction in pain and articular index at 6 months with olive oil." Brzeski M, Madhok R, Capell HA. Evening primrose oil in patients with rheumatoid arthritis and side-effects of non-steroidal anti-inflammatory drugs. *Br J Rheumatol*. 1991 Oct;30(5):370-2

[129] Rothman D, DeLuca P, Zurier RB. Botanical lipids: effects on inflammation, immune responses, and rheumatoid arthritis. *Semin Arthritis Rheum*. 1995 Oct;25(2):87-96

[130] Adam O, Beringer C, Kless T, Lemmen C, Adam A, Wiseman M, Adam P, Klimmek R, Forth W. Anti-inflammatory effects of a low arachidonic acid diet and fish oil in patients with rheumatoid arthritis. *Rheumatol Int*. 2003 Jan;23(1):27-36

[131] Lau CS, Morley KD, Belch JJ. Effects of fish oil supplementation on non-steroidal anti-inflammatory drug requirement in patients with mild rheumatoid arthritis--a double-blind placebo controlled study. *Br J Rheumatol*. 1993 Nov;32(11):982-9

[132] Kremer JM, Jubiz W, Michalek A, Rynes RI, Bartholomew LE, Bigaouette J, Timchalk M, Beeler D, Lininger L. Fish-oil fatty acid supplementation in active rheumatoid arthritis. A double-blinded, controlled, crossover study. *Ann Intern Med*. 1987 Apr;106(4):497-503

[133] Walton AJ, Snaith ML, Locniskar M, Cumberland AG, Morrow WJ, Isenberg DA. Dietary fish oil and the severity of symptoms in patients with systemic lupus erythematosus. *Ann Rheum Dis*. 1991 Jul;50(7):463-6

[134] Duffy EM, Meenagh GK, McMillan SA, Strain JJ, Hannigan BM, Bell AL. The clinical effect of dietary supplementation with omega-3 fish oils and/or copper in systemic lupus erythematosus. *J Rheumatol*. 2004 Aug;31(8):1551-6

[135] Vasquez A. Reducing Pain and Inflammation Naturally. Part 2: New Insights into Fatty Acid Supplementation and Its Effect on Eicosanoid Production and Genetic Expression. *Nutritional Perspectives* 2005; January: 5-16 http://optimalhealthresearch.com/part2

- Vitamin D3 supplementation with physiologic doses and/or tailored to serum 25(OH)D levels:
  Vitamin D deficiency is common in the general population and is even more common in patients with chronic illness and chronic musculoskeletal pain.[136] **At least 50% of patients with SLE are deficient in vitamin D.[137]** Correction of vitamin D deficiency supports normal immune function against infection and provides a clinically significant anti-inflammatory[138] and analgesic benefit in patients with back pain[139] and limb pain.[140] Reasonable daily doses for children and adults are 2,000 and 4,000 IU, respectively, as defined by Vasquez, et al.[141] Deficiency and response to treatment are monitored with serum 25(OH)vitamin D while safety is monitored with serum calcium; inflammatory granulomatous diseases and certain drugs such as

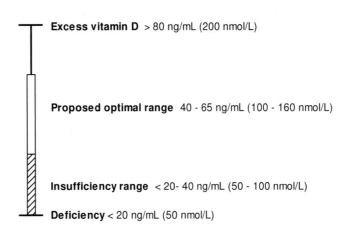

Excess vitamin D > 80 ng/mL (200 nmol/L)

Proposed optimal range 40 - 65 ng/mL (100 - 160 nmol/L)

Insufficiency range < 20- 40 ng/mL (50 - 100 nmol/L)

Deficiency < 20 ng/mL (50 nmol/L)

Proposed normal and optimal ranges for serum 25(OH)D levels

  hydrochlorothiazide greatly increase the propensity for hypercalcemia and warrant increment dosing and frequent monitoring of serum calcium.

- Assessment and treatment for dysbiosis: **Dysbiotic loci should be investigated as discussed previously in Chapter 4.** Recall that **patients with lupus have abnormal gastrointestinal bacteria** (decreased colonization resistance[142]), and some evidence suggests that **gastrointestinal bacteria in these patients may translocate into the systemic circulation to induce formation of antibodies that cross-react with double-stranded DNA to produce the clinical manifestations of the disease.[143,144]** Each cause—each contributor to disease—may in itself be "clinically insignificant" but when numerous "insignificant" additive and synergistic influences coalesce, we find ourselves confronted with an "idiopathic disease." We must then decide between the only two available options: 1) despair in the failure of our "one cause, one disease, one drug" paradigm, or 2) appreciate that numerous influences work together to disrupt physiologic function and produce the biologic dysfunction that we experience as disease. **Experimental evidence shows that exposure to single-stranded bacterial DNA can provoke formation of antibodies to single-stranded mammalian DNA. Human patients with SLE have a reduced ability to bind bacterial DNA with antibodies, thus allowing bacterial DNA to provoke an ongoing inflammatory response.[145]** Recall from Chapter 4 that stimulation of inflammation by bacterial DNA is one of the 17 pathomechanisms of autoimmune/inflammation induction by multifocal dysbiosis.

---

[136] Plotnikoff GA, Quigley JM. Prevalence of severe hypovitaminosis D in patients with persistent, nonspecific musculoskeletal pain. *Mayo Clin Proc*. 2003 Dec;78(12):1463-70

[137] "CONCLUSION: Half the SLE and FM patients had 25(OH)-vitamin D levels < 50 nmol/l, a level at which PTH stimulation occurs. Our data suggest that in SLE patients HCQ might inhibit conversion of 25(OH)-vitamin D to 1,25(OH)2-vitamin D." Huisman AM, White KP, Algra A, Harth M, Vieth R, Jacobs JW, Bijlsma JW, Bell DA. Vitamin D levels in women with systemic lupus erythematosus and fibromyalgia. *J Rheumatol*. 2001 Nov;28(11):2535-9

[138] Timms PM, Mannan N, Hitman GA, Noonan K, Mills PG, Syndercombe-Court D, Aganna E, Price CP, Boucher BJ. Circulating MMP9, vitamin D and variation in the TIMP-1 response with VDR genotype: mechanisms for inflammatory damage in chronic disorders? *QJM*. 2002 Dec;95(12):787-96 http://qjmed.oxfordjournals.org/cgi/content/full/95/12/787

[139] Al Faraj S, Al Mutairi K. Vitamin D deficiency and chronic low back pain in Saudi Arabia. *Spine*. 2003 Jan 15;28(2):177-9

[140] Masood H, Narang AP, Bhat IA, Shah GN. Persistent limb pain and raised serum alkaline phosphatase the earliest markers of subclinical hypovitaminosis D in Kashmir. *Indian J Physiol Pharmacol*. 1989 Oct-Dec;33(4):259-61

[141] Vasquez A, Manso G, Cannell J. The clinical importance of vitamin D (cholecalciferol): a paradigm shift with implications for all healthcare providers. *Altern Ther Health Med*. 2004 Sep-Oct;10(5):28-36 http://optimalhealthresearch.com/monograph04

[142] "Colonization Resistance (CR)...tended to be lower in active SLE patients than in healthy individuals. This could indicate that in SLE more and different bacteria translocate across the gut wall due to a lower CR. Some of these may serve as polyclonal B cell activators or as antigens cross-reacting with DNA." Apperloo-Renkema HZ, Bootsma H, Mulder BI, Kallenberg CG, van der Waaij D. Host-microflora interaction in systemic lupus erythematosus (SLE): colonization resistance of the indigenous bacteria of the intestinal tract. *Epidemiol Infect*. 1994;112(2):367-73

[143] "The lower IgG antibacterial antibody titres in active SLE might possibly result from sequestration of these IgG antibodies in immune complexes, indicating a possible role for antibacterial antibodies in exacerbations of SLE." Apperloo-Renkema HZ, Bootsma H, Mulder BI, Kallenberg CG, van der Waaij D. Host-microflora interaction in systemic lupus erythematosus (SLE): circulating antibodies to the indigenous bacteria of the intestinal tract. *Epidemiol Infect*. 1995 Feb;114(1):133-41

[144] Pisetsky DS. Antibody responses to DNA in normal immunity and aberrant immunity. *Clin Diagn Lab Immunol*. 1998 Jan;5(1):1-6 http://cdli.asm.org/cgi/content/full/5/1/1

[145] Pisetsky DS. Antibody responses to DNA in normal immunity and aberrant immunity. *Clin Diagn Lab Immunol*. 1998 Jan;5(1):1-6 http://cdli.asm.org/cgi/content/full/5/1/1

- Sinorespiratory/nasopharyngeal and dermal dysbiosis: **Increased nasal colonization with *Staphylococcus aureus* has been noted in patients with SLE.**[146]
- Gastrointestinal dysbiosis: Yeast, bacteria, and parasites are treated as indicated based on identification and sensitivity results from comprehensive parasitology assessments.
- Antimicrobial treatments for (gastrointestinal) dysbiosis commonly include but are not limited to the following: Combination therapy generally allows for lower doses of each intervention to be used. Severe dysbiosis often requires weeks or months of treatment. Drugs are not necessarily more effective than natural treatments; in fact, often the botanicals work when the pharmaceuticals do not. Doses listed are for adults.
  - Oregano oil: Emulsified oil of oregano in a time-released tablet is proven effective in the eradication of harmful gastrointestinal microbes, including *Blastocystis hominis, Entamoeba hartmanni,* and *Endolimax nana.*[147] An *in vitro* study[148] and clinical experience support the use of emulsified oregano against *Candida albicans* and various bacteria. The common dose is 600 mg per day in divided doses for 6 weeks.[149]
  - Berberine: Berberine is an alkaloid found in *Hydrastis canadensis* (goldenseal), *Coptis chinensis* (Coptis, goldenthread), *Berberis/Mahonia aquifolium* (Oregon grape), *Berberis vulgaris* (barberry), and *Berberis aristata* (tree turmeric)[150], and it shows effectiveness against *Giardia, Candida,* and *Streptococcus* in addition to its direct anti-inflammatory and antidiarrheal actions. Oral dose of 400-800 mg per day in divided doses is common for adults.[151]
  - *Artemisia annua*: Artemisinin has been safely used for centuries in Asia for the treatment of malaria, and it also has effectiveness against anaerobic bacteria due to the pro-oxidative sesquiterpene endoperoxide.[152,153] I commonly use artemisinin at 200 mg per day in divided doses for adults with dysbiosis.
  - St. John's Wort (*Hypericum perforatum*): Hyperforin from *Hypericum perforatum* also shows impressive antibacterial action, particularly against gram-positive bacteria such as *Staphylococcus aureus, Streptococcus pyogenes, Streptococcus agalactiae*[154] and perhaps *Helicobacter pylori.*[155] Up to 600 mg three times per day of a 3% hyperforin standardized extract is customary in the treatment of depression.
  - Bismuth: Bismuth is commonly used in the empiric treatment of diarrhea (e.g., "Pepto-Bismol") and is generally combined with other antimicrobial agents to reduce drug resistance and increase antibiotic effectiveness.[156]
  - Undecylenic acid: Derived from castor bean oil, undecylenic acid has antifungal properties and is commonly indicated by sensitivity results obtained by stool culture. Common dosages are 150-250 mg tid (up to 750 mg per day).[157]
  - Peppermint (*Mentha piperita*): Peppermint shows antimicrobial and antispasmodic actions and has demonstrated clinical effectiveness in patients with bacterial overgrowth of the small bowel.

[146] Medline abstract from Polish research: "In 9 from 14 patients with (64.3%) a.b. very massive growth of Staphylococcus aureus in culture from vestibulae of the nose swab was, in other cultures very massive growth of physiological flora was seen. ...clinical significance of asymptomatic bacteriuria and pathogenic bacteria colonisation of nostrils as a precedence to symptomatic infections needs further investigations." Koseda-Dragan M, Hebanowski M, Galinski J, Krzywinska E, Bakowska A. [Asymptomatic bacteriuria in women diagnosed with systemic lupus erythematosus (SLE)] *Pol Arch Med Wewn.* 1998 Oct;100(4):321-30.
[147] Force M, Sparks WS, Ronzio RA. Inhibition of enteric parasites by emulsified oil of oregano in vivo. *Phytother Res.* 2000 May;14(3):213-4
[148] Stiles JC, Sparks W, Ronzio RA. The inhibition of Candida albicans by oregano. *J Applied Nutr* 1995;47:96–102
[149] Force M, Sparks WS, Ronzio RA. Inhibition of enteric parasites by emulsified oil of oregano in vivo. *Phytother Res.* 2000 May;14(3):213-4
[150] [No authors listed] Berberine. *Altern Med Rev.* 2000 Apr;5(2):175-7 http://www.thorne.com/altmedrev/.fulltext/5/2/175.pdf
[151] [No authors listed] Berberine. *Altern Med Rev.* 2000 Apr;5(2):175-7 http://www.thorne.com/altmedrev/.fulltext/5/2/175.pdf
[152] Dien TK, de Vries PJ, Khanh NX, Koopmans R, Binh LN, Duc DD, Kager PA, van Boxtel CJ. Effect of food intake on pharmacokinetics of oral artemisinin in healthy Vietnamese subjects. *Antimicrob Agents Chemother.* 1997 May;41(5):1069-72
[153] Giao PT, Binh TQ, Kager PA, Long HP, Van Thang N, Van Nam N, de Vries PJ. Artemisinin for treatment of uncomplicated falciparum malaria: is there a place for monotherapy? *Am J Trop Med Hyg.* 2001 Dec;65(6):690-5
[154] Schempp CM, Pelz K, Wittmer A, Schopf E, Simon JC. Antibacterial activity of hyperforin from St John's wort, against multiresistant Staphylococcus aureus and gram-positive bacteria. *Lancet.* 1999 Jun 19;353(9170):2129
[155] "A butanol fraction of St. John's Wort revealed anti-Helicobacter pylori activity with MIC values ranging between 15.6 and 31.2 microg/ml." Reichling J, Weseler A, Saller R. A current review of the antimicrobial activity of Hypericum perforatum L. *Pharmacopsychiatry.* 2001 Jul;34 Suppl 1:S116-8
[156] Veldhuyzen van Zanten SJ, Sherman PM, Hunt RH. Helicobacter pylori: new developments and treatments. *CMAJ.* 1997;156(11):1565-74 http://www.cmaj.ca/cgi/reprint/156/11/1565.pdf
[157] "Adult dosage is usually 450-750 mg undecylenic acid daily in three divided doses." Undecylenic acid. Monograph. *Altern Med Rev.* 2002 Feb;7(1):68-70 http://www.thorne.com/altmedrev/.fulltext/7/1/68.pdf

- **Commonly used antibiotic/antifungal drugs**: The most commonly employed drugs for intestinal bacterial overgrowth are described here.[158] Treatment duration is generally at least 2 weeks and up to 8 weeks, depending on clinical response and the severity and diversity of the intestinal overgrowth. With all anti*bacterial* treatments, use empiric anti*fungal* treatment to prevent yeast overgrowth; some patients benefit from antifungal treatment that is continued for *months* and occasionally *years*. Drugs can generally be coadministered with natural antibiotics/antifungals for improved efficacy. Treatment can be guided by identification of the dysbiotic microbes and the results of culture and sensitivity tests. Effectiveness of treatment is based overall clinical response and repeat testing.

  ⇒ Metronidazole: 250-500 mg BID-QID (generally limit to 1.5 g/d); metronidazole has systemic bioavailability and effectiveness against a wide range of dysbiotic microbes, including protozoans, amebas/Giardia, *H. pylori, Clostridium difficile* and most anaerobic gram-negative bacilli.[159] Adverse effects are generally limited to stomatitis, nausea, diarrhea, and—rarely and/or with long-term use—peripheral neuropathy, dizziness, and metallic taste; the drug must not be consumed with alcohol.

  ⇒ Erythromycin: 250-500 mg TID-QID; this drug is a widely used antibiotic that also has intestinal promotility benefits (thus making it an ideal treatment for intestinal bacterial overgrowth associated with or caused by intestinal dysmotility/hypomotility such as seen in scleroderma[160,161]). Do not combine erythromycin with the promotility drug **cisapride** due to risk for serious cardiac arrhythmia.

  ⇒ Tetracycline: 250-500 mg QID

  ⇒ Ciproflaxacin: 500 mg BID

  ⇒ Cephalexin/kelfex: 250 mg QID

  ⇒ Minocycline: Minocycline (200 mg/day)[162] has received the most attention in the treatment of rheumatoid arthritis due to its superior response (65%) over placebo (13%)[163]; in addition to its antibacterial action, the drug is also immunomodulatory and anti-inflammatory. Ironically, minocycline can cause drug-induced autoimmunity, especially lupus.[164,165]

  ⇒ Nystatin: Nystatin 500,000 units bid with food; duration of treatment begins with a minimum duration of 2-4 weeks and may continue as long as the patient is deriving benefit.

  ⇒ Ketoconazole: As a systemically bioavailable antifungal drug, ketoconazole has inherent anti-inflammatory benefits which may be helpful; however the drug inhibits androgen formation and may lead to

---

[158] Saltzman JR, Russell RM. Nutritional consequences of intestinal bacterial overgrowth. *Compr Ther*. 1994;20(9):523-30

[159] Tierney ML. McPhee SJ, Papadakis MA. Current Medical Diagnosis and Treatment 2006. 45th edition. New York; Lange Medical Books: 2006, pages 1578-1577

[160] "Prokinetic agents effective in pseudoobstruction include metoclopramide, domperidone, cisapride, octreotide, and erythromycin. ... The combination of octreotide and erythromycin may be particularly effective in systemic sclerosis." Sjogren RW. Gastrointestinal features of scleroderma. *Curr Opin Rheumatol*. 1996 Nov;8(6):569-75

[161] "CONCLUSIONS: Erythromycin accelerates gastric and gallbladder emptying in scleroderma patients and might be helpful in the treatment of gastrointestinal motor abnormalities in these patients." Fiorucci S, Distrutti E, Bassotti G, Gerli R, Chiucchiu S, Betti C, Santucci L, Morelli A. Effect of erythromycin administration on upper gastrointestinal motility in scleroderma patients. *Scand J Gastroenterol*. 1994 Sep;29(9):807-13

[162] "...48-week trial of oral minocycline (200 mg/d) or placebo." Tilley BC, Alarcon GS, Heyse SP, Trentham DE, Neuner R, Kaplan DA, Clegg DO, Leisen JC, Buckley L, Cooper SM, Duncan H, Pillemer SR, Tuttleman M, Fowler SE. Minocycline in rheumatoid arthritis. A 48-week, double-blind, placebo-controlled trial. MIRA Trial Group. *Ann Intern Med*. 1995 Jan 15;122(2):81-9

[163] "In patients with early seropositive RA, therapy with minocycline is superior to placebo." O'Dell JR, Haire CE, Palmer W, Drymalski W, Wees S, Blakely K, Churchill M, Eckhoff PJ, Weaver A, Doud D, Erikson N, Dietz F, Olson R, Maloley P, Klassen LW, Moore GF. Treatment of early rheumatoid arthritis with minocycline or placebo: results of a randomized, double-blind, placebo-controlled trial. *Arthritis Rheum*. 1997 May;40(5):842-8

[164] "...many cases of drug-induced lupus related to minocycline have been reported. Some of those reports included pulmonary lupus..." Christodoulou CS, Emmanuel P, Ray RA, Good RA, Schnapf BM, Cawkwell GD. Respiratory distress due to minocycline-induced pulmonary lupus." *Chest*. 1999 May;115(5):1471-3 http://www.chestjournal.org/cgi/content/full/115/5/1471

[165] Lawson TM, Amos N, Bulgen D, Williams BD.Minocycline-induced lupus: clinical features and response to rechallenge. *Rheumatology* (Oxford). 2001 Mar;40(3):329-35 http://rheumatology.oxfordjournals.org/cgi/content/full/40/3/329

exacerbation of the hypoandrogenism that is commonly seen in autoimmune patients and which contributes to the immune dysfunction.

- ▪ <u>Probiotics</u>: Live cultures in the form of tablets, capsules, yogurt, or kefir can be used per patient preference and tolerance. Obviously, dairy-based products should be avoided by patients with dairy allergy.

- ▪ *Saccharomyces boulardii*: A non-colonizing, non-pathogenic yeast that increases sIgA production and can aid in the elimination of pathogenic/dysbiotic yeast, bacteria, and parasites. It is particularly useful during antibiotic treatment to help prevent secondary Candidal infections. Common dose is 250 mg thrice daily.

- ▪ <u>Supplemented Paleo-Mediterranean diet / Specific Carbohydrate Diet</u>: The specifications of the *specific carbohydrate diet* (SCD) detailed by Gottschall[166] are met with adherence to the Paleo diet by Cordain.[167] The combination of both approaches and books will give patients an excellent combination of informational understanding and culinary versatility.

- ▪ <u>Topical antimicrobials</u>: Treating the dermal lesions of psoriatic arthritis may help break the vicious cycles of (super)antigen absorption which perpetuates immune dysfunction. A variety of botanical and pharmaceutical creams are available. *In vitro* evidence supports the use of equal parts honey, olive oil, and beeswax against *Staph aureus* and *Candida albicans*.[168] As mentioned previously, topical *Mahonia/Berberis* is effective for dermal psoriasis[169], probably due to the combination of its anti-inflammatory and antifungal/antibacterial actions. Topical honey is better than acyclovir against oral and genital herpes; apply *qid* for 15 minutes.[170]

- • <u>Orthoendocrinology</u>: Assess melatonin, prolactin, cortisol, DHEA, free and total testosterone, serum estradiol, and thyroid status (e.g., TSH, T4, *and* anti-thyroid peroxidase antibodies).

  - o <u>Melatonin</u>: Melatonin is a pineal hormone with well-known sleep-inducing and immunomodulatory properties, and it is commonly administered in doses of 1-40 mg in the evening, before bedtime. Starting with a relatively low dose (e.g., 1-5 mg) and increasing as tolerated is recommended. Melatonin (20 mg hs) appears to have cured two patients with drug-resistant sarcoidosis[171] and 3 mg provided immediate short-term benefit to a patient with multiple sclerosis.[172]

  - o <u>Prolactin (excess)</u>: **Prolactin has proinflammatory and immunodysregulatory actions and is commonly elevated—either overtly or latently—in patients with inflammatory/autoimmune disease.** Accordingly prolactin-lowering treatment shows safety and effectiveness in the treatment of numerous inflammatory/autoimmune diseases; often these results are noted even when the patient's prolactin level was not initially elevated, suggesting the alleviation of latent hyperprolactinemia and/or an inherent anti-inflammatory action of the prolactin-lowering treatment. According to clinical trials with small numbers of patients, whether prolactin levels are high or not, prolactin-lowering treatment (such as bromocriptine[173]) appears highly beneficial when

---

[166] Gotschall E. <u>Breaking the Vicious Cycle: Intestinal health though diet</u>. Kirkton Press; Rev edition (August, 1994) http://www.scdiet.com/ http://www.breakingthevicouscycle.info/

[167] Cordain L. <u>The Paleo Diet: Lose weight and get healthy by eating the food you were designed to eat</u>. John Wiley & Sons Inc., New York 2002 http://thepaleodiet.com/

[168] "Honey, beeswax and olive oil mixture (1:1:1, v/v) is useful in the treatment of diaper dermatitis, psoriasis and eczema... CONCLUSIONS: Honey and honey mixture apparently could inhibit growth of S. aureus or C. albicans." Al-Waili NS. Mixture of honey, beeswax and olive oil inhibits growth of Staphylococcus aureus and Candida albicans. Arch Med Res. 2005 Jan-Feb;36(1):10-3

[169] "Taken together, these clinical studies conducted by several investigators in several countries indicate that Mahonia aquifolium is a safe and effective treatment of patients with mild to moderate psoriasis." Gulliver WP, Donsky HJ. A report on three recent clinical trials using Mahonia aquifolium 10% topical cream and a review of the worldwide clinical experience with Mahonia aquifolium for the treatment of plaque psoriasis. Am J Ther. 2005 Sep-Oct;12(5):398-406

[170] Al-Waili NS. Topical honey application vs. acyclovir for the treatment of recurrent herpes simplex lesions. *Med Sci Monit*. 2004 Aug;10(8):MT94-8. Epub 2004 Jul 23 http://www.medscimonit.com/pub/vol_10/no_8/4431.pdf

[171] Cagnoni ML, Lombardi A, Cerinic MC, Dedola GL, Pignone A. Melatonin for treatment of chronic refractory sarcoidosis. *Lancet*. 1995 Nov 4;346(8984):1229-30

[172] "...administration of melatonin (3 mg, orally) at 2:00 p.m., when the patient experienced severe blurring of vision, resulted within 15 minutes in a dramatic improvement in visual acuity and in normalization of the visual evoked potential latency after stimulation of the left eye." Sandyk R. Diurnal variations in vision and relations to circadian melatonin secretion in multiple sclerosis. *Int J Neurosci*. 1995 Nov;83(1-2):1-6

[173] "In 2 cases of psoriatic arthritis, adding bromocriptine to gold salts and nonsteroidal anti-inflammatory drug was followed by a drastic efficacy with spectacular improvement in clinical, biological and occupational status. Because none of the cases had hyperprolactinaemia, bromocriptine acted probably had an intrinic anti-inflammatory effect independent of its antiprolactinic effect." Eulry F, Mayaudon H, Bauduceau B, Lechevalier D, Crozes P, Magnin J, Claude-Berthelot C. [Blood prolactin under the effect of protirelin in spondylarthropathies. Treatment trial of 4 cases of reactive arthritis and 2 cases of psoriatic arthritis with bromocriptine] *Ann Med Interne* (Paris). 1996;147(1):15-9. French.

used with other anti-rheumatic treatments ("...drastic efficacy with spectacular improvement in clinical, biological and occupational status..."[174]) in patients with psoriatic arthritis. Serum prolactin is the standard assessment of prolactin status. Since elevated prolactin may be a sign of pituitary tumor, assessment for headaches, visual deficits, other abnormalities of pituitary hormones (e.g., GH and TSH) should be performed and CT or MRI must be considered. Patients with prolactin levels less than 100 ng/mL and normal CT/MRI findings can be managed conservatively with effective prolactin-lowering treatment and annual radiologic assessment (less necessary with favorable serum response).[175, see review 176] **Patients with RA and SLE have higher basal and stress-induced levels of prolactin compared with normal controls.**[177,178] A normal serum prolactin level does not necessarily exclude the use of prolactin-lowering intervention, especially since many autoimmune patients have **latent hyperprolactinemia** which may not be detected with random serum measurement of prolactin. Specific treatment options include the following:

- Thyroid hormone: Hypothyroidism frequently causes hyperprolactinemia which is reversible upon effective treatment of hypothyroidism. Obviously therefore, thyroid status should be evaluated in all patients with hyperprolactinemia. Thyroid assessment and treatment is reviewed later in this section.

- *Vitex astus-cagnus* and other supporting botanicals and nutrients: **Vitex lowers serum prolactin in humans**[179,180] **via a dopaminergic effect.**[181] Vitex is considered safe for clinical use; mild and reversible adverse effects possibly associated with Vitex include nausea, headache, gastrointestinal disturbances, menstrual disorders, acne, pruritus and erythematous rash. No drug interactions are known, but given the herb's dopaminergic effect it should probably be used with some caution in patients treated with dopamine antagonists such as the so-called antipsychotic drugs (most of which do not work very well and/or carry intolerable adverse effects[182,183]). In a recent review, Bone[184] stated that daily doses of *Vitex* can range from 500 mg to 2,000 mg DHE (dry herb equivalent) and can be tailored to the suppression of prolactin. Due at least in part to its content of L-dopa, *Mucuna pruriens* **shows clinical dopaminergic activity** as evidenced by its effectiveness in Parkinson's disease[185]; up to 15-30 gm/d of mucuna has been used clinically but doses will be dependent on preparation and phytoconcentration. **Triptolide and other extracts from** *Tripterygium wilfordii* **Hook F exert clinically significant anti-inflammatory action in patients with rheumatoid arthritis**[186,187] **and also offer protection to dopaminergic**

---

[174] Abstract from article in French: "In 2 cases of psoriatic arthritis, adding bromocriptine to gold salts and nonsteroidal anti-inflammatory drug was followed by a drastic efficacy with spectacular improvement in clinical, biological and occupational status. Because none of the cases had hyperprolactinaemia, bromocriptine acted probably had an intrinic anti-inflammatory effect independent of its antiprolactinic effect." Eulry F, Mayaudon H, Bauduceau B, Lechevalier D, Crozes P, Magnin J, Claude-Berthelot C. [Blood prolactin under the effect of protirelin in spondylarthropathies. Treatment trial of 4 cases of reactive arthritis and 2 cases of psoriatic arthritis with bromocriptine] *Ann Med Interne* (Paris). 1996;147(1):15-9. French

[175] Beers MH, Berkow R (eds). The Merck Manual. Seventeenth Edition. Whitehouse Station; Merck Research Laboratories 1999 Page 77-78

[176] Serri O, Chik CL, Ur E, Ezzat S. Diagnosis and management of hyperprolactinemia. *CMAJ*. 2003 Sep 16;169(6):575-81 http://www.cmaj.ca/cgi/content/full/169/6/575

[177] Dostal C, Moszkorzova L, Musilova L, Lacinova Z, Marek J, Zvarova J. Serum prolactin stress values in patients with systemic lupus erythematosus. *Ann Rheum Dis*. 2003 May;62(5):487-8 http://ard.bmjjournals.com/cgi/content/full/62/5/487

[178] "RESULTS: A significantly higher rate of elevated PRL levels was found in SLE patients (40.0%) compared with the healthy controls (14.8%). No proof was found of association with the presence of anti-ds-DNA or with specific organ involvement. Similarly, elevated PRL levels were found in RA patients (39.3%)." Moszkorzova L, Lacinova Z, Marek J, Musilova L, Dohnalova A, Dostal C. Hyperprolactinaemia in patients with systemic lupus erythematosus. *Clin Exp Rheumatol*. 2002 Nov-Dec;20(6):807-12

[179] "Since AC extracts were shown to have beneficial effects on premenstrual mastodynia serum prolactin levels in such patients were also studied in one double-blind, placebo-controlled clinical study. Serum prolactin levels were indeed reduced in the patients treated with the extract." Wuttke W, Jarry H, Christoffel V, Spengler B, Seidlova-Wuttke D. Chaste tree (Vitex agnus-castus)--pharmacology and clinical indications. *Phytomedicine*. 2003 May;10(4):348-57

[180] German abstract from Medline: "The prolactin release was reduced after 3 months, shortened luteal phases were normalised and deficits in the luteal progesterone synthesis were eliminated." Milewicz A, Gejdel E, Sworen H, Sienkiewicz K, Jedrzejak J, Teucher T, Schmitz H. [Vitex agnus castus extract in the treatment of luteal phase defects due to latent hyperprolactinemia. Results of a randomized placebo-controlled double-blind study] *Arzneimittelforschung*. 1993 Jul;43(7):752-6

[181] "Our results indicate a dopaminergic effect of Vitex agnus-castus extracts and suggest additional pharmacological actions via opioid receptors." Meier B, Berger D, Hoberg E, Sticher O, Schaffner W. Pharmacological activities of Vitex agnus-castus extracts in vitro. *Phytomedicine*. 2000 Oct;7(5):373-81

[182] "The majority of patients in each group discontinued their assigned treatment owing to inefficacy or intolerable side effects or for other reasons." Lieberman JA, Stroup TS, McEvoy JP, Swartz MS, Rosenheck RA, Perkins DO, Keefe RS, Davis SM, Davis CE, Lebowitz BD, Severe J, Hsiao JK; Clinical Antipsychotic Trials of Intervention Effectiveness (CATIE) Investigators. Effectiveness of antipsychotic drugs in patients with chronic schizophrenia. *N Engl J Med*. 2005 Sep 22;353(12):1209-23

[183] Whitaker R. The case against antipsychotic drugs: a 50-year record of doing more harm than good. *Med Hypotheses*. 2004;62(1):5-13

[184] "In conditions such as endometriosis and fibroids, for which a significant estrogen antagonist effect is needed, doses of at least 2 g/day DHE may be required and typically are used by professional herbalists." Bone K. New Insights Into Chaste Tree. *Nutritional Wellness* 2005 November http://www.nutritionalwellness.com/archives/2005/nov/11_bone.php

[185] "CONCLUSIONS: The rapid onset of action and longer on time without concomitant increase in dyskinesias on mucuna seed powder formulation suggest that this natural source of L-dopa might possess advantages over conventional L-dopa preparations in the long term management of PD." Katzenschlager R, Evans A, Manson A, Patsalos PN, Ratnaraj N, Watt H, Timmermann L, Van der Giessen R, Lees AJ. Mucuna pruriens in Parkinson's disease: a double blind clinical and pharmacological study. *J Neurol Neurosurg Psychiatry*. 2004 Dec;75(12):1672-7

[186] "The ethanol/ethyl acetate extract of TWHF shows therapeutic benefit in patients with treatment-refractory RA. At therapeutic dosages, the TWHF extract was well tolerated by most patients in this study." Tao X, Younger J, Fan FZ, Wang B, Lipsky PE. Benefit of an extract of Tripterygium Wilfordii Hook F in patients with rheumatoid arthritis: a double-blind, placebo-controlled study. *Arthritis Rheum*. 2002 Jul;46(7):1735-43

neurons.[188,189] Ironically, even though tyrosine is the nutritional precursor to dopamine with evidence of clinical effectiveness (e.g., narcolepsy[190], enhancement of memory[191] and cognition[192]), **supplementation with tyrosine appears to actually increase rather than decrease prolactin levels[193]; therefore tyrosine should be used cautiously if at all in patients with systemic inflammation.** Furthermore, the finding that **high-protein meals stimulate prolactin release[194]** may partly explain the benefits of vegetarian diets in the treatment of systemic inflammation; since vegetarian diets are comparatively low in protein compared to omnivorous diets, they may lead to a relative reduction in prolactin production due to lack of stimulation.

- Bromocriptine: Bromocriptine has long been considered the pharmacologic treatment of choice for elevated prolactin.[195] Typical dose is 2.5 mg per day (effective against SLE[196]); gastrointestinal upset and sedation are common.[197] **Clinical intervention with bromocriptine appears warranted in patients with RA, SLE, Reiter's syndrome, psoriatic arthritis, and probably multiple sclerosis and uveitis.[198]** A normal serum prolactin level does not necessarily exclude the use of prolactin-lowering intervention, especially since many autoimmune patients have latent hyperprolactinemia which may not be detected with random serum measurement of prolactin.

- Cabergoline/Dostinex: Cabergoline/Dostinex is a newer dopamine agonist with few adverse effects; typical dose starts at 0.5 mg per week (0.25 mg twice per week).[199] Several studies have indicated that cabergoline is safer and more effective than bromocriptine for reducing prolactin levels[200] and the dose can often be reduced after successful prolactin reduction, allowing for reductions in cost and adverse effects.[201] Although fewer studies have been published supporting the antirheumatic benefits of cabergoline than those supporting bromocriptine; its antirheumatic benefits have indeed been documented.[202]

o Estrogen (excess): A hormonal contribution to the immune dysfunction that underlies SLE is strongly suggested by the strong tendency of this disease to affect women, and by the timing of the onset of the disease during the years of highest estrogen levels and variability—generally *after menarche* and *before menopause.* **Men with rheumatoid**

[187] "CONCLUSION: The EA extract of TWHF at dosages up to 570 mg/day appeared to be safe, and doses > 360 mg/day were associated with clinical benefit in patients with RA." Tao X, Cush JJ, Garret M, Lipsky PE. A phase I study of ethyl acetate extract of the chinese antirheumatic herb Tripterygium wilfordii hook F in rheumatoid arthritis. *J Rheumatol.* 2001 Oct;28(10):2160-7
[188] "Our data suggests that triptolide may protect dopaminergic neurons from LPS-induced injury and its efficiency in inhibiting microglia activation may underlie the mechanism." Li FQ, Lu XZ, Liang XB, Zhou HF, Xue B, Liu XY, Niu DB, Han JS, Wang XM. Triptolide, a Chinese herbal extract, protects dopaminergic neurons from inflammation-mediated damage through inhibition of microglial activation. *J Neuroimmunol.* 2004 Mar;148(1-2):24-31
[189] "Moreover, tripchlorolide markedly prevented the decrease in amount of dopamine in the striatum of model rats. Taken together, our data provide the first evidence that tripchlorolide acts as a neuroprotective molecule that rescues MPP+ or axotomy-induced degeneration of dopaminergic neurons, which may imply its therapeutic potential for Parkinson's disease." Li FQ, Cheng XX, Liang XB, Wang XH, Xue B, He QH, Wang XM, Han JS. Neurotrophic and neuroprotective effects of tripchlorolide, an extract of Chinese herb Tripterygium wilfordii Hook F, on dopaminergic neurons. *Exp Neurol.* 2003 Jan;179(1):28-37
[190] "Of twenty-eight visual analogue scales rating mood and arousal, the subjects' ratings in the tyrosine treatment (9 g daily) and placebo periods differed significantly for only three (less tired, less drowsy, more alert)." Elwes RD, Crewes H, Chesterman LP, Summers B, Jenner P, Binnie CD, Parkes JD. Treatment of narcolepsy with L-tyrosine: double-blind placebo-controlled trial. *Lancet.* 1989 Nov 4;2(8671):1067-9
[191] "Ten men and 10 women subjects underwent these batteries 1 h after ingesting 150 mg/kg of l-tyrosine or placebo. Administration of tyrosine significantly enhanced accuracy and decreased frequency of list retrieval on the working memory task during the multiple task battery compared with placebo." Thomas JR, Lockwood PA, Singh A, Deuster PA. Tyrosine improves working memory in a multitasking environment. *Pharmacol Biochem Behav.* 1999 Nov;64(3):495-500
[192] "Ten subjects received five daily doses of a protein-rich drink containing 2 g tyrosine, and 11 subjects received a carbohydrate rich drink with the same amount of calories (255 kcal)." Deijen JB, Wientjes CJ, Vullinghs HF, Cloin PA, Langefeld JJ. Tyrosine improves cognitive performance and reduces blood pressure in cadets after one week of a combat training course. *Brain Res Bull.* 1999 Jan 15;48(2):203-9
[193] "Tyrosine (when compared to placebo) had no effect on any sleep related measure, but it did stimulate prolactin release." Waters WF, Magill RA, Bray GA, Volaufova J, Smith SR, Lieberman HR, Rood J, Hurry M, Anderson T, Ryan DH. A comparison of tyrosine against placebo, phentermine, caffeine, and D-amphetamine during sleep deprivation. *Nutr Neurosci.* 2003;6(4):221-35
[194] "Whereas carbohydrate meals had no discernible effects, high protein meals induced a large increase in both PRL and cortisol; high fat meals caused selective release of PRL." Ishizuka B, Quigley ME, Yen SS. Pituitary hormone release in response to food ingestion: evidence for neuroendocrine signals from gut to brain. *J Clin Endocrinol Metab.* 1983 Dec;57(6):1111-6
[195] Beers MH, Berkow R (eds). The Merck Manual. Seventeenth Edition. Whitehouse Station; Merck Research Laboratories 1999 Page 77-78
[196] "A prospective, double-blind, randomized, placebo-controlled study compared BRC at a fixed daily dosage of 2.5 mg with placebo... Long term treatment with a low dose of BRC appears to be a safe and effective means of decreasing SLE flares in SLE patients." Alvarez-Nemegyei J, Cobarrubias-Cobos A, Escalante-Triay F, Sosa-Munoz J, Miranda JM, Jara LJ. Bromocriptine in systemic lupus erythematosus: a double-blind, randomized, placebo-controlled study. *Lupus.* 1998;7(6):414-9
[197] Serri O, Chik CL, Ur E, Ezzat S. Diagnosis and management of hyperprolactinemia. *CMAJ.* 2003 Sep 16;169(6):575-81 http://www.cmaj.ca/cgi/content/full/169/6/575
[198] "...clinical observations and trials support the use of bromocriptine as a nonstandard primary or adjunctive treatment of recalcitrant RA, SLE, Reiter's syndrome, and psoriatic arthritis and associated conditions unresponsive to traditional approaches." McMurray RW. Bromocriptine in rheumatic and autoimmune diseases. *Semin Arthritis Rheum.* 2001 Aug;31(1):21-32
[199] Serri O, Chik CL, Ur E, Ezzat S. Diagnosis and management of hyperprolactinemia. *CMAJ.* 2003 Sep 16;169(6):575-81 http://www.cmaj.ca/cgi/content/full/169/6/575
[200] "CONCLUSION: These data indicate that cabergoline is a very effective agent for lowering the prolactin levels in hyperprolactinemic patients and that it appears to offer considerable advantage over bromocriptine in terms of efficacy and tolerability." Sabuncu T, Arikan E, Tasan E, Hatemi H. Comparison of the effects of cabergoline and bromocriptine on prolactin levels in hyperprolactinemic patients. *Intern Med.* 2001 Sep;40(9):857-61
[201] "Cabergoline also normalized PRL in the majority of patients with known bromocriptine intolerance or -resistance. Once PRL secretion was adequately controlled, the dose of cabergoline could often be significantly decreased, which further reduced costs of therapy." Verhelst J, Abs R, Maiter D, van den Bruel A, Vandeweghe M, Velkeniers B, Mockel J, Lamberigts G, Petrossians P, Coremans P, Mahler C, Stevenaert A, Verlooy J, Raftopoulos C, Beckers A. Cabergoline in the treatment of hyperprolactinemia: a study in 455 patients. *J Clin Endocrinol Metab.* 1999 Jul;84(7):2518-22 http://jcem.endojournals.org/cgi/content/full/84/7/2518
[202] Erb N, Pace AV, Delamere JP, Kitas GD. Control of unremitting rheumatoid arthritis by the prolactin antagonist cabergoline. *Rheumatology* (Oxford). 2001 Feb;40(2):237-9 http://rheumatology.oxfordjournals.org/cgi/content/full/40/2/237

arthritis show an excess of estradiol and a decrease in DHEA, and the **excess estrogen is proportional to the degree of inflammation**.[203] Serum estradiol is commonly used to assess estrogen status; estrogens can also be measured in 24-hour urine samples. Beyond looking at estrogens from a *quantitative* standpoint, they can also be *qualitatively* analyzed with respect to the ratio of estrone:estradiol:estriol as well as the balance between the "good" 2-hydroxyestrone relative to the purportedly carcinogenic and proinflammatory 16-alpha-hydroxyestrone. Interventions to combat high estrogen levels may include any effective combination of the following:

- Weight loss and weight optimization: In overweight patients, *weight loss* is the means to attaining the goal of *weight optimization*; the task is not complete until the body mass index is normalized/optimized. Excess adiposity and obesity raise estrogen levels due to high levels of aromatase (the hormone that makes estrogens from androgens) in adipose tissue; weight optimization and loss of excess fat helps normalize hormone levels and reduce inflammation.

- Avoidance of ethanol: Estrogen production is stimulated by ethanol intake.

- Consider surgical correction of varicocele in affected men: Men with varicocele have higher estrogen levels due to temperature-induced alterations in enzyme function in the testes; surgical correction of the varicocele lowers estrogen levels.

- "Anti-estrogen diet": Foods and supplements such as green tea, diindolylmethane (DIM), indole-3-carbinol (I3C), licorice, and a high-fiber crucifer-based "anti-estrogenic diet" can also be used; monitoring clinical status and serum estradiol will prove or disprove efficacy. Whereas 16-alpha-hydroxyestrone is pro-inflammatory and immunodysregulatory, 2-hydroxyestrone has anti-inflammatory action[204] and been described as "the good estrogen"[205] due to its anticancer and comparatively health-preserving qualities. **In a recent short-term study using I3C in patients with SLE, I3C supplementation at 375 mg per day was well tolerated and resulted in modest treatment-dependent clinical improvement as well as favorable modification of estrogen metabolism away from 16-alpha-hydroxyestrone and toward 2-hydroxyestrone.**[206]

- Anastrozole/Arimidex: In our office, we commonly measure serum estradiol in men and administer the aromatase inhibitor anastrozole/arimidex 1 mg (2-3 doses per week) to men whose estradiol level is greater than 32 picogram/mL. The Life Extension Foundation[207] advocates that the optimal serum estradiol level for a man is 10-30 picogram/mL. Clinical studies using anastrozole/arimidex in men have shown that aromatase blockade lowers estradiol and raises testosterone[208]; generally speaking, this is exactly the result that we want in patients with severe systemic autoimmunity. Frequency of dosing is based on serum and clinical response.

o Cortisol (insufficiency): Cortisol has immunoregulatory and "immunosuppressive" actions at physiological concentrations. Low adrenal function is common in patients with chronic inflammation.[209,210,211] Assessment of cortisol production and adrenal

---

[203] "RESULTS: DHEAS and estrone concentrations were lower and estradiol was higher in patients compared with healthy controls. DHEAS differed between RF positive and RF negative patients. Estrone did not correlate with any disease variable, whereas estradiol correlated strongly and positively with all measured indices of inflammation." Tengstrand B, Carlstrom K, Fellander-Tsai L, Hafstrom I. Abnormal levels of serum dehydroepiandrosterone, estrone, and estradiol in men with rheumatoid arthritis: high correlation between serum estradiol and current degree of inflammation. *J Rheumatol*. 2003 Nov;30(11):2338-43

[204] "Micromolar concentrations of beta-estradiol, estrone, 16-alpha-hydroxyestrone and estriol enhance the oxidative metabolism of activated human PMNL's. The corresponding 2-hydroxylated estrogens 2-OH-estradiol, 2-OH-estrone and 2-OH-estriol act on the contrary as powerful inhibitors of cell activity." Jansson G. Oestrogen-induced enhancement of myeloperoxidase activity in human polymorphonuclear leukocytes--a possible cause of oxidative stress in inflammatory cells. *Free Radic Res Commun*. 1991;14(3):195-208

[205] "Even more dramatically, in the case of laryngeal papillomas induction of 2-hydroxylation with indole-3-carbinol (I3C) has resulted in inhibition of tumor growth during the time that the patients continue to take I3C or vegetables rich in this compound." Bradlow HL, Telang NT, Sepkovic DW, Osborne MP. 2-hydroxyestrone: the 'good' estrogen. *J Endocrinol*. 1996 Sep;150 Suppl:S259-65

[206] "Women with SLE can manifest a metabolic response to I3C and might benefit from its antiestrogenic effects." McAlindon TE, Gulin J, Chen T, Klug T, Lahita R, Nuite M. Indole-3-carbinol in women with SLE: effect on estrogen metabolism and disease activity. *Lupus*. 2001;10(11):779-83

[207] Male Hormone Modulation Therapy, Page 4 Of 7: http://www.lef.org/protocols/prtcl-130c.shtml Accessed October 30, 2005

[208] "These data demonstrate that aromatase inhibition increases serum bioavailable and total testosterone levels to the youthful normal range in older men with mild hypogonadism." Leder BZ, Rohrer JL, Rubin SD, Gallo J, Longcope C. Effects of aromatase inhibition in elderly men with low or borderline-low serum testosterone levels. *J Clin Endocrinol Metab*. 2004 Mar;89(3):1174-80 http://jcem.endojournals.org/cgi/reprint/89/3/1174

[209] "Yet evidence that patients with rheumatoid arthritis improved with small, physiologic dosages of cortisol or cortisone acetate was reported over 25 years ago, and that patients with chronic allergic disorders or unexplained chronic fatigue also improved with administration of such small dosages was reported over 15 years ago..." Jefferies WM. Mild adrenocortical deficiency, chronic allergies, autoimmune disorders and the chronic fatigue syndrome: a continuation of the cortisone story. *Med Hypotheses*. 1994 Mar;42(3):183-9 http://www.thebuteykocentre.com/Irish_%20Buteykocenter_files/further_studies/med_hyp2.pdf http://members.westnet.com.au/pkolb/med_hyp2.pdf

function was detailed in Chapter 4 under the section of Orthoendocrinology. Supplementation with 20 mg per day of cortisol/Cortef is physiologic; my preference is to dose 10 mg first thing in the morning, then 5 mg in late morning and 5 mg in midafternoon in an attempt to replicate the diurnal variation and normal morning peak of cortisol levels. In patients with hypoadrenalism, administration of pregnenolone in doses of 10-60 mg in the morning may also be beneficial.

- Testosterone (insufficiency): Androgen deficiencies predispose to, are exacerbated by, and contribute to autoimmune/inflammatory disorders. A large proportion of men with SLE or RA have low testosterone[212] and suffer the effects of hypogonadism: fatigue, weakness, depression, slow healing, low libido, and difficulties with sexual performance. Testosterone levels may rise following DHEA supplementation (especially in women) and can be elevated in men by the use of anastrozole/arimidex. Otherwise, transdermal testosterone such as Androgel or Testim can be applied as indicated. Wright[213] previously recommended 5-10 mg/day for females, 50-100 mg/day for males, if testosterone levels were low.

- DHEA: DHEA is an anti-inflammatory and immunoregulatory hormone that is commonly deficient in patients with autoimmunity, including polymyalgia rheumatica, SLE, RA, and inflammatory arthritis.[214,215] DHEA levels are suppressed by prednisone[216], and DHEA has been shown to reverse the osteoporosis and loss of bone mass induced by corticosteroid treatment.[217] DHEA shows no acute or subacute toxicity even when used in supraphysiologic doses, even when used in sick patients. For example, in a study of 32 patients with HIV, DHEA doses of 750 mg – 2,250 mg per day were well-tolerated and produced no dose-limiting adverse effects.[218] This lack of toxicity compares favorably with any and all so-called "antirheumatic" drugs, nearly all of which show impressive comparable toxicity. **High-dose supplemental DHEA has benefits in the treatment of SLE that are comparable to those obtained with antimalarial drugs.[219]** When used at doses of 200 mg per day, DHEA safely provides clinical benefit for patients with various autoimmune diseases, including ulcerative colitis, Crohn's disease[220], and SLE.[221] In patients with SLE, DHEA supplementation allows for reduced dosing of prednisone (thus avoiding its adverse effects) while providing symptomatic improvement.[222] Optimal clinical response appears to correlate with serum levels that are supraphysiologic[223], and therefore treatment may be implemented with little regard for initial/baseline DHEA levels provided that the patient is free of contraindications,

[210] "The etiology of rheumatoid arthritis ...explained by a combination of three factors: (i) a relatively mild deficiency of cortisol, …, (ii) a deficiency of DHEA, …and (iii) infection by organisms such as mycoplasma,..." Jefferies WM. The etiology of rheumatoid arthritis. Med Hypotheses. 1998 Aug;51(2):111-4

[211] Jefferies W McK. Safe Uses of Cortisol. Second Edition. Springfield, CC Thomas, 1996

[212] Karagiannis A, Harsoulis F. Gonadal dysfunction in systemic diseases. Eur J Endocrinol. 2005 Apr;152(4):501-13 http://www.eje-online.org/cgi/content/full/152/4/501

[213] Gaby A, Wright JV. Nutritional Protocols. 1998 Nutrition Seminars

[214] "The low levels found in patients with PM:TA are in accordance with those previously reported in immune-mediated diseases such as systemic lupus erythematosus (SLE) and rheumatoid arthritis, suggesting that diminution of DHEAS is a constant endocrinologic feature in these categories of patients." Nilsson E, de la Torre B, Hedman M, Goobar J, Thorner A. Blood dehydroepiandrosterone sulphate (DHEAS) levels in polymyalgia rheumatica/giant cell arteritis and primary fibromyalgia. Clin Exp Rheumatol. 1994 Jul-Aug;12(4):415-7

[215] "DHEAS concentrations were significantly decreased in both women and men with inflammatory arthritis (IA) (P < 0.001)." Dessein PH, Joffe BI, Stanwix AE, Moomal Z. Hyposecretion of the adrenal androgen dehydroepiandrosterone sulfate and its relation to clinical variables in inflammatory arthritis. Arthritis Res. 2001;3(3):183-8. Epub 2001 Feb 21. http://arthritis-research.com/content/3/3/183

[216] "Basal serum DHEA and DHEAS concentrations were suppressed to a greater degree than was cortisol during both daily and alternate day prednisone treatments. ...Thus, adrenal androgen secretion was more easily suppressed than was cortisol secretion by this low dose of glucocorticoid, but there was no advantage to alternate day therapy." Rittmaster RS, Givner ML. Effect of daily and alternate day low dose prednisone on serum cortisol and adrenal androgens in hirsute women. J Clin Endocrinol Metab. 1988 Aug;67(2):400-3

[217] "CONCLUSION: Prasterone treatment prevented BMD loss and significantly increased BMD at both the lumbar spine and total hip in female patients with SLE receiving exogenous glucocorticoids." Mease PJ, Ginzler EM, Gluck OS, Schiff M, Goldman A, Greenwald M, Cohen S, Egan R, Quarles BJ, Schwartz KE. Effects of prasterone on bone mineral density in women with systemic lupus erythematosus receiving chronic glucocorticoid therapy. J Rheumatol. 2005 Apr;32(4):616-21

[218] "Thirty-one subjects were evaluated and monitored for safety and tolerance. The oral drug was administered three times daily in doses ranging from 750 mg/day to 2,250 mg/day for 16 weeks. ... The drug was well tolerated and no dose-limiting side effects were noted." Dyner TS, Lang W, Geaga J, Golub A, Stites D, Winger E, Galmarini M, Masterson J, Jacobson MA. An open-label dose-escalation trial of oral dehydroepiandrosterone tolerance and pharmacokinetics in patients with HIV disease. J Acquir Immune Defic Syndr. 1993 May;6(5):459-65

[219] Tierney ML. McPhee SJ, Papadakis MA. Current Medical Diagnosis and Treatment 2006. 45th edition. New York; Lange Medical Books: 2006, pages 833-837

[220] "CONCLUSIONS: In a pilot study, dehydroepiandrosterone was effective and safe in patients with refractory Crohn's disease or ulcerative colitis." Andus T, Klebl F, Rogler G, Bregenzer N, Scholmerich J, Straub RH. Patients with refractory Crohn's disease or ulcerative colitis respond to dehydroepiandrosterone: a pilot study. Aliment Pharmacol Ther. 2003 Feb;17(3):409-14

[221] "CONCLUSION: The overall results confirm that DHEA treatment was well-tolerated, significantly reduced the number of SLE flares, and improved patient's global assessment of disease activity." Chang DM, Lan JL, Lin HY, Luo SF. Dehydroepiandrosterone treatment of women with mild-to-moderate systemic lupus erythematosus: a multicenter randomized, double-blind, placebo-controlled trial. Arthritis Rheum. 2002 Nov;46(11):2924-7

[222] "CONCLUSION: Among women with lupus disease activity, reducing the dosage of prednisone to < or = 7.5 mg/day for a sustained period of time while maintaining stabilization or a reduction of disease activity was possible in a significantly greater proportion of patients treated with oral prasterone, 200 mg once daily, compared with patients treated with placebo." Petri MA, Lahita RG, Van Vollenhoven RF, Merrill JT, Schiff M, Ginzler EM, Strand V, Kunz A, Gorelick KJ, Schwartz KE; GL601 Study Group. Effects of prasterone on corticosteroid requirements of women with systemic lupus erythematosus: a double-blind, randomized, placebo-controlled trial. Arthritis Rheum. 2002 Jul;46(7):1820-9

[223] "CONCLUSION: The clinical response to DHEA was not clearly dose dependent. Serum levels of DHEA and DHEAS correlated only weakly with lupus outcomes, but suggested an optimum serum DHEAS of 1000 microg/dl." Barry NN, McGuire JL, van Vollenhoven RF. Dehydroepiandrosterone in systemic lupus erythematosus: relationship between dosage, serum levels, and clinical response. J Rheumatol. 1998 Dec;25(12):2352-6

particularly high risk for sex-hormone-dependent malignancy. Other than mild adverse effects predictable with any androgen (namely voice deepening, transient acne, and increased facial hair), DHEA supplementation does not cause serious adverse effects[224], and it is appropriate for routine clinical use particularly when 1) the dose of DHEA is kept as low as possible, 2) duration is kept as short as possible, 3) other interventions are used to address the underlying cause of the disease, 4) the patient is deriving benefit, and 5) the risk-to-benefit ratio is favorable.

- o <u>Thyroid (insufficiency or autoimmunity)</u>: Overt or imminent hypothyroidism is suggested by TSH greater than 2 mU/L[225] or 3 mU/L[226], low T4 or T3, and/or the presence of anti-thyroid peroxidase antibodies.[227] Hypothyroidism can cause an inflammatory myopathy that can resemble polymyositis, and hypothyroidism is a frequent complication of any and all autoimmune diseases. Specific treatment considerations include the following:
  - <u>Selenium</u>: Supplementation with either selenomethonine[228] or sodium selenite[229,230] can reduce thyroid autoimmunity and improve peripheral conversion of T4 to T3. Selenium may be started at 500-800 mcg per day and tapered to 200-400 mcg per day for maintenance.[231]
  - <u>L-thyroxine/levothyroxine/Synthroid—prescription synthetic T4</u>: 25-50 mcg per day is a common starting dose which can be adjusted based on clinical and laboratory response. Thyroid hormone supplements must be consumed separately from soy products (by at least 1-2 hours) and preferably on an empty stomach to avoid absorption interference by food, fiber, and minerals, especially calcium. Doses are generally started at one-half of the daily dose for the first 10 days after which the full dose is used. Caution must be applied in patients with adrenal insufficiency and/or those with cardiovascular disease.
  - <u>Armour thyroid—prescription natural T4 and T3 from cow/pig thyroid gland</u>: 60 mg (one grain) is a common starting and maintenance dose. Due to the exacerbating effect on thyroid autoimmunity, Armour thyroid is never used in patients with thyroid autoimmunity.
  - <u>Thyrolar/Liotrix—prescription synthetic T4 with T3</u>: Dosed as "1", "2", or "3." This product has been difficult to obtain for the past few years due to manufacturing problems (http://thyrolar.com/); previously it was my treatment of choice due to the combination of T4 and T3 and the lack of antigenicity compared to gland-derived products.
  - <u>Liothyronine, Cytomel®</u>: Cytomel is prescription synthetic T3. Except in patients with myxedema for whom the appropriate starting dose is 5 mcg per day, treatment generally starts with 25 mcg per day and can be increased to 75 mcg per day; dose is adjusted based on clinical and laboratory response.[232] As stated previously, thyroid hormone supplements must be consumed separately from

[224] Tierney ML. McPhee SJ, Papadakis MA. <u>Current Medical Diagnosis and Treatment 2006, 45th edition</u>. New York; Lange Medical Books: 2006, page 1721

[225] Weetman AP. Hypothyroidism: screening and subclinical disease. *BMJ*. 1997 Apr 19;314(7088):1175-8 http://bmj.bmjjournals.com/cgi/content/full/314/7088/1175

[226] "Now AACE encourages doctors to consider treatment for patients who test outside the boundaries of a narrower margin based on a target TSH level of 0.3 to 3.0. AACE believes the new range will result in proper diagnosis for millions of Americans who suffer from a mild thyroid disorder, but have gone untreated until now." American Association of Clinical Endocrinologists (AACE). 2003 Campaign Encourages Awareness of Mild Thyroid Failure, Importance of Routine Testing http://www.aace.com/pub/tam2003/press.php November 26, 2005

[227] Beers MH, Berkow R (eds). <u>The Merck Manual. Seventeenth Edition</u>. Whitehouse Station; Merck Research Laboratories 1999 Page 96

[228] Duntas LH, Mantzou E, Koutras DA. Effects of a six month treatment with selenomethionine in patients with autoimmune thyroiditis. *Eur J Endocrinol*. 2003 Apr;148(4):389-93 http://eje-online.org/cgi/reprint/148/4/389

[229] Gartner R, Gasnier BC, Dietrich JW, Krebs B, Angstwurm MW. Selenium supplementation in patients with autoimmune thyroiditis decreases thyroid peroxidase antibodies concentrations. *J Clin Endocrinol Metab*. 2002 Apr;87(4):1687-91 http://jcem.endojournals.org/cgi/content/full/87/4/1687

[230] "We recently conducted a prospective, placebo-controlled clinical study, where we could demonstrate, that a substitution of 200 wg sodium selenite for three months in patients with autoimmune thyroiditis reduced thyroid peroxidase antibody (TPO-Ab) concentrations significantly." Gartner R, Gasnier BC. Selenium in the treatment of autoimmune thyroiditis. *Biofactors*. 2003;19(3-4):165-70

[231] Bruns F, Micke O, Bremer M. Current status of selenium and other treatments for secondary lymphedema. *J Support Oncol*. 2003 Jul-Aug;1(2):121-30 http://www.supportiveoncology.net/journal/articles/0102121.pdf

[232] http://www.kingpharm.com/uploads/pdf_inserts/Cytomel_Web_PI.pdf

soy products (by at least 1-2 hours) and preferably on an empty stomach to avoid absorption interference by food, fiber, and minerals, especially calcium.

- **Thyroid glandular—nonprescription T3**: Producers of nutritional products are able to distribute T3 because it is not listed by the FDA as a prescription item. Nutritional supplement companies may start with Armour thyroid, remove the T4, and sell the thyroid glandular with active T3 thereby providing a nonprescription source of active thyroid hormone. For many patients, one tablet per day is at least as effective as a prescription source of thyroid hormone. Since it is derived from a glandular and therefore potentially antigenic source, thyroid glandular is not used in patients with thyroid autoimmunity due to its ability to induce increased production of anti-thyroid antibodies.

- **L-tyrosine and iodine**: Some patients with mild hypothyroidism respond to supplementation with L-tyrosine and iodine. Tyrosine is commonly used in doses of 4-9 grams per day in divided doses. According to Abraham and Wright[233], doses of iodine may be as high as 12.5 milligrams (12,500 micrograms), which is slightly less than the average daily intake in Japan at 13.8 mg per day.

- <u>Oral enzyme therapy with proteolytic/pancreatic enzymes</u>: Polyenzyme supplementation is used to ameliorate the pathophysiology induced by immune complexes, such as the related condition rheumatoid arthritis.[234]

- <u>CoQ10 (antihypertensive, renoprotective, and probably immunomodulatory)</u>: CoQ10 is a powerful antioxidant with a wide margin of safety and excellent clinical tolerability. **At least four studies have documented its powerful blood-pressure-lowering ability, which often surpasses the clinical effectiveness of antihypertensive drugs.[235,236,237,238] Furthermore, at least two published papers[239,240] and one case report[241] advocate that CoQ10 has powerful renoprotective benefits.** CoQ10 levels are low in patients with allergies[242], and the symptomatic relief that many allergic patients experience following supplementation with CoQ10 suggests that CoQ10 has an immunomodulatory effect. Common doses start at > 100 mg per day with food; doses of 200 mg per day are not uncommon, and doses up to 1,000 mg per day are clinically well tolerated though the high financial toll resembles that of many pharmaceutical drugs.

- *Uncaria tomentosa, Uncaria guianensis*: Cat's claw has been safely and successfully used in the treatment of osteoarthritis[243] and rheumatoid arthritis.[244] High-quality extractions from reputable manufacturers used according to directions are recommended. Most products contain between 250-500 mg and are standardized to 3.0% alkaloids and 15% total polyphenols; QD-TID po dosing should be sufficient as *part* of a comprehensive plan.

- *Harpagophytum procumbens*: Harpagophytum is a moderately effective botanical analgesic for musculoskeletal pain.[245,246,247,248,249] Products are generally standardized for the content of harpagosides, with a target dose of 60 mg harpagoside per day.[250]

[233] Wright JV. Why you need 83 times more of this essential, cancer-fighting nutrient than the "experts" say you do. *Nutrition and Healing* 2005; volume 12, issue 4.

[234] Galebskaya LV, Ryumina EV, Niemerovsky VS, Matyukov AA. Human complement system state after wobenzyme intake. *VESTNIK MOSKOVSKOGO UNIVERSITETA. KHIMIYA*. 2000. Vol. 41, No. 6. Supplement. Pages 148-149

[235] Burke BE, Neuenschwander R, Olson RD. Randomized, double-blind, placebo-controlled trial of coenzyme Q10 in isolated systolic hypertension. *South Med J*. 2001 Nov;94(11):1112-7

[236] Singh RB, Niaz MA, Rastogi SS, Shukla PK, Thakur AS. Effect of hydrosoluble coenzyme Q10 on blood pressures and insulin resistance in hypertensive patients with coronary artery disease. *J Hum Hypertens*. 1999 Mar;13(3):203-8

[237] Digiesi V, Cantini F, Oradei A, Bisi G, Guarino GC, Brocchi A, Bellandi F, Mancini M, Littarru GP. Coenzyme Q10 in essential hypertension. *Mol Aspects Med*. 1994;15 Suppl:s257-63

[238] Langsjoen P, Langsjoen P, Willis R, Folkers K. Treatment of essential hypertension with coenzyme Q10. *Mol Aspects Med*. 1994;15 Suppl:S265-72

[239] Singh RB, Khanna HK, Niaz MA. Randomized, double-blind placebo-controlled trial of coenzyme Q10 in chronic renal failure: discovery of a new role. *J Nutr Environ Med* 2000;10:281-8

[240] Singh RB, Kumar A, Naiz MA, Singh RG, Gujrati S, Singh VP, Singh M, Singh UP, Taneja C, AND Rastogi SS. Randomized, Double-blind, Placebo-controlled Trial of Coenzyme Q10 in Patients with End-stage Renal Failure. *J Nutr Environ Med* 2003; Volume 13, Number 1: 13–22

[241] Singh RB, Singh MM. Effects of CoQ10 in new indications with antioxidant vitamin deficiency. *J Nutr Environ Med* 1999; 9:223-228

[242] Ye CQ, Folkers K, Tamagawa H, Pfeiffer C. A modified determination of coenzyme Q10 in human blood and CoQ10 blood levels in diverse patients with allergies. *Biofactors*. 1988 Dec;1(4):303-6

[243] Piscoya J, Rodriguez Z, Bustamante SA, Okuhama NN, Miller MJ, Sandoval M. Efficacy and safety of freeze-dried cat's claw in osteoarthritis of the knee: mechanisms of action of the species Uncaria guianensis. *Inflamm Res*. 2001 Sep;50(9):442-8

[244] "This small preliminary study demonstrates relative safety and modest benefit to the tender joint count of a highly purified extract from the pentacyclic chemotype of UT in patients with active RA taking sulfasalazine or hydroxychloroquine." Mur E, Hartig F, Eibl G, Schirmer M. Randomized double blind trial of an extract from the pentacyclic alkaloid-chemotype of uncaria tomentosa for the treatment of rheumatoid arthritis. *J Rheumatol*. 2002 Apr;29(4):678-81

[245] Chrubasik S, Thanner J, Kunzel O, Conradt C, Black A, Pollak S. Comparison of outcome measures during treatment with the proprietary Harpagophytum extract doloteffin in patients with pain in the lower back, knee or hip. *Phytomedicine* 2002 Apr;9(3):181-94

[246] Chantre P, Cappelaere A, Leblan D, Guedon D, Vandermander J, Fournie B. Efficacy and tolerance of Harpagophytum procumbens versus diacerhein in treatment of osteoarthritis. *Phytomedicine* 2000 Jun;7(3):177-83

[247] Leblan D, Chantre P, Fournie B. Harpagophytum procumbens in the treatment of knee and hip osteoarthritis. Four-month results of a prospective, multicenter, double-blind trial versus diacerhein. *Joint Bone Spine* 2000;67(5):462-7

- <u>Willow bark</u>: Extracts from willow bark have proven safe and effective in the alleviation of moderate/severe low-back pain.[251,252] The mechanism of action appears to be inhibition of prostaglandin formation via inhibition of cyclooxygenase-2 gene transcription[253] by salicylates, phytonutrients which are widely present in fruits, vegetables, herbs and spices and which are partly responsible for the anti-cancer, anti-inflammatory, and health-promoting benefits of plant consumption.[254,255] According to a letter by Vasquez and Muanza[256], the only adverse effect that has been documented in association with willow bark was a single case of anaphylaxis in a patient previously sensitized to acetylsalicylic acid.

- *Boswellia serrata*: *Boswellia* shows clear anti-inflammatory and analgesic action via inhibition of 5-lipoxygenase[257] and clinical benefits have been demonstrated in patients with osteoarthritis of the knees[258] as well as asthma[259] and ulcerative colitis.[260] Products are generally standardized to contain 37.5–65% boswellic acids, with a target dose of approximately 150 mg of boswellic acids TID; dose and number of capsules/tablets will vary depending upon the concentration found in differing products. A German study showing that *Boswellia* was ineffective for rheumatoid arthritis[261] was poorly conducted, with inadequate follow-up, inadequate controls, and abnormal dosing of the herb.

- <u>Phytonutritional modulation of NF-kappaB</u>: As a stimulator of pro-inflammatory gene transcription, NF-kappaB is almost universally activated in conditions associated with inflammation.[262,263] Nutrients and botanicals which either directly or indirectly inhibit NF-kappaB for an anti-inflammatory benefit include vitamin D[264,265], curcumin[266] (requires piperine for absorption[267]), lipoic acid[268], green tea[269], ursolic acid[270] from rosemary[271], grape seed extract[272],

[248] "…subgroup analyses suggested that the effect was confined to patients with more severe and radiating pain accompanied by neurological deficit. …a slightly different picture, with the benefits seeming, if anything, to be greatest in the H600 group and in patients without more severe pain, radiation or neurological deficit." Chrubasik S, Junck H, Breitschwerdt H, Conradt C, Zappe H. Effectiveness of Harpagophytum extract WS 1531 in the treatment of exacerbation of low back pain: a randomized, placebo-controlled, double-blind study. *Eur J Anaesthesiol* 1999 Feb;16(2):118-29
[249] Chrubasik S, Model A, Black A, Pollak S. A randomized double-blind pilot study comparing Doloteffin and Vioxx in the treatment of low back pain. *Rheumatology* (Oxford). 2003 Jan;42(1):141-8
[250] "They took an 8-week course of Doloteffin at a dose providing 60 mg harpagoside per day… Doloteffin is well worth considering for osteoarthritic knee and hip pain and nonspecific low back pain." Chrubasik S, Thanner J, Kunzel O, Conradt C, Black A, Pollak S. Comparison of outcome measures during treatment with the proprietary Harpagophytum extract doloteffin in patients with pain in the lower back, knee or hip. *Phytomedicine* 2002 Apr;9(3):181-94
[251] Chrubasik S, Eisenberg E, Balan E, Weinberger T, Luzzati R, Conradt C. Treatment of low-back pain exacerbations with willow bark extract: a randomized double-blind study. *Am J Med.* 2000;109:9-14
[252] Chrubasik S, Kunzel O, Model A, Conradt C, Black A. Treatment of low-back pain with a herbal or synthetic anti-rheumatic: a randomized controlled study. Willow bark extract for low-back pain. *Rheumatology* (Oxford). 2001;40:1388-93
[253] Hare LG, Woodside JV, Young IS. Dietary salicylates. *J Clin Pathol* 2003 Sep;56(9):649-50
[254] Lawrence JR, Peter R, Baxter GJ, Robson J, Graham AB, Paterson JR. Urinary excretion of salicyluric and salicylic acids by non-vegetarians, vegetarians, and patients taking low dose aspirin. *J Clin Pathol.* 2003 Sep;56(9):651-3
[255] Paterson JR, Lawrence JR. Salicylic acid: a link between aspirin, diet and the prevention of colorectal cancer. *QJM.* 2001 Aug;94(8):445-8
[256] Vasquez A, Muanza DN. Evaluation of Presence of Aspirin-Related Warnings with Willow Bark: Comment on the Article by Clauson et al. *Ann Pharmacotherapy* 2005 Oct;39(10):1763
[257] Wildfeuer A, Neu IS, Safayhi H, Metzger G, Wehrmann M, Vogel U, Ammon HP. Effects of boswellic acids extracted from a herbal medicine on the biosynthesis of leukotrienes and the course of experimental autoimmune encephalomyelitis. *Arzneimittelforschung* 1998 Jun;48(6):668-74
[258] Kimmatkar N, Thawani V, Hingorani L, Khiyani R. Efficacy and tolerability of Boswellia serrata extract in treatment of osteoarthritis of knee--a randomized double blind placebo controlled trial. *Phytomedicine.* 2003 Jan;10(1):3-7
[259] Gupta I, Gupta V, Parihar A, Gupta S, Ludtke R, Safayhi H, Ammon HP. Effects of Boswellia serrata gum resin in patients with bronchial asthma: results of a double-blind, placebo-controlled, 6-week clinical study. *Eur J Med Res.* 1998 Nov 17;3(11):511-4
[260] Gupta I, Parihar A, Malhotra P, Singh GB, Ludtke R, Safayhi H, Ammon HP. Effects of Boswellia serrata gum resin in patients with ulcerative colitis. *Eur J Med Res.* 1997 Jan;2(1):37-43
[261] Sander O, Herborn G, Rau R. [Is H15 (resin extract of Boswellia serrata, "incense") a useful supplement to established drug therapy of chronic polyarthritis? Results of a double-blind pilot study] [Article in German] *Z Rheumatol.* 1998 Feb;57(1):11-6
[262] Tak PP, Firestein GS. NF-kappaB: a key role in inflammatory diseases. *J Clin Invest.* 2001 Jan;107(1):7-11 http://www.jci.org/cgi/content/full/107/1/7
[263] D'Acquisto F, May MJ, Ghosh S. Inhibition of Nuclear Factor KappaB (NF-B): An Emerging Theme in Anti-Inflammatory Therapies. *Mol Interv.* 2002 Feb;2(1):22-35 http://molinterv.aspetjournals.org/cgi/content/abstract/2/1/22
[264] "1Alpha,25-dihydroxyvitamin D3 (1,25-(OH)2-D3), the active metabolite of vitamin D, can inhibit NF-kappaB activity in human MRC-5 fibroblasts, targeting DNA binding of NF-kappaB but not translocation of its subunits p50 and p65." Harant H, Wolff B, Lindley IJ. 1Alpha,25-dihydroxyvitamin D3 decreases DNA binding of nuclear factor-kappaB in human fibroblasts. *FEBS Lett.* 1998 Oct 9;436(3):329-34
[265] "Thus, 1,25(OH)₂D₃ may negatively regulate IL-12 production by downregulation of NF-kB activation and binding to the p40-kB sequence." D'Ambrosio D, Cippitelli M, Cocciolo MG, Mazzeo D, Di Lucia P, Lang R, Sinigaglia F, Panina-Bordignon P. Inhibition of IL-12 production by 1,25-dihydroxyvitamin D3. Involvement of NF-kappaB downregulation in transcriptional repression of the p40 gene. *J Clin Invest.* 1998 Jan 1;101(1):252-62
[266] "Curcumin, EGCG and resveratrol have been shown to suppress activation of NF-kappa B." Surh YJ, Chun KS, Cha HH, Han SS, Keum YS, Park KK, Lee SS. Molecular mechanisms underlying chemopreventive activities of anti-inflammatory phytochemicals: down-regulation of COX-2 and iNOS through suppression of NF-kappa B activation. *Mutat Res.* 2001 Sep 1;480-481:243-68
[267] Shoba G, Joy D, Joseph T, Majeed M, Rajendran R, Srinivas PS. Influence of piperine on the pharmacokinetics of curcumin in animals and human volunteers. *Planta Med.* 1998 May;64(4):353-6
[268] "ALA reduced the TNF-alpha-stimulated ICAM-1 expression in a dose-dependent manner, to levels observed in unstimulated cells. Alpha-lipoic acid also reduced NF-kappaB activity in these cells in a dose-dependent manner." Lee HA, Hughes DA.Alpha-lipoic acid modulates NF-kappaB activity in human monocytic cells by direct interaction with DNA. *Exp Gerontol.* 2002 Jan-Mar;37(2-3):401-10
[269] "In conclusion, EGCG is an effective inhibitor of IKK activity. This may explain, at least in part, some of the reported anti-inflammatory and anticancer effects of green tea." Yang F, Oz HS, Barve S, de Villiers WJ, McClain CJ, Varilek GW. The green tea polyphenol (-)-epigallocatechin-3-gallate blocks nuclear factor-kappa B activation by inhibiting I kappa B kinase activity in the intestinal epithelial cell line IEC-6. *Mol Pharmacol.* 2001 Sep;60(3):528-33
[270] Shishodia S, Majumdar S, Banerjee S, Aggarwal BB. Ursolic acid inhibits nuclear factor-kappaB activation induced by carcinogenic agents through suppression of IkappaBalpha kinase and p65 phosphorylation: correlation with down-regulation of cyclooxygenase 2, matrix metalloproteinase 9, and cyclin D1. *Cancer Res.* 2003 Aug 1;63(15):4375-83 http://cancerres.aacrjournals.org/cgi/content/full/63/15/4375
[271] "These results suggest that carnosol suppresses the NO production and iNOS gene expression by inhibiting NF-kappaB activation, and provide possible mechanisms for its anti-inflammatory and chemopreventive action." Lo AH, Liang YC, Lin-Shiau SY, Ho CT, Lin JK. Carnosol, an antioxidant in rosemary, suppresses inducible nitric oxide synthase through down-regulating nuclear factor-kappaB in mouse macrophages. *Carcinogenesis.* 2002 Jun;23(6):983-91

propolis[273], zinc[274], high-dose selenium[275], indole-3-carbinol[276,277], N-acetyl-L-cysteine[278], resveratrol[279,280], isohumulones[281], GLA via PPAR-gamma[282] and EPA via PPAR-alpha.[283] I have reviewed the phytonutritional modulation of NF-kappaB later in this text and elsewhere.[284] Several phytonutritional products targeting NF-kappaB are commercially available.

- <u>Sunscreen</u>: Sunscreen, long-sleeve shirts, and hats can be used to protect against photosensitivity; vitamin D needs can be met with supplementation at physiologic doses, generally 2,000-10,000 IU per day for adults.[285]

- <u>Avoidance of *Echinacea*</u>: *Echinacea* refers to a species of immunostimulating herbs with several valid clinical indications. However, its use has been anecdotally associated with flares of lupus nephritis in patients with previously quiescent lupus.[286]

[272] "Constitutive and TNFalpha-induced NF-kappaB DNA binding activity was inhibited by GSE at doses > or =50 microg/ml and treatments for > or =12 h." Dhanalakshmi S, Agarwal R, Agarwal C. Inhibition of NF-kappaB pathway in grape seed extract-induced apoptotic death of human prostate carcinoma DU145 cells. *Int J Oncol.* 2003 Sep;23(3):721-7

[273] "Caffeic acid phenethyl ester (CAPE) is an anti-inflammatory component of propolis (honeybee resin). CAPE is reportedly a specific inhibitor of nuclear factor-kappaB (NF-kappaB)." Fitzpatrick LR, Wang J, Le T. Caffeic acid phenethyl ester, an inhibitor of nuclear factor-kappaB, attenuates bacterial peptidoglycan polysaccharide-induced colitis in rats. *J Pharmacol Exp Ther.* 2001 Dec;299(3):915-20

[274] "Our results suggest that zinc supplementation may lead to downregulation of the inflammatory cytokines through upregulation of the negative feedback loop A20 to inhibit induced NF-kappaB activation." Prasad AS, Bao B, Beck FW, Kucuk O, Sarkar FH. Antioxidant effect of zinc in humans. *Free Radic Biol Med.* 2004 Oct 15;37(8):1182-90

[275] Note that the patients in this study received a very high dose of selenium: 960 micrograms per day. This is at the top—and some would say over the top—of the safe and reasonable dose for long-term supplementation. In this case, the study lasted for three months. "In patients receiving selenium supplementation, selenium NF-kappaB activity was significantly reduced, reaching the same level as the nondiabetic control group. CONCLUSION: In type 2 diabetic patients, activation of NF-kappaB measured in peripheral blood monocytes can be reduced by selenium supplementation, confirming its importance in the prevention of cardiovascular diseases." Faure P, Ramon O, Favier A, Halimi S. Selenium supplementation decreases nuclear factor-kappa B activity in peripheral blood mononuclear cells from type 2 diabetic patients. *Eur J Clin Invest.* 2004 Jul;34(7):475-81

[276] Takada Y, Andreeff M, Aggarwal BB. Indole-3-carbinol suppresses NF-{kappa}B and I{kappa}B{alpha} kinase activation causing inhibition of expression of NF-{kappa}B-regulated antiapoptotic and metastatic gene products and enhancement of apoptosis in myeloid and leukemia cells. *Blood.* 2005 Apr 5; [Epub ahead of print]

[277] "Overall, our results indicated that indole-3-carbinol inhibits NF-kappaB and NF-kappaB-regulated gene expression and that this mechanism may provide the molecular basis for its ability to suppress tumorigenesis." Takada Y, Andreeff M, Aggarwal BB. Indole-3-carbinol suppresses NF-kappaB and IkappaBalpha kinase activation, causing inhibition of expression of NF-kappaB-regulated antiapoptotic and metastatic gene products and enhancement of apoptosis in myeloid and leukemia cells. *Blood.* 2005 Jul 15;106(2):641-9. Epub 2005 Apr 5.

[278] "CONCLUSIONS: Administration of N-acetylcysteine results in decreased nuclear factor-kappa B activation in patients with sepsis, associated with decreases in interleukin-8 but not interleukin-6 or soluble intercellular adhesion molecule-1. These pilot data suggest that antioxidant therapy with N-acetylcysteine may be useful in blunting the inflammatory response to sepsis." Paterson RL, Galley HF, Webster NR. The effect of N-acetylcysteine on nuclear factor-kappa B activation, interleukin-6, interleukin-8, and intercellular adhesion molecule-1 expression in patients with sepsis. *Crit Care Med.* 2003 Nov;31(11):2574-8

[279] "Resveratrol's anticarcinogenic, anti-inflammatory, and growth-modulatory effects may thus be partially ascribed to the inhibition of activation of NF-kappaB and AP-1 and the associated kinases." Manna SK, Mukhopadhyay A, Aggarwal BB. Resveratrol suppresses TNF-induced activation of nuclear transcription factors NF-kappa B, activator protein-1, and apoptosis: potential role of reactive oxygen intermediates and lipid peroxidation. *J Immunol.* 2000 Jun 15;164(12):6509-19

[280] "Both resveratrol and quercetin inhibited NF-kappaB-, AP-1- and CREB-dependent transcription to a greater extent than the glucocorticosteroid, dexamethasone." Donnelly LE, Newton R, Kennedy GE, Fenwick PS, Leung RH, Ito K, Russell RE, Barnes PJ. Anti-inflammatory Effects of Resveratrol in Lung Epithelial Cells: Molecular Mechanisms. *Am J Physiol Lung Cell Mol Physiol.* 2004 Jun 4 [Epub ahead of print]

[281] Yajima H, Ikeshima E, Shiraki M, Kanaya T, Fujiwara D, Odai H, Tsuboyama-Kasaoka N, Ezaki O, Oikawa S, Kondo K. Isohumulones, bitter acids derived from hops, activate both peroxisome proliferator-activated receptor alpha and gamma and reduce insulin resistance. *J Biol Chem.* 2004 Aug 6;279(32):33456-62. Epub 2004 Jun 3. http://www.jbc.org/cgi/content/full/279/32/33456

[282] "Thus, PPAR gamma serves as the receptor for GLA in the regulation of gene expression in breast cancer cells. " Jiang WG, Redfern A, Bryce RP, Mansel RE. Peroxisome proliferator activated receptor-gamma (PPAR-gamma) mediates the action of gamma linolenic acid in breast cancer cells. *Prostaglandins Leukot Essent Fatty Acids.* 2000 Feb;62(2):119-27

[283] "...EPA requires PPARalpha for its inhibitory effects on NF-kappaB." Mishra A, Chaudhary A, Sethi S. Oxidized omega-3 fatty acids inhibit NF-kappaB activation via a PPARalpha-dependent pathway. *Arterioscler Thromb Vasc Biol.* 2004 Sep;24(9):1621-7. Epub 2004 Jul 1. http://atvb.ahajournals.org/cgi/content/full/24/9/1621

[284] "Indeed, the previous view that nutrients only interact with human physiology at the metabolic/post-transcriptional level must be updated in light of current research showing that nutrients can, in fact, modify human physiology and phenotype at the genetic/pre-transcriptional level." Vasquez A. Reducing pain and inflammation naturally - part 4: nutritional and botanical inhibition of NF-kappaB, the major intracellular amplifier of the inflammatory cascade. A practical clinical strategy exemplifying anti-inflammatory nutrigenomics. *Nutritional Perspectives,* July 2005:5-12. www.OptimalHealthResearch.com/part4

[285] Vasquez A, Manso G, Cannell J. The clinical importance of vitamin D (cholecalciferol): a paradigm shift with implications for all healthcare providers. *Altern Ther Health Med.* 2004 Sep-Oct;10(5):28-36 http://optimalhealthresearch.com/monograph04

[286] Manzi S. Epidemiology of systemic lupus erythematosus. *Am J Manag Care.* 2001 Oct;7(16 Suppl):S474-9 http://www.ajmc.com/files/articlefiles/A01_131_2001octManziS474_9.pdf

Scleroderma
Systemic Sclerosis
Progressive Systemic Sclerosis

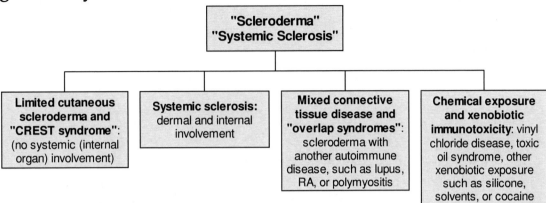

"Scleroderma"
"Systemic Sclerosis"

| **Limited cutaneous scleroderma and "CREST syndrome"**: (no systemic (internal organ) involvement) | **Systemic sclerosis:** dermal and internal involvement | **Mixed connective tissue disease and "overlap syndromes"**: scleroderma with another autoimmune disease, such as lupus, RA, or polymyositis | **Chemical exposure and xenobiotic immunotoxicity**: vinyl chloride disease, toxic oil syndrome, other xenobiotic exposure such as silicone, solvents, or cocaine |

<u>Description/pathophysiology</u>:

- Generally considered "idiopathic." The terms *scleroderma* and *systemic sclerosis* are used somewhat interchangeably; yet, as these terms suggest, *scleroderma* is properly assigned to disease that is limited to the skin, while *systemic sclerosis* denotes visceral involvement in addition to skin changes. *Scleroderma* will be the default term in this section for linguistic expediency.
- **Characterized by fibrosis of the skin and internal organs, including the esophagus, intestines, lung, heart, and kidneys.**
- <u>Four subtypes</u>:
    1. <u>Limited cutaneous scleroderma</u>: Only affecting the skin, especially of the fingers and face; relatively benign; **CREST syndrome**: calcinosis, Raynaud's phenomenon, esophageal dysmotility/dysfunction, sclerodactyly, telangiectasia
    2. <u>Diffuse systemic sclerosis</u>: Characterized by systemic fibrosis and degeneration of the skin (scleroderma) and internal organs; may rapidly progress to death.
    3. <u>Mixed connective tissue disease and "overlap syndromes"</u>: Combination of scleroderma with another autoimmune disease, such as with dermatomyositis (sclerodermatomyositis) or with RA, SLE, or Sjogren's syndrome.
    4. <u>Scleroderma secondary to xenobiotic immunotoxicity</u>: Scleroderma can result from exposure to vinyl chloride, silicone, petroleum products, toxic oil syndrome, solvents, cocaine, and pesticides.
- The condition can be mild and limited to the skin only or can be systemic and rapidly fatal due to internal organ involvement.
- Patients with scleroderma have evidence of **increased oxidative stress** demonstrated by a doubling of urinary isoprostane excretion.[1] Oxidative stress *results from* and *contributes to* systemic inflammation because 1) increased immune activity results in elaboration of oxidants, and 2) oxidative stress upregulates NF-kappaB (and other pathways) for additive immune activation.

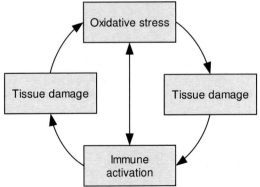

Oxidative stress

Tissue damage

Tissue damage

Immune activation

---

[1] "CONCLUSION: This study provides evidence of enhanced lipid peroxidation in both SSc and UCTD, and suggests a rationale for antioxidant treatment of SSc." Cracowski JL, Marpeau C, Carpentier PH, Imbert B, Hunt M, Stanke-Labesque F, Bessard G. Enhanced in vivo lipid peroxidation in scleroderma spectrum disorders. *Arthritis Rheum* 2001 May;44(5):1143-8

Clinical presentations:

- 4x more common in women, general age of onset is 20-40 years.
- **Raynaud's phenomenon**: Seen in 90% of patients and often precedes sclerodermatous manifestations by a period of up to 5 years.
- **Swelling and thickening of the fingers: sclerodactyly.**
- **Polyarthralgia**: Affects 90% of patients; flexion contractures of the joints due to fibrosis is also common.
- **Skin changes: hyperpigmentation, tightness, tightness and thickening of the face results in "mask-like face"**, telangiectasia, may also have depigmentation; dermal ulceration of fingertips and extensor surfaces as skin loses elasticity.
- Pulmonary: Dyspnea.
- Cardiac: Arrhythmias, CHF, hypertension, ECG abnormalities—may be fatal.
- Soft tissue calcification: Especially in the hands; systemic calcification is also seen.
- GI disturbances:
  - Esophageal dysfunction and dysphagia eventually occur in most patients
  - Heartburn, GERD: Greatly increased risk for Barrett's esophagus (33% of all scleroderma patients) with a remarkably low risk of esophageal adenocarcinoma.
  - Histologic/biopsy examination reveals degeneration of intestinal nerves, vessels, and smooth muscle.[2]
  - Slow intestinal transit—intestinal hypomotility in scleroderma promotes bacterial overgrowth of the small bowel, which probably contributes to the pathogenesis of the disease via the pro-inflammatory and immune activating effects discussed in Chapter 4. Treatment of bacterial overgrowth with antibiotics (ciprofloxacin 500 mg bid[3]) or promotility drugs (octreotide[4]) is effective treatment for scleroderma according to published case reports; **such research supports the hypothesis that intestinal dysbiosis— namely bacterial overgrowth—is an important contributor to the perpetuation of scleroderma.** Thus, part of the pathophysiology of scleroderma as related to bacterial overgrowth may be represented as follows:

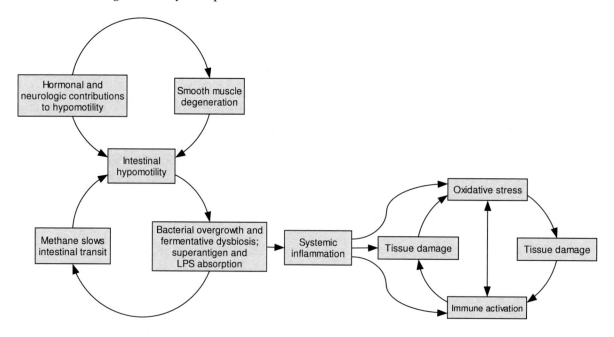

---

[2] "We found ultrastructural signs of axonal degeneration and cytoskeletal abnormalities in the bundles of unmyelinated fibers. There was also focal degeneration of smooth muscle cells, often in association with the presence of partially degranulated mast cells." Malandrini A, Selvi E, Villanova M, Berti G, Sabadini L, Salvadori C, Gambelli S, De Stefano R, Vernillo R, Marcolongo R, Guazzi G. Autonomic nervous system and smooth muscle cell involvement in systemic sclerosis: ultrastructural study of 3 cases. *J Rheumatol*. 2000 May;27(5):1203-6

[3] Over KE, Bucknall RC. Regression of skin changes in a patient with systemic sclerosis following treatment for bacterial overgrowth with ciprofloxacin. *Br J Rheumatol*. 1998 Jun;37(6):696 http://rheumatology.oxfordjournals.org/cgi/reprint/37/6/696a

[4] "After 8 months of treatment, normal weight was obtained and skin induration was spectacularly reduced and pigmentation returned to a normal state." Descamps V, Duval X, Crickx B, Bouscarat F, Coffin B, Belaich S. Global improvement of systemic scleroderma under long-term administration of octreotide. *Eur J Dermatol* 1999 Sep;9(6):446-8

Major differential diagnoses:

- Parkinson's disease: mask-like face
- Vinyl chloride disease: exposure to vinyl chloride (VC) monomer, a volatile substance mostly used for polyvinyl chloride (PVC) synthesis produces a scleroderma-like disorder that may be complicated by vasculitic and neurologic sequelae.[5,6,7]
- Toxic oil syndrome: A syndrome of incapacitating myalgias, marked peripheral eosinophilia, pulmonary infiltrates, and increased prevalence of scleroderma and neurologic disorders following widespread consumption of contaminated oil.[8]
- Other autoimmune disorder(s)
- Systemic infection

Clinical assessments:

- **History/subjective**:
  - Symptoms and complications from dermal induration/hardening and fibrosis
  - Intestinal and digestive complaints
  - Areas affected, ROM, ADL, QOL
  - Xenobiotic exposure: Occupational exposure to silica is associated with scleroderma; some cases appear to be linked to silicone breast implants[9] (controversial[10]) and anti-silicate antibodies may be valuable for documenting humoral response to silicone.[11] Clinicians should ask about any history of iatrogenic, occupational, recreational or domestic xenobiotic exposure, such as to organic solvents[12], pesticides, epoxy resins[13], and other immunotoxins.[14] Use of cocaine can cause or exacerbate scleroderma.[15]
- **Physical examination/objective**: routine, including the following:
  - Symptoms and complications from dermal induration/hardening, swelling, and fibrosis: swollen fingers, tight skin on face and hands, dermal ulcerations and hypopigmentation
  - Assess skin and ROM (limited range of motion is characteristic)
  - Abdominal exam, gastrointestinal motility
  - Pulmonary examination and auscultation
  - **Assessment for hypertension is mandatory**
- **Laboratory assessments**: *lab assessments are only minimally supportive for the diagnosis, but are helpful to monitor for complications*
  - Urinalysis to screen for renal compromise
  - Chemistry panel: assess for renal and liver status, electrolytes, etc.

[5] "Occupational exposure to vinyl chloride monomers is known to induce Raynaud's phenomenon, periportal fibrosis, liver angiosarcoma and scleroderma-like syndrome." Serratrice J, Granel B, Pache X, Disdier P, De Roux-Serratrice C, Pellissier JF, Weiller PJ. A case of polymyositis with anti-histidyl-t-RNA synthetase (Jo-1) antibody syndrome following extensive vinyl chloride exposure. *Clin Rheumatol.* 2001;20(5):379-82

[6] "An unusual case of systemic sclerosis occurring in a patient exposed to the vinyl chloride monomer (VCM) is presented." Ostlere LS, Harris D, Buckley C, Black C, Rustin MH. Atypical systemic sclerosis following exposure to vinyl chloride monomer. A case report and review of the cutaneous aspects of vinyl chloride disease. *Clin Exp Dermatol.* 1992 May;17(3):208-10

[7] "Angiosarcoma of the liver, Raynaud's phenomenon, scleroderma-like lesions, acroosteolysis and neuritis are known to be typical vinyl chloride-associated manifestations (VC disease)." Magnavita N, Bergamaschi A, Garcovich A, Giuliano G. Vasculitic purpura in vinyl chloride disease: a case report. *Angiology.* 1986 May;37(5):382-8

[8] "In 1981, in Spain, the ingestion of an oil fraudulently sold as olive oil caused an outbreak of a previously unrecorded condition, later known as toxic oil syndrome (TOS), clinically characterized by intense incapacitating myalgias, marked peripheral eosinophilia, and pulmonary infiltrates." Gelpi E, de la Paz MP, Terracini B, Abaitua I, de la Camara AG, Kilbourne EM, Lahoz C, Nemery B, Philen RM, Soldevilla L, Tarkowski S; WHO/CISAT Scientific Committee for the Toxic Oil Syndrome. Centro de Investigacion para el Sindrome del Aceite Toxico. The Spanish toxic oil syndrome 20 years after its onset: a multidisciplinary review of scientific knowledge. *Environ Health Perspect.* 2002 May;110(5):457-64 http://ehp.niehs.nih.gov/members/2002/110p457-464gelpi/gelpi-full.html

[9] "...idiopathic form of scleroderma and related conditions. CONCLUSION. These findings suggest that ANA positivity is relatively common in individuals with silicone breast implants, and may support the existence of autoimmune mechanisms in the pathogenesis of the clinical manifestations seen in this population." Cuellar ML, Scopelitis E, Tenenbaum SA, Garry RF, Silveira LH, Cabrera G, Espinoza LR. Serum antinuclear antibodies in women with silicone breast implants. *J Rheumatol.* 1995 Feb;22(2):236-40

[10] "Neither the case-control studies nor the other epidemiologic data support the hypothesis that scleroderma is associated with or causally related to breast implants." Whorton D, Wong O. Scleroderma and silicone breast implants. West J Med 1997 Sep;167(3):159-65

[11] Shen GQ, Ojo-Amaize EA, Agopian MS, Peter JB.Silicate antibodies in women with silicone breast implants: development of an assay for detection of humoral immunity. *Clin Diagn Lab Immunol.* 1996 Mar;3(2):162-6 http://cdli.asm.org/cgi/reprint/3/2/162?view=reprint&pmid=8991630

[12] "We describe a sclerodermatous syndrome in a middle-aged man who had worked with a wide variety of organic solvents over a prolonged period." Bottomley WW, Sheehan-Dare RA, Hughes P, Cunliffe WJ. A sclerodermatous syndrome with unusual features following prolonged occupational exposure to organic solvents. *Br J Dermatol* 1993 Feb;128(2):203-6

[13] "A new occupational disorder characterized by skin sclerosis is described. This disease developed acutely in workmen exposed to the vapor of epoxy resins." Yamakage A, Ishikawa H, Saito Y, Hattori A. Occupational scleroderma-like disorder occurring in men engaged in the polymerization of epoxy resins. *Dermatologica.* 1980;161(1):33-44

[14] "There is growing concern about the association between systemic sclerosis and certain environmental and occupational risk factors, including exposures to vinyl chloride, adulterated cooking oils, L-tryptophan, silica, silicone breast implants, organic solvents, and other agents such as epoxy resins, pesticides, and hand/arm vibration." Nietert PJ, Silver RM. Systemic sclerosis: environmental and occupational risk factors. *Curr Opin Rheumatol* 2000 Nov;12(6):520-6

[15] "It has been reported that cocaine may initiate scleroderma in an already susceptible individual or unmask it at an earlier age in subclinical disease." Attoussi S, Faulkner ML, Oso A, Umoru B. Cocaine-induced scleroderma and scleroderma renal crisis. *South Med J* 1998 Oct;91(10):961-3

- CBC: May reveal anemia due to malabsorption-induced deficiencies of B12, folate, iron, hypoproliferation due to inflammation (i.e., the anemia of chronic disease).
- Rheumatoid factor: positive in 33%
- Breath hydrogen/methane: This test is used to assess for bacterial overgrowth
- Lactulose and mannitol assay for "leaky gut" and malabsorption: Abnormal results are likely due to bacterial overgrowth and/or celiac disease with resultant malabsorption and increased intestinal permeability.[16]
- Leukocyte antigens: Increased prevalence of HLA-DR5 and HLA-DR1
- *Helicobacter pylori* detection: Given the increased prevalence of *Helicobacter pylori* infection[17,18], the addition of antigen testing onto a comprehensive stool analysis and comprehensive parasitology examination is recommended.
- Comprehensive stool analysis and comprehensive parasitology: essential
- **ANA: positive in up to 96% of patients with scleroderma**
- **Anticentromere antibody: positive in 50% with CREST; specific for scleroderma;** portends disease course limited to dermal involvement[19]
- **Anti-SCL-70 antibodies: positive in 20-30% of patients; specific for scleroderma;** portends disease course with internal organ involvement, particularly of the lungs
- Antifibrillarin antibodies: seen in a small portion (~4%) of patients with scleroderma and correlates with internal organ involvement[20]

- **Imaging**:
  - ECG abnormalities are common and can include ventricular ectopy, which is correlated with sudden cardiac death
  - Radiography, pulmonary function tests, and CT imaging may be used to detect fibrosing alveolitis and scleroderma-associated pulmonary decline
- **Establishing the diagnosis**:
  - Clinical assessment is sufficient in patients with classic full-blown disease
  - Combination of serologic evidence of autoimmunity and dermal induration

Complications:

- 33% of patients will develop **Barrett's esophagus** and are at increased risk for cancer; periodic endoscopic surveillance is warranted; referral to gastroenterologist is recommended. To the extent possible, acid-blocking (proton pump-inhibiting) drugs should be avoided because the iatrogenic hypochlorhydria will exacerbate the small bowel bacterial overgrowth and thereby perpetuate the systemic inflammatory state.
- **Malabsorption** and resultant **malnutrition** due to intestinal hypomotility and dysbiosis
- **Sudden cardiac death**
- **Pulmonary hypertension and pulmonary failure**
- **Increased incidence of breast and lung cancer**
- **Hypertension,** secondary to scleroderma-induced renal damage

Clinical management:

- Referral if clinical outcome is unsatisfactory or if serious complications are possible/evident.
- Treat complications such as HTN and GERD as you would normally—see Treatment section.

---

[16] "Coeliac disease may account for malabsorption in scleroderma patients even when test suggest bacterial overgrowth." Marguerie C, Kaye S, Vyse T, Mackworth-Young C, Walport MJ, Black C. Malabsorption caused by coeliac disease in patients who have scleroderma. *Br J Rheumatol.* 1995 Sep;34(9):858-61

[17] "Thus, the risk for gastric diseases caused by HP infection is enhanced in patients with systemic sclerosis compared with white healthy, asymptomatic persons examined in other studies." Reinauer S, Goerz G, Ruzicka T, Susanto F, Humfeld S, Reinauer H. Helicobacter pylori in patients with systemic sclerosis: detection with the 13C-urea breath test and eradication. *Acta Derm Venereol.* 1994 Sep;74(5):361-3

[18] "Patients with SSc have H. pylori infection at a higher prevalence than the general population." Yazawa N, Fujimoto M, Kikuchi K, Kubo M, Ihn H, Sato S, Tamaki T, Tamaki K. High seroprevalence of Helicobacter pylori infection in patients with systemic sclerosis: association with esophageal involvement. *J Rheumatol.* 1998 Apr;25(4):650-3

[19] Ho KT, Reveille JD. The clinical relevance of autoantibodies in scleroderma. Arthritis Res Ther. 2003;5(2):80-93. Epub 2003 Feb 12 http://arthritis-research.com/content/5/2/80

[20] "AFA identifies young SSc patients with frequent internal organ involvement, especially pulmonary hypertension, myositis and renal disease." Tormey VJ, Bunn CC, Denton CP, Black CM. Anti-fibrillarin antibodies in systemic sclerosis. *Rheumatology* (Oxford). 2001 Oct;40(10):1157-62 http://rheumatology.oxfordjournals.org/cgi/content/full/40/10/1157

Treatments:

> Drug treatments: "Treatment of progressive systemic sclerosis is symptomatic and supportive. ... Prednisone has little or no role in the treatment of scleroderma."[21] Other allopathic treatments have recently been reviewed in an article available for free on-line.[22]
> - Prednisone or other corticosteroid is used for myositis, MCTD, and arthritis
> - Penicillamine started at 250 mg/d and gradually increased to 0.5-1.0 g/d can reduce dermal and systemic involvement
> - Tetracycline one gram per day for bacterial overgrowth[23]
> - ACE inhibitors are the drugs of choice for scleroderma renal disease and hypertension

- Supplemented Paleo-Mediterranean diet: The health-promoting diet of choice for the majority of people is a diet based on abundant consumption of fruits, vegetables, seeds, nuts, omega-3 and monounsaturated fatty acids, and lean sources of protein such as lean meats, fatty cold-water fish, soy and whey proteins. This diet obviates overconsumption of chemical preservatives, artificial sweeteners, and carbohydrate-dominant foods such as candies, pastries, breads, potatoes, grains, and other foods with a high glycemic load and high glycemic index. This "Paleo-Mediterranean Diet" is a combination of the "Paleolithic" or "Paleo diet" and the well-known "Mediterranean diet", both of which are well described in peer-reviewed journals and the lay press. (See Chapter 2 and my other publications[24,25] for details). Although this diet is the most-nutrient dense diet available, rational supplementation with vitamins, minerals, and health promoting fatty acids (i.e., ALA, GLA, EPA, DHA) makes this the best practical diet that can possibly be conceived and implemented. For scleroderma patients whose diets have habitually been low in fiber, dietary improvement which increases fiber consumption should be implemented slowly to avoid phytobezoar formation and intestinal obstruction.[26]

- Daily use of a broad-spectrum high-potency multivitamin and multimineral supplement: **Vitamin and mineral supplementation is important for patients with scleroderma.** Vitamin supplementation (particularly with pyridoxine and riboflavin) appears warranted in patients with systemic sclerosis based on a small (n=5) study that documented the normalization of aberrant tryptophan metabolism in most patients following the administration of pyridoxine with riboflavin; the authors concluded that this was evidence of combined vitamin deficiency in patients with scleroderma.[27] This combined deficiency is not surprising given the high incidence of bacterial overgrowth and malabsorption in scleroderma patients. Deficiencies of ascorbate and selenium have also been documented in patients with scleroderma.[28] Reduced folate and cobalamin and elevated homocysteine have also been noted in patients with scleroderma.[29]

- Avoidance of proinflammatory foods: Proinflammatory foods act *directly* or *indirectly*; direct mechanisms include activating Toll-like receptors or NF-kappaB or inducing oxidative stress, while indirect mechanisms include depleting the body of anti-inflammatory nutrients and displacing more nutritious anti-inflammatory foods. Arachidonic acid (found in beef, liver, pork, and cow's milk) is the direct precursor to proinflammatory prostaglandins and leukotrienes[30] and pain-promoting isoprostanes.[31] Saturated fats promote inflammation by activating/enabling

[21] Tierney ML. McPhee SJ, Papadakis MA (eds). Current Medical Diagnosis and Treatment. 35th edition. Stamford: Appleton and Lange, 1996 page 747
[22] Sapadin AN, Fleischmajer R. Treatment of scleroderma. *Arch Dermatol.* 2002 Jan;138(1):99-105. http://archderm.ama-assn.org/cgi/content/full/138/1/99 Accessed December 16, 2005
[23] Beers MH, Berkow R (eds). The Merck Manual. Seventeenth Edition. Whitehouse Station; Merck Research Laboratories 1999 Page 433
[24] Vasquez A. A Five-Part Nutritional Protocol that Produces Consistently Positive Results. *Nutritional Wellness* 2005 September Available in the printed version and on-line at http://www.nutritionalwellness.com/archives/2005/sep/09_vasquez.php and http://optimalhealthresearch.com/protocol
[25] Vasquez A. Implementing the Five-Part Nutritional Wellness Protocol for the Treatment of Various Health Problems. *Nutritional Wellness* 2005 November. Available on-line at http://www.nutritionalwellness.com/archives/2005/nov/11_vasquez.php and http://optimalhealthresearch.com/protocol
[26] Gough A, Sheeran T, Bacon P, Emery P. Dietary advice in systemic sclerosis: the dangers of a high fibre diet. *Ann Rheum Dis.* 1998;57(11):641-2 http://ard.bmjjournals.com/cgi/content/full/57/11/641
[27] "But the simultaneous administration of pyridoxine and nicotinamide to three of these patients normalized the excretory picture after tryptophan loading." De Antoni A, Muggeo M, Costa C, Allegri G, Crepaldi G. Tryptophan metabolism "via" nicotimic acid in patients with scleroderma. *Acta Vitaminol Enzymol.* 1976;30(4-6):134-9
[28] "Plasma ascorbic acid was reduced in all 3 groups of patients: median level 10.6 mg/l in controls, 4.8 mg/l in PRP (p < 0.01), 2.5 mg/l in ISSc (p < 0.01) and 6.8 mg/l in dSSc (p < 0.05). A reduction in serum selenium was especially found in dSSc (median 75 micrograms/l compared to 100 micrograms/l in controls, p < 0.05)." Herrick AL, Rieley F, Schofield D, Hollis S, Braganza JM, Jayson MI. Micronutrient antioxidant status in patients with primary Raynaud's phenomenon and systemic sclerosis. *J Rheumatol.* 1994 Aug;21(8):1477-83
[29] "Patients with SSc had higher Hcy and vWF concentrations than those with RP or controls. Folic acid and vitamin B12 were lower in SSc than in RP or controls." Marasini B, Casari S, Bestetti A, Maioli C, Cugno M, Zeni S, Turri O, Guagnellini E, Biondi ML. Homocysteine concentration in primary and systemic sclerosis associated Raynaud's phenomenon. *J Rheumatol.* 2000 Nov;27(11):2621-3
[30] Vasquez A. Reducing Pain and Inflammation Naturally. Part 2: New Insights into Fatty Acid Supplementation and Its Effect on Eicosanoid Production and Genetic Expression. *Nutritional Perspectives* 2005; January: 5-16 www.optimalhealthresearch.com/part2
[31] Evans AR, Junger H, Southall MD, Nicol GD, Sorkin LS, Broome JT, Bailey TW, Vasko MR. Isoprostanes, novel eicosanoids that produce nociception and sensitize rat sensory neurons. *J Pharmacol Exp Ther.* 2000 Jun;293(3):912-20

proinflammatory Toll-like receptors.[32] Consumption of saturated fat in the form of cream creates marked oxidative stress and lipid peroxidation that lasts for at least 3 hours postprandially.[33] Corn oil rapidly activates NF-kappaB (in hepatic Kupffer cells) for a proinflammatory effect[34]; similarly, consumption of PUFA and linoleic acid promotes antioxidant depletion and may thus promote oxidation-mediated inflammation via activation of NF-kappaB; linoleic acid causes intracellular oxidative stress and calcium influx and results in increased transcription of NF-kappaB activated pro-inflammatory genes.[35] High glycemic foods cause oxidative stress[36,37] and inflammation via activation of NF-kappaB and other mechanisms—*white bread causes inflammation.*[38] High glycemic foods suppress immune function[39,40] and thus perpetuate and promote infection/dysbiosis. Delivery of a high carbohydrate load to the gastrointestinal lumen promotes bacterial overgrowth[41,42], which is inherently proinflammatory[43,44] and which appears to be myalgenic in humans.[45] Consumption of grains, potatoes, and manufactured foods displaces phytonutrient-dense foods such as fruits, vegetables, nuts, seeds, and berries which in sum contain more than 8,000 phytonutrients, many of which have antioxidant and thus anti-inflammatory actions.[46,47]

- <u>Avoidance of allergenic foods</u>: Any patient may be allergic to any food, even if the food is generally considered a health-promoting food. Generally speaking, the most notorious allergens are wheat, citrus (especially juice due to the industrial use of fungal hemicellulases), cow's milk, eggs, peanuts, chocolate, and yeast-containing foods; according to a study in patients with migraine, some patients will have to avoid as many as 10 specific foods in order to become symptom-free.[48] **Celiac disease is not uncommon in patients with scleroderma, and their scleroderma diagnosis may precede the recognition of celiac disease by many years.**[49,50] Clinicians must explain to their patients that celiac disease and wheat allergy are two different clinical entities and that exclusion of one does not exclude the other, and in neither case does mutual exclusion obviate the **promotion of intestinal bacterial overgrowth (i.e., proinflammatory dysbiosis) by indigestible wheat oligosaccharides.** Rapid implementation of high fiber diets may precipitate bowel obstruction.[51]

- <u>Vitamin E</u>: Morelli et al[52] describe a 60-year-old woman with systemic sclerosis complicated by hypertension, renal failure, and heart failure; although allopathic drug treatments were of no benefit, **the addition of "vitamin E (600 mg daily)" lead to rapid and significant clinical**

[32] Lee JY, Sohn KH, Rhee SH, Hwang D. Saturated fatty acids, but not unsaturated fatty acids, induce the expression of cyclooxygenase-2 mediated through Toll-like receptor 4. *J Biol Chem.* 2001 May 18;276(20):16683-9. Epub 2001 Mar 2 http://www.jbc.org/cgi/content/full/276/20/16683

[33] "CONCLUSIONS: Both fat and protein intakes stimulate ROS generation. The increase in ROS generation lasted 3 h after cream intake and 1 h after protein intake. Cream intake also caused a significant and prolonged increase in lipid peroxidation." Mohanty P, Ghanim H, Hamouda W, Aljada A, Garg R, Dandona P. Both lipid and protein intakes stimulate increased generation of reactive oxygen species by polymorphonuclear leukocytes and mononuclear cells. *Am J Clin Nutr.* 2002 Apr;75(4):767-72 http://www.ajcn.org/cgi/content/full/75/4/767

[34] Rusyn I, Bradham CA, Cohn L, Schoonhoven R, Swenberg JA, Brenner DA, Thurman RG. Corn oil rapidly activates nuclear factor-kappaB in hepatic Kupffer cells by oxidant-dependent mechanisms. *Carcinogenesis.* 1999 Nov;20(11):2095-100 http://carcin.oxfordjournals.org/cgi/content/full/20/11/2095

[35] "Exposing endothelial cells to 90 micromol linoleic acid/L for 6 h resulted in a significant increase in lipid hydroperoxides that coincided with an increase in intracellular calcium concentrations." Hennig B, Toborek M, Joshi-Barve S, Barger SW, Barve S, Mattson MP, McClain CJ. Linoleic acid activates nuclear transcription factor-kappa B (NF-kappa B) and induces NF-kappa B-dependent transcription in cultured endothelial cells. *Am J Clin Nutr.* 1996 Mar;63(3):322-8 http://www.ajcn.org/cgi/reprint/63/3/322

[36] Mohanty P, Hamouda W, Garg R, Aljada A, Ghanim H, Dandona P. Glucose challenge stimulates reactive oxygen species (ROS) generation by leucocytes. *J Clin Endocrinol Metab.* 2000 Aug;85(8):2970-3 http://jcem.endojournals.org/cgi/content/full/85/8/2970 Glucose/carbohydrate and saturated fat consumption appear to be the two biggest offenders in the food-stimulated production of oxidative stress. The effect by protein is much less. "CONCLUSIONS: Both fat and protein intakes stimulate ROS generation. The increase in ROS generation lasted 3 h after cream intake and 1 h after protein intake. Cream intake also caused a significant and prolonged increase in lipid peroxidation." Mohanty P, Ghanim H, Hamouda W, Aljada A, Garg R, Dandona P. Both lipid and protein intakes stimulate increased generation of reactive oxygen species by polymorphonuclear leukocytes and mononuclear cells. *Am J Clin Nutr.* 2002 Apr;75(4):767-72 http://www.ajcn.org/cgi/content/full/75/4/767

[37] Koska J, Blazicek P, Marko M, Grna JD, Kvetnansky R, Vigas M. Insulin, catecholamines, glucose and antioxidant enzymes in oxidative damage during different loads in healthy humans. *Physiol Res.* 2000;49 Suppl 1:S95-100 http://www.biomed.cas.cz/physiolres/pdf/2000/49_S95.pdf

[38] "Conclusion - The present study shows that high GI carbohydrate, but not low GI carbohydrate, mediates an acute proinflammatory process as measured by NF-kappaB activity." Dickinson S, Hancock DP, Petocz P, Brand-Miller JC. High glycemic index carbohydrate mediates an acute proinflammatory process as measured by NF-kappaB activation. *Asia Pac J Clin Nutr.* 2005;14 Suppl:S120

[39] Sanchez A, Reeser JL, Lau HS, et al. Role of sugars in human neutrophilic phagocytosis. *Am J Clin Nutr.* 1973 Nov;26(11):1180-4

[40] "Postoperative infusion of carbohydrate solution leads to moderate fall in the serum concentration of inorganic phosphate. ... The hypophosphatemia was associated with significant reduction of neutrophil phagocytosis, intracellular killing, generation of oxygen and generation of superoxide during phagocytosis." Rasmussen A, Segel E, Hessov I, Borregaard N. Reduced function of neutrophils during routine postoperative glucose infusion. *Acta Chir Scand.* 1988 Jul-Aug;154(7-8):429-33

[41] Ramakrishnan T, Stokes P. Beneficial effects of fasting and low carbohydrate diet in D-lactic acidosis associated with short-bowel syndrome. *JPEN J Parenter Enteral Nutr.* 1985 May-Jun;9(3):361-3

[42] Gottschall E. *Breaking the Vicious Cycle: Intestinal Health Through Diet.* Kirkton Press; Rev edition (August 1, 1994)

[43] Lin HC. Small intestinal bacterial overgrowth: a framework for understanding irritable bowel syndrome. *JAMA.* 2004 Aug 18;292(7):852-8

[44] Lichtman SN, Wang J, Sartor RB, Zhang C, Bender D, Dalldorf FG, Schwab JH. Reactivation of arthritis induced by small bowel bacterial overgrowth in rats: role of cytokines, bacteria, and bacterial polymers. *Infect Immun.* 1995 Jun;63(6):2295-301

[45] Pimentel M, et al. A link between irritable bowel syndrome and fibromyalgia may be related to findings on lactulose breath testing. *Ann Rheum Dis.* 2004 Apr;63(4):450-2

[46] "We propose that the additive and synergistic effects of phytochemicals in fruit and vegetables are responsible for their potent antioxidant and anticancer activities, and that the benefit of a diet rich in fruit and vegetables is attributed to the complex mixture of phytochemicals present in whole foods." Liu RH. Health benefits of fruit and vegetables are from additive and synergistic combinations of phytochemicals. *Am J Clin Nutr.* 2003 Sep;78(3 Suppl):517S-520S

[47] Seaman DR. The diet-induced proinflammatory state: a cause of chronic pain and other degenerative diseases? *J Manipulative Physiol Ther.* 2002;25(3):168-79

[48] Grant EC. Food allergies and migraine. *Lancet.* 1979 May 5;1(8123):966-9

[49] Gomez-Puerta JA, Gil V, Cervera R, Miquel R, Jimenez S, Ramos-Casals M, Font J. Coeliac disease associated with systemic sclerosis. *Ann Rheum Dis.* 2004 Jan;63(1):104-5 http://ard.bmjjournals.com/cgi/content/full/63/1/104

[50] "Coeliac disease may account for malabsorption in scleroderma patients even when test suggest bacterial overgrowth." Marguerie C, Kaye S, Vyse T, Mackworth-Young C, Walport MJ, Black C. Malabsorption caused by coeliac disease in patients who have scleroderma. *Br J Rheumatol.* 1995 Sep;34(9):858-61

[51] Gough A, Sheeran T, Bacon P, Emery P. Dietary advice in systemic sclerosis: the dangers of a high fibre diet. *Ann Rheum Dis.* 1998 Nov;57(11):641-2 http://ard.bmjjournals.com/cgi/content/full/57/11/641

[52] "Casually, vitamin E (600 mg daily) was added. After 6 months, clinical manifestations of heart failure were disappeared and the echocardiogram showed a normally-sized left ventricle with normal wall motion." Morelli S, Sgreccia A, Bernardo ML, Gurgo Di Castelmenardo A, Petrilli AC, De Leva R, Nuccio F, Calvieri S. Systemic sclerosis (scleroderma). A case of recovery of cardiomyopathy after vitamin E treatment. *Minerva Cardioangiol.* 2001 Apr;49(2):127-30

improvement. Ayres and Mihan[53] wrote that vitamin E was effective in the clinical management of scleroderma, discoid lupus erythematosus[54], porphyria cutanea tarda, several types of vasculitis, and polymyositis.[55] Given that vitamin E is not a single compound but rather a family of closely related tocopherols, most clinicians prefer to use a source of "mixed tocopherols" inclusive of alpha, beta, delta, and—perhaps most importantly—gamma tocopherol.[56] Vitamin E has a wide margin of safety and although daily doses are kept in the range of 400-1200 IU, doses up to 3,200 IU are generally considered non-toxic.

- <u>Vitamin D3 supplementation with physiologic doses and/or tailored to serum 25(OH)D and serum calcium levels</u> : Vitamin D deficiency is common in the general population and is even more common in patients with chronic illness and chronic musculoskeletal pain.[57] Correction of vitamin D deficiency provides a clinically significant anti-inflammatory and immunomodulatory benefit.[58] **Oral administration of active vitamin D3 (1,25-dihydroxyvitamin D) has lead to clinical improvement in patients with scleroderma.**[59] Reasonable daily doses for children and adults are 2,000 and 4,000 IU, respectively, as defined by Vasquez, et al.[60] Deficiency and response to treatment are monitored with serum 25(OH)vitamin D while safety is monitored with serum calcium; inflammatory granulomatous diseases and certain drugs such as hydrochlorothiazide greatly increase the propensity for hypercalcemia and warrant increment dosing and frequent monitoring of serum calcium.

- <u>CoQ10</u>: CoQ10 is a powerful antioxidant with a wide margin of safety and excellent clinical tolerability. **At least four studies have documented its powerful blood-pressure-lowering ability, which often surpasses the clinical effectiveness of antihypertensive drugs.**[61,62,63,64] **Furthermore, at least two published papers**[65,66] **and one case report**[67] **advocate that CoQ10 has powerful renoprotective benefits.** CoQ10 levels are low in patients with allergies[68], and the symptomatic relief that many allergic patients experience following supplementation with CoQ10 suggests that CoQ10 has an immunomodulatory effect. Common doses start at > 100 mg per day with food; doses of 200 mg per day are not uncommon, and doses up to 1,000 mg per day are clinically well tolerated though the high financial toll approximates that of many pharmaceutical drugs.

- <u>N-acetyl-cysteine (NAC)</u>: **Oxidative stress promotes a fibrotic phenotype in scleroderma fibroblasts, which was normalized by administration of NAC** *in vitro*.[69] NAC is well-tolerated, inhibits NF-kappaB, functions as an antioxidant, and promotes detoxification via hepatoprotection and glutathione conjugation.

- <u>Comprehensive antioxidation</u>: As previously mentioned, patients with scleroderma have evidence of increased oxidative stress demonstrated by a doubling of urinary isoprostane

[53] "Among the diseases that were successfully controlled were a number in the autoimmune category, including scleroderma, discoid lupus erythematosus, porphyria cutanea tarda, several types of vasculitis, and polymyositis." Ayres S Jr, Mihan R. Is vitamin E involved in the autoimmune mechanism? *Cutis.* 1978 Mar;21(3):321-5

[54] "Despite conflicting opinions, our personal experience and a number of reviewed clinical reports indicate that vitamin E, properly administered in adequate doses, is a safe and effective treatment for chronic discoid lupus erythematosus, and may be of value in treating other types of the disease." Ayres S Jr, Mihan R. Lupus erythematosus and vitamin E: an effective and nontoxic therapy. *Cutis.* 1979;23(1):49-52, 54

[55] "She then made a dramatic improvement when large doses of vitamin E (d, alpha-tocopheryl acetate) were administered." Killeen RN, Ayres S Jr, Mihan R. Polymyositis: response to vitamin E. *South Med J.* 1976 Oct;69(10):1372-4

[56] Jiang Q, Christen S, Shigenaga MK, Ames BN. gamma-tocopherol, the major form of vitamin E in the US diet, deserves more attention. *Am J Clin Nutr.* 2001 Dec;74(6):714-22 http://www.ajcn.org/cgi/content/full/74/6/714

[57] Plotnikoff GA, Quigley JM. Prevalence of severe hypovitaminosis D in patients with persistent, nonspecific musculoskeletal pain. *Mayo Clin Proc.* 2003 Dec;78(12):1463-70

[58] Timms PM, Mannan N, Hitman GA, Noonan K, Mills PG, Syndercombe-Court D, Aganna E, Price CP, Boucher BJ. Circulating MMP9, vitamin D and variation in the TIMP-1 response with VDR genotype: mechanisms for inflammatory damage in chronic disorders? *QJM.* 2002 Dec;95(12):787-96 http://qjmed.oxfordjournals.org/cgi/content/full/95/12/787

[59] "After the treatment period (6 months to 3 years), a significant improvement, as compared with baseline values, was observed. No serious side-effects were observed." Humbert P, Dupond JL, Agache P, Laurent R, Rochefort A, Drobacheff C, de Wazieres B, Aubin F. Treatment of scleroderma with oral 1,25-dihydroxyvitamin D3: evaluation of skin involvement using non-invasive techniques. Results of an open prospective trial. *Acta Derm Venereol.* 1993 Dec;73(6):449-51

[60] Vasquez A, Manso G, Cannell J. The clinical importance of vitamin D (cholecalciferol): a paradigm shift with implications for all healthcare providers. *Altern Ther Health Med.* 2004 Sep-Oct;10(5):28-36 http://optimalhealthresearch.com/monograph04

[61] Burke BE, Neuenschwander R, Olson RD. Randomized, double-blind, placebo-controlled trial of coenzyme Q10 in isolated systolic hypertension. *South Med J.* 2001 Nov;94(11):1112-7

[62] Singh RB, Niaz MA, Rastogi SS, Shukla PK, Thakur AS. Effect of hydrosoluble coenzyme Q10 on blood pressures and insulin resistance in hypertensive patients with coronary artery disease. *J Hum Hypertens.* 1999 Mar;13(3):203-8

[63] Digiesi V, Cantini F, Oradei A, Bisi G, Guarino GC, Brocchi A, Bellandi F, Mancini M, Littarru GP. Coenzyme Q10 in essential hypertension. *Mol Aspects Med.* 1994;15 Suppl:s257-63

[64] Langsjoen P, Langsjoen P, Willis R, Folkers K. Treatment of essential hypertension with coenzyme Q10. *Mol Aspects Med.* 1994;15 Suppl:S265-72

[65] Singh RB, Khanna HK, Niaz MA. Randomized, double-blind placebo-controlled trial of coenzyme Q10 in chronic renal failure: discovery of a new role. *J Nutr Environ Med* 2000;10:281-8

[66] Singh RB, Kumar A, Naiz MA, Singh RG, Gujrati S, Singh VP, Singh M, Singh UP, Taneja C, AND Rastogi SS. Randomized, Double-blind, Placebo-controlled Trial of Coenzyme Q10 in Patients with End-stage Renal Failure. *J Nutr Environ Med* 2003; Volume 13, Number 1: 13–22

[67] Singh RB, Singh MM. Effects of CoQ10 in new indications with antioxidant vitamin deficiency. *J Nutr Environ Med* 1999; 9:223-228

[68] Ye CQ, Folkers K, Tamagawa H, Pfeiffer C. A modified determination of coenzyme Q10 in human blood and CoQ10 blood levels in diverse patients with allergies. *Biofactors.* 1988 Dec;1(4):303-6

[69] "In contrast, treatment of SSc fibroblasts with the membrane-permeant antioxidant N-acetyl-L-cysteine inhibited ROS production, and this was accompanied by decreased proliferation of these cells and down-regulation of alpha1(I) and alpha2(I) collagen messenger RNA." Sambo P, Baroni SS, Luchetti M, Paroncini P, Dusi S, Orlandini G, Gabrielli A. Oxidative stress in scleroderma: maintenance of scleroderma fibroblast phenotype by the constitutive up-regulation of reactive oxygen species generation through the NADPH oxidase complex pathway. *Arthritis Rheum* 2001 Nov;44(11):2653-64

excretion.[70] Oxidative stress results from and contributes to systemic inflammation because 1) increased immune activity results in elaboration of oxidants, and 2) oxidative stress upregulates NF-kappaB (and other pathways) for additive immune activation. *Antioxidant supplementation alone is clinically and biochemically inferior to a comprehensive program* that includes both antioxidant supplementation and dietary modification (i.e., the supplemented Paleo-Mediterranean diet, as described previously) that includes heavy reliance upon fruits, vegetables, low-glycemic juices, nuts, seeds, and berries for their additive and synergistic antioxidant benefits.[71]

- Broad-spectrum fatty acid therapy with ALA, EPA, DHA, GLA and oleic acid: "Sophisticated manipulation of EFA metabolism" may prove clinically beneficial for scleroderma patients according to a review by the late David Horrobin[72]; however, a six-month clinical trial of fatty acid supplementation showed no benefit[73], thus proving the ineffectiveness of one-dimensional intervention and of fatty acid supplementation in a condition known to have a high prevalence of untreated malabsorption. Nonetheless, as part of a *comprehensive program*, fatty acid supplementation should be delivered in the form of combination therapy with ALA, GLA, DHA, and EPA. Given at doses of 3,000 – 9,000 mg per day, ALA from flax oil has impressive anti-inflammatory benefits demonstrated by its ability to halve prostaglandin production in humans.[74] Numerous studies have demonstrated the benefit of GLA in the treatment of rheumatoid arthritis when used at doses between 500 mg – 4,000 mg per day.[75,76] Fish oil provides EPA and DHA which have well-proven anti-inflammatory benefits in rheumatoid arthritis[77,78,79] and lupus.[80,81] ALA, EPA, DHA, and GLA need to be provided in the form of supplements; when using high doses of therapeutic oils, liquid supplements that can be mixed in juice or a smoothie are generally more convenient and palatable than capsules. Therapeutic amounts of oleic acid can be obtained from generous use of olive oil, preferably on fresh vegetables. Supplementation with polyunsaturated fatty acids warrants increased intake of antioxidants from diet, fruit and vegetable juices, and properly formulated supplements; since patients with systemic inflammation are generally in a pro-oxidative state, consideration must be given to the timing and starting dose of fatty acid supplementation and the need for antioxidant protection. See chapter on Therapeutics for more details and biochemical pathways. Clinicians must realize that fatty acids are not clinically or biochemically interchangeable and that one fatty acid does not substitute for another; each of the fatty acids must be supplied in order for its benefits to be obtained.[82]

- Octreotide (prescription drug): Descamps et al[83] describe the case of a 53-year-old black woman with progressive and severe systemic scleroderma, with diffuse skin sclerosis, myositis with intestinal pseudo-obstruction and bacterial overgrowth who experienced a "spectacular" normalization of clinical status and skin induration following several months of octreotide (75 mug/d). This drug is a somatostatin analog used in the treatment of acromegaly[84] and it also

[70] "CONCLUSION: This study provides evidence of enhanced lipid peroxidation in both SSc and UCTD, and suggests a rationale for antioxidant treatment of SSc." Cracowski JL, Marpeau C, Carpentier PH, Imbert B, Hunt M, Stanke-Labesque F, Bessard G. Enhanced in vivo lipid peroxidation in scleroderma spectrum disorders. *Arthritis Rheum* 2001 May;44(5):1143-8
[71] Liu RH. Health benefits of fruit and vegetables are from additive and synergistic combinations of phytochemicals. *Am J Clin Nutr.* 2003 Sep;78(3 Suppl):517S-520S http://www.ajcn.org/cgi/content/full/78/3/517S
[72] "Controlled clinical trials of supplementation with gamma-linolenic acid (GLA) as evening primrose oil (Efamol) in both primary Sjogren's syndrome and systemic sclerosis have given positive results." Horrobin DF. Essential fatty acid and prostaglandin metabolism in Sjogren's syndrome, systemic sclerosis and rheumatoid arthritis. *Scand J Rheumatol* Suppl 1986;61:242-5
[73] "Dietary essential fatty acids have no role in the treatment of vascular symptoms in established systemic sclerosis." Stainforth JM, Layton AM, Goodfield MJ. Clinical aspects of the use of gamma linolenic acid in systemic sclerosis. *Acta Derm Venereol* 1996 Mar;76(2):144-6
[74] Adam O, Wolfram G, Zollner N. Effect of alpha-linolenic acid in the human diet on linoleic acid metabolism and prostaglandin biosynthesis. *J Lipid Res.* 1986 Apr;27(4):421-6 http://www.jlr.org/cgi/reprint/27/4/421
[75] "Other results showed a significant reduction in morning stiffness with gamma-linolenic acid at 3 months and reduction in pain and articular index at 6 months with olive oil." Brzeski M, Madhok R, Capell HA. Evening primrose oil in patients with rheumatoid arthritis and side-effects of non-steroidal anti-inflammatory drugs. *Br J Rheumatol.* 1991 Oct;30(5):370-2
[76] Rothman D, DeLuca P, Zurier RB. Botanical lipids: effects on inflammation, immune responses, and rheumatoid arthritis. *Semin Arthritis Rheum.* 1995 Oct;25(2):87-96
[77] Adam O, Beringer C, Kless T, Lemmen C, Adam A, Wiseman M, Adam P, Klimmek R, Forth W. Anti-inflammatory effects of a low arachidonic acid diet and fish oil in patients with rheumatoid arthritis. *Rheumatol Int.* 2003 Jan;23(1):27-36
[78] Lau CS, Morley KD, Belch JJ. Effects of fish oil supplementation on non-steroidal anti-inflammatory drug requirement in patients with mild rheumatoid arthritis--a double-blind placebo controlled study. *Br J Rheumatol.* 1993 Nov;32(11):982-9
[79] Kremer JM, Jubiz W, Michalek A, Rynes RI, Bigaouette J, Timchalk M, Beeler D, Lininger L. Fish-oil fatty acid supplementation in active rheumatoid arthritis. A double-blinded, controlled, crossover study. *Ann Intern Med.* 1987 Apr;106(4):497-503
[80] Walton AJ, Snaith ML, Locniskar M, Cumberland AG, Morrow WJ, Isenberg DA. Dietary fish oil and the severity of symptoms in patients with systemic lupus erythematosus. *Ann Rheum Dis.* 1991 Jul;50(7):463-6
[81] Duffy EM, Meenagh GK, McMillan SA, Strain JJ, Hannigan BM, Bell AL. The clinical effect of dietary supplementation with omega-3 fish oils and/or copper in systemic lupus erythematosus. *J Rheumatol.* 2004 Aug;31(8):1551-6
[82] Vasquez A. Reducing Pain and Inflammation Naturally. Part 2: New Insights into Fatty Acid Supplementation and Its Effect on Eicosanoid Production and Genetic Expression. *Nutritional Perspectives* 2005; January: 5-16 http://optimalhealthresearch.com/part2
[83] "After 8 months of treatment, normal weight was obtained and skin induration was spectacularly reduced and pigmentation returned to a normal state." Descamps V, Duval X, Crickx B, Bouscarat F, Coffin B, Belaich S. Global improvement of systemic scleroderma under long-term administration of octreotide. *Eur J Dermatol* 1999 Sep;9(6):446-8
[84] http://www.us.sandostatin.com/info/about/home.jsp Accessed December 16, 2005

promotes intestinal motility and thus reduces dysbiotic intestinal bacterial overgrowth in patients with scleroderma.[85] Efficacy of octreotide in improving clinical manifestations of scleroderma is probably mediated *at least in part* by reducing the pro-inflammatory effects of dysbiotic intestinal bacterial overgrowth, which can be addressed by other means as well.

- Assessment for dermal and gastrointestinal dysbiosis: A growing body of literature implicates infectious agents in the etiology of scleroderma.[86] Regarding dermal dysbiosis, several articles by Cantwell et al[87,88] suggest epidermal and/or intradermal dysbiosis with pleomorphic bacteria, specifically acid-fast cell-wall-deficient mycobacteria. Regarding gastrointestinal dysbiosis, at the very least, we must acknowledge that 1) **bacterial overgrowth of the small bowel is common (33%) in patients with scleroderma**[89] due to impaired gastrointestinal motility, 2) **scleroderma patients show increased levels of deconjugating bacteria**[90], which inactivate bile acids and promote enterohepatic recirculation of endogenous and exogenous toxins, 3) **these patients have a high incidence of *Helicobacter pylori* infection (66% of patients with scleroderma, 78% of patients with scleroderma and Sicca syndrome**[91]), and 4) approximately **44% of scleroderma patients have esophageal overgrowth of *Candida albicans*.**[92] For these and other reasons (detailed in Chapter 4), **patients with scleroderma are presumed to have gastrointestinal dysbiosis until proven otherwise by the combination of 1) three-sample comprehensive parasitology examinations performed by a specialty laboratory and 2) clinical response to at least two 2-4 week courses of broad-spectrum antimicrobial treatment.** Yeast, bacteria, and parasites are treated as indicated based on identification and sensitivity results from comprehensive parasitology assessments. Breath hydrogen/methane testing is inferior to stool testing because it does not allow for identification and sensitivity testing of microbes. Other dysbiotic loci should be investigated as discussed in Chapter 4 in the section on multifocal dysbiosis. Attentive readers may have already surmised that treatment of gastrointestinal dysbiosis in patients with long-standing scleroderma is likely to be particularly difficult due to the neuropathic and myopathic **intestinal dysmotility**[93] **that will serve to perpetuate bacterial overgrowth and dysbiosis, thus necessitating vigilant and long-term treatment**; understanding and due persistence on the part of physician and patient are necessary to see this treatment through to completion—a combination of pharmaceutical/botanical antimicrobials and promotility agents, including the universally safe and effective osmotic laxative magnesium, is reasonable.

  o Gastrointestinal dysbiosis: Treatment for gastrointestinal dysbiosis should be guided by specific findings and sensitivity results from stool testing; the following are commonly employed treatments for dysbiosis:

    ▪ **Ciprofloxacin: Over and Bucknall**[94] **published a case report of a progressive scleroderma patient who experienced marked clinical improvement and biopsy-**

[85] "Octreotide stimulates intestinal motility in normal subjects and in patients with scleroderma. In such patients, the short-term administration of octreotide reduces bacterial overgrowth and improves abdominal symptoms." Soudah HC, Hasler WL, Owyang C. Effect of octreotide on intestinal motility and bacterial overgrowth in scleroderma. *N Engl J Med.* 1991 Nov 21;325(21):1461-7

[86] "…increasing evidence has accumulated to implicate infectious agents in the etiology of systemic sclerosis (SSc)… …increased antibody titers, a preponderance of specific strains in patients with SSc, and evidence of molecular mimicry inducing autoimmune responses suggest mechanisms by which infectious agents may contribute to the development and progression of SSc." Hamamdzic D, Kasman LM, LeRoy EC. The role of infectious agents in the pathogenesis of systemic sclerosis. *Curr Opin Rheumatol.* 2002 Nov;14(6):694-8

[87] Disabling pansclerotic morphea (DPM): "The organism could be identified as Staphylococcus epidermidis, but it also had stages of growth with morphologic forms more characteristic of a Corynebacterium-like or actinomycetelike microbe." Cantwell AR Jr, Jones JE, Kelso DW. Pleomorphic, variably acid-fast bacteria in an adult patient with disabling pansclerotic morphea. *Arch Dermatol.* 1984 May;120(5):656-61

[88] "Variably acid-fast coccoid forms, suggestive of cell wall deficient forms of mycobacteria, were observed in the dermis in microscopic sections of skin from six patients with generalized scleroderma, 10 patients with localized scleroderma (morphea), and four patients with lichen sclerosus et atrophicus (LSA)." Cantwell AR Jr. Histologic observations of pleomorphic, variably acid-fast bacteria in scleroderma, morphea, and lichen sclerosus et atrophicus. *Int J Dermatol.* 1984 Jan-Feb;23(1):45-52

[89] "Eight patients (33%) had significant bacterial counts: > 10(5) colony forming units per ml (cfu/ml) of jejunal fluid." Kaye SA, Lim SG, Taylor M, Patel S, Gillespie S, Black CM. Small bowel bacterial overgrowth in systemic sclerosis: detection using direct and indirect methods and treatment outcome. *Br J Rheumatol.* 1995 Mar;34(3):265-9

[90] "CONCLUSIONS: Our results demonstrated that some of the bacterial species that overgrow in the upper small intestine of patients with progressive systemic sclerosis can deconjugate bile acids, and that a shift to neutral pH in gastric juice, may promote the bacterial overgrowth related to their impaired peristaltic activity." Shindo K, Machida M, Koide K, Fukumura M, Yamazaki R. Deconjugation ability of bacteria isolated from the jejunal fluid of patients with progressive systemic sclerosis and its gastric pH. *Hepatogastroenterology.* 1998 Sep-Oct;45(23):1643-50

[91] "Urease test demonstrated the presence of HP in 23 patients out of 35 (66%); 12 of them were negative to colonization. A Sicca syndrome, with abnormal Schirmers test and dry mouth was detected in 66% of the patients. 78% of the patients with Sicca syndrome had a concomitant HP infection..." Farina G, Rosato E, Francia C, Proietti M, Donato G, Ammendolea C, Pisarri S, Salsano F. High incidence of Helicobacter pylori infection in patients with systemic sclerosis: association with Sicca Syndrome. *Int J Immunopathol Pharmacol.* 2001 May;14(2):81-85

[92] "Esophageal mucosal brushings from 51 consecutive patients with progressive systemic sclerosis (PSS) (group I), 18 PSS patients continuously treated with high-dose ranitidine or omeprazole (group II), 34 controls referred to the outpatient clinic for endoscopy (group III), and 10 patients receiving long-term potent antireflux therapy for idiopathic gastroesophageal reflux (group IV) were cultured for Candida albicans. There were 44%, 89%, 9%, and 0% Candida albicans culture-positive patients in groups I through IV, respectively." Hendel L, Svejgaard E, Walsoe I, Kieffer M, Stenderup A. Esophageal candidosis in progressive systemic sclerosis: occurrence, significance, and treatment with fluconazole. *Scand J Gastroenterol.* 1988 Dec;23(10):1182-6

[93] "We found ultrastructural signs of axonal degeneration and cytoskeletal abnormalities in the bundles of unmyelinated fibers. There was also focal degeneration of smooth muscle cells, often in association with the presence of partially degranulated mast cells." Malandrini A, Selvi E, Villanova M, Berti G, Sabadini L, Salvadori C, Gambelli S, De Stefano R, Vernillo R, Marcolongo R, Guazzi G. Autonomic nervous system and smooth muscle cell involvement in systemic sclerosis: ultrastructural study of 3 cases. *J Rheumatol.* 2000 May;27(5):1203-6

[94] Over KE, Bucknall RC. Regression of skin changes in a patient with systemic sclerosis following treatment for bacterial overgrowth with ciprofloxacin. *Br J Rheumatol.* 1998 Jun;37(6):696 http://rheumatology.oxfordjournals.org/cgi/reprint/37/6/696a

proven regression of skin changes following administration of ciprofloxacin 500 mg bid which was eventually reduced to 250 mg/d. This case report strongly supports the theory that intestinal dysbiosis is a major contributor to scleroderma. As with all antibacterial treatments, use empiric antifungal treatment with Nystatin 500,000 units bid and/or emulsified oregano 150 mg tid-qid.[95,96]

- Oregano oil: Emulsified oil of oregano in a time-released tablet is proven effective in the eradication of harmful gastrointestinal microbes, including *Blastocystis hominis, Entamoeba hartmanni*, and *Endolimax nana*.[97] An *in vitro* study[98] and clinical experience support the use of emulsified oregano against *Candida albicans* and various bacteria. The common dose is 600 mg per day in divided doses for at least 6 weeks.[99]

- Berberine: Berberine is an alkaloid extracted from plants such as *Berberis vulgaris*, and *Hydrastis canadensis*, and it shows effectiveness against *Giardia, Candida,* and *Streptococcus* in addition to its direct anti-inflammatory and antidiarrheal actions. Oral dose of 400 mg per day is common for adults.[100]

- *Artemisia annua*: Artemisinin has been safely used for centuries in Asia for the treatment of malaria, and it also has effectiveness against anaerobic bacteria due to the pro-oxidative sesquiterpene endoperoxide.[101,102] I commonly use artemisinin at 200 mg per day in divided doses for adults with dysbiosis. Evidence of past/current *H. pylori* infection is common (~40-60%) in patients with scleroderma[103], and some doctors have reported anecdotally that *Artemisia annua* helps eradicate *H. pylori*.

- St. John's Wort (*Hypericum perforatum*): Hyperforin from *Hypericum perforatum* also shows impressive antibacterial action, particularly against gram-positive bacteria such as *Staphylococcus aureus, Streptococcus pyogenes, Streptococcus agalactiae*[104] and perhaps *Helicobacter pylori*.[105] Up to 600 mg three times per day of a 3% hyperforin standardized extract is customary in the treatment of depression.

- Bismuth: Bismuth is commonly used in the empiric treatment of diarrhea (e.g., "Pepto-Bismol") and is commonly combined with other antimicrobial agents to reduce drug resistance and increase antibiotic effectiveness.[106]

- Undecylenic acid: Derived from castor bean oil, undecylenic acid has antifungal properties and is commonly indicated by sensitivity results obtained by stool culture. Common dosages are 150-250 mg tid (up to 750 mg per day).[107]

- Peppermint (*Mentha piperita*): Peppermint shows antimicrobial and antispasmodic actions and has demonstrated clinical effectiveness in patients with bacterial overgrowth of the small bowel.

- Commonly used antibiotic/antifungal drugs: The most commonly employed drugs for intestinal bacterial overgrowth are described here.[108] Treatment duration is generally at least 2 weeks and up to 8 weeks, depending on clinical response and the severity and diversity of the intestinal overgrowth. With all anti*bacterial* treatments, use empiric anti*fungal* treatment to prevent yeast overgrowth; some patients benefit from antifungal treatment that is continued for *months* and occasionally *years*. Drugs can generally be coadministered with natural antibiotics/antifungals for improved

[95] Stiles JC, Sparks W, Ronzio RA. The inhibition of Candida albicans by oregano. *J Applied Nutr* 1995;47:96–102
[96] Force M, Sparks WS, Ronzio RA. Inhibition of enteric parasites by emulsified oil of oregano in vivo. *Phytother Res.* 2000 May;14(3):213-4
[97] Force M, Sparks WS, Ronzio RA. Inhibition of enteric parasites by emulsified oil of oregano in vivo. *Phytother Res.* 2000 May;14(3):213-4
[98] Stiles JC, Sparks W, Ronzio RA. The inhibition of Candida albicans by oregano. *J Applied Nutr* 1995;47:96–102
[99] Force M, Sparks WS, Ronzio RA. Inhibition of enteric parasites by emulsified oil of oregano in vivo. *Phytother Res.* 2000 May;14(3):213-4
[100] Berberine. Altern Med Rev. 2000 Apr;5(2):175-7 http://www.thorne.com/altmedrev/.fulltext/5/2/175.pdf
[101] Dien TK, de Vries PJ, Khanh NX, Koopmans R, Binh LN, Duc DD, Kager PA, van Boxtel CJ. Effect of food intake on pharmacokinetics of oral artemisinin in healthy Vietnamese subjects. *Antimicrob Agents Chemother.* 1997 May;41(5):1069-72
[102] Giao PT, Binh TQ, Kager PA, Long HP, Van Thang N, Van Nam N, de Vries PJ. Artemisinin for treatment of uncomplicated falciparum malaria: is there a place for monotherapy? *Am J Trop Med Hyg.* 2001 Dec;65(6):690-5
[103] "Patients with SSc have H. pylori infection at a higher prevalence than the general population." Yazawa N, Fujimoto M, Kikuchi K, Kubo M, Ihn H, Sato S, Tamaki T, Tamaki K. High seroprevalence of Helicobacter pylori infection in patients with systemic sclerosis: association with esophageal involvement. *J Rheumatol.* 1998 Apr;25(4):650-3
[104] Schempp CM, Pelz K, Wittmer A, Schopf E, Simon JC. Antibacterial activity of hyperforin from St John's wort, against multiresistant Staphylococcus aureus and gram-positive bacteria. *Lancet.* 1999 Jun 19;353(9170):2129
[105] "A butanol fraction of St. John's Wort revealed anti-Helicobacter pylori activity with MIC values ranging between 15.6 and 31.2 microg/ml." Reichling J, Weseler A, Saller R. A current review of the antimicrobial activity of Hypericum perforatum L. *Pharmacopsychiatry.* 2001 Jul;34 Suppl 1:S116-8
[106] Veldhuyzen van Zanten SJ, Sherman PM, Hunt RH. Helicobacter pylori: new developments and treatments." *CMAJ.* 1997;156(11):1565-74 http://www.cmaj.ca/cgi/reprint/156/11/1565.pdf
[107] "Adult dosage is usually 450-750 mg undecylenic acid daily in three divided doses." Undecylenic acid. Monograph. *Altern Med Rev.* 2002 Feb;7(1):68-70 http://www.thorne.com/altmedrev/.fulltext/7/1/68.pdf
[108] Saltzman JR, Russell RM. Nutritional consequences of intestinal bacterial overgrowth. *Compr Ther.* 1994;20(9):523-30

efficacy. Treatment can be guided by identification of the dysbiotic microbes and the results of culture and sensitivity tests.

⇒ Metronidazole: 250-500 mg BID-QID (generally limit to 1.5 g/d); metronidazole has systemic bioavailability and effectiveness against a wide range of dysbiotic microbes, including protozoans, amebas/Giardia, *H. pylori*, *Clostridium difficile* and most anaerobic gram-negative bacilli.[109] Adverse effects are generally limited to stomatitis, nausea, diarrhea, and—rarely and/or with long-term use—peripheral neuropathy, dizziness, and metallic taste; the drug must not be consumed with alcohol. Metronidazole resistance by *Blastocystis hominis* and other parasites has been noted.

⇒ Erythromycin: 250-500 mg TID-QID; this drug is a widely used antibiotic that also has intestinal promotility benefits (thus making it an ideal treatment for intestinal bacterial overgrowth associated with or caused by intestinal dysmotility/hypomotility such as seen in scleroderma[110,111]). Do not combine erythromycin with the promotility drug **cisapride** due to risk for serious cardiac arrhythmia.

⇒ Tetracycline: 250-500 mg QID

⇒ Ciproflaxacin: 500 mg BID

⇒ Cephalexin/kelfex: 250 mg QID

⇒ Minocycline: Minocycline (200 mg/day)[112] has received the most attention in the treatment of rheumatoid arthritis due to its superior response (65%) over placebo (13%)[113]; in addition to its antibacterial action, the drug is also immunomodulatory and anti-inflammatory. Ironically, minocycline can cause drug-induced autoimmunity, especially lupus.[114,115]

⇒ Nystatin: Nystatin 500,000 units bid with food; duration of treatment begins with a minimum duration of 2-4 weeks and may continue as long as the patient is deriving benefit.

⇒ Ketoconazole: As a systemically bioavailable antifungal drug, ketoconazole has inherent anti-inflammatory benefits which may be helpful; however the drug inhibits androgen formation and may lead to exacerbation of the hypoandrogenism that is commonly seen in autoimmune patients and which contributes to the immune dysfunction.

- Probiotics: Live cultures in the form of tablets, capsules, yogurt, or kefir can be used per patient preference and tolerance. Obviously, dairy-based products should be avoided by patients with dairy allergy.

- Supplemented Paleo-Mediterranean diet / specific carbohydrate diet: The specifications of the specific carbohydrate diet detailed by Gottschall[116] are met with adherence to the Paleo diet by Cordain.[117] The combination of both approaches will give patients an excellent combination of informational understanding and culinary versatility. In accord with both of these dietary programs, the diet must remain free of gluten-containing grains such as wheat, since **some patients with scleroderma**

[109] Tierney ML. McPhee SJ, Papadakis MA. Current Medical Diagnosis and Treatment 2006. 45th edition. New York; Lange Medical Books: 2006, pages 1578-1577

[110] "Prokinetic agents effective in pseudoobstruction include metoclopramide, domperidone, cisapride, octreotide, and erythromycin. ... The combination of octreotide and erythromycin may be particularly effective in systemic sclerosis." Sjogren RW. Gastrointestinal features of scleroderma. *Curr Opin Rheumatol.* 1996 Nov;8(6):569-75

[111] "CONCLUSIONS: Erythromycin accelerates gastric and gallbladder emptying in scleroderma patients and might be helpful in the treatment of gastrointestinal motor abnormalities in these patients." Fiorucci S, Distrutti E, Bassotti G, Gerli R, Chiucchiu S, Betti C, Santucci L, Morelli A. Effect of erythromycin administration on upper gastrointestinal motility in scleroderma patients. *Scand J Gastroenterol.* 1994 Sep;29(9):807-13

[112] "...48-week trial of oral minocycline (200 mg/d) or placebo." Tilley BC, Alarcon GS, Heyse SP, Trentham DE, Neuner R, Kaplan DA, Clegg DO, Leisen JC, Buckley L, Cooper SM, Duncan H, Pillemer SR, Tuttleman M, Fowler SE. Minocycline in rheumatoid arthritis. A 48-week, double-blind, placebo-controlled trial. MIRA Trial Group. *Ann Intern Med.* 1995 Jan 15;122(2):81-9

[113] "In patients with early seropositive RA, therapy with minocycline is superior to placebo." O'Dell JR, Haire CE, Palmer W, Drymalski W, Wees S, Blakely K, Churchill M, Eckhoff PJ, Weaver A, Doud D, Erikson N, Dietz F, Olson R, Maloley P, Klassen LW, Moore GF. Treatment of early rheumatoid arthritis with minocycline or placebo: results of a randomized, double-blind, placebo-controlled trial. *Arthritis Rheum.* 1997 May;40(5):842-8

[114] "...many cases of drug-induced lupus related to minocycline have been reported. Some of those reports included pulmonary lupus..." Christodoulou CS, Emmanuel P, Ray RA, Good RA, Schnapf BM, Cawkwell GD. Respiratory distress due to minocycline-induced pulmonary lupus. *Chest.* 1999 May;115(5):1471-3 http://www.chestjournal.org/cgi/content/full/115/5/1471

[115] Lawson TM, Amos N, Bulgen D, Williams BD.Minocycline-induced lupus: clinical features and response to rechallenge. *Rheumatology* (Oxford). 2001 Mar;40(3):329-35 http://rheumatology.oxfordjournals.org/cgi/content/full/40/3/329

[116] Gotschall E. Breaking the Vicious Cycle: Intestinal health though diet. Kirkton Press; Rev edition (August, 1994) http://www.scdiet.com/

[117] Cordain L: The Paleo Diet: Lose weight and get healthy by eating the food you were designed to eat. John Wiley & Sons Inc., New York 2002 http://thepaleodiet.com/

have celiac disease[118,119], and since **wheat, like most grains (except rice), promotes bacterial overgrowth of the intestine due to its high quantity of indigestible oligosaccharides.**[120]

- Orthoendocrinology: Assess **prolactin**, cortisol, **DHEA**, free and total testosterone, serum estradiol, and thyroid status (e.g., TSH, T4, free T3, *and* anti-thyroid peroxidase antibodies).

  o Melatonin: **In a recent *in vitro* study with fibroblasts from normal and scleroderma patients, melatonin was shown to inhibit fibroblast proliferation**[121]; future trials may demonstrate that melatonin has an antifibrotic/antisclerodermatous benefit. Melatonin is a pineal hormone with well-known sleep-inducing and immunomodulatory properties, and it is commonly administered in doses of 1-40 mg in the evening, before bedtime. Its exceptional safety is well documented. In contrast to implementing treatment with high doses of 20-40 mg, starting with a relatively low dose (e.g., 1-5 mg) and increasing as tolerated is recommended. Melatonin (20 mg hs) appears to have cured two patients with drug-resistant sarcoidosis[122] and 3 mg provided immediate short-term benefit to a patient with multiple sclerosis.[123] Immunostimulatory anti-infective action of melatonin was demonstrated in a clinical trial wherein septic newborns administered 20 mg melatonin showed significantly increased survival over nontreated controls[124]; **given that scleroderma is associated with subclinical "infections", melatonin may provide therapeutic benefit by virtue of its anti-infective properties.**

  o Prolactin (excess): Serum prolactin is the standard assessment of prolactin status. Since elevated prolactin may be a sign of pituitary tumor, assessment for headaches, visual deficits, other abnormalities of pituitary hormones (e.g., GH and TSH) should be performed and CT or MRI must be considered. Patients with prolactin levels less than 100 ng/mL and normal CT/MRI findings can be managed conservatively with effective prolactin-lowering treatment and annual radiologic assessment (less necessary with favorable serum response).[125,126] Patients with

> "The altered hormonal status could result in relative immunological hyperactivity contributing to enhance tissue damage and disease severity."
>
> Mirone, Barini, Barini. **Androgen and prolactin levels in systemic sclerosis: relationship to disease severity.** *Ann N Y Acad Sci* 2006

RA and SLE have higher basal and stress-induced levels of prolactin compared with normal controls.[127,128] **Prolactin levels are high and DHEA levels are low in patients with scleroderma.**[129,130] Specific treatment options include the following:

  ▪ Thyroid hormone: Hypothyroidism frequently causes hyperprolactinemia which is reversible upon effective treatment of hypothyroidism. Therefore, thyroid status should be evaluated in all patients with hyperprolactinemia. Thyroid assessment and treatment is reviewed later in this section.

[118] "Coeliac disease may account for malabsorption in scleroderma patients even when test suggest bacterial overgrowth." Marguerie C, Kaye S, Vyse T, Mackworth-Young C, Walport MJ, Black C. Malabsorption caused by coeliac disease in patients who have scleroderma. *Br J Rheumatol*. 1995 Sep;34(9):858-61
[119] Gomez-Puerta JA, Gil V, Cervera R, Miquel R, Jimenez S, Ramos-Casals M, Font J. Coeliac disease associated with systemic sclerosis. *Ann Rheum Dis*. 2004 Jan;63(1):104-5 http://ard.bmjjournals.com/cgi/content/full/63/1/104
[120] "Short-chain fructooligosaccharides occur in a number of edible plants, such as chicory, onions, asparagus, wheat... Short-chain fructooligosaccharides, to a large extent, escape digestion in the human upper intestine and reach the colon where they are totally fermented mostly to lactate, short chain fatty acids (acetate, propionate and butyrate), and gas, like dietary fibres." Bornet FR, Brouns F, Tashiro Y, Duvillier V. Nutritional aspects of short-chain fructooligosaccharides: natural occurrence, chemistry, physiology and health implications. *Dig Liver Dis*. 2002 Sep;34 Suppl 2:S111-20
[121] "These results suggest that MLT, at higher dosages, is a potent inhibitor of the proliferation of fibroblasts derived from the skin of healthy and SSc patients." Carossino AM, Lombardi A, Matucci-Cerinic M, Pignone A, Cagnoni M. Effect of melatonin on normal and sclerodermic skin fibroblast proliferation. *Clin Exp Rheumatol*. 1996 Sep-Oct;14(5):493-8.
[122] Cagnoni ML, Lombardi A, Cerinic MC, Dedola GL, Pignone A. Melatonin for treatment of chronic refractory sarcoidosis. *Lancet*. 1995 Nov 4;346(8984):1229-30
[123] "...administration of melatonin (3 mg, orally) at 2:00 p.m., when the patient experienced severe blurring of vision, resulted within 15 minutes in a dramatic improvement in visual acuity and in normalization of the visual evoked potential latency after stimulation of the left eye." Sandyk R. Diurnal variations in vision and relations to circadian melatonin secretion in multiple sclerosis. *Int J Neurosci*. 1995 Nov;83(1-2):1-6
[124] Gitto E, Karbownik M, Reiter RJ, Tan DX, Cuzzocrea S, Chiurazzi P, Cordaro S, Corona G, Trimarchi G, Barberi I. Effects of melatonin treatment in septic newborns. *Pediatr Res*. 2001 Dec;50(6):756-60 http://www.pedresearch.org/cgi/content/full/50/6/756
[125] Beers MH, Berkow R (eds). The Merck Manual. Seventeenth Edition. Whitehouse Station; Merck Research Laboratories 1999 Page 77-78
[126] Serri O, Chik CL, Ur E, Ezzat S. Diagnosis and management of hyperprolactinemia. *CMAJ*. 2003 Sep 16;169(6):575-81 http://www.cmaj.ca/cgi/content/full/169/6/575
[127] Dostal C, Moszkorzova L, Musilova L, Lacinova Z, Marek J, Zvarova J. Serum prolactin stress values in patients with systemic lupus erythematosus. *Ann Rheum Dis*. 2003 May;62(5):487-8 http://ard.bmjjournals.com/cgi/content/full/62/5/487
[128] "RESULTS: A significantly higher rate of elevated PRL levels was found in SLE patients (40.0%) compared with the healthy controls (14.8%). No proof was found of association with the presence of anti-ds-DNA or with specific organ involvement. Similarly, elevated PRL levels were found in RA patients (39.3%)." Moszkorzova L, Lacinova Z, Marek J, Musilova L, Dohnalova A, Dostal C. Hyperprolactinaemia in patients with systemic lupus erythematosus. *Clin Exp Rheumatol*. 2002 Nov-Dec;20(6):807-12
[129] "Compared to SSc with <9 disease manifestations, patients with > or =9 disease manifestations had higher PRL, higher soluble interleukin 2 receptor and vascular cell adhesion molecule, and lower DHEAS (P = 0.029)." Straub RH, Zeuner M, Lock G, Scholmerich J, Lang B. High prolactin and low dehydroepiandrosterone sulphate serum levels in patients with severe systemic sclerosis. *Br J Rheumatol*. 1997 Apr;36(4):426-32 http://rheumatology.oxfordjournals.org/cgi/reprint/36/4/426
[130] "The dysregulation of adrenal (DHEAS) and hypothalamic-pituitary function (Prl) is a characteristic feature of immune diseases." Mirone L, Barini A, Barini A. Androgen and prolactin (Prl) levels in systemic sclerosis (SSc): relationship to disease severity. *Ann N Y Acad Sci*. 2006 Jun;1069:257-62

- *Vitex astus-cagnus* and other supporting botanicals and nutrients: **Vitex lowers serum prolactin in humans[131,132] via a dopaminergic effect.[133]** Vitex is considered safe for clinical use; mild and reversible adverse effects possibly associated with Vitex include nausea, headache, gastrointestinal disturbances, menstrual disorders, acne, pruritus and erythematous rash. No drug interactions are known, but given the herb's dopaminergic effect it should probably be used with some caution in patients treated with dopamine antagonists such as the so-called antipsychotic drugs (most of which do not work very well and/or carry intolerable adverse effects[134,135]). In a recent review, Bone[136] stated that daily doses can range from 500 mg to 2,000 mg DHE (dry herb equivalent) and can be tailored to the suppression of prolactin. Due at least in part to its content of L-dopa, *Mucuna pruriens* **shows clinical dopaminergic activity** as evidenced by its effectiveness in Parkinson's disease[137]; up to 15-30 gm/d of mucuna has been used clinically but doses will be dependent on preparation and phytoconcentration. **Triptolide and other extracts from *Tripterygium wilfordii* Hook F exert clinically significant anti-inflammatory action in patients with rheumatoid arthritis[138,139] and also offer protection to dopaminergic neurons.[140,141]** Ironically, even though tyrosine is the nutritional precursor to dopamine with evidence of clinical effectiveness (e.g., narcolepsy[142], enhancement of memory[143] and cognition[144]), **supplementation with tyrosine appears to actually increase rather than decrease prolactin levels[145]; therefore tyrosine should be used cautiously if at all in patients with systemic inflammation.** Furthermore, the finding that **high-protein meals stimulate prolactin release[146]** may partly explain the benefits of vegetarian diets in the treatment of systemic inflammation; since vegetarian diets are comparatively low in protein compared to omnivorous diets, they may lead to a relative reduction in prolactin production due to lack of stimulation.
- Bromocriptine: Bromocriptine has long been considered the pharmacologic treatment of choice for elevated prolactin.[147] Typical dose is 2.5 mg per day (effective against

---

[131] "Since AC extracts were shown to have beneficial effects on premenstrual mastodynia serum prolactin levels in such patients were also studied in one double-blind, placebo-controlled clinical study. Serum prolactin levels were indeed reduced in the patients treated with the extract." Wuttke W, Jarry H, Christoffel V, Spengler B, Seidlova-Wuttke D. Chaste tree (Vitex agnus-castus)--pharmacology and clinical indications. *Phytomedicine.* 2003 May;10(4):348-57

[132] German abstract from Medline: "The prolactin release was reduced after 3 months, shortened luteal phases were normalised and deficits in the luteal progesterone synthesis were eliminated." Milewicz A, Gejdel E, Sworen H, Sienkiewicz K, Jedrzejak J, Teucher T, Schmitz H. [Vitex agnus castus extract in the treatment of luteal phase defects due to latent hyperprolactinemia. Results of a randomized placebo-controlled double-blind study] *Arzneimittelforschung.* 1993 Jul;43(7):752-6

[133] "Our results indicate a dopaminergic effect of Vitex agnus-castus extracts and suggest additional pharmacological actions via opioid receptors." Meier B, Berger D, Hoberg E, Sticher O, Schaffner W. Pharmacological activities of Vitex agnus-castus extracts in vitro. *Phytomedicine.* 2000 Oct;7(5):373-81

[134] "The majority of patients in each group discontinued their assigned treatment owing to inefficacy or intolerable side effects or for other reasons." Lieberman JA, Stroup TS, McEvoy JP, Swartz MS, Rosenheck RA, Perkins DO, Keefe RS, Davis SM, Davis CE, Lebowitz BD, Severe J, Hsiao JK; Clinical Antipsychotic Trials of Intervention Effectiveness (CATIE) Investigators. Effectiveness of antipsychotic drugs in patients with chronic schizophrenia. *N Engl J Med.* 2005 Sep 22;353(12):1209-23

[135] Whitaker R. The case against antipsychotic drugs: a 50-year record of doing more harm than good. *Med Hypotheses.* 2004;62(1):5-13

[136] "In conditions such as endometriosis and fibroids, for which a significant estrogen antagonist effect is needed, doses of at least 2 g/day DHE may be required and typically are used by professional herbalists." Bone K. New Insights Into Chaste Tree. *Nutritional Wellness* 2005 November http://www.nutritionalwellness.com/archives/2005/nov/11_bone.php

[137] "CONCLUSIONS: The rapid onset of action and longer on time without concomitant increase in dyskinesias on mucuna seed powder formulation suggest that this natural source of L-dopa might possess advantages over conventional L-dopa preparations in the long term management of PD." Katzenschlager R, Evans A, Manson A, Patsalos PN, Ratnaraj N, Watt H, Timmermann L, Van der Giessen R, Lees AJ. Mucuna pruriens in Parkinson's disease: a double blind clinical and pharmacological study. *J Neurol Neurosurg Psychiatry.* 2004 Dec;75(12):1672-7

[138] "The ethanol/ethyl acetate extract of TWHF shows therapeutic benefit in patients with treatment-refractory RA. At therapeutic dosages, the TWHF extract was well tolerated by most patients in this study." Tao X, Younger J, Fan FZ, Wang B, Lipsky PE. Benefit of an extract of Tripterygium Wilfordii Hook F in patients with rheumatoid arthritis: a double-blind, placebo-controlled study. *Arthritis Rheum.* 2002 Jul;46(7):1735-43

[139] "CONCLUSION: The EA extract of TWHF at dosages up to 570 mg/day appeared to be safe, and doses > 360 mg/day were associated with clinical benefit in patients with RA." Tao X, Cush JJ, Garret M, Lipsky PE. A phase I study of ethyl acetate extract of the chinese antirheumatic herb Tripterygium wilfordii hook F in rheumatoid arthritis. *J Rheumatol.* 2001 Oct;28(10):2160-7

[140] "Our data suggests that triptolide may protect dopaminergic neurons from LPS-induced injury and its efficiency in inhibiting microglia activation may underlie the mechanism." Li FQ, Lu XZ, Liang XB, Zhou HF, Xue B, Liu XY, Niu DB, Han JS, Wang XM. Triptolide, a Chinese herbal extract, protects dopaminergic neurons from inflammation-mediated damage through inhibition of microglial activation. *J Neuroimmunol.* 2004 Mar;148(1-2):24-31

[141] "Moreover, tripchlorolide markedly prevented the decrease in amount of dopamine in the striatum of model rats. Taken together, our data provide the first evidence that tripchlorolide acts as a neuroprotective molecule that rescues MPP+ or axotomy-induced degeneration of dopaminergic neurons, which may imply its therapeutic potential for Parkinson's disease." Li FQ, Cheng XX, Liang XB, Wang XH, Xue B, He QH, Wang XM, Han JS. Neurotrophic and neuroprotective effects of tripchlorolide, an extract of Chinese herb Tripterygium wilfordii Hook F, on dopaminergic neurons. *Exp Neurol.* 2003 Jan;179(1):28-37

[142] "Of twenty-eight visual analogue scales rating mood and arousal, the subjects' ratings in the tyrosine treatment (9 g daily) and placebo periods differed significantly for only three (less tired, less drowsy, more alert)." Elwes RD, Crewes H, Chesterman LP, Summers B, Jenner P, Binnie CD, Parkes JD. Treatment of narcolepsy with L-tyrosine: double-blind placebo-controlled trial. *Lancet.* 1989 Nov 4;2(8671):1067-9

[143] "Ten men and 10 women subjects underwent these batteries 1 h after ingesting 150 mg/kg of l-tyrosine or placebo. Administration of tyrosine significantly enhanced accuracy and decreased frequency of list retrieval on the working memory task during the multiple task battery compared with placebo." Thomas JR, Lockwood PA, Singh A, Deuster PA. Tyrosine improves working memory in a multitasking environment. *Pharmacol Biochem Behav.* 1999 Nov;64(3):495-500

[144] "Ten subjects received five daily doses of a protein-rich drink containing 2 g tyrosine, and 11 subjects received a carbohydrate rich drink with the same amount of calories (255 kcal)." Deijen JB, Wientjes CJ, Vullinghs HF, Cloin PA, Langefeld JJ. Tyrosine improves cognitive performance and reduces blood pressure in cadets after one week of a combat training course. *Brain Res Bull.* 1999 Jan 15;48(2):203-9

[145] "Tyrosine (when compared to placebo) had no effect on any sleep related measure, but it did stimulate plasma prolactin release." Waters WF, Magill RA, Bray GA, Volaufova J, Smith SR, Lieberman HR, Rood J, Hurry M, Anderson T, Ryan DH. A comparison of tyrosine against placebo, phentermine, caffeine, and D-amphetamine during sleep deprivation. *Nutr Neurosci.* 2003;6(4):221-35

[146] "Whereas carbohydrate meals had no discernible effects, high protein meals induced a large increase in both PRL and cortisol; high fat meals caused selective release of PRL." Ishizuka B, Quigley ME, Yen SS. Pituitary hormone release in response to food ingestion: evidence for neuroendocrine signals from gut to brain. *J Clin Endocrinol Metab.* 1983 Dec;57(6):1111-6

[147] Beers MH, Berkow R (eds). The Merck Manual. Seventeenth Edition. Whitehouse Station; Merck Research Laboratories 1999 Page 77-78

lupus[148]); gastrointestinal upset and sedation are common.[149] Clinical intervention with bromocriptine appears warranted in patients with RA, SLE, Reiter's syndrome, psoriatic arthritis, and probably multiple sclerosis and uveitis.[150]

- Cabergoline/Dostinex: Cabergoline/Dostinex is a newer dopamine agonist with few adverse effects; typical dose starts at 0.5 mg per week (0.25 mg twice per week).[151] Several studies have indicated that cabergoline is safer and more effective than bromocriptine for reducing prolactin levels[152] and the dose can often be reduced after successful prolactin reduction, allowing for reductions in cost and adverse effects.[153] Although fewer studies have been published supporting the antirheumatic benefits of cabergoline than those supporting bromocriptine; its antirheumatic benefits have indeed been documented.[154]

o Estrogen (excess): **Research suggests that estrogen is immunodysregulatory and an important contributor to autoimmune disease**, perhaps explaining the greatly higher incidence of autoimmune diseases in women compared to men. So-called **"estrogen-replacement therapy" used in postmenopausal women increases the risk for lupus and scleroderma**.[155] Men with rheumatoid arthritis show an excess of estradiol and a decrease in DHEA, and the excess estrogen is proportional to the degree of inflammation.[156] Serum estradiol is commonly used to assess estrogen status; estrogens can also be measured in 24-hour urine samples. Interventions to combat high estrogen levels may include any effective combination of the following:

- Weight loss and weight optimization: In overweight patients, weight loss is the means to attaining the goal of weight optimization; the task is not complete until the body mass index is normalized/optimized. Excess adiposity and obesity raise estrogen levels due to high levels of aromatase (the hormone that makes estrogen) in adipose tissue; weight optimization and loss of excess fat helps normalize hormone levels and reduce inflammation.

- Avoidance of ethanol: Estrogen production is stimulated by ethanol intake.

- Consider surgical correction of varicocele in affected men: Men with varicocele have higher estrogen levels due to temperature-induced alterations in enzyme function in the testes; surgical correction of the varicocele lowers estrogen levels.

- "Anti-estrogen diet": Foods and supplements such as green tea, DIM, I3C, licorice, and a high-fiber "anti-estrogenic diet" can also be used; monitoring clinical status and serum estradiol will prove or disprove efficacy.

- Anastrozole/Arimidex: In our office, we commonly measure serum estradiol in men and administer the aromatase inhibitor anastrozole/arimidex 1 mg (2-3 doses per week) to men whose estradiol level is greater than 32 picogram/mL; we consider estradiol 10-24 picogram/mL to be optimal for a man.[157] Clinical studies using anastrozole/arimidex in men have shown that aromatase blockade lowers

---

[148] "A prospective, double-blind, randomized, placebo-controlled study compared BRC at a fixed daily dosage of 2.5 mg with placebo... Long term treatment with a low dose of BRC appears to be a safe and effective means of decreasing SLE flares in SLE patients." Alvarez-Nemegyei J, Cobarrubias-Cobos A, Escalante-Triay F, Sosa-Munoz J, Miranda JM, Jara LJ. Bromocriptine in systemic lupus erythematosus: a double-blind, randomized, placebo-controlled study. *Lupus*. 1998;7(6):414-9
[149] Serri O, Chik CL, Ur E, Ezzat S. Diagnosis and management of hyperprolactinemia. *CMAJ*. 2003 Sep 16;169(6):575-81 http://www.cmaj.ca/cgi/content/full/169/6/575
[150] "...clinical observations and trials support the use of bromocriptine as a nonstandard primary or adjunctive therapy in the treatment of recalcitrant RA, SLE, Reiter's syndrome, and psoriatic arthritis and associated conditions unresponsive to traditional approaches." McMurray RW. Bromocriptine in rheumatic and autoimmune diseases. *Semin Arthritis Rheum*. 2001 Aug;31(1):21-32
[151] Serri O, Chik CL, Ur E, Ezzat S. Diagnosis and management of hyperprolactinemia. *CMAJ*. 2003 Sep 16;169(6):575-81 http://www.cmaj.ca/cgi/content/full/169/6/575
[152] "CONCLUSION: These data indicate that cabergoline is a very effective agent for lowering the prolactin levels in hyperprolactinemic patients and that it appears to offer considerable advantage over bromocriptine in terms of efficacy and tolerability." Sabuncu T, Arikan E, Tasan E, Hatemi H. Comparison of the effects of cabergoline and bromocriptine on prolactin levels in hyperprolactinemic patients. *Intern Med*. 2001 Sep;40(9):857-61
[153] "Cabergoline also normalized PRL in the majority of patients with known bromocriptine intolerance or -resistance. Once PRL secretion was adequately controlled, the dose of cabergoline could often be significantly decreased, which further reduced costs of therapy." Verhelst J, Abs R, Maiter D, van den Bruel A, Vandeweghe M, Velkeniers B, Mockel J, Lamberigts G, Petrossians P, Coremans P, Mahler C, Stevenaert A, Verlooy J, Raftopoulos C, Beckers A. Cabergoline in the treatment of hyperprolactinemia: a study in 455 patients. *J Clin Endocrinol Metab*. 1999 Jul;84(7):2518-22 http://jcem.endojournals.org/cgi/content/full/84/7/2518
[154] Erb N, Pace AV, Delamere JP, Kitas GD. Control of unremitting rheumatoid arthritis by the prolactin antagonist cabergoline. *Rheumatology* (Oxford). 2001 Feb;40(2):237-9 http://rheumatology.oxfordjournals.org/cgi/content/full/40/2/237
[155] "These studies indicate that estrogen replacement therapy in postmenopausal women increases the risk of developing lupus, scleroderma, and Raynaud disease..." Mayes MD. Epidemiologic studies of environmental agents and systemic autoimmune diseases. *Environ Health Perspect*. 1999 Oct;107 Suppl 5:743-8
[156] "RESULTS: DHEAS and estrone concentrations were lower and estradiol was higher in patients compared with healthy controls. DHEAS differed between RF positive and RF negative patients. Estrone did not correlate with any disease variable, whereas estradiol correlated strongly and positively with all measured indices of inflammation." Tengstrand B, Carlstrom K, Fellander-Tsai L, Hafstrom I. Abnormal levels of serum dehydroepiandrosterone, estrone, and estradiol in men with rheumatoid arthritis: high correlation between serum estradiol and current degree of inflammation. *J Rheumatol*. 2003 Nov;30(11):2338-43
[157] Male Hormone Modulation Therapy, Page 4 Of 7: http://www.lef.org/protocols/prtcl-130c.shtml Accessed October 30, 2005

estradiol and raises testosterone[158]; generally speaking, this is exactly the result that we want in patients with severe systemic autoimmunity. Frequency of dosing is based on serum and clinical response.

- Cortisol (insufficiency): Cortisol has immunoregulatory and "immunosuppressive" actions at physiological concentrations. Low adrenal function is common in patients with chronic inflammation[159,160,161] Assessment of cortisol production and adrenal function was detailed in Chapter 4 under the section of Orthoendocrinology. Supplementation with 20 mg per day of cortisol/Cortef is physiologic; my preference is to dose 10 mg first thing in the morning, then 5 mg in late morning and 5 mg in midafternoon in an attempt to replicate the diurnal variation and normal morning peak of cortisol levels. In patients with hypoadrenalism, administration of pregnenolone in doses of 10-60 mg in the morning may also be beneficial.

- Testosterone (insufficiency): Androgen deficiencies predispose to, are exacerbated by, and contribute to autoimmune/inflammatory disorders. A large proportion of men with lupus or RA have low testosterone[162] and suffer the effects of hypogonadism: fatigue, weakness, depression, slow healing, low libido, and difficulties with sexual performance. Testosterone levels may rise following DHEA supplementation (especially in women) and can be elevated in men by the use of anastrozole/arimidex. Otherwise, transdermal testosterone such as Androgel or Testim can be applied as indicated.

- DHEA (insufficiency / supraphysiologic supplementation): **Prolactin levels are high and DHEA levels are low in patients with scleroderma.**[163] DHEA is an anti-inflammatory and immunoregulatory hormone that is commonly deficient in patients with autoimmunity and inflammatory arthritis.[164] DHEA levels are suppressed by prednisone[165], and DHEA has been shown to reverse the osteoporosis and loss of bone mass induced by corticosteroid treatment.[166] DHEA shows no acute or subacute toxicity even when used in supraphysiologic doses, even when used in sick patients. For example, in a study of 32 patients with HIV, DHEA doses of 750 mg – 2,250 mg per day were well tolerated and produced no dose-limiting adverse effects.[167] This lack of toxicity compares favorably with any and all so-called "antirheumatic" drugs, nearly all of which show impressive comparable toxicity. When used at doses of 200 mg per day, DHEA safely provides clinical benefit for patients with various autoimmune diseases, including ulcerative colitis, Crohn's disease[168], and SLE.[169] In patients with SLE, DHEA supplementation allows for reduced dosing of prednisone (thus avoiding its adverse effects) while providing symptomatic improvement.[170] Optimal clinical response appears to correlate with serum levels that are

[158] "These data demonstrate that aromatase inhibition increases serum bioavailable and total testosterone levels to the youthful normal range in older men with mild hypogonadism." Leder BZ, Rohrer JL, Rubin SD, Gallo J, Longcope C. Effects of aromatase inhibition in elderly men with low or borderline-low serum testosterone levels. *J Clin Endocrinol Metab.* 2004 Mar;89(3):1174-80 http://jcem.endojournals.org/cgi/reprint/89/3/1174
[159] "Yet evidence that patients with rheumatoid arthritis improved with small, physiologic dosages of cortisol or cortisone acetate was reported over 25 years ago, and that patients with chronic allergic disorders or unexplained chronic fatigue also improved with administration of such small dosages was reported over 15 years ago..." Jefferies WM. Mild adrenocortical deficiency, chronic allergies, autoimmune disorders and the chronic fatigue syndrome: a continuation of the cortisone story. *Med Hypotheses.* 1994 Mar;42(3):183-9 http://www.thebuteykocentre.com/Irish_%20Buteykocenter_files/further_studies/med_hyp2.pdf http://members.westnet.com.au/pkolb/med_hyp2.pdf
[160] "The etiology of rheumatoid arthritis ...explained by a combination of three factors: (i) a relatively mild deficiency of cortisol, ..., (ii) a deficiency of DHEA, ...and (iii) infection by organisms such as mycoplasma,..." Jefferies WM. The etiology of rheumatoid arthritis. *Med Hypotheses.* 1998 Aug;51(2):111-4
[161] Jefferies W McK. Safe Uses of Cortisol. Second Edition. Springfield, CC Thomas, 1996
[162] Karagiannis A, Harsoulis F. Gonadal dysfunction in systemic diseases. *Eur J Endocrinol.* 2005 Apr;152(4):501-13 http://www.eje-online.org/cgi/content/full/152/4/501
[163] "Compared to SSc with <9 disease manifestations, patients with > or =9 disease manifestations had higher PRL, higher soluble interleukin 2 receptor and vascular cell adhesion molecule, and lower DHEAS (P = 0.029)." Straub RH, Zeuner M, Lock G, Scholmerich J, Lang B. High prolactin and low dehydroepiandrosterone sulphate serum levels in patients with severe systemic sclerosis. *Br J Rheumatol.* 1997 Apr;36(4):426-32 http://rheumatology.oxfordjournals.org/cgi/reprint/36/4/426 and http://rheumatology.oxfordjournals.org/cgi/content/abstract/36/4/426
[164] "DHEAS concentrations were significantly decreased in both women and men with inflammatory arthritis (IA) (P < 0.001)." Dessein PH, Joffe BI, Stanwix AE, Moomal Z. Hyposecretion of the adrenal androgen dehydroepiandrosterone sulfate and its relation to clinical variables in inflammatory arthritis. *Arthritis Res.* 2001;3(3):183-8. Epub 2001 Feb 21. http://arthritis-research.com/content/3/3/183
[165] "Basal serum DHEA and DHEAS concentrations were suppressed to a greater degree than was cortisol during both daily and alternate day prednisone treatments. ...Thus, adrenal androgen secretion was more easily suppressed than was cortisol secretion by this low dose of glucocorticoid, but there was no advantage to alternate day therapy." Rittmaster RS, Givner ML. Effect of daily and alternate day low dose prednisone on serum cortisol and adrenal androgens in hirsute women. *J Clin Endocrinol Metab.* 1988 Aug;67(2):400-3
[166] "CONCLUSION: Prasterone treatment prevented BMD loss and significantly increased BMD at both the lumbar spine and total hip in female patients with SLE receiving exogenous glucocorticoids." Mease PJ, Ginzler EM, Gluck OS, Schiff M, Goldman A, Greenwald M, Cohen S, Egan R, Quarles BJ, Schwartz KE. Effects of prasterone on bone mineral density in women with systemic lupus erythematosus receiving chronic glucocorticoid therapy. *J Rheumatol.* 2005 Apr;32(4):616-21
[167] "Thirty-one subjects were evaluated and monitored for safety and tolerance. The oral drug was administered three times daily in doses ranging from 750 mg/day to 2,250 mg/day for 16 weeks. ... The drug was well tolerated and no dose-limiting side effects were noted." Dyner TS, Lang W, Geaga J, Golub A, Stites D, Winger E, Galmarini M, Masterson J, Jacobson MA. An open-label dose-escalation trial of oral dehydroepiandrosterone tolerance and pharmacokinetics in patients with HIV disease. *J Acquir Immune Defic Syndr.* 1993 May;6(5):459-65
[168] "CONCLUSIONS: In a pilot study, dehydroepiandrosterone was effective and safe in patients with refractory Crohn's disease or ulcerative colitis." Andus T, Klebl F, Rogler G, Bregenzer N, Scholmerich J, Straub RH. Patients with refractory Crohn's disease or ulcerative colitis respond to dehydroepiandrosterone: a pilot study. *Aliment Pharmacol Ther.* 2003 Feb;17(3):409-14
[169] "CONCLUSION: The overall results confirm that DHEA treatment was well-tolerated, significantly reduced the number of SLE flares, and improved patient's global assessment of disease activity." Chang DM, Lan JL, Lin HY, Luo SF. Dehydroepiandrosterone treatment of women with mild-to-moderate systemic lupus erythematosus: a multicenter randomized, double-blind, placebo-controlled trial. *Arthritis Rheum.* 2002 Nov;46(11):2924-7
[170] "CONCLUSION: Among women with lupus disease activity, reducing the dosage of prednisone to < or = 7.5 mg/day for a sustained period of time while maintaining stabilization or a reduction of disease activity was possible in a significantly greater proportion of patients treated with oral prasterone, 200 mg once daily, compared with patients treated with placebo." Petri MA, Lahita RG, Van Vollenhoven RF,

supraphysiologic[171], treatment may be implemented with little regard for initial DHEA levels, particularly when 1) the dose of DHEA is kept as low as possible, 2) duration is kept as short as possible, 3) other interventions are used to address the underlying cause of the disease, 4) the patient is deriving benefit and the risk-to-benefit ratio is favorable.

- o Thyroid (insufficiency or autoimmunity): Overt or imminent hypothyroidism is suggested by TSH greater than 2 mU/L[172] or 3 mU/L[173], low T4 or T3, and/or the presence of anti-thyroid peroxidase antibodies.[174] Hypothyroidism can cause an inflammatory myopathy that can resemble polymyositis, and hypothyroidism is a frequent complication of any and all autoimmune diseases. Specific treatment considerations include the following:

  - Selenium: Supplementation with either selenomethonine[175] or sodium selenite[176,177] can reduce thyroid autoimmunity and improve peripheral conversion of T4 to T3. Selenium may be started at 500-800 mcg per day and tapered to 200-400 mcg per day for maintenance.

  - L-thyroxine/levothyroxine/Synthroid—prescription synthetic T4: 25-50 mcg per day is a common starting dose which can be adjusted based on clinical and laboratory response. All thyroid hormone supplements must be taken away from soy products and preferably on an empty stomach. Doses are generally started at one-half of the daily dose for the first 10 days after which the full dose is used. Caution must be applied in patients with adrenal insufficiency and/or those with cardiovascular disease.

  - Armour thyroid—prescription natural T4 and T3 from cow/pig thyroid gland: 60 mg (one grain) is a common starting and maintenance dose. Due to the exacerbating effect on thyroid autoimmunity, Armour thyroid is never used in patients with thyroid autoimmunity.

  - Thyrolar/Liotrix—prescription synthetic T4 with T3: Dosed as "1" (low), "2" (intermediate), or "3" (high). Although this product has been difficult to obtain for the past few years due to manufacturing problems (http://thyrolar.com/), it has been my treatment of choice due to the combination of T4 and T3 and the lack of antigenicity compared to gland-derived products.

  - Thyroid glandular—nonprescription T3: Apparently, producers of nutritional products are able to distribute T3 because it is not listed by the FDA as a prescription item. A better nutritional company will start from Armour thyroid, remove the T4, and sell the thyroid glandular with active T3. For many patients, one tablet per day is at least as effective as a prescription source of thyroid hormone. Since it is derived from a glandular and therefore potentially antigenic source, thyroid glandular is not used in patients with thyroid autoimmunity.

- Xenobiotic immunotoxicity: Given that **antifibrillarin antibodies are specifically seen in patients with scleroderma**[178] and that **mercury exposure induces antifibrillarin autoimmunity in susceptible mice**[179], clinicians may be justified in searching for and treating evidence of mercury exposure in patients with autoimmunity in general and scleroderma in particular.

Merrill JT, Schiff M, Ginzler EM, Strand V, Kunz A, Gorelick KJ, Schwartz KE; GL601 Study Group. Effects of prasterone on corticosteroid requirements of women with systemic lupus erythematosus: a double-blind, randomized, placebo-controlled trial. *Arthritis Rheum*. 2002 Jul;46(7):1820-9

[171] "CONCLUSION: The clinical response to DHEA was not clearly dose dependent. Serum levels of DHEA and DHEAS correlated only weakly with lupus outcomes, but suggested an optimum serum DHEAS of 1000 microg/dl." Barry NN, McGuire JL, van Vollenhoven RF. Dehydroepiandrosterone in systemic lupus erythematosus: relationship between dosage, serum levels, and clinical response. *J Rheumatol*. 1998 Dec;25(12):2352-6

[172] Weetman AP. Hypothyroidism: screening and subclinical disease. *BMJ*. 1997 Apr 19;314(7088):1175-8 http://bmj.bmjjournals.com/cgi/content/full/314/7088/1175

[173] "Now AACE encourages doctors to consider treatment for patients who test outside the boundaries of a narrower margin based on a target TSH level of 0.3 to 3.0. AACE believes the new range will result in proper diagnosis for millions of Americans who suffer from a mild thyroid disorder, but have gone untreated until now." American Association of Clinical Endocrinologists (AACE). 2003 Campaign Encourages Awareness of Mild Thyroid Failure, Importance of Routine Testing http://www.aace.com/pub/tam2003/press.php November 26, 2005

[174] Beers MH, Berkow R (eds). The Merck Manual. Seventeenth Edition. Whitehouse Station; Merck Research Laboratories 1999 Page 96

[175] Duntas LH, Mantzou E, Koutras DA. Effects of a six month treatment with selenomethionine in patients with autoimmune thyroiditis. *Eur J Endocrinol*. 2003 Apr;148(4):389-93 http://eje-online.org/cgi/reprint/148/4/389

[176] Gartner R, Gasnier BC, Dietrich JW, Krebs B, Angstwurm MW. Selenium supplementation in patients with autoimmune thyroiditis decreases thyroid peroxidase antibodies concentrations. *J Clin Endocrinol Metab*. 2002 Apr;87(4):1687-91 http://jcem.endojournals.org/cgi/content/full/87/4/1687

[177] "We recently conducted a prospective, placebo-controlled clinical study, where we could demonstrate, that a substitution of 200 wg sodium selenite for three months in patients with autoimmune thyroiditis reduced thyroid peroxidase antibody (TPO-Ab) concentrations significantly." Gartner R, Gasnier BC. Selenium in the treatment of autoimmune thyroiditis. *Biofactors*. 2003;19(3-4):165-70

[178] "Since anti-fibrillarin antibodies are specific markers of scleroderma, the present animal model may be valuable for studies of the immunological aberrations which are likely to induce this autoimmune response." Hultman P, Enestrom S, Pollard KM, Tan EM. Anti-fibrillarin autoantibodies in mercury-treated mice. *Clin Exp Immunol*. 1989 Dec;78(3):470-7

[179] Nielsen JB, Hultman P. Mercury-induced autoimmunity in mice. Environ Health Perspect. 2002 Oct;110 Suppl 5:877-81 http://ehp.niehs.nih.gov/docs/2002/suppl-5/877-881nielsen/abstract.html

Detailed history, dental examination for mercury-containing amalgams, and post-DMSA urine metal analysis are suggested.

- Oral enzyme therapy with proteolytic/pancreatic enzymes: Polyenzyme supplementation is used to ameliorate the pathophysiology induced by immune complexes.[180] Immune complexes are detected in the majority of patients with scleroderma[181] and correlate with disease severity and visceral involvement.[182] Orally administered polyenzyme preparations have an "immune stimulating" action[183] and promote degradation of microbial biofilms and increased immune and antimicrobial penetration into infectious foci.[184] Given that maldigestion, malabsorption, and pancreatic insufficiency are not uncommon in patients with scleroderma[185], enzymes may be given with food for optimal benefit.

- PABA—para-amino benzoic acid: **Ninety percent of patients treated with PABA experience clinical benefit, namely skin softening.**[186] **PABA therapy prolongs survival in patients with scleroderma.**[187] "Potaba" is a well-tolerated prescription form of PABA.[188] Wright and Gaby[189] recommend "PABA, 2-3 g, 4 times a day." Adverse effects attributable to PABA are dose-dependent and include low blood sugar, rash, fever, and liver damage. Adverse effects may be seen with doses approximating or exceeding eight grams per day; thus serial serum chemistries (e.g., monthly at first, then bimonthly, then quarterly) are warranted, especially when using such high doses.

- *Centella asiatica* (Gotu cola): This botanical has been reported to favorably influence scleroderma.[190] Available forms include teas, tinctures, standardized capsules/tablets, topical ointments, and injectable preparations. The proprietary product "Madecassol" containing madecassic acid, asiatic acid and asiaticoside has been used in several studies and has demonstrated clinical benefit in scleroderma[191]; some preparations of this product apparently contain nitrofural, a topically and orally active antibiotic. Contact dermatitis has been reported.

- Phytonutritional modulation of NF-kappaB: As a stimulator of pro-inflammatory gene transcription, NF-kappaB is almost universally activated in autoimmune/inflammatory conditions.[192,193] Nutrients and botanicals which either directly or indirectly inhibit NF-kappaB for an anti-inflammatory benefit include vitamin D[194,195], curcumin[196] (requires piperine for absorption[197]), lipoic acid[198], green tea[199], rosemary[200], grape seed extract[201], propolis[202], zinc[203],

[180] Galebskaya LV, Ryumina EV, Niemerovsky VS, Matyukov AA. Human complement system state after wobenzyme intake. *VESTNIK MOSKOVSKOGO UNIVERSITETA. KHIMIYA.* 2000. Vol. 41, No. 6. Supplement. Pages 148-149

[181] "Serum immune complexes were measured in 92 patients with progressive systemic sclerosis, and elevated levels were found as follows: Raji cell assay 72% (59% after pronase treatment of Raji cell), agarose gel electrophoresis 52%, and C1q binding 24%." Seibold JR, Medsger TA Jr, Winkelstein A, Kelly RH, Rodnan GP. Immune complexes in progressive systemic sclerosis (scleroderma). *Arthritis Rheum.* 1982 Oct;25(10):1167-73

[182] "Patients with SS showed an incidence of circulating immune complexes comparable to that found in SLE, with 20 patients (58.5%),… …associated with both elevation of serum IgG and IgA levels and extensive visceral involvement by the disease." Hughes P, Cunningham J, Day M, Fitzgerald JC, French MA, Wright JK, Rowell NR. Immune complexes in systemic sclerosis; detection by C1q binding, K-cell inhibition and Raji cell radioimmunoassays. *J Clin Lab Immunol.* 1983 Mar;10(3):133-8

[183] Zavadova E, Desser L, Mohr T. Stimulation of reactive oxygen species production and cytotoxicity in human neutrophils in vitro and after oral administration of a polyenzyme preparation. *Cancer Biother.* 1995 Summer;10(2):147-52

[184] "The enzymes were shown to inhibit the biofilm formation. When appliled to the formed associations, the enzymes potentiated the effect of antibiotics on the bacteria located in them." Tets VV, Knorring GIu, Artemenko NK, Zaslavskaia NV, Artemenko KL. [Impact of exogenic proteolytic enzymes on bacteria][Article in Russian] *Antibiot Khimioter.* 2004;49(12):9-13

[185] Of 20 patients: "Three patients had very low levels of tryptic activity in their intestinal juice and only nine had results which were unequivocally normal." Cobden I, Axon AT, Rowell NR. Pancreatic exocrine function in systemic sclerosis. *Br J Dermatol* 1981 Aug;105(2):189-93

[186] "Ninety percent of 224 patients treated with KPAB experienced mild, moderate, or marked skin softening." Zarafonetis CJ, Dabich L, Skovronski JJ, DeVol EB, Negri D, Yuan W, Wolfe R. Retrospective studies in scleroderma: skin response to potassium para-aminobenzoate therapy. *Clin Exp Rheumatol.* 1988 Jul-Sep;6(3):261-8

[187] "For the entire group an estimated 81.4% survived 5 years from diagnosis and 69.4% survived 10 years. …adequate treatment with potassium para-aminobenzoate (Potaba KPAB) was associated with improved survival (p less than 0.01); 88.5% 5 year survival rate and 76.6% 10 year survival rate for adequately treated patients." Zarafonetis CJ, Dabich L, Negri D, Skovronski JJ, DeVol EB, Wolfe R. Retrospective studies in scleroderma: effect of potassium para-aminobenzoate on survival. *J Clin Epidemiol.* 1988;41(2):193-205

[188] http://www.glenwood-llc.com/potaba.html

[189] Gaby A, Wright JV. Nutritional Protocols. © 1998 by Nutrition Seminars.

[190] "Titrated extract of Centella asiatica (TECA) contains three principal ingredients, asiaticoside (AS), asiatic acid (AA), and madecassic acid (MA). These components are known to be clinically effective on systemic scleroderma, abnormal scar formation, and keloids." Hong SS, Kim JH, Li H, Shim CK. Advanced formulation and pharmacological activity of hydrogel of the titrated extract of C. asiatica. *Arch Pharm Res.* 2005 Apr;28(4):502-8

[191] "Madecassol is effective and well tolerated and therefore recommended for oral and local use in combined treatment of SS adn FS." Guseva NG, Starovoitova MN, Mach ES. [Madecassol treatment of systemic and localized scleroderma]. *Ter Arkh.* 1998;70(5):58-61. Russian.

[192] Tak PP, Firestein GS. NF-kappaB: a key role in inflammatory diseases. *J Clin Invest.* 2001 Jan;107(1):7-11 http://www.jci.org/cgi/content/full/107/1/7

[193] D'Acquisto F, May MJ, Ghosh S. Inhibition of Nuclear Factor KappaB (NF-B): An Emerging Theme in Anti-Inflammatory Therapies. *Mol Interv.* 2002 Feb;2(1):22-35 http://molinterv.aspetjournals.org/cgi/content/abstract/2/1/22

[194] "1Alpha,25-dihydroxyvitamin D3 (1,25-(OH)2-D3), the active metabolite of vitamin D, can inhibit NF-kappaB activity in human MRC-5 fibroblasts, targeting DNA binding of NF-kappaB but not translocation of its subunits p50 and p65." Harant H, Wolff B, Lindley IJ. 1Alpha,25-dihydroxyvitamin D3 decreases DNA binding of nuclear factor-kappaB in human fibroblasts. *FEBS Lett.* 1998 Oct 9;436(3):329-34

[195] "Thus, 1,25(OH)₂D₃ may negatively regulate IL-12 production by downregulation of NF-kB activation and binding to the p40-kB sequence." D'Ambrosio D, Cippitelli M, Cocciolo MG, Mazzeo D, Di Lucia P, Lang R, Sinigaglia F, Panina-Bordignon P. Inhibition of IL-12 production by 1,25-dihydroxyvitamin D3. Involvement of NF-kappaB downregulation in transcriptional repression of the p40 gene. *J Clin Invest.* 1998 Jan 1;101(1):252-62

[196] "Curcumin, EGCG and resveratrol have been shown to suppress activation of NF-kappa B." Surh YJ, Chun KS, Cha HH, Han SS, Keum YS, Park KK, Lee SS. Molecular mechanisms underlying chemopreventive activities of anti-inflammatory phytochemicals: down-regulation of COX-2 and iNOS through suppression of NF-kappa B activation. *Mutat Res.* 2001 Sep 1;480-481:243-68

[197] Shoba G, Joy D, Joseph T, Majeed M, Rajendran R, Srinivas PS. Influence of piperine on the pharmacokinetics of curcumin in animals and human volunteers. *Planta Med.* 1998 May;64(4):353-6

[198] "ALA reduced the TNF-alpha-stimulated ICAM-1 expression in a dose-dependent manner, to levels observed in unstimulated cells. Alpha-lipoic acid also reduced NF-kappaB activity in these cells in a dose-dependent manner." Lee HA, Hughes DA. Alpha-lipoic acid modulates NF-kappaB activity in human monocytic cells by direct interaction with DNA. *Exp Gerontol.* 2002 Jan-Mar;37(2-3):401-10

high-dose selenium[204], indole-3-carbinol[205,206], N-acetyl-L-cysteine[207], resveratrol[208,209], isohumulones[210], GLA via PPAR-gamma[211] and EPA via PPAR-alpha.[212] I have reviewed the phytonutritional modulation of NF-kappaB later in this text and elsewhere.[213] Several phytonutritional products targeting NF-kappaB are available.

- Raynaud's phenomenon—specific treatments: Treatment of Raynaud's phenomenon should not be trivialized as merely symptomatic; the pain experienced by some patients with Raynaud's phenomenon is truly excruciating. Additionally, a wonderfully insightful comment by Simonini et al[214] stated that the tissue ischemia induced by Raynaud's phenomenon is *pathogenic* because it promotes oxidative stress and the vicious cycle of inflammation; the recurrent ischemia and reperfusion of hypoxic Raynaud's phenomenon could be thought of somewhat as a "recurrent, mild heart attack of the hands." Thus, treatments to maintain vasodilation and quench the free radicals resultant from recurrent hypoxic events are necessary. Antioxidants have been discussed previously and should be common knowledge to readers of this text. Vasodilation in Raynaud's phenomenon can be supported with any/all of the following:

  o Inositol hexaniacinate: 3,000-4,000 mg/d in divided doses[215,216,217]

  o *Ginkgo biloba*: Ginkgo reduces the number of daily Raynaud's attacks in patients with primary Raynaud's disease[218], and it is also an excellent antioxidant with potent anti-inflammatory benefits.

  o Magnesium: 300-500 mg/d or bowel tolerance

  o Combination fatty acid therapy: must include GLA (minimum 500 mg) and EPA (minimum 2,000 mg)

[199] "In conclusion, EGCG is an effective inhibitor of IKK activity. This may explain, at least in part, some of the reported anti-inflammatory and anticancer effects of green tea." Yang F, Oz HS, Barve S, de Villiers WJ, McClain CJ, Varilek GW. The green tea polyphenol (-)-epigallocatechin-3-gallate blocks nuclear factor-kappa B activation by inhibiting I kappa B kinase activity in the intestinal epithelial cell line IEC-6. *Mol Pharmacol*. 2001 Sep;60(3):528-33

[200] "These results suggest that carnosol suppresses the NO production and iNOS gene expression by inhibiting NF-kappaB activation, and provide possible mechanisms for its anti-inflammatory and chemopreventive action." Lo AH, Liang YC, Lin-Shiau SY, Ho CT, Lin JK. Carnosol, an antioxidant in rosemary, suppresses inducible nitric oxide synthase through down-regulating nuclear factor-kappaB in mouse macrophages. *Carcinogenesis*. 2002 Jun;23(6):983-91

[201] "Constitutive and TNFalpha-induced NF-kappaB DNA binding activity was inhibited by GSE at doses > or =50 microg/ml and treatments for > or =12 h." Dhanalakshmi S, Agarwal R, Agarwal C. Inhibition of NF-kappaB pathway in grape seed extract-induced apoptotic death of human prostate carcinoma DU145 cells. *Int J Oncol*. 2003 Sep;23(3):721-7

[202] "Caffeic acid phenethyl ester (CAPE) is an anti-inflammatory component of propolis (honeybee resin). CAPE is reportedly a specific inhibitor of nuclear factor-kappaB (NF-kappaB)." Fitzpatrick LR, Wang J, Le T. Caffeic acid phenethyl ester, an inhibitor of nuclear factor-kappaB, attenuates bacterial peptidoglycan polysaccharide-induced colitis in rats. *J Pharmacol Exp Ther*. 2001 Dec;299(3):915-20

[203] "Our results suggest that zinc supplementation may lead to downregulation of the inflammatory cytokines through upregulation of the negative feedback loop A20 to inhibit induced NF-kappaB activation." Prasad AS, Bao B, Beck FW, Kucuk O, Sarkar FH. Antioxidant effect of zinc in humans. *Free Radic Biol Med*. 2004 Oct 15;37(8):1182-90

[204] Note that the patients in this study received a very high dose of selenium: 960 micrograms per day. This is at the top—and some would say over the top—of the safe and reasonable dose for long-term supplementation. In this case, the study lasted for three months. "In patients receiving selenium supplementation, selenium NF-kappaB activity was significantly reduced, reaching the same level as the nondiabetic control group. CONCLUSION: In type 2 diabetic patients, activation of NF-kappaB measured in peripheral blood monocytes can be reduced by selenium supplementation, confirming its importance in the prevention of cardiovascular diseases." Faure P, Ramon O, Favier A, Halimi S. Selenium supplementation decreases nuclear factor-kappa B activity in peripheral blood mononuclear cells from type 2 diabetic patients. *Eur J Clin Invest*. 2004 Jul;34(7):475-81

[205] Takada Y, Andreeff M, Aggarwal BB. Indole-3-carbinol suppresses NF-{kappa}B and I{kappa}B{alpha} kinase activation causing inhibition of expression of NF-{kappa}B-regulated antiapoptotic and metastatic gene products and enhancement of apoptosis in myeloid and leukemia cells. *Blood*. 2005 Apr 5; [Epub ahead of print]

[206] "Overall, our results indicated that indole-3-carbinol inhibits NF-kappaB and NF-kappaB-regulated gene expression and that this mechanism may provide the molecular basis for its ability to suppress tumorigenesis." Takada Y, Andreeff M, Aggarwal BB. Indole-3-carbinol suppresses NF-kappaB and IkappaBalpha kinase activation, causing inhibition of expression of NF-kappaB-regulated antiapoptotic and metastatic gene products and enhancement of apoptosis in myeloid and leukemia cells. *Blood*. 2005 Jul 15;106(2):641-9. Epub 2005 Apr 5.

[207] "CONCLUSIONS: Administration of N-acetylcysteine results in decreased nuclear factor-kappa B activation in patients with sepsis, associated with decreases in interleukin-8 but not interleukin-6 or soluble intercellular adhesion molecule-1. These pilot data suggest that antioxidant therapy with N-acetylcysteine may be useful in blunting the inflammatory response to sepsis." Paterson RL, Galley HF, Webster NR. The effect of N-acetylcysteine on nuclear factor-kappa B activation, interleukin-6, interleukin-8, and intercellular adhesion molecule-1 expression in patients with sepsis. *Crit Care Med*. 2003 Nov;31(11):2574-8

[208] "Resveratrol's anticarcinogenic, anti-inflammatory, and growth-modulatory effects may thus be partially ascribed to the inhibition of activation of NF-kappaB and AP-1 and the associated kinases." Manna SK, Mukhopadhyay A, Aggarwal BB. Resveratrol suppresses TNF-induced activation of nuclear transcription factors NF-kappa B, activator protein-1, and apoptosis: potential role of reactive oxygen intermediates and lipid peroxidation. *J Immunol*. 2000 Jun 15;164(12):6509-19

[209] "Both resveratrol and quercetin inhibited NF-kappaB-, AP-1- and CREB-dependent transcription to a greater extent than the glucocorticosteroid, dexamethasone." Donnelly LE, Newton R, Kennedy GE, Fenwick PS, Leung RH, Ito K, Russell RE, Barnes PJ.Anti-inflammatory Effects of Resveratrol in Lung Epithelial Cells: Molecular Mechanisms. *Am J Physiol Lung Cell Mol Physiol*. 2004 Jun 4 [Epub ahead of print]

[210] Yajima H, Ikeshima E, Shiraki M, Kanaya T, Fujiwara D, Odai H, Tsuboyama-Kasaoka N, Ezaki O, Oikawa S, Kondo K. Isohumulones, bitter acids derived from hops, activate both peroxisome proliferator-activated receptor alpha and gamma and reduce insulin resistance. *J Biol Chem*. 2004 Aug 6;279(32):33456-62. Epub 2004 Jun 3. http://www.jbc.org/cgi/content/full/279/32/33456

[211] "Thus, PPAR gamma serves as the receptor for GLA in the regulation of gene expression in breast cancer cells. " Jiang WG, Redfern A, Bryce RP, Mansel RE. Peroxisome proliferator activated receptor-gamma (PPAR-gamma) mediates the action of gamma linolenic acid in breast cancer cells. *Prostaglandins Leukot Essent Fatty Acids*. 2000 Feb;62(2):119-27

[212] "...EPA requires PPARalpha for its inhibitory effects on NF-kappaB." Mishra A, Chaudhary A, Sethi S. Oxidized omega-3 fatty acids inhibit NF-kappaB activation via a PPARalpha-dependent pathway. *Arterioscler Thromb Vasc Biol*. 2004 Sep;24(9):1621-7. Epub 2004 Jul 1. http://atvb.ahajournals.org/cgi/content/full/24/9/1621

[213] "Indeed, the previous view that nutrients only interact with human physiology at the metabolic/post-transcriptional level must be updated in light of current research showing that nutrients can, in fact, modify human physiology and phenotype at the genetic/pre-transcriptional level." Vasquez A. Reducing pain and inflammation naturally - part 4: nutritional and botanical inhibition of NF-kappaB, the major intracellular amplifier of the inflammatory cascade. A practical clinical strategy exemplifying anti-inflammatory nutrigenomics. *Nutritional Perspectives*, July 2005:5-12. www.OptimalHealthResearch.com/part4

[214] "...daily episodes of hypoxia-reperfusion injury, produces several episodes of free radicals-mediated endothelial derangement. These events results in a positive feedback effect of luminal narrowing and ischemia and therefore to the birth of a vicious cycle of oxygen free radicals (OFR) generation, leading to endothelial damage, intimal thickening and fibrosis." Simonini G, Pignone A, Generini S, Falcini F, Cerinic MM. Emerging potentials for an antioxidant therapy as a new approach to the treatment of systemic sclerosis. *Toxicology*. 2000 Nov 30;155(1-3):1-15

[215] "It appears to be a safe and well tolerated drug, which, together with other symptomatic measures, merits to be used in the management of vasospastic disease of the extremities even in the presence of partial obliteration of the microcirculation." Holti G. An experimentally controlled evaluation of the effect of inositol nicotinate upon the digital blood flow in patients with Raynaud's phenomenon. *J Int Med Res*. 1979;7(6):473-83

[216] "Although the mechanism of action remains unclear Hexopal is safe and is effective in reducing the vasospasm of primary Raynaud's disease during the winter months." Sunderland GT, Belch JJ, Sturrock RD, Forbes CD, McKay AJ. A double blind randomised placebo controlled trial of hexopal in primary Raynaud's disease. *Clin Rheumatol*. 1988 Mar;7(1):46-9

[217] "It is suggested that long-term treatment with nicotinate acid derivatives may produce improvement in the peripheral circulation by a different mechanism than the transient effect detected by short-term studies." Ring EF, Bacon PA. Quantitative thermographic assessment of inositol nicotinate therapy in Raynaud's phenomena. J Int Med Res 1977;5(4):217-22

[218] "Ginkgo biloba phytosome may be effective in reducing the number of Raynaud's attacks per week in patients suffering from Raynaud's phenomena." Muir AH, Robb R, McLaren M, Daly F, Belch JJ. The use of Ginkgo biloba in Raynaud's disease: a double-blind placebo-controlled trial. *Vasc Med*. 2002;7(4):265-7

- o <u>L-arginine</u>: L-arginine is the biochemical precursor to nitric oxide, which has vasodilating actions. L-arginine supplementation in patients with Raynaud's phenomenon showed benefit in one study[219] and no benefit in another.[220] However, arginine supplementation was tremendously beneficial in 4 case reports of scleroderma patients with Raynaud's-induced digital necrosis.[221] Excess arginine supplementation may lead to an overproduction of nitric oxide, which can be harmful in excess due to its free radical behavior and its contribution to peroxynitrite.
- o <u>Acupuncture, biofeedback, counseling, stress reduction, cold avoidance, smoking cessation</u>: Since stressful events, cold exposure, and cigarette smoking are all vasoconstrictive, these should be avoided/modified to the highest extent possible. Stress reduction and modification of inter- and intra-personal socioemotional exchange would be beneficial for anyone.

- <u>Esophageal dysfunction and GERD—specific treatments</u>:
  - o <u>Low carbohydrate diet, specific carbohydrate diet</u>: The gastroesophageal dysfunction that contributes to the high incidence of Barrett's esophagus is likely the result of a confluence of different factors: neurogenic, myogenic, and dysbiotic. With regard to the latter, clinicians must be diligent in the eradication of small intestine bacterial overgrowth, since microbial products of fermentation lead to relaxation of the so-called lower esophageal sphincter.[222,223] This is why diets low in carbohydrate and fermentable fibers (such as those found in grains)—in other words: "**low fermentation diets**"—are effective in the treatment of esophageal reflux; low-carbohydrate diets deprive gut microbes of substrate for fermentation into metabolites that relax the lower esophageal sphincter and thereby contribute to symptomatic improvement in patients with gastroesophageal reflux.[224] This is part of the reason why the diet for these patients must be as low as possible in the difficult-to-digest and easy-to-ferment carbohydrates that are common in the Standard American Diet (SAD) from corn, potatoes, wheat, oats, and disaccharides such as lactose and sucrose; see *Breaking the Vicious Cycle*[225] by the late Elaine Gottschall for more details and recipes for the specific carbohydrate diet. Similarly, a low-carbohydrate Atkins-type low-carbohydrate diet[226] might also be considered, particularly for short-term use and particularly if modified away from proinflammatory saturated fats and arachidonic acid.
  - o <u>Alginate</u>: Alginate is a processed extract from seaweed that is the active ingredient in the FDA-approved OTC anti-heartburn drug Gaviscon.[227] When mixed with stomach acid, alginate forms a foam "raft" that creates a barrier of protection for the esophagus, and it significantly reduces the number of acidic reflux events. Clinical studies have proven the effectiveness of alginate for treating GERD; however pure supplements of sodium alginate may be preferred over Gaviscon due to the latter's inclusion of aluminum (hydroxide)[228], a metal correlated with adverse effects and increased risk for neurologic disease. Alginate is

---

[219] "After therapy, patients with Raynaud's phenomenon secondary to systemic sclerosis showed: (1) higher digital vasodilation after local warming, (2) cold-induced digital vasodilation, and (3) increase of plasma levels of tissue-type plasminogen activator." Agostoni A, Marasini B, Biondi ML, Bassani C, Cazzaniga A, Bottasso B, Cugno M. L-arginine therapy in Raynaud's phenomenon? *Int J Clin Lab Res*. 1991;21(2):202-3

[220] "L-arginine supplementation, however, had no significant effect on vascular responses to acetylcholine and sodium nitroprusside." Khan F, Belch JJ. Skin blood flow in patients with systemic sclerosis and Raynaud's phenomenon: effects of oral L-arginine supplementation. *J Rheumatol*. 1999 Nov;26(11):2389-94

[221] "We report two cases in which oral L-arginine reversed digital necrosis in Raynaud's phenomenon and two additional cases in which the symptoms of severe Raynaud's phenomenon were improved with oral L-arginine." Rembold CM, Ayers CR. Oral L-arginine can reverse digital necrosis in Raynaud's phenomenon. *Mol Cell Biochem*. 2003 Feb;244(1-2):139-41

[222] "Colonic fermentation of indigestible carbohydrates increases the rate of TLESRs [transient lower esophageal sphincter relaxations], the number of acid reflux episodes, and the symptoms of GERD." Piche T, des Varannes SB, Sacher-Huvelin S, Holst JJ, Cuber JC, Galmiche JP. Colonic fermentation influences lower esophageal sphincter function in gastroesophageal reflux disease. *Gastroenterology*. 2003 Apr;124(4):894-902

[223] Piche T, Zerbib F, Varannes SB, Cherbut C, Anini Y, Roze C, le Quellec A, Galmiche JP. Modulation by colonic fermentation of LES function in humans. *Am J Physiol Gastrointest Liver Physiol*. 2000 Apr;278(4):G578-84 http://ajpgi.physiology.org/cgi/content/full/278/4/G578

[224] "The 5 individuals described in these case reports experienced resolution of GERD symptoms after self-initiation of a low-carbohydrate diet." Yancy WS Jr, Provenzale D, Westman EC. Improvement of gastroesophageal reflux disease after initiation of a low-carbohydrate diet: five brief case reports. *Altern Ther Health Med*. 2001 Nov-Dec;7(6):120, 116-9

[225] Gotschall E. Breaking the Vicious Cycle: Intestinal health though diet. Kirkton Press; Rev edition (August, 1994) http://www.scdiet.com/

[226] Atkins, RC. Dr. Atkins' New Diet Revolution (revised and updated). New York: Avon Books, 1999

[227] "For this population, sodium alginate was assessed as significantly superior by both investigators and patients at week two (p < 0.001 and p = 0.004, respectively) and at week four (p = 0.001 and p < 0.001, respectively)." Chatfield S. A comparison of the efficacy of the alginate preparation, Gaviscon Advance, with placebo in the treatment of gastro-oesophageal reflux disease. *Curr Med Res Opin*. 1999;15(3):152-9

[228] http://www.gaviscon.com/info.htm

also said to bind toxic metals and may therefore reduce enterohepatic recirculation of these proinflammatory immunotoxins.

- o **Betaine hydrochloric acid (betaine HCL)**: Many patients with gastroesophageal reflux are cured with the administration of supplemental HCL. Although the addition of acid rather than the suppression of acid goes against the well-funded acid-blocking drug paradigm, the truth remains that—*physiologically*—gastric emptying is promoted by acidification and—*clinically*—the treatment works for a significant number of patients with GERD. Furthermore, correction of hypochlorhydria by supplementation with betaine HCL helps to reduce bacterial/yeast counts in the stomach and upper small intestine, thereby alleviating GERD by reducing the bacteria/yeast available for fermentation; recall that microbial fermentation is one of the primary driving influences for gastroesophageal reflux.[229]

- o **GLA**: Numerous studies have documented the anti-cancer effects of GLA, and these have specifically been documented in esophageal cancer cell lines.[230] Thus, GLA consumption may help protect against the development of esophageal cancer, in addition to its important anti-inflammatory and vasodilating actions.

- o **Vitamin B12**: Vitamin B-12 levels are low in patients with malabsorption, and vitamin B-12 administration (4,000 mcg/d orally, or 1,000-2,000 mcg intramuscularly/ 2-3 times weekly) promotes intestinal motility.

Notes:

_____
_____
_____
_____
_____
_____
_____
_____
_____
_____
_____
_____
_____
_____
_____
_____
_____
_____
_____
_____
_____
_____

---

[229] "Colonic fermentation of indigestible carbohydrates increases the rate of TLESRs [transient lower esophageal sphincter relaxations], the number of acid reflux episodes, and the symptoms of GERD." Piche T, des Varannes SB, Sacher-Huvelin S, Holst JJ, Cuber JC, Galmiche JP. Colonic fermentation influences lower esophageal sphincter function in gastroesophageal reflux disease. *Gastroenterology*. 2003 Apr;124(4):894-902
[230] "A statistically highly significant growth-suppressive effect of the prostaglandin precursor gamma-linolenic acid (GLA) on MG63 human osteogenic sarcoma and oesophageal carcinoma cells in culture was found." Booyens J, Dippenaar N, Fabbri D, Engelbrecht P, Katzeff IE. The effect of gamma-linolenic acid on the growth of human osteogenic sarcoma and oesophageal carcinoma cells in culture. *S Afr Med J*. 1984 Feb 18;65(7):240-2

Psoriasis
Psoriatic Arthritis
Psoriatic Arthropathy

Description/pathophysiology:

- Psoriatic arthritis is an inflammatory arthropathy seen in patients with psoriasis that can have both peripheral (e.g., hands and feet) and axial (i.e., spine and sacroiliac joints) manifestations. This condition has frequently been referred to as *psoriatic rheumatism* or *rheumatic psoriasis*.

- Similar to reactive arthritis and rheumatoid arthritis; strongly associated with streptococcal infections as well as staphylococcal infections.[1] Although many researchers have contributed to the literature which establishes psoriasis as a disease of multifocal dysbiosis, to the best of my knowledge the work of Patricia W. Noah PhD is exceptionally noteworthy; her 1990 review published in *Seminars in Dermatology*[2] is required reading for doctors wishing to gain independent *peer-reviewed* confirmation that **multifocal dysbiosis is the major initiator and perpetuator of this systemic autoimmunity-inflammatory disorder.** In this particular article, she documents the experience of her group at the College of Medicine at the University of Tennessee and their anti-dysbiosis protocol and it success in the treatment of psoriasis.

> "We have repeatedly observed psoriatic flares associated with microbial infection, sequestered antigen, and colonization.
>
> **Removal of these microbial foci results in clearing of the disease.**"
>
> Patricia Noah PhD from University of Tennessee College of Medicine. *Semin Dermatol.* 1990;9:269

- Psoriasis and psoriatic arthritis must be considered an autoimmune diseases based on the findings of autoantibodies directed against dermal structures—stratum corneum[3] and keratinocytes[4]—and antibody-dependent and antibody-independent immune-mediated tissue destruction. Although stratum corneum antibodies are found in healthy patients without consequence, what makes them uniquely pathogenic in psoriasis is their tissue penetration in lesioned skin, their ability to bind with autoantigens, and their activation of complement.[5,6]

- *Comment*: Given the **overwhelming basic science and clinical research** implicating multifocal dysbiosis as the primary initiator of psoriasis—and by extension, psoriatic arthritis—it seems impossible that major allopathic textbooks such as *The Merck Manual*[7] and the widely read *Principles of Dermatology*[8] and *Current Medical Diagnosis and Treatment*[9] would perpetuate the myth that the condition is "idiopathic" so that no cure can be hoped for other than additive, endless, and perpetually "new" medicalization; but there we have it. This is clearly an example of medical practice being incongruent with biomedical research.

---

[1] Klippel JH (ed). Primer on the Rheumatic Diseases. 11th Edition. Atlanta: Arthritis Foundation. 1997 page 176

[2] **Noah PW. The role of microorganisms in psoriasis. Semin Dermatol. 1990 Dec;9(4):269-76**

[3] "… titers of IgG anti-SC autoantibodies in psoriatic patients were not specifically higher than in normal controls but were more variable, indicating that their circulating levels are dependent on a delicate balance between consumption at inflammatory sites and a secondary increase due to SC-antigen release following inflammation." Tagami H, Iwatsuki K, Yamada M. Profile of anti-stratum corneum autoantibodies in psoriatic patients. Arch Dermatol Res. 1983;275(2):71-5

[4] "It seems that autoantibodies, although they do not appear to participate in the pathogenesis of psoriasis, are an important feature, and that skin antigens, which appear in lesional immature keratinocytes, cross-react with S. pyogenes and contribute to the autoimmune process in psoriasis." Perez-Lorenzo R, Zambrano-Zaragoza JF, Saul A, Jimenez-Zamudio L, Reyes-Maldonado E, Garcia-Latorre E. Autoantibodies to autologous skin in guttate and plaque forms of psoriasis and cross-reaction of skin antigens with streptococcal antigens. Int J Dermatol. 1998 Jul;37(7):524-31. The authors found that all psoriais paitents had dermal autoantiboes and that these antibodies reacted specifically with endogenous dermal antigens; thus their finding that "Deposits of immunoglobulin G (IgG) were not detected in the lesions" is unexpected and inexplicable. This statement from their research is inconsistent with the findings of other research groups, and—specifically—must be placed in a context of other articles, most notably "… titers of IgG anti-SC autoantibodies in psoriatic patients were not specifically higher than in normal controls but were more variable, indicating that their circulating levels are dependent on a delicate balance between consumption at inflammatory sites and a secondary increase due to SC-antigen release following inflammation." Tagami H, Iwatsuki K, Yamada M. Profile of anti-stratum corneum autoantibodies in psoriatic patients. Arch Dermatol Res. 1983;275(2):71-5.

[5] "The stratum corneum (SC) antibodies are present in all human sera as seen by indirect immunofluorescent (IF) staining… IF tests with proper controls showed that the SC antigen in psoriatic scales is coated not only with IgG but in a majority of the lesions also with complement." Beutner EH, Jarzabek-Chorzelska M, Jablonska S, Chorzelski TP, Rzesa G. Autoimmunity in psoriasis. A complement immunofluorescence study. Arch Dermatol Res. 1978 Apr 7;261(2):123-34

[6] "Indirect immunofluorescent (IF) tests on sections of normal human skin reveal the presence of antibodies to the stratum corneum in most normal human sera. …Direct IF tests of psoriatic lesions revealed the presence of in vivo bound IgG as well as other immunoglobulins and complement in the stratum corneum." Beutner EH, Jablonska S, Jarzabek-Chorzelska M, Marciejowska E, Rzesa G, Chorzelski TP. Studies in immunodermatology. VI. IF studies of autoantibodies to the stratum corneum and of in vivo fixed IgG in stratum corneum of psoriatic lesions. Int Arch Allergy Appl Immunol. 1975;48(3):301-23

[7] Beers MH, Berkow R (eds). The Merck Manual. Seventeenth Edition. Whitehouse Station; Merck Research Laboratories 1999 pages 448 and 816

[8] Lookingbill DP, Marks JG, eds. Principles of dermatology. Philadelphia: W.B. Saunders, 1986: 138

[9] Tierney LM, McPhee SJ Papadakis MA (eds). Current Medical Diagnosis and Treatment. 35th edition. New York: Lange; 1996, page 101

Clinical presentations:

- Dermal lesions are generally described as well demarcated erythematous patches with silvery scales. Lesions may be widespread or comparatively minor. Patients may have *hidden* dermal lesions on scalp or in gluteal cleft; clinical examination in patients with oligoarthritis can search for dermal psoriatic lesions while assessing for cutaneous dysbiosis. Rarely, nail pitting is the only cutaneous lesion.
- Chronologic association of *dermal psoriasis* with *psoriatic arthritis*:
  - 7-30% of patients with (dermal) psoriasis develop psoriatic arthritis
  - In 70% of patients, *dermal psoriasis* precedes *psoriatic arthritis* by several years
  - In 15% of patients, *dermal psoriasis* and *psoriatic arthritis* occur at the same time
  - In 15% of patients, *psoriatic arthritis* precedes *dermal psoriasis*—this 'reverse presentation' is particularly common in children
- Onset may be gradual (70%) or acute (30%)
- In some patients the onset and disease can be of such severity that hospitalization is required.
- Peripheral joint involvement is more common in women; spinal involvement is more common in men, particularly in association with HLA-B27
- Peak onset age 30-55 years
- Musculoskeletal manifestations: prevalence: hands > feet > sacroiliac > spine
  - Oligoarticular peripheral arthropathy—distal interphalangeal (DIP) joints are notably affected
  - Peripheral polyarthritis: distribution may be symmetric or asymmetric
  - Arthritis mutilans: total destruction of the phalanges and meta-tarsals/carpals
  - Spinal and sacroiliac involvement: may affect any portion of the spine in a random fashion—lumbar spondylitis and sacroiliitis are more common than atlantoaxial instability; spinal involvement is more common in patients positive for HLA-B27
  - Enthesitis: inflammation at the junction of tendons to bones, especially at the insertion of the Achilles tendon
- Systemic manifestations and complications
  - Conjunctivitis, uveitis: seen in 30%
  - Nail pitting may or may not be present; other findings may include transverse ridging, thickening, flaking and brittleness
  - Aortic insufficiency
  - Pulmonary fibrosis
  - Swelling of the fingers and hands

Major differential diagnoses:

- <u>Ankylosing spondylitis</u>: does not occur with dermal psoriatic lesions
- <u>Rheumatoid arthritis</u>: differentiated from rheumatoid arthritis by 1) skin lesions, 2) absence of rheumatoid nodules, 3) negative rheumatoid factor
- <u>Hemochromatosis</u>: non-inflammatory peripheral arthropathy
- <u>Reactive arthritis</u>: does not classically occur with dermal psoriatic lesions
- <u>Septic arthritis</u>: e.g., infected psoriatic skin lesion predisposing to septicemia with resultant joint infection
- <u>HIV infection</u>: increased prevalence of psoriasis[10] especially associated with "an explosive onset of psoriasis and psoriatic arthritis" [11]

Clinical assessments:

- **History/subjective:**
  - Inquire about the clinical presentations listed above
  - Family and personal history of psoriasis is often positive
  - Historical risk factors for psoriasis include bacterial pharyngitis and stressful life events[12]

---

[10] Beers MH, Berkow R (eds). <u>The Merck Manual. Seventeenth Edition</u>. Whitehouse Station; Merck Research Laboratories 1999 page 448
[11] Klippel JH (ed). <u>Primer on the Rheumatic Diseases. 11th Edition</u>. Atlanta: Arthritis Foundation. 1997 page 176

- **Physical examination/objective**:
  - **Psoriasis—sharply demarcated erythematous plaque with silver scales**
  - Neuromusculoskeletal examination as indicated—see *Integrative Orthopedics*[13]
  - Assess blood pressure and perform screening physical examination
- **Laboratory assessments**:
  - <u>ANA</u>: Antinuclear antibodies are present in 47% of patients with psoriatic arthritis, further supporting the "autoimmune" description of this disease.[14]
  - <u>Rheumatoid factor</u>: RF is negative: positive RF suggests concomitant RA along with psoriasis.
  - <u>Chemistry/metabolic panel with uric acid</u>: Assess for overall status and elevated uric acid, the latter may be increased due to rapid skin turnover.
  - <u>Ferritin</u>: Assess ferritin preferably with transferrin saturation and CRP to exclude iron overload.
  - <u>CRP</u>: Generally elevated; can be used to track progression/remission of the disease
  - <u>HLA-B27</u>: Present in 40% of patients with psoriatic arthritis; correlates with increased severity of disease, including increased CRP, increased propensity for sacroiliitis, and more extensive joint destruction.[15]
  - <u>HIV serologic testing</u>: Especially for patients with severe disease and/or sudden onset.
  - <u>Lactulose/mannitol assay for "leaky gut"</u>: Patients with psoriasis have increased intestinal permeability.[16]
  - <u>Dysbiosis assessments</u>
    - **<u>Gastrointestinal dysbiosis</u>: Comprehensive stool and parasitology testing must include bacterial/yeast culture; antigen or antibody testing for *H. pylori* is recommended**; patients with psoriasis have shown a greatly increased prevalence of *H. pylori* compared with controls[17], and the authors of this study suggested a causal association; likewise intestinal colonization with yeasts including *Candida albicans* and *Geotrichum candidum* are found much more commonly in psoriatics than controls.[18] Stressing the importance of this association, Waldman et al[19] wrote, "Our results reinforce the hypothesis that *C. albicans* is one of the triggers to both exacerbation and persistence of psoriasis. We propose that in psoriatics with a significant quantity of *Candida* in faeces, an antifungal treatment should be considered as an adjuvant treatment of psoriasis."
    - <u>Dermal dysbiosis</u>: Skin/nail culture, Giemsa staining, culture lesioned skin on blood agar, MacConkey agar, Sabouraud plates.[20]
    - <u>Sinorespiratory dysbiosis</u>: Nasal swab and culture, throat culture for bacteria and yeasts.[21]

---

[12] "The study confirmed that recent pharyngeal infection is a risk factor for guttate psoriasis… Finally, the study added evidence to the belief that stressful life events may represent risk factors for the onset of psoriasis." Naldi L, Peli L, Parazzini F, Carrel CF; Psoriasis Study Group of the Italian Group for Epidemiological Research in Dermatology. Family history of psoriasis, stressful life events, and recent infectious disease are risk factors for a first episode of acute guttate psoriasis: results of a case-control study. *J Am Acad Dermatol.* 2001 Mar;44(3):433-8

[13] Vasquez A. <u>Integrative Orthopedics—The Art of Creating Wellness While Effectively Managing Acute and Chronic Musculoskeletal Disorders</u>. 2004: www.OptimalHealthResearch.com

[14] "RESULTS: 44/94 (47%) patients with PsA were ANA positive (>/=1/40); 13/94 (14%) had a clinically significant titre of >/=1/80. Three per cent had dsDNA antibodies, 2% had RF and anti-Ro antibodies, 1% had anti-RNP antibodies, and none had anti-La or anti-Smith antibodies." Johnson SR, Schentag CT, Gladman DD. Autoantibodies in biological agent naive patients with psoriatic arthritis. *Ann Rheum Dis.* 2005 May;64(5):770-2

[15] Tsai YG, Chang DM, Kuo SY, Wang WM, Chen YC, Lai JH. Relationship between human lymphocyte antigen-B27 and clinical features of psoriatic arthritis. *J Microbiol Immunol Infect.* 2003 Jun;36(2):101-4 http://www.jmii.org/content/abstracts/v36n2p101.php

[16] "The 24-h urine excretion of 51Cr-EDTA from psoriatic patients was 2.46 +/- 0.81%. These results differed significantly from controls (1.95 +/- 0.36%; P less than 0.05)." Humbert P, Bidet A, Treffel P, Drobacheff C, Agache P. Intestinal permeability in patients with psoriasis. *J Dermatol Sci.* 1991 Jul;2(4):324-6

[17] "In the current study, 20 (40%), psoriatic patients and 5 (10%) patients of control group demonstrated H. pylori antibodies... Although our study supports a causal role of H. pylori in the pathogenesis of psoriasis, a large scale study is needed to confirm the findings." Qayoom S, Ahmad QM. Psoriasis and helicobacter pylori. *Indian J Dermatol Venereol Leprol* 2003;69:133-134 http://www.ijdvl.com/

[18] Candida albicans (and other yeasts) was detected in 68% of psoriatics, 70% of eczematics, 54% of the controls. Qualitative analysis revealed a predominance of Candida albicans. Geotrichum candidum occurred in 22% of psoriatics, 10% of eczematics, and 3% of controls. Buslau M, Menzel I, Holzmann H. Fungal flora of human faeces in psoriasis and atopic dermatitis. *Mycoses.* 1990 Feb;33(2):90-4

[19] "Our results reinforce the hypothesis that C. albicans is one of the triggers to both exacerbation and persistence of psoriasis. We propose that in psoriatics with a significant quantity of Candida in faeces, an antifungal treatment should be considered as an adjuvant treatment of psoriasis." Waldman A, Gilhar A, Duek L, Berdicevsky I. Incidence of Candida in psoriasis--a study on the fungal flora of psoriatic patients. *Mycoses.* 2001 May;44(3-4):77-8

[20] Noah PW. The role of microorganisms in psoriasis. *Semin Dermatol.* 1990 Dec;9(4):269-76

[21] Noah PW. The role of microorganisms in psoriasis. *Semin Dermatol.* 1990 Dec;9(4):269-76

- ▪ <u>Genitourinary dysbiosis</u>: Culture and sensitivity testing for all organisms from clean catch specimens; assessment of sexual partners is advised.[22]
- ▪ <u>Orodental dysbiosis</u>: Culture of dentures and oral cavity for yeast and bacteria.
- ▪ <u>Environmental dysbiosis</u>: Examination, culture, and/or thorough cleaning of wigs, shoes, furniture, whirlpool/pool water.[23]

- • **<u>Imaging</u>**:
  - o Radiographic findings are characteristic and can aid in differential diagnosis; findings such as the osteolytic "pencil-in-cup" and "marginal erosions" are characteristic and differentiate psoriatic arthropathy from other conditions.
  - o Radiographic changes in the spine may be severe even when the patient has mild or no symptoms—assess the spine radiographically before initiating spinal manipulative therapy. Note that inflammatory changes such as facet ankylosis and atlantoaxial instability may occur and could potentially complicate manipulative therapy.[24] Myelocompressive atlantoaxial subluxation has been reported as the presenting manifestation of psoriatic arthropathy.[25] Remarkably, Lee and Lui[26] published that, "...atlantoaxial subluxation without high cervical myelopathy has been reported in 45% of cases of psoriatic spondylitis."

- • **<u>Establishing the diagnosis</u>**:
  - o Pattern recognition: psoriasis with arthritis after the exclusion of RA, iron overload, AS, and HIV

<u>Complications</u>:

- • Infection of skin lesions, may progress to septicemia or septic arthritis
- • Atlantoaxial instability
- • Cosmetic and functional deformity
- • Pain
- • Destructive and crippling arthritis
- • Depression, social isolation, pain, reduced quality of life: **"Patients with psoriasis reported reduction in physical functioning and mental functioning comparable to that seen in cancer, arthritis, hypertension, heart disease, diabetes, and depression."[27]**

<u>Clinical management</u>:

- • Referral if clinical outcome is unsatisfactory or if serious complications are evident.

<u>Treatments</u>:

<u>Medical treatments</u>: The goal of medical treatment is to suppress inflammation and dermal proliferation; no consideration is given to searching for and addressing the underlying cause(s) of the disorder because the disease is considered idiopathic.[28] Medical textbooks describe the treatment as merely targeted toward the symptoms, e.g., "Treatment [of psoriatic arthritis] is symptomatic."[29]

For dermal psoriasis:
- • Prescription topical steroids
- • Topical coal tars and hydrocarbons: carcinogenic
- • UV-B radiation
- • PUVA: psoralen with UV-A radiation; may result in cataracts and skin cancer
- • Methotrexate
- • Etretinate: a **severely teratogenic** retinoid

[22] **Noah PW. The role of microorganisms in psoriasis. *Semin Dermatol*. 1990 Dec;9(4):269-76**
[23] **Noah PW. The role of microorganisms in psoriasis. *Semin Dermatol*. 1990 Dec;9(4):269-76**
[24] Laiho K, Kauppi M. The cervical spine in patients with psoriatic arthritis. *Ann Rheum Dis*. 2002 Jul;61(7):650-2 http://ard.bmjjournals.com/cgi/content/full/61/7/650
[25] "We report severe upward axial dislocation and acquired basilar impression as a presenting manifestation of psoriatic arthropathy." Kaplan JG, Rosenberg RS, DeSouza T, Post KD, Freilich MD, Salamon O, Lantos G, Reinitz E. Atlantoaxial subluxation in psoriatic arthropathy. *Ann Neurol*. 1988 May;23(5):522-4
[26] "...atlantoaxial subluxation without high cervical myelopathy has been reported in 45% of cases of psoriatic spondylitis." Lee ST, Lui TN. Psoriatic arthritis with C-1-C-2 subluxation as a neurosurgical complication. *Surg Neurol*. 1986 Nov;26(5):428-30
[27] "Patients with psoriasis reported reduction in physical functioning and mental functioning comparable to that seen in cancer, arthritis, hypertension, heart disease, diabetes, and depression." Rapp SR, Feldman SR, Exum ML, Fleischer AB Jr, Reboussin DM. Psoriasis causes as much disability as other major medical diseases. *J Am Acad Dermatol* 1999 Sep;41(3 Pt 1):401-7
[28] Lookingbill DP, Marks JG, eds. Principles of dermatology. Philadelphia: W.B. Saunders, 1986: 138
[29] Tierney ML. McPhee SJ, Papadakis MA. Current Medical Diagnosis and Treatment 2006. 45th edition. New York; Lange Medical Books: 2006, pages 851-855

> *For psoriatic arthritis*: Allopathic treatments for psoriatic arthritis are essentially the same as for rheumatoid arthritis[30] and are generally noncurative and "symptomatic."[31]
> - Etretinate: a **severely teratogenic** retinoid
> - PUVA: psoralen with UV-A radiation; may result in cataracts and skin cancer
> - Corticosteroids are not highly effective
> - Antimalarial drugs (commonly used against systemic lupus erythematosus) frequently exacerbate psoriasis
> - Methotrexate: Used for recalcitrant psoriatic arthritis.[32]
> - TNF inhibitors: Etanercept 25 mg subcutaneously twice weekly, or infliximab 5 mg/kg every other month. These drugs are clinically effective from the perspective of anti-inflammation, but they are associated with increased risks for lymphoma, infections, congestive heart failure, demyelinating diseases, and systemic lupus erythematosus.

- Avoidance of proinflammatory foods: Proinflammatory foods act *directly* or *indirectly*; direct mechanisms include activating Toll-like receptors or NF-kappaB or inducing oxidative stress, while indirect mechanisms include depleting the body of anti-inflammatory nutrients and displacing more nutritious anti-inflammatory foods. Arachidonic acid (found in beef, liver, pork, and cow's milk) is the direct precursor to proinflammatory prostaglandins and leukotrienes[33] and pain-promoting isoprostanes.[34] Saturated fats promote inflammation by activating/enabling proinflammatory Toll-like receptors.[35] Consumption of saturated fat in the form of cream creates marked oxidative stress and lipid peroxidation that lasts for at least 3 hours postprandially.[36] Corn oil rapidly activates NF-kappaB (in hepatic Kupffer cells) for a proinflammatory effect[37]; similarly, consumption of PUFA and linoleic acid promotes antioxidant depletion and may thus promote oxidation-mediated inflammation via activation of NF-kappaB; linoleic acid causes intracellular oxidative stress and calcium influx and results in increased transcription of NF-kappaB activated pro-inflammatory genes.[38] High glycemic foods cause oxidative stress[39,40] and inflammation via activation of NF-kappaB and other mechanisms—*white bread causes inflammation*.[41] High glycemic foods suppress immune function[42,43] and thus perpetuate and promote infection/dysbiosis. Delivery of a high carbohydrate load to the gastrointestinal lumen promotes bacterial overgrowth[44,45], which is inherently proinflammatory[46,47] and which appears to

[30] Beers MH, Berkow R (eds). The Merck Manual. Seventeenth Edition. Whitehouse Station; Merck Research Laboratories 1999 page 448
[31] Tierney ML. McPhee SJ, Papadakis MA. Current Medical Diagnosis and Treatment 2006. 45th edition. New York; Lange Medical Books: 2006, pages 851-855
[32] Tierney ML. McPhee SJ, Papadakis MA. Current Medical Diagnosis and Treatment 2006. 45th edition. New York; Lange Medical Books: 2006, pages 851-855
[33] Vasquez A. Reducing Pain and Inflammation Naturally. Part 2: New Insights into Fatty Acid Supplementation and Its Effect on Eicosanoid Production and Genetic Expression. *Nutritional Perspectives* 2005; January: 5-16 www.optimalhealthresearch.com/part2
[34] Evans AR, Junger H, Southall MD, Nicol GD, Sorkin LS, Broome JT, Bailey TW, Vasko MR. Isoprostanes, novel eicosanoids that produce nociception and sensitize rat sensory neurons. *J Pharmacol Exp Ther*. 2000 Jun;293(3):912-20
[35] Lee JY, Sohn KH, Rhee SH, Hwang D. Saturated fatty acids, but not unsaturated fatty acids, induce the expression of cyclooxygenase-2 mediated through Toll-like receptor 4. *J Biol Chem*. 2001 May 18;276(20):16683-9. Epub 2001 Mar 2 http://www.jbc.org/cgi/content/full/276/20/16683
[36] "CONCLUSIONS: Both fat and protein intakes stimulate ROS generation. The increase in ROS generation lasted 3 h after cream intake and 1 h after protein intake. Cream intake also caused a significant and prolonged increase in lipid peroxidation." Mohanty P, Ghanim H, Hamouda W, Aljada A, Garg R, Dandona P. Both lipid and protein intakes stimulate increased generation of reactive oxygen species by polymorphonuclear leukocytes and mononuclear cells. *Am J Clin Nutr*. 2002 Apr;75(4):767-72 http://www.ajcn.org/cgi/content/full/75/4/767
[37] Rusyn I, Bradham CA, Cohn L, Schoonhoven R, Swenberg JA, Brenner DA, Thurman RG. Corn oil rapidly activates nuclear factor-kappaB in hepatic Kupffer cells by oxidant-dependent mechanisms. *Carcinogenesis*. 1999 Nov;20(11):2095-100 http://carcin.oxfordjournals.org/cgi/content/full/20/11/2095
[38] "Exposing endothelial cells to 90 micromol linoleic acid/L for 6 h resulted in a significant increase in lipid hydroperoxides that coincided with an increase in intracellular calcium concentrations." Hennig B, Toborek M, Joshi-Barve S, Barger SW, Barve S, Mattson MP, McClain CJ. Linoleic acid activates nuclear transcription factor-kappa B (NF-kappa B) and induces NF-kappa B-dependent transcription in cultured endothelial cells. *Am J Clin Nutr*. 1996 Mar;63(3):322-8 http://www.ajcn.org/cgi/reprint/63/3/322
[39] Mohanty P, Hamouda W, Garg R, Aljada A, Ghanim H, Dandona P. Glucose challenge stimulates reactive oxygen species (ROS) generation by leucocytes. *J Clin Endocrinol Metab*. 2000 Aug;85(8):2970-3 http://jcem.endojournals.org/cgi/content/full/85/8/2970 Glucose/carbohydrate and saturated fat consumption appear to be the two biggest offenders in the food-stimulated production of oxidative stress. The effect by protein is much less. "CONCLUSIONS: Both fat and protein intakes stimulate ROS generation. The increase in ROS generation lasted 3 h after cream intake and 1 h after protein intake. Cream intake also caused a significant and prolonged increase in lipid peroxidation." Mohanty P, Ghanim H, Hamouda W, Aljada A, Garg R, Dandona P. Both lipid and protein intakes stimulate increased generation of reactive oxygen species by polymorphonuclear leukocytes and mononuclear cells. *Am J Clin Nutr*. 2002 Apr;75(4):767-72 http://www.ajcn.org/cgi/content/full/75/4/767
[40] Koska J, Blazicek P, Marko M, Grna JD, Kvetnansky R, Vigas M. Insulin, catecholamines, glucose and antioxidant enzymes in oxidative damage during different loads in healthy humans. *Physiol Res*. 2000;49 Suppl 1:S95-100 http://www.biomed.cas.cz/physiolres/pdf/2000/49_S95.pdf
[41] "Conclusion - The present study shows that high GI carbohydrate, but not low GI carbohydrate, mediates an acute proinflammatory process as measured by NF-kappaB activity." Dickinson S, Hancock DP, Petocz P, Brand-Miller JC..High glycemic index carbohydrate mediates an acute proinflammatory process as measured by NF-kappaB activation. *Asia Pac J Clin Nutr*. 2005;14 Suppl:S120
[42] Sanchez A, Reeser JL, Lau HS, et al. Role of sugars in human neutrophilic phagocytosis. *Am J Clin Nutr*. 1973 Nov;26(11):1180-4
[43] "Postoperative infusion of carbohydrate solution leads to moderate fall in the serum concentration of inorganic phosphate. ... The hypophosphatemia was associated with significant reduction of neutrophil phagocytosis, intracellular killing, consumption of oxygen and generation of superoxide during phagocytosis." Rasmussen A, Segel E, Hessov I, Borregaard N. Reduced function of neutrophils during routine postoperative glucose infusion. *Acta Chir Scand*. 1988 Jul-Aug;154(7-8):429-33
[44] Ramakrishnan T, Stokes P. Beneficial effects of fasting and low carbohydrate diet in D-lactic acidosis associated with short-bowel syndrome. *JPEN J Parenter Enteral Nutr*. 1985 May-Jun;9(3):361-3
[45] Gottschall E. Breaking the Vicious Cycle: Intestinal Health Through Diet. Kirkton Press; Rev edition (August 1, 1994)
[46] Lin HC. Small intestinal bacterial overgrowth: a framework for understanding irritable bowel syndrome. *JAMA*. 2004 Aug 18;292(7):852-8

be myalgenic in humans.[48] Consumption of grains, potatoes, and manufactured foods displaces phytonutrient-dense foods such as fruits, vegetables, nuts, seeds, and berries which in sum contain more than 8,000 phytonutrients, many of which have anti-oxidant and thus anti-inflammatory actions.[49,50]

- Avoidance of allergenic foods: Any patient may be allergic to any food, even if the food is generally considered a health-promoting food. Generally speaking, the most notorious allergens are wheat, citrus (especially juice due to the industrial use of fungal hemicellulases), cow's milk, eggs, peanuts, chocolate, and yeast-containing foods; according to a study in patients with migraine, some patients will have to avoid as many as 10 specific foods in order to become symptom-free.[51] In 2005 I reported the remarkably successful treatment of a young woman with head-to-toe psoriasis who achieved complete and permanent remission of her "untreatable" "idiopathic" drug-resistant disease by diet modification, nutritional supplementation, and avoidance of offending allergens—in her case, chicken broth.[52] **Patients with psoriasis and psoriatic arthritis show elevated prevalences of occult celiac disease and "wheat allergy" (identified by anti-gliadin antibodies), and therefore the diet program for such patients should exclude wheat and other gluten-containing grains.**[53] Celiac disease can present with inflammatory oligoarthritis that resembles rheumatoid arthritis and which remits with avoidance of wheat/gluten; the inflammatory arthropathy of celiac disease has preceded bowel symptoms and/or an accurate diagnosis by as many as 3-15 years.[54,55] **Antibody patterns characteristic of celiac disease (IgG and IgA antigliadin antibodies, IgA antitransglutaminase antibody, IgA antiendomysial antibody) correlate with disease activity in patients with psoriasis[56], and gluten-free diets can lead to rapid resolution of skin lesions in patients with psoriasis.**[57] Clinicians must explain to their patients that celiac disease and wheat allergy are two different clinical entities and that exclusion of one does not exclude the other, and in neither case does mutual exclusion obviate the promotion of intestinal bacterial overgrowth (i.e., proinflammatory dysbiosis) by indigestible wheat oligosaccharides.

- Supplemented Paleo-Mediterranean diet: The health-promoting diet of choice for the majority of people is a diet based on abundant consumption of fruits, vegetables, seeds, nuts, omega-3 and monounsaturated fatty acids, and lean sources of protein such as lean meats, fatty cold-water fish, soy and whey proteins. This diet obviates overconsumption of chemical preservatives, artificial sweeteners, and carbohydrate-dominant foods such as candies, pastries, breads, potatoes, grains, and other foods with a high glycemic load and high glycemic index. This "Paleo-Mediterranean Diet" is a combination of the "Paleolithic" or "Paleo diet" and the well-known "Mediterranean diet", both of which are well described in peer-reviewed journals and the lay press. (See Chapter 2 and my other publications[58,59] for details). Although this diet is the most-nutrient dense diet available, rational supplementation with vitamins, minerals, and health

---

[47] Lichtman SN, Wang J, Sartor RB, Zhang C, Bender D, Dalldorf FG, Schwab JH. Reactivation of arthritis induced by small bowel bacterial overgrowth in rats: role of cytokines, bacteria, and bacterial polymers. *Infect Immun.* 1995 Jun;63(6):2295-301

[48] Pimentel M, et al. A link between irritable bowel syndrome and fibromyalgia may be related to findings on lactulose breath testing. *Ann Rheum Dis.* 2004 Apr;63(4):450-2

[49] "We propose that the additive and synergistic effects of phytochemicals in fruit and vegetables are responsible for their potent antioxidant and anticancer activities, and that the benefit of a diet rich in fruit and vegetables is attributed to the complex mixture of phytochemicals present in whole foods." Liu RH. Health benefits of fruit and vegetables are from additive and synergistic combinations of phytochemicals. *Am J Clin Nutr.* 2003 Sep;78(3 Suppl):517S-520S

[50] Seaman DR. The diet-induced proinflammatory state: a cause of chronic pain and other degenerative diseases? *J Manipulative Physiol Ther.* 2002;25(3):168-79

[51] Grant EC. Food allergies and migraine. *Lancet.* 1979 May 5;1(8123):966-9

[52] Vasquez A. Implementing the Five-Part Nutritional Wellness Protocol for the Treatment of Various Health Problems. *Nutritional Wellness* 2005 November. Available on-line at http://www.nutritionalwellness.com/archives/2005/nov/11_vasquez.php and http://optimalhealthresearch.com/protocol

[53] "Patients with PsoA have an increased prevalence of raised serum IgA [anti-gliadin antibodies] and of coeliac disease. Patients with raised IgA AGA seem to have more pronounced inflammation than those with a low IgA AGA concentration." Lindqvist U, Rudsander A, Bostrom A, Nilsson B, Michaelsson G. IgA antibodies to gliadin and coeliac disease in psoriatic arthritis. *Rheumatology* (Oxford). 2002 Jan;41(1):31-7 http://rheumatology.oxfordjournals.org/cgi/content/full/41/1/31

[54] "We report six patients with coeliac disease in whom arthritis was prominent at diagnosis and who improved with dietary therapy. Joint pain preceded diagnosis by up to three years in five patients and 15 years in one patient." Bourne JT, Kumar P, Huskisson EC, Mageed R, Unsworth DJ, Wojtulewski JA. Arthritis and coeliac disease. *Ann Rheum Dis.* 1985 Sep;44(9):592-8

[55] "A 15-year-old girl, with synovitis of the knees and ankles for 3 years before a diagnosis of gluten-sensitive enteropathy, is described." Pinals RS. Arthritis associated with gluten-sensitive enteropathy. *J Rheumatol.* 1986 Feb;13(1):201-4

[56] "The presence of CD-associated antibodies in psoriasis patients correlates with greater disease activity." Woo WK, McMillan SA, Watson RG, McCluggage WG, Sloan JM, McMillan JC. Coeliac disease-associated antibodies correlate with psoriasis activity. *Br J Dermatol.* 2004 Oct;151(4):891-4

[57] "The present case supports the association between CD and psoriasis and the concept that psoriasis in CD patients can be improved by GFD." Addolorato G, Parente A, de Lorenzi G, D'angelo Di Paola ME, Abenavoli L, Leggio L, Capristo E, De Simone C, Rotoli M, Rapaccini GL, Gasbarrini G. Rapid regression of psoriasis in a coeliac patient after gluten-free diet. A case report and review of the literature. *Digestion.* 2003;68(1):9-12. Epub 2003 Aug 29

[58] Vasquez A. A Five-Part Nutritional Protocol that Produces Consistently Positive Results. *Nutritional Wellness* 2005 September Available in the printed version and on-line at http://www.nutritionalwellness.com/archives/2005/sep/09_vasquez.php and http://optimalhealthresearch.com/protocol

[59] Vasquez A. Implementing the Five-Part Nutritional Wellness Protocol for the Treatment of Various Health Problems. *Nutritional Wellness* 2005 November. Available on-line at http://www.nutritionalwellness.com/archives/2005/nov/11_vasquez.php and http://optimalhealthresearch.com/protocol

promoting fatty acids (i.e., ALA, GLA, EPA, DHA) makes this the best practical diet that can possibly be conceived and implemented.

- Folic acid 5-20 mg per day: Patients with psoriasis have reduced folate status and elevated homocysteine levels.[60] Wright and Gaby recommended 50-150 mg per day of folic acid for psoriatics.[61] Folic acid has antiproliferative and anti-inflammatory effects mediated by nutrigenomic mechanisms. Folic acid, along with other vitamins and nutrients, may also help alleviate the biochemical aspect of the depression that is common in patients with psoriasis. Always supplement with vitamin B-12 in form of hydroxocobalamin or methylcobalamin (e.g., 2,000 mcg per day) when using high-dose folic acid.

- Alcohol/ethanol avoidance: Consumption of alcoholic beverages—even in low doses—increases intestinal permeability and exacerbates psoriasis. Psoriatics should avoid ethanol consumption.[62]

- Gluten-free vegetarian diet: Vegetarian/vegan diets have a place in the treatment plan of all patients with autoimmune/inflammatory disorders[63]--including psoriasis and psoriatic arthritis[64]; this is also true for patients for whom long-term exclusive reliance on a meat-free vegetarian diet is either not appropriate or not appealing. No legitimate scientist or literate clinician doubts the antirheumatic power and anti-inflammatory advantages of vegetarian diets, whether used short-term or long term.[65] The benefits of gluten-free vegetarian diets are well documented, and the mechanisms of action are well elucidated, including reduced intake of proinflammatory linoleic[66] and arachidonic acids[67], iron[68], common food antigens[69], gluten[70] and gliadin[71,72], proinflammatory sugars[73] and increased intake of omega-3 fatty acids and micronutrients[74], and anti-inflammatory and anti-oxidant phytonutrients[75]; vegetarian diets also effect profound changes—both *qualitative* and *quantitative*—in intestinal flora[76,77] that correlate with clinical improvement.[78] Patients who rely on the Paleo-Mediterranean Diet can use vegetarian meals, on a daily basis or for days at a time, for example, by having a daily vegetarian meal, or one week per month of vegetarianism. Of course, some (not all) patients can use a purely vegetarian diet long-term provided that nutritional needs (especially protein and cobalamin) are consistently met. **One particular advantage to low-protein diets in psoriasis is that the relative reduction in amino acid**

---

[60] "The mean levels of serum tHcy, fibrinogen, fibronectin, sICAM, PAI-1 and AuAb-oxLDL were increased in patients whereas tPA, vitamin B(12) and folate levels were decreased significantly." Vanizor Kural B, Orem A, Cimsit G, Uydu HA, Yandi YE, Alver A. Plasma homocysteine and its relationships with atherothrombotic markers in psoriatic patients. *Clin Chim Acta*. 2003 Jun;332(1-2):23-30

[61] Gaby A, Wright JV. Nutritional Protocols. 1998 Nutrition Seminars

[62] "We recommend that clinicians discourage patients with psoriasis from consuming alcohol, especially during periods of disease exacerbation." Behnam SM, Behnam SE, Koo JY. Alcohol as a risk factor for plaque-type psoriasis. *Cutis*. 2005 Sep;76(3):181-5

[63] "After four weeks at the health farm the diet group showed a significant improvement in number of tender joints, Ritchie's articular index, number of swollen joints, pain score, duration of morning stiffness, grip strength, erythrocyte sedimentation rate, C-reactive protein, white blood cell count, and a health assessment questionnaire score." Kjeldsen-Kragh J, Haugen M, Borchgrevink CF, Laerum E, Eek M, Mowinkel P, Hovi K, Forre O. Controlled trial of fasting and one-year vegetarian diet in rheumatoid arthritis. *Lancet*. 1991 Oct 12;338(8772):899-902

[64] "During the vegan diet, both signs and symptoms returned in most patients, with the exception of some patients with psoriasis who experienced an improvement." Lithell H, Bruce A, Gustafsson IB, Hoglund NJ, Karlstrom B, Ljunghall K, Sjolin K, Venge P, Werner I, Vessby B. A fasting and vegetarian diet treatment trial on chronic inflammatory disorders. *Acta Derm Venereol*. 1983;63(5):397-403

[65] "For the patients who were randomised to the vegetarian diet there was a significant decrease in platelet count, leukocyte count, calprotectin, total IgG, IgM rheumatoid factor (RF), C3-activation products, and the complement components C3 and C4 after one month of treatment." Kjeldsen-Kragh J, Mellbye OJ, Haugen M, Mollnes TE, Hammer HB, Sioud M, Forre O. Changes in laboratory variables in rheumatoid arthritis patients during a trial of fasting and one-year vegetarian diet. *Scand J Rheumatol*. 1995;24(2):85-93

[66] Rusyn I, Bradham CA, Cohn L, Schoonhoven R, Swenberg JA, Brenner DA, Thurman RG. Corn oil rapidly activates nuclear factor-kappaB in hepatic Kupffer cells by oxidant-dependent mechanisms. *Carcinogenesis*. 1999 Nov;20(11):2095-100 http://carcin.oxfordjournals.org/content/full/20/11/2095

[67] Vasquez A. Reducing Pain and Inflammation Naturally. Part 2: New Insights into Fatty Acid Supplementation and Its Effect on Eicosanoid Production and Genetic Expression. *Nutritional Perspectives* 2005; January: 5-16 http://optimalhealthresearch.com/part2

[68] Dabbagh AJ, Trenam CW, Morris CJ, Blake DR. Iron in joint inflammation. *Ann Rheum Dis*. 1993 Jan;52(1):67-73

[69] Hafstrom I, Ringertz B, Spangberg A, von Zweigbergk L, Brannemark S, Nylander I, Ronnelid J, Laasonen L, Klareskog L. A vegan diet free of gluten improves the signs and symptoms of rheumatoid arthritis: the effects on arthritis correlate with a reduction in antibodies to food antigens. *Rheumatology* (Oxford). 2001 Oct;40(10):1175-9 http://rheumatology.oxfordjournals.org/cgi/reprint/40/10/1175

[70] "The data provide evidence that dietary modification may be of clinical benefit for certain RA patients, and that this benefit may be related to a reduction in immunoreactivity to food antigens eliminated by the change in diet." Hafstrom I, Ringertz B, Spangberg A, von Zweigbergk L, Brannemark S, Nylander I, Ronnelid J, Laasonen L, Klareskog L. A vegan diet free of gluten improves the signs and symptoms of rheumatoid arthritis: the effects on arthritis correlate with a reduction in antibodies to food antigens. *Rheumatology* (Oxford). 2001 Oct;40(10):1175-9

[71] "Despite the increased AGA [antigliadin antibodies] positivity found distinctively in patients with recent-onset RA, none of the RA patients showed clear evidence of coeliac disease." Paimela L, Kurki P, Leirisalo-Repo M, Piirainen H. Gliadin immune reactivity in patients with rheumatoid arthritis. *Clin Exp Rheumatol*. 1995 Sep-Oct;13(5):603-7

[72] "The median IgA antigliadin ELISA index was 7.1 (range 2.1-22.4) for the RA group and 3.1 (range 0.3-34.9) for the controls (p = 0.0001)." Koot VC, Van Straaten M, Hekkens WT, Collee G, Dijkmans BA. Elevated level of IgA gliadin antibodies in patients with rheumatoid arthritis. *Clin Exp Rheumatol*. 1989 Nov-Dec;7(6):623-6

[73] Seaman DR. The diet-induced proinflammatory state: a cause of chronic pain and other degenerative diseases? *J Manipulative Physiol Ther*. 2002 Mar-Apr;25(3):168-79

[74] Hagfors L, Nilsson I, Skoldstam L, Johansson G. Fat intake and composition of fatty acids in serum phospholipids in a randomized, controlled, Mediterranean dietary intervention study on patients with rheumatoid arthritis. *Nutr Metab* (Lond). 2005 Oct 10;2:26 http://www.nutritionandmetabolism.com/content/2/1/26

[75] Liu RH. Health benefits of fruit and vegetables are from additive and synergistic combinations of phytochemicals. *Am J Clin Nutr* 2003;78(3 Suppl):517S-520S http://www.ajcn.org/cgi/content/full/78/3/517S

[76] "Significant alteration in the intestinal flora was observed when the patients changed from omnivorous to vegan diet. ... This finding of an association between intestinal flora and disease activity may have implications for our understanding of how diet can affect RA." Peltonen R, Kjeldsen-Kragh J, Haugen M, Tuominen J, Toivanen P, Forre O, Eerola E. Changes of faecal flora in rheumatoid arthritis during fasting and one-year vegetarian diet. *Br J Rheumatol*. 1994 Jul;33(7):638-43

[77] Toivanen P, Eerola E. A vegan diet changes the intestinal flora. *Rheumatology* (Oxford). 2002 Aug;41(8):950-1 http://rheumatology.oxfordjournals.org/cgi/reprint/41/8/950

[78] "We conclude that a vegan diet changes the faecal microbial flora in RA patients, and changes in the faecal flora are associated with improvement in RA activity." Peltonen R, Nenonen M, Helve T, Hanninen O, Toivanen P, Eerola E. Faecal microbial flora and disease activity in rheumatoid arthritis during a vegan diet. *Br J Rheumatol*. 1997 Jan;36(1):64-8 http://rheumatology.oxfordjournals.org/cgi/reprint/36/1/64

---

availability should serve to reduce polyamine formation. Formed from amino acids via ornithine decarboxylase and other enzymes, **polyamines stimulate dermal hyperproliferation and are elevated in patients with psoriasis.**[79] Effective psoriasis treatments are associated with a reduction in dermal/urinary polyamine levels, and, conversely, reducing polyamine formation—via either dietary manipulation or antibiologic/pharmaceutical drugs—is associated with clinical improvements in patients with psoriasis.

- <u>Short-term fasting</u>: Whether the foundational diet is Paleo-Mediterranean, vegetarian, vegan, or a combination of all of these, autoimmune/inflammatory patients will still benefit from periodic fasting, whether on a weekly (e.g., every Saturday), monthly (every first week or weekend of the month, or every other month), or yearly (1-2 weeks of the year) basis. Since consumption of food—particularly unhealthy foods—induces an inflammatory effect[80], abstinence from food provides a relative anti-oxidative and anti-inflammatory benefit[81] with many of the antioxidant benefits beginning within 24 hours of the initiation of the fast.[82] Fasting indeed provides a distinct anti-inflammatory benefit and may help "re-calibrate" metabolic and homeostatic mechanisms by breaking self-perpetuating "vicious cycles"[83] that autonomously promote inflammation independent from proinflammatory stimuli. Of course, water-only fasting is completely hypoallergenic (assuming that the patient is not sensitive to chlorine, fluoride, or other contaminants), and subsequent re-introduction of foods provides the ideal opportunity to identify offending foods. Fasting deprives intestinal microbes of substrate[84], stimulates intestinal B-cell immunity[85], improves the bactericidal action of neutrophils[86], reduces lysozyme release and leukotriene formation[87], and ameliorates intestinal hyperpermeability.[88] In case reports and/or clinical trials, short-term fasting (or protein-sparing fasting) has been documented as safe and effective treatment for SLE[89], RA[90], and non-rheumatic diseases such as chronic severe hypertension[91], moderate hypertension[92], obesity[93,94], type-2 diabetes[95], and epilepsy.[96]

---

[79] "Psoriasis lesions showed increased ornithine decarboxylase activity compared with uninvolved skin." Lowe NJ, Breeding J, Russell D. Cutaneous polyamines in psoriasis. *Br J Dermatol.* 1982 Jul;107(1):21-5

[80] Aljada A, Mohanty P, Ghanim H, Abdo T, Tripathy D, Chaudhuri A, Dandona P. Increase in intranuclear nuclear factor kappaB and decrease in inhibitor kappaB in mononuclear cells after a mixed meal: evidence for a proinflammatory effect. *Am J Clin Nutr.* 2004 Apr;79(4):682-90 http://www.ajcn.org/cgi/content/full/79/4/682

[81] "This is the first demonstration of ...a decrease in reactive oxygen species generation by leukocytes and oxidative damage to lipids, proteins, and amino acids after dietary restriction and weight loss in the obese over a short period." Dandona P, Mohanty P, Ghanim H, Aljada A, Browne R, Hamouda W, Prabhala A, Afzal A, Garg R. The suppressive effect of dietary restriction and weight loss in the obese on the generation of reactive oxygen species by leukocytes, lipid peroxidation, and protein carbonylation. *J Clin Endocrinol Metab.* 2001 Jan;86(1):355-62 http://jcem.endojournals.org/cgi/content/full/86/1/355

[82] "Thus, a 48h fast may reduce ROS generation, total oxidative load and oxidative damage to amino acids." Dandona P, Mohanty P, Hamouda W, Ghanim H, Aljada A, Garg R, Kumar V. Inhibitory effect of a two day fast on reactive oxygen species (ROS) generation by leucocytes and plasma ortho-tyrosine and meta-tyrosine concentrations. *J Clin Endocrinol Metab.* 2001 Jun;86(6):2899-902 http://jcem.endojournals.org/cgi/content/abstract/86/6/2899

[83] "The ability of therapeutic fasts to break metabolic vicious cycles may also contribute to the efficacy of fasting in the treatment of type 2 diabetes and autoimmune disorders." McCarty MF. A preliminary fast may potentiate response to a subsequent low-salt, low-fat vegan diet in the management of hypertension - fasting as a strategy for breaking metabolic vicious cycles. *Med Hypotheses.* 2003 May;60(5):624-33

[84] Ramakrishnan T, Stokes P. Beneficial effects of fasting and low carbohydrate diet in D-lactic acidosis associated with short-bowel syndrome. *JPEN J Parenter Enteral Nutr.* 1985 May-Jun;9(3):361-3

[85] Trollmo C, Verdrengh M, Tarkowski A. Fasting enhances mucosal antigen specific B cell responses in rheumatoid arthritis. *Ann Rheum Dis.* 1997 Feb;56(2):130-4 http://ard.bmjjournals.com/cgi/content/full/56/2/130

[86] "An association was found between improvement in inflammatory activity of the joints and enhancement of neutrophil bactericidal capacity. Fasting appears to improve the clinical status of patients with RA." Uden AM, Trang L, Venizelos N, Palmblad J. Neutrophil functions and clinical performance after total fasting in patients with rheumatoid arthritis. *Ann Rheum Dis.* 1983 Feb;42(1):45-51

[87] "We thus conclude that a reduced ability to generate cytotaxins, reduced release of enzyme, and reduced leukotriene formation from RA neutrophils, together with an altered fatty acid composition of membrane phospholipids, may be mechanisms for the decrease of inflammatory symptoms that results from fasting." Hafstrom I, Ringertz B, Gyllenhammar H, Palmblad J, Harms-Ringdahl M. Effects of fasting on disease activity, neutrophil function, fatty acid composition, and leukotriene biosynthesis in patients with rheumatoid arthritis. *Arthritis Rheum.* 1988 May;31(5):585-92

[88] "The results indicate that, unlike lactovegetarian diet, fasting may ameliorate the disease activity and reduce both the intestinal and the non-intestinal permeability in rheumatoid arthritis." Sundqvist T, Lindstrom F, Magnusson KE, Skoldstam L, Stjernstrom I, Tagesson C. Influence of fasting on intestinal permeability and disease activity in patients with rheumatoid arthritis. *Scand J Rheumatol.* 1982;11(1):33-8

[89] Fuhrman J, Sarter B, Calabro DJ. Brief case reports of medically supervised, water-only fasting associated with remission of autoimmune disease. *Altern Ther Health Med.* 2002 Jul-Aug;8(4):112, 110-1

[90] "An association was found between improvement in inflammatory activity of the joints and enhancement of neutrophil bactericidal capacity. Fasting appears to improve the clinical status of patients with RA." Uden AM, Trang L, Venizelos N, Palmblad J. Neutrophil functions and clinical performance after total fasting in patients with rheumatoid arthritis. *Ann Rheum Dis.* 1983 Feb;42(1):45-51

[91] "The average reduction in blood pressure was 37/13 mm Hg, with the greatest decrease being observed for subjects with the most severe hypertension. Patients with stage 3 hypertension (those with systolic blood pressure greater than 180 mg Hg, diastolic blood pressure greater than 110 mg Hg, or both) had an average reduction of 60/17 mm Hg at the conclusion of treatment." Goldhamer A, Lisle D, Parpia B, Anderson SV, Campbell TC. Medically supervised water-only fasting in the treatment of hypertension. *J Manipulative Physiol Ther.* 2001 Jun;24(5):335-9 http://www.healthpromoting.com/335-339Goldhamer115263.QXD.pdf

[92] "RESULTS: Approximately 82% of the subjects achieved BP at or below 120/80 mm Hg by the end of the treatment program. The mean BP reduction was 20/7 mm Hg, with the greatest decrease being observed for subjects with the highest baseline BP." Goldhamer AC, Lisle DJ, Sultana P, Anderson SV, Parpia B, Hughes D, Campbell TC. Medically supervised water-only fasting in the treatment of borderline hypertension. *J Altern Complement Med.* 2002 Oct;8(5):643-50 http://www.healthpromoting.com/Articles/articles/study%202/acmpaper5.pdf

[93] Vertes V, Genuth SM, Hazelton IM. Supplemented fasting as a large-scale outpatient program. *JAMA.* 1977 Nov 14;238(20):2151-3

[94] Bauman WA, Schwartz E, Rose HG, Eisenstein HN, Johnson DW. Early and long-term effects of acute caloric deprivation in obese diabetic patients. *Am J Med.* 1988 Jul;85(1):38-46

[95] Goldhamer AC. Initial cost of care results in medically supervised water-only fasting for treating high blood pressure and diabetes. *J Altern Complement Med.* 2002 Dec;8(6):696-7 http://www.healthpromoting.com/Articles/pdf/Study%2032.pdf

[96] "The ketogenic diet should be considered as alternative therapy for children with difficult-to-control seizures. It is more effective than many of the new anticonvulsant medications and is well tolerated by children and families when it is effective." Freeman JM, Vining EP, Pillas DJ, Pyzik PL, Casey JC, Kelly LM. The efficacy of the ketogenic diet-1998: a prospective evaluation of intervention in 150 children. *Pediatrics.* 1998 Dec;102(6):1358-63 http://pediatrics.aappublications.org/cgi/reprint/102/6/1358

- Broad-spectrum fatty acid therapy with ALA, EPA, DHA, GLA and oleic acid: **Fish oil supplementation (especially in combination with a low-fat, low-arachidonate diet[97]) has been shown to help alleviate dermal psoriasis.[98,99,100] Fish oil supplementation has also been shown to protect psoriasis patients against the iatrogenic nephrotoxicity of cyclosporin.[101]** Fatty acid supplementation should be delivered in the form of combination therapy with ALA, GLA, DHA, and EPA. Given at doses of 3,000 – 9,000 mg per day, ALA from flax oil has impressive anti-inflammatory benefits demonstrated by its ability to halve prostaglandin production in humans.[102] Numerous studies have demonstrated the benefit of GLA in the treatment of rheumatoid arthritis when used at doses between 500 mg – 4,000 mg per day.[103,104] Fish oil provides EPA and DHA which have well-proven anti-inflammatory benefits in rheumatoid arthritis[105,106,107] and lupus.[108,109] ALA, EPA, DHA, and GLA need to be provided in the form of supplements; when using high doses of therapeutic oils, liquid supplements that can be mixed in juice or a smoothie are generally more convenient and palatable than capsules. Therapeutic amounts of oleic acid can be obtained from generous use of olive oil, preferably on fresh vegetables. Supplementation with polyunsaturated fatty acids warrants increased intake of antioxidants from diet, fruit and vegetable juices, and properly formulated supplements; since patients with systemic inflammation are generally in a pro-oxidative state, consideration must be given to the timing and starting dose of fatty acid supplementation and the need for anti-oxidant protection. See chapter on Therapeutics for more details and biochemical pathways. Clinicians must realize that fatty acids are not clinically or biochemically interchangeable and that one fatty acid does not substitute for another; each of the fatty acids must be supplied in order for its benefits to be obtained.[110]

- Vitamin D3 supplementation with physiologic doses and/or tailored to serum 25(OH)D levels: Vitamin D deficiency is common in the general population and is even more common in patients with chronic illness and chronic musculoskeletal pain.[111] **Vitamin D3 can be applied topically and is about as effective as topical steroids in the treatment of psoriatic skin lesions.[112]** Correction of vitamin D deficiency supports normal immune function against infection and provides a clinically significant anti-inflammatory[113] and analgesic benefit in patients with back pain[114] and limb pain.[115] Reasonable daily doses for children and adults are 2,000 and 4,000 IU,

[97] "Moderate or excellent improvement was observed in 58% of the patients, while mild improvement or no change was observed in 19% and 23%, respectively." Kragballe K, Fogh K. A low-fat diet supplemented with dietary fish oil (Max-EPA) results in improvement of psoriasis and in formation of leukotriene B5. *Acta Derm Venereol* 1989;69(1):23-8
[98] A clinical trial of 13 psoriatic patients: "Global clinical evaluation showed that eight patients demonstrated mild to moderate improvement in their psoriatic lesions. Improved clinical response correlated with high EPA/DCHA ratios attained in epidermal tissue specimens." Ziboh VA, Cohen KA, Ellis CN, Miller C, Hamilton TA, Kragballe K, Hydrick CR, Voorhees JJ. Effects of dietary supplementation of fish oil on neutrophil and epidermal fatty acids. Modulation of clinical course of psoriatic subjects. *Arch Dermatol* 1986 Nov;122(11):1277-82
[99] "Although its effects are modest, it is nontoxic and its favorable effect appears to continue for the duration of its usage, indicating that EPA could be beneficial for the long-term treatment of psoriasis." Kojima T, Terano T, Tanabe E, Okamoto S, Tamura Y, Yoshida S. Long-term administration of highly purified eicosapentaenoic acid provides improvement of psoriasis. *Dermatologica* 1991;182(4):225-30
[100] "In conclusion, modulation of eicosanoid metabolism by intravenous n-3 fatty acid supplementation appears to exert a rapid beneficial effect on inflammatory skin lesions in acute guttate psoriasis." Grimminger F, Mayser P, Papavassilis C, Thomas M, Schlotzer E, Heuer KU, Fuhrer D, Hinsch KD, Walmrath D, Schill WB, et al. A double-blind, randomized, placebo-controlled trial of n-3 fatty acid based lipid infusion in acute, extended guttate psoriasis. Rapid improvement of clinical manifestations and changes in neutrophil leukotriene profile. *Clin Investig* 1993 Aug;71(8):634-43
[101] "The results of this pilot study suggest that fish oil can reduce CyA-associated renal dysfunction in psoriasis patients." Stoof TJ, Korstanje MJ, Bilo HJ, Starink TM, Hulsmans RF, Donker AJ. Does fish oil protect renal function in cyclosporin-treated psoriasis patients? *J Intern Med* 1989 Dec;226(6):437-41
[102] Adam O, Wolfram G, Zollner N. Effect of alpha-linolenic acid in the human diet on linoleic acid metabolism and prostaglandin biosynthesis. *J Lipid Res.* 1986 Apr;27(4):421-6 http://www.jlr.org/cgi/reprint/27/4/421
[103] "Other results showed a significant reduction in morning stiffness with gamma-linolenic acid at 3 months and reduction in pain and articular index at 6 months with olive oil." Brzeski M, Madhok R, Capell HA. Evening primrose oil in patients with rheumatoid arthritis and side-effects of non-steroidal anti-inflammatory drugs. *Br J Rheumatol.* 1991 Oct;30(5):370-2
[104] Rothman D, DeLuca P, Zurier RB. Botanical lipids: effects on inflammation, immune responses, and rheumatoid arthritis. *Semin Arthritis Rheum.* 1995 Oct;25(2):87-96
[105] Adam O, Beringer C, Kless T, Lemmen C, Adam A, Wiseman M, Adam P, Klimmek R, Forth W. Anti-inflammatory effects of a low arachidonic acid diet and fish oil in patients with rheumatoid arthritis. *Rheumatol Int.* 2003 Jan;23(1):27-36
[106] Lau CS, Morley KD, Belch JJ. Effects of fish oil supplementation on non-steroidal anti-inflammatory drug requirement in patients with mild rheumatoid arthritis--a double-blind placebo controlled study. *Br J Rheumatol.* 1993 Nov;32(11):982-9
[107] Kremer JM, Jubiz W, Michalek A, Rynes RI, Bartholomew LE, Bigaouette J, Timchalk M, Beeler D, Lininger L. Fish-oil fatty acid supplementation in active rheumatoid arthritis. A double-blinded, controlled, crossover study. *Ann Intern Med.* 1987 Apr;106(4):497-503
[108] Walton AJ, Snaith ML, Locniskar M, Cumberland AG, Morrow WJ, Isenberg DA. Dietary fish oil and the severity of symptoms in patients with systemic lupus erythematosus. *Ann Rheum Dis.* 1991 Jul;50(7):463-6
[109] Duffy EM, Meenagh GK, McMillan SA, Strain JJ, Hannigan BM, Bell AL. The clinical effect of dietary supplementation with omega-3 fish oils and/or copper in systemic lupus erythematosus. *J Rheumatol.* 2004 Aug;31(8):1551-6
[110] Vasquez A. Reducing Pain and Inflammation Naturally. Part 2: New Insights into Fatty Acid Supplementation and Its Effect on Eicosanoid Production and Genetic Expression. *Nutritional Perspectives* 2005; January: 5-16 http://optimalhealthresearch.com/part2
[111] Plotnikoff GA, Quigley JM. Prevalence of severe hypovitaminosis D in patients with persistent, nonspecific musculoskeletal pain. *Mayo Clin Proc.* 2003 Dec;78(12):1463-70
[112] Lookingbill DP, Marks JG, eds. Principles of dermatology. Philadelphia: W.B. Saunders, 1986: 141
[113] Timms PM, Mannan N, Hitman GA, Noonan K, Mills PG, Syndercombe-Court D, Aganna E, Price CP, Boucher BJ. Circulating MMP9, vitamin D and variation in the TIMP-1 response with VDR genotype: mechanisms for inflammatory damage in chronic disorders? *QJM.* 2002 Dec;95(12):787-96 http://qjmed.oxfordjournals.org/cgi/content/full/95/12/787
[114] Al Faraj S, Al Mutairi K. Vitamin D deficiency and chronic low back pain in Saudi Arabia. *Spine.* 2003 Jan 15;28(2):177-9
[115] Masood H, Narang AP, Bhat IA, Shah GN. Persistent limb pain and raised serum alkaline phosphatase the earliest markers of subclinical hypovitaminosis D in Kashmir. *Indian J Physiol Pharmacol.* 1989 Oct-Dec;33(4):259-61

respectively, as defined by Vasquez, et al.[116] Deficiency and response to treatment are monitored with serum 25(OH)vitamin D while safety is monitored with serum calcium; inflammatory granulomatous diseases and certain drugs such as hydrochlorothiazide greatly increase the propensity for hypercalcemia and warrant increment dosing and frequent monitoring of serum calcium.

- Assessment for dysbiosis: **All dysbiotic loci should be investigated as discussed previously in this chapter and in Chapter 4 in the section on multifocal dysbiosis.** In a very intensive investigation into the role of bacteria, yeast/fungi, and viruses in the pathogenesis of psoriasis, Noah[117] assessed microflora of 297 psoriasis patients by culture and serologic tests. Culture samples for aerobic bacteria, yeast, and dermatophytes were taken from the throat, urine, and skin surfaces from scalp, ears, chest, face, axillary, submammary, umbilical, upper back, inguinal crease, gluteal-fold, perirectal, vaginal, pubis, penis, scrotal, leg, hands, feet, finger, and toenail areas. More than 15 different microbes were causatively associated with exacerbation of psoriasis; this finding is entirely logical and is consistent with the 'idiopathic' nature of the illness and why Koch-indoctrinated researchers and clinicians have failed to understand the microbial contribution to autoimmune/inflammatory diseases. Given that each of the microbes listed (see shaded box on upcoming page) is a *common*—but not necessarily *optimal*—inhabitant of human surfaces and orifices, it is possible to see how their synergism *particularly in a genetically susceptible patient with hormonal imbalances and a proinflammatory lifestyle/diet* could tip the scales in favor of systemic inflammation and the picture/illusion of autoimmunity. Of the more than 15 categories/subspecies listed as causative microbes, what if only seven of these common "commensals" were present in a systemically-genetically-nutritionally-hormonally-emotionally predisposed patient, and each contributed only 5% to the pathophysiology of a patient's psoriasis? We would have already arrived at 35% of the psoriatic pathogenesis, leaving 10% each for hormones, diet, allergy, nutrition, xenobiotic accumulation (present in everyone[118,119]). While these numbers and percentages are purely speculative, I left 15% for "idiopathic" to keep researchers and clinicians alert to new possibilities and to placate the therapeutic and epidemiologic nihilists that have so far dominated the field of rheumatology with their "unknown cause" rhetoric. **Each cause—each contributor to disease—may in itself be "clinically insignificant" but when additive and synergistic influences coalesce, we find ourselves confronted with an "idiopathic disease" and the decision to choose between the only two available options: 1) despair in the failure of our "one cause, one disease, one drug" paradigm, or 2) appreciate that numerous influences work together to disrupt physiologic function and produce the biologic dysfunction that we experience as disease.**

  - Sinorespiratory/nasopharyngeal and dermal dysbiosis: **Sinorespiratory and dermal dysbiosis in patients with psoriasis is *qualitatively* (increased prevalence in psoriatics compared with healthy controls) and *quantitatively* (increased prevalence of toxin-producing strains compared to those found in controls) associated with the severity of the disease.[120]** Patients with psoriasis show an increased rate of nasal/dermal colonization with *Staphylococcus aureus*[121,122], a microbe known to produce several powerfully inflammatory antigens, toxins, and superantigens, and nasal colonization with which appears causally associated with the inflammatory/autoimmune disorder

[116] Vasquez A, Manso G, Cannell J. The clinical importance of vitamin D (cholecalciferol): a paradigm shift with implications for all healthcare providers. *Altern Ther Health Med*. 2004 Sep-Oct;10(5):28-36 http://optimalhealthresearch.com/monograph04
[117] **Noah PW. The role of microorganisms in psoriasis. *Semin Dermatol*. 1990 Dec;9(4):269-76**
[118] "Although the use of HCB as a fungicide has virtually been eliminated, detectable levels of HCB are still found in nearly all people in the USA." Robinson PE, Leczynski BA, Kutz FW, Remmers JC. An evaluation of hexachlorobenzene body-burden levels in the general population of the USA. *IARC Sci Publ* 1986;(77):183-92
[119] "Many U.S. residents carry toxic pesticides in their bodies above government assessed "acceptable" levels." Pesticide Action Network North America (PANNA). Chemical Trespass: Pesticides in Our Bodies and Corporate Accountability. http://www.panna.org/campaigns/docsTrespass/chemicalTrespass2004.dv.html
[120] "In this study, S aureus was present in more than 50% of patients with AD and PS. We found that the severity of AD and PS significantly correlated to enterotoxin production of the isolated S aureus strains." Tomi NS, Kranke B, Aberer E. Staphylococcal toxins in patients with psoriasis, atopic dermatitis, and erythroderma, and in healthy control subjects. *J Am Acad Dermatol*. 2005 Jul;53(1):67-72
[121] "In this study, S aureus was present in more than 50% of patients with AD and PS. We found that the severity of AD and PS significantly correlated to enterotoxin production of the isolated S aureus strains." Tomi NS, Kranke B, Aberer E. Staphylococcal toxins in patients with psoriasis, atopic dermatitis, and erythroderma, and in healthy control subjects. *J Am Acad Dermatol*. 2005 Jul;53(1):67-72
[122] "The nasal carriage rate of Staphylococcus aureus in psoriatics was higher than the control groups." Singh G, Rao DJ. Bacteriology of psoriatic plaques. *Dermatologica*. 1978;157(1):21-7

Wegener's granulomatosis.[123,124] A study by Bartenjev et al[125] showed that subclinical streptococcal/staphylococcal infections were detected in 68% of psoriasis patients and in only 11 % of the control group; these authors encouraged searching for and eliminating microbial infections as an important aspect of the management of psoriasis. Supportively, other researchers[126] have found that infection with *S pyogenes* can initiate and/or exacerbate guttate psoriasis; therefore streptococcal throat infections should be treated assertively and early to avoid triggering an exacerbation of psoriasis.[127] *Streptococcus pyogenes* is a very likely trigger of psoriasis[128]; **chronic penicillin treatment leads to clinical improvement of recalcitrant psoriasis.**[129] Patients with guttate psoriasis have increased oropharyngeal colonization with *Streptococcus hemolyticus* compared with controls.[130] Similar to Behcet's disease[131], the dermal lesions of psoriasis are commonly colonized by proinflammatory microbes including *Staphylococcus aureus*.[132] More conclusively, research by Villeda-Gabriel et al[133] and Perez-Lorenzo et al[134] has clearly shown that antibodies against *Streptococcus pyogenes* cross-react (perhaps via molecular mimicry or epitope spreading) with dermal antigens; additionally, the work of Muto et al[135] showed that antibodies against streptococcal cell wall proteins could bind with nuclei and cytoplasm of cells from skin and synovium. **Thus, psoriasis is indeed a microbe-induced autoimmune disease by virtue of these cross-reacting endogenous antibodies that bind with nuclear, dermal, and articular antigens. Patients with psoriasis have elevated serum levels of antibodies against streptococcal M12 protein[136], and patients with psoriatic arthritis have a heightened inflammatory response to staphylococcal superantigens.**[137]

---

[123] Brons RH, Bakker HI, Van Wijk RT, Van Dijk NW, Muller Kobold AC, Limburg PC, Manson WL, Kallenberg CG, Tervaert JW. Staphylococcal acid phosphatase binds to endothelial cells via charge interaction; a pathogenic role in Wegener's granulomatosis? *Clin Exp Immunol.* 2000 Mar;119(3):566-73 http://www.blackwell-synergy.com/doi/abs/10.1046/j.1365-2249.2000.01172.x

[124] Popa ER, Stegeman CA, Kallenberg CG, Tervaert JW. Staphylococcus aureus and Wegener's granulomatosis. *Arthritis Res.* 2002;4(2):77-9 http://arthritis-research.com/content/4/2/77

[125] "Subclinical streptococcal and/or staphylococcal infections were detected in 68 % of tested patients and in only 11 % of the control group. The results of this study indicate that subclinical bacterial infections of the upper respiratory tract may be an important factor in provoking a new relapse of chronic plaque psoriasis. Searching for, and eliminating, microbial infections could be of importance in the treatment of psoriasis." Bartenjev I, Rogl Butina M, Potocnik M. Subclinical microbial infection in patients with chronic plaque psoriasis. *Acta Derm Venereol Suppl* (Stockh). 2000;(211):17-8

[126] "CONCLUSIONS--This study confirms the strong association between prior infection with S pyogenes and guttate psoriasis but suggests that the ability to trigger guttate psoriasis is not serotype specific." Telfer NR, Chalmers RJ, Whale K, Colman G. The role of streptococcal infection in the initiation of guttate psoriasis. *Arch Dermatol.* 1992 Jan;128(1):39-42

[127] "CONCLUSIONS: This study confirms anecdotal and retrospective reports that streptococcal throat infections can cause exacerbation of chronic plaque psoriasis." Gudjonsson JE, Thorarinsson AM, Sigurgeirsson B, Kristinsson KG, Valdimarsson H. Streptococcal throat infections and exacerbation of chronic plaque psoriasis: a prospective study. *Br J Dermatol.* 2003 Sep;149(3):530-4

[128] "These findings justify the hypothesis that S pyogenes infections are more important in the pathogenesis of chronic plaque psoriasis than has previously been recognized, and indicate the need for further controlled therapeutic trials of antibacterial measures in this common skin disease." El-Rachkidy RG, Hales JM, Freestone PP, Young HS, Griffiths CE, Camp RD. Increased Blood Levels of IgG Reactive with Secreted Streptococcus pyogenes Proteins in Chronic Plaque Psoriasis. *J Invest Dermatol.* 2007 Mar 8; [Epub ahead of print]

[129] "Total duration of the study was two years. Initially benzathine penicillin 1.2 million units, was given I.M. AST fortnightly. After 24 weeks benzathine penicillin was reduced to 1.2 million units once a month... Significant improvement in the PASI score was noted from 12 weeks onwards. All patients showed excellent improvement at 2 years." Saxena VN, Dogra J. Long-term use of penicillin for the treatment of chronic plaque psoriasis. *Eur J Dermatol.* 2005 Sep-Oct;15(5):359-62 http://www.john-libbey-eurotext.fr/en/revues/medecine/ejd/e-docs/00/04/10/A4/article.md?type=text.html

[130] "A high incidence of Streptococcus hemolyticus culture was observed in the guttate psoriatic group compared with the plaque psoriasis and control groups." Zhao G, Feng X, Na A, Yongqiang J, Cai Q, Kong J, Ma H. Acute guttate psoriasis patients have positive streptococcus hemolyticus throat cultures and elevated antistreptococcal M6 protein titers. *J Dermatol.* 2005;32(2):91-6

[131] "At least one type of microorganism was grown from each pustule. Staphylococcus aureus (41/70, 58.6%, p = 0.008) and Prevotella spp (17/70, 24.3%, p = 0.002) were significantly more common in pustules from BS patients, and coagulase negative staphylococci (17/37, 45.9%, p = 0.007) in pustules from acne patients. CONCLUSIONS: The pustular lesions of BS are not usually sterile." Hatemi G, Bahar H, Uysal S, Mat C, Gogus F, Masatlioglu S, Altas K, Yazici H. The pustular skin lesions in Behcet's syndrome are not sterile. *Ann Rheum Dis.* 2004 Nov;63(11):1450-2

[132] "In this study, S aureus was present in more than 50% of patients with AD and PS. We found that the severity of AD and PS significantly correlated to enterotoxin production of the isolated S aureus strains." Tomi NS, Kranke B, Aberer E. Staphylococcal toxins in patients with psoriasis, atopic dermatitis, and erythroderma, and in healthy control subjects. *J Am Acad Dermatol.* 2005 Jul;53(1):67-72

[133] "The recognition by immunoblot of streptococcal antigens by serum of guttate psoriasis patients, the presence of autoantibodies against their own skin, and recognition of the same skin antigens by anti-streptococcal rabbit antibodies confirm the participation of the immune system and of streptococcal infections in guttate psoriasis." Villeda-Gabriel G, Santamaria-Cogollos LC, Perez-Lorenzo R, Reyes-Maldonado E, Saul A, Jurado-Santacruz F, Jimenez-Zamudio L, Garcia-Latorre E. Recognition of Streptococcus pyogenes and skin autoantigens in guttate psoriasis. *Arch Med Res.* 1998 Summer;29(2):143-8

[134] "It seems that autoantibodies, although they do not appear to participate in the pathogenesis of psoriasis, are an important feature, and that skin antigens, which appear in lesional immature keratinocytes, cross-react with S. pyogenes and contribute to the autoimmune process in psoriasis." Perez-Lorenzo R, Zambrano-Zaragoza JF, Saul A, Jimenez-Zamudio L, Reyes-Maldonado E, Garcia-Latorre E. Autoantibodies to autologous skin in guttate and plaque forms of psoriasis and cross-reaction of skin antigens with streptococcal antigens. *Int J Dermatol.* 1998 Jul;37(7):524-31. The authors found that all psoriasis paitents had dermal autoantiboes and that these antibodies reacted specifically with endogenous dermal antigens; thus their finding that "Deposits of immunoglobulin G (IgG) were not detected in the lesions" is unexpected and inexplicable. This statement from their research is inconsistent with the findings of other research groups, and— specifically—must be placed in a context of other articles, most notably "... titers of IgG anti-SC autoantibodies in psoriatic patients were not specifically higher than in normal controls but were more variable, indicating that their circulating levels are dependent on a delicate balance between consumption at inflammatory sites and a secondary increase due to SC-antigen release following inflammation." Tagami H, Iwatsuki K, Yamada M. Profile of anti-stratum corneum autoantibodies in psoriatic patients. *Arch Dermatol Res.* 1983;275(2):71-5

[135] "Monoclonal antibodies directed against type 12 Group A streptococcal cell wall antigens cross-react with nuclei and cytoplasm of cells from skin and synovium from controls, uninvolved skin of psoriatics and psoriatic plaques." Muto M, Fujikura Y, Hamamoto Y, Ichimiya M, Ohmura A, Sasazuki T, Fukumoto T, Asagami C. Immune response to Streptococcus pyogenes and the susceptibility to psoriasis. *Australas J Dermatol.* 1996 May;37 Suppl 1:S54-5

[136] "Patients with psoriasis had high serum titres of antibody against the M12 (C-region) streptococcal antigen compared to controls." Muto M, Fujikura Y, Hamamoto Y, Ichimiya M, Ohmura A, Sasazuki T, Fukumoto T, Asagami C. Immune response to Streptococcus pyogenes and the susceptibility to psoriasis. *Australas J Dermatol.* 1996 May;37 Suppl 1:S54-5

[137] "Our data raised the possibility that staphylococcal superantigens may also play an exacerbating role in PA." Yamamoto T, Katayama I, Nishioka K. Peripheral blood mononuclear cell proliferative response against staphylococcal superantigens in patients with psoriasis arthropathy. *Eur J Dermatol.* 1999 Jan-Feb;9(1):17-21 http://www.john-libbey-eurotext.fr/en/revues/medecine/ejd/e-docs/00/01/87/C8/resume.md

Microbes and Mechanistic Pathways in Psoriatogenic Multifocal Dysbiosis

Microorganisms causally associated with psoriasis:
- streptococcal groups A (including **Streptococcus pyogenes**), B, C, D, F, G, *S viridans, S pneumoniae*
- *Klebsiella pneumoniae, oxytoca*
- *Escherichia coli*
- *Enterobacter cloacae, E aerogenes, E agglomerans*
- *Proteus mirabilis, P vulgaris*
- *Citrobacter freundii, C diversus*
- *Morganella morganii*
- *Pseudomonas aeruginosa, P maltiphilia, P putida*
- *Serratia marcescens*
- *Acinetobacter calbio aceticus, A luoffi;*
- *Flavobacterium* specie
- CDC groups Ve-1, Ve-2, E-o2
- *Bacillus subtilis, B cereus*
- **Staphylococcus aureus**
- **Candida albicans**, *C parapsilosis*
- *Torulopsis/Candida glabrata*
- *Rhodotorula* spp.
- *H. pylori**

See **Noah. Semin Dermatol. 1990;9:269**
* Qayoom S, Ahmad QM. *Indian J Dermatol Venereol Leprol* 2003;69:133

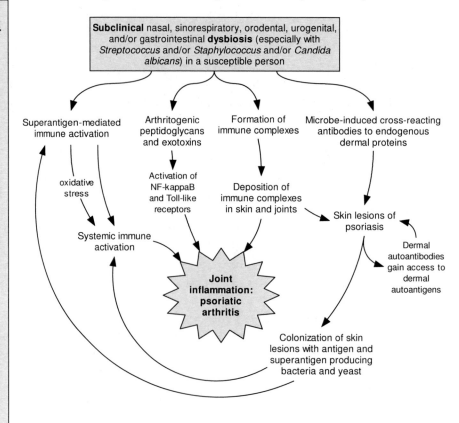

- o <u>Gastrointestinal dysbiosis</u>: **All patients with psoriatic arthritis should be considered to have gastrointestinal dysbiosis until proven otherwise. A three-sample comprehensive parasitology examination performed by a specialty laboratory is strongly recommended as a minimal component of basic care. In lieu of a comprehensive parasitology test, patients can be treated for 4-8 weeks with broad-spectrum antimicrobial treatment that is effective against gram-positive and gram-negative bacteria, aerobes and anaerobes, yeast, protozoa and amebas.** For additional details, see the Section on *multifocal dysbiosis* in Chapter 4. **Patients with psoriasis have shown a greatly increased prevalence of *H. pylori*[138] and *Candida albicans*[139] and *Geotrichum candidum*.[140]**

- o <u>Antimicrobial treatments for (gastrointestinal) dysbiosis commonly include but are not limited to the following</u>: Doses listed are for adults. Combination therapy generally allows for lower doses of each intervention to be used. Severe dysbiosis often requires weeks or months of treatment. Drugs are not necessarily more effective than natural treatments; in fact, often the botanicals work when the pharmaceuticals do not.

  - ▪ <u>Oregano oil</u>: Emulsified oil of oregano in a time-released tablet is proven effective in the eradication of harmful gastrointestinal microbes, including *Blastocystis hominis, Entamoeba hartmanni,* and *Endolimax nana*.[141] An *in vitro*

---

[138] "In the current study, 20 (40%), psoriatic patients and 5 (10%) patients of control group demonstrated H. pylori antibodies... Although our study supports a causal role of H. pylori in the pathogenesis of psoriasis, a large scale study is needed to confirm the findings." Qayoom S, Ahmad QM. Psoriasis and helicobacter pylori. *Indian J Dermatol Venereol Leprol* 2003;69:133-134 http://www.ijdvl.com/

[139] "Our results reinforce the hypothesis that C. albicans is one of the triggers to both exacerbation and persistence of psoriasis. We propose that in psoriatics with a significant quantity of Candida in faeces, an antifungal treatment should be considered as an adjuvant treatment of psoriasis." Waldman A, Gilhar A, Duek L, Berdicevsky I. Incidence of Candida in psoriasis--a study on the fungal flora of psoriatic patients. *Mycoses.* 2001 May;44(3-4):77-8

[140] Candida albicans (and other yeasts) was detected in 68% of psoriatics, 70% of eczematics, 54% of the controls. Qualitative analysis revealed a predominance of Candida albicans. Geotrichum candidum occurred in 22% of psoriatics, 10% of eczematics, and 3% of controls. Buslau M, Menzel I, Holzmann H. Fungal flora of human faeces in psoriasis and atopic dermatitis. *Mycoses.* 1990 Feb;33(2):90-4

[141] Force M, Sparks WS, Ronzio RA. Inhibition of enteric parasites by emulsified oil of oregano in vivo. *Phytother Res.* 2000 May;14(3):213-4

study[142] and clinical experience support the use of emulsified oregano against *Candida albicans* and various bacteria. The common dose is 600 mg per day in divided doses for 6 weeks.[143]

- <u>Berberine</u>: Berberine is an alkaloid found in *Hydrastis canadensis* (goldenseal), *Coptis chinensis* (Coptis, goldenthread), *Berberis/Mahonia aquifolium* (Oregon grape), *Berberis vulgaris* (barberry), and *Berberis aristata* (tree turmeric)[144], and it shows effectiveness against *Giardia, Candida,* and *Streptococcus* in addition to its direct anti-inflammatory and antidiarrheal actions. Oral dose of 400-800 mg per day in divided doses is common for adults.[145] **Berberine-containing botanicals may provide additional benefit in the treatment of psoriatic disease due to the antiproliferative[146] and anti-inflammatory/antileukotriene[147] characteristics of berberine and other phytoconstituents.** Berberine-containing plants have also been traditionally used for jaundice, an application supported by a recent animal study showing increased bilirubin excretion in rats following berberine administration.[148] Topical *Berberis/Mahonia* is effective for dermal psoriasis.[149]

- *Artemisia annua*: Artemisinin has been safely used for centuries in Asia for the treatment of malaria, and it also has effectiveness against anaerobic bacteria due to the pro-oxidative sesquiterpene endoperoxide.[150,151] I commonly use artemisinin at 200 mg per day in divided doses for adults with dysbiosis.

- <u>St. John's Wort</u> (*Hypericum perforatum*): *Hypericum* **may prove to be an ideal botanical for the treatment of psoriasis due to the combination of its antidepressant and antimicrobial benefits.** Hyperforin from *Hypericum perforatum* also shows impressive antibacterial action, particularly against gram-positive bacteria such as *Staphylococcus aureus, Streptococcus pyogenes, Streptococcus agalactiae*[152] and perhaps *Helicobacter pylori*.[153] Up to 600 mg three times per day of a 3% hyperforin standardized extract is customary in the treatment of depression.

- <u>Bismuth</u>: Bismuth is commonly used in the empiric treatment of diarrhea (e.g., "Pepto-<u>Bis</u>mol") and is commonly combined with other antimicrobial agents to reduce drug resistance and increase antibiotic effectiveness.[154]

- <u>Undecylenic acid</u>: Derived from castor bean oil, undecylenic acid has antifungal properties and is commonly indicated by sensitivity results obtained by stool culture. Common dosages are 150-250 mg tid (up to 750 mg per day).[155]

---

[142] Stiles JC, Sparks W, Ronzio RA. The inhibition of Candida albicans by oregano. *J Applied Nutr* 1995;47:96–102

[143] Force M, Sparks WS, Ronzio RA. Inhibition of enteric parasites by emulsified oil of oregano in vivo. *Phytother Res.* 2000 May;14(3):213-4

[144] [No authors listed] Berberine. *Altern Med Rev.* 2000 Apr;5(2):175-7 http://www.thorne.com/altmedrev/.fulltext/5/2/175.pdf

[145] [No authors listed] Berberine. *Altern Med Rev.* 2000 Apr;5(2):175-7 http://www.thorne.com/altmedrev/.fulltext/5/2/175.pdf

[146] "The extract of the bark of Mahonia aquifolium is an inhibitor of keratinocyte growth with an IC50 of 35 microM. Of its main alkaloids tested, berberine inhibited cell growth to the same extent as did the Mahonia extract, while the benzylisoquinoline alkaloids berbamine and oxyacanthine were more potent inhibitors by a factor of three." Muller K, Ziereis K, Gawlik I. The antipsoriatic *Mahonia aquifolium* and its active constituents; II. Antiproliferative activity against cell growth of human keratinocytes. *Planta Med* 1995 Feb;61(1):74-

[147] "Inhibition of lipoxygenase by these compounds may contribute to the therapeutic effect of M. aquifolium extracts in the treatment of psoriasis." Misik V, Bezakova L, Malekova L, Kostalova D. Lipoxygenase inhibition and antioxidant properties of protoberberine and aporphine alkaloids isolated from Mahonia aquifolium. *Planta Med* 1995 Aug;61(4):372-3

[148] "Acute doses of berberine were found to increase the secretion of bilirubin in experimental hyperbilrubinemia without affecting the UDP-glucuronyltransferase activity and BSP clearance. Continuous treatment abolished this effect. This apparent tolerance could be attributed to the inhibitory action of chronic berberine treatment on UDP-glucuronyltransferase activity…" Chan MY. The effect of berberine on bilirubin excretion in the rat. *Comp Med East West.* 1977 Summer;5(2):161-8

[149] "Taken together, these clinical studies conducted by several investigators in several countries indicate that Mahonia aquifolium is a safe and effective treatment of patients with mild to moderate psoriasis." Gulliver WP, Donsky HJ. A report on three recent clinical trials using Mahonia aquifolium 10% topical cream and a review of the worldwide clinical experience with Mahonia aquifolium for the treatment of plaque psoriasis. *Am J Ther.* 2005 Sep-Oct;12(5):398-406

[150] Dien TK, de Vries PJ, Khanh NX, Koopmans R, Binh LN, Duc DD, Kager PA, van Boxtel CJ. Effect of food intake on pharmacokinetics of oral artemisinin in healthy Vietnamese subjects. *Antimicrob Agents Chemother.* 1997 May;41(5):1069-72

[151] Giao PT, Binh TQ, Kager PA, Long HP, Van Thang N, Van Nam N, de Vries PJ. Artemisinin for treatment of uncomplicated falciparum malaria: is there a place for monotherapy? *Am J Trop Med Hyg.* 2001 Dec;65(6):690-5

[152] Schempp CM, Pelz K, Wittmer A, Schopf E, Simon JC. Antibacterial activity of hyperforin from St John's wort, against multiresistant Staphylococcus aureus and gram-positive bacteria. *Lancet.* 1999 Jun 19;353(9170):2129

[153] "A butanol fraction of St. John's Wort revealed anti-Helicobacter pylori activity with MIC values ranging between 15.6 and 31.2 microg/ml." Reichling J, Weseler A, Saller R. A current review of the antimicrobial activity of Hypericum perforatum L. *Pharmacopsychiatry.* 2001 Jul;34 Suppl 1:S116-8

[154] Veldhuyzen van Zanten SJ, Sherman PM, Hunt RH. Helicobacter pylori: new developments and treatments. *CMAJ.* 1997;156(11):1565-74 http://www.cmaj.ca/cgi/reprint/156/11/1565.pdf

[155] "Adult dosage is usually 450-750 mg undecylenic acid daily in three divided doses." Undecylenic acid. Monograph. *Altern Med Rev.* 2002 Feb;7(1):68-70 http://www.thorne.com/altmedrev/.fulltext/7/1/68.pdf

- Peppermint *(Mentha piperita)*: Peppermint shows antimicrobial and antispasmodic actions and has demonstrated clinical effectiveness in patients with bacterial overgrowth of the small bowel.

- Probiotics: Live cultures in the form of tablets, capsules, yogurt, or kefir can be used per patient preference and tolerance. Obviously, dairy-based products should be avoided by patients with dairy allergy.

- Supplemented Paleo-Mediterranean diet / specific carbohydrate diet: The specifications of the specific carbohydrate diet detailed by Gottschall[156] are met with adherence to the Paleo diet by Cordain.[157] The combination of both approaches and books will give patients an excellent combination of informational understanding and culinary versatility.

- Topical antimicrobials: Treating the dermal lesions of psoriatic arthritis may help break the vicious cycles of (super)antigen absorption which perpetuates immune dysfunction. A variety of botanical and pharmaceutical creams are available. *In vitro* evidence supports the use of equal parts honey, olive oil, and beeswax against *Staph aureus* and *Candida albicans*.[158] As mentioned previously, topical *Mahonia/Berberis* is effective for dermal psoriasis.[159] A topical gel containing artemesinin is also available for clinical use, and animal studies have demonstrated systemic absorption from topical application[160]; its use in humans with psoriasis has not been studied. Topical honey is better than acyclovir against oral and genital herpes; apply *qid* for 15 minutes.[161]

- Commonly used antibiotic/antifungal drugs: The most commonly employed drugs for intestinal bacterial overgrowth are described here.[162] Treatment duration is generally at least 2 weeks and up to 8 weeks, depending on clinical response and the severity and diversity of the intestinal overgrowth. With all anti*bacterial* treatments, use empiric anti*fungal* treatment to prevent yeast overgrowth; some patients benefit from antifungal treatment that is continued for *months* and occasionally *years*. Drugs can generally be coadministered with natural antibiotics/antifungals for improved efficacy. Treatment can be guided by identification of the dysbiotic microbes and the results of culture and sensitivity tests.

  ⇒ **Penicillin: Chronic penicillin treatment leads to clinical improvement of recalcitrant psoriasis; benefits are seen when treatment is continued for at least 12 weeks, according to a clinical trial of treatment lasting for two years.[163]**

  ⇒ Metronidazole: 250-500 mg BID-QID (generally limit to 1.5 g/d); metronidazole has systemic bioavailability and effectiveness against a wide range of dysbiotic microbes, including protozoans, amebas/Giardia, *H. pylori*, *Clostridium difficile* and most anaerobic gram-negative bacilli.[164] Adverse effects are generally limited to stomatitis, nausea, diarrhea,

[156] Gotschall E. Breaking the Vicious Cycle: Intestinal health though diet. Kirkton Press; Rev edition (August, 1994) http://www.scdiet.com/ http://www.breakingtheviciouscycle.info/
[157] Cordain L: The Paleo Diet: Lose weight and get healthy by eating the food you were designed to eat. John Wiley & Sons Inc., New York 2002 http://thepaleodiet.com/
[158] "Honey, beeswax and olive oil mixture (1:1:1, v/v) is useful in the treatment of diaper dermatitis, psoriasis and eczema... CONCLUSIONS: Honey and honey mixture apparently could inhibit growth of S. aureus or C. albicans." Al-Waili NS. Mixture of honey, beeswax and olive oil inhibits growth of Staphylococcus aureus and Candida albicans. *Arch Med Res*. 2005 Jan-Feb;36(1):10-3
[159] "Taken together, these clinical studies conducted by several investigators in several countries indicate that Mahonia aquifolium is a safe and effective treatment of patients with mild to moderate psoriasis." Gulliver WP, Donsky HJ. A report on three recent clinical trials using Mahonia aquifolium 10% topical cream and a review of the worldwide clinical experience with Mahonia aquifolium for the treatment of plaque psoriasis. *Am J Dermatol*. 2005 Sep-Oct;12(5):398-406
[160] "This paper reports results of pharmacokinetic studies of this preparation when applied onto a fixed area of the shaved skin of mice and rabbits. ..The drug was found to be easily absorbed from the skin." Zhao KC, Xuan WY, Zhao Y, Song ZY. [The pharmacokinetics of a transdermal preparation of artesunate in mice and rabbits] [Article in Chinese] Yao Xue Xue Bao. 1989;24(11):813-6
[161] Al-Waili NS. Topical honey application vs. acyclovir for the treatment of recurrent herpes simplex lesions. *Med Sci Monit*. 2004 Aug;10(8):MT94-8. Epub 2004 Jul 23 http://www.medscimonit.com/pub/vol_10/no_8/4431.pdf
[162] Saltzman JR, Russell RM. Nutritional consequences of intestinal bacterial overgrowth. *Compr Ther*. 1994;20(9):523-30
[163] "Total duration of the study was two years. Initially benzathine penicillin 1.2 million units, was given I.M. AST fortnightly. After 24 weeks benzathine penicillin was reduced to 1.2 million units once a month... Significant improvement in the PASI score was noted from 12 weeks onwards. All patients showed excellent improvement at 2 years." Saxena VN, Dogra J. Long-term use of penicillin for the treatment of chronic plaque psoriasis. *Eur J Dermatol*. 2005 Sep-Oct;15(5):359-62 http://www.john-libbey-eurotext.fr/en/revues/medecine/ejd/e-docs/00/04/10/A4/article.md?type=text.html
[164] Tierney ML. McPhee SJ, Papadakis MA. Current Medical Diagnosis and Treatment 2006. 45th edition. New York; Lange Medical Books: 2006, pages 1578-1577

and—rarely and/or with long-term use—peripheral neuropathy, dizziness, and metallic taste; the drug must not be consumed with alcohol. Metronidazole resistance by *Blastocystis hominis* and other parasites has been noted.

⇒ Erythromycin: 250-500 mg TID-QID; this drug is a widely used antibiotic that also has intestinal promotility benefits (thus making it an ideal treatment for intestinal bacterial overgrowth associated with or caused by intestinal dysmotility/hypomotility such as seen in scleroderma[165,166]). Do not combine erythromycin with the promotility drug **cisapride** due to risk for serious cardiac arrhythmia.

⇒ Tetracycline: 250-500 mg QID

⇒ Ciproflaxacin: 500 mg BID

⇒ Cephalexin/kelfex: 250 mg QID

⇒ Minocycline: Minocycline (200 mg/day)[167] has received the most attention in the treatment of rheumatoid arthritis due to its superior response (65%) over placebo (13%)[168]; in addition to its antibacterial action, the drug is also immunomodulatory and anti-inflammatory. Ironically, minocycline can cause drug-induced autoimmunity, especially lupus.[169,170]

⇒ Nystatin: Nystatin 500,000 units bid with food; duration of treatment begins with a minimum duration of 2-4 weeks and may continue as long as the patient is deriving benefit.

⇒ Ketoconazole: As a systemically bioavailable antifungal drug, ketoconazole has inherent anti-inflammatory benefits which may be helpful; however the drug inhibits androgen formation and may lead to exacerbation of the hypoandrogenism that is commonly seen in autoimmune patients and which contributes to the immune dysfunction.

- Orthoendocrinology: Assess melatonin, prolactin, cortisol, DHEA, free and total testosterone, serum estradiol, and thyroid status (e.g., TSH, T4, *and* anti-thyroid peroxidase antibodies).
  - Melatonin: Melatonin is a pineal hormone with well-known sleep-inducing and immunomodulatory properties, and it is commonly administered in doses of 1-40 mg in the evening, before bedtime. Its exceptional safety is well documented. **Although psoriatic patients appear to have lost the physiologic nocturnal peak of melatonin[171], the role of supplemental melatonin in the treatment of patients with psoriasis has not been researched**; however clinicians may reasonably decide to add this to their patients' treatment plan as appropriate. In contrast to implementing treatment with high doses of 20-40 mg, starting with a relatively low dose (e.g., 1-5 mg) and increasing as tolerated is recommended. Melatonin (20 mg hs) appears to have cured two patients with drug-resistant sarcoidosis[172] and 3 mg provided immediate short-term benefit to a patient with

[165] "Prokinetic agents effective in pseudoobstruction include metoclopramide, domperidone, cisapride, octreotide, and erythromycin. ... The combination of octreotide and erythromycin may be particularly effective in systemic sclerosis." Sjogren RW. Gastrointestinal features of scleroderma. *Curr Opin Rheumatol.* 1996 Nov;8(6):569-75

[166] "CONCLUSIONS: Erythromycin accelerates gastric and gallbladder emptying in scleroderma patients and might be helpful in the treatment of gastrointestinal motor abnormalities in these patients." Fiorucci S, Distrutti E, Bassotti G, Gerli R, Chiucchiu S, Betti C, Santucci L, Morelli A. Effect of erythromycin administration on upper gastrointestinal motility in scleroderma patients. *Scand J Gastroenterol.* 1994 Sep;29(9):807-13

[167] "...48-week trial of oral minocycline (200 mg/d) or placebo." Tilley BC, Alarcon GS, Heyse SP, Trentham DE, Neuner R, Kaplan DA, Clegg DO, Leisen JC, Buckley L, Cooper SM, Duncan H, Pillemer SR, Tuttleman M, Fowler SE. Minocycline in rheumatoid arthritis. A 48-week, double-blind, placebo-controlled trial. MIRA Trial Group. *Ann Intern Med.* 1995 Jan 15;122(2):81-9

[168] "In patients with early seropositive RA, therapy with minocycline is superior to placebo." O'Dell JR, Haire CE, Palmer W, Drymalski W, Wees S, Blakely K, Churchill M, Eckhoff PJ, Weaver A, Doud D, Erikson N, Dietz F, Olson R, Maloley P, Klassen LW, Moore GF. Treatment of early rheumatoid arthritis with minocycline or placebo: results of a randomized, double-blind, placebo-controlled trial. *Arthritis Rheum.* 1997 May;40(5):842-8

[169] "...many cases of drug-induced lupus related to minocycline have been reported. Some of those reports included pulmonary lupus..." Christodoulou CS, Emmanuel P, Ray RA, Good RA, Schnapf BM, Cawkwell GD. Respiratory distress due to minocycline-induced pulmonary lupus. *Chest.* 1999 May;115(5):1471-3 http://www.chestjournal.org/cgi/content/full/115/5/1471

[170] Lawson TM, Amos N, Bulgen D, Williams BD.Minocycline-induced lupus: clinical features and response to rechallenge. *Rheumatology* (Oxford). 2001 Mar;40(3):329-35 http://rheumatology.oxfordjournals.org/cgi/content/full/40/3/329

[171] "Our results show that psoriatic patients had lost the nocturnal peak and usual circadian rhythm of melatonin secretion. Levels of melatonin were significantly lower than in controls at 2 a.m., and higher at 6 and 8 a.m. and at 12 noon." Mozzanica N, Tadini G, Radaelli A, Negri M, Pigatto P, Morelli M, Frigerio U, Finzi A, Esposti G, Rossi D, et al. Plasma melatonin levels in psoriasis. *Acta Derm Venereol.* 1988;68(4):312-6

[172] Cagnoni ML, Lombardi A, Cerinic MC, Dedola GL, Pignone A. Melatonin for treatment of chronic refractory sarcoidosis. *Lancet.* 1995 Nov 4;346(8984):1229-30

multiple sclerosis.[173]   Immunostimulatory anti-infective action of melatonin was demonstrated in a clinical trial wherein septic newborns administered 20 mg melatonin showed significantly increased survival over nontreated controls[174]; **given that psoriasis is associated with many subclinical infections, melatonin may provide therapeutic benefit by virtue of its anti-infective properties**.

- o Prolactin (excess): According to clinical trials with small numbers of patients, **whether prolactin levels are high or not, treatment with prolactin-lowering treatment (such as bromocriptine[175]) appears beneficial in patients with psoriatic arthritis.** Serum prolactin is the standard assessment of prolactin status. Since elevated prolactin may be a sign of pituitary tumor, assessment for headaches, visual deficits, other abnormalities of pituitary hormones (e.g., GH and TSH) should be performed and CT or MRI must be considered. Patients with prolactin levels less than 100 ng/mL and normal CT/MRI findings can be managed conservatively with effective prolactin-lowering treatment and annual radiologic assessment (less necessary with favorable serum response).[176, see review 177] Patients with RA and SLE have higher basal and stress-induced levels of prolactin compared with normal controls.[178,179]   A normal serum prolactin level does not necessarily exclude the use of prolactin-lowering intervention, especially since many autoimmune patients have latent hyperprolactinemia which may not be detected with random serum measurement of prolactin. Specific treatment options include the following:

  - ▪ Thyroid hormone: Hypothyroidism frequently causes hyperprolactinemia which is reversible upon effective treatment of hypothyroidism. Obviously therefore, thyroid status should be evaluated in all patients with hyperprolactinemia. Thyroid assessment and treatment is reviewed later in this section.

  - ▪ *Vitex astus-cagnus* and other supporting botanicals and nutrients: **Vitex lowers serum prolactin in humans[180,181] via a dopaminergic effect.[182]**   Vitex is considered safe for clinical use; mild and reversible adverse effects possibly associated with Vitex include nausea, headache, gastrointestinal disturbances, menstrual disorders, acne, pruritus and erythematous rash. No drug interactions are known, but given the herb's dopaminergic effect it should probably be used with some caution in patients treated with dopamine antagonists such as the so-called antipsychotic drugs (most of which do not work very well and/or carry intolerable adverse effects[183,184]). In a recent review, Bone[185] stated that daily doses can range from 500 mg to 2,000 mg DHE (dry herb equivalent) and can be tailored to the suppression of prolactin. Due at least in part to its content of L-

---

[173] "…administration of melatonin (3 mg, orally) at 2:00 p.m., when the patient experienced severe blurring of vision, resulted within 15 minutes in a dramatic improvement in visual acuity and in normalization of the visual evoked potential latency after stimulation of the left eye." Sandyk R. Diurnal variations in vision and relations to circadian melatonin secretion in multiple sclerosis. *Int J Neurosci.* 1995 Nov;83(1-2):1-6

[174] Gitto E, Karbownik M, Reiter RJ, Tan DX, Cuzzocrea S, Chiurazzi P, Cordaro S, Corona G, Trimarchi G, Barberi I. Effects of melatonin treatment in septic newborns. *Pediatr Res.* 2001 Dec;50(6):756-60 http://www.pedresearch.org/cgi/content/full/50/6/756

[175] "In 2 cases of psoriatic arthritis, adding bromocriptine to gold salts and nonsteroidal anti-inflammatory drug was followed by a drastic efficacy with spectacular improvement in clinical, biological and occupational status. Because none of the cases had hyperprolactinaemia, bromocriptine acted probably had an intrinic anti-inflammatory effect independent of its antiprolactinic effect." Eulry F, Mayaudon H, Bauduceau B, Lechevalier D, Crozes P, Magnin J, Claude-Berthelot C. [Blood prolactin under the effect of protirelin in spondylarthropathies. Treatment trial of 4 cases of reactive arthritis and 2 cases of psoriatic arthritis with bromocriptine] *Ann Med Interne* (Paris). 1996;147(1):15-9. French.

[176] Beers MH, Berkow R (eds). The Merck Manual. Seventeenth Edition. Whitehouse Station; Merck Research Laboratories 1999 Page 77-78

[177] Serri O, Chik CL, Ur E, Ezzat S. Diagnosis and management of hyperprolactinemia. *CMAJ.* 2003 Sep 16;169(6):575-81 http://www.cmaj.ca/cgi/content/full/169/6/575

[178] Dostal C, Moszkorzova L, Musilova L, Lacinova Z, Marek J, Zvarova J. Serum prolactin stress values in patients with systemic lupus erythematosus. *Ann Rheum Dis.* 2003 May;62(5):487-8 http://ard.bmjjournals.com/cgi/content/full/62/5/487

[179] "RESULTS: A significantly higher rate of elevated PRL levels was found in SLE patients (40.0%) compared with the healthy controls (14.8%). No proof was found of association with the presence of anti-ds-DNA or with specific organ involvement. Similarly, elevated PRL levels were found in RA patients (39.3%)." Moszkorzova L, Lacinova Z, Marek J, Musilova L, Dohnalova A, Dostal C. Hyperprolactinaemia in patients with systemic lupus erythematosus. *Clin Exp Rheumatol.* 2002 Nov-Dec;20(6):807-12

[180] "Since AC extracts were shown to have beneficial effects on premenstrual mastodynia serum prolactin levels in such patients were also studied in one double-blind, placebo-controlled clinical study. Serum prolactin levels were indeed reduced in the patients treated with the extract." Wuttke W, Jarry H, Christoffel V, Spengler B, Seidlova-Wuttke D. Chaste tree (Vitex agnus-castus)--pharmacology and clinical indications. *Phytomedicine.* 2003 May;10(4):348-57

[181] German abstract from Medline: "The prolactin release was reduced after 3 months, shortened luteal phases were normalised and deficits in the luteal progesterone synthesis were eliminated." Milewicz A, Gejdel E, Sworen H, Sienkiewicz K, Jedrzejak J, Teucher T, Schmitz H. [Vitex agnus castus extract in the treatment of luteal phase defects due to latent hyperprolactinemia. Results of a randomized placebo-controlled double-blind study] *Arzneimittelforschung.* 1993 Jul;43(7):752-6

[182] "Our results indicate a dopaminergic effect of Vitex agnus-castus extracts and suggest additional pharmacological actions via opioid receptors." Meier B, Berger D, Hoberg E, Sticher O, Schaffner W. Pharmacological activities of Vitex agnus-castus extracts in vitro. *Phytomedicine.* 2000 Oct;7(5):373-81

[183] "The majority of patients in each group discontinued their assigned treatment owing to inefficacy or intolerable side effects or for other reasons." Lieberman JA, Stroup TS, McEvoy JP, Swartz MS, Rosenheck RA, Perkins DO, Keefe RS, Davis SM, Davis CE, Lebowitz BD, Severe J, Hsiao JK; Clinical Antipsychotic Trials of Intervention Effectiveness (CATIE) Investigators. Effectiveness of antipsychotic drugs in patients with chronic schizophrenia. *N Engl J Med.* 2005 Sep 22;353(12):1209-23

[184] Whitaker R. The case against antipsychotic drugs: a 50-year record of doing more harm than good. *Med Hypotheses.* 2004;62(1):5-13

[185] "In conditions such as endometriosis and fibroids, for which a significant estrogen antagonist effect is needed, doses of at least 2 g/day DHE may be required and typically are used by professional herbalists." Bone K. New Insights Into Chaste Tree. *Nutritional Wellness* 2005 November http://www.nutritionalwellness.com/archives/2005/nov/11_bone.php

dopa, *Mucuna pruriens* **shows clinical dopaminergic activity** as evidenced by its effectiveness in Parkinson's disease[186]; up to 15-30 gm/d of mucuna has been used clinically but doses will be dependent on preparation and phytoconcentration. **Triptolide and other extracts from *Tripterygium wilfordii* Hook F exert clinically significant anti-inflammatory action in patients with rheumatoid arthritis[187,188] and also offer protection to dopaminergic neurons.**[189,190] Ironically, even though tyrosine is the nutritional precursor to dopamine with evidence of clinical effectiveness (e.g., narcolepsy[191], enhancement of memory[192] and cognition[193]), **supplementation with tyrosine appears to actually increase rather than decrease prolactin levels[194]; therefore tyrosine should be used cautiously if at all in patients with systemic inflammation.** Furthermore, the finding that **high-protein meals stimulate prolactin release**[195] may partly explain the benefits of vegetarian diets in the treatment of systemic inflammation; since vegetarian diets are comparatively low in protein compared to omnivorous diets, they may lead to a relative reduction in prolactin production due to lack of stimulation.

- Bromocriptine: Bromocriptine has long been considered the pharmacologic treatment of choice for elevated prolactin.[196] **Bromocriptine appears to benefit most patients with psoriasis/psoriatic arthritis, according to a small Italian study[197] and three case reports in the French literature.**[198] Typical dose is 2.5 mg per day (effective against lupus[199]); gastrointestinal upset and sedation are common.[200] Clinical intervention with bromocriptine appears warranted in patients with RA, SLE, Reiter's syndrome, psoriatic arthritis, and probably multiple sclerosis and uveitis.[201] A normal serum prolactin level does not necessarily exclude the use of prolactin-lowering intervention, especially since many autoimmune patients have latent hyperprolactinemia which may not be detected with random serum measurement of prolactin.

- Cabergoline/Dostinex: Cabergoline/Dostinex is a newer dopamine agonist with few adverse effects; typical dose starts at 0.5 mg per week (0.25 mg twice per

[186] "CONCLUSIONS: The rapid onset of action and longer on time without concomitant increase in dyskinesias on mucuna seed powder formulation suggest that this natural source of L-dopa might possess advantages over conventional L-dopa preparations in the long term management of PD." Katzenschlager R, Evans A, Manson A, Patsalos PN, Ratnaraj N, Watt H, Timmermann L, Van der Giessen R, Lees AJ. Mucuna pruriens in Parkinson's disease: a double blind clinical and pharmacological study. *J Neurol Neurosurg Psychiatry*. 2004 Dec;75(12):1672-7

[187] "The ethanol/ethyl acetate extract of TWHF shows therapeutic benefit in patients with treatment-refractory RA. At therapeutic dosages, the TWHF extract was well tolerated by most patients in this study." Tao X, Younger J, Fan FZ, Wang B, Lipsky PE. Benefit of an extract of Tripterygium Wilfordii Hook F in patients with rheumatoid arthritis: a double-blind, placebo-controlled study. *Arthritis Rheum*. 2002 Jul;46(7):1735-43

[188] "CONCLUSION: The EA extract of TWHF at dosages up to 570 mg/day appeared to be safe, and doses > 360 mg/day were associated with clinical benefit in patients with RA." Tao X, Cush JJ, Garret M, Lipsky PE. A phase I study of ethyl acetate extract of the chinese antirheumatic herb Tripterygium wilfordii hook F in rheumatoid arthritis. *J Rheumatol*. 2001 Oct;28(10):2160-7

[189] "Our data suggests that triptolide may protect dopaminergic neurons from LPS-induced injury and its efficiency in inhibiting microglia activation may underlie the mechanism." Li FQ, Lu XZ, Liang XB, Zhou HF, Xue B, Liu XY, Niu DB, Han JS, Wang XM. Triptolide, a Chinese herbal extract, protects dopaminergic neurons from inflammation-mediated damage through inhibition of microglial activation. *J Neuroimmunol*. 2004 Mar;148(1-2):24-31

[190] "Moreover, tripchlorolide markedly prevented the decrease in amount of dopamine in the striatum of model rats. Taken together, our data provide the first evidence that tripchlorolide acts as a neuroprotective molecule that rescues MPP+ or axotomy-induced degeneration of dopaminergic neurons, which may imply its therapeutic potential for Parkinson's disease." Li FQ, Cheng XX, Liang XB, Wang XH, Xue B, He QH, Wang XM, Han JS. Neurotrophic and neuroprotective effects of tripchlorolide, an extract of Chinese herb Tripterygium wilfordii Hook F, on dopaminergic neurons. *Exp Neurol*. 2003 Jan;179(1):28-37

[191] "Of twenty-eight visual analogue scales rating mood and arousal, the subjects' ratings in the tyrosine treatment (9 g daily) and placebo periods differed significantly for only three (less tired, less drowsy, more alert)." Elwes RD, Crewes H, Chesterman LP, Summers B, Jenner P, Binnie CD, Parkes JD. Treatment of narcolepsy with L-tyrosine: double-blind placebo-controlled trial. *Lancet*. 1989 Nov 4;2(8671):1067-9

[192] "Ten men and 10 women subjects underwent these batteries 1 h after ingesting 150 mg/kg of l-tyrosine or placebo. Administration of tyrosine significantly enhanced accuracy and decreased frequency of list retrieval on the working memory task during the multiple task battery compared with placebo." Thomas JR, Lockwood PA, Singh A, Deuster PA. Tyrosine improves working memory in a multitasking environment. *Pharmacol Biochem Behav*. 1999 Nov;64(3):495-500

[193] "Ten subjects received five daily doses of a protein-rich drink containing 2 g tyrosine, and 11 subjects received a carbohydrate rich drink with the same amount of calories (255 kcal)." Deijen JB, Wientjes CJ, Vullinghs HF, Cloin PA, Langefeld JJ. Tyrosine improves cognitive performance and reduces blood pressure in cadets after one week of a combat training course. *Brain Res Bull*. 1999 Jan 15;48(2):203-9

[194] "Tyrosine (when compared to placebo) had no effect on any sleep related measure, but it did stimulate prolactin release." Waters WF, Magill RA, Bray GA, Volaufova J, Smith SR, Lieberman HR, Rood J, Hurry M, Anderson T, Ryan DH. A comparison of tyrosine against placebo, phentermine, caffeine, and D-amphetamine during sleep deprivation. *Nutr Neurosci*. 2003;6(4):221-35

[195] "Whereas carbohydrate meals had no discernible effects, high protein meals induced a large increase in both PRL and cortisol; high fat meals caused selective release of PRL." Ishizuka B, Quigley ME, Yen SS. Pituitary hormone release in response to food ingestion: evidence for neuroendocrine signals from gut to brain. *J Clin Endocrinol Metab*. 1983 Dec;57(6):1111-6

[196] Beers MH, Berkow R (eds). The Merck Manual. Seventeenth Edition. Whitehouse Station; Merck Research Laboratories 1999 Page 77-78

[197] "Bromocriptin was shown to be effective in 13 of our 18 psoriatic patients." Valentino A, Fimiani M, Bilenchi R, Castelli A, Francini G, Gonnelli S, Gennari C, Andreassi L. [Therapy with bromocriptine and behavior of various hormones in psoriasis patients] *Boll Soc Ital Biol Sper*. 1984 Oct 30;60(10):1841-4. Italian.

[198] "All three were treated with bromocriptine (5 mg/d in 2 doses) after verification of normal baseline and protirelin-stimulation prolactin levels. There was a beneficial effect in nocturnal pain relief, morning stiffness, the Lee and Ritchie scores and biological markers of inflammation." Eulry F, Mayaudon H, Lechevalier D, Bauduceau B, Ariche L, Ouakil H, Crozes P, Magnin J. [Treatment of rheumatoid psoriasis with bromocriptine] *Presse Med*. 1995 Nov 18;24(35):1642-4. French.

[199] "A prospective, double-blind, randomized, placebo-controlled study compared BRC at a fixed daily dosage of 2.5 mg with placebo... Long term treatment with a low dose of BRC appears to be a safe and effective means of decreasing SLE flares in SLE patients." Alvarez-Nemegyei J, Cobarrubias-Cobos A, Escalante-Triay F, Sosa-Munoz J, Miranda JM, Jara LJ. Bromocriptine in systemic lupus erythematosus: a double-blind, randomized, placebo-controlled study. *Lupus*. 1998;7(6):414-9

[200] Serri O, Chik CL, Ur E, Ezzat S. Diagnosis and management of hyperprolactinemia. *CMAJ*. 2003 Sep 16;169(6):575-81 http://www.cmaj.ca/cgi/content/full/169/6/575

[201] "...clinical observations and trials support the use of bromocriptine as a nonstandard primary or adjunctive therapy in the treatment of recalcitrant RA, SLE, Reiter's syndrome, and psoriatic arthritis and associated conditions unresponsive to traditional approaches." McMurray RW. Bromocriptine in rheumatic and autoimmune diseases. *Semin Arthritis Rheum*. 2001 Aug;31(1):21-32

week).[202]   Several studies have indicated that cabergoline is safer and more effective than bromocriptine for reducing prolactin levels[203] and the dose can often be reduced after successful prolactin reduction, allowing for reductions in cost and adverse effects.[204]   Although fewer studies have been published supporting the antirheumatic benefits of cabergoline than those supporting bromocriptine; its antirheumatic benefits have indeed been documented.[205]

o   Estrogen (excess): Although the classic pattern in patients with autoimmunity is elevated estrogen (generally considered immunodysregulatory) and reduced testosterone (generally considered anti-inflammatory and immunoregulatory), data in patients with psoriatic arthritis is inadequate to extend this otherwise consistent and successful generalization to this group. On the contrary, Stevens et al[206] published a case report of a woman with recalcitrant psoriasis and psoriatic arthritis who responded very well to anti-estrogen treatment. The small amount of data available actually suggests that estrogen may be beneficial (reduction in skin lesions with pregnancy) and that testosterone (in one woman who developed psoriasis following a testosterone-containing hormonal implant following oophorectomy) could exacerbate the disease. Estrogen and testosterone should be measured in serum and modulated appropriately as described in Chapter 4 (Orthoendocrinology) on a *per patient* basis.

> **"We report a patient with severe psoriatic arthritis in whom the severity of both the arthritis and psoriasis fluctuated with the menstrual cycle. These features failed to improve with standard therapy, but there was a prompt response to treatment which suppressed estrogen secretion."**
>
> Stevens et al Cyclical psoriatic arthritis responding to anti-oestrogen therapy. *Br J Dermatol.* 1993

o   Cortisol (insufficiency): Cortisol has immunoregulatory and "immunosuppressive" actions at physiological concentrations. Low adrenal function is common in patients with chronic inflammation[207,208,209] Assessment of cortisol production and adrenal function was detailed in Chapter 4 under the section of Orthoendocrinology. Supplementation with 20 mg per day of cortisol/Cortef is physiologic; my preference is to dose 10 mg first thing in the morning, then 5 mg in late morning and 5 mg in midafternoon in an attempt to replicate the diurnal variation and normal morning peak of cortisol levels. In patients with hypoadrenalism, administration of pregnenolone in doses of 10-60 mg in the morning may also be beneficial.

o   Testosterone (insufficiency): Androgen deficiencies predispose to, are exacerbated by, and contribute to autoimmune/inflammatory disorders. **Female patients with psoriasis have lower levels of testosterone compared to those seen in healthy controls.**[210] A large proportion of men with lupus or RA have low testosterone[211] and suffer the effects of hypogonadism: fatigue, weakness, depression, slow healing, low libido, and difficulties

[202] Serri O, Chik CL, Ur E, Ezzat S. Diagnosis and management of hyperprolactinemia. *CMAJ*. 2003 Sep 16;169(6):575-81 http://www.cmaj.ca/cgi/content/full/169/6/575
[203] "CONCLUSION: These data indicate that cabergoline is a very effective agent for lowering the prolactin levels in hyperprolactinemic patients and that it appears to offer considerable advantage over bromocriptine in terms of efficacy and tolerability." Sabuncu T, Arikan E, Tasan E, Hatemi H. Comparison of the effects of cabergoline and bromocriptine on prolactin levels in hyperprolactinemic patients. *Intern Med*. 2001 Sep;40(9):857-61
[204] "Cabergoline also normalized PRL in the majority of patients with known bromocriptine intolerance or -resistance. Once PRL secretion was adequately controlled, the dose of cabergoline could often be significantly decreased, which further reduced costs of therapy." Verhelst J, Abs R, Maiter D, van den Bruel A, Vandeweghe M, Velkeniers B, Mockel J, Lamberigts G, Petrossians P, Coremans P, Mahler C, Stevenaert A, Verlooy J, Raftopoulos C, Beckers A. Cabergoline in the treatment of hyperprolactinemia: a study in 455 patients. *J Clin Endocrinol Metab*. 1999 Jul;84(7):2518-22 http://jcem.endojournals.org/cgi/content/full/84/7/2518
[205] Erb N, Pace AV, Delamere JP, Kitas GD. Control of unremitting rheumatoid arthritis by the prolactin antagonist cabergoline. *Rheumatology* (Oxford). 2001 Feb;40(2):237-9 http://rheumatology.oxfordjournals.org/cgi/content/full/40/2/237
[206] "We report a patient with severe psoriatic arthritis in whom the severity of both the arthritis and psoriasis fluctuated with the menstrual cycle. These features failed to improve with standard therapy, but there was a prompt response to treatment which suppressed oestrogen secretion." Stevens HP, Ostlere LS, Black CM, Jacobs HS, Rustin MH. Cyclical psoriatic arthritis responding to anti-oestrogen therapy. *Br J Dermatol*. 1993 Oct;129(4):458-60
[207] "Yet evidence that patients with rheumatoid arthritis improved with small, physiologic dosages of cortisol or cortisone acetate was reported over 25 years ago, and that patients with chronic allergic disorders or unexplained chronic fatigue also improved with administration of such small dosages was reported over 15 years ago..." Jefferies WM. Mild adrenocortical deficiency, chronic allergies, autoimmune disorders and the chronic fatigue syndrome: a continuation of the cortisone story. *Med Hypotheses*. 1994 Mar;42(3):183-9 http://www.thebuteykocentre.com/Irish_%20Buteykocenter_files/further_studies/med_hyp2.pdf http://members.westnet.com.au/pkolb/med_hyp2.pdf
[208] "The etiology of rheumatoid arthritis ...explained by a combination of three factors: (i) a relatively mild deficiency of cortisol, …, (ii) a deficiency of DHEA, …and (iii) infection by organisms such as mycoplasma,..." Jefferies WM. The etiology of rheumatoid arthritis. *Med Hypotheses*. 1998 Aug;51(2):111-4
[209] Jefferies W McK. Safe Uses of Cortisol. Second Edition. Springfield, CC Thomas, 1996
[210] "The testosterone levels and LH/FSH ratio were significantly lower in the psoriatic group." Pietrzak A, Lecewicz-Torun B, Jakimiuk A. Lipid and hormone profile in psoriatic females. *Ann Univ Mariae Curie Sklodowska* [Med]. 2002;57(2):478-83
[211] Karagiannis A, Harsoulis F. Gonadal dysfunction in systemic diseases. *Eur J Endocrinol*. 2005 Apr;152(4):501-13 http://www.eje-online.org/cgi/content/full/152/4/501

with sexual performance. Testosterone levels may rise following DHEA supplementation (especially in women) and can be elevated in men by the use of anastrozole/arimidex. Otherwise, transdermal testosterone such as Androgel or Testim can be applied as indicated.

o DHEA: DHEA is an anti-inflammatory and immunoregulatory hormone that is commonly deficient in patients with autoimmunity and inflammatory arthritis.[212] However, the role of DHEA in psoriatic arthritis *en masse* is unclear due to conflicting data. One study showed that patients with psoriasis did not show evidence of DHEA insufficiency[213], while other studies—especially in the German literature—have consistently documented low serum and intracellular levels of DHEA.[214] **DHEA levels should be measured in these patients—especially those with severe disease, deficiencies should be treated unless contraindicated, and therapeutic trials are not unreasonable.** DHEA is an anti-inflammatory and immunoregulatory hormone which is commonly deficient in patients with autoimmunity, including polymyalgia rheumatica, lupus, and rheumatoid arthritis.[215] DHEA levels are suppressed by prednisone[216], and DHEA has been shown to reverse the osteoporosis and loss of bone mass induced by corticosteroid treatment.[217] DHEA shows no acute or subacute toxicity even when used in supraphysiologic doses, even when used in sick patients. For example, in a study of 32 patients with HIV, DHEA doses of 750 mg – 2,250 mg per day were well tolerated and produced no dose-limiting adverse effects.[218] This lack of toxicity compares favorably with any and all so-called "antirheumatic" drugs, nearly all of which show impressive comparable toxicity. When used at doses of 200 mg per day, DHEA safely provides clinical benefit for patients with various autoimmune diseases, including ulcerative colitis, Crohn's disease[219], and SLE.[220] In patients with SLE, DHEA supplementation allows for reduced dosing of prednisone (thus avoiding its adverse effects) while providing symptomatic improvement.[221] Optimal clinical response appears to correlate with serum levels that are supraphysiologic[222], treatment may be implemented with little regard for initial DHEA levels, particularly when 1) the dose of DHEA is kept as low as possible, 2) duration is kept as short as possible, 3) other interventions are used to address the underlying cause of the disease, 4) the patient is deriving benefit and the risk-to-benefit ratio is favorable.

[212] "DHEAS concentrations were significantly decreased in both women and men with inflammatory arthritis (IA) (P < 0.001)." Dessein PH, Joffe BI, Stanwix AE, Moomal Z. Hyposecretion of the adrenal androgen dehydroepiandrosterone sulfate and its relation to clinical variables in inflammatory arthritis. *Arthritis Res.* 2001;3(3):183-8. Epub 2001 Feb 21. http://arthritis-research.com/content/3/3/183

[213] "Assessing the patients by group, the mean DHEAS level was markedly lower in the pemphigoid/pemphigus than in the psoriasis and OA patients (geometric mean 600 vs. 2130 and 2100 nmol/l, respectively; p < 0.001)." de la Torre B, Fransson J, Scheynius A. Blood dehydroepiandrosterone sulphate (DHEAS) levels in pemphigoid/pemphigus and psoriasis. *Clin Exp Rheumatol.* 1995 May-Jun;13(3):345-8

[214] "The effects of this dehydroepiandrosterone deficiency are changes in the humoral regulation of events in growth and proliferation in patients with psoriasis." Holzmann H, Benes P, Morsches B. [Dehydroepiandrosterone deficiency in psoriasis. Hypothesis on the etiopathogenesis of this disease] *Hautarzt.* 1980 Feb;31(2):71-5. Review. German.

[215] "The low levels found in patients with PM:TA are in accordance with those previously reported in immune-mediated diseases such as systemic lupus erythematosus (SLE) and rheumatoid arthritis, suggesting that diminution of DHEAS is a constant endocrinologic feature in these categories of patients." Nilsson E, de la Torre B, Hedman M, Goobar J, Thorner A. Blood dehydroepiandrosterone sulphate (DHEAS) levels in polymyalgia rheumatica/giant cell arteritis and primary fibromyalgia. *Clin Exp Rheumatol.* 1994 Jul-Aug;12(4):415-7

[216] "Basal serum DHEA and DHEAS concentrations were suppressed to a greater degree than was cortisol during both daily and alternate day prednisone treatments. ...Thus, adrenal androgen secretion was more easily suppressed than was cortisol secretion by this low dose of glucocorticoid, but there was no advantage to alternate day therapy." Rittmaster RS, Givner ML. Effect of daily and alternate day low dose prednisone on serum cortisol and adrenal androgens in hirsute women. *J Clin Endocrinol Metab.* 1988 Aug;67(2):400-3

[217] "CONCLUSION: Prasterone treatment prevented BMD loss and significantly increased BMD at both the lumbar spine and total hip in female patients with SLE receiving exogenous glucocorticoids." Mease PJ, Ginzler EM, Gluck OS, Schiff M, Goldman A, Greenwald M, Cohen S, Egan R, Quarles BJ, Schwartz KE. Effects of prasterone on bone mineral density in women with systemic lupus erythematosus receiving chronic glucocorticoid therapy. *J Rheumatol.* 2005 Apr;32(4):616-21

[218] "Thirty-one subjects were evaluated and monitored for safety and tolerance. The oral drug was administered three times daily in doses ranging from 750 mg/day to 2,250 mg/day for 16 weeks. ... The drug was well tolerated and no dose-limiting side effects were noted." Dyner TS, Lang W, Geaga J, Golub A, Stites D, Winger E, Galmarini M, Masterson J, Jacobson MA. An open-label dose-escalation trial of oral dehydroepiandrosterone tolerance and pharmacokinetics in patients with HIV disease. *J Acquir Immune Defic Syndr.* 1993 May;6(5):459-65

[219] "CONCLUSIONS: In a pilot study, dehydroepiandrosterone was effective and safe in patients with refractory Crohn's disease or ulcerative colitis." Andus T, Klebl F, Rogler G, Bregenzer N, Scholmerich J, Straub RH. Patients with refractory Crohn's disease or ulcerative colitis respond to dehydroepiandrosterone: a pilot study. *Aliment Pharmacol Ther.* 2003 Feb;17(3):409-14

[220] "CONCLUSION: The overall results confirm that DHEA treatment was well-tolerated, significantly reduced the number of SLE flares, and improved patient's global assessment of disease activity." Chang DM, Lan JL, Lin HY, Luo SF. Dehydroepiandrosterone treatment of women with mild-to-moderate systemic lupus erythematosus: a multicenter randomized, double-blind, placebo-controlled trial. *Arthritis Rheum.* 2002 Nov;46(11):2924-7

[221] "CONCLUSION: Among women with lupus disease activity, reducing the dosage of prednisone to < or = 7.5 mg/day for a sustained period of time while maintaining stabilization or a reduction of disease activity was possible in a significantly greater proportion of patients treated with oral prasterone, 200 mg once daily, compared with patients treated with placebo." Petri MA, Lahita RG, Van Vollenhoven RF, Merrill JT, Schiff M, Ginzler EM, Strand V, Kunz A, Gorelick KJ, Schwartz KE; GL601 Study Group. Effects of prasterone on corticosteroid requirements of women with systemic lupus erythematosus: a double-blind, randomized, placebo-controlled trial. *Arthritis Rheum.* 2002 Jul;46(7):1820-9

[222] "CONCLUSION: The clinical response to DHEA was not clearly dose dependent. Serum levels of DHEA and DHEAS correlated only weakly with lupus outcomes, but suggested an optimum serum DHEAS of 1000 microg/dl." Barry NN, McGuire JL, van Vollenhoven RF. Dehydroepiandrosterone in systemic lupus erythematosus: relationship between dosage, serum levels, and clinical response. *J Rheumatol.* 1998 Dec;25(12):2352-6

o <u>Thyroid (insufficiency or autoimmunity)</u>: Overt or imminent hypothyroidism is suggested by TSH greater than 2 mU/L[223] or 3 mU/L[224], low T4 or T3, and/or the presence of anti-thyroid peroxidase antibodies.[225] Hypothyroidism can cause an inflammatory myopathy that can resemble polymyositis, and hypothyroidism is a frequent complication of any and all autoimmune diseases. Specific treatment considerations include the following:

- <u>Selenium</u>: Supplementation with either selenomethonine[226] or sodium selenite[227,228] can reduce thyroid autoimmunity and improve peripheral conversion of T4 to T3. Selenium may be started at 500-800 mcg per day and tapered to 200-400 mcg per day for maintenance.

- <u>L-thyroxine/levothyroxine/Synthroid—prescription synthetic T4</u>: 25-50 mcg per day is a common starting dose which can be adjusted based on clinical and laboratory response. All thyroid hormone supplements must be taken away from soy products and preferably on an empty stomach. Doses are generally started at one-half of the daily dose for the first 10 days after which the full dose is used. Caution must be applied in patients with adrenal insufficiency and/or those with cardiovascular disease.

- <u>Armour thyroid—prescription natural T4 and T3 from cow/pig thyroid gland</u>: 60 mg (one grain) is a common starting and maintenance dose. Due to the exacerbating effect on thyroid autoimmunity, Armour thyroid is never used in patients with thyroid autoimmunity.

- <u>Thyrolar/Liotrix—prescription synthetic T4 with T3</u>: Dosed as "1" (low), "2" (intermediate), or "3" (high). Although this product has been difficult to obtain for the past few years due to manufacturing problems (http://thyrolar.com/), it has been my treatment of choice due to the combination of T4 and T3 and the lack of antigenicity compared to gland-derived products.

- <u>Thyroid glandular—nonprescription T3</u>: Apparently, producers of nutritional products are able to distribute T3 because it is not listed by the FDA as a prescription item. A better nutritional company will start from Armour thyroid, remove the T4, and sell the thyroid glandular with active T3. For many patients, one tablet per day is at least as effective as a prescription source of thyroid hormone. Since it is derived from a glandular and therefore potentially antigenic source, thyroid glandular is not used in patients with thyroid autoimmunity.

- <u>Oral enzyme therapy with proteolytic/pancreatic enzymes</u>: Polyenzyme supplementation is used to ameliorate the pathophysiology induced by immune complexes, such as the related condition rheumatoid arthritis.[229]

- <u>*Uncaria tomentosa, Uncaria guianensis*</u>: Cat's claw has been safely and successfully used in the treatment of osteoarthritis[230] and rheumatoid arthritis.[231] **Since serum nitric oxide levels are 5x higher in patients with psoriasis (157) than controls (32)[232], the nitric oxide inhibiting action of**

[223] Weetman AP. Hypothyroidism: screening and subclinical disease. *BMJ*. 1997 Apr 19;314(7088):1175-8 http://bmj.bmjjournals.com/cgi/content/full/314/7088/1175
[224] "Now AACE encourages doctors to consider treatment for patients who test outside the boundaries of a narrower margin based on a target TSH level of 0.3 to 3.0. AACE believes the new range will result in proper diagnosis for millions of Americans who suffer from a mild thyroid disorder, but have gone untreated until now." American Association of Clinical Endocrinologists (AACE). 2003 Campaign Encourages Awareness of Mild Thyroid Failure, Importance of Routine Testing http://www.aace.com/pub/tam2003/press.php November 26, 2005
[225] Beers MH, Berkow R (eds). The Merck Manual. Seventeenth Edition. Whitehouse Station; Merck Research Laboratories 1999 Page 96
[226] Duntas LH, Mantzou E, Koutras DA. Effects of a six month treatment with selenomethionine in patients with autoimmune thyroiditis. *Eur J Endocrinol*. 2003 Apr;148(4):389-93 http://eje-online.org/cgi/reprint/148/4/389
[227] Gartner R, Gasnier BC, Dietrich JW, Krebs B, Angstwurm MW. Selenium supplementation in patients with autoimmune thyroiditis decreases thyroid peroxidase antibodies concentrations. *J Clin Endocrinol Metab*. 2002 Apr;87(4):1687-91 http://jcem.endojournals.org/cgi/content/full/87/4/1687
[228] "We recently conducted a prospective, placebo-controlled clinical study, where we could demonstrate, that a substitution of 200 wg sodium selenite for three months in patients with autoimmune thyroiditis reduced thyroid peroxidase antibody (TPO-Ab) concentrations significantly." Gartner R, Gasnier BC. Selenium in the treatment of autoimmune thyroiditis. *Biofactors*. 2003;19(3-4):165-70
[229] Galebskaya LV, Ryumina EV, Niemerovsky VS, Matyukov AA. Human complement system state after wobenzyme intake. *VESTNIK MOSKOVSKOGO UNIVERSITETA. KHIMIYA*. 2000. Vol. 41, No. 6. Supplement. Pages 148-149
[230] Piscoya J, Rodriguez Z, Bustamante SA, Okuhama NN, Miller MJ, Sandoval M.Efficacy and safety of freeze-dried cat's claw in osteoarthritis of the knee: mechanisms of action of the species Uncaria guianensis. *Inflamm Res*. 2001 Sep;50(9):442-8
[231] "This small preliminary study demonstrates relative safety and modest benefit to the tender joint count of a highly purified extract from the pentacyclic chemotype of UT in patients with active RA taking sulfasalazine or hydroxychloroquine." Mur E, Hartig F, Eibl G, Schirmer M. Randomized double blind trial of an extract from the pentacyclic alkaloid-chemotype of uncaria tomentosa for the treatment of rheumatoid arthritis. *J Rheumatol*. 2002 Apr;29(4):678-81
[232] "The mean NO level in the psoriatic group was 157.7 with SD 50.4 while in the control group it was 32.8 with SD 4.03." Gokhale NR, Belgaumkar VA, Pandit DP, Deshpande S, Damle DK. A study of serum nitric oxide levels in psoriasis. *Indian J Dermatol Venereol Leprol* 2005;71:175-178 http://www.ijdvl.com/

***Uncaria* may be particularly helpful, particularly if used with a low-arginine diet.** However, the clinician must never waiver from attempts to identify the *cause* of the inflammation, rather than merely seeking to quench the *mediators* of inflammation. High-quality extractions from reputable manufacturers used according to directions are recommended. Most products contain between 250-500 mg and are standardized to 3.0% alkaloids and 15% total polyphenols; QD-TID po dosing should be sufficient as *part* of a comprehensive plan.

- *Harpagophytum procumbens*: Harpagophytum is a moderately effective botanical analgesic for musculoskeletal pain.[233,234,235,236,237] Products are generally standardized for the content of harpagosides, with a target dose of 60 mg harpagoside per day.[238]

- Willow bark: Extracts from willow bark have proven safe and effective in the alleviation of moderate/severe low-back pain.[239,240] The mechanism of action appears to be inhibition of prostaglandin formation via inhibition of cyclooxygenase-2 gene transcription[241] by salicylates, phytonutrients which are widely present in fruits, vegetables, herbs and spices and which are partly responsible for the anti-cancer, anti-inflammatory, and health-promoting benefits of plant consumption.[242,243] According to a letter by Vasquez and Muanza[244], the only adverse effect that has been documented in association with willow bark was a single case of anaphylaxis in a patient previously sensitized to acetylsalicylic acid.

- *Boswellia serrata*: *Boswellia* shows clear anti-inflammatory and analgesic action via inhibition of 5-lipoxygenase[245] and clinical benefits have been demonstrated in patients with osteoarthritis of the knees[246] as well as asthma[247] and ulcerative colitis.[248] A German study showing that *Boswellia* was ineffective for rheumatoid arthritis[249] was poorly conducted, with inadequate follow-up, inadequate controls, and abnormal dosing of the herb. Products are generally standardized to contain 37.5–65% boswellic acids, with a target dose is approximately 150 mg of boswellic acids TID; dose and number of capsules/tablets will vary depending upon the concentration found in differing products.

- Phytonutritional modulation of NF-kappaB: As a stimulator of pro-inflammatory gene transcription, NF-kappaB is almost universally activated in conditions associated with inflammation.[250,251] As we would expect, **NF-kappaB plays a central role in the pathogenesis of synovitis and joint destruction seen in RA and psoriatic arthritis.**[252] Nutrients and botanicals

[233] Chrubasik S, Thanner J, Kunzel O, Conradt C, Black A, Pollak S. Comparison of outcome measures during treatment with the proprietary Harpagophytum extract doloteffin in patients with pain in the lower back, knee or hip. *Phytomedicine* 2002 Apr;9(3):181-94

[234] Chantre P, Cappelaere A, Leblan D, Guedon D, Vandermander J, Fournie B. Efficacy and tolerance of Harpagophytum procumbens versus diacerhein in treatment of osteoarthritis. *Phytomedicine* 2000 Jun;7(3):177-83

[235] Leblan D, Chantre P, Fournie B. Harpagophytum procumbens in the treatment of knee and hip osteoarthritis. Four-month results of a prospective, multicenter, double-blind trial versus diacerhein. *Joint Bone Spine* 2000;67(5):462-7

[236] "...subgroup analyses suggested that the effect was confined to patients with more severe and radiating pain accompanied by neurological deficit. ...a slightly different picture, with the benefits seeming, if anything, to be greatest in the H600 group and in patients without more severe pain, radiation or neurological deficit." Chrubasik S, Junck H, Breitschwerdt H, Conradt C, Zappe H. Effectiveness of Harpagophytum extract WS 1531 in the treatment of exacerbation of low back pain: a randomized, placebo-controlled, double-blind study. *Eur J Anaesthesiol* 1999 Feb;16(2):118-29

[237] Chrubasik S, Model A, Black A, Pollak S. A randomized double-blind pilot study comparing Doloteffin and Vioxx in the treatment of low back pain. *Rheumatology* (Oxford). 2003 Jan;42(1):141-8

[238] "They took an 8-week course of Doloteffin at a dose providing 60 mg harpagoside per day... Doloteffin is well worth considering for osteoarthritic knee and hip pain and nonspecific low back pain." Chrubasik S, Thanner J, Kunzel O, Conradt C, Black A, Pollak S. Comparison of outcome measures during treatment with the proprietary Harpagophytum extract doloteffin in patients with pain in the lower back, knee or hip. *Phytomedicine* 2002 Apr;9(3):181-94

[239] Chrubasik S, Eisenberg E, Balan E, Weinberger T, Luzzati R, Conradt C. Treatment of low-back pain exacerbations with willow bark extract: a randomized double-blind study. *Am J Med.* 2000;109:9-14

[240] Chrubasik S, Kunzel O, Model A, Conradt C, Black A. Treatment of low-back pain with a herbal or synthetic anti-rheumatic: a randomized controlled study. Willow bark extract for low-back pain. *Rheumatology* (Oxford). 2001;40:1388-93

[241] Hare LG, Woodside JV, Young IS. Dietary salicylates. *J Clin Pathol* 2003 Sep;56(9):649-50

[242] Lawrence JR, Peter R, Baxter GJ, Robson J, Graham AB, Paterson JR. Urinary excretion of salicyluric and salicylic acids by non-vegetarians, vegetarians, and patients taking low dose aspirin. *J Clin Pathol.* 2003 Sep;56(9):651-3

[243] Paterson JR, Lawrence JR. Salicylic acid: a link between aspirin, diet and the prevention of colorectal cancer. *QJM.* 2001 Aug;94(8):445-8

[244] Vasquez A, Muanza DN. Evaluation of Presence of Aspirin-Related Warnings with Willow Bark: Comment on the Article by Clauson et al. *Ann Pharmacotherapy* 2005 Oct;39(10):1763

[245] Wildfeuer A, Neu IS, Safayhi H, Metzger G, Wehrmann M, Vogel U, Ammon HP. Effects of boswellic acids extracted from a herbal medicine on the biosynthesis of leukotrienes and the course of experimental autoimmune encephalomyelitis. *Arzneimittelforschung* 1998 Jun;48(6):668-74

[246] Kimmatkar N, Thawani V, Hingorani L, Khiyani R. Efficacy and tolerability of Boswellia serrata extract in treatment of osteoarthritis of knee--a randomized double blind placebo controlled trial. *Phytomedicine.* 2003 Jan;10(1):3-7

[247] Gupta I, Gupta V, Parihar A, Gupta S, Ludtke R, Safayhi H, Ammon HP. Effects of Boswellia serrata gum resin in patients with bronchial asthma: results of a double-blind, placebo-controlled, 6-week clinical study. *Eur J Med Res.* 1998 Nov 17;3(11):511-4

[248] Gupta I, Parihar A, Malhotra P, Singh GB, Ludtke R, Safayhi H, Ammon HP. Effects of Boswellia serrata gum resin in patients with ulcerative colitis. *Eur J Med Res.* 1997 Jan;2(1):37-43

[249] Sander O, Herborn G, Rau R. [Is H15 (resin extract of Boswellia serrata, "incense") a useful supplement to established drug therapy of chronic polyarthritis? Results of a double-blind pilot study] [Article in German] *Z Rheumatol.* 1998 Feb;57(1):11-6

[250] Tak PP, Firestein GS. NF-kappaB: a key role in inflammatory diseases. *J Clin Invest.* 2001 Jan;107(1):7-11 http://www.jci.org/cgi/content/full/107/1/7

[251] D'Acquisto F, May MJ, Ghosh S. Inhibition of Nuclear Factor KappaB (NF-B): An Emerging Theme in Anti-Inflammatory Therapies. *Mol Interv.* 2002 Feb;2(1):22-35 http://molinterv.aspetjournals.org/cgi/content/abstract/2/1/22

[252] "NF-B plays a central role in the pathogenesis of synovitis in RA and PsA." Foell D, Kane D, Bresnihan B, Vogl T, Nacken W, Sorg C, Fitzgerald O, Roth J. Expression of the pro-inflammatory protein S100A12 (EN-RAGE) in rheumatoid and psoriatic arthritis. *Rheumatology* (Oxford). 2003 Nov;42(11):1383-9 http://rheumatology.oxfordjournals.org/cgi/content/full/42/11/1383

which either directly or indirectly inhibit NF-kappaB for an anti-inflammatory benefit include vitamin D[253,254], curcumin[255] (requires piperine for absorption[256]), lipoic acid[257], green tea[258], ursolic acid[259] from rosemary[260], grape seed extract[261], propolis[262], zinc[263], high-dose selenium[264], indole-3-carbinol[265,266], N-acetyl-L-cysteine[267], resveratrol[268,269], isohumulones[270], GLA via PPAR-gamma[271] and EPA via PPAR-alpha.[272] I have reviewed the phytonutritional modulation of NF-kappaB later in this text and elsewhere.[273] Several phytonutritional products targeting NF-kappaB are available.

- <u>Topical *Capsicum annuum, Capsicum frutescens*</u> (Cayenne pepper, hot chili pepper): **Topical capsaicin has proven beneficial for alleviating the pruritus of psoriasis, presumably by depleting cutaneous neurons of substance P.**[274] Controlled clinical trials have conclusively demonstrated capsaicin's ability deplete sensory fibers of the neuropeptide substance P to thus reduce pain. Topical capsaicin is proven effective in relieving the pain associated with diabetic neuropathy[275], chronic low back pain[276], chronic neck pain[277], osteoarthritis[278], and rheumatoid arthritis.[279] Given the important role of neurogenic inflammation in chronic arthritis[280,281], the use

[253] "1Alpha,25-dihydroxyvitamin D3 (1,25-(OH)2-D3), the active metabolite of vitamin D, can inhibit NF-kappaB activity in human MRC-5 fibroblasts, targeting DNA binding of NF-kappaB but not translocation of its subunits p50 and p65." Harant H, Wolff B, Lindley IJ. 1Alpha,25-dihydroxyvitamin D3 decreases DNA binding of nuclear factor-kappaB in human fibroblasts. *FEBS Lett.* 1998 Oct 9;436(3):329-34

[254] "Thus, 1,25(OH)₂D₃ may negatively regulate IL-12 production by downregulation of NF-kB activation and binding to the p40-kB sequence." D'Ambrosio D, Cippitelli M, Cocciolo MG, Mazzeo D, Di Lucia P, Lang R, Sinigaglia F, Panina-Bordignon P. Inhibition of IL-12 production by 1,25-dihydroxyvitamin D3. Involvement of NF-kappaB downregulation in transcriptional repression of the p40 gene. *J Clin Invest.* 1998 Jan 1;101(1):252-62

[255] "Curcumin, EGCG and resveratrol have been shown to suppress activation of NF-kappa B." Surh YJ, Chun KS, Cha HH, Han SS, Keum YS, Park KK, Lee SS. Molecular mechanisms underlying chemopreventive activities of anti-inflammatory phytochemicals: down-regulation of COX-2 and iNOS through suppression of NF-kappa B activation. *Mutat Res.* 2001 Sep 1;480-481:243-68

[256] Shoba G, Joy D, Joseph T, Majeed M, Rajendran R, Srinivas PS. Influence of piperine on the pharmacokinetics of curcumin in animals and human volunteers. *Planta Med.* 1998 May;64(4):353-6

[257] "ALA reduced the TNF-alpha-stimulated ICAM-1 expression in a dose-dependent manner, to levels observed in unstimulated cells. Alpha-lipoic acid also reduced NF-kappaB activity in these cells in a dose-dependent manner." Lee HA, Hughes DA. Alpha-lipoic acid modulates NF-kappaB activity in human monocytic cells by direct interaction with DNA. *Exp Gerontol.* 2002 Jan-Mar;37(2-3):401-10

[258] "In conclusion, EGCG is an effective inhibitor of IKK activity. This may explain, at least in part, some of the reported anti-inflammatory and anticancer effects of green tea." Yang F, Oz HS, Barve S, de Villiers WJ, McClain CJ, Varilek GW. The green tea polyphenol (-)-epigallocatechin-3-gallate blocks nuclear factor-kappa B activation by inhibiting I kappa B kinase activity in the intestinal epithelial cell line IEC-6. *Mol Pharmacol.* 2001 Sep;60(3):528-33

[259] Shishodia S, Majumdar S, Banerjee S, Aggarwal BB. Ursolic acid inhibits nuclear factor-kappaB activation induced by carcinogenic agents through suppression of IkappaBalpha kinase and p65 phosphorylation: correlation with down-regulation of cyclooxygenase 2, matrix metalloproteinase 9, and cyclin D1. *Cancer Res.* 2003 Aug 1;63(15):4375-83 http://cancerres.aacrjournals.org/cgi/content/full/63/15/4375

[260] "These results suggest that carnosol suppresses the NO production and iNOS gene expression by inhibiting NF-kappaB activation, and provide possible mechanisms for its anti-inflammatory and chemopreventive action." Lo AH, Liang YC, Lin-Shiau SY, Ho CT, Lin JK. Carnosol, an antioxidant in rosemary, suppresses inducible nitric oxide synthase through down-regulating nuclear factor-kappaB in mouse macrophages. *Carcinogenesis.* 2002 Jun;23(6):983-91

[261] "Constitutive and TNFalpha-induced NF-kappaB DNA binding activity was inhibited by GSE at doses > or =50 microg/ml and treatments for > or =12 h." Dhanalakshmi S, Agarwal R, Agarwal C. Inhibition of NF-kappaB pathway in grape seed extract-induced apoptotic death of human prostate carcinoma DU145 cells. *Int J Oncol.* 2003 Sep;23(3):721-7

[262] "Caffeic acid phenethyl ester (CAPE) is an anti-inflammatory component of propolis (honeybee resin). CAPE is reportedly a specific inhibitor of nuclear factor-kappaB (NF-kappaB)." Fitzpatrick LR, Wang J, Le T. Caffeic acid phenethyl ester, an inhibitor of nuclear factor-kappaB, attenuates bacterial peptidoglycan polysaccharide-induced colitis in rats. *J Pharmacol Exp Ther.* 2001 Dec;299(3):915-20

[263] "Our results suggest that zinc supplementation may lead to downregulation of the inflammatory cytokines through upregulation of the negative feedback loop A20 to inhibit induced NF-kappaB activation." Prasad AS, Bao B, Beck FW, Kucuk O, Sarkar FH. Antioxidant effect of zinc in humans. *Free Radic Biol Med.* 2004 Oct 15;37(8):1182-90

[264] Note that the patients in this study received a very high dose of selenium: 960 micrograms per day. This is at the top—and some would say over the top—of the safe and reasonable dose for long-term supplementation. In this case, the study lasted for three months. "In patients receiving selenium supplementation, selenium NF-kappaB activity was significantly reduced, reaching the same level as the nondiabetic control group. CONCLUSION: In type 2 diabetic patients, activation of NF-kappaB measured in peripheral blood monocytes can be reduced by selenium supplementation, confirming its importance in the prevention of cardiovascular diseases." Faure P, Ramon O, Favier A, Halimi S. Selenium supplementation decreases nuclear factor-kappa B activity in peripheral blood mononuclear cells from type 2 diabetic patients. *Eur J Clin Invest.* 2004 Jul;34(7):475-81

[265] Takada Y, Andreeff M, Aggarwal BB. Indole-3-carbinol suppresses NF-{kappa}B and I{kappa}B{alpha} kinase activation causing inhibition of expression of NF-{kappa}B-regulated antiapoptotic and metastatic gene products and enhancement of apoptosis in myeloid and leukemia cells. *Blood.* 2005 Apr 5; [Epub ahead of print]

[266] "Overall, our results indicated that indole-3-carbinol inhibits NF-kappaB and NF-kappaB-regulated gene expression and that this mechanism may provide the molecular basis for its ability to suppress tumorigenesis." Takada Y, Andreeff M, Aggarwal BB. Indole-3-carbinol suppresses NF-kappaB and IkappaBalpha kinase activation, causing inhibition of expression of NF-kappaB-regulated antiapoptotic and metastatic gene products and enhancement of apoptosis in myeloid and leukemia cells. *Blood.* 2005 Jul 15;106(2):641-9. Epub 2005 Apr 5.

[267] "CONCLUSIONS: Administration of N-acetylcysteine results in decreased nuclear factor-kappa B activation in patients with sepsis, associated with decreases in interleukin-8 but not interleukin-6 or soluble intercellular adhesion molecule-1. These pilot data suggest that antioxidant therapy with N-acetylcysteine may be useful in blunting the inflammatory response to sepsis." Paterson RL, Galley HF, Webster NR. The effect of N-acetylcysteine on nuclear factor-kappa B activation, interleukin-6, interleukin-8, and intercellular adhesion molecule-1 expression in patients with sepsis. *Crit Care Med.* 2003 Nov;31(11):2574-8

[268] "Resveratrol's anticarcinogenic, anti-inflammatory, and growth-modulatory effects may thus be partially ascribed to the inhibition of activation of NF-kappaB and AP-1 and the associated kinases." Manna SK, Mukhopadhyay A, Aggarwal BB. Resveratrol suppresses TNF-induced activation of nuclear transcription factors NF-kappa B, activator protein-1, and apoptosis: potential role of reactive oxygen intermediates and lipid peroxidation. *J Immunol.* 2000 Jun 15;164(12):6509-19

[269] "Both resveratrol and quercetin inhibited NF-kappaB-, AP-1- and CREB-dependent transcription to a greater extent than the glucocorticosteroid, dexamethasone." Donnelly LE, Newton R, Kennedy GE, Fenwick PS, Leung RH, Ito K, Russell RE, Barnes PJ. Anti-inflammatory Effects of Resveratrol in Lung Epithelial Cells: Molecular Mechanisms. *Am J Physiol Lung Cell Mol Physiol.* 2004 Jun 4 [Epub ahead of print]

[270] Yajima H, Ikeshima E, Shiraki M, Kanaya T, Fujiwara D, Odai H, Tsuboyama-Kasaoka N, Ezaki O, Oikawa S, Kondo K. Isohumulones, bitter acids derived from hops, activate both peroxisome proliferator-activated receptor alpha and gamma and reduce insulin resistance. *J Biol Chem.* 2004 Aug 6;279(32):33456-62. Epub 2004 Jun 3. http://www.jbc.org/cgi/content/full/279/32/33456

[271] "Thus, PPAR gamma serves as the receptor for GLA in the regulation of gene expression in breast cancer cells. " Jiang WG, Redfern A, Bryce RP, Mansel RE. Peroxisome proliferator activated receptor-gamma (PPAR-gamma) mediates the action of gamma linolenic acid in breast cancer cells. *Prostaglandins Leukot Essent Fatty Acids.* 2000 Feb;62(2):119-27

[272] "...EPA requires PPARalpha for its inhibitory effects on NF-kappaB." Mishra A, Chaudhary A, Sethi S. Oxidized omega-3 fatty acids inhibit NF-kappaB activation via a PPARalpha-dependent pathway. *Arterioscler Thromb Vasc Biol.* 2004 Sep;24(9):1621-7. Epub 2004 Jul 1. http://atvb.ahajournals.org/cgi/content/full/24/9/1621

[273] "Indeed, the previous view that nutrients only interact with human physiology at the metabolic/post-transcriptional level must be updated in light of current research showing that nutrients can, in fact, modify human physiology and phenotype at the genetic/pre-transcriptional level." Vasquez A. Reducing pain and inflammation naturally - part 4: nutritional and botanical inhibition of NF-kappaB, the major intracellular amplifier of the inflammatory cascade. A practical clinical strategy exemplifying anti-inflammatory nutrigenomics. *Nutritional Perspectives*, July 2005:5-12. www.OptimalHealthResearch.com/part4

[274] "CONCLUSION: Topically applied capsaicin effectively treats pruritic psoriasis, a finding that supports a role for substance P in this disorder." Ellis CN, Berberian B, Sulica VI, Dodd WA, Jarratt MT, Katz HI, Prawer S, Krueger G, Rex IH Jr, Wolf JE. A double-blind evaluation of topical capsaicin in pruritic psoriasis. *J Am Acad Dermatol* 1993 Sep;29(3):438-42

[275] Treatment of painful diabetic neuropathy with topical capsaicin. A multicenter, double-blind, vehicle-controlled study. The Capsaicin Study Group. [No authors listed] *Arch Intern Med.* 1991 Nov;151(11):2225-9

[276] Keitel W, Frerick H, Kuhn U, Schmidt U, Kuhlmann M, Bredehorst A. Capsicum pain plaster in chronic non-specific low back pain. *Arzneimittelforschung.* 2001 Nov;51(11):896-903

[277] Mathias BJ, Dillingham TR, Zeigler DN, Chang AS, Belandres PV. Topical capsaicin for chronic neck pain. A pilot study. *Am J Phys Med Rehabil* 1995 Jan-Feb;74(1):39-44

[278] McCarthy GM, McCarty DJ. Effect of topical capsaicin in the therapy of painful osteoarthritis of the hands. *J Rheumatol.* 1992;19(4):604-7

[279] Deal CL, Schnitzer TJ, Lipstein E, Seibold JR, Stevens RM, Levy MD, Albert D, Renold F. Treatment of arthritis with topical capsaicin: a double-blind trial. *Clin Ther.* 1991 May-Jun;13(3):383-95

of topical *Capsicum* should not be viewed as merely symptomatic; by depleting neurons of substance P it has the ability to help break the vicious cycle of neurogenic-immunogenic inflammation.

- Glucosamine sulfate and chondroitin sulfate: Glucosamine and chondroitin sulfates are well tolerated and well documented in the treatment of osteoarthritis.[282,283,284,285] Since these serve as substrate for the "rebuilding" and preservation of joint cartilage, they would clearly help shift the balance toward anabolism and away from catabolism within articular tissues.

- Carnitine fumarate: Fumaric acid 250-500 mg 3 times a day was advocated by Wright and Gaby[286], who advised beginning with a low dose and slowly increasing the dose over a period of weeks. Flushing and hypoglycemia may occur; serial measurements of liver and kidney function tests are mandatory since fumarate has been reported to cause liver and/or renal damage. Carnitine appears to have anti-inflammatory action via its corticosteroid receptor agonist properties[287,288] and has been reported as beneficial in a case of psoriatic arthritis.[289]

- Spinal manipulation: Many years ago I read a published case report of a female patient who experienced acute onset of psoriasis following trauma received during a skiing accident. Her psoriasis resolved promptly following a series of treatments of chiropractic spinal manipulative therapy.

- Sarsaparilla (*Smilax* spp): **A clinical trial published in the *New England Journal of Medicine* in 1942 documented benefit of a sarsaparilla compound.**[290]

- Hydrotherapy, local hyperthermia: **Hot bath hyperthermia (or heating pads[291]) improves skin lesions and lessens pruritus in the majority of patients with psoriasis.**[292] The dermatologic improvements following hyperthermia can be objectively documented clinically and histologically/microscopically.[293]

- Detoxification support: Cytochrome P450 defects have been noted in patients with psoriasis and correlate with the severity of the disease.[294] See Chapter 4 for discussion on Detoxification and Xenobiotic Immunotoxicity.

Notes:

_____

_____

_____

_____

_____

[280] Gouze-Decaris E, Philippe L, Minn A, Haouzi P, Gillet P, Netter P, Terlain B. Neurophysiological basis for neurogenic-mediated articular cartilage anabolism alteration. *Am J Physiol Regul Integr Comp Physiol*. 2001;280(1):R115-22 http://ajpregu.physiology.org/cgi/content/full/280/1/R115

[281] Decaris E, Guingamp C, Chat M, Philippe L, Grillasca JP, Abid A, Minn A, Gillet P, Netter P, Terlain B. Evidence for neurogenic transmission inducing degenerative cartilage damage distant from local inflammation. *Arthritis Rheum*. 1999;42(9):1951-60

[282] Braham R, Dawson B, Goodman C. The effect of glucosamine supplementation on people experiencing regular knee pain. *Br J Sports Med*. 2003;37(1):45-9

[283] Nguyen P, Mohamed SE, Gardiner D, Salinas T. A randomized double-blind clinical trial of the effect of chondroitin sulfate and glucosamine hydrochloride on temporomandibular joint disorders: a pilot study. *Cranio*. 2001 Apr;19(2):130-9

[284] "...oral glucosamine therapy achieved a significantly greater improvement in articular pain score than ibuprofen, and the investigators rated treatment efficacy as 'good' in a significantly greater proportion of glucosamine than ibuprofen recipients. In comparison with piroxicam, glucosamine significantly improved arthritic symptoms after 12 weeks of therapy..." Matheson AJ, Perry CM. Glucosamine: a review of its use in the management of osteoarthritis. *Drugs Aging*. 2003; 20(14): 1041-60

[285] Muller-Fassbender H, Bach GL, Haase W, Rovati LC, Setnikar I. Glucosamine sulfate compared to ibuprofen in osteoarthritis of the knee. *Osteoarthritis Cartilage*. 1994 Mar;2(1):61-9

[286] Gaby A, Wright JV. Nutritional Protocols. © 1998 by Nutrition Seminars

[287] "Accumulating evidence from both animal and human studies indicates that pharmacologic doses of L-carnitine (LCAR) have immunomodulatory effects resembling those of glucocorticoids (GC)." Manoli I, De Martino MU, Kino T, Alesci S. Modulatory effects of L-carnitine on glucocorticoid receptor activity. *Ann N Y Acad Sci*. 2004 Nov;1033:147-57

[288] "Taken together, our results suggest that pharmacological doses of L-carnitine can activate GRalpha and, through this mechanism, regulate glucocorticoid-responsive genes, potentially sharing some of the biological and therapeutic properties of glucocorticoids." Alesci S, De Martino MU, Mirani M, Benvenga S, Trimarchi F, Kino T, Chrousos GP. L-carnitine: A nutritional modulator of glucocorticoid receptor functions. *FASEB J*. 2003 Aug;17(11):1553-5. Epub 2003 Jun 17 http://www.fasebj.org/cgi/reprint/02-1024fjev1

[289] Afeltra A, Amoroso A, Sgro P, Gandini L, Lenzi A. Clinical improvement in psoriatic arthritis symptoms during treatment for infertility with carnitine. *Clin Exp Rheumatol*. 2004 Jan-Feb;22(1):138

[290] Thurmon FM. The treatment of psoriasis with a sarsaparilla compound. *N Engl J Med* 1942; 227 (4): 128-33

[291] Urabe H, Nishitani K, Kohda H. Hyperthermia in the treatment of psoriasis. *Arch Dermatol*. 1981 Dec;117(12):770-4

[292] "These results indicate that simple repetitive water bath hyperthermia alone is effective in the treatment of psoriatic lesions in heatable locations." Boreham DR, Gasmann HC, Mitchel RE. Water bath hyperthermia is a simple therapy for psoriasis and also stimulates skin tanning in response to sunlight. *Int J Hyperthermia*. 1995 Nov-Dec;11(6):745-54

[293] "Electron microscopy of psoriatic skin prior to and after local hyperthermia revealed both temporary and gradual changes following treatment." Imayama S, Urabe H. Human psoriatic skin lesions improve with local hyperthermia: an ultrastructural study. *J Cutan Pathol*. 1984 Feb;11(1):45-52

[294] "Low CYP2C activity was associated with severe psoriasis, poor metaboliser status occurring in 50% of the severe group, but in none of the mild cases, p < 0.01." Helsby NA, Ward SA, Parslew RA, Friedmann PS, Rhodes LE. Hepatic cytochrome P450 CYP2C activity in psoriasis: studies using proguanil as a probe compound. *Acta Derm Venereol* 1998 Mar;78(2):81-3

Sjogren's Syndrome

<u>Description/pathophysiology</u>:
- **Autoimmune condition affecting the exocrine glands; mucosal surfaces become dry, irritated and prone to microbial colonization**
- Like most conditions, it is generally described as "idiopathic" by medical textbooks and journal articles[1]
- More common than SLE, less common than RA; Sjogren's syndrome is considered by some references to be as common as RA.
- Occurs in two general forms:
    1. "Primary"—only Sjogren's/Sicca syndrome *without evidence of systemic autoimmunity*
    2. "Secondary"—the occurrence of Sjogren's syndrome *along with another autoimmune disease*, especially rheumatoid arthritis, but also SLE, systemic sclerosis, primary biliary cirrhosis, polymyositis, Hashimoto's thyroiditis, polyarteritis, interstitial pulmonary fibrosis

<u>Clinical presentations</u>:
- Much more common in women—90% of patients with Sjogren's disease are female[2]
- Average age of onset is 50 years (typical range 40-60 years)
- **"Sicca syndrome"** denotes dryness of mucus membranes:
    o **Dry eyes, "keratoconjunctivitis sicca":** lymphocyte and plasma cells cause destruction of lacrimal glands; subjective complaints are more prominent than objective evidence: dry eyes, burning, itching, inability to wear contact lenses, thick mucus, photophobia, corneal ulceration
    o **Dry mouth, "xerostomia":** this is generally more problematic than keratoconjunctivitis sicca; dental carries ("cavities") are greatly increased; 33% of patients will have parotid gland tenderness (can be treated with analgesics) and fluctuations in gland size.
    o **Nose, throat, bronchi, and vagina may also be affected.**
- **Joint pain**—similar distribution to RA but less severe and nondestructive; minimal swelling: PIP and knees most common
- Classic presentation: woman (90%) aged 40-60 years with dry mouth, dry eyes, and arthritis that mimics RA
- Photosensitivity, skin rash
- Hair loss
- Mouth lesions
- Chest pain
- Raynaud's phenomenon

<u>Major differential diagnoses</u>:
- Dehydration
- Exposure to excessively dry air (furnaces, dehumidifiers, etc.)
- Another autoimmune disease may mimic or occur concomitantly: RA, SLE, scleroderma, polymyositis, autoimmune thyroid disease, arteritis
- Medication side effects (dry eyes and dry mouth are common side effects of many drugs)

---

[1] "In spite of [the fact that we have no evidence-based solutions to the etiology and pathogenesis of autoimmune diseases], consensus is often taken as a truth, which may hamper the production, funding and/or publication of new and original ideas and views." Konttinen YT, Kasna-Ronkainen L. Sjogren's syndrome: viewpoint on pathogenesis. One of the reasons I was never asked to write a textbook chapter on it. *Scand J Rheumatol Suppl* 2002;(116):15-22
[2] Tierney ML. McPhee SJ, Papadakis MA. <u>Current Medical Diagnosis and Treatment 2006. 45th edition</u>. New York; Lange Medical Books: 2006, pages 842-843

Major differential diagnoses: *continued*
- HIV
- Lymphoma
- Sarcoidosis
- Hepatitis C—may possibly induce Sjogren's syndrome[3]
- Depression
- Fibromyalgia
- Mumps
- Menopause
- Normal aging
- Salivary gland atrophy/fibrosis due to previous radiation to head and neck

Clinical assessments:
- **History/subjective**:
    - See clinical presentations
- **Physical examination/objective**:
    - Schirmer test: Use filter paper to assess adequacy of lacrimation for 5 minutes; less than 5 mm of wetness is abnormal
    - Rose Bengal staining: Used to assess the health of the cornea and to thus search for objective evidence of keratoconjunctivitis sicca
- **Laboratory assessments**:
    - ANA: positive in >95%
        - If ANA is negative, consider HIV, lymphoma, sarcoidosis, hepatitis C.
        - Supportive evidence with **anti-SS-A (anti-Ro)** and **anti-SS-B (anti-La),** neither of which are specific
        - Autoimmunity directed toward glands/tissues such as stomach, adrenal, and neurons may also be noted[4]
    - RF: positive in 70%
    - ESR: elevated in 70%
    - CBC: shows anemia (33%), leukopenia and eosinophilia (25%)
    - Thyroid disorders: Thyroid autoimmunity is common in patients with Sjogren's syndrome; test anti-thyroid peroxidase antibodies and anti-thyroglobulin antibodies along with TSH, T4, and perhaps T3
    - HLA markers: DR2 and DR3 are more common in patients who have Sjogren's syndrome *without rheumatoid arthritis*
    - Schirmer test: measures quantity of tears and thus objectively quantifies keratoconjunctivitis sicca
    - Salivary gland biopsy: not commonly performed except for atypical presentations such as unilateral involvement and to exclude malignancy
    - Assess patient as indicated for other conditions and complications.
- **Imaging**: Used as indicated per patient; generally not part of assessment
- **Establishing the diagnosis**:
    - Both of the following must be present:
        1. **Evidence of a systemic autoimmune disorder**—autoantibodies, preferably in combination with the gold standard in allopathic medicine: salivary gland biopsy—this is necessary for "definite diagnosis" but is not necessary for clinical purposes based on "probable diagnosis"
        2. **Evidence of exocrine damage: keratoconjunctivitis sicca and/or xerostomia**

---

[3] Siegel LB, Gall EP. Viral infection as a cause of arthritis. *Am Fam Physician* 1996 Nov 1;54(6):2009-15
[4] Rehman HU. Sjogren's syndrome. *Yonsei Med J*. 2003 Dec 30;44(6):947-54 http://www.eymj.org/2003/pdf/12947.pdf

Complications:

- Vision impairment
- Dental carries
- Malnutrition, especially vitamin B-12 deficiency
- Inflammatory polyarthropathy
- Salivary stones
- Pneumonia: can be fatal
- Pancreatitis
- Raynaud's phenomenon is seen in ~20%
- Sensory neuropathy, peripheral neuropathy
- Renal tubular acidosis
- Renal insufficiency and failure: can be fatal
- Nephritis (immune complex disorder)
- Vasculitis (immune complex disorder)
- Cryoglobulinemia (immune complex disorder)
- **Lymphoma: up to 3-10% of patients with Sjogren's syndrome develop lymphoma**; risk is increased in patients with severe dryness and systemic complications such as vasculitis, splenomegally, and cryoglobulinemia
- Waldenstrom's macroglobulinemia: increased risk

Clinical management:

- *Medical treatment*:
  - o "Treatment is symptomatic and supportive."[5]
  - o "There is no specific treatment for the basic process. Local manifestations can be treated symptomatically."[6]
- Referral if clinical outcome is unsatisfactory or if serious complications are possible.

Treatments:

- Drug treatments include pilocarpine (5 mg 4 times daily) and/or cevimeline (30 mg three times daily) to promote salivation
- Associated rheumatic diseases are treated as indicated

- Eye drops: consider vitamin-A-containing eye drops, available OTC or by a compounding pharmacist
- Life hygiene: Stress reduction, regular sleep, emotional housecleaning
- For dry mouth:
  - o Sip fluids throughout the day.
  - o Chew sugarless gum to promote saliva flow.
  - o Saliva substitute with carboxymethylcellulose.
  - o Fastidious oral hygiene and regular dental care are important.
  - o **Liquid folic acid** supplementation swished in the mouth may help alleviate mouth sores; likewise, **topical vitamin E** and **glutamine** may help (as they do with chemotherapy-induced mucositis); **chewable deglycyrrhizinated licorice** benefits some patients.
  - o Acupuncture improves salivary flow rates in patients with Sjogren's syndrome.[7,8]

---

[5] Tierney ML. McPhee SJ, Papadakis MA. Current Medical Diagnosis and Treatment. 35th edition. Stamford: Appleton and Lange, 1996 page 749 and Tierney ML. McPhee SJ, Papadakis MA. Current Medical Diagnosis and Treatment 2006. 45th edition. New York; Lange Medical Books: 2006, pages 842-843
[6] Beers MH, Berkow R (eds). The Merck Manual. Seventeenth Edition. Whitehouse Station; Merck Research Laboratories 1999 Page 424
[7] "CONCLUSIONS: This study shows that acupuncture treatment results in statistically significant improvements in SFR in patients with xerostomia up to 6 months. It suggests that additional acupuncture therapy can maintain this improvement in SFR for up to 3 years. "Blom M, Lundeberg T. Long-term follow-up of patients treated with acupuncture for xerostomia and the influence of additional treatment. *Oral Dis* 2000 Jan;6(1):15-24
[8] "A majority of the patients subjectively reported some improvement after treatment, and a significant increase in paraffin-stimulated saliva secretion was found after treatment." List T, Lundeberg T, Lundstrom I, Lindstrom F, Ravald N. The effect of acupuncture in the treatment of patients with primary Sjogren's syndrome. A controlled study. *Acta Odontol Scand* 1998 Apr;56(2):95-9

- <u>Avoidance of allergenic foods</u>: Any patient may be allergic to any food, even if the food is generally considered a health-promoting food. Generally speaking, the most notorious allergens are wheat, citrus (especially juice due to the industrial use of fungal hemicellulases), cow's milk, eggs, peanuts, chocolate, and yeast-containing foods; according to a study in patients with migraine, some patients will have to avoid as many as 10 specific foods in order to become symptom-free.[9] **Patients with celiac disease have an increased prevalence of Sjogren's syndrome[10], and patients with Sjogren's syndrome have an increased prevalence of celiac disease.[11] In one study, the estimated prevalence of celiac disease in Sjogren's patients was nearly 1 in 20.[12]** Celiac disease can present with inflammatory oligoarthritis that resembles rheumatoid arthritis and which remits with avoidance of wheat/gluten; the inflammatory arthropathy of celiac disease has preceded bowel symptoms and/or an accurate diagnosis by as many as 3-15 years.[13,14] Clinicians must explain to their patients that celiac disease and wheat allergy are two different clinical entities and that exclusion of one does not exclude the other, and in neither case does mutual exclusion obviate the promotion of intestinal bacterial overgrowth (i.e., proinflammatory dysbiosis) by indigestible wheat oligosaccharides.

- <u>Avoidance of proinflammatory foods</u>: Proinflammatory foods act *directly* or *indirectly*; direct mechanisms include activating Toll-like receptors or NF-kappaB or inducing oxidative stress, while indirect mechanisms include depleting the body of anti-inflammatory nutrients and displacing more nutritious anti-inflammatory foods. Arachidonic acid (found in beef, liver, pork, and cow's milk) is the direct precursor to proinflammatory prostaglandins and leukotrienes[15] and pain-promoting isoprostanes.[16] Saturated fats promote inflammation by activating/enabling proinflammatory Toll-like receptors.[17] Consumption of saturated fat in the form of cream creates marked oxidative stress and lipid peroxidation that lasts for at least 3 hours postprandially.[18] Corn oil rapidly activates NF-kappaB (in hepatic Kupffer cells) for a proinflammatory effect[19]; similarly, consumption of PUFA and linoleic acid promotes antioxidant depletion and may thus promote oxidation-mediated inflammation via activation of NF-kappaB; linoleic acid causes intracellular oxidative stress and calcium influx and results in increased transcription of NF-kappaB activated pro-inflammatory genes.[20] High glycemic foods cause oxidative stress[21,22] and inflammation via activation of NF-kappaB and other mechanisms—*white bread causes inflammation.*[23] High glycemic foods suppress immune function[24,25] and thus perpetuate and

[9] Grant EC. Food allergies and migraine. *Lancet*. 1979 May 5;1(8123):966-9

[10] "Sjogren's syndrome occurred in 3.3% of coeliac patients and in 0.3% of controls (p = 0.0059)." Collin P, Reunala T, Pukkala E, Laippala P, Keyrilainen O, Pasternack A. Coeliac disease--associated disorders and survival. *Gut*. 1994 Sep;35(9):1215-8.

[11] "Further, our study shows that anti-tTG is more prevalent in SS than in other systemic rheumatic diseases." Luft LM, Barr SG, Martin LO, Chan EK, Fritzler MJ. Autoantibodies to tissue transglutaminase in Sjogren's syndrome and related rheumatic diseases. *J Rheumatol*. 2003 Dec;30(12):2613-9

[12] "The frequency of CD in the SS population was significantly higher than in the non-SS European population (4.5:100 vs 4.5-5.5:1,000)." Szodoray P, Barta Z, Lakos G, Szakall S, Zeher M. Coeliac disease in Sjogren's syndrome--a study of 111 Hungarian patients. Rheumatol Int. 2004 Sep;24(5):278-82. Epub 2003 Sep 17.

[13] "We report six patients with coeliac disease in whom arthritis was prominent at diagnosis and who improved with dietary therapy. Joint pain preceded diagnosis by up to three years in five patients and 15 years in one patient." Bourne JT, Kumar P, Huskisson EC, Mageed R, Unsworth DJ, Wojtulewski JA. Arthritis and coeliac disease. *Ann Rheum Dis*. 1985 Sep;44(9):592-8

[14] "A 15-year-old girl, with synovitis of the knees and ankles for 3 years before a diagnosis of gluten-sensitive enteropathy, is described." Pinals RS. Arthritis associated with gluten-sensitive enteropathy. *J Rheumatol*. 1986 Feb;13(1):201-4

[15] Vasquez A. Reducing Pain and Inflammation Naturally. Part 2: New Insights into Fatty Acid Supplementation and Its Effect on Eicosanoid Production and Genetic Expression. *Nutritional Perspectives* 2005; January: 5-16 www.optimalhealthresearch.com/part2

[16] Evans AR, Junger H, Southall MD, Nicol GD, Sorkin LS, Broome JT, Bailey TW, Vasko MR. Isoprostanes, novel eicosanoids that produce nociception and sensitize rat sensory neurons. *J Pharmacol Exp Ther*. 2000 Jun;293(3):912-20

[17] Lee JY, Sohn KH, Rhee SH, Hwang D. Saturated fatty acids, but not unsaturated fatty acids, induce the expression of cyclooxygenase-2 mediated through Toll-like receptor 4. *J Biol Chem*. 2001 May 18;276(20):16683-9. Epub 2001 Mar 2 http://www.jbc.org/cgi/content/full/276/20/16683

[18] "CONCLUSIONS: Both fat and protein intakes stimulate ROS generation. The increase in ROS generation lasted 3 h after cream intake and 1 h after protein intake. Cream intake also caused a significant and prolonged increase in lipid peroxidation." Mohanty P, Ghanim H, Hamouda W, Aljada A, Garg R, Dandona P. Both lipid and protein intakes stimulate increased generation of reactive oxygen species by polymorphonuclear leukocytes and mononuclear cells. *Am J Clin Nutr*. 2002 Apr;75(4):767-72 http://www.ajcn.org/cgi/content/full/75/4/767

[19] Rusyn I, Bradham CA, Cohn L, Schoonhoven R, Swenberg JA, Brenner DA, Thurman RG. Corn oil rapidly activates nuclear factor-kappaB in hepatic Kupffer cells by oxidant-dependent mechanisms. Carcinogenesis. 1999 Nov;20(11):2095-100 http://carcin.oxfordjournals.org/cgi/content/full/20/11/2095

[20] "Exposing endothelial cells to 90 micromol linoleic acid/L for 6 h resulted in a significant increase in lipid hydroperoxides that coincided wih an increase in intracellular calcium concentrations." Hennig B, Toborek M, Joshi-Barve S, Barger SW, Barve S, Mattson MP, McClain CJ. Linoleic acid activates nuclear transcription factor-kappa B (NF-kappa B) and induces NF-kappa B-dependent transcription in cultured endothelial cells. *Am J Clin Nutr*. 1996 Mar;63(3):322-8 http://www.ajcn.org/cgi/reprint/63/3/322

[21] Mohanty P, Hamouda W, Garg R, Aljada A, Ghanim H, Dandona P. Glucose challenge stimulates reactive oxygen species (ROS) generation by leucocytes. *J Clin Endocrinol Metab*. 2000 Aug;85(8):2970-3 http://jcem.endojournals.org/cgi/content/full/85/8/2970 Glucose/carbohydrate and saturated fat consumption appear to be the two biggest offenders in the food-stimulated production of oxidative stress. The effect by protein is much less. "CONCLUSIONS: Both fat and protein intakes stimulate ROS generation. The increase in ROS generation lasted 3 h after cream intake and 1 h after protein intake. Cream intake also caused a significant and prolonged increase in lipid peroxidation." Mohanty P, Ghanim H, Hamouda W, Aljada A, Garg R, Dandona P. Both lipid and protein intakes stimulate increased generation of reactive oxygen species by polymorphonuclear leukocytes and mononuclear cells. *Am J Clin Nutr*. 2002 Apr;75(4):767-72 http://www.ajcn.org/cgi/content/full/75/4/767

[22] Koska J, Blazicek P, Marko M, Grna JD, Kvetnansky R, Vigas M. Insulin, catecholamines, glucose and antioxidant enzymes in oxidative damage during different loads in healthy humans. *Physiol Res*. 2000;49 Suppl 1:S95-100 http://www.biomed.cas.cz/physiolres/pdf/2000/49_S95.pdf

[23] "Conclusion - The present study shows that high GI carbohydrate, but not low GI carbohydrate, mediates an acute proinflammatory process as measured by NF-kappaB activity." Dickinson S, Hancock DP, Petocz P, Brand-Miller JC..High glycemic index carbohydrate mediates an acute proinflammatory process as measured by NF-kappaB activation. Asia Pac J Clin Nutr. 2005;14 Suppl:S120

[24] Sanchez A, Reeser JL, Lau HS, et al. Role of sugars in human neutrophilic phagocytosis. *Am J Clin Nutr*. 1973 Nov;26(11):1180-4

promote infection/dysbiosis. Delivery of a high carbohydrate load to the gastrointestinal lumen promotes bacterial overgrowth[26,27], which is inherently proinflammatory[28,29] and which appears to be myalgenic in humans.[30] Consumption of grains, potatoes, and manufactured foods displaces phytonutrient-dense foods such as fruits, vegetables, nuts, seeds, and berries which in sum contain more than 8,000 phytonutrients, many of which have anti-oxidant and thus anti-inflammatory actions.[31,32]

- Broad-spectrum fatty acid therapy with ALA, EPA, DHA, GLA and oleic acid: Fatty acid supplementation should be delivered in the form of combination therapy with ALA, GLA, DHA, and EPA. Given at doses of 3,000 – 9,000 mg per day, ALA from flax oil has impressive anti-inflammatory benefits demonstrated by its ability to halve prostaglandin production in humans.[33] **Patients with Sjogren's syndrome have lower levels of GLA/DGLA[34] and fatty acid supplementation—particularly with GLA (along with vitamin C)—is safe may be beneficial (positive reports[35,36], neutral report[37], negative report[38]).** Numerous studies have demonstrated the benefit of GLA in the treatment of rheumatoid arthritis when used at doses between 500 mg – 4,000 mg per day.[39,40] Fish oil provides EPA and DHA which have well-proven anti-inflammatory benefits in rheumatoid arthritis[41,42,43] and lupus.[44,45] ALA, EPA, DHA, and GLA need to be provided in the form of supplements; when using high doses of therapeutic oils, liquid supplements that can be mixed in juice or a smoothie are generally more convenient and palatable than capsules. Therapeutic amounts of oleic acid can be obtained from generous use of olive oil, preferably on fresh vegetables. Supplementation with polyunsaturated fatty acids warrants increased intake of antioxidants from diet, fruit and vegetable juices, and properly formulated supplements; since patients with systemic inflammation are generally in a pro-oxidative state, consideration must be given to the timing and starting dose of fatty acid supplementation and the need for anti-oxidant protection. See chapter on Therapeutics for more details and biochemical pathways. Clinicians must realize that fatty acids are not clinically or

[25] "Postoperative infusion of carbohydrate solution leads to moderate fall in the serum concentration of inorganic phosphate. ... The hypophosphatemia was associated with significant reduction of neutrophil phagocytosis, intracellular killing, consumption of oxygen and generation of superoxide during phagocytosis." Rasmussen A, Segel E, Hessov I, Borregaard N. Reduced function of neutrophils during routine postoperative glucose infusion. *Acta Chir Scand.* 1988 Jul-Aug;154(7-8):429-33

[26] Ramakrishnan T, Stokes P. Beneficial effects of fasting and low carbohydrate diet in D-lactic acidosis associated with short-bowel syndrome. *JPEN J Parenter Enteral Nutr.* 1985 May-Jun;9(3):361-3

[27] Gottschall E. Breaking the Vicious Cycle: Intestinal Health Through Diet. Kirkton Press; Rev edition (August 1, 1994)

[28] Lin HC. Small intestinal bacterial overgrowth: a framework for understanding irritable bowel syndrome. *JAMA.* 2004 Aug 18;292(7):852-8

[29] Lichtman SN, Wang J, Sartor RB, Zhang C, Bender D, Dalldorf FG, Schwab JH. Reactivation of arthritis induced by small bowel bacterial overgrowth in rats: role of cytokines, bacteria, and bacterial polymers. *Infect Immun.* 1995 Jun;63(6):2295-301

[30] Pimentel M, et al. A link between irritable bowel syndrome and fibromyalgia may be related to findings on lactulose breath testing. *Ann Rheum Dis.* 2004 Apr;63(4):450-2

[31] "We propose that the additive and synergistic effects of phytochemicals in fruit and vegetables are responsible for their potent antioxidant and anticancer activities, and that the benefit of a diet rich in fruit and vegetables is attributed to the complex mixture of phytochemicals present in whole foods." Liu RH. Health benefits of fruit and vegetables are from additive and synergistic combinations of phytochemicals. *Am J Clin Nutr.* 2003 Sep;78(3 Suppl):517S-520S

[32] Seaman DR. The diet-induced proinflammatory state: a cause of chronic pain and other degenerative diseases? *J Manipulative Physiol Ther.* 2002;25(3):168-79

[33] Adam O, Wolfram G, Zollner N. Effect of alpha-linolenic acid in the human diet on linoleic acid metabolism and prostaglandin biosynthesis. *J Lipid Res.* 1986 Apr;27(4):421-6
http://www.jlr.org/cgi/reprint/27/4/421

[34] "We found MD levels of 20:3n6 (dihommo-gamma-linolenic acid), and basal and indomethacin-enhanced NK cell activity significantly reduced, in 10 primary Sjogren's syndrome patients as compared with 10 healthy controls." Oxholm P, Pedersen BK, Horrobin DF.Natural killer cell functions are related to the cell membrane composition of essential fatty acids: differences in healthy persons and patients with primary Sjogren's syndrome. *Clin Exp Rheumatol.* 1992 May-Jun;10(3):229-34

[35] "An attempt to treat humans with Sjogren's syndrome by raising endogenous PGE1 production by administration of essential fatty acid PGE1 precursors, of pyridoxine and of vitamin C was successful in raising the rates of tear and saliva production." Horrobin DF, Campbell A. Sjogren's syndrome and the sicca syndrome: the role of prostaglandin E1 deficiency. Treatment with essential fatty acids and vitamin C. *Med Hypotheses.* 1980 Mar;6(3):225-32

[36] "Efamol treatment improved the Schirmer-I-test..." Manthorpe R, Hagen Petersen S, Prause JU. Primary Sjogren's syndrome treated with Efamol/Efavit. A double-blind cross-over investigation. *Rheumatol Int.* 1984;4(4):165-7. The duration of this study was ridiculously short—only 3 weeks.

[37] "The objective ocular status, evaluated by a combined ocular score, including the results from Schirmer-I test, break-up time and van Bijsterveld score, improved significantly during Efamol treatment when compared with Efamol start-values (p less than 0.05), but not when compared with placebo values (p less than 0.2)." Oxholm P, Manthorpe R, Prause JU, Horrobin D. Patients with primary Sjogren's syndrome treated for two months with evening primrose oil. *Scand J Rheumatol.* 1986;15(2):103-8

[38] "There was no significant improvement in any of the patients during the treatment period compared to assessments done pre and post treatment." McKendry RJ. Treatment of Sjogren's syndrome with essential fatty acids, pyridoxine and vitamin C. *Prostaglandins Leukot Med.* 1982 Apr;8(4):403-8

[39] "Other results showed a significant reduction in morning stiffness with gamma-linolenic acid at 3 months and reduction in pain and articular index at 6 months with olive oil." Brzeski M, Madhok R, Capell HA. Evening primrose oil in patients with rheumatoid arthritis and side-effects of non-steroidal anti-inflammatory drugs. *Br J Rheumatol.* 1991 Oct;30(5):370-2

[40] Rothman D, DeLuca P, Zurier RB. Botanical lipids: effects on inflammation, immune responses, and rheumatoid arthritis. *Semin Arthritis Rheum.* 1995 Oct;25(2):87-96

[41] Adam O, Beringer C, Kless T, Lemmen C, Adam A, Wiseman M, Adam P, Klimmek R, Forth W. Anti-inflammatory effects of a low arachidonic acid diet and fish oil in patients with rheumatoid arthritis. *Rheumatol Int.* 2003 Jan;23(1):27-36

[42] Lau CS, Morley KD, Belch JJ. Effects of fish oil supplementation on non-steroidal anti-inflammatory drug requirement in patients with mild rheumatoid arthritis--a double-blind placebo controlled study. *Br J Rheumatol.* 1993 Nov;32(11):982-9

[43] Kremer JM, Jubiz W, Michalek A, Rynes RI, Bartholomew LE, Bigaouette J, Timchalk M, Beeler D, Lininger L. Fish-oil fatty acid supplementation in active rheumatoid arthritis. A double-blinded, controlled, crossover study. *Ann Intern Med.* 1987 Apr;106(4):497-503

[44] Walton AJ, Snaith ML, Locniskar M, Cumberland AG, Morrow WJ, Isenberg DA. Dietary fish oil and the severity of symptoms in patients with systemic lupus erythematosus. *Ann Rheum Dis.* 1991 Jul;50(7):463-6

[45] Duffy EM, Meenagh GK, McMillan SA, Strain JJ, Hannigan BM, Bell AL. The clinical effect of dietary supplementation with omega-3 fish oils and/or copper in systemic lupus erythematosus. *J Rheumatol.* 2004 Aug;31(8):1551-6

biochemically interchangeable and that one fatty acid does not substitute for another; each of the fatty acids must be supplied in order for its benefits to be obtained.[46]

- Assess for and treat dysbiosis: Insufficient flow of saliva and other fluids promotes microbial colonization of mucosal surfaces, particularly the digestive and respiratory tracts. **Gastrointestinal infection/dysbiosis can cause nutrient malabsorption, and the resultant nutritional insufficiencies can exacerbate the sicca symptoms.**[47] Patients with Sjogren's syndrome may have an increased prevalence of infection/colonization with *H. pylori*[48], an organism known to incite systemic inflammation and to produce pro-inflammatory endotoxin and antigens.

- Vitamin D3 supplementation with physiologic doses and/or tailored to serum 25(OH)D levels: **Vitamin D insufficiency has been reported in patients with Sjogren's syndrome, presumably due to reduced intake and/or malabsorption.** Vitamin D deficiency is common in the general population and is even more common in patients with chronic illness and chronic musculoskeletal pain.[49] Correction of vitamin D deficiency supports normal immune function against infection and provides a clinically significant anti-inflammatory[50] and analgesic benefit in patients with back pain[51] and limb pain.[52] **Vitamin D status is inversely associated with inflammation in patients with Sjogren's syndrome.**[53,54]

Reasonable daily doses for children and adults are 2,000 and 4,000 IU, respectively, as defined by Vasquez, et al.[55] Deficiency and response to treatment are monitored with serum 25(OH)vitamin D while safety is monitored with serum calcium; inflammatory granulomatous diseases and certain drugs such as hydrochlorothiazide greatly

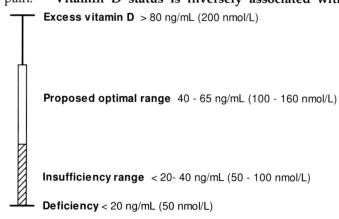

Excess vitamin D > 80 ng/mL (200 nmol/L)

Proposed optimal range 40 - 65 ng/mL (100 - 160 nmol/L)

Insufficiency range < 20- 40 ng/mL (50 - 100 nmol/L)

Deficiency < 20 ng/mL (50 nmol/L)

Proposed normal and optimal ranges for serum 25(OH)D levels

increase the propensity for hypercalcemia and warrant increment dosing and frequent monitoring of serum calcium.

- Supplemented Paleo-Mediterranean diet: The health-promoting diet of choice for the majority of people is a diet based on abundant consumption of fruits, vegetables, seeds, nuts, omega-3 and monounsaturated fatty acids, and lean sources of protein such as lean meats, fatty cold-water fish, soy and whey proteins. This diet obviates overconsumption of chemical preservatives, artificial sweeteners, and carbohydrate-dominant foods such as candies, pastries, breads, potatoes, grains, and other foods with a high glycemic load and high glycemic index. This "Paleo-Mediterranean Diet" is a combination of the "Paleolithic" or "Paleo diet" and the well-

[46] Vasquez A. Reducing Pain and Inflammation Naturally. Part 2: New Insights into Fatty Acid Supplementation and Its Effect on Eicosanoid Production and Genetic Expression. *Nutritional Perspectives* 2005; January: 5-16 http://optimalhealthresearch.com/part2

[47] Bosman C, Boldrini R, Borsetti G, Morelli S, Paglia MG, Visca P. Sicca syndrome associated with Tropheryma whipplei intestinal infection. *J Clin Microbiol.* 2002 Aug;40(8):3104-6 http://jcm.asm.org/cgi/content/full/40/8/3104?view=long&pmid=12149393

[48] "Patients with SS are more prone to have H. pylori infection in comparison to other connective tissue diseases. Serum antibody titer to H. pylori correlated with index for clinical disease manifestations, age, disease duration and CRP." El Miedany YM, Baddour M, Ahmed I, Fahmy H. Sjogren's syndrome: concomitant H. pylori infection and possible correlation with clinical parameters. *Joint Bone Spine.* 2005 Mar;72(2):135-41

[49] Plotnikoff GA, Quigley JM. Prevalence of severe hypovitaminosis D in patients with persistent, nonspecific musculoskeletal pain. *Mayo Clin Proc.* 2003 Dec;78(12):1463-70

[50] Timms PM, Mannan N, Hitman GA, Noonan K, Mills PG, Syndercombe-Court D, Aganna E, Price CP, Boucher BJ. Circulating MMP9, vitamin D and variation in the TIMP-1 response with VDR genotype: mechanisms for inflammatory damage in chronic disorders? *QJM.* 2002 Dec;95(12):787-96 http://qjmed.oxfordjournals.org/cgi/content/full/95/12/787

[51] Al Faraj S, Al Mutairi K. Vitamin D deficiency and chronic low back pain in Saudi Arabia. *Spine.* 2003 Jan 15;28(2):177-9

[52] Masood H, Narang AP, Bhat IA, Shah GN. Persistent limb pain and raised serum alkaline phosphatase the earliest markers of subclinical hypovitaminosis D in Kashmir. *Indian J Physiol Pharmacol.* 1989 Oct-Dec;33(4):259-61

[53] "In conclusion the inverse correlations found between levels of 25 OH D and measures of clinical and immunoinflammatory status support the notion that vitamin D metabolism may be involved in the pathogenesis of primary SS." Bang B, Asmussen K, Sorensen OH, Oxholm P. Reduced 25-hydroxyvitamin D levels in primary Sjogren's syndrome. Correlations to disease manifestations. *Scand J Rheumatol.* 1999;28(3):180-3

[54] "Among patients with increased concentrations of IgM rheumatoid factor there was a significant negative correlation between the serum titres of IgM rheumatoid factor and 25-OHD3 concentrations." Muller K, Oxholm P, Sorensen OH, Thymann M, Hoier-Madsen M, Bendtzen K. Abnormal vitamin D3 metabolism in patients with primary Sjogren's syndrome. *Ann Rheum Dis.* 1990 Sep;49(9):682-4

[55] **Vasquez A, Manso G, Cannell J. The clinical importance of vitamin D (cholecalciferol): a paradigm shift with implications for all healthcare providers. *Altern Ther Health Med.* 2004 Sep-Oct;10(5):28-36** http://optimalhealthresearch.com/monograph04

known "Mediterranean diet", both of which are well described in peer-reviewed journals and the lay press. (See Chapter 2 and my other publications[56,57] for details). Although this diet is the most-nutrient dense diet available, rational supplementation with vitamins, minerals, and health promoting fatty acids (i.e., ALA, GLA, EPA, DHA) makes this the best practical diet that can possibly be conceived and implemented.

- Orthoendocrinology: Assess and treat per patient. In direct contrast to the commonly observed pattern implicating a relative *excess of estrogen* and *insufficiency of testosterone* in the genesis of autoimmunity, animal models of Sjogren's syndrome have found an increased prevalence of Sjogren's in estrogen-deficient animals and a protective benefit from phytoestrogens[58], and recent human data has shown that higher testosterone levels correlate with more severe disease activity in patients with Sjogren's syndrome.[59] As noted with most other autoimmune/inflammatory diseases, patients with Sjogren's syndrome have elevated levels of pro-inflammatory prolactin that correlate with disease activity.[60]

- Raynaud's phenomenon—specific treatments: Treatment of Raynaud's phenomenon should not be trivialized as merely symptomatic; the pain experienced by some patients with Raynaud's phenomenon is truly excruciating. Vasodilation/vasostabilization in Raynaud's phenomenon can be supported with any/all of the following:
  o Inositol hexaniacinate: 3,000-4,000 mg/d in divided doses[61,62,63]
  o *Ginkgo biloba*: Ginkgo reduces the number of daily Raynaud's attacks in patients with primary Raynaud's disease[64], and it is also an excellent antioxidant with potent anti-inflammatory actions.
  o Magnesium: 300-500 mg/d or bowel tolerance
  o Combination fatty acid therapy: must include GLA (minimum 500 mg) and EPA (minimum 2,000 mg)
  o Acupuncture, biofeedback, counseling, stress reduction, cold avoidance, smoking cessation: Since stressful events, cold exposure, and cigarette smoking are all vasoconstrictive, these should be avoided/modified to the highest extent possible. Stress reduction and ongoing refinement of inter- and intra-personal socioemotional exchange is beneficial for everyone.[65,66,67]

- Green tea, green tea extract (EGCG), and other phytonutritional antioxidants and anti-inflammatories: Very interestingly, a recent *in vitro* study[68] showed that epigallocatechin gallate inhibited the expression of major autoantigens, including those which are characteristic of Sjogren's syndrome: SS-B/La, SS-A/Ro. Given its antioxidant properties and anti-inflammatory

[56] Vasquez A. A Five-Part Nutritional Protocol that Produces Consistently Positive Results. *Nutritional Wellness* 2005 September Available in the printed version and on-line at http://www.nutritionalwellness.com/archives/2005/sep/09_vasquez.php and http://optimalhealthresearch.com/protocol
[57] Vasquez A. Implementing the Five-Part Nutritional Wellness Protocol for the Treatment of Various Health Problems. *Nutritional Wellness* 2005 November. Available on-line at http://www.nutritionalwellness.com/archives/2005/nov/11_vasquez.php and http://optimalhealthresearch.com/protocol
[58] Shim GJ, Warner M, Kim HJ, Andersson S, Liu L, Ekman J, Imamov O, Jones ME, Simpson ER, Gustafsson JA. Aromatase-deficient mice spontaneously develop a lymphoproliferative autoimmune disease resembling Sjogren's syndrome. *Proc Natl Acad Sci U S A.* 2004 Aug 24;101(34):12628-33 http://www.pnas.org/cgi/content/full/101/34/12628
[59] "Higher levels of disease activity (ESR, serum protein, and focus score) were associated with higher concentrations of testosterone." Brennan MT, Sankar V, Leakan RA, Grisius MM, Collins MT, Fox PC, Baum BJ, Pillemer SR. Sex steroid hormones in primary Sjogren's syndrome. *J Rheumatol.* 2003 Jun;30(6):1267-7
[60] "Patients with primary SS have moderately increased levels of serum PRL, especially evident in patients diagnosed at a young age with active immunological disease." Haga HJ, Rygh T. The prevalence of hyperprolactinemia in patients with primary Sjogren's syndrome. *J Rheumatol.* 1999 Jun;26(6):1291-5
[61] "It appears to be a safe and well tolerated drug, which, together with other symptomatic measures, merits to be used in the management of vasospastic disease of the extremities even in the presence of partial obliteration of the microcirculation." Holti G. An experimentally controlled evaluation of the effect of inositol nicotinate upon the digital blood flow in patients with Raynaud's phenomenon. *J Int Med Res.* 1979;7(6):473-83
[62] "Although the mechanism of action remains unclear Hexopal is safe and is effective in reducing the vasospasm of primary Raynaud's disease during the winter months." Sunderland GT, Belch JJ, Sturrock RD, Forbes CD, McKay AJ. A double blind randomised placebo controlled trial of hexopal in primary Raynaud's disease. *Clin Rheumatol.* 1988 Mar;7(1):46-9
[63] "It is suggested that long-term treatment with nicotinic acid derivatives may produce improvement in the peripheral circulation by a different mechanism than the transient effect detected by short-term studies." Ring EF, Bacon PA. Quantitative thermographic assessment of inositol nicotinate therapy in Raynaud's phenomena. J Int Med Res. 1977;5(4):217-22
[64] "Ginkgo biloba phytosome may be effective in reducing the number of Raynaud's attacks per week in patients suffering from Raynaud's disease." Muir AH, Robb R, McLaren M, Daly F, Belch JJ. The use of Ginkgo biloba in Raynaud's disease: a double-blind placebo-controlled trial. *Vasc Med.* 2002;7(4):265-7
[65] Rick Brinkman ND and Rick Kirschner ND. How to Deal With Difficult People [Audio Cassette. Career Track, 1995]
[66] Bradshaw J. Healing the Shame that Binds You [Audio Cassette (April 1990) Health Communications Audio; ISBN: 1558740430]
[67] Miller A. The Drama of the Gifted Child: The Search for the True Self. Basic Books: 1981
[68] "EGCG inhibited the transcription and translation of major autoantigens, including SS-B/La, SS-A/Ro, coilin, DNA topoisomerase I, and alpha-fodrin. These findings, taken together with green tea's anti-inflammatory and antiapoptotic effects, suggest that green tea polyphenols could serve as an important component in novel approaches to combat autoimmune disorders in humans." Hsu S, Dickinson DP, Qin H, Lapp C, Lapp D, Borke J, Walsh DS, Bollag WB, Stoppler H, Yamamoto T, Osaki T, Schuster G. Inhibition of autoantigen expression by (-)-epigallocatechin-3-gallate (the major constituent of green tea) in normal human cells. *J Pharmacol Exp Ther.* 2005 Nov;315(2):805-11. Epub 2005 Jul 26

actions (specifically via inhibition of NF-kappaB[69]), green tea and related supplements may prove beneficial for patients with Sjogren's syndrome.

- <u>High-dose short-term oral vitamin A</u>: Szocsik et al[70] administered vitamin A 100,000 IU per day for two weeks and obtained improved immune function, such as improved natural killer cell function, in patients with Sjogren's syndrome.
- <u>Individualized homeopathy</u>: A small randomized placebo-controlled trial found homeopathy beneficial for xerostomia.[71]

Additional notes:

_____

_____

_____

_____

_____

_____

_____

_____

_____

_____

_____

_____

_____

_____

_____

_____

_____

_____

_____

_____

_____

_____

_____

_____

_____

_____

_____

_____

_____

_____

_____

_____

[69] "In conclusion, EGCG is an effective inhibitor of IKK activity. This may explain, at least in part, some of the reported anti-inflammatory and anti-cancer effects of green tea." Yang F, Oz HS, Barve S, de Villiers WJ, McClain CJ, Varilek GW. The green tea polyphenol (-)-epigallocatechin-3-gallate blocks nuclear factor-kappa B activation by inhibiting I kappa B kinase activity in the intestinal epithelial cell line IEC-6. *Mol Pharmacol.* 2001 Sep;60(3):528-33

[70] "Patients with Sjogren's syndrome were treated with vitamin A (100,000 U) daily during a two-week period. The vitamin treatment significantly elevated their ADCC and NK activity." Szocsik K, Gonzalez-Cabello R, Vien CV, Mezes M, Szongoth M, Gergely P. Effect of vitamin A treatment on immune reactivity and lipid peroxidation in patients with Sjogren's syndrome. *Clin Rheumatol.* 1988 Dec;7(4):514-9

[71] "Our results suggest that individually prescribed homeopathic medicine could be a valuable adjunct to the treatment of oral discomfort and xerostomic symptoms." Haila S, Koskinen A, Tenovuo J. Effects of homeopathic treatment on salivary flow rate and subjective symptoms in patients with oral dryness: a randomized trial. *Homeopathy.* 2005 Jul;94(3):175-81

Spondyloarthropathies
- **Ankylosing spondylitis**
- **Reactive arthritis (previously Reiter's syndrome)**
- **Enteropathic spondyloarthropathy, enteropathic arthritis**

<u>Description/pathophysiology</u>:
- Inflammatory arthropathies affecting the spine and sacroiliac joints are termed "spondyloarthropathies" and like other arthritic conditions are termed *seronegative* if not related to rheumatoid arthritis in general and RF positivity in particular. **The spondyloarthropathies differ in some aspects of their etiologies, affected populations, clinical presentations, and treatment; however—regarding etiology and treatment—the similarities far outnumber the differences.** Regarding clinical management, from both allopathic and integrative/naturopathic perspectives, the treatment and management of these different conditions is virtually identical, save for a few important nuances.
- Spondyloarthropathies and reactive arthritis differ from the classic pattern of other autoimmune conditions in that 1) most patients affected are male, 2) they are highly correlated with HLA-B27, 3) serologic evidence of autoimmunity is generally absent, 4) they are strongly associated with dysbiosis, infections, and/or occult or overt enteropathy.[1,2]
- Some variation exists in the conditions that are included under the heading of *Spondyloarthropathies*. Most medical textbooks include four disorders under the heading of spondyloarthropathies: 1) ankylosing spondylitis, 2) psoriatic arthritis, 3) reactive arthritis, and 4) enteropathic spondyloarthropathy (ES), while a few others go on to include 5) juvenile spondyloarthropathy, and 6) rheumatoid arthritis. Psoriatic arthritis (PsA) and rheumatoid arthritis (RA) are detailed in their own chapters in this book and therefore will not be discussed in great detail here.
- Although ankylosing spondylitis (AS) is the prototype of the spondyloarthropathies, reactive arthritis (ReA) is the best-known and most well accepted model for microbe-induced musculoskeletal autoimmunity. Despite nearly overwhelming research demonstrating that all of these conditions are triggered by exposure to microbes, major medical textbooks[3] still describe these conditions as *idiopathic*. Enteropathic arthritis and enteropathic spondyloarthropathy (EAES) demonstrate how gastrointestinal dysbiosis, hormonal imbalances, increased intestinal permeability ("leaky gut"), and non-musculoskeletal systemic inflammation can spill-over into peripheral and axial arthritis. As detailed in the separate chapter on psoriasis and psoriatic arthritis (PsA), PsA is clearly a microbe-triggered disease, and its similarity to AS suggests a common physiologic etiology. The common themes that weave these disorders together are 1) dysbiosis-induced musculoskeletal inflammation, 2) hormonal imbalances, and 3) increased intestinal/mucosal permeability—the latter is the most voluminous route of absorption of arthritogenic antigens, immunogens, and antimetabolites—see Chapter 4 for overview and details.
- All of these conditions are *systemic* inflammatory disorders that show clear evidence of immune-mediated tissue damage and are therefore worthy of being dubbed *autoimmune*. The systemic nature of these disorders carries important clinical implications because both doctor and patient need to be aware of *non-musculoskeletal* complications. Non-musculoskeletal complications of these disorders include renal failure secondary to amyloidosis[4,5], cardiovascular and pulmonary complications, and

[1] Colmegna I, Cuchacovich R, Espinoza LR. HLA-B27-associated reactive arthritis: pathogenetic and clinical considerations. *Clin Microbiol Rev.* 2004 Apr;17(2):348-69 http://cmr.asm.org/cgi/content/full/17/2/348
[2] Ringrose JH. HLA-B27 associated spondyloarthropathy, an autoimmune disease based on crossreactivity between bacteria and HLA-B27? *Ann Rheum Dis.* 1999 Oct;58(10):598-610 http://ard.bmjjournals.com/cgi/content/full/58/10/598
[3] Klippel JH (ed). Primer on the rheumatic diseases. 11th edition. Atlanta: Arthritis Foundation; 1997, page 181
[4] "The mechanism of death in these patients was secondary amyloidosis in 19, cardiovascular complications in six, fracture of the spine in one, and it was not known in one patient. Excess deaths due to circulatory, gastrointestinal and renal diseases, and violence were also observed." Lehtinen K. Mortality and causes of death in 398 patients admitted to hospital with ankylosing spondylitis. *Ann Rheum Dis.* 1993 Mar;52(3):174-6
[5] "During an outbreak of Yersinia pseudotuberculosis III, one of two HLA-B27 positive brothers developed reactive arthritis (ReA), mild at first, but later severely destructive and ultimately fatal. The reactivation of ReA was possibly triggered by an oral polio vaccine. The cause of death was severe secondary amyloidosis." Yli-Kerttula T, Mottonen T, Toivanen A. Different course of reactive arthritis in two HLA-B27 positive brothers with fatal outcome in one. *J Rheumatol.* 1997 Oct;24(10):2047-50

increased risk of trauma, violent death, poisonings, and alcohol misuse.[6,7,8] Not surprisingly, the risk of pulmonary, renal, neurologic, ocular and cardiac complications is increased in patients with long-standing and severe disease.

Differentiating Characteristics of the Spondyloarthropathies

Condition	Etiological distinctions	Unique presentation	Specific emphasis
Ankylosing spondylitis	• *Allopathic*: idiopathic • *Integrative*: dysbiosis is paramount	• Insidious onset of low-back pain in young patient • Ankylosis begins in lumbopelvis and can progress to thorax, neck, hips and knees. • 90% positive HLA-B27	• *Allopathic*: anti-inflammatory drugs • *Integrative*: Antidysbiosis and orthoendocrinology are treatment cornerstones
Reactive arthritis (previously Reiter's syndrome[9])	• *Allopathic*: infection-triggered arthritis • *Integrative*: infection-triggered arthritis in a patient with dietary and endocrinologic predispositions.	• Classically associated with a recent infection, particularly a genitourinary infection or gastrointestinal infection. • Inflammation is characteristically located at the low-back, iris, and heels. • 75% positive HLA-B27	• Antimicrobial treatment for acute and chronic infections is the mainstay of treatment although in a large percentage of patients the arthropathy continues despite apparent clearance of the primary infection.
Enteropathic spondylo-arthropathy, enteropathic arthritis	• *Allopathic*: idiopathic • *Integrative*: dysbiosis-triggered arthritis in a patient with dietary and endocrinologic predispositions	• Arthropathy of the peripheral joints and/or spine in a patient with inflammatory bowel disease—Crohn's disease or ulcerative colitis • 50% positive HLA-B27	• *Allopathic*: anti-inflammatory drugs • *Integrative*: Antidysbiosis and orthoendocrinology are treatment cornerstones • Treatment is similar to other treatments except with a greater focus on addressing the intestinal lesions
Juvenile spondylo-arthropathy	• *Allopathic*: idiopathic • *Integrative*: dysbiosis[10]	• Generally occurs in boys aged 8-18 years • Peripheral arthritis (90%) is more common than spondylitis (50%)	• *Allopathic*: anti-inflammatory drugs • *Integrative*: Antidysbiosis
Psoriatic arthritis (See Chapter 9 on psoriasis)	• *Allopathic*: idiopathic • *Integrative*: Food allergies and dysbiosis are paramount	• Arthropathy of the peripheral joints and/or spine in a patient with psoriasis • 50% positive HLA-B27	• *Allopathic*: anti-inflammatory drugs • *Integrative*: Antidysbiosis and orthoendocrinology are treatment cornerstones
Rheumatoid arthritis	• *Allopathic*: idiopathic • *Integrative*: dysbiosis-triggered arthritis in a patient with dietary and endocrinologic predisposition	• Inflammatory peripheral arthropathy generally precedes axial joints • Sacroiliac joints are generally spared • RF is frequently positive	• *Allopathic*: anti-inflammatory drugs • *Integrative*: Antidysbiosis and orthoendocrinology are treatment cornerstones

[6] "A marked sex-associated effect was noted among deaths caused by injuries/poisoning, since 6 of the deaths occurred in men and only 1 was in a woman. CONCLUSION: Patients with PsA are at an increased risk of death compared with the general population." Gladman DD, Farewell VT, Wong K, Husted J.Mortality studies in psoriatic arthritis: results from a single outpatient center. II. Prognostic indicators for death. *Arthritis Rheum.* 1998 Jun;41(6):1103-10

[7] "The 4 leading causes of death were diseases of the circulatory (36.2%) or respiratory (21.3%) system, malignant neoplasms (17.0%), and injuries/poisoning (14.9%). The SMR for the female cohort was 1.59, and for the men, it was 1.65, indicating a 59% and 65% increase in the death rate, respectively. Deaths due to respiratory causes were particularly increased in these patients." Wong K, Gladman DD, Husted J, Long JA, Farewell VT. Mortality studies in psoriatic arthritis: results from a single outpatient clinic. I. Causes and risk of death. *Arthritis Rheum.* 1997 Oct;40(10):1868-72

[8] "Subjects with ankylosing spondylitis (AS) have an increased incidence of deaths from accidents and violence, which is due in part, but perhaps not entirely, to the vulnerability of the affected spine to fractures… Uncontrolled use of alcohol is an important determinant in the surplus of deaths from accidents and violence in Finnish patients with AS." Myllykangas-Luosujarvi R, Aho K, Lehtinen K, Kautiainen H, Hakala M. Increased incidence of alcohol-related deaths from accidents and violence in subjects with ankylosing spondylitis. *Br J Rheumatol.* 1998 Jun;37(6):688-90 http://rheumatology.oxfordjournals.org/cgi/reprint/37/6/688

[9] The term "Reiter's syndrome" has fallen out of favor due to the increasing acknowledgement that Dr Hans Reiter was affiliated with Nazi atrocities during World War II. See the following for additional information: "During World War II, Reiter, a physician leader of the Nazi party, authorized medical experiments on concentration camp prisoners." Lu DW, Katz KA. Declining use of the eponym "Reiter's syndrome" in the medical literature, 1998-2003. *J Am Acad Dermatol.* 2005 Oct;53(4):720-3 and "There is more than ample evidence that Hans Reiter, whose name has been eponymously linked to a rheumatologic syndrome, was a Nazi war criminal. He was responsible for heinous atrocities that violated the precepts of humanity, ethics, and professionalism." Panush RS, Paraschiv D, Dorff RE. The tainted legacy of Hans Reiter. *Semin Arthritis Rheum.* 2003 Feb;32(4):231-6

[10] "Our findings provide clear evidence of ReA diagnosis following an acute M. pneumoniae infection in that in four patients progressed to chronic jSpA. Our results suggest that detecting M. pneumoniae-specific antibodies in serological screening of jSpA patients might be useful." Harjacek M, Ostojic J, Djakovic Rode O. Juvenile spondyloarthropathies associated with Mycoplasma pneumoniae infection. *Clin Rheumatol.* 2006 Jan 4;:1-6

Clinical presentations:

- Musculoskeletal:
  - Pain and limited motion in the low-back sacroiliac joints: This is an aspect of all of the spondyloarthropathies, especially AS and ReA. Back pain is generally worse in the morning and alleviated by motion, including passive motion such as spinal manipulation.
  - Thoracic spine pain and decreased rib expansion/excursion: Although it typically begins in the lumbar spine and sacroiliac joints, AS commonly progresses to involve the thoracic spine and rib cage. Decreased mobility of the ribs limit respiration, and thus respirometry is used in the clinical assessment of patients with AS.
  - Neck pain: particularly common in RA and AS, two conditions associated with spontaneous atlantoaxial instability
  - Atlantoaxial instability: May be the presenting manifestation of AS[11] and is a common long-term complication of RA. Particularly in patients with neck pain and/or long-standing inflammation, cervical radiographs including APOM and measurement of the atlantodental interval should be performed before the clinical use of forceful cervical spine manipulation as well as esophageal/tracheal endoscopy.
  - Enthesopathies: Inflammation at the site of ligament insertion into bone—classically seen at the insertion of the Achilles' tendon at the calcaneus—is a characteristic finding and complaint in patients with ReA.
  - Non-erosive asymmetrical peripheral arthritis: 50% of patients with AS experience a temporary peripheral arthritis, while in 25% of patients the peripheral arthritis is permanent.
- Pulmonary: Pleurisy (painful inflammation of the pleural lining of the internal thoracic cavity) may be a complication of nearly all rheumatic/inflammatory disorders. Patients with AS may develop pulmonary fibrosis.
- Cardiac: "Spondylitic heart disease" is seen in patients with AS and commonly includes atrioventricular conduction defects and aortic regurgitation.[12]
- GI tract: oral ulcers, intestinal inflammation, increased intestinal permeability
- Skin/mucosal lesions: Dermal lesions are particularly common in patients with ReA and PsA. Psoriatic lesions are typically well-demarcated erythematous patches with white/silvery scales. Dermal lesions of ReA can include pustular lesions on the feet and hands (palmoplantar pustulosis) in addition to genital lesions in patients with sexually transmitted diseases.
- Renal complications: These can be seen in nearly all rheumatic disorders, either as a result of the systemic inflammation (particularly immune complexes), amyloidosis, or as a result of NSAIDs or other pharmaceutical drugs.
- Neurological complications: Cerebral necrosis, corticosteroid psychosis, and transverse myelitis may occur. Atlantoaxial subluxation can present with myelopathic signs.
- Ocular complications: Anterior uveitis is seen in ~25% of patients with AS and is a characteristic finding in patients with ReA.

---

[11] Thompson GH, Khan MA, Bilenker RM. Spontaneous atlantoaxial subluxation as a presenting manifestation of juvenile ankylosing spondylitis. A case report. *Spine* 1982 Jan-Feb;7(1):78-9
[12] Tierney ML. McPhee SJ, Papadakis MA (eds). Current Medical Diagnosis and Treatment 2006. 45th edition. New York; Lange Medical Books: 2006, pages 851-855

Low Back Pain: Differential Diagnostic Considerations

	DDX Category	Examples:
V	Vascular	Aortic aneurysm
	Visceral referral	Pancreatic disease/cancer
I	Infectious	Ankylosing spondylitis, Reiter's syndrome
	Inflammatory	Rheumatoid arthritis
	Immunologic	Psoriatic arthritis
		Enteropathic spondyloarthropathy
		Lymphoma, leukemia
		Bone/ tissue infections
		Gastrointestinal disease
		Kidney infection
		Psoriatic arthritis
		Herpes zoster
N	Neurologic	Metastatic disease
	Nutritional	Primary bone tumors
	New growth: neoplasia or	Multiple myeloma
	pregnancy	Herpes zoster
		Cauda equina syndrome
D	Deficiency	Degenerative joint/spine disease
	Degenerative	Congenital malformations of bones/ viscera
	Developmental	Scoliosis
		Postural syndromes
		Disc herniation
		Varicose veins in the leg mimicking sciatica
I	Iatrogenic (drug related)	Anticoagulants predispose to epidural or spinal cord bleeding[13]
	Intoxication	Prednisone use promotes osteoporosis and spinal fractures
	Idiosyncratic	Excess alcohol consumption[14]
C	Congenital	Congenital malformations of bones: hemivertebrae, leg length inequality, etc.
A	Allergy	Ankylosing spondylitis
	Autoimmune	Fractures, injuries
	Abuse	
T	Trauma	Fractures: injuries to vertebrae, ribs, muscles
E	Endocrine	Diabetes mellitus
	Exposure	
S	Subluxation	Segmental dysfunction of lumbar spine and pelvis
	Structural	Muscle tension
	Stress	
	Secondary gain	
M	Mental	Anxiety
	Malpractice	Depression
	Mental disorder	Endometriosis, hematocolpos[15]
	Malignancy	Ovarian tumor
	Metabolic disease	Nephrolithiasis
	Menstrual	Metastasis to spine
	Myofascial	Myofascial trigger points in quadratus lumborum, piriformis, iliacus, psoas

---

[13] Souza TA. Differential Diagnosis for the Chiropractor: Protocols and Algorithms. Gaithersburg: Aspen Publications. 1997 page 110
[14] "Alcohol abuse was significantly more frequent among the male low back patients." Sandstrom J, Andersson GB, Wallerstedt S. The role of alcohol abuse in working disability in patients with low back pain. *Scand J Rehabil Med.* 1984;16(4):147-9
[15] London NJ, Sefton GK. Hematocolpos. An unusual cause of sciatica in an adolescent girl. *Spine.* 1996 Jun 1;21(11):1381-2

Algorithm for the Assessment and Management of Low Back Complaints

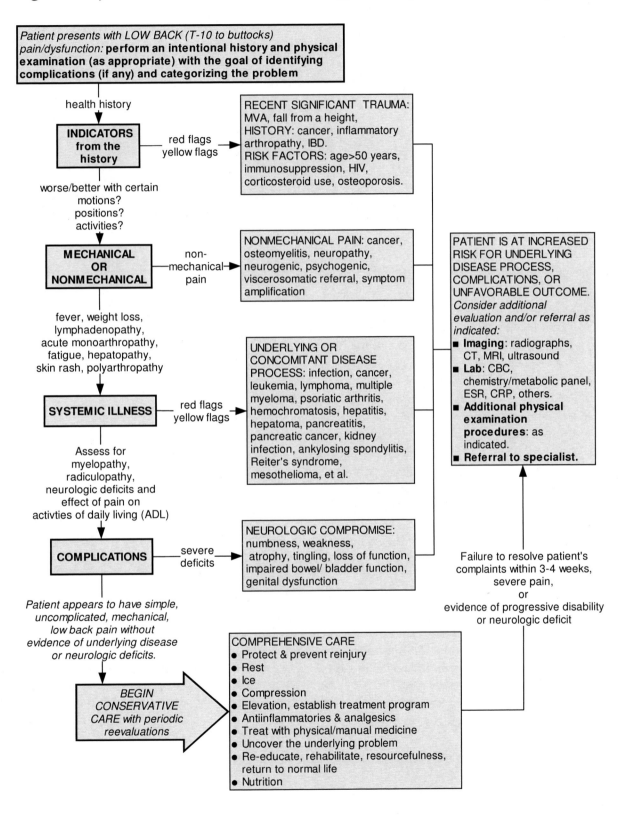

High-Risk Pain Patients

When a patient has musculoskeletal pain and any of the following characteristics, radiographs should be considered as an appropriate component of comprehensive evaluation. These considerations are particularly—though not exclusively—relevant for spine and low back pain.[16]

1. **More than 50 years of age**
2. **Physical trauma** (accident, fall, etc.)
3. **Pain at night**
4. **Back pain not relieved by lying supine**
5. **Neurologic deficits** (motor or sensory)
6. **Unexplained weight loss**
7. **Documentation or suspicion of inflammatory arthropathy**[17]
    - **Ankylosing spondylitis**
    - **Lupus**
    - **Rheumatoid arthritis**
    - **Juvenile rheumatoid arthritis**
    - **Psoriatic arthritis**
8. **Drug or alcohol abuse** (increased risk of infection, nutritional deficiencies, anesthesia)
9. **History of cancer**
10. **Intravenous drug use**
11. **Immunosuppression, due to illness (e.g., HIV) or medications (e.g., steroids or cyclosporine)**
12. **History of corticosteroid use** (causes osteoporosis and increased risk for infection)
13. **Fever above 100° F or suspicion of septic arthritis or osteomyelitis**
14. **Diabetes** (increased risk of infection, nutritional deficiencies, anesthesia)
15. **Hypertension** (abdominal aneurysm: low back pain, nausea, pulsatile abdominal mass)
16. **Recent visit for same problem and not improved**
17. **Patient seeking compensation for pain/ injury** (increased need for documentation)
18. **Skin lesion** (psoriasis, melanoma, dermatomyositis, the butterfly rash of lupus, scars from previous surgery, accident, etc.…)
19. **Deformity or immobility**
20. **Lymphadenopathy** (suggests cancer or infection)
21. **Elevated ESR/CRP** (cancer, infection, inflammatory disorder)
22. **Elevated WBC count**
23. **Elevated alkaline phosphatase** (bone lesions, metabolic bone disease, hepatopathy)
24. **Elevated acid phosphatase** (occasionally used to monitor prostate cancer)
25. **Positive rheumatoid factor and/or CCP—cyclic citrullinated protein antibodies**
26. **Positive HLA-B27** (propensity for inflammatory arthropathies)
27. **Serum gammopathy** (multiple myeloma is the most common primary bone tumor)
28. **High-risk for disease:** *examples:*
    - Long-term heavy smoking of cigarettes
    - Long-term exposure to radiation
    - Obesity
29. **Strong family history of inflammatory, musculoskeletal, or malignant disease**

> Strongly consider the possibility of **osteoporotic fracture** in any patient—regardless of age or gender—who presents with spinal pain following multi-year use of **corticosteroids/prednisone** as treatment for a chronic inflammatory disorder.
>
> This applies both to *new patients with a previous history of long-term* pain as well as *long-term patients with new pain.*
>
> This continues to apply to patients for months and a few years after they have stopped multi-year use of **corticosteroids/prednisone.**

---

[16] Remember that metastasis often travel first from the primary site to bone, therefore bone pain may be an early manifestation of occult cancer. Most of the above are from "Table 1: The high-risk patient: clinical indications for radiography in low back pain patients." J Taylor, DC, DACBR, D Resnick, MD. Imaging decisions in the management of low back pain. Advances in Chiropractic. Mosby Year Book. 1994; 1-28

[17] Radiographs are often essential for diagnosis or to rule out complications of the disease. For example, in patients with inflammatory arthropathies such as these, spontaneous rupture of the transverse ligament (at the odontoid process) has been reported; although rare, this complication could be life-threatening if mismanaged or undiagnosed.

Major differential diagnoses:

- Initial evaluation of patients with spondyloarthropathy must include consideration of numerous differential diagnoses which may mimic or co-exist with inflammatory spondyloarthropathy. See table of *Differential Diagnoses* at the end of this chapter, as well as *algorithm for patient assessment and management*. Useful categories during the evaluation of low-back pain include the following:

    1. <u>Serious organic diseases requiring immediate attention</u>: Metastatic disease, viscerosomatic referral, osteomyelitis/discitis, aortic aneurysm.

    2. <u>Serious musculoskeletal disorders requiring immediate attention</u>: Recent fracture (pathologic fracture, osteoporosis, compression fracture, fall from a height, major motor vehicle accident), cauda equina syndrome, and severe radiculopathy (i.e., severe pain or progressive muscular deficits).

    3. <u>Rheumatologic disorders affecting the low back and pelvis</u>: Ankylosing spondylitis, reactive arthritis, enteropathic spondyloarthropathy, psoriatic arthritis, rheumatoid arthritis, and fibromyalgia.

    4. <u>Psychogenic</u>: Emotional overlay, symptom amplification, secondary gain, depression.

    5. <u>Benign musculoskeletal disorders requiring conservative treatment and monitoring</u>: Muscle spasm, facet irritation, disc injuries causing radiculitis or radiculopathy, self-limiting inflammation due to injury.

    6. <u>Functional, metabolic, allergic or nutritional causes of low-back pain</u>: Food allergies, obesity leading to a systemic inflammatory state as well as biomechanical stress on the lumbar spine, vitamin D deficiency[18], acidifying diet[19] (i.e., the Standard American Diet[20,21]).

<u>Specific differential diagnoses</u>

- <u>Mechanical low back pain</u>
- <u>Traumatic low back pain, spinal strain/sprain</u>
- <u>Cauda equina syndrome</u>
- <u>Vitamin D deficiency</u>: Vitamin D deficiency causes inflammation and low-back pain. Measure 25(OH)vitamin D in serum or supplement with 4,000-10,000 IU daily for at least three months[22] unless contraindicated by drugs (e.g., hydrochlorothiazide) or hypercalcemic condition (e.g., sarcoidosis, cancer, or hyperparathyroidism, etc.).[23]
- <u>Spinal degeneration, degenerative arthritis of the spine</u>
- <u>Spinal fracture</u>: Patients with AS may experience fracture following trivial "injury" such as rolling over in bed: "Fracture should be suspected when ever a patient complains of new back pain."[24]
- <u>Osteitis condensans ilii</u>
- <u>Cancer, malignant disease</u>
- <u>Vertebral osteomyelitis, infectious discitis</u>
- <u>Muscle spasm</u>
- <u>Developmental/congenital sacralization of the lumbar vertebrae</u>
- <u>Other autoimmune disease</u>
- <u>Lung disease</u>: asthma, COPD, bronchitis, tuberculosis
- <u>Iron overload</u>: Hemochromatosis may resemble ankylosing spondylitis clinically and radiographically.[25]
- <u>Fibromyalgia</u>: ESR, CRP, thyroid tests, ANA and most other 'basic' tests are normal; assess and treat for bacterial overgrowth of the small bowel.[26]

---

[18] Al Faraj S, Al Mutairi K. Vitamin D deficiency and chronic low back pain in Saudi Arabia. *Spine*. 2003 Jan 15;28(2):177-9

[19] "The results show that a disturbed acid-base balance may contribute to the symptoms of low back pain. The simple and safe addition of an alkaline multimineral preparate was able to reduce the pain symptoms in these patients with chronic low back pain." Vormann J,Worlitschek M,Goedecke T,Silver B. Supplementation with alkaline minerals reduces symptoms in patients with chronic low back pain. *J Trace Elem Med Biol.* 2001;15(2-3):179-83

[20] Seaman DR. The diet-induced proinflammatory state: a cause of chronic pain and other degenerative diseases? *J Manipulative Physiol Ther.* 2002 Mar-Apr;25(3):168-79

[21] Cordain L: *The Paleo Diet*. John Wiley & Sons Inc., New York 2002

[22] Al Faraj S, Al Mutairi K. Vitamin D deficiency and chronic low back pain in Saudi Arabia. *Spine*. 2003 Jan 15;28(2):177-9

[23] Vasquez A, Manso G, Cannell J. The clinical importance of vitamin D (cholecalciferol): a paradigm shift with implications for all healthcare providers. *Altern Ther Health Med.* 2004 Sep-Oct;10(5):28-36 http://optimalhealthresearch.com/monograph04

[24] Harley JB, Scofield RH. The spectrum of ankylosing spondylitis. *Hosp Pract (Off Ed)* 1995 Jul 15;30(7):37-43, 46

[25] Bywaters EGL, Hamilton EBD, Williams R. The spine in idiopathic hemochromatosis. *Ann Rheum Dis* 1971; 30: 453-65

[26] Pimentel M, et al. A link between irritable bowel syndrome and fibromyalgia may be related to findings on lactulose breath testing. *Ann Rheum Dis.* 2004 Apr;63(4):450-2

- Diffuse idiopathic skeletal hyperostosis (DISH): DISH generally affects the longitudinal ligaments of the spine rather than the intervertebral discs. Cervical involvement generally precedes that of the lumbar spine, and the condition is strongly associated with diabetes mellitus.

Clinical assessments:
- History/subjective: See clinical presentations
  - **Typical presentation is that of dull achy pain in the low-back—worse in the morning and improving as the day progresses and/or with activity.**
  - **Systemic manifestations may or may not be present in the early stages of disease.**
- Physical examination/objective:
  - ROM, neurologic assessments; orthopedic assessments
  - Specialty examinations may be indicated:
    - Eye exam: for retinal and anterior chamber abnormalities; external exam for scleritis
    - Genital examination and/or assessment for UTI and STDs: Indicated in patients with ReA due to high association with sexually transmitted diseases. Urethral swab for culture and DNA probes are commonly indicated.
    - Cardiopulmonary assessment: common considerations include auscultation, measurement of thoracic excursion, and spirometry. Chest radiographs may be indicated.
    - Neurologic examination: A screening neurologic examination should be performed as part of the initial assessment of all patients and more detailed examinations are carried out when indicated.
    - Schober test: Draw a line over the spinous process of L5, then mark a line 10 cm above and 5 cm below; with lumbar flexion, the total distance should increase from 15 cm to 20 cm—less than 5 cm excursion indicates spinal rigidity, consistent with AS.
    - Occiput-to-wall distance: This assessment can be used to quantify progression/regression of cervical flexion in patients with AS.
    - Chest expansion: Use tape measure around lower thorax; measure chest circumference before and after inhalation; use along with spirometry to monitor thoracic stiffness in patients with AS.
- Laboratory assessments:
  - ESR or CRP: These are generally elevated, and neither test is superior to the other in the assessment of patients with AS. One study[27] used a unique approach to differentiate active disease from inactive disease in patients with AS; they added the ESR value (measured in mm/h) and CRP value (measured in mg/L) and classified patients as having active inflammatory disease if the total was greater than thirty (30).
  - Rheumatoid factor (RF): Characteristically **negative** *by definition* in patients with sero**negative** spondyloarthropathies. Positivity suggests rheumatoid spondylitis or concomitant RA with another spondyloarthropathy.
  - CBC: Look for evidence of true *infection* (in contrast to *dysbiosis*); also assess for anemia, which may be secondary to renal failure, NSAID gastropathy, chronic inflammation, or nutritional inadequacy.
  - Comprehensive metabolic panel: Assess as indicated for complications and concomitant disease.
  - Comprehensive stool analysis with comprehensive parasitology: **All patients with AS, RA, and PsA have gastrointestinal dysbiosis until proven otherwise.** Use of comprehensive stool tests should be the standard of care for all patients with AS, RA, PsA, and of course those with enteropathic spondyloarthropathy. Patients with ReA due to gastroenteritis or those whose primary infection has not been identified/eliminated are also obvious candidates for stool testing; the most commonly implicated microbes are *Salmonella, Shigella,* and *Yersinia.* Regarding the etiopathogenesis of AS, the most commonly implicated microbes are *Klebsiella*

---

[27] Maki-Ikola O, Lehtinen K, Nissila M, Granfors K. IgM, IgA and IgG class serum antibodies against Klebsiella pneumoniae and Escherichia coli lipopolysaccharides in patients with ankylosing spondylitis. *Br J Rheumatol* 1994 Nov;33(11):1025-9

and *E. coli*. However, it is more accurate to see that microbes incite autoimmunity/inflammation by numerous mechanisms and that exposure to numerous microbes—each one of which *in isolation* may be innocuous—in combination leads to additive and synergistic proinflammatory effects, as reviewed in Chapter 4 in the section on multifocal dysbiosis and elsewhere in a recent publication by the current author.[28]

o <u>Serologic and genital tests for sexually transmitted diseases</u>: These tests are particularly indicated in patients with ReA due to the frequent association of this disorder with genitourinary infections, particularly those caused by *Chlamydia*. Numerous articles have shown that patients with long-term idiopathic oligoarthritis harbor "silent infections"—otherwise known as dysbiosis—in the genitourinary and gastrointestinal tracts; the most commonly identified organisms are *Chlamydia trachomatis*, yersinia, salmonella, *Mycoplasma*, and *Ureaplasma*.[29,30]

o <u>Serum vitamin D</u>: Measure 25(OH)vitamin D in all patients and/or begin empiric treatment with physiologic doses of vitamin D3. Emulsified cholecalciferol is particularly efficacious in older patients and those with malabsorption due to enteropathy.[31] According to research by Falkenbach et al[32], **"Patients with ankylosing spondylitis may have extremely low levels of 25(OH)D."** Vitamin D deficiency appears common in patients with low-back pain[33], limb pain[34], chronic persistent musculoskeletal pain[35], and in general medical patients.[36] [37] In our review of the literature[38], we concluded that **optimal serum 25(OH)-vitamin D levels should be defined as 40 – 65 ng/mL (100 - 160 nmol/L)** and that, "Until proven otherwise, the balance of the research clearly indicates that oral supplementation in the range of 1,000 IU per day for infants, 2,000 IU per day for children and **4,000 IU per day for adults** is safe and reasonable to meet physiologic requirements, to promote optimal health, and to reduce the risk of several serious diseases. Safety and effectiveness of supplementation are assured by periodic monitoring of serum 25(OH)D and serum calcium." For additional research on the importance and safety of vitamin D, see the articles by Vieth[39], Heaney et al[40], Holick[41], and Vasquez, Manso, and Cannell.[42] Vitamin D supplementation

Microorganisms clinically or molecularly associated with induction of seronegative spondyloarthropathy, ankylosing spondylitis, and reactive arthritis
• *Campylobacter* spp
• *Chlamydia trachomatis*
• *Citrobacter freundii*
• *E. coli*
• *Giardia lamblia*
• *Helicobacter pylori*
• *Klebsiella pneumoniae*
• *Mycoplasma* spp
• *Proteus mirabilis*
• *Salmonella typhimurium*
• *Shigella flexneri*
• *Shigella sonnei*
• *Staphylococcus aureus*
• *Streptococcus pyogenes*
• *Ureaplasma* spp
• *Yersinia enterocolitica*

[28] Vasquez A. Reducing Pain and Inflammation Naturally. Part 6: Nutritional and Botanical Treatments Against "Silent Infections" and Gastrointestinal Dysbiosis, Commonly Overlooked Causes of Neuromusculoskeletal Inflammation and Chronic Health Problems. *Nutritional Perspectives* 2006; January http://optimalhealthresearch.com/part6

[29] "Urogenital swab cultures showed a microbial infection in 44% of the patients with oligoarthritis (15% Chlamydia, 14% Mycoplasma, 28% Ureaplasma), whereas in the control group only 26% had a positive result (4% Chlamydia, 7% Mycoplasma, 21% Ureaplasma)." Erlacher L, Wintersberger W, Menschik M, Benke-Studnicka A, Machold K, Stanek G, Soltz-Szots J, Smolen J, Graninger W. Reactive arthritis: urogenital swab culture is the only useful diagnostic method for the detection of the arthritogenic infection in extra-articularly asymptomatic patients with undifferentiated oligoarthritis. *Br J Rheumatol.* 1995 Sep;34(9):838-42

[30] Fendler C, Laitko S, Sorensen H, Gripenberg-Lerche C, Groh A, Uksila J, Granfors K, Braun J, Sieper J. Frequency of triggering bacteria in patients with reactive arthritis and undifferentiated oligoarthritis and the relative importance of the tests used for diagnosis. *Ann Rheum Dis.* 2001 Apr;60(4):337-43 http://ard.bmjjournals.com/cgi/content/full/60/4/337

[31] Vasquez A. Subphysiologic Doses of Vitamin D are Subtherapeutic: Comment on the Study by The Record Trial Group. *The Lancet* Published on-line May 6, 2005 http://optimalhealthresearch.com/reprints/Vasquez-Lancet-refined.pdf

[32] "Patients with ankylosing spondylitis may have extremely low levels of 25(OH)D." Falkenbach A, Tripathi R, Sedlmeyer A, Staudinger M, Herold M. Serum 25-hydroxyvitamin D and parathyroid hormone in patients with ankylosing spondylitis before and after a three-week rehabilitation treatment at high altitude during winter and spring. *Wien Klin Wochenschr.* 2001 Apr 30;113(9):328-32

[33] Al Faraj S, Al Mutairi K. Vitamin D deficiency and chronic low back pain in Saudi Arabia. *Spine.* 2003 Jan 15;28(2):177-9

[34] Masood H, Narang AP, Bhat IA, Shah GN. Persistent limb pain and raised serum alkaline phosphatase the earliest markers of subclinical hypovitaminosis D in Kashmir. *Indian J Physiol Pharmacol.* 1989 Oct-Dec;33(4):259-61

[35] Plotnikoff GA, Quigley JM. Prevalence of severe hypovitaminosis D in patients with persistent, nonspecific musculoskeletal pain. *Mayo Clin Proc.* 2003 Dec;78(12):1463-70

[36] Thomas MK, Lloyd-Jones DM, Thadhani RI, Shaw AC, Deraska DJ, Kitch BT, Vamvakas EC, Dick IM, Prince RL, Finkelstein JS. Hypovitaminosis D in medical inpatients. *N Engl J Med.* 1998 Mar 19;338(12):777-83

[37] Kauppinen-Makelin R, Tahtela R, Loyttyniemi E, Karkkainen J, Valimaki MJ. A high prevalence of hypovitaminosis D in Finnish medical in- and outpatients. *J Intern Med.* 2001 Jun;249(6):559-63

[38] Vasquez A, Manso G, Cannell J. The Clinical Importance of Vitamin D (Cholecalciferol): A Paradigm Shift with Implications for All Healthcare Providers. *Alternative Therapies in Health and Medicine* and *Integrative Medicine: A Clinician's Journal* In press: See www.optimalhealthresearch.com/monograph04

[39] Vieth R. Vitamin D supplementation, 25-hydroxyvitamin D concentrations, and safety. *Am J Clin Nutr.* 1999 May;69(5):842-56

[40] Heaney RP, Davies KM, Chen TC, Holick MF, Barger-Lux MJ. Human serum 25-hydroxycholecalciferol response to extended oral dosing with cholecalciferol. *Am J Clin Nutr.* 2003 Jan;77(1):204-10

[41] Holick MF. Vitamin D: importance in the prevention of cancers, type 1 diabetes, heart disease, and osteoporosis. *Am J Clin Nutr.* 2004 Mar;79(3):362-71

[42] Vasquez A, Manso G, Cannell J. The Clinical Importance of Vitamin D (Cholecalciferol): A Paradigm Shift with Implications for All Healthcare Providers. *Alternative Therapies in Health and Medicine* and *Integrative Medicine: A Clinician's Journal* In press: See www.optimalhealthresearch.com/monograph04

5,000 – 10,000 IU per day for adults was shown to alleviate low-back pain after 3 months in nearly all patients with low initial serum levels of vitamin D.[43]

- o Testing for multifocal dysbiosis: If the intestinal and genitourinary tracts appear clear of infection following direct testing, then empiric antimicrobial treatment should be considered. Following this, searching for other loci of infection—namely the mouth, throat, nose, sinuses, lungs, and skin—should be pursued as discussed in Chapter 4.
- o HLA-B27: This marker is seen with increased prevalence in patients with AS and ReA. The test can be used to support the diagnosis, particularly early in the course of the illness when radiographs are *negative*.
- o Hormone assessments: These should be performed as detailed in Chapter 4 and/or as indicated per patient.
- **Imaging**:
  - o Plain radiographs: In contrast to most of the other rheumatic disorders wherein radiographs are generally unnecessary in early stages of the disease, plain radiographs are of tremendous value in the assessment of spondylitis and sacroiliitis and are generally diagnostic once the diagnostic threshold has been crossed; i.e., they may be negative in early disease, but become positive after a given amount of time, which varies per patient and per disease. Characteristic initial findings in AS are lumbar syndesmophytes and sacroiliitis.
  - o MRI and CT imaging: Generally reserved for the evaluation of spinal stenosis and inflammatory myelopathy. **CT imaging is more sensitive than plain radiography for the initial evaluation of sacroiliitis.**[44] Also used for assessment of other complications as indicated.
- **Establishing the diagnosis**:
  - o Inflammatory spondyloarthropathy as a general term can be diagnosed with a combination of serologic, clinical, and radiographic findings. The subtype of spondyloarthropathy—AS, ReA, PsA, RA, ES, etc—is then distinguished based on the details of the clinical history (e.g., inflammatory bowel disease or recent infection), presentation, clinical findings, serologic tests, and radiographic characteristics.

Complications:

- Chronic pain, significant physical limitations and significant morbidity
- Renal failure, secondary to amyloidosis or medications such as sulfasalazine or NSAID's
- Spinal fracture (in patients with spinal ankylosis following minor trauma)
- Respiratory insufficiency
- Immobility
- Permanent disability due to rigid spinal flexion secondary to bony ankylosis resulting in loss of spinal motion
- Neurologic compromise: due to spinal stenosis, transverse myelopathy, atlantoaxial subluxation, cauda equina fibrosis[45], or cauda equina syndrome

Clinical management:

- Referral if clinical outcome is unsatisfactory or as otherwise indicated.

Treatments:

> *Drug treatments*[46]
> - NSAIDs, especially indomethacin 25-50 mg thrice daily—"side effects" of indomethacin include headache, giddiness, psychosis, depression, nausea, vomiting, gastric ulcer, and renal impairment. Sulfasalazine: 1,000 mg twice daily.
> - Corticosteroids are notably ineffective in the treatment of spondyloarthropathy, though they are commonly used against complications such as uveitis.

---

[43] Al Faraj S, Al Mutairi K. Vitamin D deficiency and chronic low back pain in Saudi Arabia. *Spine*. 2003 Jan 15;28(2):177-9
[44] Tierney ML. McPhee SJ, Papadakis MA. Current Medical Diagnosis and Treatment 2006. 45th edition. New York; Lange Medical Books: 2006, pages 851-855
[45] Tierney ML. McPhee SJ, Papadakis MA. Current Medical Diagnosis and Treatment 2006. 45th edition. New York; Lange Medical Books: 2006, page 852
[46] Tierney ML. McPhee SJ, Papadakis MA. Current Medical Diagnosis and Treatment 2006. 45th edition. New York; Lange Medical Books: 2006, pages 851-855

- **TNF inhibitors:** <u>Etanercept</u> 25 mg subcutaneously twice weekly, or <u>infliximab</u> 5 mg/kg every other month. These drugs are clinically effective from the perspective of anti-inflammation, but they are associated with increased risks for lymphoma, serious infections including pulmonary tuberculosis, congestive heart failure, demyelinating diseases, and systemic lupus erythematosus.
- <u>Methotrexate</u>: Used for recalcitrant psoriatic arthritis.[47]

- <u>Avoidance of pro-inflammatory foods</u>: Pro-inflammatory foods act *directly* and *indirectly* to promote and exacerbate systemic inflammation. *Direct* mechanisms include the activation of Toll-like receptors and NF-kappaB, while *indirect* mechanisms include depleting the body of anti-inflammatory nutrients and dietary displacement of more nutrient-dense anti-inflammatory foods. Arachidonic acid (found in cow's milk, beef, liver, pork, and lamb) is the direct precursor to pro-inflammatory prostaglandins and leukotrienes[48] and pain-promoting isoprostanes.[49] Saturated fats promote inflammation by activating/enabling pro-inflammatory Toll-like receptors, which are otherwise "specific" for inducing pro-inflammatory responses to microorganisms.[50] Consumption of saturated fat in the form of cream creates marked oxidative stress and lipid peroxidation that lasts for at least 3 hours postprandially.[51] Corn oil rapidly activates NF-kappaB (in hepatic Kupffer cells) for a pro-inflammatory effect[52]; similarly, consumption of PUFA and linoleic acid promotes antioxidant depletion and may thus promote oxidation-mediated inflammation via activation of NF-kappaB. Linoleic acid causes intracellular oxidative stress and calcium influx and results in increased NF-kappaB-stimulated transcription of pro-inflammatory genes.[53] High glycemic foods cause oxidative stress[54,55] and inflammation via activation of NF-kappaB and other mechanisms—e.g., *white bread causes inflammation*[56] as does *a high-fat high-carbohydrate fast-food-style breakfast*.[57] High glycemic foods suppress immune function[58,59] and thus promote the perpetuation of infection/dysbiosis. Delivery of a high carbohydrate load to the gastrointestinal lumen promotes bacterial overgrowth[60,61], which is inherently pro-inflammatory[62,63] and which appears to be myalgenic in humans[64] at least in part due to the ability of endotoxin to impair muscle function.[65] Overconsumption of high-carbohydrate low-phytonutrient grains, potatoes, and manufactured foods displaces phytonutrient-dense foods such as

[47] Tierney ML. McPhee SJ, Papadakis MA. <u>Current Medical Diagnosis and Treatment 2006. 45th edition</u>. New York; Lange Medical Books: 2006, pages 851-855

[48] Vasquez A. Reducing Pain and Inflammation Naturally. Part 2: New Insights into Fatty Acid Supplementation and Its Effect on Eicosanoid Production and Genetic Expression. *Nutritional Perspectives* 2005; January: 5-16 www.optimalhealthresearch.com/part2

[49] Evans AR, Junger H, Southall MD, Nicol GD, Sorkin LS, Broome JT, Bailey TW, Vasko MR. Isoprostanes, novel eicosanoids that produce nociception and sensitize rat sensory neurons. *J Pharmacol Exp Ther*. 2000 Jun;293(3):912-20

[50] Lee JY, Sohn KH, Rhee SH, Hwang D. Saturated fatty acids, but not unsaturated fatty acids, induce the expression of cyclooxygenase-2 mediated through Toll-like receptor 4. *J Biol Chem*. 2001 May 18;276(20):16683-9. Epub 2001 Mar 2 http://www.jbc.org/cgi/content/full/276/20/16683

[51] "CONCLUSIONS: Both fat and protein intakes stimulate ROS generation. The increase in ROS generation lasted 3 h after cream intake and 1 h after protein intake. Cream intake also caused a significant and prolonged increase in lipid peroxidation." Mohanty P, Ghanim H, Hamouda W, Aljada A, Garg R, Dandona P. Both lipid and protein intakes stimulate increased generation of reactive oxygen species by polymorphonuclear leukocytes and mononuclear cells. *Am J Clin Nutr*. 2002 Apr;75(4):767-72 http://www.ajcn.org/cgi/content/full/75/4/767

[52] Rusyn I, Bradham CA, Cohn L, Schoonhoven R, Swenberg JA, Brenner DA, Thurman RG. Corn oil rapidly activates nuclear factor-kappaB in hepatic Kupffer cells by oxidant-dependent mechanisms. *Carcinogenesis*. 1999 Nov;20(11):2095-100 http://carcin.oxfordjournals.org/cgi/content/full/20/11/2095

[53] "Exposing endothelial cells to 90 micromol linoleic acid/L for 6 h resulted in a significant increase in lipid hydroperoxides that coincided wih an increase in intracellular calcium concentrations." Hennig B, Toborek M, Joshi-Barve S, Barger SW, Barve S, Mattson MP, McClain CJ. Linoleic acid activates nuclear transcription factor-kappa B (NF-kappa B) and induces NF-kappa B-dependent transcription in cultured endothelial cells. *Am J Clin Nutr*. 1996 Mar;63(3):322-8 http://www.ajcn.org/cgi/reprint/63/3/322

[54] Mohanty P, Hamouda W, Garg R, Aljada A, Ghanim H, Dandona P. Glucose challenge stimulates reactive oxygen species (ROS) generation by leucocytes. *J Clin Endocrinol Metab*. 2000 Aug;85(8):2970-3 http://jcem.endojournals.org/cgi/content/full/85/8/2970 Glucose/carbohydrate and saturated fat consumption appear to be the two biggest offenders in the food-stimulated production of oxidative stress. The effect by protein is much less. "CONCLUSIONS: Both fat and protein intakes stimulate ROS generation. The increase in ROS generation lasted 3 h after cream intake and 1 h after protein intake. Cream intake also caused a significant and prolonged increase in lipid peroxidation." Mohanty P, Ghanim H, Hamouda W, Aljada A, Garg R, Dandona P. Both lipid and protein intakes stimulate increased generation of reactive oxygen species by polymorphonuclear leukocytes and mononuclear cells. *Am J Clin Nutr*. 2002 Apr;75(4):767-72 http://www.ajcn.org/cgi/content/full/75/4/767

[55] Koska J, Blazicek P, Marko M, Grna JD, Kvetnansky R, Vigas M. Insulin, catecholamines, glucose and antioxidant enzymes in oxidative damage during different loads in healthy humans. *Physiol Res*. 2000;49 Suppl 1:S95-100 http://www.biomed.cas.cz/physiolres/pdf/2000/49_S95.pdf

[56] "Conclusion - The present study shows that high GI carbohydrate, but not low GI carbohydrate, mediates an acute proinflammatory process as measured by NF-kappaB activity." Dickinson S, Hancock DP, Petocz P, Brand-Miller JC..High glycemic index carbohydrate mediates an acute proinflammatory process as measured by NF-kappaB activation. *Asia Pac J Clin Nutr*. 2005;14 Suppl:S120

[57] Aljada A, Mohanty P, Ghanim H, Abdo T, Tripathy D, Chaudhuri A, Dandona P. Increase in intranuclear nuclear factor kappaB and decrease in inhibitor kappaB in mononuclear cells after a mixed meal: evidence for a proinflammatory effect. *Am J Clin Nutr*. 2004 Apr;79(4):682-90 http://www.ajcn.org/cgi/content/full/79/4/682

[58] Sanchez A, Reeser JL, Lau HS, et al. Role of sugars in human neutrophilic phagocytosis. *Am J Clin Nutr*. 1973 Nov;26(11):1180-4

[59] "Postoperative infusion of carbohydrate solution leads to moderate fall in the serum concentration of inorganic phosphate. ... The hypophosphatemia was associated with significant reduction of neutrophil phagocytosis, intracellular killing, consumption of oxygen and generation of superoxide during phagocytosis." Rasmussen A, Segel E, Hessov I, Borregaard N. Reduced function of neutrophils during routine postoperative glucose infusion. *Acta Chir Scand*. 1988 Jul-Aug;154(7-8):429-33

[60] Ramakrishnan T, Stokes P. Beneficial effects of fasting and low carbohydrate diet in D-lactic acidosis associated with short-bowel syndrome. *JPEN J Parenter Enteral Nutr*. 1985 May-Jun;9(3):361-3

[61] Gottschall E. <u>Breaking the Vicious Cycle: Intestinal Health Through Diet</u>. Kirkton Press; Rev edition (August 1, 1994)

[62] Lin HC. Small intestinal bacterial overgrowth: a framework for understanding irritable bowel syndrome. *JAMA*. 2004 Aug 18;292(7):852-8

[63] Lichtman SN, Wang J, Sartor RB, Zhang C, Bender D, Dalldorf FG, Schwab JH. Reactivation of arthritis induced by small bowel bacterial overgrowth in rats: role of cytokines, bacteria, and bacterial polymers. *Infect Immun*. 1995 Jun;63(6):2295-301

[64] Pimentel M, et al. A link between irritable bowel syndrome and fibromyalgia may be related to findings on lactulose breath testing. *Ann Rheum Dis*. 2004 Apr;63(4):450-2

[65] Bundgaard H, Kjeldsen K, Suarez Krabbe K, van Hall G, Simonsen L, Qvist J, Hansen CM, Moller K, Fonsmark L, Lav Madsen P, Klarlund Pedersen B. Endotoxemia stimulates skeletal muscle Na+-K+-ATPase and raises blood lactate under aerobic conditions in humans. *Am J Physiol Heart Circ Physiol*. 2003 Mar;284(3):H1028-34. Epub 2002 Nov 21 http://ajpheart.physiology.org/cgi/reprint/284/3/H1028

fruits, vegetables, nuts, seeds, and berries which contain more than 8,000 phytonutrients, many of which have antioxidant and thus anti-inflammatory actions.[66,67]

- <u>Supplemented Paleo-Mediterranean diet</u>: The health-promoting diet of choice for the majority of people is a diet based on abundant consumption of fruits, vegetables, seeds, nuts, omega-3 and monounsaturated fatty acids, and lean sources of protein such as lean meats, fatty cold-water fish, soy and whey proteins. This diet obviates overconsumption of chemical preservatives, artificial sweeteners, and carbohydrate-dominant foods such as candies, pastries, breads, potatoes, grains, and other foods with a high glycemic load and high glycemic index. This "Paleo-Mediterranean Diet" is a combination of the "Paleolithic" or "Paleo diet" and the well-known "Mediterranean diet", both of which are well described in peer-reviewed journals and the lay press. (See Chapter 2 and my other publications[68,69] for details). This diet is the most nutrient-dense diet available, and its benefits are further enhanced by supplementation with vitamins, minerals, and the health-promoting fatty acids: ALA, GLA, EPA, DHA.

- <u>Avoidance of allergenic foods</u>: Any patient may be allergic to any food, even if the food is generally considered a health-promoting food. Generally speaking, the most notorious allergens are wheat, citrus (especially juice due to the industrial use of fungal hemicellulases), cow's milk, eggs, peanuts, chocolate, and yeast-containing foods. According to a study in patients with migraine, some patients will have to avoid as many as 10 specific foods in order to become symptom-free.[70] Celiac disease can present with inflammatory oligoarthritis that resembles rheumatoid arthritis and which remits with avoidance of wheat/gluten. The inflammatory arthropathy of celiac disease has preceded bowel symptoms and/or an accurate diagnosis by as many as 3-15 years.[71,72] Clinicians must explain to their patients that celiac disease and wheat allergy are two different clinical entities and that exclusion of one does not exclude the other, and in neither case does mutual exclusion obviate the promotion of intestinal bacterial overgrowth (i.e., pro-inflammatory dysbiosis) by indigestible wheat oligosaccharides.

- <u>Gluten-free vegetarian/vegan diet</u>: Vegetarian/vegan diets have a place in the treatment plan of all patients with autoimmune/inflammatory disorders[73,74,75,76]; this is also true for patients for whom long-term exclusive reliance on a meat-free vegetarian diet is either not appropriate or not appealing. No scientist or clinician familiar with the research literature doubts the antirheumatic power and anti-inflammatory advantages of vegetarian diets, whether used short-term or long term.[77] The benefits of gluten-free vegetarian diets are well documented, and the mechanisms of action are well elucidated, including reduced intake of pro-inflammatory linoleic[78] and arachidonic acids[79], iron[80], common food

---

[66] "We propose that the additive and synergistic effects of phytochemicals in fruit and vegetables are responsible for their potent antioxidant and anticancer activities, and that the benefit of a diet rich in fruit and vegetables is attributed to the complex mixture of phytochemicals present in whole foods." Liu RH. Health benefits of fruit and vegetables are from additive and synergistic combinations of phytochemicals. *Am J Clin Nutr.* 2003 Sep;78(3 Suppl):517S-520S

[67] Seaman DR. The diet-induced proinflammatory state: a cause of chronic pain and other degenerative diseases? *J Manipulative Physiol Ther.* 2002;25(3):168-79

[68] Vasquez A. A Five-Part Nutritional Protocol that Produces Consistently Positive Results. *Nutritional Wellness* 2005 September Available in the printed version and on-line at http://www.nutritionalwellness.com/archives/2005/sep/09_vasquez.php and http://optimalhealthresearch.com/protocol

[69] Vasquez A. Implementing the Five-Part Nutritional Wellness Protocol for the Treatment of Various Health Problems. *Nutritional Wellness* 2005 November. Available on-line at http://www.nutritionalwellness.com/archives/2005/nov/11_vasquez.php and http://optimalhealthresearch.com/protocol

[70] Grant EC. Food allergies and migraine. *Lancet.* 1979 May 5;1(8123):966-9

[71] "We report six patients with coeliac disease in whom arthritis was prominent at diagnosis and who improved with dietary therapy. Joint pain preceded diagnosis by up to three years in five patients and 15 years in one patient." Bourne JT, Kumar P, Huskisson EC, Mageed R, Unsworth DJ, Wojtulewski JA. Arthritis and coeliac disease. *Ann Rheum Dis.* 1985 Sep;44(9):592-8

[72] "A 15-year-old girl, with synovitis of the knees and ankles for 3 years before a diagnosis of gluten-sensitive enteropathy, is described." Pinals RS. Arthritis associated with gluten-sensitive enteropathy. *J Rheumatol.* 1986 Feb;13(1):201-4

[73] "The immunoglobulin G (IgG) antibody levels against gliadin and beta-lactoglobulin decreased in the responder subgroup in the vegan diet-treated patients, but not in the other analysed groups." Hafstrom I, Ringertz B, Spangberg A, von Zweigbergk L, Brannemark S, Nylander I, Ronnelid J, Laasonen L, Klareskog L. A vegan diet free of gluten improves the signs and symptoms of rheumatoid arthritis: the effects on arthritis correlate with a reduction in antibodies to food antigens. *Rheumatology* (Oxford). 2001 Oct;40(10):1175-9 http://rheumatology.oxfordjournals.org/cgi/content/abstract/40/10/1175

[74] "After four weeks at the health farm the diet group showed a significant improvement in number of tender joints, Ritchie's articular index, number of swollen joints, pain score, duration of morning stiffness, grip strength, erythrocyte sedimentation rate, C-reactive protein, white blood cell count, and a health assessment questionnaire score." Kjeldsen-Kragh J, Haugen M, Borchgrevink CF, Laerum E, Eek M, Mowinkel P, Hovi K, Forre O. Controlled trial of fasting and one-year vegetarian diet in rheumatoid arthritis. *Lancet.* 1991 Oct 12;338(8772):899-902

[75] "During fasting, arthralgia was less intense in many subjects. In some types of skin diseases (pustulosis palmaris et plantaris and atopic eczema) an improvement could be demonstrated during the fast. During the vegan diet, both signs and symptoms returned in most patients, with the exception of some patients with psoriasis who experienced an improvement." Lithell H, Bruce A, Gustafsson IB, Hoglund NJ, Karlstrom B, Ljunghall K, Sjolin K, Venge P, Werner I, Vessby B. A fasting and vegetarian diet treatment trial on chronic inflammatory disorders. *Acta Derm Venereol.* 1983;63(5):397-403

[76] Tanaka T, Kouda K, Kotani M, Takeuchi A, Tabei T, Masamoto Y, Nakamura H, Takigawa M, Suemura M, Takeuchi H, Kouda M. Vegetarian diet ameliorates symptoms of atopic dermatitis through reduction of the number of peripheral eosinophils and of PGE2 synthesis by monocytes. *J Physiol Anthropol Appl Human Sci.* 2001 Nov;20(6):353-61 http://www.jstage.jst.go.jp/article/jpa/20/6/20_353/_article/-char/en

[77] "For the patients who were randomised to the vegetarian diet there was a significant decrease in platelet count, leukocyte count, calprotectin, total IgG, IgM rheumatoid factor (RF), C3-activation products, and the complement components C3 and C4 after one month of treatment." Kjeldsen-Kragh J, Mellbye OJ, Haugen M, Mollnes TE, Hammer HB, Sioud M, Forre O. Changes in laboratory variables in rheumatoid arthritis patients during a trial of fasting and one-year vegetarian diet. *Scand J Rheumatol.* 1995;24(2):85-93

[78] Rusyn I, Bradham CA, Cohn L, Schoonhoven R, Swenberg JA, Brenner DA, Thurman RG. Corn oil rapidly activates nuclear factor-kappaB in hepatic Kupffer cells by oxidant-dependent mechanisms. *Carcinogenesis.* 1999 Nov;20(11):2095-100 http://carcin.oxfordjournals.org/cgi/content/full/20/11/2095

[79] Vasquez A. Reducing Pain and Inflammation Naturally. Part 2: New Insights into Fatty Acid Supplementation and Its Effect on Eicosanoid Production and Genetic Expression. *Nutritional Perspectives* 2005; January: 5-16 http://optimalhealthresearch.com/part2

[80] Dabbagh AJ, Trenam CW, Morris CJ, Blake DR. Iron in joint inflammation. *Ann Rheum Dis.* 1993 Jan;52(1):67-73

antigens[81], gluten[82] and gliadin[83,84], pro-inflammatory sugars[85] and increased intake of omega-3 fatty acids, micronutrients[86], and anti-inflammatory and antioxidant phytonutrients.[87] Vegetarian diets also effect subtle yet biologically and clinically important changes—both *qualitative* and *quantitative*—in intestinal flora[88,89] that correlate with clinical improvement.[90]   Patients who rely on the Paleo-Mediterranean diet (which is inherently omnivorous) can use vegetarian *meals* on a daily basis or for days at a time—for example, by having a daily vegetarian meal, or one week per month of vegetarianism.   Some (not all) patients can use a purely vegetarian diet long-term provided that nutritional needs (especially protein and cobalamin) are consistently met.

- Short-term fasting: Whether the foundational diet is Paleo-Mediterranean, vegetarian, vegan, or a combination of all of these, autoimmune/inflammatory patients will still benefit from periodic fasting, whether on a weekly (e.g., every Saturday), monthly (every first week or weekend of the month, or every other month), or yearly (1-2 weeks of the year) basis.   Since consumption of food—particularly unhealthy foods—induces an inflammatory effect[91], abstinence from food provides a relative anti-inflammatory effect.   Fasting indeed provides a distinct anti-inflammatory benefit and may help "re-calibrate" metabolic and homeostatic mechanisms by breaking self-perpetuating "vicious cycles"[92] that autonomously promote inflammation independent of pro-inflammatory stimuli.   Water-only fasting is completely hypoallergenic (assuming that the patient is not sensitive to chlorine, fluoride, or other contaminants), and subsequent re-introduction of foods provides the ideal opportunity to identify offending foods.   Fasting deprives intestinal microbes of substrate[93], stimulates intestinal B-cell immunity[94], improves the bactericidal action of neutrophils[95], reduces lysozyme release and leukotriene formation[96], and ameliorates intestinal hyperpermeability.[97]   In case reports and clinical trials, short-term fasting (or protein-sparing fasting) has been documented as safe and effective treatment for SLE[98], RA[99], and non-rheumatic diseases such as chronic severe hypertension[100], moderate hypertension[101], obesity[102,103], type-2 diabetes[104], and epilepsy.[105]

---

[81] Hafstrom I, Ringertz B, Spangberg A, von Zweigbergk L, Brannemark S, Nylander I, Ronnelid J, Laasonen L, Klareskog L. A vegan diet free of gluten improves the signs and symptoms of rheumatoid arthritis: the effects on arthritis correlate with a reduction in antibodies to food antigens. *Rheumatology* (Oxford). 2001 Oct;40(10):1175-9 http://rheumatology.oxfordjournals.org/cgi/reprint/40/10/1175

[82] "The data provide evidence that dietary modification may be of clinical benefit for certain RA patients, and that this benefit may be related to a reduction in immunoreactivity to food antigens eliminated by the change in diet." Hafstrom I, Ringertz B, Spangberg A, von Zweigbergk L, Brannemark S, Nylander I, Ronnelid J, Laasonen L, Klareskog L. A vegan diet free of gluten improves the signs and symptoms of rheumatoid arthritis: the effects on arthritis correlate with a reduction in antibodies to food antigens. *Rheumatology* (Oxford). 2001 Oct;40(10):1175-9

[83] "Despite the increased AGA [antigliadin antibodies] positivity found distinctively in patients with recent-onset RA, none of the RA patients showed clear evidence of coeliac disease." Paimela L, Kurki P, Leirisalo-Repo M, Piirainen H.   Gliadin immune reactivity in patients with rheumatoid arthritis. Clin Exp Rheumatol. 1995 Sep-Oct;13(5):603-7

[84] "The median IgA antigliadin ELISA index was 7.1 (range 2.1-22.4) for the RA group and 3.1 (range 0.3-34.9) for the controls (p = 0.0001)." Koot VC, Van Straaten M, Hekkens WT, Collee G, Dijkmans BA. Elevated level of IgA gliadin antibodies in patients with rheumatoid arthritis. Clin Exp Rheumatol. 1989 Nov-Dec;7(6):623-6

[85] Seaman DR. The diet-induced proinflammatory state: a cause of chronic pain and other degenerative diseases? *J Manipulative Physiol Ther*. 2002 Mar-Apr;25(3):168-79

[86] Hagfors L, Nilsson I, Skoldstam L, Johansson G. Fat intake and composition of fatty acids in serum phospholipids in a randomized, controlled, Mediterranean dietary intervention study on patients with rheumatoid arthritis. *Nutr Metab* (Lond). 2005 Oct 10;2:26 http://www.nutritionandmetabolism.com/content/2/1/26

[87] Liu RH. Health benefits of fruit and vegetables are from additive and synergistic combinations of phytochemicals. *Am J Clin Nutr* 2003;78(3 Suppl):517S-520S http://www.ajcn.org/cgi/content/full/78/3/517S

[88] "Significant alteration in the intestinal flora was observed when the patients changed from omnivorous to vegan diet. ... This finding of an association between intestinal flora and disease activity may have implications for our understanding of how diet can affect RA." Peltonen R, Kjeldsen-Kragh J, Haugen M, Tuominen J, Toivanen P, Forre O, Eerola E. Changes of faecal flora in rheumatoid arthritis during fasting and one-year vegetarian diet. Br J Rheumatol. 1994 Jul;33(7):638-43

[89] Toivanen P, Eerola E. A vegan diet changes the intestinal flora. *Rheumatology* (Oxford). 2002 Aug;41(8):950-1 http://rheumatology.oxfordjournals.org/cgi/reprint/41/8/950

[90] "We conclude that a vegan diet changes the faecal microbial flora in RA patients, and changes in the faecal flora are associated with improvement in RA activity." Peltonen R, Nenonen M, Helve T, Hanninen O, Toivanen P, Eerola E. Faecal microbial flora and disease activity in rheumatoid arthritis during a vegan diet. Br J Rheumatol. 1997 Jan;36(1):64-8 http://rheumatology.oxfordjournals.org/cgi/reprint/36/1/64

[91] Aljada A, Mohanty P, Ghanim H, Abdo T, Tripathy D, Chaudhuri A, Dandona P. Increase in intranuclear nuclear factor kappaB and decrease in inhibitor kappaB in mononuclear cells after a mixed meal: evidence for a proinflammatory effect. *Am J Clin Nutr*. 2004 Apr;79(4):682-90 http://www.ajcn.org/cgi/content/full/79/4/682

[92] "The ability of therapeutic fasts to break metabolic vicious cycles may also contribute to the efficacy of fasting in the treatment of type 2 diabetes and autoimmune disorders." McCarty MF. A preliminary fast may potentiate response to a subsequent low-salt, low-fat vegan diet in the management of hypertension - fasting as a strategy for breaking metabolic vicious cycles. *Med Hypotheses*. 2003 May;60(5):624-33

[93] Ramakrishnan T, Stokes P. Beneficial effects of fasting and low carbohydrate diet in D-lactic acidosis associated with short-bowel syndrome. *JPEN J Parenter Enteral Nutr*. 1985 May-Jun;9(3):361-3

[94] Trollmo C, Verdrengh M, Tarkowski A. Fasting enhances mucosal antigen specific B cell responses in rheumatoid arthritis. *Ann Rheum Dis*. 1997 Feb;56(2):130-4 http://ard.bmjjournals.com/cgi/content/full/56/2/130

[95] "An association was found between improvement in inflammatory activity of the joints and enhancement of neutrophil bactericidal capacity. Fasting appears to improve the clinical status of patients with RA." Uden AM, Trang L, Venizelos N, Palmblad J. Neutrophil functions and clinical performance after total fasting in patients with rheumatoid arthritis. *Ann Rheum Dis*. 1983 Feb;42(1):45-51

[96] "We thus conclude that a reduced ability to generate cytotaxins, reduced release of enzyme, and reduced leukotriene formation from RA neutrophils, together with an altered fatty acid composition of membrane phospholipids, may be mechanisms for the decrease of inflammatory symptoms that results from fasting." Hafstrom I, Ringertz B, Gyllenhammar H, Palmblad J, Harms-Ringdahl M. Effects of fasting on disease activity, neutrophil function, fatty acid composition, and leukotriene biosynthesis in patients with rheumatoid arthritis. *Arthritis Rheum*. 1988 May;31(5):585-92

[97] "The results indicate that, unlike lactovegetarian diet, fasting may ameliorate the disease activity and reduce both the intestinal and the non-intestinal permeability in rheumatoid arthritis." Sundqvist T, Lindstrom F, Magnusson KE, Skoldstam L, Stjernstrom I, Tagesson C. Influence of fasting on intestinal permeability and disease activity in patients with rheumatoid arthritis. *Scand J Rheumatol*. 1982;11(1):33-8

[98] Fuhrman J, Sarter B, Calabro DJ. Brief case reports of medically supervised, water-only fasting associated with remission of autoimmune disease. *Altern Ther Health Med*. 2002 Jul-Aug;8(4):112, 110-1

[99] "An association was found between improvement in inflammatory activity of the joints and enhancement of neutrophil bactericidal capacity. Fasting appears to improve the clinical status of patients with RA." Uden AM, Trang L, Venizelos N, Palmblad J. Neutrophil functions and clinical performance after total fasting in patients with rheumatoid arthritis. *Ann Rheum Dis*. 1983 Feb;42(1):45-51

[100] "The average reduction in blood pressure was 37/13 mm Hg, with the greatest decrease being observed for subjects with the most severe hypertension. Patients with stage 3 hypertension (those with systolic blood pressure greater than 180 mg Hg, diastolic blood pressure greater than 110 mg Hg, or both) had an average reduction of 60/17 mm Hg at the conclusion of treatment."

- <u>Broad-spectrum fatty acid therapy with ALA, EPA, DHA, GLA and oleic acid</u>: Fatty acid supplementation should be delivered in the form of combination therapy with ALA, GLA, DHA, and EPA. Given at doses of 3,000 – 9,000 mg per day, ALA from flaxseed oil has impressive anti-inflammatory benefits demonstrated by its ability to halve prostaglandin production in humans.[106] Numerous studies have demonstrated the benefit of GLA in the treatment of rheumatoid arthritis when used at doses between 500 mg – 4,000 mg per day.[107,108] Fish oil provides EPA and DHA which have well-proven anti-inflammatory benefits in rheumatoid arthritis[109,110,111] and lupus.[112,113] ALA, EPA, DHA, and GLA need to be provided in the form of supplements; when using high doses of therapeutic oils, *liquid* supplements that can be mixed in juice or a smoothie are generally more convenient and palatable than are *capsules*. For example, at the upper end of oral fatty acid administration, the patient may be consuming as much as one-quarter cup per day of fatty acid supplementation; this same dose administered in the form of pills would require at least 72 capsules to attain the equivalent doses of ALA, EPA, DHA, and GLA. Therapeutic amounts of oleic acid can be obtained from generous use of olive oil, preferably on fresh vegetables. Supplementation with polyunsaturated fatty acids warrants increased intake of antioxidants from diet, from fruit and vegetable juices, and from properly formulated supplements. Since patients with systemic inflammation are generally in a pro-oxidative state, consideration must be given to the timing and starting dose of fatty acid supplementation and the need for antioxidant protection; some patients should start with a low dose of fatty acid supplementation until inflammation and the hyperoxidative state have been reduced; see the final chapter in this text on Therapeutics for more fatty acid details and biochemical pathways. Clinicians must realize that fatty acids are not clinically or biochemically interchangeable and that one fatty acid does not substitute for another; each of the fatty acids must be supplied in order for its benefits to be obtained.[114]

- <u>Vitamin D3 supplementation with physiologic doses and/or tailored to serum 25(OH)D levels</u>: Vitamin D deficiency is common in the general population and is even more common in patients with chronic illness and chronic musculoskeletal pain.[115] Correction of vitamin D deficiency supports normal immune function against infection and provides a clinically significant anti-inflammatory[116] and analgesic benefit in patients with back pain[117] and limb pain.[118] Reasonable daily doses for children and adults are 1,000-2,000 and 4,000 IU, respectively.[119] Deficiency and response to treatment are monitored with serum 25(OH)vitamin D while safety is monitored with serum calcium; inflammatory granulomatous diseases and certain drugs such as hydrochlorothiazide greatly increase the propensity for hypercalcemia and warrant increment dosing and frequent monitoring of serum

Goldhamer A, Lisle D, Parpia B, Anderson SV, Campbell TC. Medically supervised water-only fasting in the treatment of hypertension. *J Manipulative Physiol Ther.* 2001 Jun;24(5):335-9 http://www.healthpromoting.com/335-339Goldhamer115263.QXD.pdf

[101] "RESULTS: Approximately 82% of the subjects achieved BP at or below 120/80 mm Hg by the end of the treatment program. The mean BP reduction was 20/7 mm Hg, with the greatest decrease being observed for subjects with the highest baseline BP." Goldhamer AC, Lisle DJ, Sultana P, Anderson SV, Parpia B, Hughes B, Campbell TC. Medically supervised water-only fasting in the treatment of borderline hypertension. *J Altern Complement Med.* 2002 Oct;8(5):643-50 http://www.healthpromoting.com/Articles/articles/study%202/acmpaper5.pdf

[102] Vertes V, Genuth SM, Hazelton IM. Supplemented fasting as a large-scale outpatient program. *JAMA.* 1977 Nov 14;238(20):2151-3

[103] Bauman WA, Schwartz E, Rose HG, Eisenstein HN, Johnson DW. Early and long-term effects of acute caloric deprivation in obese diabetic patients. *Am J Med.* 1988 Jul;85(1):38-46

[104] Goldhamer AC. Initial cost of care results in medically supervised water-only fasting for treating high blood pressure and diabetes. *J Altern Complement Med.* 2002 Dec;8(6):696-7 http://www.healthpromoting.com/Articles/pdf/Study%2032.pdf

[105] "The ketogenic diet should be considered as alternative therapy for children with difficult-to-control seizures. It is more effective than many of the new anticonvulsant medications and is well tolerated by children and families when it is effective." Freeman JM, Vining EP, Pillas DJ, Pyzik PL, Casey JC, Kelly LM. The efficacy of the ketogenic diet-1998: a prospective evaluation of intervention in 150 children. *Pediatrics.* 1998 Dec;102(6):1358-63 http://pediatrics.aappublications.org/cgi/reprint/102/6/1358

[106] Adam O, Wolfram G, Zollner N. Effect of alpha-linolenic acid in the human diet on linoleic acid metabolism and prostaglandin biosynthesis. *J Lipid Res.* 1986 Apr;27(4):421-6 http://www.jlr.org/cgi/reprint/27/4/421

[107] "Other results showed a significant reduction in morning stiffness with gamma-linolenic acid at 3 months and reduction in pain and articular index at 6 months with olive oil." Brzeski M, Madhok R, Capell HA. Evening primrose oil in patients with rheumatoid arthritis and side-effects of non-steroidal anti-inflammatory drugs. *Br J Rheumatol.* 1991 Oct;30(5):370-2

[108] Rothman D, DeLuca P, Zurier RB. Botanical lipids: effects on inflammation, immune responses, and rheumatoid arthritis. *Semin Arthritis Rheum.* 1995 Oct;25(2):87-96

[109] Adam O, Beringer C, Kless T, Lemmen C, Adam A, Wiseman M, Adam P, Klimmek R, Forth W. Anti-inflammatory effects of a low arachidonic acid diet and fish oil in patients with rheumatoid arthritis. *Rheumatol Int.* 2003 Jan;23(1):27-36

[110] Lau CS, Morley KD, Belch JJ. Effects of fish oil supplementation on non-steroidal anti-inflammatory drug requirement in patients with mild rheumatoid arthritis--a double-blind placebo controlled study. *Br J Rheumatol.* 1993 Nov;32(11):982-9

[111] Kremer JM, Jubiz W, Michalek A, Rynes RI, Bartholomew LE, Bigaouette J, Timchalk M, Beeler D, Lininger L. Fish-oil fatty acid supplementation in active rheumatoid arthritis. A double-blinded, controlled, crossover study. *Ann Intern Med.* 1987 Apr;106(4):497-503

[112] Walton AJ, Snaith ML, Locniskar M, Cumberland AG, Morrow WJ, Isenberg DA. Dietary fish oil and the severity of symptoms in patients with systemic lupus erythematosus. *Ann Rheum Dis.* 1991 Jul;50(7):463-6

[113] Duffy EM, Meenagh GK, McMillan SA, Strain JJ, Hannigan BM, Bell AL. The clinical effect of dietary supplementation with omega-3 fish oils and/or copper in systemic lupus erythematosus. *J Rheumatol.* 2004 Aug;31(8):1551-6

[114] Vasquez A. Reducing Pain and Inflammation Naturally. Part 2: New Insights into Fatty Acid Supplementation and Its Effect on Eicosanoid Production and Genetic Expression. *Nutritional Perspectives* 2005; January: 5-16 http://optimalhealthresearch.com/part2

[115] Plotnikoff GA, Quigley JM. Prevalence of severe hypovitaminosis D in patients with persistent, nonspecific musculoskeletal pain. *Mayo Clin Proc.* 2003 Dec;78(12):1463-70

[116] Timms PM, Mannan N, Hitman GA, Noonan K, Mills PG, Syndercombe-Court D, Aganna E, Price CP, Boucher BJ. Circulating MMP9, vitamin D and variation in the TIMP-1 response with VDR genotype: mechanisms for inflammatory damage in chronic disorders? *QJM.* 2002 Dec;95(12):787-96 http://qjmed.oxfordjournals.org/cgi/content/full/95/12/787

[117] Al Faraj S, Al Mutairi K. Vitamin D deficiency and chronic low back pain in Saudi Arabia. *Spine.* 2003 Jan 15;28(2):177-9

[118] Masood H, Narang AP, Bhat IA, Shah GN. Persistent limb pain and raised serum alkaline phosphatase the earliest markers of subclinical hypovitaminosis D in Kashmir. *Indian J Physiol Pharmacol.* 1989 Oct-Dec;33(4):259-61

[119] Vasquez A, Manso G, Cannell J. The clinical importance of vitamin D (cholecalciferol): a paradigm shift with implications for all healthcare providers. *Altern Ther Health Med.* 2004 Sep-Oct;10(5):28-36 http://optimalhealthresearch.com/monograph04

calcium. Vitamin D2 (ergocalciferol) is not a human nutrient and should not be used in clinical practice.

- **Assessment for dysbiosis: All patients with spondyloarthropathy and reactive arthritis have dysbiosis until proven otherwise by the combination of 1) three-sample comprehensive parasitology examinations performed by a specialty laboratory and 2) clinical response to at least two 2-4 week courses of broad-spectrum antimicrobial treatment.** Yeast, bacteria, and parasites are treated as indicated based on identification and sensitivity results from comprehensive parasitology assessments. Patients taking immunosuppressant drugs such as corticosteroids/prednisone have increased risk of intestinal bacterial overgrowth and translocation.[120,121] Other dysbiotic loci should be investigated as discussed in Chapter 4 in the section on multifocal dysbiosis.

  o Gastrointestinal dysbiosis: Additionally or empirically, treatment for gastrointestinal dysbiosis may include the following:

    ▪ Oregano oil: Emulsified oil of oregano in a time-released tablet is proven effective in the eradication of harmful gastrointestinal microbes, including *Blastocystis hominis*, *Entamoeba hartmanni*, and *Endolimax nana*.[122] An *in vitro* study[123] and clinical experience support the use of emulsified oregano against *Candida albicans* and various bacteria. The common dose is 600 mg per day in divided doses for 6 weeks.[124]

    ▪ Berberine: Berberine is an alkaloid extracted from plants such as *Berberis vulgaris*, and *Hydrastis canadensis*, and it shows effectiveness against *Giardia*, *Candida*, and *Streptococcus* in addition to its direct anti-inflammatory and antidiarrheal actions. Oral dose of 400 mg per day is common for adults.[125]

    ▪ *Artemisia annua*: Artemisinin has been safely used for centuries in Asia for the treatment of malaria, and it also has effectiveness against anaerobic bacteria due to the pro-oxidative sesquiterpene endoperoxide.[126,127] I commonly use artemisinin at 200 mg per day in divided doses for adults with dysbiosis.

    ▪ St. John's Wort (*Hypericum perforatum*): Hyperforin from *Hypericum perforatum* also shows impressive antibacterial action, particularly against gram-positive bacteria such as *Staphylococcus aureus*, *Streptococcus pyogenes*, *Streptococcus agalactiae*[128] and perhaps *Helicobacter pylori*.[129] Up to 600 mg three times per day of a 3% hyperforin standardized extract is customary in the treatment of depression.

    ▪ Bismuth: Bismuth is commonly used in the empiric treatment of diarrhea (e.g., "Pepto-Bismol") and is commonly combined with other antimicrobial agents to reduce drug resistance and increase antibiotic effectiveness.[130]

    ▪ Undecylenic acid: Derived from castor bean oil, undecylenic acid has antifungal properties and is commonly indicated by sensitivity results obtained by stool culture. Common dosages are 150-250 mg tid (up to 750 mg per day).[131]

    ▪ Peppermint (*Mentha piperita*): Peppermint shows antimicrobial and antispasmodic actions and has demonstrated clinical effectiveness in patients with bacterial overgrowth of the small bowel.

---

[120] "A 63-year-old man with systemic lupus erythematosus and selective IgA deficiency developed intractable diarrhoea the day after treatment with prednisone, 50 mg daily, was started. The diarrhoea was considered to be caused by bacterial overgrowth and was later successfully treated with doxycycline." Denison H, Wallerstedt S. Bacterial overgrowth after high-dose corticosteroid treatment. *Scand J Gastroenterol*. 1989 Jun;24(5):561-4

[121] "These bacteria also translocated to the mesenteric lymph nodes in mice injected with cyclophosphamide or prednisone." Berg RD, Wommack E, Deitch EA. Immunosuppression and intestinal bacterial overgrowth synergistically promote bacterial translocation. *Arch Surg*. 1988 Nov;123(11):1359-64

[122] Force M, Sparks WS, Ronzio RA. Inhibition of enteric parasites by emulsified oil of oregano in vivo. *Phytother Res*. 2000 May;14(3):213-4

[123] Stiles JC, Sparks W, Ronzio RA. The inhibition of Candida albicans by oregano. *J Applied Nutr* 1995;47:96–102

[124] Force M, Sparks WS, Ronzio RA. Inhibition of enteric parasites by emulsified oil of oregano in vivo. *Phytother Res*. 2000 May;14(3):213-4

[125] Berberine. Altern Med Rev. 2000 Apr;5(2):175-7 http://www.thorne.com/altmedrev/.fulltext/5/2/175.pdf

[126] Dien TK, de Vries PJ, Khanh NX, Koopmans R, Binh LN, Duc DD, Kager PA, van Boxtel CJ. Effect of food intake on pharmacokinetics of oral artemisinin in healthy Vietnamese subjects. *Antimicrob Agents Chemother*. 1997 May;41(5):1069-72

[127] Giao PT, Binh TQ, Kager PA, Long HP, Van Thang N, Van Nam N, de Vries PJ. Artemisinin for treatment of uncomplicated falciparum malaria: is there a place for monotherapy? *Am J Trop Med Hyg*. 2001 Dec;65(6):690-5

[128] Schempp CM, Pelz K, Wittmer A, Schopf E, Simon JC. Antibacterial activity of hyperforin from St John's wort, against multiresistant Staphylococcus aureus and gram-positive bacteria. *Lancet*. 1999 Jun 19;353(9170):2129

[129] "A butanol fraction of St. John's Wort revealed anti-Helicobacter pylori activity with MIC values ranging between 15.6 and 31.2 microg/ml." Reichling J, Weseler A, Saller R. A current review of the antimicrobial activity of Hypericum perforatum L. *Pharmacopsychiatry*. 2001 Jul;34 Suppl 1:S116-9

[130] Veldhuyzen van Zanten SJ, Sherman PM, Hunt RH. Helicobacter pylori: new developments and treatments. *CMAJ*. 1997;156(11):1565-74 http://www.cmaj.ca/cgi/reprint/156/11/1565.pdf

[131] "Adult dosage is usually 450-750 mg undecylenic acid daily in three divided doses." Undecylenic acid. Monograph. *Altern Med Rev*. 2002 Feb;7(1):68-70 http://www.thorne.com/altmedrev/.fulltext/7/1/68.pdf

- **Commonly used antibiotic/antifungal drugs:** The most commonly employed drugs for intestinal bacterial overgrowth are described here.[132] Treatment duration is generally at least 2 weeks and up to 8 weeks, depending on clinical response and the severity and diversity of the intestinal overgrowth. With all anti*bacterial* treatments, use empiric anti*fungal* treatment to prevent yeast overgrowth; some patients benefit from antifungal treatment that is continued for *months* and occasionally *years*. Drugs can generally be coadministered with natural antibiotics/antifungals for improved efficacy. Treatment can be guided by identification of the dysbiotic microbes and the results of culture and sensitivity tests.

  ⇒ Metronidazole: 250-500 mg BID-QID (generally limit to 1.5 g/d); metronidazole has systemic bioavailability and effectiveness against a wide range of dysbiotic microbes, including protozoans, amebas/Giardia, *H. pylori*, *Clostridium difficile* and most anaerobic gram-negative bacilli.[133] Adverse effects are generally limited to stomatitis, nausea, diarrhea, and—rarely and/or with long-term use—peripheral neuropathy, dizziness, and metallic taste; the drug must not be consumed with alcohol. Metronidazole resistance by *Blastocystis hominis* and other parasites has been noted.

  ⇒ Erythromycin: 250-500 mg TID-QID; this drug is a widely used antibiotic that also has intestinal promotility benefits (thus making it an ideal treatment for intestinal bacterial overgrowth associated with or caused by intestinal dysmotility/hypomotility such as seen in scleroderma[134,135]). Do not combine erythromycin with the promotility drug **cisapride** due to risk for serious cardiac arrhythmia.

  ⇒ Tetracycline: 250-500 mg QID

  ⇒ Ciproflaxacin: 500 mg BID

  ⇒ Cephalexin/kelfex: 250 mg QID

  ⇒ Minocycline: Minocycline (200 mg/day)[136] has received the most attention in the treatment of rheumatoid arthritis due to its superior response (65%) over placebo (13%)[137]; in addition to its antibacterial action, the drug is also immunomodulatory and anti-inflammatory. Ironically, minocycline can cause drug-induced autoimmunity, especially lupus.[138,139]

  ⇒ **Nystatin:** Nystatin 500,000 units bid with food; duration of treatment begins with a minimum duration of 2-4 weeks and may continue as long as the patient is deriving benefit.

  ⇒ Ketoconazole: As a systemically bioavailable antifungal drug, ketoconazole has inherent anti-inflammatory benefits which may be helpful; however the drug inhibits androgen formation and may lead to exacerbation of the hypoandrogenism that is commonly seen in autoimmune patients and which contributes to the immune dysfunction.

- Probiotics: Live cultures in the form of tablets, capsules, yogurt, or kefir can be used per patient preference and tolerance. Obviously, dairy-based products should be avoided by patients with dairy allergy.

- *Saccharomyces boulardii*: A non-colonizing, non-pathogenic yeast that increases sIgA production and can aid in the elimination of pathogenic/dysbiotic yeast, bacteria, and

---

[132] Saltzman JR, Russell RM. Nutritional consequences of intestinal bacterial overgrowth. *Compr Ther*. 1994;20(9):523-30

[133] Tierney ML. McPhee SJ, Papadakis MA. Current Medical Diagnosis and Treatment 2006. 45th edition. New York; Lange Medical Books: 2006, pages 1578-1577

[134] "Prokinetic agents effective in pseudoobstruction include metoclopramide, domperidone, cisapride, octreotide, and erythromycin. ... The combination of octreotide and erythromycin may be particularly effective in systemic sclerosis." Sjogren RW. Gastrointestinal features of scleroderma. *Curr Opin Rheumatol*. 1996 Nov;8(6):569-75

[135] "CONCLUSIONS: Erythromycin accelerates gastric and gallbladder emptying in scleroderma patients and might be helpful in the treatment of gastrointestinal motor abnormalities in these patients." Fiorucci S, Distrutti E, Bassotti G, Gerli R, Chiucchiu S, Betti C, Santucci L, Morelli A. Effect of erythromycin administration on upper gastrointestinal motility in scleroderma patients. *Scand J Gastroenterol*. 1994 Sep;29(9):807-13

[136] "...48-week trial of oral minocycline (200 mg/d) or placebo." Tilley BC, Alarcon GS, Heyse SP, Trentham DE, Neuner R, Kaplan DA, Clegg DO, Leisen JC, Buckley L, Cooper SM, Duncan H, Pillemer SR, Tuttleman M, Fowler SE. Minocycline in rheumatoid arthritis. A 48-week, double-blind, placebo-controlled trial. MIRA Trial Group. *Ann Intern Med*. 1995 Jan 15;122(2):81-9

[137] "In patients with early seropositive RA, therapy with minocycline is superior to placebo." O'Dell JR, Haire CE, Palmer W, Drymalski W, Wees S, Blakely K, Churchill M, Eckhoff PJ, Weaver A, Doud D, Erikson N, Dietz F, Olson R, Maloley P, Klassen LW, Moore GF. Treatment of early rheumatoid arthritis with minocycline or placebo: results of a randomized, double-blind, placebo-controlled trial. *Arthritis Rheum*. 1997 May;40(5):842-8

[138] "...many cases of drug-induced lupus related to minocycline have been reported. Some of those reports included pulmonary lupus..." Christodoulou CS, Emmanuel P, Ray RA, Good RA, Schnapf BM, Cawkwell GD. Respiratory distress due to minocycline-induced pulmonary lupus. *Chest*. 1999 May;115(5):1471-3 http://www.chestjournal.org/cgi/content/full/115/5/1471

[139] Lawson TM, Amos N, Bulgen D, Williams BD.Minocycline-induced lupus: clinical features and response to rechallenge. *Rheumatology* (Oxford). 2001 Mar;40(3):329-35 http://rheumatology.oxfordjournals.org/cgi/content/full/40/3/329

parasites. It is particularly useful during antibiotic treatment to help prevent secondary Candidal infections. Common dose is 250 mg thrice daily.

- Supplemented Paleo-Mediterranean diet / Specific Carbohydrate Diet: The specifications of the *specific carbohydrate diet* (SCD) detailed by Gottschall[140] are met with adherence to the Paleo diet by Cordain.[141] The combination of both approaches and books will give patients an excellent combination of informational understanding and culinary versatility.

- Orthoendocrinology: Assess prolactin, cortisol, DHEA, free and total testosterone, serum estradiol, and thyroid status (e.g., TSH, T4, *and* anti-thyroid peroxidase antibodies).

  o Prolactin (excess): Prolactin is a proinflammatory hormone that is commonly elevated in patients with inflammatory disorders[142,143,144,145] Serum prolactin is the standard assessment of prolactin status. Since elevated prolactin may be a sign of pituitary tumor, assessment for headaches, visual deficits, and other abnormalities of pituitary hormones (e.g., GH and TSH) should be performed; CT or MRI must be considered. Patients with prolactin levels less than 100 ng/mL and normal CT/MRI findings can be managed conservatively with effective prolactin-lowering treatment and annual radiologic assessment (less necessary with favorable serum response).[146, see review 147] Specific treatment options include the following:

    - Thyroid hormone: Hypothyroidism frequently causes hyperprolactinemia which is reversible upon effective treatment of hypothyroidism. Obviously therefore, thyroid status should be evaluated in all patients with hyperprolactinemia. Thyroid assessment and treatment is reviewed later in this section.

    - *Vitex astus-cagnus* and other supporting botanicals and nutrients: **Vitex lowers serum prolactin in humans[148,149] via a dopaminergic effect.**[150] Vitex is considered safe for clinical use; mild and reversible adverse effects possibly associated with Vitex include nausea, headache, gastrointestinal disturbances, menstrual disorders, acne, pruritus and erythematous rash. No drug interactions are known, but given the herb's dopaminergic effect it should probably be used with some caution in patients treated with dopamine antagonists such as the so-called antipsychotic drugs (most of which do not work very well and/or carry intolerable adverse effects[151,152]). In a recent review, Bone[153] stated that daily doses can range from 500 mg to 2,000 mg DHE (dry herb equivalent) and can be tailored to the suppression of prolactin. Due at least in part to its content of L-dopa, *Mucuna pruriens* **shows clinical dopaminergic activity** as evidenced by its effectiveness in Parkinson's disease[154]; up to 15-30 gm/d of

[140] Gotschall E. Breaking the Vicious Cycle: Intestinal health though diet. Kirkton Press; Rev edition (August, 1994) http://www.scdiet.com/

[141] Cordain L: The Paleo Diet: Lose weight and get healthy by eating the food you were designed to eat. John Wiley & Sons Inc., New York 2002 http://thepaleodiet.com/

[142] Dostal C, Moszkorzova L, Musilova L, Lacinova Z, Marek J, Zvarova J. Serum prolactin stress values in patients with systemic lupus erythematosus. *Ann Rheum Dis*. 2003 May;62(5):487-8 http://ard.bmjjournals.com/cgi/content/full/62/5/487

[143] "RESULTS: A significantly higher rate of elevated PRL levels was found in SLE patients (40.0%) compared with the healthy controls (14.8%). No proof was found of association with the presence of anti-ds-DNA or with specific organ involvement. Similarly, elevated PRL levels were found in RA patients (39.3%)." Moszkorzova L, Lacinova Z, Marek J, Musilova L, Dohnalova A, Dostal C. Hyperprolactinaemia in patients with systemic lupus erythematosus. *Clin Exp Rheumatol*. 2002 Nov-Dec;20(6):807-12

[144] "CONCLUSION: Men with RA have high serum PRL levels and concentrations increase with longer disease evolution and worse functional stage." Mateo L, Nolla JM, Bonnin MR, Navarro MA, Roig-Escofet D. High serum prolactin levels in men with rheumatoid arthritis. *J Rheumatol*. 1998 Nov;25(11):2077-82

[145] "Male patients affected by RA showed high serum PRL levels. The serum PRL concentration was found to be increased in relation to the duration and the activity of the disease. Serum PRL levels do not seem to have any relationship with the BMD, at least in RA." Seriolo B, Ferretti V, Sulli A, Fasciolo D, Cutolo M. Serum prolactin concentrations in male patients with rheumatoid arthritis. *Ann N Y Acad Sci*. 2002 Jun;966:258-62

[146] Beers MH, Berkow R (eds). The Merck Manual. Seventeenth Edition. Whitehouse Station; Merck Research Laboratories 1999 Page 77-78

[147] Serri O, Chik CL, Ur E, Ezzat S. Diagnosis and management of hyperprolactinemia. *CMAJ*. 2003 Sep 16;169(6):575-81 http://www.cmaj.ca/cgi/content/full/169/6/575

[148] "Since AC extracts were shown to have beneficial effects on premenstrual mastodynia serum prolactin levels in such patients were also studied in one double-blind, placebo-controlled clinical study. Serum prolactin levels were indeed reduced in the patients treated with the extract." Wuttke W, Jarry H, Christoffel V, Spengler B, Seidlova-Wuttke D. Chaste tree (Vitex agnus-castus)--pharmacology and clinical indications. *Phytomedicine*. 2003 May;10(4):348-57

[149] German abstract from Medline: "The prolactin release was reduced after 3 months, shortened luteal phases were normalised and deficits in the luteal progesterone synthesis were eliminated." Milewicz A, Gejdel E, Sworen H, Sienkiewicz K, Jedrzejak J, Teucher T, Schmitz H. [Vitex agnus castus extract in the treatment of luteal phase defects due to latent hyperprolactinemia. Results of a randomized placebo-controlled double-blind study] *Arzneimittelforschung*. 1993 Jul;43(7):752-6

[150] "Our results indicate a dopaminergic effect of Vitex agnus-castus extracts and suggest additional pharmacological actions via opioid receptors." Meier B, Berger D, Hoberg E, Sticher O, Schaffner W. Pharmacological activities of Vitex agnus-castus extracts in vitro. *Phytomedicine*. 2000 Oct;7(5):373-81

[151] "The majority of patients in each group discontinued their assigned treatment owing to inefficacy or intolerable side effects or for other reasons." Lieberman JA, Stroup TS, McEvoy JP, Swartz MS, Rosenheck RA, Perkins DO, Keefe RS, Davis SM, Davis CE, Lebowitz BD, Severe J, Hsiao JK; Clinical Antipsychotic Trials of Intervention Effectiveness (CATIE) Investigators. Effectiveness of antipsychotic drugs in patients with chronic schizophrenia. *N Engl J Med*. 2005 Sep 22;353(12):1209-23

[152] Whitaker R. The case against antipsychotic drugs: a 50-year record of doing more harm than good. *Med Hypotheses*. 2004;62(1):5-13

[153] "In conditions such as endometriosis and fibroids, for which a significant estrogen antagonist effect is needed, doses of at least 2 g/day DHE may be required and typically are used by professional herbalists." Bone K. New Insights Into Chaste Tree. *Nutritional Wellness* 2005 November http://www.nutritionalwellness.com/archives/2005/nov/11_bone.php

[154] "CONCLUSIONS: The rapid onset of action and longer on time without concomitant increase in dyskinesias on mucuna seed powder formulation suggest that this natural source of L-dopa might possess advantages over conventional L-dopa preparations in the long term management of PD." Katzenschlager R, Evans A, Manson A, Patsalos PN, Ratnaraj N, Watt H, Timmermann L, Van der Giessen R, Lees AJ. Mucuna pruriens in Parkinson's disease: a double blind clinical and pharmacological study. *J Neurol Neurosurg Psychiatry*. 2004 Dec;75(12):1672-7

mucuna has been used clinically but doses will be dependent on preparation and phytoconcentration. **Triptolide and other extracts from *Tripterygium wilfordii* Hook F exert clinically significant anti-inflammatory action in patients with rheumatoid arthritis[155,156] and also offer protection to dopaminergic neurons.**[157,158] Ironically, even though tyrosine is the nutritional precursor to dopamine with evidence of clinical effectiveness (e.g., narcolepsy[159], enhancement of memory[160] and cognition[161]), **supplementation with tyrosine appears to actually increase rather than decrease prolactin levels[162]; therefore tyrosine should be used cautiously (if at all) in patients with systemic inflammation and elevated prolactin.** Furthermore, the finding that **high-protein meals stimulate prolactin release[163]** may partly explain the benefits of vegetarian diets in the treatment of systemic inflammation; since vegetarian diets are comparatively low in protein compared to omnivorous diets, they may lead to a relative reduction in prolactin production due to lack of stimulation.

- Bromocriptine: Bromocriptine has long been considered the pharmacologic treatment of choice for elevated prolactin.[164] Typical dose is 2.5 mg per day (effective against lupus[165]); gastrointestinal upset and sedation are common.[166] Clinical intervention with bromocriptine appears warranted in patients with RA, SLE, Reiter's syndrome, psoriatic arthritis, and probably multiple sclerosis and uveitis.[167]

- Cabergoline/Dostinex: Cabergoline/Dostinex is a newer dopamine agonist with few adverse effects; typical dose starts at 0.5 mg per week (0.25 mg twice per week).[168] Several studies have indicated that cabergoline is safer and more effective than bromocriptine for reducing prolactin levels[169] and the dose can often be reduced after successful prolactin reduction, allowing for reductions in cost and adverse effects.[170] Although fewer studies have been published supporting the antirheumatic benefits of cabergoline than bromocriptine, its antirheumatic benefits have been documented.[171]

  o Estrogen (excess): Estrogen in general and 16-alpha-hydroxyestrone in particular appear to be at least somewhat proinflammatory and immunodysregulatory. Men with rheumatoid arthritis show an excess of estradiol and a decrease in DHEA, and the excess estrogen is

[155] "The ethanol/ethyl acetate extract of TWHF shows therapeutic benefit in patients with treatment-refractory RA. At therapeutic dosages, the TWHF extract was well tolerated by most patients in this study." Tao X, Younger J, Fan FZ, Wang B, Lipsky PE. Benefit of an extract of Tripterygium Wilfordii Hook F in patients with rheumatoid arthritis: a double-blind, placebo-controlled study. *Arthritis Rheum.* 2002 Jul;46(7):1735-43

[156] "CONCLUSION: The EA extract of TWHF at dosages up to 570 mg/day appeared to be safe, and doses > 360 mg/day were associated with clinical benefit in patients with RA." Tao X, Cush JJ, Garret M, Lipsky PE. A phase I study of ethyl acetate extract of the chinese antirheumatic herb Tripterygium wilfordii hook F in rheumatoid arthritis. *J Rheumatol.* 2001 Oct;28(10):2160-7

[157] "Our data suggests that triptolide may protect dopaminergic neurons from LPS-induced injury and its efficiency in inhibiting microglia activation may underlie the mechanism." Li FQ, Lu XZ, Liang XB, Zhou HF, Xue B, Liu XY, Niu DB, Han JS, Wang XM. Triptolide, a Chinese herbal extract, protects dopaminergic neurons from inflammation-mediated damage through inhibition of microglial activation. *J Neuroimmunol.* 2004 Mar;148(1-2):24-31

[158] "Moreover, tripchlorolide markedly prevented the decrease in amount of dopamine in the striatum of model rats. Taken together, our data provide the first evidence that tripchlorolide acts as a neuroprotective molecule that rescues MPP+ or axotomy-induced degeneration of dopaminergic neurons, which may imply its therapeutic potential for Parkinson's disease." Li FQ, Cheng XX, Liang XB, Wang XH, Xue B, He QH, Wang XM, Han JS. Neurotrophic and neuroprotective effects of tripchlorolide, an extract of Chinese herb Tripterygium wilfordii Hook F, on dopaminergic neurons. *Exp Neurol.* 2003 Jan;179(1):28-37

[159] "Of twenty-eight visual analogue scales rating mood and arousal, the subjects' ratings in the tyrosine treatment (9 g daily) and placebo periods differed significantly for only three (less tired, less drowsy, more alert)." Elwes RD, Crewes H, Chesterman LP, Summers B, Jenner P, Binnie CD, Parkes JD. Treatment of narcolepsy with L-tyrosine: double-blind placebo-controlled trial. *Lancet.* 1989 Nov 4;2(8671):1067-9

[160] "Ten men and 10 women subjects underwent these batteries 1 h after ingesting 150 mg/kg of l-tyrosine or placebo. Administration of tyrosine significantly enhanced accuracy and decreased frequency of list retrieval on the working memory task during the multiple task battery compared with placebo." Thomas JR, Lockwood PA, Singh A, Deuster PA. Tyrosine improves working memory in a multitasking environment. *Pharmacol Biochem Behav.* 1999 Nov;64(3):495-500

[161] "Ten subjects received five daily doses of a protein-rich drink containing 2 g tyrosine, and 11 subjects received a carbohydrate rich drink with the same amount of calories (255 kcal)." Deijen JB, Wientjes CJ, Vullinghs HF, Cloin PA, Langefeld JJ. Tyrosine improves cognitive performance and reduces blood pressure in cadets after one week of a combat training course. *Brain Res Bull.* 1999 Jan 15;48(2):203-9

[162] "Tyrosine (when compared to placebo) had no effect on any sleep related measure, but it did stimulate prolactin release." Waters WF, Magill RA, Bray GA, Volaufova J, Smith SR, Lieberman HR, Rood J, Hurry M, Anderson T, Ryan DH. A comparison of tyrosine against placebo, phentermine, caffeine, and D-amphetamine during sleep deprivation. *Nutr Neurosci.* 2003;6(4):221-35

[163] "Whereas carbohydrate meals had no discernible effects, high protein meals induced a large increase in both PRL and cortisol; high fat meals caused selective release of PRL." Ishizuka B, Quigley ME, Yen SS. Pituitary hormone release in response to food ingestion: evidence for neuroendocrine signals from gut to brain. *J Clin Endocrinol Metab.* 1983 Dec;57(6):1111-6

[164] Beers MH, Berkow R (eds). The Merck Manual. Seventeenth Edition. Whitehouse Station; Merck Research Laboratories 1999 Page 77-78

[165] "A prospective, double-blind, randomized, placebo-controlled study compared BRC at a fixed daily dosage of 2.5 mg with placebo... Long term treatment with a low dose of BRC appears to be a safe and effective means of decreasing SLE flares in SLE patients." Alvarez-Nemegyei J, Cobarrubias-Cobos A, Escalante-Triay F, Sosa-Munoz J, Miranda JM, Jara LJ. Bromocriptine in systemic lupus erythematosus: a double-blind, randomized, placebo-controlled study. *Lupus.* 1998;7(6):414-9

[166] Serri O, Chik CL, Ur E, Ezzat S. Diagnosis and management of hyperprolactinemia. *CMAJ.* 2003 Sep 16;169(6):575-81 http://www.cmaj.ca/cgi/content/full/169/6/575

[167] "...clinical observations and trials support the use of bromocriptine as a nonstandard primary or adjunctive therapy in the treatment of recalcitrant RA, SLE, Reiter's syndrome, and psoriatic arthritis and associated conditions unresponsive to traditional approaches." McMurray RW. Bromocriptine in rheumatic and autoimmune diseases. *Semin Arthritis Rheum.* 2001 Aug;31(1):21-32

[168] Serri O, Chik CL, Ur E, Ezzat S. Diagnosis and management of hyperprolactinemia. *CMAJ.* 2003 Sep 16;169(6):575-81 http://www.cmaj.ca/cgi/content/full/169/6/575

[169] "CONCLUSION: These data indicate that cabergoline is a very effective agent for lowering the prolactin levels in hyperprolactinemic patients and that it appears to offer considerable advantage over bromocriptine in terms of efficacy and tolerability." Sabuncu T, Arikan E, Tasan E, Hatemi H. Comparison of the effects of cabergoline and bromocriptine on prolactin levels in hyperprolactinemic patients. *Intern Med.* 2001 Sep;40(9):857-61

[170] "Cabergoline also normalized PRL in the majority of patients with known bromocriptine intolerance or -resistance. Once PRL secretion was adequately controlled, the dose of cabergoline could often be significantly decreased, which further reduced costs of therapy." Verhelst J, Abs R, Maiter D, van den Bruel A, Vandeweghe M, Velkeniers B, Mockel J, Lamberigts G, Petrossians P, Coremans P, Mahler C, Stevenaert A, Verlooy J, Raftopoulos C, Beckers A. Cabergoline in the treatment of hyperprolactinemia: a study in 455 patients. *J Clin Endocrinol Metab.* 1999 Jul;84(7):2518-22 http://jcem.endojournals.org/cgi/content/full/84/7/2518

[171] Erb N, Pace AV, Delamere JP, Kitas GD. Control of unremitting rheumatoid arthritis by the prolactin antagonist cabergoline. *Rheumatology* (Oxford). 2001 Feb;40(2):237-9 http://rheumatology.oxfordjournals.org/cgi/content/full/40/2/237

proportional to the degree of inflammation.[172] Serum estradiol is commonly used to assess estrogen status; estrogens can also be measured in 24-hour urine samples. Beyond looking at estrogens from a *quantitative* standpoint, they can also be *qualitatively* analyzed with respect to the ratio of estrone:estradiol:estriol as well as the balance between the "good" 2-hydroxyestrone relative to the purportedly carcinogenic and proinflammatory 16-alpha-hydroxyestrone. Interventions to combat high estrogen levels may include any effective combination of the following:

- <u>Weight loss and weight optimization</u>: In overweight patients, *weight loss* is the means to attaining the goal of *weight optimization*; the task is not complete until the body mass index is normalized/optimized. Excess adiposity and obesity raise estrogen levels due to high levels of aromatase (the hormone that makes estrogens from androgens) in adipose tissue; weight optimization and loss of excess fat helps normalize hormone levels and reduce inflammation.

- <u>Avoidance of ethanol</u>: Estrogen production is stimulated by ethanol intake.

- <u>Consider surgical correction of varicocele in affected men</u>: Men with varicocele have higher estrogen levels due to temperature-induced alterations in enzyme function in the testes; surgical correction of the varicocele lowers estrogen levels.

- <u>"Anti-estrogen diet"</u>: Foods and supplements such as green tea, diindolylmethane (DIM), indole-3-carbinol (I3C), licorice, and a high-fiber crucifer-based "anti-estrogenic diet" can also be used; monitoring clinical status and serum estradiol will prove or disprove efficacy. Whereas 16-alpha-hydroxyestrone is pro-inflammatory and immunodysregulatory, 2-hydroxyestrone has anti-inflammatory action[173] and been described as "the good estrogen"[174] due to its anticancer and comparatively health-preserving qualities. In a recent short-term study using I3C in patients with SLE, I3C supplementation at 375 mg per day was well tolerated and resulted in modest treatment-dependent clinical improvement as well as favorable modification of estrogen metabolism away from 16-alpha-hydroxyestrone and toward 2-hydroxyestrone.[175]

- <u>Anastrozole/Arimidex</u>: In our office, we commonly measure serum estradiol in men and administer the aromatase inhibitor anastrozole/arimidex 1 mg (2-3 doses per week) to men whose estradiol level is greater than 32 picogram/mL. The Life Extension Foundation[176] advocates that the optimal serum estradiol level for a man is 10-30 picogram/mL. Clinical studies using anastrozole/arimidex in men have shown that aromatase blockade lowers estradiol and raises testosterone[177]; generally speaking, this is exactly the result that we want in patients with severe systemic autoimmunity. Frequency of dosing is based on serum and clinical response.

o <u>Cortisol (insufficiency)</u>: Cortisol has immunoregulatory and "immunosuppressive" actions at physiological concentrations. Low adrenal function is common in patients with chronic inflammation.[178,179,180] Assessment of cortisol production and adrenal function was detailed in

---

[172] "RESULTS: DHEAS and estrone concentrations were lower and estradiol was higher in patients compared with healthy controls. DHEAS differed between RF positive and RF negative patients. Estrone did not correlate with any disease variable, whereas estradiol correlated strongly and positively with all measured indices of inflammation." Tengstrand B, Carlstrom K, Fellander-Tsai L, Hafstrom I. Abnormal levels of serum dehydroepiandrosterone, estrone, and estradiol in men with rheumatoid arthritis: high correlation between serum estradiol and current degree of inflammation. *J Rheumatol.* 2003 Nov;30(11):2338-43

[173] "Micromolar concentrations of beta-estradiol, estrone, 16-alpha-hydroxyestrone and estriol enhance the oxidative metabolism of activated human PMNL's. The corresponding 2-hydroxylated estrogens 2-OH-estradiol, 2-OH-estrone and 2-OH-estriol act on the contrary as powerful inhibitors of cell activity." Jansson G. Oestrogen-induced enhancement of myeloperoxidase activity in human polymorphonuclear leukocytes--a possible cause of oxidative stress in inflammatory cells. *Free Radic Res Commun.* 1991;14(3):195-208

[174] "Even more dramatically, in the case of laryngeal papillomas induction of 2-hydroxylation with indole-3-carbinol (I3C) has resulted in inhibition of tumor growth during the time that the patients continue to take I3C or vegetables rich in this compound." Bradlow HL, Telang NT, Sepkovic DW, Osborne MP. 2-hydroxyestrone: the 'good' estrogen. *J Endocrinol.* 1996 Sep;150 Suppl:S259-65

[175] "Women with SLE can manifest a metabolic response to I3C and might benefit from its antiestrogenic effects." McAlindon TE, Gulin J, Chen T, Klug T, Lahita R, Nuite M. Indole-3-carbinol in women with SLE: effect on estrogen metabolism and disease activity. *Lupus.* 2001;10(11):779-83

[176] Male Hormone Modulation Therapy, Page 4 Of 7: http://www.lef.org/protocols/prtcl-130c.shtml Accessed October 30, 2005

[177] "These data demonstrate that aromatase inhibition increases serum bioavailable and total testosterone levels to the youthful normal range in older men with mild hypogonadism." Leder BZ, Rohrer JL, Rubin SD, Gallo J, Longcope C. Effects of aromatase inhibition in elderly men with low or borderline-low serum testosterone levels. *J Clin Endocrinol Metab.* 2004 Mar;89(3):1174-80 http://jcem.endojournals.org/cgi/reprint/89/3/1174

[178] "Yet evidence that patients with rheumatoid arthritis improved with small, physiologic dosages of cortisol or cortisone acetate was reported over 25 years ago, and that patients with chronic allergic disorders or unexplained chronic fatigue also improved with administration of such small dosages was reported over 15 years ago..." Jefferies WM. Mild adrenocortical deficiency, chronic allergies, autoimmune disorders and the chronic fatigue syndrome: a continuation of the cortisone story. *Med Hypotheses.* 1994 Mar;42(3):183-9 http://www.thebuteykocentre.com/Irish_%20Buteykocenter_files/further_studies/med_hyp2.pdf http://members.westnet.com.au/pkolb/med_hyp2.pdf

Chapter 4 under the section of Orthoendocrinology. Supplementation with 20 mg per day of cortisol/Cortef is physiologic; my preference is to dose 10 mg first thing in the morning, then 5 mg in late morning and 5 mg in midafternoon in an attempt to replicate the diurnal variation and normal morning peak of cortisol levels. In patients with hypoadrenalism, administration of pregnenolone in doses of 10-60 mg in the morning may also be beneficial.

- Testosterone (insufficiency): Androgen deficiencies predispose to, are exacerbated by, and contribute to autoimmune/inflammatory disorders. A large proportion of men with lupus or RA have low testosterone[181] and suffer the effects of hypogonadism: fatigue, weakness, depression, slow healing, low libido, and difficulties with sexual performance. Testosterone levels may rise following DHEA supplementation (especially in women) and can be elevated in men by the use of anastrozole/arimidex. Otherwise, transdermal testosterone such as Androgel or Testim can be applied as indicated.

- DHEA (insufficiency / supraphysiologic supplementation): DHEA is an anti-inflammatory and immunoregulatory hormone that is commonly deficient in patients with autoimmunity and inflammatory arthritis.[182] DHEA levels are suppressed by prednisone[183], and DHEA supplementation has been shown to reverse the osteoporosis and loss of bone mass induced by corticosteroid treatment.[184] DHEA shows no acute or subacute toxicity even when used in supraphysiologic doses, even when used in sick patients. For example, in a study of 32 patients with HIV, DHEA doses of 750 mg – 2,250 mg per day were well-tolerated and produced no dose-limiting adverse effects.[185] This lack of toxicity compares favorably with any and all so-called "antirheumatic" drugs, nearly all of which show impressive comparable toxicity. When used at doses of 200 mg per day, DHEA safely provides clinical benefit for patients with various autoimmune diseases, including ulcerative colitis, Crohn's disease[186], and SLE.[187] In patients with SLE, DHEA supplementation allows for reduced dosing of prednisone (thus avoiding its adverse effects) while providing symptomatic improvement.[188] Optimal clinical response appears to correlate with serum levels that are supraphysiologic[189], and therefore treatment may be implemented with little regard for initial/baseline DHEA levels provided that the patient is free of contraindications, particularly high risk for sex-hormone-dependent malignancy. Other than mild adverse effects predictable with any androgen (namely voice deepening, transient acne, and increased facial hair), DHEA supplementation does not cause serious adverse effects[190], and it is appropriate for routine clinical use particularly when 1) the dose of DHEA is kept as low as possible, 2) duration is kept as short as possible, 3) other interventions are used to address the underlying cause of the disease, 4) the patient is deriving benefit, and 5) the risk-to-benefit ratio is favorable.

- Thyroid (insufficiency or autoimmunity): Overt or imminent hypothyroidism is suggested by TSH greater than 2 mU/L[191] or 3 mU/L[192], low T4 or T3, and/or the presence of anti-thyroid

---

[179] "The etiology of rheumatoid arthritis …explained by a combination of three factors: (i) a relatively mild deficiency of cortisol, …, (ii) a deficiency of DHEA, …and (iii) infection by organisms such as mycoplasma,..." Jefferies WM. The etiology of rheumatoid arthritis. *Med Hypotheses.* 1998 Aug;51(2):111-4

[180] Jefferies W McK. Safe Uses of Cortisol. Second Edition. Springfield, CC Thomas, 1996

[181] Karagiannis A, Harsoulis F. Gonadal dysfunction in systemic diseases. *Eur J Endocrinol.* 2005 Apr;152(4):501-13 http://www.eje-online.org/cgi/content/full/152/4/501

[182] "DHEAS concentrations were significantly decreased in both women and men with inflammatory arthritis (IA) (P < 0.001)." Dessein PH, Joffe BI, Stanwix AE, Moomal Z. Hyposecretion of the adrenal androgen dehydroepiandrosterone sulfate and its relation to clinical variables in inflammatory arthritis. *Arthritis Res.* 2001;3(3):183-8. Epub 2001 Feb 21. http://arthritis-research.com/content/3/3/183

[183] "Basal serum DHEA and DHEAS concentrations were suppressed to a greater degree than was cortisol during both daily and alternate day prednisone treatments. ...Thus, adrenal androgen secretion was more easily suppressed than was cortisol secretion by this low dose of glucocorticoid, but there was no advantage to alternate day therapy." Rittmaster RS, Givner ML. Effect of daily and alternate day low dose prednisone on serum cortisol and adrenal androgens in hirsute women. *J Clin Endocrinol Metab.* 1988 Aug;67(2):400-3

[184] "CONCLUSION: Prasterone treatment prevented BMD loss and significantly increased BMD at both the lumbar spine and total hip in female patients with SLE receiving exogenous glucocorticoids." Mease PJ, Ginzler EM, Gluck OS, Schiff M, Goldman A, Greenwald M, Cohen S, Egan R, Quarles BJ, Schwartz KE. Effects of prasterone on bone mineral density in women with systemic lupus erythematosus receiving chronic glucocorticoid therapy. *J Rheumatol.* 2005 Apr;32(4):616-21

[185] "Thirty-one subjects were evaluated and monitored for safety and tolerance. The oral drug was administered three times daily in doses ranging from 750 mg/day to 2,250 mg/day for 16 weeks. ... The drug was well tolerated and no dose-limiting side effects were noted." Dyner TS, Lang W, Geaga J, Golub A, Stites D, Winger E, Galmarini M, Masterson J, Jacobson MA. An open-label dose-escalation trial of oral dehydroepiandrosterone tolerance and pharmacokinetics in patients with HIV disease. *J Acquir Immune Defic Syndr.* 1993 May;6(5):459-65

[186] "CONCLUSIONS: In a pilot study, dehydroepiandrosterone was effective and safe in patients with refractory Crohn's disease or ulcerative colitis." Andus T, Klebl F, Rogler G, Bregenzer N, Scholmerich J, Straub RH. Patients with refractory Crohn's disease or ulcerative colitis respond to dehydroepiandrosterone: a pilot study. *Aliment Pharmacol Ther.* 2003 Feb;17(3):409-14

[187] "CONCLUSION: The overall results confirm that DHEA treatment was well-tolerated, significantly reduced the number of SLE flares, and improved patient's global assessment of disease activity." Chang DM, Lan JL, Lin HY, Luo SF. Dehydroepiandrosterone treatment of women with mild-to-moderate systemic lupus erythematosus: a multicenter randomized, double-blind, placebo-controlled trial. *Arthritis Rheum.* 2002 Nov;46(11):2924-7

[188] "CONCLUSION: Among women with lupus disease activity, reducing the dosage of prednisone to < or = 7.5 mg/day for a sustained period of time while maintaining stabilization or a reduction of disease activity was possible in a significantly greater proportion of patients treated with oral prasterone, 200 mg once daily, compared with patients treated with placebo." Petri MA, Lahita RG, Van Vollenhoven RF, Merrill JT, Schiff M, Ginzler EM, Strand V, Kunz A, Gorelick KJ, Schwartz KE; GL601 Study Group. Effects of prasterone on corticosteroid requirements of women with systemic lupus erythematosus: a double-blind, randomized, placebo-controlled trial. *Arthritis Rheum.* 2002 Jul;46(7):1820-9

[189] "CONCLUSION: The clinical response to DHEA was not clearly dose dependent. Serum levels of DHEA and DHEAS correlated only weakly with lupus outcomes, but suggested an optimum serum DHEAS of 1000 microg/dl." Barry NN, McGuire JL, van Vollenhoven RF. Dehydroepiandrosterone in systemic lupus erythematosus: relationship between dosage, serum levels, and clinical response. *J Rheumatol.* 1998 Dec;25(12):2352-6

[190] Tierney ML. McPhee SJ, Papadakis MA. Current Medical Diagnosis and Treatment 2006. 45th edition. New York; Lange Medical Books; 2006, page 1721

[191] Weetman AP. Hypothyroidism: screening and subclinical disease. *BMJ.* 1997 Apr 19;314(7088):1175-8 http://bmj.bmjjournals.com/cgi/content/full/314/7088/1175

peroxidase antibodies.[193] Hypothyroidism can cause an inflammatory myopathy that can resemble polymyositis, and hypothyroidism is a frequent complication of any and all autoimmune diseases. Specific treatment considerations include the following:

- Selenium: Supplementation with either selenomethonine[194] or sodium selenite[195,196] can reduce thyroid autoimmunity and improve peripheral conversion of T4 to T3. Selenium may be started at 500-800 mcg per day and tapered to 200-400 mcg per day for maintenance.[197]

- L-thyroxine/levothyroxine/Synthroid—prescription synthetic T4: 25-50 mcg per day is a common starting dose which can be adjusted based on clinical and laboratory response. Thyroid hormone supplements must be consumed separately from soy products (by at least 1-2 hours) and preferably on an empty stomach to avoid absorption interference by food, fiber, and minerals, especially calcium. Doses are generally started at one-half of the daily dose for the first 10 days after which the full dose is used. Caution must be applied in patients with adrenal insufficiency and/or those with cardiovascular disease.

- Armour thyroid—prescription natural T4 and T3 from cow/pig thyroid gland: 60 mg (one grain) is a common starting and maintenance dose. Due to the exacerbating effect on thyroid autoimmunity, Armour thyroid is never used in patients with thyroid autoimmunity.

- Thyrolar/Liotrix—prescription synthetic T4 with T3: Dosed as "1" (low), "2" (intermediate), or "3" (high). Although this product has been difficult to obtain for the past few years due to manufacturing problems (http://thyrolar.com/), it has been my treatment of choice due to the combination of T4 and T3 and the lack of antigenicity compared to gland-derived products.

- Thyroid glandular—nonprescription T3: Producers of nutritional products are able to distribute T3 because it is not listed by the FDA as a prescription item. Nutritional supplement companies may start with Armour thyroid, remove the T4, and sell the thyroid glandular with active T3 thereby providing a nonprescription source of active thyroid hormone. For many patients, one tablet per day is at least as effective as a prescription source of thyroid hormone. Since it is derived from a glandular and therefore potentially antigenic source, thyroid glandular is not used in patients with thyroid autoimmunity due to its ability to induce increased production of anti-thyroid antibodies.

- L-tyrosine and iodine: Some patients with mild hypothyroidism respond to supplementation with L-tyrosine and iodine. Tyrosine is commonly used in doses of 4-9 grams per day in divided doses. According to Abraham and Wright[198], doses of iodine may be as high as 12.5 milligrams (12,500 micrograms), which is slightly less than the average daily intake in Japan at 13.8 mg per day.

- Oral enzyme therapy with proteolytic/pancreatic enzymes: Polyenzyme supplementation is used to ameliorate the pathophysiology induced by immune complexes, such as rheumatoid arthritis.[199]
- Anti-inflammatory botanicals:
    - *Uncaria tomentosa, Uncaria guianensis*: Cat's claw has been safely and successfully used in the treatment of osteoarthritis[200] and rheumatoid arthritis.[201] High-quality extractions from reputable

[192] "Now AACE encourages doctors to consider treatment for patients who test outside the boundaries of a narrower margin based on a target TSH level of 0.3 to 3.0. AACE believes the new range will result in proper diagnosis for millions of Americans who suffer from a mild thyroid disorder, but have gone untreated until now." American Association of Clinical Endocrinologists (AACE). 2003 Campaign Encourages Awareness of Mild Thyroid Failure, Importance of Routine Testing http://www.aace.com/pub/tam2003/press.php November 26, 2005
[193] Beers MH, Berkow R (eds). The Merck Manual. Seventeenth Edition. Whitehouse Station; Merck Research Laboratories 1999 Page 96
[194] Duntas LH, Mantzou E, Koutras DA. Effects of a six month treatment with selenomethionine in patients with autoimmune thyroiditis. *Eur J Endocrinol.* 2003 Apr;148(4):389-93 http://eje-online.org/cgi/reprint/148/4/389
[195] Gartner R, Gasnier BC, Dietrich JW, Krebs B, Angstwurm MW. Selenium supplementation in patients with autoimmune thyroiditis decreases thyroid peroxidase antibodies concentrations. *J Clin Endocrinol Metab.* 2002 Apr;87(4):1687-91 http://jcem.endojournals.org/cgi/content/full/87/4/1687
[196] "We recently conducted a prospective, placebo-controlled clinical study, where we could demonstrate, that a substitution of 200 wg sodium selenite for three months in patients with autoimmune thyroiditis reduced thyroid peroxidase antibody (TPO-Ab) concentrations significantly." Gartner R, Gasnier BC. Selenium in the treatment of autoimmune thyroiditis. *Biofactors.* 2003;19(3-4):165-70
[197] Bruns F, Micke O, Bremer M. Current status of selenium and other treatments for secondary lymphedema. *J Support Oncol.* 2003 Jul-Aug;1(2):121-30 http://www.supportiveoncology.net/journal/articles/0102121.pdf
[198] Wright JV. Why you need 83 times more of this essential, cancer-fighting nutrient than the "experts" say you do. *Nutrition and Healing* 2005; volume 12, issue 4.
[199] Galebskaya LV, Ryumina EV, Niemerovsky VS, Matyukov AA. Human complement system state after wobenzyme intake. *VESTNIK MOSKOVSKOGO UNIVERSITETA. KHIMIYA.* 2000. Vol. 41, No. 6. Supplement. Pages 148-149
[200] Piscoya J, Rodriguez Z, Bustamante SA, Okuhama NN, Miller MJ, Sandoval M.Efficacy and safety of freeze-dried cat's claw in osteoarthritis of the knee: mechanisms of action of the species Uncaria guianensis. *Inflamm Res.* 2001 Sep;50(9):442-8
[201] "This small preliminary study demonstrates relative safety and modest benefit to the tender joint count of a highly purified extract from the pentacyclic chemotype of UT in patients with active RA taking sulfasalazine or hydroxychloroquine." Mur E, Hartig F, Eibl G, Schirmer M. Randomized double blind trial of an extract from the pentacyclic alkaloid-chemotype of uncaria tomentosa for the treatment of rheumatoid arthritis. *J Rheumatol.* 2002 Apr;29(4):678-81

manufacturers used according to directions are recommended. Most products contain between 250-500 mg and are standardized to 3.0% alkaloids and 15% total polyphenols; QD-TID po dosing should be sufficient as *part* of a comprehensive plan.

- o *Harpagophytum procumbens*: Harpagophytum is a moderately effective botanical analgesic.[202,203,204,205,206] Products are generally standardized for the content of harpagosides, with a target dose of 60 mg harpagoside per day.[207]

- o Willow bark: Extracts from willow bark have proven safe and effective in the alleviation of moderate/severe low-back pain.[208,209] The mechanism of action appears to be inhibition of prostaglandin formation via inhibition of cyclooxygenase-2 gene transcription[210] by salicylates, phytonutrients which are widely present in fruits, vegetables, herbs and spices and which are partly responsible for the anti-cancer, anti-inflammatory, and health-promoting benefits of plant consumption.[211,212] According to a letter by Vasquez and Muanza[213], the only adverse effect that has been documented in association with willow bark was a single case of anaphylaxis in a patient previously sensitized to acetylsalicylic acid.

- o *Boswellia serrata*: *Boswellia* shows clear anti-inflammatory and analgesic action via inhibition of 5-lipoxygenase[214] and clinical benefits have been demonstrated in patients with osteoarthritis of the knees[215] as well as asthma[216] and ulcerative colitis.[217] Products are generally standardized to contain 37.5–65% boswellic acids, with a target dose is approximately 150 mg of boswellic acids TID; dose and number of capsules/tablets will vary depending upon the concentration found in differing products. A German study showing that *Boswellia* was ineffective for rheumatoid arthritis[218] was poorly conducted, with inadequate follow-up, inadequate controls, and abnormal dosing of the herb.

- Phytonutritional modulation of NF-kappaB: As a stimulator of pro-inflammatory gene transcription, NF-kappaB is almost universally activated in conditions associated with inflammation.[219,220] As we would expect, NF-kappaB plays a central role in the pathogenesis of synovitis and joint destruction seen in RA.[221] Nutrients and botanicals which either directly or indirectly inhibit NF-kappaB for an anti-inflammatory benefit include vitamin D[222,223], curcumin[224] (requires piperine for absorption[225]), lipoic acid[226], green tea[227], rosemary[228], grape seed extract[229], propolis[230], zinc[231], high-dose selenium[232], indole-3-carbinol[233,234], N-acetyl-

[202] Chrubasik S, Thanner J, Kunzel O, Conradt C, Black A, Pollak S. Comparison of outcome measures during treatment with the proprietary Harpagophytum extract doloteffin in patients with pain in the lower back, knee or hip. *Phytomedicine* 2002 Apr;9(3):181-94

[203] Chantre P, Cappelaere A, Leblan D, Guedon D, Vandermander J, Fournie B. Efficacy and tolerance of Harpagophytum procumbens versus diacerhein in treatment of osteoarthritis. *Phytomedicine* 2000 Jun;7(3):177-83

[204] Leblan D, Chantre P, Fournie B. Harpagophytum procumbens in the treatment of knee and hip osteoarthritis. Four-month results of a prospective, multicenter, double-blind trial versus diacerhein. *Joint Bone Spine* 2000;67(5):462-7

[205] "...subgroup analyses suggested that the effect was confined to patients with more severe and radiating pain accompanied by neurological deficit. ...a slightly different picture, with the benefits seeming, if anything, to be greatest in the H600 group and in patients without more severe pain, radiation or neurological deficit." Chrubasik S, Junck H, Breitschwerdt H, Conradt C, Zappe H. Effectiveness of Harpagophytum extract WS 1531 in the treatment of exacerbation of low back pain: a randomized, placebo-controlled, double-blind study. *Eur J Anaesthesiol* 1999 Feb;16(2):118-29

[206] Chrubasik S, Model A, Black A, Pollak S. A randomized double-blind pilot study comparing Doloteffin and Vioxx in the treatment of low back pain. *Rheumatology* (Oxford). 2003 Jan;42(1):141-8

[207] "They took an 8-week course of Doloteffin at a dose providing 60 mg harpagoside per day... Doloteffin is well worth considering for osteoarthritic knee and hip pain and nonspecific low back pain." Chrubasik S, Thanner J, Kunzel O, Conradt C, Black A, Pollak S. Comparison of outcome measures during treatment with the proprietary Harpagophytum extract doloteffin in patients with pain in the lower back, knee or hip. *Phytomedicine* 2002 Apr;9(3):181-94

[208] Chrubasik S, Eisenberg E, Balan E, Weinberger T, Luzzati R, Conradt C. Treatment of low-back pain exacerbations with willow bark extract: a randomized double-blind study. *Am J Med*. 2000;109:9-14

[209] Chrubasik S, Kunzel O, Model A, Conradt C, Black A. Treatment of low-back pain with a herbal or synthetic anti-rheumatic: a randomized controlled study. Willow bark extract for low-back pain. *Rheumatology* (Oxford). 2001;40:1388-93

[210] Hare LG, Woodside JV, Young IS. Dietary salicylates. *J Clin Pathol* 2003 Sep;56(9):649-50

[211] Lawrence JR, Peter R, Baxter GJ, Robson J, Graham AB, Paterson JR. Urinary excretion of salicyluric and salicylic acids by non-vegetarians, vegetarians, and patients taking low dose aspirin. *J Clin Pathol*. 2003 Sep;56(9):651-3

[212] Paterson JR, Lawrence JR. Salicylic acid: a link between aspirin, diet and the prevention of colorectal cancer. *QJM*. 2001 Aug;94(8):445-8

[213] Vasquez A, Muanza DN. Evaluation of Presence of Aspirin-Related Warnings with Willow Bark: Comment on the Article by Clauson et al. *Ann Pharmacotherapy* 2005 Oct;39(10):1763

[214] Wildfeuer A, Neu IS, Safayhi H, Metzger G, Wehrmann M, Vogel U, Ammon HP. Effects of boswellic acids extracted from a herbal medicine on the biosynthesis of leukotrienes and the course of experimental autoimmune encephalomyelitis. *Arzneimittelforschung* 1998 Jun;48(6):668-74

[215] Kimmatkar N, Thawani V, Hingorani L, Khiyani R. Efficacy and tolerability of Boswellia serrata extract in treatment of osteoarthritis of knee--a randomized double blind placebo controlled trial. *Phytomedicine*. 2003 Jan;10(1):3-7

[216] Gupta I, Gupta V, Parihar A, Gupta S, Ludtke R, Safayhi H, Ammon HP. Effects of Boswellia serrata gum resin in patients with bronchial asthma: results of a double-blind, placebo-controlled, 6-week clinical study. *Eur J Med Res*. 1998 Nov 17;3(11):511-4

[217] Gupta I, Parihar A, Malhotra P, Singh GB, Ludtke R, Safayhi H, Ammon HP. Effects of Boswellia serrata gum resin in patients with ulcerative colitis. *Eur J Med Res*. 1997 Jan;2(1):37-43

[218] Sander O, Herborn G, Rau R. [Is H15 (resin extract of Boswellia serrata, "incense") a useful supplement to established drug therapy of chronic polyarthritis? Results of a double-blind pilot study] [Article in German] *Z Rheumatol*. 1998 Feb;57(1):11-6

[219] Tak PP, Firestein GS. NF-kappaB: a key role in inflammatory diseases. *J Clin Invest*. 2001 Jan;107(1):7-11 http://www.jci.org/cgi/content/full/107/1/7

[220] D'Acquisto F, May MJ, Ghosh S. Inhibition of Nuclear Factor KappaB (NF-B): An Emerging Theme in Anti-Inflammatory Therapies. *Mol Interv*. 2002 Feb;2(1):22-35 http://molinterv.aspetjournals.org/cgi/content/abstract/2/1/22

[221] "NF-B plays a central role in the pathogenesis of synovitis in RA and PsA." Foell D, Kane D, Bresnihan B, Vogl T, Nacken W, Sorg C, Fitzgerald O, Roth J. Expression of the pro-inflammatory protein S100A12 (EN-RAGE) in rheumatoid and psoriatic arthritis. *Rheumatology* (Oxford). 2003 Nov;42(11):1383-9 http://rheumatology.oxfordjournals.org/cgi/content/full/42/11/1383

[222] "1Alpha,25-dihydroxyvitamin D3 (1,25-(OH)2-D3), the active metabolite of vitamin D, can inhibit NF-kappaB activity in human MRC-5 fibroblasts, targeting DNA binding of NF-kappaB but not translocation of its subunits p50 and p65." Harant H, Wolff B, Lindley IJ. 1Alpha,25-dihydroxyvitamin D3 decreases DNA binding of nuclear factor-kappaB in human fibroblasts. *FEBS Lett*. 1998 Oct 9;436(3):329-34

[223] "Thus, 1,25(OH)2D3 may negatively regulate IL-12 production by downregulation of NF-kB activation and binding to the p40-kB sequence." D'Ambrosio D, Cippitelli M, Cocciolo MG, Mazzeo D, Di Lucia P, Lang R, Sinigaglia F, Panina-Bordignon P. Inhibition of IL-12 production by 1,25-dihydroxyvitamin D3. Involvement of NF-kappaB downregulation in transcriptional repression of the p40 gene. *J Clin Invest*. 1998 Jan 1;101(1):252-62

[224] "Curcumin, EGCG and resveratrol have been shown to suppress activation of NF-kappa B." Surh YJ, Chun KS, Cha HH, Han SS, Keum YS, Park KK, Lee SS. Molecular mechanisms underlying chemopreventive activities of anti-inflammatory phytochemicals: down-regulation of COX-2 and iNOS through suppression of NF-kappa B activation. *Mutat Res*. 2001 Sep 1;480-481:243-68

[225] Shoba G, Joy D, Joseph T, Majeed M, Rajendran R, Srinivas PS. Influence of piperine on the pharmacokinetics of curcumin in animals and human volunteers. *Planta Med*. 1998 May;64(4):353-6

[226] "ALA reduced the TNF-alpha-induced ICAM-1 expression in a dose-dependent manner, to levels observed in unstimulated cells. Alpha-lipoic acid also reduced NF-kappaB activity in these cells in a dose-dependent manner." Lee HA, Hughes DA. Alpha-lipoic acid modulates NF-kappaB activity in human monocytic cells by direct interaction with DNA. *Exp Gerontol*. 2002 Jan-Mar;37(2-3):401-10

[227] "In conclusion, EGCG is an effective inhibitor of IKK activity. This may explain, at least in part, some of the reported anti-inflammatory and anticancer effects of green tea." Yang F, Oz HS, Barve S, de Villiers WJ, McClain CJ, Varilek GW. The green tea polyphenol (-)-epigallocatechin-3-gallate blocks nuclear factor-kappa B activation by inhibiting I kappa B kinase activity in the intestinal epithelial cell line IEC-6. *Mol Pharmacol*. 2001 Sep;60(3):528-33

[228] "These results suggest that carnosol suppresses the NO production and iNOS gene expression by inhibiting NF-kappaB activation, and provide possible mechanisms for its anti-inflammatory and chemopreventive action." Lo AH, Liang YC, Lin-Shiau SY, Ho CT, Lin JK. Carnosol, an antioxidant in rosemary, suppresses inducible nitric oxide synthase through down-regulating nuclear factor-kappaB in mouse macrophages. *Carcinogenesis*. 2002 Jun;23(6):983-91

L-cysteine[235], resveratrol[236,237], isohumulones[238], GLA via PPAR-gamma[239] and EPA via PPAR-alpha.[240] I have reviewed the phytonutritional modulation of NF-kappaB later in this text and elsewhere.[241] Several phytonutritional products targeting NF-kappaB are available.

- <u>Glucosamine sulfate and chondroitin sulfate</u>: Glucosamine and chondroitin sulfates are well tolerated and well documented in the treatment of osteoarthritis.[242,243,244,245] Since these serve as substrate for the "rebuilding" and preservation of joint cartilage, they would clearly help shift the balance toward anabolism and away from catabolism within articular tissues.

- <u>Topical *Capsicum annuum, Capsicum frutescens* (Cayenne pepper, hot chili pepper)</u>: Controlled clinical trials have conclusively demonstrated capsaicin's ability to deplete sensory fibers of the neuropeptide **substance P** and to thus reduce pain. Topical capsaicin has been proven effective in relieving the pain associated with diabetic neuropathy[246], chronic low back pain[247], chronic neck pain[248], osteoarthritis[249], and rheumatoid arthritis.[250] Given the important role of neurogenic inflammation in chronic arthritis[251,252], the use of topical *Capsicum* should not be viewed as merely symptomatic; by depleting neurons of substance P it has the ability to help break the vicious cycle of neurogenic-immunogenic inflammation.

Notes:

_____

_____

_____

_____

_____

_____

_____

_____

[229] "Constitutive and TNFalpha-induced NF-kappaB DNA binding activity was inhibited by GSE at doses > or =50 microg/ml and treatments for > or =12 h." Dhanalakshmi S, Agarwal R, Agarwal C. Inhibition of NF-kappaB pathway in grape seed extract-induced apoptotic death of human prostate carcinoma DU145 cells. *Int J Oncol.* 2003 Sep;23(3):721-7

[230] "Caffeic acid phenethyl ester (CAPE) is an anti-inflammatory component of propolis (honeybee resin). CAPE is reportedly a specific inhibitor of nuclear factor-kappaB (NF-kappaB)." Fitzpatrick LR, Wang J, Le T. Caffeic acid phenethyl ester, an inhibitor of nuclear factor-kappaB, attenuates bacterial peptidoglycan polysaccharide-induced colitis in rats. *J Pharmacol Exp Ther.* 2001 Dec;299(3):915-20

[231] "Our results suggest that zinc supplementation may lead to downregulation of the inflammatory cytokines through upregulation of the negative feedback loop A20 to inhibit induced NF-kappaB activation." Prasad AS, Bao B, Beck FW, Kucuk O, Sarkar FH. Antioxidant effect of zinc in humans. *Free Radic Biol Med.* 2004 Oct 15;37(8):1182-90

[232] Note that the patients in this study received a very high dose of selenium: 960 micrograms per day. This is at the top—and some would say over the top—of the safe and reasonable dose for long-term supplementation. In this case, the study lasted for three months. "In patients receiving selenium supplementation, selenium NF-kappaB activity was significantly reduced, reaching the same level as the nondiabetic control group. CONCLUSION: In type 2 diabetic patients, activation of NF-kappaB measured in peripheral blood monocytes can be reduced by selenium supplementation, confirming its importance in the prevention of cardiovascular diseases." Faure P, Ramon O, Favier A, Halimi S. Selenium supplementation decreases nuclear factor-kappa B activity in peripheral blood mononuclear cells from type 2 diabetic patients. *Eur J Clin Invest.* 2004 Jul;34(7):475-81

[233] Takada Y, Andreeff M, Aggarwal BB. Indole-3-carbinol suppresses NF-{kappa}B and I{kappa}B{alpha} kinase activation causing inhibition of expression of NF-{kappa}B-regulated antiapoptotic and metastatic gene products and enhancement of apoptosis in myeloid and leukemia cells. *Blood.* 2005 Apr 5; [Epub ahead of print]

[234] "Overall, our results indicated that indole-3-carbinol inhibits NF-kappaB and NF-kappaB-regulated gene expression and that this mechanism may provide the molecular basis for its ability to suppress tumorigenesis." Takada Y, Andreeff M, Aggarwal BB. Indole-3-carbinol suppresses NF-kappaB and IkappaBalpha kinase activation, causing inhibition of expression of NF-kappaB-regulated antiapoptotic and metastatic gene products and enhancement of apoptosis in myeloid and leukemia cells. *Blood.* 2005 Jul 15;106(2):641-9. Epub 2005 Apr 5.

[235] "CONCLUSIONS: Administration of N-acetylcysteine results in decreased nuclear factor-kappa B activation in patients with sepsis, associated with decreases in interleukin-8 but not interleukin-6 or soluble intercellular adhesion molecule-1. These pilot data suggest that antioxidant therapy with N-acetylcysteine may be useful in blunting the inflammatory response to sepsis." Paterson RL, Galley HF, Webster NR. The effect of N-acetylcysteine on nuclear factor-kappa B activation, interleukin-6, interleukin-8, and intercellular adhesion molecule-1 expression in patients with sepsis. *Crit Care Med.* 2003 Nov;31(11):2574-8

[236] "Resveratrol's anticarcinogenic, anti-inflammatory, and growth-modulatory effects may thus be partially ascribed to the inhibition of activation of NF-kappaB and AP-1 and the associated kinases." Manna SK, Mukhopadhyay A, Aggarwal BB. Resveratrol suppresses TNF-induced activation of nuclear transcription factors NF-kappa B, activator protein-1, and apoptosis: potential role of reactive oxygen intermediates and lipid peroxidation. *J Immunol.* 2000 Jun 15;164(12):6509-19

[237] "Both resveratrol and quercetin inhibited NF-kappaB-, AP-1- and CREB-dependent transcription to a greater extent than the glucocorticosteroid, dexamethasone." Donnelly LE, Newton R, Kennedy GE, Fenwick PS, Leung RH, Ito K, Russell RE, Barnes PJ. Anti-inflammatory Effects of Resveratrol in Lung Epithelial Cells: Molecular Mechanisms. *Am J Physiol Lung Cell Mol Physiol.* 2004 Jun 4 [Epub ahead of print]

[238] Yajima H, Ikeshima E, Shiraki M, Kanaya T, Fujiwara D, Odai H, Tsuboyama-Kasaoka N, Ezaki O, Oikawa S, Kondo K. Isohumulones, bitter acids derived from hops, activate both peroxisome proliferator-activated receptor alpha and gamma and reduce insulin resistance. *J Biol Chem.* 2004 Aug 6;279(32):33456-62. Epub 2004 Jun 3. http://www.jbc.org/cgi/content/full/279/32/33456

[239] "Thus, PPAR gamma serves as the receptor for GLA in the regulation of gene expression in breast cancer cells. " Jiang WG, Redfern A, Bryce RP, Mansel RE. Peroxisome proliferator activated receptor-gamma (PPAR gamma) mediates the action of gamma linolenic acid in breast cancer cells. *Prostaglandins Leukot Essent Fatty Acids.* 2000 Feb;62(2):119-27

[240] "...EPA requires PPARalpha for its inhibitory effects on NF-kappaB." Mishra A, Chaudhary A, Sethi S. Oxidized omega-3 fatty acids inhibit NF-kappaB activation via a PPARalpha-dependent pathway. *Arterioscler Thromb Vasc Biol.* 2004 Sep;24(9):1621-7. Epub 2004 Jul 1. http://atvb.ahajournals.org/cgi/content/full/24/9/1621

[241] "Indeed, the previous view that nutrients only interact with human physiology at the metabolic/post-transcriptional level must be updated in light of current research showing that nutrients can, in fact, modify human physiology and phenotype at the genetic/pre-transcriptional level." Vasquez A. Reducing pain and inflammation naturally - part 4: nutritional and botanical inhibition of NF-kappaB, the major intracellular amplifier of the inflammatory cascade. A practical clinical strategy exemplifying anti-inflammatory nutrigenomics. *Nutritional Perspectives,* July 2005:5-12. www.OptimalHealthResearch.com/part4

[242] Braham R, Dawson B, Goodman C. The effect of glucosamine supplementation on people experiencing regular knee pain. *Br J Sports Med.* 2003;37(1):45-9

[243] Nguyen P, Mohamed SE, Gardiner D, Salinas T. A randomized double-blind clinical trial of the effect of chondroitin sulfate and glucosamine hydrochloride on temporomandibular joint disorders: a pilot study. *Cranio.* 2001 Apr;19(2):130-9

[244] "...oral glucosamine therapy achieved a significantly greater improvement in articular pain score than ibuprofen, and the investigators rated treatment efficacy as 'good' in a significantly greater proportion of glucosamine than ibuprofen recipients. ...while glucosamine significantly improved arthritic symptoms after 12 weeks of therapy..." Matheson AJ, Perry CM. Glucosamine: a review of its use in the management of osteoarthritis. *Drugs Aging.* 2003; 20(14): 1041-60

[245] Muller-Fassbender H, Bach GL, Haase W, Rovati LC, Setnikar I. Glucosamine sulfate compared to ibuprofen in osteoarthritis of the knee. *Osteoarthritis Cartilage.* 1994 Mar;2(1):61-9

[246] Treatment of painful diabetic neuropathy with topical capsaicin. A multicenter, double-blind, vehicle-controlled study. The Capsaicin Study Group. [No authors listed] *Arch Intern Med.* 1991 Nov;151(11):2225-9

[247] Keitel W, Frerick H, Kuhn U, Schmidt U, Kuhlmann M, Bredehorst A. Capsicum pain plaster in chronic non-specific low back pain. *Arzneimittelforschung.* 2001 Nov;51(11):896-903

[248] Mathias BJ, Dillingham TR, Zeigler DN, Chang AS, Belandres PV. Topical capsaicin for chronic neck pain. A pilot study. *Am J Phys Med Rehabil* 1995 Jan-Feb;74(1):39-44

[249] McCarthy GM, McCarty DJ. Effect of topical capsaicin in the therapy of painful osteoarthritis of the hands. *J Rheumatol.* 1992;19(4):604-7

[250] Deal CL, Schnitzer TJ, Lipstein E, Seibold JR, Stevens RM, Levy MD, Albert D, Renold F. Treatment of arthritis with topical capsaicin: a double-blind trial. *Clin Ther.* 1991 May-Jun;13(3):383-95

[251] Gouze-Decaris E, Philippe L, Minn A, Haouzi P, Gillet P, Netter P, Terlain B. Neurophysiological basis for neurogenic-mediated articular cartilage anabolism alteration. *Am J Physiol Regul Integr Comp Physiol.* 2001;280(1):R115-22 http://ajpregu.physiology.org/cgi/content/full/280/1/R115

[252] Decaris E, Guingamp C, Chat M, Philippe L, Grillasca JP, Abid A, Minn A, Gillet P, Netter P, Terlain B. Evidence for neurogenic transmission inducing degenerative cartilage damage distant from local inflammation. *Arthritis Rheum.* 1999;42(9):1951-60

Vertebral Osteomyelitis
Infectious Discitis

Description/pathophysiology:
- Bacterial or fungal infection of the spine
- Back pain is common; spinal infection is relatively rare. Spinal infections are "a rare cause of common symptoms."[253]

Clinical presentations:
- Classic presentation: "...the diagnosis is suggested by the clinical findings: a sick patient with severe pain, a rigid back, fever, and a raised WBC and sedimentation rate."[254]
  - Patient generally appears sick with systemic manifestations: fatigue, sweats, anorexia, fever
  - Back/neck/spine pain (90%): Most common region for spinal osteomyelitis is the lumbar spine, followed by the thoracic spine, then the cervical spine. Cervical spine infections are more common in IV drug abusers
  - Pain may be acute, subacute, or chronic:
    - 30% of patients with vertebral osteomyelitis have had pain for 3 weeks to 3 months at time of diagnosis
    - 50% of patients with vertebral osteomyelitis have had pain for more than 3 months at time of diagnosis
  - Pain is continuous, intermittent, and/or "throbbing" and often worse at night
  - Pain is unrelated to motion or position (non-mechanical)
  - Localized stiffness
  - Elevated ESR/CRP
  - Vertebral osteomyelitis is more common in patients with a history of recurrent urinary tract infections and diabetes mellitus
- Atypical presentations: as many as 15% of affected patients
  - Little or no fever
  - Little or no back or neck pain
  - Little or no local tenderness
  - Cervical osteomyelitis may present with headache, dysphagia, sore throat rather than febrile neck pain
  - Vertebral osteomyelitis of the thoracic and lumbar spine may present with pain in the chest, shoulder, abdominal, hip or leg
  - Risk factors: IV drug use, DM, history of septicemia, spinal trauma, pulmonary tuberculosis, urinary tract infections, surgery, older men

Major differential diagnoses:
- Benign neck or back pain
- Degenerative disc disease
- Tumor
- Fracture
- Spondyloarthropathies: In particular, reactive arthritis is a difficult differential in this situation because of the concomitant infection (perhaps with fever and systemic symptoms) and back pain. Differentiation may be difficult, but is generally possible based on the severity of the systemic manifestations and local examination findings. Patients with *focal pain*—particularly that which is exacerbated by vertebral percussion—should be further evaluated for osteomyelitis, fracture, or acute disc herniation

---

[253] Strausbaugh LJ. Vertebral osteomyelitis. How to differentiate it from other causes of back and neck pain. *Postgrad Med* 1995 Jun;97(6):147-8, 151-4
[254] Macnab I, McCulloch J. Backache. Second Edition. Williams and Wilkins: Baltimore, 1990

Clinical assessment:

- **History/subjective**:
  - o Spinal pain
  - o Malaise: may or may not have systemic symptoms
- **Physical examination/objective**:
  - o Mild local tenderness
  - o Paravertebral muscle spasm with limited ROM
  - o Fever (50%)
  - o Neurologic signs (20-40%)
  - o Spinal percussion is positive for pain
  - o May have painful and limited SLR due to hamstring spasm
- **Imaging & laboratory assessments**:
  - o High ESR—elevated to 20-100 mm/hr in 90% of patients. ESR was considered "the most useful test for monitoring the disease activity and the efficacy of treatment." [255]
  - o 50% have slight elevation of WBC.
  - o The disc space is the first structure destroyed—the clinician and radiologist must not misinterpret early signs of infection with "degenerative disc disease."
  - o **MRI has a sensitivity and specificity of >90% and also helps to assess epidural abscess.**
  - o Radiographs are positive in 80% after the condition has been present for at least 10-14 days.
  - o Bone scan is diagnostic in 90% of cases.
  - o "Computed tomography is the imaging study of choice for preoperative evaluation and biopsy procedures. It is not a good screening test..." [256] and is generally used after routine radiographs and/or bone scan.

Establishing the diagnosis:

- Diagnosis is established based on a consistent spectrum of clinical signs and symptoms and is confirmed with imaging and/or biopsy, aspiration, and/or blood cultures

Complications:

- Abscesses
- Meningitis
- Vertebral collapse, fracture
- Neurologic injury: paralysis
- Septicemia and death

Clinical management:

- Immediate/urgent referral for diagnostic procedures, IV and oral antimicrobials, and surgery if needed

Treatments:

- **Antimicrobial drugs: Organism-specific IV/oral antimicrobials are generally administered on an in-patient basis.**
- Rest: Bed rest, bracing, activity limitation
- Surgery: Surgery for debridement and complications such as cord compression, vertebral collapse or instability.
- **Immunonutrition:** Immunonutritional considerations are listed below; doses listed are for adults. Although studies have not been performed specifically in patients with bone/joint infections, general benefits derived from the use of immunonutrition are reductions in severity/frequency/duration of major infections, abbreviated hospitalization (i.e., early discharge due to expedited healing and

---

[255] Macnab I, McCulloch J. Backache. Second Edition. Williams and Wilkins: Baltimore, 1990
[256] Strausbaugh LJ. Vertebral osteomyelitis. How to differentiate it from other causes of back and neck pain. Postgrad Med 1995 Jun;97(6):147-8, 151-4

recovery), reductions in the need for medications, significant improvements in survival, and hospital savings.[257,258,259,260,261,262,263]

- o Paleo-Mediterranean diet: As detailed later in this text and elsewhere[264,265]
- o Vitamin and mineral supplementation: anti-infective benefits shown in elderly diabetics[266]
- o High-dose vitamin A: Vitamin A shows potent immunosupportive benefits, and vitamin A stores are depleted by the stress of infection and injury. Consider 200,000-300,000 IU per day of retinol palmitate for 1-4 weeks, then taper; reduce dose or discontinue with onset of toxicity symptoms such as skin problems (dry skin, flaking skin, chapped or split lips, red skin rash, hair loss), joint pain, bone pain, headaches, anorexia (loss of appetite), edema (water retention, weight gain, swollen ankles, difficulty breathing), fatigue, and/or liver damage.
- o Arginine: Dose for adults is in the range of 5-10 grams daily
- o Fatty acid supplementation: In contrast to the higher doses used to provide an anti-inflammatory effect in patients with autoimmune/inflammatory disorders, doses used for immunosupportive treatments should be kept rather modest to avoid the *relative* immunosuppression that has been controversially reported in patients treated with EPA and DHA. Reasonable doses are in the following ranges for adults: EPA+DHA: 500-1,500, and GLA: 300-500 mg.
- o Glutamine: Glutamine enhances bacterial killing by neutrophils[267], and administration of 18 grams per day in divided doses to patients in intensive care units was shown to improve survival, expedite hospital discharge, and reduce total healthcare costs.[268] Another study using glutamine 12-18 grams per day showed no benefit in overall mortality but significant benefits in terms of reduced healthcare costs (-30%) and significantly reduced need for medical interventions.[269] After administering glutamine 26 grams/d to severely burned patients, Garrel et al[270] concluded that glutamine reduced the risk of infection by 3-fold and that oral glutamine "may be a life-saving intervention" in patients with severe burns. A dose of 30 grams/d was used in a recent clinical trial showing hemodynamic benefit in patients with sickle cell anemia.[271] The highest glutamine dose that the current author is aware of is the study by Scheltinga et al[272] who used 0.57 gm/kg/day in cancer patients following chemotherapy administration; for a 220-lb-pt, this would be approximately 57 grams of glutamine per day.
- o Melatonin: 20-40 mg hs (*hora somni*—Latin: sleep time). Immunostimulatory anti-infective action of melatonin was demonstrated in a small clinical trial wherein septic newborns administered 20 mg melatonin showed significantly increased survival over nontreated controls.[273]

[257] "To evaluate the metabolic and immune effects of dietary arginine, glutamine and omega-3 fatty acids (fish oil) supplementation, we performed a prospective study... CONCLUSIONS: The feeding of Neomune in critically injured patients was well tolerated as Traumacal and significant improvement was observed in serum protein. Shorten ICU stay and wean-off respirator day may benefit from using the immunonutrient formula." Chuntrasakul C, Siltham S, Sarasombath S, Sittapairochana C, Leowattana W, Chockvivatananavanit S, Bunnak A. Comparison of a immunonutrition formula enriched arginine, glutamine and omega-3 fatty acid, with a currently high-enriched enteral nutrition for trauma patients. *J Med Assoc Thai*. 2003 Jun;86(6):552-6
[258] "CONCLUSIONS: In conclusion, arginine-enhanced formula improves fistula rates in postoperative head and neck cancer patients and decreases length of stay." de Luis DA, Izaola O, Cuellar L, Terroba MC, Aller R. Randomized clinical trial with an enteral arginine-enhanced formula in early postsurgical head and neck cancer patients. *Eur J Clin Nutr*. 2004;58(11):1505-8
[259] "In this prospective, randomised, double-blind, placebo-controlled study, we randomly assigned 50 patients who were scheduled to undergo coronary artery bypass to receive either an oral immune-enhancing nutritional supplement containing L-arginine, omega3 polyunsaturated fatty acids, and yeast RNA (n=25), or a control (n=25) for a minimum of 5 days... Intake of an oral immune-enhancing nutritional supplement for a minimum of 5 days before surgery can improve outlook in high-risk patients who are undergoing elective cardiac surgery." Tepaske R, Velthuis H, Oudemans-van Straaten HM, Heisterkamp SH, van Deventer SJ, Ince C, Eysman L, Kesecioglu J. Effect of preoperative oral immune-enhancing nutritional supplement on patients at high risk of infection after cardiac surgery: a randomised placebo-controlled trial. *Lancet*. 2001 Sep 1;358(9283):696-701
[260] "The feeding of IMMUNE FORMULA was well tolerated and significant improvement was observed in nutritional and immunologic parameters as in other immunoenhancing diets. Further clinical trials of prospective double-blind randomized design are necessary to address the so that the necessity of using immunonutrition in critically ill patients will be clarified." Chuntrasakul C, Siltharm S, Sarasombath S, Sittapairochana C, Leowattana W, Chockvivatananavanit S, Bunnak A. Metabolic and immune effects of dietary arginine, glutamine and omega-3 fatty acids supplementation in immunocompromised patients. *J Med Assoc Thai*. 1998 May;81(5):334-43
[261] "enteral diet supplemented with arginine, dietary nucleotides, and omega-3 fatty acids (IMPACT, Sandoz Nutrition, Bern, Switzerland)" Senkal M, Mumme A, Eickhoff U, Geier B, Spath G, Wulfert D, Joosten U, Frei A, Kemen M. Early postoperative enteral immunonutrition: clinical outcome and cost-comparison analysis in surgical patients. *Crit Care Med* 1997;25(9):1489-96
[262] "supplemented diet with glutamine, arginine and omega-3-fatty acids... It was clearly established in this study that early postoperative enteral feeding is safe in patients who have undergone major operations for gastrointestinal cancer. Supplementation of enteral nutrition with glutamine, arginine, and omega-3-fatty acids positively modulated postsurgical immunosuppressive and inflammatory responses." Wu GH, Zhang YW, Wu ZH. Modulation of postoperative immune and inflammatory response by immune-enhancing enteral diet in gastrointestinal cancer patients. *World J Gastroenterol*. 2001 Jun;7(3):357-62 http://www.wjgnet.com/1007-9327/7/357.pdf
[263] "using a formula supplemented with arginine, mRNA, and omega-3 fatty acids from fish oil (Impact)... CONCLUSIONS: Immune-enhancing enteral nutrition resulted in a significant reduction in the mortality rate and infection rate in septic patients admitted to the ICU. These benefits were greater for patients with less severe illness." Galban C, Montejo JC, Mesejo A, Marco P, Celaya S, Sanchez-Segura JM, Farre M, Bryg DJ. An immune-enhancing enteral diet reduces mortality rate and episodes of bacteremia in septic intensive care unit patients. *Crit Care Med*. 2000 Mar;28(3):643-8
[264] Vasquez A. A Five-Part Nutritional Protocol that Produces Consistently Positive Results. *Nutritional Wellness* 2005 September http://www.nutritionalwellness.com/archives/2005/sep/09_vasquez.php
[265] Vasquez A. Implementing the Five-Part Nutritional Wellness Protocol for the Treatment of Various Health Problems. *Nutritional Wellness* 2005 November. http://www.nutritionalwellness.com/archives/2005/nov/11_vasquez.php
[266] "CONCLUSIONS: A multivitamin and mineral supplement reduced the incidence of participant-reported infection and related absenteeism in a sample of participants with type 2 diabetes mellitus and a high prevalence of subclinical micronutrient deficiency." Barringer TA, Kirk JK, Santaniello AC, Foley KL, Michielutte R. Effect of a multivitamin and mineral supplement on infection and quality of life. A randomized, double-blind, placebo-controlled trial. *Ann Intern Med*. 2003 Mar 4;138(5):365-71 http://www.annals.org/cgi/reprint/138/5/365
[267] Furukawa S, Saito H, Fukatsu K, Hashiguchi Y, Inaba T, Lin MT, Inoue T, Han I, Matsuda T, Muto T. Glutamine-enhanced bacterial killing by neutrophils from postoperative patients. *Nutrition* 1997;13(10):863-9. *In vitro study*.
[268] Griffiths RD, Jones C, Palmer TE. Six-month outcome of critically ill patients given glutamine-supplemented parenteral nutrition. *Nutrition* 1997 Apr;13(4):295-302
[269] "There was no mortality difference between those patients receiving glutamine-containing enteral feed and the controls. However, there was a significant reduction in the median postintervention ICU and hospital patient costs in the glutamine recipients $23 000 versus $30 900 in the control patients." Jones C, Palmer TE, Griffiths RD. Randomized clinical outcome study of critically ill patients given glutamine-supplemented enteral nutrition. *Nutrition*. 1999 Feb;15(2):108-15
[270] The glutamine dose in this study was "a total of 26 g/day" administered in four divided doses. CONCLUSION: "The results of this prospective randomized clinical trial show that enteral G reduces blood culture positivity, particularly with P. aeruginosa, in adults with severe burns and may be a life-saving intervention." Garrel D, Patenaude J, Nedelec B, Samson L, Dorais J, Champoux J, D'Elia M, Bernier J. Decreased mortality and infectious morbidity in adult burn patients given enteral glutamine supplements: a prospective, controlled, randomized clinical trial. *Crit Care Med*. 2003 Oct;31(10):2444-9
[271] Niihara Y, Matsui NM, Shen YM, Akiyama DA, Johnson CS, Sunga MA, Magpayo J, Embury SH, Kalra VK, Cho SH, Tanaka KR. L-glutamine therapy reduces endothelial adhesion of sickle red blood cells to human umbilical vein endothelial cells. *BMC Blood Disord*. 2005 Jul 25;5:4 http://www.biomedcentral.com.proxy.hsc.unt.edu/1471-2326/5/4
[272] "Subjects with hematological malignancies in remission underwent a standard treatment of high-dose chemotherapy and total body irradiation before bone marrow transplantation. After completion of this regimen, they were randomized to receive either standard parenteral nutrition (STD, n = 10) or an isocaloric, isonitrogenous nutrient solution enriched with crystalline L-glutamine (0.57 g/kg/day, GLN, n = 10)." Scheltinga MR, Young LS, Benfell K, Bye RL, Ziegler TR, Santos AA, Antin JH, Schloerb PR, Wilmore DW. Glutamine-enriched intravenous feedings attenuate extracellular fluid expansion after a standard stress. *Ann Surg*. 1991 Oct;214(4):385-93; discussion 393-5 http://www.pubmedcentral.nih.gov/articlerender.fcgi?tool=pubmed&pubmedid=1953094 For additional review, see Ziegler TR. Glutamine supplementation in cancer patients receiving bone marrow transplantation and high dose chemotherapy. *J Nutr*. 2001 Sep;131(9 Suppl):2578S-84S http://jn.nutrition.org/cgi/content/full/131/9/2578S
[273] Gitto E, Karbownik M, Reiter RJ, Tan DX, Cuzzocrea S, Chiurazzi P, Cordaro S, Corona G, Trimarchi G, Barberi I. Effects of melatonin treatment in septic newborns. *Pediatr Res*. 2001 Dec;50(6):756-60 http://www.pedresearch.org/cgi/content/full/50/6/756

Sarcoidosis

<u>Description/pathophysiology</u>:
- A multisystem granulomatous disease; symptoms are dependent upon the site of involvement, most common of which is the mediastinum as well as central and peripheral lymph nodes.
- Sarcoidosis is not a *classic* autoimmune disease except that 1) endogenous immune mechanisms contribute to tissue destruction and clinical manifestations, and 2) approximately 20% of patients have endocrine autoimmunity.[1]
- Spontaneous improvement and resolution may occur in as many as 50-80% of patients.
- Allopaths have traditionally considered this condition "idiopathic"[2] yet new research is showing that occult infections (i.e., dysbiosis) are the underlying trigger.[3] The proposal that the condition has an infectious etiology is somewhat supported by cure of the disease in two case reports following administration of melatonin[4], which has potent immunostimulatory and anti-infective actions.[5]

<u>Clinical presentations</u>:
- Typical age of onset is between 20-40 years
- More common in Northern Europeans and African Americans (two groups with pandemic vitamin D deficiency)
- Typical autoimmune systemic manifestations: fatigue, malaise, low-grade fever, anorexia, and weight loss
- Hypercalcemia—due to a combination of hyperparathyroidism and granulomatous conversion of 25-hydroxycholecalciferol (the less active form of vitamin D) to 1,25-dihydroxycholecalciferol (the much more active form of vitamin D)
- Hyperparathyroidism
- Lymphadenopathy
- Dermal plaques and nodules in chronic disease
- Erythema nodosum—a nonspecific dermatologic manifestation characterized by erythema and subcutaneous nodules—this is considered a positive/beneficial finding in sarcoidosis because it is the best predictor of benign course of disease
- Hepatic granulomas are found in 70% of patients and may be present despite normal levels of serum liver enzymes
- **Granulomatous uveitis occurs in 15% of patients and can result in bilateral blindness—this must be treated as a medically urgent condition**
- Cardiac involvement—seen in 5-10% of patients—can result in heart failure
- Peripheral polyarthropathy or oligoarthropathy
- CNS involvement and cranial nerve palsies: **neurosarcoidosis has been associated with a 10% mortality[6] and must therefore be treated as a medically urgent condition.**

<u>Major differential diagnoses</u>:
- Lymphoma
- Tuberculosis
- **Fungal infection of the lungs: histoplasmosis, coccidioidomycosis, aspergillosis, cryptococcosis—** appropriate management of sarcoidosis requires exclusion of these conditions before the administration of prednisone or other immunosuppressants.
- Rheumatoid arthritis with pulmonary involvement
- Idiopathic pulmonary fibrosis

[1] "In conclusion, a high frequency of endocrine autoimmunity in patients with sarcoidosis, occurring in about 20% of the cases, was demonstrated. Thyroid autoimmunity and polyglandular autoimmune syndromes occurred most frequently." Papadopoulos KI, Hornblad Y, Liljebladh H, Hallengren B. High frequency of endocrine autoimmunity in patients with sarcoidosis. *Eur J Endocrinol* 1996 Mar;134(3):331-336
[2] Beers MH, Berkow R (eds). The Merck Manual. Seventeenth Edition. Whitehouse Station; Merck Research Laboratories: 1999, pages 2482-85
[3] "But now the inflammation of sarcoidosis has succumbed to antibiotics in two independent studies. This review examines the cell wall deficient (antibiotic resistant) bacteria which have been found in tissue from patients with sarcoidosis." Marshall TG, Marshall FE. Sarcoidosis succumbs to antibiotics--implications for autoimmune disease. *Autoimmun Rev.* 2004 Jun;3(4):295-300
[4] Cagnoni ML, Lombardi A, Cerinic MC, Dedola GL, Pignone A. **Melatonin for treatment of chronic refractory sarcoidosis.** *Lancet.* 1995 Nov 4;346(8984):1229-30
[5] Gitto E, Karbownik M, Reiter RJ, Tan DX, Cuzzocrea S, Chiurazzi P, Cordaro S, Corona G, Trimarchi G, Barberi I. Effects of melatonin treatment in septic newborns. *Pediatr Res.* 2001 Dec;50(6):756-60 http://www.pedresearch.org/cgi/content/full/50/6/756
[6] "Neurosarcoidosis carries a mortality of 10 per cent, over twice that of sarcoidosis overall." James DG.Life-threatening situations in sarcoidosis. *Sarcoidosis Vasc Diffuse Lung Dis* 1998 Sep;15(2):134-9

Clinical assessments:

- **History/subjective:** See clinical presentations.
- **Physical examination/objective:**
  - As indicated—see clinical presentations
  - Skin examination
  - Cardiopulmonary examination
- **Laboratory assessments:**
  - Leukopenia: common
  - Elevated serum uric acid: without gout
  - Alkaline phosphatase and GGT: elevated with liver involvement
  - Assessment for any and all types of dysbiosis and/or the implementation of empiric clinical trials of systemic antimicrobial treatments appears warranted based on emerging evidence that occult infections are a primary perpetuating factor in this disease.[7]
  - Creatine kinase: may be elevated in patients with sarcoid myopathy
  - Intestinal permeability (IP) assessment with lactulose and mannitol: Increased intestinal permeability in patients with active sarcoidosis has been documented.[8] The clinical implications of this are not perfectly clear, since the increased mucosal permeability may simply reflect systemic inflammation and does not necessarily point to an enterogenic problem. However, as discussed previously in Chapter 4, increased intestinal permeability alone is sufficient to perpetuate systemic inflammation via increased antigen absorption and bacterial translocation. Some doctors use IP testing as a barometer of overall health and thus IP testing can be used to objectively quantify overall health.
  - Endocrine autoimmunity is very common (20%) in patients with sarcoidosis[9] and is detected by appropriate serologic tests and clinical assessments:
    - Hashimoto's thyroiditis: elevated anti-thyroid peroxidase enzymes, normal or elevated TSH
    - Grave's disease: elevated thyrotropin-receptor antibodies; suppressed TSH, elevated T4
    - Addison's disease: increased ACTH, low cortisol, failure to increase cortisol production following ACTH injection, anti-adrenal antibodies[10]
    - Insulin-dependent diabetes mellitus: hyperglycemia with hypoinsulinemia
    - Premature ovarian failure: anovulation, hypoestrogenemia, infertility, elevated FSH and LH
- **Imaging and biopsy:**
  - **Chest radiographs are abnormal in 90% of patients and are an excellent and commonly employed screening test—characteristic findings include mediastinal lymphadenopathy and "ground glass" pulmonary infiltration**
  - **Biopsy results** of pulmonary nodules, liver, or lymph nodes
  - **Whole-body gallium scanning shows pathognomonic signs**—false negative results due to prednisone/immunosuppression should be avoided
- **Establishing the diagnosis:** any one of the following:
  - Characteristic radiographic findings and clinical presentation
  - Biopsy results of pulmonary nodules (50-80% positive), liver (70% positive), or palpable lymph nodes (> 85% positive)
  - Pathognomonic signs with whole-body gallium scanning
- **Complications:** 10% of patients develop serious disability, including or due to pulmonary insufficiency, cardiac insufficiency, blindness, fatigue and debility. Granulomatous uveitis occurs in 15% of patients with sarcoidosis and can result in bilateral blindness—this must be managed as a medically urgent condition.

---

[7] "But now the inflammation of sarcoidosis has succumbed to antibiotics in two independent studies. This review examines the cell wall deficient (antibiotic resistant) bacteria which have been found in tissue from patients with sarcoidosis." Marshall TG, Marshall FE. Sarcoidosis succumbs to antibiotics--implications for autoimmune disease. *Autoimmun Rev.* 2004 Jun;3(4):295-300

[8] "Patients with active pulmonary sarcoidosis exhibited a marked increased IP to 51Cr-EDTA (4 +/- 0.54%), which was not found in patients with inactive sarcoidosis." Wallaert B, Colombel JF, Adenis A, Marchandise X, Hallgren R, Janin A, Tonnel AB. Increased intestinal permeability in active pulmonary sarcoidosis. *Am Rev Respir Dis.* 1992 Jun;145(6):1440-5

[9] "In conclusion, a high frequency of endocrine autoimmunity in patients with sarcoidosis, occurring in about 20% of the cases, was demonstrated. Thyroid autoimmunity and polyglandular autoimmune syndromes occurred most frequently." Papadopoulos KI, Hornblad Y, Liljebladh H, Hallengren B. High frequency of endocrine autoimmunity in patients with sarcoidosis. *Eur J Endocrinol* 1996 Mar;134(3):331-336

[10] "Autoantibodies in patients with isolated Addison's disease are directed against the enzymes involved in steroid synthesis, P45oc21, P45oscc and P45oc17." Martin Martorell P, Roep BO, Smit JW. Autoimmunity in Addison's disease. *Neth J Med.* 2002 Aug;60(7):269-75. Review. Erratum in: Neth J Med. 2002 Oct;60(9):378 http://www.zuidencomm.nl/njm/getpdf.php?id=159

Clinical management:

- Serial pulmonary function tests are recommended—consider referral to pulmonologist or other specialist.
- **Pulmonary fungal infections should be conclusively excluded—referral to pulmonologist or other specialist is advised.**
- **Granulomatous uveitis occurs in 15% of patients with sarcoidosis and can result in bilateral blindness**—this must be managed as a medically urgent condition.
- Referral if clinical outcome is unsatisfactory or if serious complications are evident.

Therapeutic considerations:

> Drug treatments[11]:
> - Prednisone may be initiated at 20-60 mg/d po and tapered to 5 mg/d po for relief of symptoms; this treatment does not alter long-term outcome. **Prednisone and any immunosuppressant medication must only be employed following exclusion of an infectious differential diagnosis—administration of corticosteroids to a patient with occult pulmonary infections could result in a fatal outcome.**
> - Methotrexate at 2.5 mg per week can be initiated in patients unresponsive to prednisone; CBC and liver enzymes are measured every six weeks

- Avoidance of proinflammatory foods: Proinflammatory foods act *directly* or *indirectly*; direct mechanisms include activating Toll-like receptors or NF-kappaB or inducing oxidative stress, while indirect mechanisms include depleting the body of anti-inflammatory nutrients and displacing more nutritious anti-inflammatory foods. Arachidonic acid (found in beef, liver, pork, and cow's milk) is the direct precursor to proinflammatory prostaglandins and leukotrienes[12] and pain-promoting isoprostanes.[13] Saturated fats promote inflammation by activating/enabling proinflammatory Toll-like receptors.[14] Consumption of saturated fat in the form of cream creates marked oxidative stress and lipid peroxidation that lasts for at least 3 hours postprandially.[15] Corn oil rapidly activates NF-kappaB (in hepatic Kupffer cells) for a proinflammatory effect[16]; similarly, consumption of PUFA and linoleic acid promotes antioxidant depletion and may thus promote oxidation-mediated inflammation via activation of NF-kappaB; linoleic acid causes intracellular oxidative stress and calcium influx and results in increased transcription of NF-kappaB activated pro-inflammatory genes.[17] High glycemic foods cause oxidative stress[18,19] and inflammation via activation of NF-kappaB and other mechanisms—*white bread causes inflammation.*[20] High glycemic foods suppress immune function[21,22] and thus perpetuate and promote infection/dysbiosis. Delivery of a high carbohydrate load to the gastrointestinal lumen promotes bacterial overgrowth[23,24], which is inherently proinflammatory[25,26] and which appears to be myalgenic in humans.[27] Consumption of grains, potatoes, and manufactured

[11] Beers MH, Berkow R (eds). The Merck Manual. Seventeenth Edition. Whitehouse Station; Merck Research Laboratories: 1999, pages 2482-85
[12] Vasquez A. Reducing Pain and Inflammation Naturally. Part 2: New Insights into Fatty Acid Supplementation and Its Effect on Eicosanoid Production and Genetic Expression. Nutritional Perspectives 2005; January: 5-16 www.optimalhealthresearch.com/part2
[13] Evans AR, Junger H, Southall MD, Nicol GD, Sorkin LS, Broome JT, Bailey TW, Vasko MR. Isoprostanes, novel eicosanoids that produce nociception and sensitize rat sensory neurons. J Pharmacol Exp Ther. 2000 Jun;293(3):912-20
[14] Lee JY, Sohn KH, Rhee SH, Hwang D. Saturated fatty acids, but not unsaturated fatty acids, induce the expression of cyclooxygenase-2 mediated through Toll-like receptor 4. J Biol Chem. 2001 May 18;276(20):16683-9. Epub 2001 Mar 2 http://www.jbc.org/cgi/content/full/276/20/16683
[15] "CONCLUSIONS: Both fat and protein intakes stimulate ROS generation. The increase in ROS generation lasted 3 h after cream intake and 1 h after protein intake. Cream intake also caused a significant and prolonged increase in lipid peroxidation." Mohanty P, Ghanim H, Hamouda W, Aljada A, Garg R, Dandona P. Both lipid and protein intakes stimulate increased generation of reactive oxygen species by polymorphonuclear leukocytes and mononuclear cells. Am J Clin Nutr. 2002 Apr;75(4):767-72 http://www.ajcn.org/cgi/content/full/75/4/767
[16] Rusyn I, Bradham CA, Cohn L, Schoonhoven R, Swenberg JA, Brenner DA, Thurman RG. Corn oil rapidly activates nuclear factor-kappaB in hepatic Kupffer cells by oxidant-dependent mechanisms. Carcinogenesis. 1999 Nov;20(11):2095-100 http://carcin.oxfordjournals.org/cgi/content/full/20/11/2095
[17] "Exposing endothelial cells to 90 micromol linoleic acid/L for 6 h resulted in a significant increase in lipid hydroperoxides that coincided wih an increase in intracellular calcium concentrations." Hennig B, Toborek M, Joshi-Barve S, Barger SW, Barve S, Mattson MP, McClain CJ. Linoleic acid activates nuclear transcription factor-kappa B (NF-kappa B) and induces NF-kappa B-dependent transcription in cultured endothelial cells. Am J Clin Nutr. 1996 Mar;63(3):322-8 http://www.ajcn.org/cgi/reprint/63/3/322
[18] Mohanty P, Hamouda W, Garg R, Aljada A, Ghanim H, Dandona P. Glucose challenge stimulates reactive oxygen species (ROS) generation by leucocytes. J Clin Endocrinol Metab. 2000 Aug;85(8):2970-3 http://jcem.endojournals.org/cgi/content/full/85/8/2970 Glucose/carbohydrate and saturated fat consumption appear to be the two biggest offenders in the food-stimulated production of oxidative stress. The effect by protein is much less. "CONCLUSIONS: Both fat and protein intakes stimulate ROS generation. The increase in ROS generation lasted 3 h after cream intake and 1 h after protein intake. Cream intake also caused a significant and prolonged increase in lipid peroxidation." Mohanty P, Ghanim H, Hamouda W, Aljada A, Garg R, Dandona P. Both lipid and protein intakes stimulate increased generation of reactive oxygen species by polymorphonuclear leukocytes and mononuclear cells. Am J Clin Nutr. 2002 Apr;75(4):767-72 http://www.ajcn.org/cgi/content/full/75/4/767
[19] Koska J, Blazicek P, Marko M, Grna JD, Kvetnansky R, Vigas M. Insulin, catecholamines, glucose and antioxidant enzymes in oxidative damage during different loads in healthy humans. Physiol Res. 2000;49 Suppl 1:S95-100 http://www.biomed.cas.cz/physiolres/pdf/2000/49_S95.pdf
[20] "Conclusion - The present study shows that high GI carbohydrate, but not low GI carbohydrate, mediates an acute proinflammatory process as measured by NF-kappaB activity." Dickinson S, Hancock DP, Petocz P, Brand-Miller JC..High glycemic index carbohydrate mediates an acute proinflammatory process as measured by NF-kappaB activation. Asia Pac J Clin Nutr. 2005;14 Suppl:S120
[21] Sanchez A, Reeser JL, Lau HS, et al. Role of sugars in human neutrophilic phagocytosis. Am J Clin Nutr. 1973 Nov;26(11):1180-4
[22] "Postoperative infusion of carbohydrate solution leads to moderate fall in the serum concentration of inorganic phosphate. ... The hypophosphatemia was associated with significant reduction of neutrophil phagocytosis, intracellular killing, consumption of oxygen and generation of superoxide during phagocytosis." Rasmussen A, Segel E, Hessov I, Borregaard N. Reduced function of neutrophils during routine postoperative glucose infusion. Acta Chir Scand. 1988 Jul-Aug;154(7-8):429-33
[23] Ramakrishnan T, Stokes P. Beneficial effects of fasting and low carbohydrate diet in D-lactic acidosis associated with short-bowel syndrome. JPEN J Parenter Enteral Nutr. 1985 May-Jun;9(3):361-3
[24] Gottschall E. Breaking the Vicious Cycle: Intestinal Health Through Diet. Kirkton Press; Rev edition (August 1, 1994)
[25] Lin HC. Small intestinal bacterial overgrowth: a framework for understanding irritable bowel syndrome. JAMA. 2004 Aug 18;292(7):852-8
[26] Lichtman SN, Wang J, Sartor RB, Zhang C, Bender D, Dalldorf FG, Schwab JH. Reactivation of arthritis induced by small bowel bacterial overgrowth in rats: role of cytokines, bacteria, and bacterial polymers. Infect Immun. 1995 Jun;63(6):2295-301
[27] Pimentel M, et al. A link between irritable bowel syndrome and fibromyalgia may be related to findings on lactulose breath testing. Ann Rheum Dis. 2004 Apr;63(4):450-2

foods displaces phytonutrient-dense foods such as fruits, vegetables, nuts, seeds, and berries which in sum contain more than 8,000 phytonutrients, many of which have anti-oxidant and thus anti-inflammatory actions.[28,29]

- <u>Avoidance of allergenic foods</u>: Any patient may be allergic to any food, even if the food is generally considered a health-promoting food. Generally speaking, the most notorious allergens are wheat, citrus (especially juice due to the industrial use of fungal hemicellulases), cow's milk, eggs, peanuts, chocolate, and yeast-containing foods; according to a study in patients with migraine, some patients will have to avoid as many as 10 specific foods in order to become symptom-free.[30]

- <u>Supplemented Paleo-Mediterranean diet</u>: The health-promoting diet of choice for the majority of people is a diet based on abundant consumption of fruits, vegetables, seeds, nuts, omega-3 and monounsaturated fatty acids, and lean sources of protein such as lean meats, fatty cold-water fish, soy and whey proteins. This diet obviates overconsumption of chemical preservatives, artificial sweeteners, and carbohydrate-dominant foods such as candies, pastries, breads, potatoes, grains, and other foods with a high glycemic load and high glycemic index. This "Paleo-Mediterranean Diet" is a combination of the "Paleolithic" or "Paleo diet" and the well-known "Mediterranean diet", both of which are well described in peer-reviewed journals and the lay press. (See Chapter 2 for details). **Habitual avoidance of refined sugars and other immunosuppressing foods is essential when treating chronic systemic infections**.

- <u>Short-term fasting</u>: Whether the foundational diet is Paleo-Mediterranean, vegetarian, vegan, or a combination of all of these, autoimmune/inflammatory patients will still benefit from periodic fasting, whether on a weekly (e.g., every Saturday), monthly (every first week or weekend of the month, or every other month), or yearly (1-2 weeks of the year) basis. Since consumption of food—particularly unhealthy foods—induces an inflammatory effect[31], abstinence from food provides a relative anti-inflammatory effect. Fasting indeed provides a distinct anti-inflammatory benefit and may help "re-calibrate" metabolic and homeostatic mechanisms by breaking self-perpetuating "vicious cycles"[32] that autonomously promote inflammation independent from pro-inflammatory stimuli. Of course, water-only fasting is completely hypoallergenic (assuming that the patient is not sensitive to chlorine, fluoride, or other contaminants), and subsequent re-introduction of foods provides the ideal opportunity to identify offending foods. Fasting deprives intestinal microbes of substrate[33], stimulates intestinal B-cell immunity[34], improves the bactericidal action of neutrophils[35], reduces lysozyme release and leukotriene formation[36], and ameliorates intestinal hyperpermeability.[37] In case reports and/or clinical trials, short-term fasting (or protein-sparing fasting) has been documented as safe and effective treatment for SLE[38], RA[39], and non-rheumatic diseases such as chronic severe hypertension[40], moderate hypertension[41], obesity[42,43], type-2 diabetes[44], and epilepsy.[45]

[28] "We propose that the additive and synergistic effects of phytochemicals in fruit and vegetables are responsible for their potent antioxidant and anticancer activities, and that the benefit of a diet rich in fruit and vegetables is attributed to the complex mixture of phytochemicals present in whole foods." Liu RH. Health benefits of fruit and vegetables are from additive and synergistic combinations of phytochemicals. Am J Clin Nutr. 2003 Sep;78(3 Suppl):517S-520S

[29] Seaman DR. The diet-induced proinflammatory state: a cause of chronic pain and other degenerative diseases? J Manipulative Physiol Ther. 2002;25(3):168-79

[30] Grant EC. Food allergies and migraine. Lancet. 1979 May 5;1(8123):966-9

[31] Aljada A, Mohanty P, Ghanim H, Abdo T, Tripathy D, Chaudhuri A, Dandona P. Increase in intranuclear nuclear factor kappaB and decrease in inhibitor kappaB in mononuclear cells after a mixed meal: evidence for a proinflammatory effect. Am J Clin Nutr. 2004 Apr;79(4):682-90 http://www.ajcn.org/cgi/content/full/79/4/682

[32] "The ability of therapeutic fasts to break metabolic vicious cycles may also contribute to the efficacy of fasting in the treatment of type 2 diabetes and autoimmune disorders." McCarty MF. A preliminary fast may potentiate response to a subsequent low-salt, low-fat vegan diet in the management of hypertension - a strategy for breaking metabolic vicious cycles. Med Hypotheses. 2003 May;60(5):624-33

[33] Ramakrishnan T, Stokes P. Beneficial effects of fasting and low carbohydrate diet in D-lactic acidosis associated with short-bowel syndrome. JPEN J Parenter Enteral Nutr. 1985 May-Jun;9(3):361-3

[34] Trollmo C, Verdrengh M, Tarkowski A. Fasting enhances mucosal antigen specific B cell responses in rheumatoid arthritis. Ann Rheum Dis. 1997 Feb;56(2):130-4 http://ard.bmjjournals.com/cgi/content/full/56/2/130

[35] "An association was found between improvement in inflammatory activity of the joints and enhancement of neutrophil bactericidal capacity. Fasting appears to improve the clinical status of patients with RA." Uden AM, Trang L, Venizelos N, Palmblad J. Neutrophil functions and clinical performance after total fasting in patients with rheumatoid arthritis. Ann Rheum Dis. 1983 Feb;42(1):45-51

[36] "We thus conclude that a reduced ability to generate cytotaxins, reduced release of enzyme, and reduced leukotriene formation from RA neutrophils, together with an altered fatty acid composition of membrane phospholipids, may be mechanisms for the decrease of inflammatory symptoms that results from fasting." Hafstrom I, Ringertz B, Gyllenhammar H, Palmblad J, Harms-Ringdahl M. Effects of fasting on disease activity, neutrophil function, fatty acid composition, and leukotriene biosynthesis in patients with rheumatoid arthritis. Arthritis Rheum. 1988 May;31(5):585-92

[37] "The results indicate that, unlike lactovegetarian diet, fasting may ameliorate the disease activity and reduce both the intestinal and the non-intestinal permeability in rheumatoid arthritis." Sundqvist T, Lindstrom F, Magnusson KE, Skoldstam L, Stjernstrom I, Tagesson C. Influence of fasting on intestinal permeability and disease activity in patients with rheumatoid arthritis. Scand J Rheumatol. 1982;11(1):33-8

[38] Fuhrman J, Sarter B, Calabro DJ. Brief case reports of medically supervised, water-only fasting associated with remission of autoimmune disease. Altern Ther Health Med. 2002 Jul-Aug;8(4):112, 110-1

[39] "An association was found between improvement in inflammatory activity of the joints and enhancement of neutrophil bactericidal capacity. Fasting appears to improve the clinical status of patients with RA." Uden AM, Trang L, Venizelos N, Palmblad J. Neutrophil functions and clinical performance after total fasting in patients with rheumatoid arthritis. Ann Rheum Dis. 1983 Feb;42(1):45-51

[40] "The average reduction in blood pressure was 37/13 mm Hg, with the greatest decrease being observed for subjects with the most severe hypertension. Patients with stage 3 hypertension (those with systolic blood pressure greater than 180 mg Hg, diastolic blood pressure greater than 110 mg Hg, or both) had an average reduction of 60/17 mm Hg at the conclusion of treatment." Goldhamer A, Lisle D, Parpia B, Anderson SV, Campbell TC. Medically supervised water-only fasting in the treatment of hypertension. J Manipulative Physiol Ther. 2001 Jun;24(5):335-9 http://www.healthpromoting.com/335-339Goldhamer115263.QXD.pdf

[41] "RESULTS: Approximately 82% of the subjects achieved BP at or below 120/80 mm Hg by the end of the treatment program. The mean BP reduction was 20/7 mm Hg, with the greatest decrease being observed for subjects with the highest baseline BP." Goldhamer AC, Lisle DJ, Sultana P, Anderson SV, Parpia B, Hughes B, Campbell TC. Medically supervised water-only fasting in the treatment of borderline hypertension. J Altern Complement Med. 2002 Oct;8(5):643-50 http://www.healthpromoting.com/Articles/articles/study%202/acmpaper5.pdf

[42] Vertes V, Genuth SM, Hazelton IM. Supplemented fasting as a large-scale outpatient program. JAMA. 1977 Nov 14;238(20):2151-3

[43] Bauman WA, Schwartz E, Rose HG, Eisenstein HN, Johnson DW. Early and long-term effects of acute caloric deprivation in obese diabetic patients. Am J Med. 1988 Jul;85(1):38-46

[44] Goldhamer AC. Initial cost of care results in medically supervised water-only fasting for treating high blood pressure and diabetes. J Altern Complement Med. 2002 Dec;8(6):696-7 http://www.healthpromoting.com/Articles/pdf/Study%2032.pdf

[45] "The ketogenic diet should be considered as alternative therapy for children with difficult-to-control seizures. It is more effective than many of the new anticonvulsant medications and is well tolerated by children and families when it is effective." Freeman JM, Vining EP, Pillas DJ, Pyzik PL, Casey JC, Kelly LM. The efficacy of the ketogenic diet-1998: a prospective evaluation of intervention in 150 children. Pediatrics. 1998 Dec;102(6):1358-63 http://pediatrics.aappublications.org/cgi/reprint/102/6/1358

- <u>Broad-spectrum fatty acid therapy with ALA, EPA, DHA, GLA and oleic acid</u>:   Fatty acid supplementation should be delivered in the form of combination therapy with ALA, GLA, DHA, and EPA. Given at doses of 3,000 – 9,000 mg per day, ALA from flax oil has impressive anti-inflammatory benefits demonstrated by its ability to halve prostaglandin production in humans.[46] Numerous studies have demonstrated the benefit of GLA in the treatment of rheumatoid arthritis when used at doses between 500 mg – 4,000 mg per day.[47,48] Fish oil provides EPA and DHA which have well-proven anti-inflammatory benefits in rheumatoid arthritis[49,50,51] and lupus.[52,53] ALA, EPA, DHA, and GLA need to be provided in the form of supplements; when using high doses of therapeutic oils, liquid supplements that can be mixed in juice or a smoothie are generally more convenient and palatable than capsules. Therapeutic amounts of oleic acid can be obtained from generous use of olive oil, preferably on fresh vegetables. Supplementation with polyunsaturated fatty acids warrants increased intake of antioxidants from diet, fruit and vegetable juices, and properly formulated supplements; since patients with systemic inflammation are generally in a pro-oxidative state, consideration must be given to the timing and starting dose of fatty acid supplementation and the need for anti-oxidant protection. See chapter on Therapeutics for more details and biochemical pathways. Clinicians must realize that fatty acids are not clinically or biochemically interchangeable and that one fatty acid does not substitute for another; each of the fatty acids must be supplied in order for its benefits to be obtained.[54]

- <u>Vitamin D3 supplementation tailored to serum 25(OH)D levels and serum calcium levels</u>: **Sarcoidosis is the classic exemplification of a granulomatous disease that can cause hypercalcemia due to "vitamin D hypersensitivity."** [55,56] **Vitamin D supplementation—if used at all in these patients—must be supervised with extreme care to avoid hypercalcemia.** Deficiency and response to treatment are monitored with serum 25(OH)vitamin D while **safety is monitored with serum calcium;** **inflammatory granulomatous diseases**—*sarcoidosis being the classic example*—**and certain drugs such as hydrochlorothiazide greatly increase the propensity for hypercalcemia and warrant increment dosing and frequent monitoring of serum calcium.**

- <u>Orthoendocrinology</u>: No characteristic patterns of hormonal abnormalities have been described nor researched in patients with sarcoidosis. However, on an individual basis, clinicians and patients may find it valuable to assess prolactin, cortisol, DHEA, free and total testosterone, serum estradiol, and thyroid status (e.g., TSH, T4, *and* anti-thyroid peroxidase antibodies). **Melatonin (20 mg hs) appears to have cured two patients with drug-resistant sarcoidosis[57] and 3 mg provided immediate short-term benefit to a patient with multiple sclerosis.[58] Immunostimulatory anti-infective action of melatonin was demonstrated in a clinical trial wherein septic newborns administered 20 mg melatonin showed significantly increased survival over nontreated controls[59]; given that sarcoidosis is associated with many subclinical infections, melatonin may provide therapeutic benefit by virtue of its anti-infective properties.**

- <u>Antibacterial therapies with systemic bioavailability</u>: The 2004 monograph by Marshall and Marshall[60] reviewed research implicating cell wall deficient (antibiotic resistant) bacteria as the major causative

[46] Adam O, Wolfram G, Zollner N. Effect of alpha-linolenic acid in the human diet on linoleic acid metabolism and prostaglandin biosynthesis. *J Lipid Res.* 1986 Apr;27(4):421-6 http://www.jlr.org/cgi/reprint/27/4/421
[47] "Other results showed a significant reduction in morning stiffness with gamma-linolenic acid at 3 months and reduction in pain and articular index at 6 months with olive oil." Brzeski M, Madhok R, Capell HA. Evening primrose oil in patients with rheumatoid arthritis and side-effects of non-steroidal anti-inflammatory drugs. *Br J Rheumatol.* 1991 Oct;30(5):370-2
[48] Rothman D, DeLuca P, Zurier RB. Botanical lipids: effects on inflammation, immune responses, and rheumatoid arthritis. *Semin Arthritis Rheum.* 1995 Oct;25(2):87-96
[49] Adam O, Beringer C, Kless T, Lemmen C, Adam A, Wiseman M, Adam P, Klimmek R, Forth W. Anti-inflammatory effects of a low arachidonic acid diet and fish oil in patients with rheumatoid arthritis. *Rheumatol Int.* 2003 Jan;23(1):27-36
[50] Lau CS, Morley KD, Belch JJ. Effects of fish oil supplementation on non-steroidal anti-inflammatory drug requirement in patients with mild rheumatoid arthritis--a double-blind placebo controlled study. *Br J Rheumatol.* 1993 Nov;32(11):982-9
[51] Kremer JM, Jubiz W, Michalek A, Rynes RI, Bartholomew LE, Bigaouette J, Timchalk M, Beeler D, Lininger L. Fish-oil fatty acid supplementation in active rheumatoid arthritis. A double-blinded, controlled, crossover study. *Ann Intern Med.* 1987 Apr;106(4):497-503
[52] Walton AJ, Snaith ML, Locniskar M, Cumberland AG, Morrow WJ, Isenberg DA. Dietary fish oil and the severity of symptoms in patients with systemic lupus erythematosus. *Ann Rheum Dis.* 1991 Jul;50(7):463-6
[53] Duffy EM, Meenagh GK, McMillan SA, Strain JJ, Hannigan BM, Bell AL. The clinical effect of dietary supplementation with omega-3 fish oils and/or copper in systemic lupus erythematosus. *J Rheumatol.* 2004 Aug;31(8):1551-6
[54] Vasquez A. Reducing Pain and Inflammation Naturally. Part 2: New Insights into Fatty Acid Supplementation and Its Effect on Eicosanoid Production and Genetic Expression. *Nutritional Perspectives* 2005; January: 5-16 http://optimalhealthresearch.com/part2
[55] Vasquez A, Manso G, Cannell J. The clinical importance of vitamin D (cholecalciferol): a paradigm shift with implications for all healthcare providers. *Altern Ther Health Med.* 2004 Sep-Oct;10(5):28-36 http://optimalhealthresearch.com/monograph04
[56] Sharma OP. Vitamin D, calcium, and sarcoidosis. *Chest.* 1996 Feb;109(2):535-9 http://www.chestjournal.org/cgi/reprint/109/2/535
[57] Cagnoni ML, Lombardi A, Cerinic MC, Dedola GL, Pignone A. Melatonin for treatment of chronic refractory sarcoidosis. *Lancet.* 1995 Nov 4;346(8984):1229-30
[58] "...administration of melatonin (3 mg, orally) at 2:00 p.m., when the patient experienced severe blurring of vision, resulted within 15 minutes in a dramatic improvement in visual acuity and in normalization of the visual evoked potential latency after stimulation of the left eye." Sandyk R. Diurnal variations in vision and relations to circadian melatonin secretion in multiple sclerosis. *Int J Neurosci.* 1995 Nov;83(1-2):1-6
[59] Gitto E, Karbownik M, Reiter RJ, Tan DX, Cuzzocrea S, Chiurazzi P, Cordaro S, Corona G, Trimarchi G, Barberi I. Effects of melatonin treatment in septic newborns. *Pediatr Res.* 2001 Dec;50(6):756-60 http://www.pedresearch.org/cgi/content/full/50/6/756
[60] "But now the inflammation of sarcoidosis has succumbed to antibiotics in two independent studies. This review examines the cell wall deficient (antibiotic resistant) bacteria which have been found in tissue from patients with sarcoidosis." Marshall TG, Marshall FE. Sarcoidosis succumbs to antibiotics--implications for autoimmune disease. *Autoimmun Rev.* 2004 Jun;3(4):295-300

factor in sarcoidosis, evidenced by remission of the disease following antimicrobial treatment and the incitement of a rather **severe Jarisch-Herxheimer reaction** as the bacteria increase their production of endotoxin in response to exposure to antimicrobial agents. Also in 2004, Bachelez et al[61] published results of a small clinical trail using minocycline and/or doxycycline in 12 patients with sarcoidosis—ten of twelve patients showed a positive response.

- <u>Minocycline</u>: **The study by Bachelez et al[62] used 200 mg/d minocycline for 12 months for the treatment of sarcoidosis.**

- <u>Doxycycline</u>: **Alternate treatment by Bachelez et al[63] was 200 mg/d doxycycline for the treatment of sarcoidosis.**

- *Artemisia annua*: Artemisinin has been safely used for centuries in Asia for the treatment of malaria, and it also has effectiveness against anaerobic bacteria due to the pro-oxidative sesquiterpene endoperoxide.[64,65] I commonly use artemisinin at 200 mg per day in divided doses for adults with dysbiosis. Whether from dried herb, teas, or standardized extracts, **artemisinin is systemically bioavailable** and has an excellent record of safety. However, its usefulness in sarcoidosis based on the treatment of occult infections has not been documented.

- St. John's Wort (*Hypericum perforatum*): Hyperforin from *Hypericum perforatum* shows *in vitro* antibacterial action, particularly against gram-positive bacteria such as *Staphylococcus aureus*, *Streptococcus pyogenes, Streptococcus agalactiae*[66] and perhaps *Helicobacter pylori*.[67] Up to 600 mg three times per day of a 3% hyperforin standardized extract is customary in the treatment of depression, and such **high doses may result in serum hyperforin levels that are systemically antimicrobial.** The safety and antidepressant effectiveness of Hypericum extracts are exceedingly well documented. The usefulness of hyperforin in sarcoidosis based on the treatment of occult infections has not been documented.

- <u>Fumaric acid esters</u>: **Three patients with drug-resistant cutaneous sarcoidosis were successfully treated with fumaric acid esters** (Fumaderm®).[68] Adverse effects of oral fumarate have been reported, namely renal failure.[69]

- <u>Oral enzyme therapy with proteolytic/pancreatic enzymes</u>: Polyenzyme supplementation is used to ameliorate the pathophysiology induced by immune complexes.[70] Approximately 60% of sarcoid patients have CIC (circulating immune complexes)[71] and these are particularly relevant in patients with concomitant vasculitis.[72] Importantly, orally administered polyenzyme preparations have an "immune stimulating" action[73] and promote degradation of microbial biofilms and increased immune and antimicrobial penetration into infectious foci.[74]

[61] Bachelez H, Senet P, Cadranel J, Kaoukhov A, Dubertret L. The use of tetracyclines for the treatment of sarcoidosis. *Arch Dermatol*. 2001 Jan;137(1):69-73 Sign on for free full-text at http://archderm.ama-assn.org/cgi/content/full/137/1/69

[62] Bachelez H, Senet P, Cadranel J, Kaoukhov A, Dubertret L. The use of tetracyclines for the treatment of sarcoidosis. *Arch Dermatol*. 2001 Jan;137(1):69-73 Sign on for free full-text at http://archderm.ama-assn.org/cgi/content/full/137/1/69

[63] Bachelez H, Senet P, Cadranel J, Kaoukhov A, Dubertret L. The use of tetracyclines for the treatment of sarcoidosis. *Arch Dermatol*. 2001 Jan;137(1):69-73 Sign on for free full-text at http://archderm.ama-assn.org/cgi/content/full/137/1/69

[64] Dien TK, de Vries PJ, Khanh NX, Koopmans R, Binh LN, Duc DD, Kager PA, van Boxtel CJ. Effect of food intake on pharmacokinetics of oral artemisinin in healthy Vietnamese subjects. *Antimicrob Agents Chemother*. 1997 May;41(5):1069-72

[65] Giao PT, Binh TQ, Kager PA, Long HP, Van Thang N, Van Nam N, de Vries PJ. Artemisinin for treatment of uncomplicated falciparum malaria: is there a place for monotherapy? *Am J Trop Med Hyg*. 2001 Dec;65(6):690-5

[66] Schempp CM, Pelz K, Wittmer A, Schopf E, Simon JC. Antibacterial activity of hyperforin from St John's wort, against multiresistant Staphylococcus aureus and gram-positive bacteria. *Lancet*. 1999 Jun 19;353(9170):2129

[67] "A butanol fraction of St. John's Wort revealed anti-Helicobacter pylori activity with MIC values ranging between 15.6 and 31.2 microg/ml." Reichling J, Weseler A, Saller R. A current review of the antimicrobial activity of Hypericum perforatum L. *Pharmacopsychiatry*. 2001 Jul;34 Suppl 1:S116-8

[68] "CONCLUSIONS: On the basis of our findings FAE therapy seems to be a safe and effective regimen for patients with recalcitrant cutaneous sarcoidosis."Nowack U, Gambichler T, Hanefeld C, Kastner U, Altmeyer P. Successful treatment of recalcitrant cutaneous sarcoidosis with fumaric acid esters. *BMC Dermatol* 2002 Dec 24;2(1):15 http://www.biomedcentral.com/1471-5945/2/15

[69] "The case of a 38 year old woman who was treated with fumaric acid (420 mg bid) for 5 years before she complained of fatigue and weakness. According to clinical laboratory she had developed severe proximal tubular damage." Raschka C, Koch HJ. Longterm treatment of psoriasis using fumaric acid preparations can be associated with severe proximal tubular damage. *Hum Exp Toxicol* 1999 Dec;18(12):738-9

[70] Galebskaya LV, Ryumina EV, Niemerovsky VS, Matyukov AA. Human complement system state after wobenzyme intake. *VESTNIK MOSKOVSKOGO UNIVERSITETA. KHIMIYA*. 2000. Vol. 41, No. 6. Supplement. Pages 148-149

[71] "Complexes were detected in 29 (58%) patients." Johnson NM, NcNicol MW, Burton-Kee JE, Mowbray JF. Circulating immune complexes in sarcoidosis. *Thorax*. 1980 Apr;35(4):286-9

[72] "Circulating immune complexes were demonstrated and may have been important in the pathogenesis of both types of skin lesion." Johnston C, Kennedy C. Cutaneous leucocytoclastic vasculitis associated with acute sarcoidosis. *Postgrad Med J*. 1984 Summer;60(706):549-50

[73] Zavadova E, Desser L, Mohr T. Stimulation of reactive oxygen species production and cytotoxicity in human neutrophils in vitro and after oral administration of a polyenzyme preparation. *Cancer Biother*. 1995 Summer;10(2):147-52

[74] "The enzymes were shown to inhibit the biofilm formation. When applilied to the formed associations, the enzymes potentiated the effect of antibiotics on the bacteria located in them." Tets VV, Knorring Glu, Artemenko NK, Zaslavskaia NV, Artemenko KL. [Impact of exogenic proteolytic enzymes on bacteria][Article in Russian] *Antibiot Khimioter*. 2004;49(12):9-13

Polymyositis
Dermatomyositis
Dermatopolymyositis
Dermatomyositis sine myositis

Description/pathophysiology:

- **Autoimmune disease associated with immune complexes, autoantibodies, and cell-mediated muscle destruction.** Although both conditions are characterized by polymyopathy, skin involvement is a characteristic of **dermatomyositis (DM)** and not **polymyositis (PM)**. Unless articles/textbooks specifically refer to either PM or DM, the hyphenation PM-DM will be used to acknowledge that data probably applies to both conditions. The term **dermatopolymyositis** is somewhat outdated and not commonly used in contemporary literature. **Dermatomyositis sine myositis** is a rare variant of dermatomyositis characterized by inflammation of the skin *without overt myopathy*. Endogenous antigens targeted for autoimmune attack include human **Glycyl-tRNA synthetase**[1] and—not surprisingly—**myosin** from skeletal muscle.[2]

- Tissue damage is caused in large part by muscle infiltration by lymphocytes and macrophages. Lymphocytes from patients with PM-DM produce a "lymphotoxin" that causes muscle necrosis.[3]

- Despite the *idiopathic* label which is inappropriately applied to these disorders, several medical textbooks and numerous journal articles readily acknowledge that underlying viral infections[4,5], bacterial infections[6], parasitic infections[7], and malignancy[8] can contribute to the development of PM-DM. Interestingly and specifically supportive of the hypothesis that dysbiosis plays an etiologic role in the development of PM-DM, two of the endogenous autoantigens in PM share amino acid homology (molecular mimicry) with **histidyl-tRNA synthetase** and **alanyl-RNA synthetase** from *E. coli*.[9]

> **Microorganisms causatively or molecularly associated with induction of polymyositis/dermatomyositis**
> - *Streptococcus pyogenes*
> - *Staphylococcus aureus*
> - *Toxoplasma gondii*
> - *Mycoplasma pneumoniae*
> - *Borrelia burgdorferi*
> - Coxsackie B virus
> - *Mycoplasma hominis*
> - *Haemophilus influenzae*
> - *Helicobacter pylori*
> - *Escherichia coli*
> - *Bacillus subtilis*

Furthermore, myosin in human skeletal muscle shares amino acid homology with M5 protein from *Streptococcus pyogenes*.[10] Limited evidence suggests that DM may be triggered or exacerbated by bacterial infections/dysbiosis—particularly with *Staphylococcus aureus*[11,12] and *Streptococcus pyogenes*.[13,14] Patients with DM have an exaggerated response to streptococcal M5

---

[1] Ge Q, Trieu EP, Targoff IN. Primary structure and functional expression of human Glycyl-tRNA synthetase, an autoantigen in myositis. *J Biol Chem*. 1994 Nov 18;269(46):28790-7 http://www.jbc.org/cgi/reprint/269/46/28790

[2] Massa M, Costouros N, Mazzoli F, De Benedetti F, La Cava A, Le T, De Kleer I, Ravelli A, Liotta M, Roord S, Berry C, Pachman LM, Martini A, Albani S. Self epitopes shared between human skeletal myosin and Streptococcus pyogenes M5 protein are targets of immune responses in active juvenile dermatomyositis. *Arthritis Rheum*. 2002 Nov;46(11):3015-25

[3] Ichimiya M, Yasui H, Hirota Y, Ohmura A, Muto M. Association between elevated serum antibody levels to streptococcal M12 protein and susceptibility to dermatomyositis. *Arch Dermatol Res*. 1998 Apr;290(4):229-30

[4] Beers MH, Berkow R (eds). The Merck Manual. Seventeenth Edition. Whitehouse Station; Merck Research Laboratories 1999 Page 434

[5] Siegel LB, Gall EP. Viral infection as a cause of arthritis. *Am Fam Physician* 1996 Nov 1;54(6):2009-15

[6] Massa M, Costouros N, Mazzoli F, De Benedetti F, La Cava A, Le T, De Kleer I, Ravelli A, Liotta M, Roord S, Berry C, Pachman LM, Martini A, Albani S. Self epitopes shared between human skeletal myosin and Streptococcus pyogenes M5 protein are targets of immune responses in active juvenile dermatomyositis. *Arthritis Rheum*. 2002 Nov;46(11):3015-

[7] "We report a case of polymyositis and myocarditis in a 13-year old immunocompetent girl with toxoplasmosis. The patient presented with proximal muscle weakness, dysphagia, palms and soles rash and elevated serum levels of muscle enzymes, with liver and myocardial involvement." Paspalaki PK, Mihailidou EP, Bitsori M, Tsagkaraki D, Mantzouranis E. Polyomyositis and myocarditis associated with acquired toxoplasmosis in an immunocompetent girl. *BMC Musculoskelet Disord*. 2001;2:8. Epub 2001 Nov 20 http://www.biomedcentral.com/1471-2474/2/8

[8] Tierney ML. McPhee SJ, Papadakis MA (eds). Current Medical Diagnosis and Treatment 2006. 45th edition. New York; Lange Medical Books: 2006, pages 840-842

[9] "The amino acid sequences of Escherichia coli histidyl-tRNA synthetase and alanyl-tRNA synthetase, two proteins recently identified as autoantigens in polymyositis, were compared by a computer alignment procedure with those of the 3600 proteins tabulated in the National Biomedical Research Foundation protein sequence database. Both proteins contain sequences long enough to function as epitopes that match sequences on viral and muscle proteins." Walker EJ, Jeffrey PD. Polymyositis and molecular mimicry, a mechanism of autoimmunity. *Lancet*. 1986 Sep 13;2(8507):605-7

[10] Massa M, Costouros N, Mazzoli F, De Benedetti F, La Cava A, Le T, De Kleer I, Ravelli A, Liotta M, Roord S, Berry C, Pachman LM, Martini A, Albani S. Self epitopes shared between human skeletal myosin and Streptococcus pyogenes M5 protein are targets of immune responses in active juvenile dermatomyositis. *Arthritis Rheum*. 2002 Nov;46(11):3015-25

[11] Lane S, Doherty M, Powell RJ. Dermatomyositis following chronic staphylococcal joint sepsis. *Ann Rheum Dis*. 1990 Jun;49(6):405-6

[12] Moore EC, Cohen F, Douglas SD, Gutta V. Staphylococcal infections in childhood dermatomyositis--association with the development of calcinosis, raised IgE concentrations and granulocyte chemotactic defect. *Ann Rheum Dis*. 1992 Mar;51(3):378-83

[13] Massa M, Costouros N, Mazzoli F, De Benedetti F, La Cava A, Le T, De Kleer I, Ravelli A, Liotta M, Roord S, Berry C, Pachman LM, Martini A, Albani S. Self epitopes shared between human skeletal myosin and Streptococcus pyogenes M5 protein are targets of immune responses in active juvenile dermatomyositis. *Arthritis Rheum*. 2002 Nov;46(11):3015-25

[14] Ichimiya M, Yasui H, Hirota Y, Ohmura A, Muto M. Association between elevated serum antibody levels to streptococcal M12 protein and susceptibility to dermatomyositis. *Arch Dermatol Res*. 1998 Apr;290(4):229-30

protein[15] as well as streptococcal M12 protein.[16] Streptococcal infections may precipitate or exacerbate DM via mechanisms including molecular mimicry[17,18]; furthermore, streptococcal M protein acts as a superantigen and may enhance expression of endogenous autoantigens.[19] Young patients with calcific dermatomyositis have at least one immune defect (impaired granulocyte chemotaxis) that impairs their ability to fight *Staphylococcus aureus* infections/colonization/dysbiosis; this defect in chemotaxis is associated with and may be caused by elevations in serum IgE, some of which is specific for *Staphylococcus aureus*.[20] A relatively complete list of microorganisms associated with induction of PM-DM in humans includes *Staphylococcus aureus*[21,22], *Streptococcus pyogenes*[23,24], *Toxoplasma gondii*[25,26,27,28], *Mycoplasma pneumoniae*[29,30], *Borrelia burgdorferi*[31,32], and Coxsackie B virus.[33] Microorganisms that share amino acid homology with human skeletal muscle myosin include *Streptococcus pyogenes, Borrelia burgdorferi, Mycoplasma hominis, Haemophilus influenzae, Helicobacter pylori, Escherichia coli,* and *Bacillus subtilis.*[34]

- Like other disorders, PM-DM may occur with other autoimmune diseases, in which case it is described as an **overlap syndrome**. This is not surprising since the underlying characteristic of all autoimmune disorders is *immune dysfunction*; the protean consequences of immune dysfunction can morph without regard for the anthropocentric labels that we affix to different patterns of disordered expression. As with all autoimmune disorders, the course is variable and marked by exacerbations and remissions; yet the general trend is one of progressive decline. Spontaneous remission may occur, but should not be depended upon in lieu of proactive intervention.

- *Comment*: These conditions are commonly described as "idiopathic." In fact, the 2006 edition of <u>Current Medical Diagnosis and Treatment</u> refers to these two disorders as "idiopathic inflammatory myopathies"—a title no longer worthy of codification since 1) we have clear evidence of microbial induction/exacerbation of these disorders, 2) the hormonal aspects of these disorders (like most other autoimmune disorders) is increasingly recognized (for the most recent example, see Sereda and Werth[35]), and 3) the intentional overuse of the term *idiopathic* is leveraged by drug companies and

[15] Massa M, Costouros N, Mazzoli F, De Benedetti F, La Cava A, Le T, De Kleer I, Ravelli A, Liotta M, Roord S, Berry C, Pachman LM, Martini A, Albani S. Self epitopes shared between human skeletal myosin and Streptococcus pyogenes M5 protein are targets of immune responses in active juvenile dermatomyositis. *Arthritis Rheum.* 2002 Nov;46(11):3015-25

[16] Ichimiya M, Yasui H, Hirota Y, Ohmura A, Muto M. Association between elevated serum antibody levels to streptococcal M12 protein and susceptibility to dermatomyositis. *Arch Dermatol Res.* 1998 Apr;290(4):229-30

[17] Ichimiya M, Yasui H, Hirota Y, Ohmura A, Muto M. Association between elevated serum antibody levels to streptococcal M12 protein and susceptibility to dermatomyositis. *Arch Dermatol Res.* 1998 Apr;290(4):229-30

[18] Ichimiya M, Yasui H, Hirota Y, Ohmura A, Muto M. Association between elevated serum antibody levels to streptococcal M12 protein and susceptibility to dermatomyositis. *Arch Dermatol Res.* 1998 Apr;290(4):229-30

[19] Ichimiya M, Yasui H, Hirota Y, Ohmura A, Muto M. Association between elevated serum antibody levels to streptococcal M12 protein and susceptibility to dermatomyositis. *Arch Dermatol Res.* 1998 Apr;290(4):229-30

[20] Moore EC, Cohen F, Douglas SD, Gutta V. Staphylococcal infections in childhood dermatomyositis--association with the development of calcinosis, raised IgE concentrations and granulocyte chemotactic defect. *Ann Rheum Dis.* 1992 Mar;51(3):378-83

[21] Lane S, Doherty M, Powell RJ. Dermatomyositis following chronic staphylococcal joint sepsis. *Ann Rheum Dis.* 1990 Jun;49(6):405-6

[22] Moore EC, Cohen F, Douglas SD, Gutta V. Staphylococcal infections in childhood dermatomyositis--association with the development of calcinosis, raised IgE concentrations and granulocyte chemotactic defect. *Ann Rheum Dis.* 1992 Mar;51(3):378-83

[23] Massa M, Costouros N, Mazzoli F, De Benedetti F, La Cava A, Le T, De Kleer I, Ravelli A, Liotta M, Roord S, Berry C, Pachman LM, Martini A, Albani S. Self epitopes shared between human skeletal myosin and Streptococcus pyogenes M5 protein are targets of immune responses in active juvenile dermatomyositis. *Arthritis Rheum.* 2002 Nov;46(11):3015-25

[24] Ichimiya M, Yasui H, Hirota Y, Ohmura A, Muto M. Association between elevated serum antibody levels to streptococcal M12 protein and susceptibility to dermatomyositis. *Arch Dermatol Res.* 1998 Apr;290(4):229-30

[25] "The case of a patient who developed an acute dermatomyositis-like syndrome upon infection by Toxoplasma gondii is reported." Saberin A, Lutgen C, Humbel RL, Hentges F. Dermatomyositis-like syndrome following acute toxoplasmosis. *Bull Soc Sci Med Grand Duche Luxemb.* 2004;(2):109-19

[26] "We report a case of polymyositis and myocarditis in a 13-year old immunocompetent girl with toxoplasmosis. The patient presented with proximal muscle weakness, dysphagia, palms and soles rash and elevated serum levels of muscle enzymes, with liver and myocardial involvement." Paspalaki PK, Mihailidou EP, Bitsori M, Tsagkaraki D, Mantzouranis E. Polyomyositis and myocarditis associated with acquired toxoplasmosis in an immunocompetent girl. *BMC Musculoskelet Disord.* 2001;2:8. Epub 2001 Nov 20 http://www.biomedcentral.com/1471-2474/2/8

[27] "The patient improved over the next six months and has been followed for approximately a five year period. During this time, antibody levels to the toxoplasma antigen have significantly decreased but the patient has developed a chronic myositis indistinguishable from polymyositis." Adams EM, Hafez GR, Carnes M, Wiesner JK, Graziano FM. The development of polymyositis in a patient with toxoplasmosis: clinical and pathologic findings and review of literature. *Clin Exp Rheumatol.* 1984 Jul-Sep;2(3):205-8

[28] "The serologic data suggested that inflammatory muscle disease was associated with recent active toxoplasma infection in certain patients." Phillips PE, Kassan SS, Kagen LJ. Increased toxoplasma antibodies in idiopathic inflammatory muscle disease. A case-controlled study. *Arthritis Rheum.* 1979 Mar;22(3):209-14

[29] "We describe the case of a 10-year-old girl who developed polymyositis associated with a Mycoplasma pneumoniae infection." Aihara Y, Mori M, Kobayashi T, Yokota S. A pediatric case of polymyositis associated with Mycoplasma pneumoniae infection. *Scand J Rheumatol.* 1997;26(6):480-1

[30] "Polymyositis, transverse myelitis, ascending polyneuritis, bilateral optic neuritis, and hearing loss developed in a patient with high complement-fixing antibody titers to Mycoplasma pneumoniae." Rothstein TL, Kenny GE. Cranial neuropathy, myeloradiculopathy, and myositis: complications of Mycoplasma pneumoniae infection. *Arch Neurol.* 1979 Aug;36(8):476-7

[31] "Lyme disease with muscle involvement can mimic or trigger dermatomyositis and should be considered in the differential diagnosis of dermatomyositis." Hoffmann JC, Stichtenoth DO, Zeidler H, Follmann M, Brandis A, Stanek G, Wollenhaupt J. Lyme disease in a 74-year-old forest owner with symptoms of dermatomyositis. *Arthritis Rheum.* 1995 Aug;38(8):1157-60

[32] "We report the first case of dermatomyositis that appears to have been triggered by B. burgdorferi. This case involved an individual from Westchester County, NY, who presented with skin lesions suggestive of erythema migrans and who was seropositive for Lyme disease. He soon developed a clinical syndrome suggestive of dermatomyositis: periorbital edema, dysphagia, proximal muscle weakness, and a markedly elevated level of creatine phosphokinase." Horowitz HW, Sanghera K, Goldberg N, Pechman D, Kamer R, Duray P, Weinstein A. Dermatomyositis associated with Lyme disease: case report and review of Lyme myositis. *Clin Infect Dis.* 1994 Feb;18(2):166-71

[33] "These data suggest that the host response to coxsackie B virus might be related to the pathophysiology of JDM." Christensen ML, Pachman LM, Schneiderman R, Patel DC, Friedman JM. Prevalence of Coxsackie B virus antibodies in patients with juvenile dermatomyositis. *Arthritis Rheum.* 1986 Nov;29(11):1365-70

[34] Massa M, Costouros N, Mazzoli F, De Benedetti F, La Cava A, Le T, De Kleer I, Ravelli A, Liotta M, Roord S, Berry C, Pachman LM, Martini A, Albani S. Self epitopes shared between human skeletal myosin and Streptococcus pyogenes M5 protein are targets of immune responses in active juvenile dermatomyositis. *Arthritis Rheum.* 2002 Nov;46(11):3015-25

[35] "Using antiestrogen medication in women with DM may result in a significant improvement in their rash, possibly via the inhibition of TNF-alpha production by immune or other cells." Sereda D, Werth VP. Improvement in dermatomyositis rash associated with the use of antiestrogen medication. *Arch Dermatol.* 2006 Jan;142(1):70-2

other pharmaceutical/medical interests to justify endless medicalization in lieu of more profound assessments and effective treatments. One of the consequences of the pharmaceutically-influenced *idiopathicization* of otherwise understandable and treatable diseases is that doctors are no longer trained to *cure* disease by addressing the underlying problems; rather, they are trained to *medicate* disease indefinitely by *additive and infinite pharmacotherapy* and **symptom exchange**—trading symptoms of the disease for the side effects of the drugs used to treat the disease.[36,37] Consequently, the top questions that doctors ask themselves during clinical encounters are 1) "What is the cause of symptom X?", 2) "What is the dose of the 'appropriate' drug?", and 3) "How should I manage disease or finding X?"[38] Notice that the internal dialogue of the allopathically trained physicians in this study centers on symptoms, drugs, and management rather than any attempt to discover and address the underlying cause(s) of the symptoms or any attempt at authentic cure. Convincing doctors that *endless additive medicalization* is synonymous with *effective patient care* has been the major goal of the pharmaceutical companies[39] and is one that they accomplish by influencing medical school curricula[40,] sources of biomedical information[41], and by 'educating' doctors and patients with an incessant barrage of infomercials.[42]

Clinical presentations:

- **Bilateral symmetrical proximal muscle weakness most commonly affecting the shoulders, neck, and hips:** This weakness is reflective of the underlying autoimmune myopathy and may not be markedly present at the beginning of the disease process although it is eventually noted in all PM-DM patients. Characteristic difficulties include rising from a chair or squatting position (indicating weakness of glutei, quadriceps, and other intrinsic hip muscles), and upholding the arms or lifting objects overhead (deltoids and rotator cuff muscles).
- **Skin/dermatologic abnormalities:**
  - **Heliotrope/purple facial/cheek rash:** "Periorbital edema with a heliotrope hue (purplish appearance) is pathognomonic."[43]
  - **Gottron's sign:** scaly patches over the metacarpophalangeal (MCP) and PIP joints of the hands—considered highly suggestive (not quite pathognomonic) of the disease.
  - Generalized skin rash and erythema, particularly over the shoulders ("shawl sign") and eyelids
  - Cuticular telangiectasias
  - Photosensitivity
- Polyarthralgia: pain and swelling, generally mild
- Muscle tenderness
- Raynaud's phenomenon: most commonly in patients with other autoimmune disease
- Fatigue
- Weight loss
- Soft tissue calcification: seen in PM-DM and scleroderma
- Cardiac involvement
- 2:1 more common in women than in men

---

[36] "It begins on the first day of medical school... It starts slowly and insidiously, like an addiction, and can end up influencing the very nature of medical decision-making and practice... Attempts to influence the judgment of doctors by commercial interests serving the medical industrial complex are nothing if not thorough." Editorial. Drug-company influence on medical education in USA. *Lancet.* 2000 Sep 2;356(9232):781

[37] "...despite lush advertisements from companies with obvious vested interests, and authoritative testimonials from biased investigators who presumably believe in their own work to the point of straining credulity and denying common sense... (translate: economic improvement, not biological superiority)." Stevens CW, Glatstein E. Beware the Medical-Industrial Complex. *Oncologist* 1996;1(4):IV-V   http://theoncologist.alphamedpress.org/cgi/reprint/1/4/190-iv.pdf

[38] ""What is the cause of symptom X?" "What is the dose of drug X?" and "How should I manage disease or finding X?"" Ely JW, Osheroff JA, Ebell MH, Bergus GR, Levy BT, Chambliss ML, Evans ER. Analysis of questions asked by family doctors regarding patient care. BMJ. 1999 Aug 7;319(7206):358-61 http://bmj.bmjjournals.com/cgi/content/full/319/7206/358

[39] Angell M. The Truth About the Drug Companies: How They Deceive Us and What to Do About it. Random House; August 2004

[40] "It begins on the first day of medical school... It starts slowly and insidiously, like an addiction, and can end up influencing the very nature of medical decision-making and practice... Attempts to influence the judgment of doctors by commercial interests serving the medical industrial complex are nothing if not thorough." Editorial. Drug-company influence on medical education in USA. *Lancet.* 2000 Sep 2;356(9232):781

[41] "...despite lush advertisements from companies with obvious vested interests, and authoritative testimonials from biased investigators who presumably believe in their own work to the point of straining credulity and denying common sense... (translate: economic improvement, not biological superiority)." Stevens CW, Glatstein E. Beware the Medical-Industrial Complex. *Oncologist* 1996;1(4):IV-V   http://theoncologist.alphamedpress.org/cgi/reprint/1/4/190-iv.pdf

[42] "...many ads may be targeted specifically at women and older viewers. Our findings suggest that Americans who watch average amounts of television may be exposed to more than 30 hours of direct-to-consumer drug advertisements each year, far surpassing their exposure to other forms of health communication." Brownfield ED, Bernhardt JM, Phan JL, Williams MV, Parker RM. Direct-to-consumer drug advertisements on network television: an exploration of quantity, frequency, and placement. *J Health Commun.* 2004 Nov-Dec;9(6):491-7

[43] Beers MH, Berkow R (eds). The Merck Manual. Seventeenth Edition. Whitehouse Station; Merck Research Laboratories 1999 Page 435

- More common in persons of African descent, which is probably due at least in part to the higher incidence of vitamin D deficiency in this population. Vitamin D insufficiency predisposes toward inflammation, immune dysfunction, autoimmunity, and increased susceptibility to infections.[44,45,46,47]
- Seen in children (5-15 years: "juvenile dermatomyositis/polymyositis") and adults (40-60 years)
- Rapid or slow onset
- Often preceded by infection

Major differential diagnoses:
- **Inclusion body myositis (IBM):** Earlier editions of some medical books discussed inclusion body myositis as a subset of polymyositis; more recent editions clearly distinguish inclusion body myositis as a distinct entity, hence its inclusion here under the category of differential diagnoses. Clinically, **IBM tends to present with *distal* muscle involvement rather than the *proximal* localization of early PM-DM.** Furthermore, muscle involvement is likely to be *asymmetrical* with IBM, differentiating IBM from PM-DM in which muscle involvement is typically symmetric.
- Hypothyroidism: Hypothyroidism can almost perfectly mimic PM-DM with periorbital edema, dermatitis, and "hypothyroid myopathy" with proximal muscle weakness, and elevated CK.[48]
- SLE: Both SLE and DM can present with systemic inflammation, fatigue, butterfly heliotrope facial rash, and positive ANA. Elevated CK and aldolase are characteristic of DM but are uncommon in SLE.
- Myasthenia gravis (MG): Presents with muscle weakness; however MG presents with facial and ocular weakness which are not characteristic of PM-DM; caused by auto-antibodies directed to neuromuscular junction (acetylcholine receptor of the motor end plate).
- Polymyalgia rheumatica: In these patients, muscle pain predominates over muscle weakness.
- Hepatitis and viral hepatitis: Elevated AST and ALT may be seen in PM-DM and hepatitis.
- Infection: viral infection, bacterial infection, toxoplasmosis, "HIV polymyositis."
- Postviral rhabdomyolysis
- Neuropathy and radiculopathy: Both can cause muscle weakness that can mimic PM-DM.
- Cancer: All patients with PM-DM must be screened for cancer.
- Lambert-Eaton myasthenic syndrome: A disorder with pathophysiology similar to myasthenia gravis—auto-antibodies directed to neuromuscular junction (voltage-gated calcium channels at terminal of alpha motor neuron); clinical presentation similar to PM-DM with proximal limb weakness. May also present with dry mouth and dry eyes (DDX: **Sjogren's syndrome**), eye ptosis and diplopia (DDX: **myasthenia gravis**), and exacerbations caused by heat (DDX: **multiple sclerosis**). Lambert-Eaton myasthenia is like PM-DM commonly associated with occult malignancy (especially small cell lung cancer) and therefore all patients with Lambert-Eaton myasthenia must be comprehensively screened for cancer. Diagnosis of Lambert-Eaton myasthenia is performed with serum tests for antibodies, supported by EMG, and followed with comprehensive cancer screening, which should include CT of lungs and biopsy of suspicious lung lesions.
- Myocardial infarction: both MI and PM-DM have elevated CK-MB.
- Multiple sclerosis: Diagnosis based on clinical presentation, findings such as internuclear ophthalmoplegia and optic neuritis, and characteristic MRI brain lesions. DDX: celiac encephalopathy.
- Drug toxicity: Numerous drugs can cause muscle weakness and elevated serum levels of muscle enzymes. All of the following drugs can cause proximal muscle weakness, and the drugs that are

---

[44] Cantorna MT. Vitamin D and autoimmunity: is vitamin D status an environmental factor affecting autoimmune disease prevalence? *Proc Soc Exp Biol Med.* 2000;223(3):230-3

[45] Timms PM, Mannan N, Hitman GA, Noonan K, Mills PG, Syndercombe-Court D, Aganna E, Price CP, Boucher BJ. Circulating MMP9, vitamin D and variation in the TIMP-1 response with VDR genotype: mechanisms for inflammatory damage in chronic disorders? *QJM.* 2002;95:787-96 http://qjmed.oxfordjournals.org/cgi/content/full/95/12/787

[46] Van den Berghe G, Van Roosbroeck D, Vanhove P, Wouters PJ, De Pourcq L, Bouillon R. Bone turnover in prolonged critical illness: effect of vitamin D. *J Clin Endocrinol Metab.* 2003;88(10):4623-32

[47] "Children who regularly took the recommended dose of vitamin D (2000 IU daily) had a RR of 0.22 (0.05-0.89) compared with those who regularly received less than the recommended amount." Hypponen E, Laara E, Reunanen A, Jarvelin MR, Virtanen SM. Intake of vitamin D and risk of type 1 diabetes: a birth-cohort study. *Lancet.* 2001;358(9292):1500-3

[48] Bowman CA, Jeffcoate WJ, Pattrick M, Doherty M. Bilateral adhesive capsulitis, oligoarthritis and proximal myopathy as presentation of hypothyroidism. *Br J Rheumatol* 1988;27(1):62-4

underlined can also cause elevated muscle enzymes: corticosteroids, alcohol, clofibrate, penicillamine (very commonly reported cause of polymyositis), hydroxychloroquine, colchicine (especially in older patients with renal failure), HMG-CoA reductase inhibitors, especially when combined with gemfibrozil, cyclosporine, niacin, erythromycin, azole antifungals, and protease inhibitors, Zidovudine, and AZT.

Clinical assessments:
- **History/subjective**: See clinical presentations
- **Physical examination/objective**:
  - Assess muscle strength:
    - Shoulders: flexion and abduction.
    - Neck: flexion, extension, and lateral bending.
    - Hips: use a combination of direct muscle testing as well as functional assessments such as "squat and rise" and rising from a chair.
- **Laboratory assessments**:
  - ESR/CRP: Normal in 50% of patients.
  - CBC: Assess for anemia (uncommon), infection, and possible nutritional deficiencies
  - Metabolic/chemistry panel: Elevated AST and ALT may be seen and can be confused with hepatitis.
  - **Muscle enzymes: These are useful for establishing the diagnosis and monitoring the course of disease and response to treatment.** Both tests should be performed together, especially at the initial evaluation.
    - **Creatine kinase (CK) (previously called creatine phosphokinase (CPK):** CK is generally elevated but may normalize in patients with active disease and widespread muscle atrophy[49] in a manner similar to the reduction of liver enzymes with the progression of hepatic cirrhosis.
    - **Aldolase**
  - ANA: Positive in many patients[50] especially those with another autoimmune disorder— overlap syndrome.[51]
  - Anti-Jo-1: Seen mostly with lung disease.
  - Serum IgE: Young DM patients affected by calcinosis have elevated serum IgE.[52]
  - Serologic testing for *Toxoplasma gondii*: Serologic testing for *Toxoplasma gondii* has been recommended because of the association between this infection and the development of PM-DM.[53]
  - Testing for celiac disease: This is especially important in PM-DM patients who have malabsorption.[54]
  - Dysbiosis testing: Assess for multifocal dysbiosis.

---

[49] Klippel JH (ed). Primer on the Rheumatic Diseases. 11th Edition. Atlanta: Arthritis Foundation. 1997, page 277

[50] Tierney ML. McPhee SJ, Papadakis MA (eds). Current Medical Diagnosis and Treatment 2006. 45th edition. New York; Lange Medical Books: 2006, pages 840-842

[51] Tierney LM. Saint S, Whooley MA (Eds). Current Essentials of Medicine. Third Edition. New York; Lange Medical Books: 2005, page 165

[52] Moore EC, Cohen F, Douglas SD, Gutta V. Staphylococcal infections in childhood dermatomyositis--association with the development of calcinosis, raised IgE concentrations and granulocyte chemotactic defect. *Ann Rheum Dis.* 1992 Mar;51(3):378-83

[53] "We report a case of polymyositis and myocarditis in a 13-year old immunocompetent girl with toxoplasmosis. The patient presented with proximal muscle weakness, dysphagia, palms and soles rash and elevated serum levels of muscle enzymes, with liver and myocardial involvement." Paspalaki PK, Mihailidou EP, Bitsori M, Tsagkaraki D, Mantzouranis E. Polyomyositis and myocarditis associated with acquired toxoplasmosis in an immunocompetent girl. *BMC Musculoskelet Disord.* 2001;2:8. Epub 2001 Nov 20 http://www.biomedcentral.com/1471-2474/2/8

[54] "Based on our findings, we further emphasize that an evaluation for celiac disease, including anti-gliadin antibodies, anti-endomysium antibody and tissue trans-glutaminase antibodies should be considered in PM/DM patients presenting with unusual and unexplained gastrointestinal features." Marie I, Lecomte F, Hachulla E, Antonietti M, Francois A, Levesque H, Courtois H. An uncommon association: celiac disease and dermatomyositis in adults. *Clin Exp Rheumatol.* 2001 Mar-Apr;19(2):201-3

- **Imaging and biopsy**:
  - o **Skin/muscle biopsy is necessary for definitive diagnosis**.
  - o Imaging is not generally indicated except when looking for complications or concomitant disease, such as chest radiographs for associated interstitial lung disease.
  - o Electromyographic assessment may be used to support the diagnosis and to exclude/evaluate concomitant disorders; this is generally unnecessary.
- **Establishing the diagnosis**:
  - o The following should be present:
    - Proximal muscle weakness
    - Skin rash
    - Increased levels of muscle enzymes in serum
    - Muscle biopsy findings—specific, mandatory for definite diagnosis
    - EMG abnormalities are supportive

Complications:

- **Occult malignancy—up to 25% of patients with dermatomyositis have an occult malignancy. Evaluation for underlying/occult malignancy is mandatory in all adult patients with dermatomyositis.**[55] Assessment for malignancy should include complete physical examination and routine blood tests (CBC, chemistry/metabolic panel, serum protein electrophoresis, serum ferritin); additional assessments are chosen per the patient's individual profile based on age, gender, family history, and other risk factors. Measuring PSA in middle aged and older men and CA-125 in adult women would be very reasonable, as would a colonoscopy in any PM-DM patient over age 40 years. Radiographs and CT imaging are warranted for any PM-DM patient with pulmonary symptoms or history of exposure to inhaled carcinogens, including asbestos and tobacco smoke.
  - o **Up to 20% of women with dermatomyositis develop ovarian cancer**
  - o **Breast cancer** and **lung cancer** are also more common
  - o Associated cancers have **poor prognosis**
  - o **Appropriate screening includes the following**[56]:
    - **History**
    - **Physical examination**
    - **CBC**
    - **Chemistry panel**
    - **Serum protein electrophoresis**
    - **Urinalysis**
    - **Age-, gender-, and risk-appropriate screening tests**
    - **Follow-up for cancers that become evident within the next few months**
- Vasculitis with necrosis of internal organs, especially intestines
- Dyspnea due to weakness of respiratory muscles may progress to respiratory failure
- Dysphagia: due to weakness of muscles of upper pharynx
- Cardiac involvement
- Renal failure secondary to rhabdomyolysis
- Intestinal ulcerations with bleeding
- Corticosteroid myopathy
- Muscle inflammation begins with weakness and progresses to fibrosis and contractures

Clinical management:

- Referral if clinical outcome is unsatisfactory or if serious complications are possible or evident.

---

[55] Tierney ML. McPhee SJ, Papadakis MA. Current Medical Diagnosis and Treatment 2006. 45th edition. New York; Lange Medical Books: 2006, pages 840-842
[56] Tierney ML. McPhee SJ, Papadakis MA. Current Medical Diagnosis and Treatment 2006. 45th edition. New York; Lange Medical Books: 2006, pages 840-842

Treatments:

> *Medical/drug treatments*[57,58]
> - <u>Prednisone</u>: Generally started at 40-60 mg/g, then tapered.
> - <u>Methotrexate</u>, <u>azathioprine</u>, or <u>intravenous immune globulin</u>: Used for patients who do not respond to corticosteroids.

- <u>Avoidance of pro-inflammatory foods</u>: Pro-inflammatory foods act *directly* and *indirectly* to promote and exacerbate systemic inflammation. *Direct* mechanisms include the activation of Toll-like receptors and NF-kappaB, while *indirect* mechanisms include depleting the body of anti-inflammatory nutrients and dietary displacement of more nutrient-dense anti-inflammatory foods. Arachidonic acid (found in beef, liver, pork, lamb, and cow's milk) is the direct precursor to pro-inflammatory prostaglandins and leukotrienes[59] and pain-promoting isoprostanes.[60] Saturated fats promote inflammation by activating/enabling pro-inflammatory Toll-like receptors, which are otherwise "specific" for inducing pro-inflammatory responses to microorganisms.[61] Consumption of saturated fat in the form of cream creates marked oxidative stress and lipid peroxidation that lasts for at least 3 hours postprandially.[62] Corn oil rapidly activates NF-kappaB (in hepatic Kupffer cells) for a pro-inflammatory effect[63]; similarly, consumption of PUFA and linoleic acid promotes antioxidant depletion and may thus promote oxidation-mediated inflammation via activation of NF-kappaB. Linoleic acid causes intracellular oxidative stress and calcium influx and results in increased NF-kappaB-stimulated transcription of pro-inflammatory genes.[64] High glycemic foods cause oxidative stress[65,66] and inflammation via activation of NF-kappaB and other mechanisms—e.g., *white bread causes inflammation*[67] as does *a high-fat high-carbohydrate fast-food-style breakfast.*[68] High glycemic foods suppress immune function[69,70] and thus promote the perpetuation of infection/dysbiosis. Delivery of a high carbohydrate load to the gastrointestinal lumen promotes bacterial overgrowth[71,72], which is inherently pro-inflammatory[73,74] and which appears to be myalgenic in humans[75] at least in part due to the ability of endotoxin to lead to impairments in muscle function.[76] Overconsumption of

[57] Tierney ML. McPhee SJ, Papadakis MA. <u>Current Medical Diagnosis and Treatment 2006. 45th edition</u>. New York; Lange Medical Books: 2006, pages 840-842

[58] Tierney LM. Saint S, Whooley MA (Eds). <u>Current Essentials of Medicine. Third Edition</u>. New York; Lange Medical Books: 2005, page 165

[59] Vasquez A. Reducing Pain and Inflammation Naturally. Part 2: New Insights into Fatty Acid Supplementation and Its Effect on Eicosanoid Production and Genetic Expression. *Nutritional Perspectives* 2005; January: 5-16 www.optimalhealthresearch.com/part2

[60] Evans AR, Junger H, Southall MD, Nicol GD, Sorkin LS, Broome JT, Bailey TW, Vasko MR. Isoprostanes, novel eicosanoids that produce nociception and sensitize rat sensory neurons. *J Pharmacol Exp Ther*. 2000 Jun;293(3):912-20

[61] Lee JY, Sohn KH, Rhee SH, Hwang D. Saturated fatty acids, but not unsaturated fatty acids, induce the expression of cyclooxygenase-2 mediated through Toll-like receptor 4. *J Biol Chem*. 2001 May 18;276(20):16683-9. Epub 2001 Mar 2 http://www.jbc.org/cgi/content/full/276/20/16683

[62] "CONCLUSIONS: Both fat and protein intakes stimulate ROS generation. The increase in ROS generation lasted 3 h after cream intake and 1 h after protein intake. Cream intake also caused a significant and prolonged increase in lipid peroxidation." Mohanty P, Ghanim H, Hamouda W, Aljada A, Garg R, Dandona P. Both lipid and protein intakes stimulate increased generation of reactive oxygen species by polymorphonuclear leukocytes and mononuclear cells. *Am J Clin Nutr*. 2002 Apr;75(4):767-72 http://www.ajcn.org/cgi/content/full/75/4/767

[63] Rusyn I, Bradham CA, Cohn L, Schoonhoven R, Swenberg JA, Brenner DA, Thurman RG. Corn oil rapidly activates nuclear factor-kappaB in hepatic Kupffer cells by oxidant-dependent mechanisms. *Carcinogenesis*. 1999 Nov;20(11):2095-100 http://carcin.oxfordjournals.org/cgi/content/full/20/11/2095

[64] "Exposing endothelial cells to 90 micromol linoleic acid/L for 6 h resulted in a significant increase in lipid hydroperoxides that coincided wih an increase in intracellular calcium concentrations." Hennig B, Toborek M, Joshi-Barve S, Barger SW, Barve S, Mattson MP, McClain CJ. Linoleic acid activates nuclear transcription factor-kappa B (NF-kappa B) and induces NF-kappa B-dependent transcription in cultured endothelial cells. *Am J Clin Nutr*. 1996 Mar;63(3):322-8 http://www.ajcn.org/cgi/reprint/63/3/322

[65] Mohanty P, Hamouda W, Garg R, Aljada A, Ghanim H, Dandona P. Glucose challenge stimulates reactive oxygen species (ROS) generation by leucocytes. *J Clin Endocrinol Metab*. 2000 Aug;85(8):2970-3 http://jcem.endojournals.org/cgi/content/full/85/8/2970 Glucose/carbohydrate and saturated fat consumption appear to be the two biggest offenders in the food-stimulated production of oxidative stress. The effect by protein is much less. "CONCLUSIONS: Both fat and protein intakes stimulate ROS generation. The increase in ROS generation lasted 3 h after cream intake and 1 h after protein intake. Cream intake also caused a significant and prolonged increase in lipid peroxidation." Mohanty P, Ghanim H, Hamouda W, Aljada A, Garg R, Dandona P. Both lipid and protein intakes stimulate increased generation of reactive oxygen species by polymorphonuclear leukocytes and mononuclear cells. *Am J Clin Nutr*. 2002 Apr;75(4):767-72 http://www.ajcn.org/cgi/content/full/75/4/767

[66] Koska J, Blazicek P, Marko M, Grna JD, Kvetnansky R, Vigas M. Insulin, catecholamines, glucose and antioxidant enzymes in oxidative damage during different loads in healthy humans. *Physiol Res*. 2000;49 Suppl 1:S95-100 http://www.biomed.cas.cz/physiolres/pdf/2000/49_S95.pdf

[67] "Conclusion - The present study shows that high GI carbohydrate, but not low GI carbohydrate, mediates an acute proinflammatory process as measured by NF-kappaB activity." Dickinson S, Hancock DP, Petocz P, Brand-Miller JC..High glycemic index carbohydrate mediates an acute proinflammatory process as measured by NF-kappaB activation. *Asia Pac J Clin Nutr*. 2005;14 Suppl:S120

[68] Aljada A, Mohanty P, Ghanim H, Abdo T, Tripathy D, Chaudhuri A, Dandona P. Increase in intranuclear nuclear factor kappaB and decrease in inhibitor kappaB in mononuclear cells after a mixed meal: evidence for a proinflammatory effect. *Am J Clin Nutr*. 2004 Apr;79(4):682-90 http://www.ajcn.org/cgi/content/full/79/4/682

[69] Sanchez A, Reeser JL, Lau HS, et al. Role of sugars in human neutrophilic phagocytosis. *Am J Clin Nutr*. 1973 Nov;26(11):1180-4

[70] "Postoperative infusion of carbohydrate solution leads to moderate fall in the serum concentration of inorganic phosphate. ... The hypophosphatemia was associated with significant reduction of neutrophil phagocytosis, intracellular killing, consumption of oxygen and generation of superoxide during phagocytosis." Rasmussen A, Segel E, Hessov I, Borregaard N. Reduced function of neutrophils during routine postoperative glucose infusion. *Acta Chir Scand*. 1988 Jul-Aug;154(7-8):429-33

[71] Ramakrishnan T, Stokes P. Beneficial effects of fasting and low carbohydrate diet in D-lactic acidosis associated with short-bowel syndrome. *JPEN J Parenter Enteral Nutr*. 1985 May-Jun;9(3):361-3

[72] Gottschall E. <u>Breaking the Vicious Cycle: Intestinal Health Through Diet</u>. Kirkton Press; Rev edition (August 1, 1994)

[73] Lin HC. Small intestinal bacterial overgrowth: a framework for understanding irritable bowel syndrome. *JAMA*. 2004 Aug 18;292(7):852-8

[74] Lichtman SN, Wang J, Sartor RB, Zhang C, Bender D, Dalldorf FG, Schwab JH. Reactivation of arthritis induced by small bowel bacterial overgrowth in rats: role of cytokines, bacteria, and bacterial polymers. *Infect Immun*. 1995 Jun;63(6):2295-301

[75] Pimentel M, et al. A link between irritable bowel syndrome and fibromyalgia may be related to findings on lactulose breath testing. *Ann Rheum Dis*. 2004 Apr;63(4):450-2

[76] Bundgaard H, Kjeldsen K, Suarez Krabbe K, van Hall G, Simonsen L, Qvist J, Hansen CM, Moller K, Fonsmark L, Lav Madsen P, Klarlund Pedersen B. Endotoxemia stimulates skeletal muscle Na+-K+-ATPase and raises blood lactate under aerobic conditions in humans. *Am J Physiol Heart Circ Physiol*. 2003 Mar;284(3):H1028-34. Epub 2002 Nov 21 http://ajpheart.physiology.org/cgi/reprint/284/3/H1028

high-carbohydrate low-phytonutrient grains, potatoes, and manufactured foods displaces phytonutrient-dense foods such as fruits, vegetables, nuts, seeds, and berries which contain more than 8,000 phytonutrients, many of which have antioxidant and thus anti-inflammatory actions.[77,78]

- <u>Supplemented Paleo-Mediterranean diet</u>: The health-promoting diet of choice for the majority of people is a diet based on abundant consumption of fruits, vegetables, seeds, nuts, omega-3 and monounsaturated fatty acids, and lean sources of protein such as lean meats, fatty cold-water fish, soy and whey proteins. This diet obviates overconsumption of chemical preservatives, artificial sweeteners, and carbohydrate-dominant foods such as candies, pastries, breads, potatoes, grains, and other foods with a high glycemic load and high glycemic index. This "Paleo-Mediterranean Diet" is a combination of the "Paleolithic" or "Paleo diet" and the well-known "Mediterranean diet", both of which are well described in peer-reviewed journals and the lay press. (See Chapter 2 and my other publications[79,80] for details). This diet is the most nutrient-dense diet available, and its benefits are further enhanced by supplementation with vitamins, minerals, and the health-promoting fatty acids: ALA, GLA, EPA, DHA.

- <u>Vitamin E</u>: Several articles have shown benefit of vitamin E supplementation in different autoimmune conditions. Conditions that may respond to vitamin E supplementation include scleroderma, discoid lupus erythematosus[81], porphyria cutanea tarda, **polymyositis**, and vasculitis.[82,83,84] Given that vitamin E is not a single compound but rather a family of closely related tocopherols, most clinicians prefer to use a source of "mixed tocopherols" inclusive of alpha, beta, delta, and—perhaps most importantly—gamma tocopherol.[85] Vitamin E has a wide margin of safety and although daily doses are kept in the range of 400-1200 IU, doses up to 3,200 IU are generally considered non-toxic.

- <u>Avoidance of allergenic foods</u>: **Celiac disease can present with a clinical picture that closely mimics polymyositis; the '"disease" remits with gluten avoidance.**[86] Any patient may be allergic to any food, even if the food is generally considered a health-promoting food. Generally speaking, the most notorious allergens are wheat, citrus (especially juice due to the industrial use of fungal hemicellulases), cow's milk, eggs, peanuts, chocolate, and yeast-containing foods. According to a study in patients with migraine, some patients will have to avoid as many as 10 specific foods in order to become symptom-free.[87] **Several cases of co-existent celiac disease with PM-DM have been reported.**[88] Regardless of the absence of allergy in a particular patient, clinicians must explain to their patients that celiac disease and wheat allergy are two different clinical entities and that exclusion of one does not exclude the other, and in neither case does mutual exclusion obviate the promotion of intestinal bacterial overgrowth (i.e., pro-inflammatory dysbiosis) by indigestible wheat oligosaccharides.

---

[77] "We propose that the additive and synergistic effects of phytochemicals in fruit and vegetables are responsible for their potent antioxidant and anticancer activities, and that the benefit of a diet rich in fruit and vegetables is attributed to the complex mixture of phytochemicals present in whole foods." Liu RH. Health benefits of fruit and vegetables are from additive and synergistic combinations of phytochemicals. *Am J Clin Nutr*. 2003 Sep;78(3 Suppl):517S-520S

[78] Seaman DR. The diet-induced proinflammatory state: a cause of chronic pain and other degenerative diseases? *J Manipulative Physiol Ther*. 2002;25(3):168-79

[79] Vasquez A. A Five-Part Nutritional Protocol that Produces Consistently Positive Results. *Nutritional Wellness* 2005 September Available in the printed version and on-line at http://www.nutritionalwellness.com/archives/2005/sep/09_vasquez.php and http://optimalhealthresearch.com/protocol

[80] Vasquez A. Implementing the Five-Part Nutritional Wellness Protocol for the Treatment of Various Health Problems. *Nutritional Wellness* 2005 November. Available on-line at http://www.nutritionalwellness.com/archives/2005/nov/11_vasquez.php and http://optimalhealthresearch.com/protocol

[81] "Despite conflicting opinions, our personal experience and a number of reviewed clinical reports indicate that vitamin E, properly administered in adequate doses, is a safe and effective treatment for chronic discoid lupus erythematosus, and may be of value in treating other types of the disease." Ayres S Jr, Mihan R. Lupus erythematosus and vitamin E: an effective and nontoxic therapy. *Cutis*. 1979 Jan;23(1):49-52, 54

[82] "She then made a dramatic improvement when large doses of vitamin E (d, alpha-tocopheryl acetate) were administered." Killeen RN, Ayres S Jr, Mihan R. Polymyositis: response to vitamin E. *South Med J*. 1976 Oct;69(10):1372-4

[83] "Casually, vitamin E (600 mg daily) was added. After 6 months, clinical manifestations of heart failure were disappeared and the echocardiogram showed a normally-sized left ventricle with normal wall motion." Morelli S, Sgreccia A, Bernardo ML, Gurgo Di Castelmenardo A, Petrilli AC, De Leva R, Nuccio F, Calvieri S. Systemic sclerosis (scleroderma). A case of recovery of cardiomyopathy after vitamin E treatment. *Minerva Cardioangiol*. 2001 Apr;49(2):127-30

[84] "Among the diseases that were successfully controlled were a number in the autoimmune category, including scleroderma, discoid lupus erythematosus, porphyria cutanea tarda, several types of vasculitis, and polymyositis." Ayres S Jr, Mihan R. Is vitamin E involved in the autoimmune mechanism? *Cutis*. 1978 Mar;21(3):321-5

[85] Jiang Q, Christen S, Shigenaga MK, Ames BN. gamma-tocopherol, the major form of vitamin E in the US diet, deserves more attention. *Am J Clin Nutr*. 2001 Dec;74(6):714-22 http://www.ajcn.org/cgi/content/full/74/6/714

[86] "Treatment with gluten-free diet resolved all clinical and laboratory abnormalities." Evron E, Abarbanel JM, Branski D, Sthoeger ZM. Polymyositis, arthritis, and proteinuria in a patient with adult celiac disease. J Rheumatol. 1996 Apr;23(4):782-3

[87] Grant EC. Food allergies and migraine. *Lancet*. 1979 May 5;1(8123):966-9

[88] "Based on our findings, we further emphasize that an evaluation for celiac disease, including anti-gliadin antibodies, anti-endomysium antibody and tissue trans-glutaminase antibodies should be considered in PM/DM patients presenting with unusual and unexplained gastrointestinal features." Marie I, Lecomte F, Hachulla E, Antonietti M, Francois A, Levesque H, Courtois H. An uncommon association: celiac disease and dermatomyositis in adults. *Clin Exp Rheumatol*. 2001 Mar-Apr;19(2):201-3

- <u>Gluten-free vegetarian/vegan diet</u>: Gluten-free vegetarian/vegan diets have a place in the treatment plan of all patients with autoimmune/inflammatory disorders.[89,90,91,92] The benefits of gluten-free vegetarian diets are well documented, and the mechanisms of action are well elucidated, including reduced intake of pro-inflammatory linoleic[93] and arachidonic acids[94], iron[95], common food antigens[96], gluten[97] and gliadin[98,99], pro-inflammatory sugars[100] and increased intake of omega-3 fatty acids, micronutrients[101], and anti-inflammatory and antioxidant phytonutrients.[102] Vegetarian diets also effect subtle yet biologically and clinically important changes—both *qualitative* and *quantitative*—in intestinal flora[103,104] that correlate with clinical improvement.[105] Patients who rely on the Paleo-Mediterranean diet (which is inherently omnivorous) can use vegetarian *meals* on a daily basis or for days at a time—for example, by having a daily vegetarian meal, or one week per month of vegetarianism. Some (not all) patients can use a purely vegetarian diet long-term provided that nutritional needs (especially protein and cobalamin) are consistently met.

- <u>Short-term fasting</u>: Whether the foundational diet is Paleo-Mediterranean, vegetarian, vegan, or a combination of all of these, autoimmune/inflammatory patients will still benefit from periodic fasting, whether on a weekly (e.g., every Saturday), monthly (every first week or weekend of the month, or every other month), or yearly (1-2 weeks of the year) basis. Since consumption of food—particularly unhealthy foods—induces an inflammatory effect[106], abstinence from food provides a relative anti-inflammatory effect. Fasting indeed provides a distinct anti-inflammatory benefit and may help "re-calibrate" metabolic and homeostatic mechanisms by breaking self-perpetuating "vicious cycles"[107] that autonomously promote inflammation independent of pro-inflammatory stimuli. Water-only fasting is completely hypoallergenic (assuming that the patient is not sensitive to chlorine, fluoride, or other contaminants), and subsequent re-introduction of foods provides the ideal opportunity to identify offending foods.

---

[89] "The immunoglobulin G (IgG) antibody levels against gliadin and beta-lactoglobulin decreased in the responder subgroup in the vegan diet-treated patients, but not in the other analysed groups." Hafstrom I, Ringertz B, Spangberg A, von Zweigbergk L, Brannemark S, Nylander I, Ronnelid J, Laasonen L, Klareskog L. A vegan diet free of gluten improves the signs and symptoms of rheumatoid arthritis: the effects on arthritis correlate with a reduction in antibodies to food antigens. *Rheumatology* (Oxford). 2001 Oct;40(10):1175-9 http://rheumatology.oxfordjournals.org/cgi/content/abstract/40/10/1175

[90] "After four weeks at the health farm the diet group showed a significant improvement in number of tender joints, Ritchie's articular index, number of swollen joints, pain score, duration of morning stiffness, grip strength, erythrocyte sedimentation rate, C-reactive protein, white blood cell count, and a health assessment questionnaire score." Kjeldsen-Kragh J, Haugen M, Borchgrevink CF, Laerum E, Eek M, Mowinkel P, Hovi K, Forre O. Controlled trial of fasting and one-year vegetarian diet in rheumatoid arthritis. *Lancet*. 1991 Oct 12;338(8772):899-902

[91] "During fasting, arthralgia was less intense in many subjects. In some types of skin diseases (pustulosis palmaris et plantaris and atopic eczema) an improvement could be demonstrated during the fast. During the vegan diet, both signs and symptoms returned in most patients, with the exception of some patients with psoriasis who experienced an improvement." Lithell H, Bruce A, Gustafsson IB, Hoglund NJ, Karlstrom B, Ljunghall K, Sjolin K, Venge P, Werner I, Vessby B. A fasting and vegetarian diet treatment trial on chronic inflammatory disorders. *Acta Derm Venereol*. 1983;63(5):397-403

[92] Tanaka T, Kouda K, Kotani M, Takeuchi A, Tabei T, Masamoto Y, Nakamura H, Takigawa M, Suemura M, Takeuchi H, Kouda M. Vegetarian diet ameliorates symptoms of atopic dermatitis through reduction of the number of peripheral eosinophils and of PGE2 synthesis by monocytes. *J Physiol Anthropol Appl Human Sci*. 2001 Nov;20(6):353-61 http://www.jstage.jst.go.jp/article/jpa/20/6/20_353/_article/-char/en

[93] Rusyn I, Bradham CA, Cohn L, Schoonhoven R, Swenberg JA, Brenner DA, Thurman RG. Corn oil rapidly activates nuclear factor-kappaB in hepatic Kupffer cells by oxidant-dependent mechanisms. *Carcinogenesis*. 1999 Nov;20(11):2095-100 http://carcin.oxfordjournals.org/cgi/content/full/20/11/2095

[94] Vasquez A. Reducing Pain and Inflammation Naturally. Part 2: New Insights into Fatty Acid Supplementation and Its Effect on Eicosanoid Production and Genetic Expression. *Nutritional Perspectives* 2005; January: 5-16 http://optimalhealthresearch.com/part2

[95] Dabbagh AJ, Trenam CW, Morris CJ, Blake DR. Iron in joint inflammation. *Ann Rheum Dis*. 1993 Jan;52(1):67-73

[96] Hafstrom I, Ringertz B, Spangberg A, von Zweigbergk L, Brannemark S, Nylander I, Ronnelid J, Laasonen L, Klareskog L. A vegan diet free of gluten improves the signs and symptoms of rheumatoid arthritis: the effects on arthritis correlate with a reduction in antibodies to food antigens. *Rheumatology* (Oxford). 2001 Oct;40(10):1175-9 http://rheumatology.oxfordjournals.org/cgi/reprint/40/10/1175

[97] "The data provide evidence that dietary modification may be of clinical benefit for certain RA patients, and that this benefit may be related to a reduction in immunoreactivity to food antigens eliminated by the change in diet." Hafstrom I, Ringertz B, Spangberg A, von Zweigbergk L, Brannemark S, Nylander I, Ronnelid J, Laasonen L, Klareskog L. A vegan diet free of gluten improves the signs and symptoms of rheumatoid arthritis: the effects on arthritis correlate with a reduction in antibodies to food antigens. *Rheumatology* (Oxford). 2001 Oct;40(10):1175-9

[98] "Despite the increased AGA [antigliadin antibodies] positivity found distinctively in patients with recent-onset RA, none of the RA patients showed clear evidence of coeliac disease." Paimela L, Kurki P, Leirisalo-Repo M, Piirainen H. Gliadin immune reactivity in patients with rheumatoid arthritis. Clin Exp Rheumatol. 1995 Sep-Oct;13(5):603-7

[99] "The median IgA antigliadin ELISA index was 7.1 (range 2.1-22.4) for the RA group and 3.1 (range 0.3-34.9) for the controls (p = 0.0001)." Koot VC, Van Straaten M, Hekkens WT, Collee G, Dijkmans BA. Elevated level of IgA gliadin antibodies in patients with rheumatoid arthritis. Clin Exp Rheumatol. 1989 Nov-Dec;7(6):623-6

[100] Seaman DR. The diet-induced proinflammatory state: a cause of chronic pain and other degenerative diseases? *J Manipulative Physiol Ther*. 2002 Mar-Apr;25(3):168-79

[101] Hagfors L, Nilsson I, Skoldstam L, Johansson G. Fat intake and composition of fatty acids in serum phospholipids in a randomized, controlled, Mediterranean dietary intervention study on patients with rheumatoid arthritis. *Nutr Metab* (Lond). 2005 Oct 10;2:26 http://www.nutritionandmetabolism.com/content/2/1/26

[102] Liu RH. Health benefits of fruit and vegetables are from additive and synergistic combinations of phytochemicals. *Am J Clin Nutr* 2003;78(3 Suppl):517S-520S http://www.ajcn.org/cgi/content/full/78/3/517S

[103] "Significant alteration in the intestinal flora was observed when the patients changed from omnivorous to vegan diet. ... This finding of an association between intestinal flora and disease activity may have implications for our understanding of how diet can affect RA." Peltonen R, Kjeldsen-Kragh J, Haugen M, Tuominen J, Toivanen P, Forre O, Eerola E. Changes of faecal flora in rheumatoid arthritis during fasting and one-year vegetarian diet. *Br J Rheumatol*. 1994 Jul;33(7):638-43

[104] Toivanen P, Eerola E. A vegan diet changes the intestinal flora. *Rheumatology* (Oxford). 2002 Aug;41(8):950-1 http://rheumatology.oxfordjournals.org/cgi/reprint/41/8/950

[105] "We conclude that a vegan diet changes the faecal microbial flora in RA patients, and changes in the faecal flora are associated with improvement in RA activity." Peltonen R, Nenonen M, Helve T, Hanninen O, Toivanen P, Eerola E. Faecal microbial flora and disease activity in rheumatoid arthritis during a vegan diet. *Br J Rheumatol*. 1997 Jan;36(1):64-8 http://rheumatology.oxfordjournals.org/cgi/reprint/36/1/64

[106] Aljada A, Mohanty P, Ghanim H, Abdo T, Tripathy D, Chaudhuri A, Dandona P. Increase in intranuclear nuclear factor kappaB and decrease in inhibitor kappaB in mononuclear cells after a mixed meal: evidence for a proinflammatory effect. *Am J Clin Nutr*. 2004 Apr;79(4):682-90 http://www.ajcn.org/cgi/content/full/79/4/682

[107] "The ability of therapeutic fasts to break metabolic vicious cycles may also contribute to the efficacy of fasting in the treatment of type 2 diabetes and autoimmune disorders." McCarty MF. A preliminary fast may potentiate response to a subsequent low-salt, low-fat vegan diet in the management of hypertension - fasting as a strategy for breaking metabolic vicious cycles. *Med Hypotheses*. 2003 May;60(5):624-33

Fasting deprives intestinal microbes of substrate[108], stimulates intestinal B-cell immunity[109], improves the bactericidal action of neutrophils[110], reduces lysozyme release and leukotriene formation[111], and ameliorates intestinal hyperpermeability.[112] In case reports and clinical trials, short-term fasting (or protein-sparing fasting) has been documented as safe and effective treatment for SLE[113], RA[114], and non-rheumatic diseases such as chronic severe hypertension[115], moderate hypertension[116], obesity[117,118], type-2 diabetes[119], and epilepsy.[120]

- <u>Broad-spectrum fatty acid therapy with ALA, EPA, DHA, GLA and oleic acid</u>: Fatty acid supplementation should be delivered in the form of combination therapy with ALA, GLA, DHA, and EPA. Given at doses of 3,000 – 9,000 mg per day, ALA from flaxseed oil has impressive anti-inflammatory benefits demonstrated by its ability to halve prostaglandin production in humans.[121] Numerous studies have demonstrated the benefit of GLA in the treatment of rheumatoid arthritis when used at doses between 500 mg – 4,000 mg per day.[122,123] Fish oil provides EPA and DHA which have well-proven anti-inflammatory benefits in rheumatoid arthritis[124,125,126] and lupus.[127,128] ALA, EPA, DHA, and GLA need to be provided in the form of supplements; when using high doses of therapeutic oils, *liquid* supplements that can be mixed in juice or a smoothie are generally more convenient and palatable than are *capsules*. For example, at the upper end of oral fatty acid administration, the patient may be consuming as much as one-quarter cup per day of fatty acid supplementation; this same dose administered in the form of pills would require at least 72 capsules to attain the equivalent doses of ALA, EPA, DHA, and GLA. Therapeutic amounts of oleic acid can be obtained from generous use of olive oil, preferably on fresh vegetables. Supplementation with polyunsaturated fatty acids warrants increased intake of antioxidants from diet, from fruit and vegetable juices, and from properly formulated supplements. Since patients with systemic inflammation are generally in a pro-oxidative state, consideration must be given to the timing and starting dose of fatty acid supplementation and the need for antioxidant protection; some patients should start with a low

---

[108] Ramakrishnan T, Stokes P. Beneficial effects of fasting and low carbohydrate diet in D-lactic acidosis associated with short-bowel syndrome. *JPEN J Parenter Enteral Nutr.* 1985 May-Jun;9(3):361-3

[109] Trollmo C, Verdrengh M, Tarkowski A. Fasting enhances mucosal antigen specific B cell responses in rheumatoid arthritis. *Ann Rheum Dis.* 1997 Feb;56(2):130-4 http://ard.bmjjournals.com/cgi/content/full/56/2/130

[110] "An association was found between improvement in inflammatory activity of the joints and enhancement of neutrophil bactericidal capacity. Fasting appears to improve the clinical status of patients with RA." Uden AM, Trang L, Venizelos N, Palmblad J. Neutrophil functions and clinical performance after total fasting in patients with rheumatoid arthritis. *Ann Rheum Dis.* 1983 Feb;42(1):45-51

[111] "We thus conclude that a reduced ability to generate cytotaxins, reduced release of enzyme, and reduced leukotriene formation from RA neutrophils, together with an altered fatty acid composition of membrane phospholipids, may be mechanisms for the decrease of inflammatory symptoms that results from fasting." Hafstrom I, Ringertz B, Gyllenhammar H, Palmblad J, Harms-Ringdahl M. Effects of fasting on disease activity, neutrophil function, fatty acid composition, and leukotriene biosynthesis in patients with rheumatoid arthritis. *Arthritis Rheum.* 1988 May;31(5):585-92

[112] "The results indicate that, unlike lactovegetarian diet, fasting may ameliorate the disease activity and reduce both the intestinal and the non-intestinal permeability in rheumatoid arthritis." Sundqvist T, Lindstrom F, Magnusson KE, Skoldstam L, Stjernstrom I, Tagesson C. Influence of fasting on intestinal permeability and disease activity in patients with rheumatoid arthritis. *Scand J Rheumatol.* 1982;11(1):33-8

[113] Fuhrman J, Sarter B, Calabro DJ. Brief case reports of medically supervised, water-only fasting associated with remission of autoimmune disease. *Altern Ther Health Med.* 2002 Jul-Aug;8(4):112, 110-1

[114] "An association was found between improvement in inflammatory activity of the joints and enhancement of neutrophil bactericidal capacity. Fasting appears to improve the clinical status of patients with RA." Uden AM, Trang L, Venizelos N, Palmblad J. Neutrophil functions and clinical performance after total fasting in patients with rheumatoid arthritis. *Ann Rheum Dis.* 1983 Feb;42(1):45-51

[115] "The average reduction in blood pressure was 37/13 mm Hg, with the greatest decrease being observed for subjects with the most severe hypertension. Patients with stage 3 hypertension (those with systolic blood pressure greater than 180 mg Hg, diastolic blood pressure greater than 110 mg Hg, or both) had an average reduction of 60/17 mm Hg at the conclusion of treatment." Goldhamer A, Lisle D, Parpia B, Anderson SV, Campbell TC. Medically supervised water-only fasting in the treatment of hypertension. *J Manipulative Physiol Ther.* 2001 Jun;24(5):335-9 http://www.healthpromoting.com/335-339Goldhamer115263.QXD.pdf

[116] "RESULTS: Approximately 82% of the subjects achieved BP at or below 120/80 mm Hg by the end of the treatment program. The mean BP reduction was 20/7 mm Hg, with the greatest decrease being observed for subjects with the highest baseline BP." Goldhamer AC, Lisle DJ, Sultana P, Anderson SV, Parpia B, Hughes B, Campbell TC. Medically supervised water-only fasting in the treatment of borderline hypertension. *J Altern Complement Med.* 2002 Oct;8(5):643-50 http://www.healthpromoting.com/Articles/articles/study%202/acmpaper5.pdf

[117] Vertes V, Genuth SM, Hazelton IM. Supplemented fasting as a large-scale outpatient program. *JAMA.* 1977 Nov 14;238(20):2151-3

[118] Bauman WA, Schwartz E, Rose HG, Eisenstein HN, Johnson DW. Early and long-term effects of acute caloric deprivation in obese diabetic patients. *Am J Med.* 1988 Jul;85(1):38-46

[119] Goldhamer AC. Initial cost of care results in medically supervised water-only fasting for treating high blood pressure and diabetes. *J Altern Complement Med.* 2002 Dec;8(6):696-7 http://www.healthpromoting.com/Articles/pdf/Study%2032.pdf

[120] "The ketogenic diet should be considered as alternative therapy for children with difficult-to-control seizures. It is more effective than many of the new anticonvulsant medications and is well tolerated by children and families when it is effective." Freeman JM, Vining EP, Pillas DJ, Pyzik PL, Casey JC, Kelly LM. The efficacy of the ketogenic diet-1998: a prospective evaluation of intervention in 150 children. *Pediatrics.* 1998 Dec;102(6):1358-63 http://pediatrics.aappublications.org/cgi/reprint/102/6/1358

[121] Adam O, Wolfram G, Zollner N. Effect of alpha-linolenic acid in the human diet on linoleic acid metabolism and prostaglandin biosynthesis. *J Lipid Res.* 1986 Apr;27(4):421-6 http://www.jlr.org/cgi/reprint/27/4/421

[122] "Other results showed a significant reduction in morning stiffness with gamma-linolenic acid at 3 months and reduction in pain and articular index at 6 months with olive oil." Brzeski M, Madhok R, Capell HA. Evening primrose oil in patients with rheumatoid arthritis and side-effects of non-steroidal anti-inflammatory drugs. *Br J Rheumatol.* 1991 Oct;30(5):370-2

[123] Rothman D, DeLuca P, Zurier RB. Botanical lipids: effects on inflammation, immune responses, and rheumatoid arthritis. *Semin Arthritis Rheum.* 1995 Oct;25(2):87-96

[124] Adam O, Beringer C, Kless T, Lemmen C, Adam A, Wiseman M, Adam P, Klimmek R, Forth W. Anti-inflammatory effects of a low arachidonic acid diet and fish oil in patients with rheumatoid arthritis. *Rheumatol Int.* 2003 Jan;23(1):27-36

[125] Lau CS, Morley KD, Belch JJ. Effects of fish oil supplementation on non-steroidal anti-inflammatory drug requirement in patients with mild rheumatoid arthritis--a double-blind placebo controlled study. *Br J Rheumatol.* 1993 Nov;32(11):982-9

[126] Kremer JM, Jubiz W, Michalek A, Rynes RI, Bartholomew LE, Bigaouette J, Timchalk M, Beeler D, Lininger L. Fish-oil fatty acid supplementation in active rheumatoid arthritis. A double-blinded, controlled, crossover study. *Ann Intern Med.* 1987 Apr;106(4):497-503

[127] Walton AJ, Snaith ML, Locniskar M, Cumberland AG, Morrow WJ, Isenberg DA. Dietary fish oil and the severity of symptoms in patients with systemic lupus erythematosus. *Ann Rheum Dis.* 1991 Jul;50(7):463-6

[128] Duffy EM, Meenagh GK, McMillan SA, Strain JJ, Hannigan BM, Bell AL. The clinical effect of dietary supplementation with omega-3 fish oils and/or copper in systemic lupus erythematosus. *J Rheumatol.* 2004 Aug;31(8):1551-6

dose of fatty acid supplementation until inflammation and the hyperoxidative state have been reduced; see the final chapter in this text on Therapeutics for more fatty acid details and biochemical pathways. Clinicians must realize that fatty acids are not clinically or biochemically interchangeable and that one fatty acid does not substitute for another; each of the fatty acids must be supplied in order for its benefits to be obtained.[129]

- Vitamin D3 supplementation with physiologic doses and/or tailored to serum 25(OH)D levels: Vitamin D deficiency is common in the general population and is even more common in patients with chronic illness and chronic musculoskeletal pain.[130] Correction of vitamin D deficiency supports normal immune function against infection and provides a clinically significant anti-inflammatory[131] and analgesic benefit in patients with back pain[132] and limb pain.[133] Reasonable daily doses for children and adults are 1,000-2,000 and 4,000 IU, respectively.[134] Deficiency and response to treatment are monitored with serum 25(OH)vitamin D while safety is monitored with serum calcium; inflammatory granulomatous diseases and certain drugs such as hydrochlorothiazide greatly increase the propensity for hypercalcemia and warrant increment dosing and frequent monitoring of serum calcium. Vitamin D2 (ergocalciferol) is not a human nutrient and should not be used in clinical practice.

Microorganisms causatively or molecularly associated with polymyositis/dermatomyositis
• *Streptococcus pyogenes*
• *Staphylococcus aureus*
• *Toxoplasma gondii*
• *Mycoplasma pneumoniae*
• *Borrelia burgdorferi*
• Coxsackie B virus
• *Mycoplasma hominis*
• *Haemophilus influenzae*
• *Helicobacter pylori*
• *Escherichia coli*
• *Bacillus subtilis*

- **Assessment for dysbiosis: Given the numerous links between PM-DM and various microorganisms, testing for and treating multifocal dysbiosis (as outlined in Chapter 4) is strongly encouraged.** Yeast, bacteria, and parasites are treated as indicated based on identification and sensitivity results from comprehensive parasitology assessments. Patients taking immunosuppressant drugs such as corticosteroids/prednisone have increased risk of intestinal bacterial overgrowth and translocation.[135,136] Other dysbiotic loci should be investigated as discussed in Chapter 4 in the section on multifocal dysbiosis.

  o Gastrointestinal dysbiosis: Treatment for gastrointestinal dysbiosis may include the following:

    ▪ Oregano oil: Emulsified oil of oregano in a time-released tablet is proven effective in the eradication of harmful gastrointestinal microbes, including *Blastocystis hominis*, *Entamoeba hartmanni*, and *Endolimax nana*.[137] An *in vitro* study[138] and clinical experience support the use of emulsified oregano against *Candida albicans* and various bacteria. The common dose is 600 mg per day in divided doses for 6 weeks.[139]

    ▪ Berberine: Berberine is an alkaloid extracted from plants such as *Berberis vulgaris*, and *Hydrastis canadensis*, and it shows effectiveness against *Giardia*, *Candida*, and

[129] Vasquez A. Reducing Pain and Inflammation Naturally. Part 2: New Insights into Fatty Acid Supplementation and Its Effect on Eicosanoid Production and Genetic Expression. *Nutritional Perspectives* 2005; January: 5-16 http://optimalhealthresearch.com/part2

[130] Plotnikoff GA, Quigley JM. Prevalence of severe hypovitaminosis D in patients with persistent, nonspecific musculoskeletal pain. *Mayo Clin Proc.* 2003 Dec;78(12):1463-70

[131] Timms PM, Mannan N, Hitman GA, Noonan K, Mills PG, Syndercombe-Court D, Aganna E, Price CP, Boucher BJ. Circulating MMP9, vitamin D and variation in the TIMP-1 response with VDR genotype: mechanisms for inflammatory damage in chronic disorders? *QJM.* 2002 Dec;95(12):787-96 http://qjmed.oxfordjournals.org/cgi/content/full/95/12/787

[132] Al Faraj S, Al Mutairi K. Vitamin D deficiency and chronic low back pain in Saudi Arabia. *Spine.* 2003 Jan 15;28(2):177-9

[133] Masood H, Narang AP, Bhat IA, Shah GN. Persistent limb pain and raised serum alkaline phosphatase the earliest markers of subclinical hypovitaminosis D in Kashmir. *Indian J Physiol Pharmacol.* 1989 Oct-Dec;33(4):259-61

[134] Vasquez A, Manso G, Cannell J. The clinical importance of vitamin D (cholecalciferol): a paradigm shift with implications for all healthcare providers. *Altern Ther Health Med.* 2004 Sep-Oct;10(5):28-36 http://optimalhealthresearch.com/monograph04

[135] "A 63-year-old man with systemic lupus erythematosus and selective IgA deficiency developed intractable diarrhoea the day after treatment with prednisone, 50 mg daily, was started. The diarrhoea was considered to be caused by bacterial overgrowth and was later successfully treated with doxycycline." Denison H, Wallerstedt S. Bacterial overgrowth after high-dose corticosteroid treatment. *Scand J Gastroenterol.* 1989 Jun;24(5):561-4

[136] "These bacteria also translocated to the mesenteric lymph nodes in mice injected with cyclophosphamide or prednisone." Berg RD, Wommack E, Deitch EA. Immunosuppression and intestinal bacterial overgrowth synergistically promote bacterial translocation. *Arch Surg.* 1988 Nov;123(11):1359-64

[137] Force M, Sparks WS, Ronzio RA. Inhibition of enteric parasites by emulsified oil of oregano in vivo. *Phytother Res.* 2000 May;14(3):213-4

[138] Stiles JC, Sparks W, Ronzio RA. The inhibition of Candida albicans by oregano. *J Applied Nutr* 1995;47:96–102

[139] Force M, Sparks WS, Ronzio RA. Inhibition of enteric parasites by emulsified oil of oregano in vivo. *Phytother Res.* 2000 May;14(3):213-4

Streptococcus in addition to its direct anti-inflammatory and antidiarrheal actions. Oral dose of 400 mg per day is common for adults.[140]

- *Artemisia annua*: Artemisinin has been safely used for centuries in Asia for the treatment of malaria, and it also has effectiveness against anaerobic bacteria due to the pro-oxidative sesquiterpene endoperoxide.[141,142] I commonly use artemisinin at 200 mg per day in divided doses for adults with dysbiosis.

- St. John's Wort (*Hypericum perforatum*): Hyperforin from *Hypericum perforatum* also shows impressive antibacterial action, particularly against gram-positive bacteria such as *Staphylococcus aureus*, *Streptococcus pyogenes*, *Streptococcus agalactiae*[143] and perhaps *Helicobacter pylori*.[144] Up to 600 mg three times per day of a 3% hyperforin standardized extract is customary in the treatment of depression.

- Bismuth: Bismuth is commonly used in the empiric treatment of diarrhea (e.g., "Pepto-Bismol") and is commonly combined with other antimicrobial agents to reduce drug resistance and increase antibiotic effectiveness.[145]

- Undecylenic acid: Derived from castor bean oil, undecylenic acid has antifungal properties and is commonly indicated by sensitivity results obtained by stool culture. Common dosages are 150-250 mg tid (up to 750 mg per day).[146]

- Peppermint (*Mentha piperita*): Peppermint shows antimicrobial and antispasmodic actions and has demonstrated clinical effectiveness in patients with bacterial overgrowth of the small bowel.

- Commonly used antibiotic/antifungal drugs: The most commonly employed drugs for intestinal bacterial overgrowth are described here.[147] Treatment duration is generally at least 2 weeks and up to 8 weeks, depending on clinical response and the severity and diversity of the intestinal overgrowth. With all anti*bacterial* treatments, use empiric anti*fungal* treatment to prevent yeast overgrowth; some patients benefit from antifungal treatment that is continued for *months* and occasionally *years*. Drugs can generally be coadministered with natural antibiotics/antifungals for improved efficacy. Treatment can be guided by identification of the dysbiotic microbes and the results of culture and sensitivity tests.

  ⇒ Metronidazole: 250-500 mg BID-QID (generally limit to 1.5 g/d); metronidazole has systemic bioavailability and effectiveness against a wide range of dysbiotic microbes, including protozoans, amebas/Giardia, *H. pylori*, *Clostridium difficile* and most anaerobic gram-negative bacilli.[148] Adverse effects are generally limited to stomatitis, nausea, diarrhea, and—rarely and/or with long-term use—peripheral neuropathy, dizziness, and metallic taste; the drug must not be consumed with alcohol.

  ⇒ Erythromycin: 250-500 mg TID-QID; this drug is a widely used antibiotic that also has intestinal promotility benefits (thus making it an ideal treatment for intestinal bacterial overgrowth associated with or caused

[140] Berberine. Altern Med Rev. 2000 Apr;5(2):175-7 http://www.thorne.com/altmedrev/.fulltext/5/2/175.pdf
[141] Dien TK, de Vries PJ, Khanh NX, Koopmans R, Binh LN, Duc DD, Kager PA, van Boxtel CJ. Effect of food intake on pharmacokinetics of oral artemisinin in healthy Vietnamese subjects. *Antimicrob Agents Chemother*. 1997 May;41(5):1069-72
[142] Giao PT, Binh TQ, Kager PA, Long HP, Van Thang N, Van Nam N, de Vries PJ. Artemisinin for treatment of uncomplicated falciparum malaria: is there a place for monotherapy? *Am J Trop Med Hyg*. 2001 Dec;65(6):690-5
[143] Schempp CM, Pelz K, Wittmer A, Schopf E, Simon JC. Antibacterial activity of hyperforin from St John's wort, against multiresistant Staphylococcus aureus and gram-positive bacteria. *Lancet*. 1999 Jun 19;353(9170):2129
[144] "A butanol fraction of St. John's Wort revealed anti-Helicobacter pylori activity with MIC values ranging between 15.6 and 31.2 microg/ml." Reichling J, Weseler A, Saller R. A current review of the antimicrobial activity of Hypericum perforatum L. *Pharmacopsychiatry*. 2001 Jul;34 Suppl 1:S116-8
[145] Veldhuyzen van Zanten SJ, Sherman PM, Hunt RH. Helicobacter pylori: new developments and treatments. *CMAJ*. 1997;156(11):1565-74 http://www.cmaj.ca/cgi/reprint/156/11/1565.pdf
[146] "Adult dosage is usually 450-750 mg undecylenic acid daily in three divided doses." Undecylenic acid. Monograph. *Altern Med Rev*. 2002 Feb;7(1):68-70 http://www.thorne.com/altmedrev/.fulltext/7/1/68.pdf
[147] Saltzman JR, Russell RM. Nutritional consequences of intestinal bacterial overgrowth. *Compr Ther*. 1994;20(9):523-30
[148] Tierney ML. McPhee SJ, Papadakis MA. Current Medical Diagnosis and Treatment 2006. 45th edition. New York; Lange Medical Books: 2006, pages 1578-1577

by intestinal dysmotility/hypomotility such as seen in scleroderma[149,150]). Do not combine erythromycin with the promotility drug **cisapride** due to risk for serious cardiac arrhythmia.

⇒ Tetracycline: 250-500 mg QID

⇒ Ciproflaxacin: 500 mg BID

⇒ Cephalexin/kelfex: 250 mg QID

⇒ Minocycline: Minocycline (200 mg/day)[151] has received the most attention in the treatment of rheumatoid arthritis due to its superior response (65%) over placebo (13%)[152]; in addition to its antibacterial action, the drug is also immunomodulatory and anti-inflammatory. Ironically, minocycline can cause drug-induced autoimmunity, especially lupus.[153,154]

⇒ Nystatin: Nystatin 500,000 units bid with food; duration of treatment begins with a minimum duration of 2-4 weeks and may continue as long as the patient is deriving benefit.

⇒ Emulsified time-released oil of oregano: The standard dose for adults is 600 mg per day in divided doses for 6-8 weeks when used as a single antimicrobial agent against various bacteria (per culture and sensitivity results), *Blastocystis hominis, Entamoeba hartmanni, Endolimax nana*[155] and *Candida albicans*.[156]

⇒ Ketoconazole: As a systemically bioavailable antifungal drug, ketoconazole has inherent anti-inflammatory benefits which may be helpful; however the drug inhibits androgen formation and may lead to exacerbation of the hypoandrogenism that is commonly seen in autoimmune patients and which contributes to the immune dysfunction.

▪ Probiotics: Live cultures in the form of tablets, capsules, yogurt, or kefir can be used per patient preference and tolerance. Obviously, dairy-based products should be avoided by patients with dairy allergy.

▪ Supplemented Paleo-Mediterranean diet / Specific Carbohydrate Diet: The specifications of the *specific carbohydrate diet* (SCD) detailed by Gottschall[157] are met with adherence to the Paleo diet by Cordain.[158] The combination of both approaches and books will give patients an excellent combination of informational understanding and culinary versatility.

• Orthoendocrinology: Assess prolactin, cortisol, DHEA, free and total testosterone, serum estradiol, and thyroid status (e.g., TSH, T4, *and* anti-thyroid peroxidase antibodies).

  o Prolactin (excess): The role of prolactin in PM-DM has not been studied. However, prolactin is increasingly well-known as a proinflammatory and immunodysregulatory hormone. **Serum levels of prolactin tend to be higher in patients with autoimmunity, and therapeutic lowering of prolactin levels results in clinically significant anti-**

---

[149] "Prokinetic agents effective in pseudoobstruction include metoclopramide, domperidone, cisapride, octreotide, and erythromycin. ... The combination of octreotide and erythromycin may be particularly effective in systemic sclerosis." Sjogren RW. Gastrointestinal features of scleroderma. *Curr Opin Rheumatol.* 1996 Nov;8(6):569-75

[150] "CONCLUSIONS: Erythromycin accelerates gastric and gallbladder emptying in scleroderma patients and might be helpful in the treatment of gastrointestinal motor abnormalities in these patients." Fiorucci S, Distrutti E, Bassotti G, Gerli R, Chiucchiu S, Betti C, Santucci L, Morelli A. Effect of erythromycin administration on upper gastrointestinal motility in scleroderma patients. *Scand J Gastroenterol.* 1994 Sep;29(9):807-13

[151] "...48-week trial of oral minocycline (200 mg/d) or placebo." Tilley BC, Alarcon GS, Heyse SP, Trentham DE, Neuner R, Kaplan DA, Clegg DO, Leisen JC, Buckley L, Cooper SM, Duncan H, Pillemer SR, Tuttleman M, Fowler SE. Minocycline in rheumatoid arthritis. A 48-week, double-blind, placebo-controlled trial. MIRA Trial Group. *Ann Intern Med.* 1995 Jan 15;122(2):81-9

[152] "In patients with early seropositive RA, therapy with minocycline is superior to placebo." O'Dell JR, Haire CE, Palmer W, Drymalski W, Wees S, Blakely K, Churchill M, Eckhoff PJ, Weaver A, Doud D, Erikson N, Dietz F, Olson R, Maloley P, Klassen LW, Moore GF. Treatment of early rheumatoid arthritis with minocycline or placebo: results of a randomized, double-blind, placebo-controlled trial. *Arthritis Rheum.* 1997 May;40(5):842-8

[153] "...many cases of drug-induced lupus related to minocycline have been reported. Some of those reports included pulmonary lupus..." Christodoulou CS, Emmanuel P, Ray RA, Good RA, Schnapf BM, Cawkwell GD. Respiratory distress due to minocycline-induced pulmonary lupus. *Chest.* 1999 May;115(5):1471-3 http://www.chestjournal.org/cgi/content/full/115/5/1471

[154] Lawson TM, Amos N, Bulgen D, Williams BD.Minocycline-induced lupus: clinical features and response to rechallenge. *Rheumatology* (Oxford). 2001 Mar;40(3):329-35 http://rheumatology.oxfordjournals.org/cgi/content/full/40/3/329

[155] Force M, Sparks WS, Ronzio RA. Inhibition of enteric parasites by emulsified oil of oregano in vivo. *Phytother Res.* 2000 May;14(3):213-4

[156] Stiles JC, Sparks W, Ronzio RA. The inhibition of Candida albicans by oregano. *J Applied Nutr* 1995;47:96–102

[157] Gottschall E. Breaking the Vicious Cycle: Intestinal health though diet. Kirkton Press; Rev edition (August, 1994) http://www.scdiet.com/

[158] Cordain L: The Paleo Diet: Lose weight and get healthy by eating the food you were designed to eat. John Wiley & Sons Inc., New York 2002 http://thepaleodiet.com/

inflammatory benefits. Among women with hyperprolactinemia, 75% of them show serologic evidence of asymptomatic autoimmunity.[159] As discussed elsewhere, patients with RA and SLE have higher basal and stress-induced levels of prolactin compared with normal controls[160,161], and men with RA have higher serum levels of prolactin that correlate with the severity and duration of the disorder.[162,163] Serum prolactin is the standard assessment of prolactin status. Since elevated prolactin may be a sign of pituitary tumor, assessment for headaches, visual deficits, and other abnormalities of pituitary hormones (e.g., GH and TSH) should be performed; CT or MRI must be considered. Patients with prolactin levels less than 100 ng/mL and normal CT/MRI findings can be managed conservatively with effective prolactin-lowering treatment and annual radiologic assessment (less necessary with favorable serum response).[164, see review 165] Specific treatment options include the following:

- Thyroid hormone: Hypothyroidism frequently causes hyperprolactinemia which is reversible upon effective treatment of hypothyroidism. Obviously therefore, thyroid status should be evaluated in all patients with hyperprolactinemia. Thyroid assessment and treatment is reviewed later in this section.

- *Vitex astus-cagnus* and other supporting botanicals and nutrients: **Vitex lowers serum prolactin in humans[166,167] via a dopaminergic effect.[168]** Vitex is considered safe for clinical use; mild and reversible adverse effects possibly associated with Vitex include nausea, headache, gastrointestinal disturbances, menstrual disorders, acne, pruritus and erythematous rash. No drug interactions are known, but given the herb's dopaminergic effect it should probably be used with some caution in patients treated with dopamine antagonists such as the so-called antipsychotic drugs (most of which do not work very well and/or carry intolerable adverse effects[169,170]). In a recent review, Bone[171] stated that daily doses can range from 500 mg to 2,000 mg DHE (dry herb equivalent) and can be tailored to the suppression of prolactin. Due at least in part to its content of L-dopa, *Mucuna pruriens* **shows clinical dopaminergic activity** as evidenced by its effectiveness in Parkinson's disease[172]; up to 15-30 gm/d of mucuna has been used clinically but doses will be dependent on preparation and phytoconcentration. **Triptolide and other extracts from *Tripterygium wilfordii* Hook F exert clinically significant anti-inflammatory action in patients with rheumatoid**

[159] "Twenty-five of 33 (75.7%) HPRL women were found to have at least one autoantibody, while none of the 19 women with normal PRL had any. Yet none of the HPRL women whose serum was found to contain high titers of autoantibodies presented with symptoms related to the respective autoimmune disorders." Buskila D, Berezin M, Gur H, Lin HC, Alosachie I, Terryberry JW, Barka N, Shen B, Peter JB, Shoenfeld Y. Autoantibody profile in the sera of women with hyperprolactinemia. *J Autoimmun.* 1995 Jun;8(3):415-24

[160] Dostal C, Moszkorzova L, Musilova L, Lacinova Z, Marek J, Zvarova J. Serum prolactin stress values in patients with systemic lupus erythematosus. *Ann Rheum Dis.* 2003 May;62(5):487-8 http://ard.bmjjournals.com/cgi/content/full/62/5/487

[161] "RESULTS: A significantly higher rate of elevated PRL levels was found in SLE patients (40.0%) compared with the healthy controls (14.8%). No proof was found of association with the presence of anti-ds-DNA or with specific organ involvement. Similarly, elevated PRL levels were found in RA patients (39.3%)." Moszkorzova L, Lacinova Z, Marek J, Musilova L, Dohnalova A, Dostal C. Hyperprolactinaemia in patients with systemic lupus erythematosus. *Clin Exp Rheumatol.* 2002 Nov-Dec;20(6):807-12

[162] "CONCLUSION: Men with RA have high serum PRL levels and concentrations increase with longer disease evolution and worse functional stage." Mateo L, Nolla JM, Bonnin MR, Navarro MA, Roig-Escofet D. High serum prolactin levels in men with rheumatoid arthritis. *J Rheumatol.* 1998 Nov;25(11):2077-82

[163] "Male patients affected by RA showed high serum PRL levels. The serum PRL concentration was found to be increased in relation to the duration and the activity of the disease. Serum PRL levels do not seem to have any relationship with the BMD, at least in RA." Seriolo B, Ferretti V, Sulli A, Fasciolo D, Cutolo M. Serum prolactin concentrations in male patients with rheumatoid arthritis. *Ann N Y Acad Sci.* 2002 Jun;966:258-62

[164] Beers MH, Berkow R (eds). The Merck Manual. Seventeenth Edition. Whitehouse Station; Merck Research Laboratories 1999 Page 77-78

[165] Serri O, Chik CL, Ur E, Ezzat S. Diagnosis and management of hyperprolactinemia. *CMAJ.* 2003 Sep 16;169(6):575-81 http://www.cmaj.ca/cgi/content/full/169/6/575

[166] "Since AC extracts were shown to have beneficial effects on premenstrual mastodynia serum prolactin levels in such patients were also studied in one double-blind, placebo-controlled clinical study. Serum prolactin levels were indeed reduced in the patients treated with the extract." Wuttke W, Jarry H, Christoffel V, Spengler B, Seidlova-Wuttke D. Chaste tree (Vitex agnus-castus)--pharmacology and clinical indications. *Phytomedicine.* 2003 May;10(4):348-57

[167] German abstract from Medline: "The prolactin release was reduced after 3 months, shortened luteal phases were normalised and deficits in the luteal progesterone synthesis were eliminated." Milewicz A, Gejdel E, Sworen H, Sienkiewicz K, Jedrzejak J, Teucher T, Schmitz H. [Vitex agnus castus extract in the treatment of luteal phase defects due to latent hyperprolactinemia. Results of a randomized placebo-controlled double-blind study] *Arzneimittelforschung.* 1993 Jul;43(7):752-6

[168] "Our results indicate a dopaminergic effect of Vitex agnus-castus extracts and suggest additional pharmacological actions via opioid receptors." Meier B, Berger D, Hoberg E, Sticher O, Schaffner W. Pharmacological activities of Vitex agnus-castus extracts in vitro. *Phytomedicine.* 2000 Oct;7(5):373-81

[169] "The majority of patients in each group discontinued their assigned treatment owing to inefficacy or intolerable side effects or for other reasons." Lieberman JA, Stroup TS, McEvoy JP, Swartz MS, Rosenheck RA, Perkins DO, Keefe RS, Davis SM, Davis CE, Lebowitz BD, Severe J, Hsiao JK; Clinical Antipsychotic Trials of Intervention Effectiveness (CATIE) Investigators. Effectiveness of antipsychotic drugs in patients with chronic schizophrenia. *N Engl J Med.* 2005 Sep 22;353(12):1209-23

[170] Whitaker R. The case against antipsychotic drugs: a 50-year record of doing more harm than good. *Med Hypotheses.* 2004;62(1):5-13

[171] "In conditions such as endometriosis and fibroids, for which a significant estrogen antagonist effect is needed, doses of at least 2 g/day DHE may be required and typically are used by professional herbalists." Bone K. New Insights Into Chaste Tree. *Nutritional Wellness* 2005 November http://www.nutritionalwellness.com/archives/2005/nov/11_bone.php

[172] "CONCLUSIONS: The rapid onset of action and longer on time without concomitant increase in dyskinesias on mucuna seed powder formulation suggest that this natural source of L-dopa might possess advantages over conventional L-dopa preparations in the long term management of PD." Katzenschlager R, Evans A, Manson A, Patsalos PN, Ratnaraj N, Watt H, Timmermann L, Van der Giessen R, Lees AJ. Mucuna pruriens in Parkinson's disease: a double blind clinical and pharmacological study. *J Neurol Neurosurg Psychiatry.* 2004 Dec;75(12):1672-7

arthritis[173,174] **and also offer protection to dopaminergic neurons.**[175,176] Ironically, even though tyrosine is the nutritional precursor to dopamine with evidence of clinical effectiveness (e.g., narcolepsy[177], enhancement of memory[178] and cognition[179]), **supplementation with tyrosine appears to actually increase rather than decrease prolactin levels**[180]; **therefore tyrosine should be used cautiously (if at all) in patients with systemic inflammation and elevated prolactin.** Furthermore, the finding that **high-protein meals stimulate prolactin release**[181] may partly explain the benefits of vegetarian diets in the treatment of systemic inflammation; since vegetarian diets are comparatively low in protein compared to omnivorous diets, they may lead to a relative reduction in prolactin production due to lack of stimulation.

- Bromocriptine: Bromocriptine has long been considered the pharmacologic treatment of choice for elevated prolactin.[182] Typical dose is 2.5 mg per day (effective against lupus[183]); gastrointestinal upset and sedation are common.[184] Clinical intervention with bromocriptine appears warranted in patients with RA, SLE, Reiter's syndrome, psoriatic arthritis, and probably multiple sclerosis and uveitis.[185]

- Cabergoline/Dostinex: Cabergoline/Dostinex is a newer dopamine agonist with few adverse effects; typical dose starts at 0.5 mg per week (0.25 mg twice per week).[186] Several studies have indicated that cabergoline is safer and more effective than bromocriptine for reducing prolactin levels[187] and the dose can often be reduced after successful prolactin reduction, allowing for reductions in cost and adverse effects.[188] Although fewer studies have been published supporting the antirheumatic benefits of cabergoline than bromocriptine, its antirheumatic benefits have been documented.[189]

- Estrogen (excess): **Men with rheumatoid arthritis show an excess of estradiol** and a decrease in DHEA, and the **excess estrogen is proportional to the degree of**

[173] "The ethanol/ethyl acetate extract of TWHF shows therapeutic benefit in patients with treatment-refractory RA. At therapeutic dosages, the TWHF extract was well tolerated by most patients in this study." Tao X, Younger J, Fan FZ, Wang B, Lipsky PE. Benefit of an extract of Tripterygium Wilfordii Hook F in patients with rheumatoid arthritis: a double-blind, placebo-controlled study. *Arthritis Rheum.* 2002 Jul;46(7):1735-43

[174] "CONCLUSION: The EA extract of TWHF at dosages up to 570 mg/day appeared to be safe, and doses > 360 mg/day were associated with clinical benefit in patients with RA." Tao X, Cush JJ, Garret M, Lipsky PE. A phase I study of ethyl acetate extract of the chinese antirheumatic herb Tripterygium wilfordii hook F in rheumatoid arthritis. *J Rheumatol.* 2001 Oct;28(10):2160-7

[175] "Our data suggests that triptolide may protect dopaminergic neurons from LPS-induced injury and its efficiency in inhibiting microglia activation may underlie the mechanism." Li FQ, Lu XZ, Liang XB, Zhou HF, Xue B, Liu XY, Niu DB, Han JS, Wang XM. Triptolide, a Chinese herbal extract, protects dopaminergic neurons from inflammation-mediated damage through inhibition of microglial activation. *J Neuroimmunol.* 2004 Mar;148(1-2):24-31

[176] "Moreover, tripchlorolide markedly prevented the decrease in amount of dopamine in the striatum of model rats. Taken together, our data provide the first evidence that tripchlorolide acts as a neuroprotective molecule that rescues MPP+ or axotomy-induced degeneration of dopaminergic neurons, which may imply its therapeutic potential for Parkinson's disease." Li FQ, Cheng XX, Liang XB, Wang XH, Xue B, He QH, Wang XM, Han JS. Neurotrophic and neuroprotective effects of tripchlorolide, an extract of Chinese herb Tripterygium wilfordii Hook F, on dopaminergic neurons. *Exp Neurol.* 2003 Jan;179(1):28-37

[177] "Of twenty-eight visual analogue scales rating mood and arousal, the subjects' ratings in the tyrosine treatment (9 g daily) and placebo periods differed significantly for only three (less tired, less drowsy, more alert)." Elwes RD, Crewes H, Chesterman LP, Summers B, Jenner P, Binnie CD, Parkes JD. Treatment of narcolepsy with L-tyrosine: double-blind placebo-controlled trial. *Lancet.* 1989 Nov 4;2(8671):1067-9

[178] "Ten men and 10 women subjects underwent these batteries 1 h after ingesting 150 mg/kg of l-tyrosine or placebo. Administration of tyrosine significantly enhanced accuracy and decreased frequency of list retrieval on the working memory task during the multiple task battery compared with placebo." Thomas JR, Lockwood PA, Singh A, Deuster PA. Tyrosine improves working memory in a multitasking environment. *Pharmacol Biochem Behav.* 1999 Nov;64(3):495-500

[179] "Ten subjects received five daily doses of a protein-rich drink containing 2 g tyrosine, and 11 subjects received a carbohydrate rich drink with the same amount of calories (255 kcal)." Deijen JB, Wientjes CJ, Vullinghs HF, Cloin PA, Langefeld JJ. Tyrosine improves cognitive performance and reduces blood pressure in cadets after one week of a combat training course. *Brain Res Bull.* 1999 Jan 15;48(2):203-9

[180] "Tyrosine (when compared to placebo) had no effect on any sleep related measure, but it did stimulate prolactin release." Waters WF, Magill RA, Bray GA, Volaufova J, Smith SR, Lieberman HR, Rood J, Hurry M, Anderson T, Ryan DH. A comparison of tyrosine against placebo, phentermine, caffeine, and D-amphetamine during sleep deprivation. *Nutr Neurosci.* 2003;6(4):221-35

[181] "Whereas carbohydrate meals had no discernible effects, high protein meals induced a large increase in both PRL and cortisol; high fat meals caused selective release of PRL." Ishizuka B, Quigley ME, Yen SS. Pituitary hormone release in response to food ingestion: evidence for neuroendocrine signals from gut to brain. *J Clin Endocrinol Metab.* 1983 Dec;57(6):1111-6

[182] Beers MH, Berkow R (eds). The Merck Manual. Seventeenth Edition. Whitehouse Station; Merck Research Laboratories 1999 Page 77-78

[183] "A prospective, double-blind, randomized, placebo-controlled study compared BRC at a fixed daily dosage of 2.5 mg with placebo... Long term treatment with a low dose of BRC appears to be a safe and effective means of decreasing SLE flares in SLE patients." Alvarez-Nemegyei J, Cobarrubias-Cobos A, Escalante-Triay F, Sosa-Munoz J, Miranda JM, Jara LJ. Bromocriptine in systemic lupus erythematosus: a double-blind, randomized, placebo-controlled study. *Lupus.* 1998;7(6):414-9

[184] Serri O, Chik CL, Ur E, Ezzat S. Diagnosis and management of hyperprolactinemia. *CMAJ.* 2003 Sep 16;169(6):575-81 http://www.cmaj.ca/cgi/content/full/169/6/575

[185] "...clinical observations and trials support the use of bromocriptine as a nonstandard primary or adjunctive therapy in the treatment of recalcitrant RA, SLE, Reiter's syndrome, and psoriatic arthritis and associated conditions unresponsive to traditional approaches." McMurray RW. Bromocriptine in rheumatic and autoimmune diseases. *Semin Arthritis Rheum.* 2001 Aug;31(1):21-32

[186] Serri O, Chik CL, Ur E, Ezzat S. Diagnosis and management of hyperprolactinemia. *CMAJ.* 2003 Sep 16;169(6):575-81 http://www.cmaj.ca/cgi/content/full/169/6/575

[187] "CONCLUSION: These data indicate that cabergoline is a very effective agent for lowering the prolactin levels in hyperprolactinemic patients and that it appears to offer considerable advantage over bromocriptine in terms of efficacy and tolerability." Sabuncu T, Arikan E, Tasan E, Hatemi H. Comparison of the effects of cabergoline and bromocriptine on prolactin levels in hyperprolactinemic patients. *Intern Med.* 2001 Sep;40(9):857-61

[188] "Cabergoline also normalized PRL in the majority of patients with known bromocriptine intolerance or -resistance. Once PRL secretion was adequately controlled, the dose of cabergoline could often be significantly decreased, which further reduced costs of therapy." Verhelst J, Abs R, Maiter D, van den Bruel A, Vandeweghe M, Velkeniers B, Mockel J, Lamberigts G, Petrossians P, Coremans P, Mahler C, Stevenaert A, Verlooy J, Raftopoulos C, Beckers A. Cabergoline in the treatment of hyperprolactinemia: a study in 455 patients. *J Clin Endocrinol Metab.* 1999 Jul;84(7):2518-22 http://jcem.endojournals.org/cgi/content/full/84/7/2518

[189] Erb N, Pace AV, Delamere JP, Kitas GD. Control of unremitting rheumatoid arthritis by the prolactin antagonist cabergoline. *Rheumatology* (Oxford). 2001 Feb;40(2):237-9 http://rheumatology.oxfordjournals.org/cgi/content/full/40/2/237

inflammation.[190] Estrogen status can be assessed using serum estradiol or a 24-hour urine sample. Interventions to combat high estrogen levels may include any effective combination of the following:

- Weight loss and weight optimization: In overweight patients, *weight loss* is the means to attaining the goal of *weight optimization*; the task is not complete until the body mass index is normalized/optimized. Excess adiposity and obesity raise estrogen levels due to high levels of aromatase (the hormone that makes estrogen) in adipose tissue; weight optimization and loss of excess fat helps normalize hormone levels and reduce inflammation.

- Avoidance of ethanol: Estrogen production is stimulated by ethanol intake.

- Consider surgical correction of varicocele in affected men: Men with varicocele have higher estrogen levels due to temperature-induced alterations in enzyme function in the testes; surgical correction of the varicocele lowers estrogen levels.

- "Anti-estrogen diet": Foods and supplements such as green tea, DIM, I3C, licorice, and a high-fiber "anti-estrogenic diet" can also be used; monitoring clinical status and serum estradiol will prove or disprove efficacy.

- Anastrozole/Arimidex: **In a recent case report, administration of anastrozole lead to clinical improvement in a woman with dermatomyositis.**[191]   In our office, we commonly measure serum estradiol in men and administer the aromatase inhibitor anastrozole/arimidex 1 mg (2-3 doses per week) to men whose estradiol level is greater than 32 picogram/mL. The Life Extension Foundation[192] advocates that the optimal serum estradiol level for a man is 10-30 picogram/mL.   Clinical studies using anastrozole/arimidex in men have shown that aromatase blockade lowers estradiol and raises testosterone[193]; generally speaking, this is exactly the result that we want in patients with severe systemic autoimmunity. Our practice has been to use the 1 (one) mg dose, with the frequency of dosing based on serum and clinical response.

> "Using **antiestrogen medication** in women with **dermatomyositis** may result in a significant improvement in their rash, possibly via the inhibition of TNF-alpha production by immune or other cells."
>
> Sereda D, Werth VP. *Arch Dermatol.* 2006 Jan;142(1):70-2

- Cortisol (insufficiency): Cortisol has immunoregulatory and "immunosuppressive" actions at physiological concentrations. Low adrenal function is common in patients with chronic inflammation.[194,195,196] Assessment of cortisol production and adrenal function was detailed in Chapter 4 under the section of Orthoendocrinology. Supplementation with 20 mg per day of cortisol/Cortef is physiologic; my preference is to dose 10 mg first thing in the morning, then 5 mg in late morning and 5 mg in midafternoon in an attempt to replicate the diurnal variation and normal morning peak of cortisol levels. In patients with hypoadrenalism, administration of pregnenolone in doses of 10-60 mg in the morning may also be beneficial.

---

[190] "RESULTS: DHEAS and estrone concentrations were lower and estradiol was higher in patients compared with healthy controls. DHEAS differed between RF positive and RF negative patients. Estrone did not correlate with any disease variable, whereas estradiol correlated strongly and positively with all measured indices of inflammation." Tengstrand B, Carlstrom K, Fellander-Tsai L, Hafstrom I. Abnormal levels of serum dehydroepiandrosterone, estrone, and estradiol in men with rheumatoid arthritis: high correlation between serum estradiol and current degree of inflammation. *J Rheumatol.* 2003 Nov;30(11):2338-43

[191] "Using antiestrogen medication in women with DM may result in a significant improvement in their rash, possibly via the inhibition of TNF-alpha production by immune or other cells." Sereda D, Werth VP. Improvement in dermatomyositis rash associated with the use of antiestrogen medication. *Arch Dermatol.* 2006 Jan;142(1):70-2

[192] Male Hormone Modulation Therapy, Page 4 Of 7: http://www.lef.org/protocols/prtcl-130c.shtml Accessed October 30, 2005

[193] "These data demonstrate that aromatase inhibition increases serum bioavailable and total testosterone levels to the youthful normal range in older men with mild hypogonadism." Leder BZ, Rohrer JL, Rubin SD, Gallo J, Longcope C. Effects of aromatase inhibition in elderly men with low or borderline-low serum testosterone levels. *J Clin Endocrinol Metab.* 2004 Mar;89(3):1174-80 http://jcem.endojournals.org/cgi/reprint/89/3/1174

[194] "Yet evidence that patients with rheumatoid arthritis improved with small, physiologic dosages of cortisol or cortisone acetate was reported over 25 years ago, and that patients with chronic allergic disorders or unexplained chronic fatigue also improved with administration of such small dosages was reported over 15 years ago..." Jefferies WM. Mild adrenocortical deficiency, chronic allergies, autoimmune disorders and the chronic fatigue syndrome: a continuation of the cortisone story. *Med Hypotheses.* 1994 Mar;42(3):183-9 http://www.thebuteykocentre.com/Irish_%20Buteykocenter_files/further_studies/med_hyp2.pdf http://members.westnet.com.au/pkolb/med_hyp2.pdf

[195] "The etiology of rheumatoid arthritis ...explained by a combination of three factors: (i) a relatively mild deficiency of cortisol, ..., (ii) a deficiency of DHEA, ...and (iii) infection by organisms such as mycoplasma,..." Jefferies WM. The etiology of rheumatoid arthritis. *Med Hypotheses.* 1998 Aug;51(2):111-4

[196] Jefferies W McK. Safe Uses of Cortisol. Second Edition. Springfield, CC Thomas, 1996

- o Testosterone (insufficiency): Androgen deficiencies predispose to, are exacerbated by, and contribute to autoimmune/inflammatory disorders. **A large proportion of men with lupus or RA have low testosterone**[197] and suffer the effects of hypogonadism: fatigue, weakness, depression, slow healing, low libido, and difficulties with sexual performance. Testosterone levels may rise following DHEA supplementation (especially in women) and can be elevated in men by the use of anastrozole/arimidex. Otherwise, transdermal testosterone such as Androgel or Testim can be applied as indicated.

- o DHEA (insufficiency / supraphysiologic supplementation): DHEA is an anti-inflammatory and immunoregulatory hormone that is commonly deficient in patients with autoimmunity and inflammatory arthritis.[198] DHEA levels are suppressed by prednisone[199], and DHEA supplementation has been shown to reverse the osteoporosis and loss of bone mass induced by corticosteroid treatment.[200] DHEA shows no acute or subacute toxicity even when used in supraphysiologic doses, even when used in sick patients. For example, in a study of 32 patients with HIV, DHEA doses of 750 mg – 2,250 mg per day were well-tolerated and produced no dose-limiting adverse effects.[201] This lack of toxicity compares favorably with any and all so-called "antirheumatic" drugs, nearly all of which show impressive comparable toxicity. When used at doses of 200 mg per day, DHEA safely provides clinical benefit for patients with various autoimmune diseases, including ulcerative colitis, Crohn's disease[202], and SLE.[203] In patients with SLE, DHEA supplementation allows for reduced dosing of prednisone (thus avoiding its adverse effects) while providing symptomatic improvement.[204] Optimal clinical response appears to correlate with serum levels that are supraphysiologic[205], and therefore treatment may be implemented with little regard for initial/baseline DHEA levels provided that the patient is free of contraindications, particularly high risk for sex-hormone-dependent malignancy. Other than mild adverse effects predictable with any androgen (namely voice deepening, transient acne, and increased facial hair), DHEA supplementation does not cause serious adverse effects[206], and it is appropriate for routine clinical use particularly when 1) the dose of DHEA is kept as low as possible, 2) duration is kept as short as possible, 3) other interventions are used to address the underlying cause of the disease, 4) the patient is deriving benefit, and 5) the risk-to-benefit ratio is favorable.

- o Thyroid (insufficiency or autoimmunity): **Because PM-DM can be convincingly mimicked by asymptomatic hyperthyroidism, hypothyroidism, and thyroid autoimmunity (including Grave's disease and Hashimoto's thyroiditis), all patients with PM-DM should receive a comprehensive thyroid evaluation including thyroid**

[197] Karagiannis A, Harsoulis F. Gonadal dysfunction in systemic diseases. *Eur J Endocrinol.* 2005 Apr;152(4):501-13 http://www.eje-online.org/cgi/content/full/152/4/501

[198] "DHEAS concentrations were significantly decreased in both women and men with inflammatory arthritis (IA) (P < 0.001)." Dessein PH, Joffe BI, Stanwix AE, Moomal Z. Hyposecretion of the adrenal androgen dehydroepiandrosterone sulfate and its relation to clinical variables in inflammatory arthritis. *Arthritis Res.* 2001;3(3):183-8. Epub 2001 Feb 21. http://arthritis-research.com/content/3/3/183

[199] "Basal serum DHEA and DHEAS concentrations were suppressed to a greater degree than was cortisol during both daily and alternate day prednisone treatments. ...Thus, adrenal androgen secretion was more easily suppressed than was cortisol secretion by this low dose of glucocorticoid, but there was no advantage to alternate day therapy." Rittmaster RS, Givner ML. Effect of daily and alternate day low dose prednisone on serum cortisol and adrenal androgens in hirsute women. *J Clin Endocrinol Metab.* 1988 Aug;67(2):400-3

[200] "CONCLUSION: Prasterone treatment prevented BMD loss and significantly increased BMD at both the lumbar spine and total hip in female patients with SLE receiving exogenous glucocorticoids." Mease PJ, Ginzler EM, Gluck OS, Schiff M, Goldman A, Greenwald M, Cohen S, Egan R, Quarles BJ, Schwartz KE. Effects of prasterone on bone mineral density in women with systemic lupus erythematosus receiving chronic glucocorticoid therapy. *J Rheumatol.* 2005 Apr;32(4):616-21

[201] "Thirty-one subjects were evaluated and monitored for safety and tolerance. The oral drug was administered three times daily in doses ranging from 750 mg/day to 2,250 mg/day for 16 weeks. ... The drug was well tolerated and no dose-limiting side effects were noted." Dyner TS, Lang W, Geaga J, Golub A, Stites D, Winger E, Galmarini M, Masterson J, Jacobson MA. An open-label dose-escalation trial of oral dehydroepiandrosterone tolerance and pharmacokinetics in patients with HIV disease. *J Acquir Immune Defic Syndr.* 1993 May;6(5):459-65

[202] "CONCLUSIONS: In a pilot study, dehydroepiandrosterone was effective and safe in patients with refractory Crohn's disease or ulcerative colitis." Andus T, Klebl F, Rogler G, Bregenzer N, Scholmerich J, Straub RH. Patients with refractory Crohn's disease or ulcerative colitis respond to dehydroepiandrosterone: a pilot study. *Aliment Pharmacol Ther.* 2003 Feb;17(3):409-14

[203] "CONCLUSION: The overall results confirm that DHEA treatment was well-tolerated, significantly reduced the number of SLE flares, and improved patient's global assessment of disease activity." Chang DM, Lan JL, Lin HY, Luo SF. Dehydroepiandrosterone treatment of women with mild-to-moderate systemic lupus erythematosus: a multicenter randomized, double-blind, placebo-controlled trial. *Arthritis Rheum.* 2002 Nov;46(11):2924-7

[204] "CONCLUSION: Among women with lupus disease activity, reducing the dosage of prednisone to < or = 7.5 mg/day for a sustained period of time while maintaining stabilization or a reduction of disease activity was possible in a significantly greater proportion of patients treated with oral prasterone, 200 mg once daily, compared with patients treated with placebo." Petri MA, Lahita RG, Van Vollenhoven RF, Merrill JT, Schiff M, Ginzler EM, Strand V, Kunz A, Gorelick KJ, Schwartz KE; GL601 Study Group. Effects of prasterone on corticosteroid requirements of women with systemic lupus erythematosus: a double-blind, randomized, placebo-controlled trial. *Arthritis Rheum.* 2002 Jul;46(7):1820-9

[205] "CONCLUSION: The clinical response to DHEA was not clearly dose dependent. Serum levels of DHEA and DHEAS correlated only weakly with lupus outcomes, but suggested an optimum serum DHEAS of 1000 microg/dl." Barry NN, McGuire JL, van Vollenhoven RF. Dehydroepiandrosterone in systemic lupus erythematosus: relationship between dosage, serum levels, and clinical response. *J Rheumatol.* 1998 Dec;25(12):2352-6

[206] Tierney ML. McPhee SJ, Papadakis MA. <u>Current Medical Diagnosis and Treatment 2006. 45th edition</u>. New York; Lange Medical Books: 2006, page 1721

gland palpation and serum measurements of TSH, T4, anti-thyroid peroxidase antibodies, and possibly free T3. Overt or imminent hypothyroidism is suggested by TSH greater than 2 mU/L[207] or 3 mU/L[208], low T4 or T3, and/or the presence of anti-thyroid peroxidase antibodies.[209] **Hypothyroidism can cause an inflammatory myopathy that can resemble polymyositis, and hypothyroidism is a frequent complication of any and all autoimmune diseases.** Specific treatment considerations include the following:

- <u>Selenium</u>: Supplementation with either selenomethonine[210] or sodium selenite[211,212] can reduce thyroid autoimmunity and improve peripheral conversion of T4 to T3. Selenium may be started at 500-800 mcg per day and tapered to 200-400 mcg per day for maintenance.[213]

- <u>L-thyroxine/levothyroxine/Synthroid—prescription synthetic T4</u>: 25-50 mcg per day is a common starting dose which can be adjusted based on clinical and laboratory response. Thyroid hormone supplements must be consumed separately from soy products (by at least 1-2 hours) and preferably on an empty stomach to avoid absorption interference by food, fiber, and minerals, especially calcium. Doses are generally started at one-half of the daily dose for the first 10 days after which the full dose is used. Caution must be applied in patients with adrenal insufficiency and/or those with cardiovascular disease.

- <u>Armour thyroid—prescription natural T4 and T3 from cow/pig thyroid gland</u>: 60 mg (one grain) is a common starting and maintenance dose. **Due to the exacerbating effect on thyroid autoimmunity, Armour thyroid is never used in patients with thyroid autoimmunity**.

- <u>Thyrolar/Liotrix—prescription synthetic T4 with T3</u>: Dosed as "1" (low), "2" (intermediate), or "3" (high). Although this product has been difficult to obtain for the past few years due to manufacturing problems (http://thyrolar.com/), it has been my treatment of choice due to the combination of T4 and T3 and the lack of antigenicity compared to gland-derived products.

- <u>Thyroid glandular—nonprescription T3</u>: Producers of nutritional products are able to distribute T3 because it is not listed by the FDA as a prescription item. Nutritional supplement companies may start with Armour thyroid, remove the T4, and sell the thyroid glandular with active T3 thereby providing a nonprescription source of active thyroid hormone. For many patients, one tablet per day is at least as effective as a prescription source of thyroid hormone. Since it is derived from a glandular and therefore potentially antigenic source, thyroid glandular is not used in patients with thyroid autoimmunity due to its ability to induce increased production of anti-thyroid antibodies.

- <u>L-tyrosine and iodine</u>: Some patients with mild hypothyroidism respond to supplementation with L-tyrosine and iodine. Tyrosine is commonly used in doses of 4-9 grams per day in divided doses. According to Abraham and Wright[214], doses of iodine may be as high as 12.5 milligrams (12,500 micrograms), which is slightly less than the average daily intake in Japan at 13.8 mg per day.

[207] Weetman AP. Hypothyroidism: screening and subclinical disease. *BMJ*. 1997 Apr 19;314(7088):1175-8 http://bmj.bmjjournals.com/cgi/content/full/314/7088/1175

[208] "Now AACE encourages doctors to consider treatment for patients who test outside the boundaries of a narrower margin based on a target TSH level of 0.3 to 3.0. AACE believes the new range will result in proper diagnosis for millions of Americans who suffer from a mild thyroid disorder, but have gone untreated until now." American Association of Clinical Endocrinologists (AACE). 2003 Campaign Encourages Awareness of Mild Thyroid.Failure, Importance of Routine Testing http://www.aace.com/pub/tam2003/press.php November 26, 2005

[209] Beers MH, Berkow R (eds). The Merck Manual. Seventeenth Edition. Whitehouse Station; Merck Research Laboratories 1999 Page 96

[210] Duntas LH, Mantzou E, Koutras DA. Effects of a six month treatment with selenomethionine in patients with autoimmune thyroiditis. *Eur J Endocrinol*. 2003 Apr;148(4):389-93 http://eje-online.org/cgi/reprint/148/4/389

[211] Gartner R, Gasnier BC, Dietrich JW, Krebs B, Angstwurm MW. Selenium supplementation in patients with autoimmune thyroiditis decreases thyroid peroxidase antibodies concentrations. *J Clin Endocrinol Metab*. 2002 Apr;87(4):1687-91 http://jcem.endojournals.org/cgi/content/full/87/4/1687

[212] "We recently conducted a prospective, placebo-controlled clinical study, where we could demonstrate, that a substitution of 200 wg sodium selenite for three months in patients with autoimmune thyroiditis reduced thyroid peroxidase antibody (TPO-Ab) concentrations significantly." Gartner R, Gasnier BC. Selenium in the treatment of autoimmune thyroiditis. *Biofactors*. 2003;19(3-4):165-70

[213] Bruns F, Micke O, Bremer M. Current status of selenium and other treatments for secondary lymphedema. *J Support Oncol*. 2003 Jul-Aug;1(2):121-30 http://www.supportiveoncology.net/journal/articles/0102121.pdf

[214] Wright JV. Why you need 83 times more of this essential, cancer-fighting nutrient than the "experts" say you do. *Nutrition and Healing* 2005; volume 12, issue 4.

- Oral enzyme therapy with proteolytic/pancreatic enzymes: Polyenzyme supplementation is used to ameliorate the pathophysiology induced by immune complexes, such as rheumatoid arthritis.[215]

- Comprehensive antioxidation: **Patients with PM-DM may have reduced antioxidant defenses amenable to antioxidant supplementation.**[216] Oxidative stress results from and contributes to systemic inflammation because 1) increased immune activity results in elaboration of oxidants, and 2) oxidative stress upregulates NF-kappaB (and other pathways) for additive immune activation. *Antioxidant supplementation* alone is clinically and biochemically inferior to a *comprehensive program* that includes both antioxidant supplementation and dietary modification (i.e., the supplemented Paleo-Mediterranean diet, as described previously) that includes heavy reliance upon fruits, vegetables, low-glycemic juices, nuts, seeds, and berries for their additive and synergistic antioxidant benefits.[217]

- Phytonutritional modulation of NF-kappaB: As a stimulator of pro-inflammatory gene transcription, NF-kappaB is almost universally activated in conditions associated with inflammation.[218,219] As we would expect, **NF-kappaB plays a central role in the pathogenesis of synovitis and joint destruction seen in RA.**[220] Nutrients and botanicals which either directly or indirectly inhibit NF-kappaB for an anti-inflammatory benefit include vitamin D[221,222], curcumin[223] (requires piperine for absorption[224]), lipoic acid[225], green tea[226], rosemary[227], grape seed extract[228], propolis[229], zinc[230], high-dose selenium[231], indole-3-carbinol[232,233], N-acetyl-L-cysteine[234],

[215] Galebskaya LV, Ryumina EV, Niemerovsky VS, Matyukov AA. Human complement system state after wobenzyme intake. *VESTNIK MOSKOVSKOGO UNIVERSITETA. KHIMIYA.* 2000. Vol. 41, No. 6. Supplement. Pages 148-149

[216] "Fifty patients with low GSH-Px levels were treated with tablets containing 0.2 mg selenium as Na2SeO3 and 10 mg tocopheryl succinate. The GSH-Px levels increased slowly within 6-8 weeks of treatment." Juhlin L, Edqvist LE, Ekman LG, Ljunghall K, Olsson M. Blood glutathione-peroxidase levels in skin diseases: effect of selenium and vitamin E treatment. *Acta Derm Venereol.* 1982;62(3):211-4

[217] Liu RH. Health benefits of fruit and vegetables are from additive and synergistic combinations of phytochemicals. *Am J Clin Nutr.* 2003 Sep;78(3 Suppl):517S-520S http://www.ajcn.org/cgi/content/full/78/3/517S

[218] Tak PP, Firestein GS. NF-kappaB: a key role in inflammatory diseases. *J Clin Invest.* 2001 Jan;107(1):7-11 http://www.jci.org/cgi/content/full/107/1/7

[219] D'Acquisto F, May MJ, Ghosh S. Inhibition of Nuclear Factor KappaB (NF-B): An Emerging Theme in Anti-Inflammatory Therapies. *Mol Interv.* 2002 Feb;2(1):22-35 http://molinterv.aspetjournals.org/cgi/content/abstract/2/1/22

[220] "NF-B plays a central role in the pathogenesis of synovitis in RA and PsA." Foell D, Kane D, Bresnihan B, Vogl T, Nacken W, Sorg C, Fitzgerald O, Roth J. Expression of the pro-inflammatory protein S100A12 (EN-RAGE) in rheumatoid and psoriatic arthritis. *Rheumatology* (Oxford). 2003 Nov;42(11):1383-9 http://rheumatology.oxfordjournals.org/cgi/content/full/42/11/1383

[221] "1 Alpha,25-dihydroxyvitamin D3 (1,25-(OH)2-D3), the active metabolite of vitamin D, can inhibit NF-kappaB activity in human MRC-5 fibroblasts, targeting DNA binding of NF-kappaB but not translocation of its subunits p50 and p65." Harant H, Wolff B, Lindley IJ. 1Alpha,25-dihydroxyvitamin D3 decreases DNA binding of nuclear factor-kappaB in human fibroblasts. *FEBS Lett.* 1998 Oct 9;436(3):329-34

[222] "Thus, 1,25(OH)2D3 may negatively regulate IL-12 production by downregulation of NF-kB activation and binding to the p40-kB sequence." D'Ambrosio D, Cippitelli M, Cocciolo MG, Mazzeo D, Di Lucia P, Lang R, Sinigaglia F, Panina-Bordignon P. Inhibition of IL-12 production by 1,25-dihydroxyvitamin D3. Involvement of NF-kappaB downregulation in transcriptional repression of the p40 gene. *J Clin Invest.* 1998 Jan 1;101(1):252-62

[223] "Curcumin, EGCG and resveratrol have been shown to suppress activation of NF-kappa B." Surh YJ, Chun KS, Cha HH, Han SS, Keum YS, Park KK, Lee SS. Molecular mechanisms underlying chemopreventive activities of anti-inflammatory phytochemicals: down-regulation of COX-2 and iNOS through suppression of NF-kappa B activation. *Mutat Res.* 2001 Sep 1;480-481:243-68

[224] Shoba G, Joy D, Joseph T, Majeed M, Rajendran R, Srinivas PS. Influence of piperine on the pharmacokinetics of curcumin in animals and human volunteers. *Planta Med.* 1998 May;64(4):353-6

[225] "ALA reduced the TNF-alpha-stimulated ICAM-1 expression in a dose-dependent manner, to levels observed in unstimulated cells. Alpha-lipoic acid also reduced NF-kappaB activity in these cells in a dose-dependent manner." Lee HA, Hughes DA.Alpha-lipoic acid modulates NF-kappaB activity in human monocytic cells by direct interaction with DNA. *Exp Gerontol.* 2002 Jan-Mar;37(2-3):401-10

[226] "In conclusion, EGCG is an effective inhibitor of IKK activity. This may explain, at least in part, some of the reported anti-inflammatory and anticancer effects of green tea." Yang F, Oz HS, Barve S, de Villiers WJ, McClain CJ, Varilek GW. The green tea polyphenol (-)-epigallocatechin-3-gallate blocks nuclear factor-kappa B activation by inhibiting I kappa B kinase activity in the intestinal epithelial cell line IEC-6. *Mol Pharmacol.* 2001 Sep;60(3):528-33

[227] "These results suggest that carnosol suppresses the NO production and iNOS gene expression by inhibiting NF-kappaB activation, and provide possible mechanisms for its anti-inflammatory and chemopreventive action." Lo AH, Liang YC, Lin-Shiau SY, Ho CT, Lin JK. Carnosol, an antioxidant in rosemary, suppresses inducible nitric oxide synthase through down-regulating nuclear factor-kappaB in mouse macrophages. *Carcinogenesis.* 2002 Jun;23(6):983-91

[228] "Constitutive and TNFalpha-induced NF-kappaB DNA binding activity was inhibited by GSE at doses > or =50 microg/ml and treatments for > or =12 h." Dhanalakshmi S, Agarwal R, Agarwal C. Inhibition of NF-kappaB pathway in grape seed extract-induced apoptotic death of human prostate carcinoma DU145 cells. *Int J Oncol.* 2003 Sep;23(3):721-7

[229] "Caffeic acid phenethyl ester (CAPE) is an anti-inflammatory component of propolis (honeybee resin). CAPE is reportedly a specific inhibitor of nuclear factor-kappaB (NF-kappaB)." Fitzpatrick LR, Wang J, Le T. Caffeic acid phenethyl ester, an inhibitor of nuclear factor-kappaB, attenuates bacterial peptidoglycan polysaccharide-induced colitis in rats. *J Pharmacol Exp Ther.* 2001 Dec;299(3):915-20

[230] "Our results suggest that zinc supplementation may lead to downregulation of the inflammatory cytokines through upregulation of the negative feedback loop A20 to inhibit induced NF-kappaB activation." Prasad AS, Bao B, Beck FW, Kucuk O, Sarkar FH. Antioxidant effect of zinc in humans. *Free Radic Biol Med.* 2004 Oct 15;37(8):1182-90

[231] Note that the patients in this study received a very high dose of selenium: 960 micrograms per day. This is at the top—and some would say over the top—of the safe and reasonable dose for long-term supplementation. In this case, the study lasted for three months. "In patients receiving selenium supplementation, selenium NF-kappaB activity was significantly reduced, reaching the same level as the nondiabetic control group. CONCLUSION: In type 2 diabetic patients, activation of NF-kappaB measured in peripheral blood monocytes can be reduced by selenium supplementation, confirming its importance in the prevention of cardiovascular diseases." Faure P, Ramon O, Favier A, Halimi S. Selenium supplementation decreases nuclear factor-kappa B activity in peripheral blood mononuclear cells from type 2 diabetic patients. *Eur J Clin Invest.* 2004 Jul;34(7):475-81

[232] Takada Y, Andreeff M, Aggarwal BB. Indole-3-carbinol suppresses NF-{kappa}B and I{kappa}B{alpha} kinase activation causing inhibition of expression of NF-{kappa}B-regulated antiapoptotic and metastatic gene products and enhancement of apoptosis in myeloid and leukemia cells. *Blood.* 2005 Apr 5; [Epub ahead of print]

[233] "Overall, our results indicated that indole-3-carbinol inhibits NF-kappaB and NF-kappaB-regulated gene expression and that this mechanism may provide the molecular basis for its ability to suppress tumorigenesis." Takada Y, Andreeff M, Aggarwal BB. Indole-3-carbinol suppresses NF-kappaB and IkappaBalpha kinase activation, causing inhibition of expression of NF-kappaB-regulated antiapoptotic and metastatic gene products and enhancement of apoptosis in myeloid and leukemia cells. *Blood.* 2005 Jul 15;106(2):641-9. Epub 2005 Apr 5.

[234] "CONCLUSIONS: Administration of N-acetylcysteine results in decreased nuclear factor-kappa B activation in patients with sepsis, associated with decreases in interleukin-8 but not interleukin-6 or soluble intercellular adhesion molecule-1. These pilot data suggest that antioxidant therapy with N-acetylcysteine may be useful in blunting the inflammatory response to sepsis." Paterson RL, Galley HF, Webster NR. The effect of N-acetylcysteine on nuclear factor-kappa B activation, interleukin-6, interleukin-8, and intercellular adhesion molecule-1 expression in patients with sepsis. *Crit Care Med.* 2003 Nov;31(11):2574-8

resveratrol[235,236], isohumulones[237], GLA via PPAR-gamma[238] and EPA via PPAR-alpha.[239] I have reviewed the phytonutritional modulation of NF-kappaB later in this text and elsewhere.[240] Several phytonutritional products targeting NF-kappaB are available.

- <u>Sunscreen</u>: To protect against photosensitivity.

Notes:

_____

_____

_____

_____

_____

_____

_____

_____

_____

_____

_____

_____

_____

_____

_____

_____

_____

_____

_____

_____

_____

_____

_____

_____

_____

_____

_____

_____

_____

_____

_____

_____

[235] "Resveratrol's anticarcinogenic, anti-inflammatory, and growth-modulatory effects may thus be partially ascribed to the inhibition of activation of NF-kappaB and AP-1 and the associated kinases." Manna SK, Mukhopadhyay A, Aggarwal BB. Resveratrol suppresses TNF-induced activation of nuclear transcription factors NF-kappa B, activator protein-1, and apoptosis: potential role of reactive oxygen intermediates and lipid peroxidation. *J Immunol*. 2000 Jun 15;164(12):6509-19

[236] "Both resveratrol and quercetin inhibited NF-kappaB-, AP-1- and CREB-dependent transcription to a greater extent than the glucocorticosteroid, dexamethasone." Donnelly LE, Newton R, Kennedy GE, Fenwick PS, Leung RH, Ito K, Russell RE, Barnes PJ.Anti-inflammatory Effects of Resveratrol in Lung Epithelial Cells: Molecular Mechanisms. *Am J Physiol Lung Cell Mol Physiol*. 2004 Jun 4 [Epub ahead of print]

[237] Yajima H, Ikeshima E, Shiraki M, Kanaya T, Fujiwara D, Odai H, Tsuboyama-Kasaoka N, Ezaki O, Oikawa S, Kondo K. Isohumulones, bitter acids derived from hops, activate both peroxisome proliferator-activated receptor alpha and gamma and reduce insulin resistance. *J Biol Chem*. 2004 Aug 6;279(32):33456-62. Epub 2004 Jun 3. http://www.jbc.org/cgi/content/full/279/32/33456

[238] "Thus, PPAR gamma serves as the receptor for GLA in the regulation of gene expression in breast cancer cells. " Jiang WG, Redfern A, Bryce RP, Mansel RE. Peroxisome proliferator activated receptor-gamma (PPAR-gamma) mediates the action of gamma linolenic acid in breast cancer cells. *Prostaglandins Leukot Essent Fatty Acids*. 2000 Feb;62(2):119-27

[239] "...EPA requires PPARalpha for its inhibitory effects on NF-kappaB." Mishra A, Chaudhary A, Sethi S. Oxidized omega-3 fatty acids inhibit NF-kappaB activation via a PPARalpha-dependent pathway. *Arterioscler Thromb Vasc Biol*. 2004 Sep;24(9):1621-7. Epub 2004 Jul 1. http://atvb.ahajournals.org/cgi/content/full/24/9/1621

[240] "Indeed, the previous view that nutrients only interact with human physiology at the metabolic/post-transcriptional level must be updated in light of current research showing that nutrients can, in fact, modify human physiology and phenotype at the genetic/pre-transcriptional level." Vasquez A. Reducing pain and inflammation naturally - part 4: nutritional and botanical inhibition of NF-kappaB, the major intracellular amplifier of the inflammatory cascade. A practical clinical strategy exemplifying anti-inflammatory nutrigenomics. *Nutritional Perspectives*, July 2005:5-12. www.OptimalHealthResearch.com/part4

Polymyalgia Rheumatica
Giant Cell Arteritis (previously Temporal Arteritis)

<u>Description/pathophysiology</u>:
- This group of tightly related and largely synonymous disorders is described as "idiopathic" by medical textbooks.
- **Polymyalgia rheumatica (PMR)**: This disorder typically presents with painful inflammation of the shoulder/neck and hip muscles along with systemic manifestations of fever, malaise, and weight loss. When present in isolation (i.e., not with giant cell arteritis), it does not lead to blindness, and the condition responds to low-dose (10-20 mg) prednisone.
- **Giant Cell Arteritis (GCA):** When treated allopathically, GCA requires higher daily doses (40-60 mg) of prednisone than PMR. GCA can result in rapid-onset blindness and therefore any evidence of ocular involvement in a patient with GCA must be treated as a medical emergency. **Indeed, the diagnosis of GCA itself is considered urgent due to ability of blindness to occur rapidly and without warning.** GCA was previously called temporal arteritis. Approximately 50% of patients with GCA have PMR.

<u>Clinical presentations</u>:
- Pain and stiffness in proximal muscle groups: shoulders, neck, and hips; weakness—if any—is secondary to pain, disuse atrophy, drug side-effect (e.g., "steroid myopathy"), or other concomitant disorder. Presentations are consistent with muscle/tissue ischemia due to the underlying panarteritis which results in vessel occlusion: head pain, jaw claudication, blindness.
- Generally presents after age 50 years. The later age of onset helps distinguish PMR from fibromyalgia, which generally affects young adult patients between the ages of 20-40 years.
- 2x more common in women than in men
- Typical autoimmune systemic manifestations: fatigue, malaise, fever, anorexia, and weight loss.
- Patients may have high fever and chills with disease initiation and/or exacerbation.

<u>Major differential diagnoses</u>:
- <u>Fibromyalgia</u>: ESR is normal, age of onset is nearly always before 50 years.
- <u>Dermatomyositis, polymyositis</u>: These conditions cause muscle weakness, which is characteristically absent in patients with PMR. Muscle enzymes are elevated in patients with dermatomyositis/polymyositis but are normal in patients with PMR.
- <u>Cancer, particularly multiple myeloma</u>
- <u>Hypothyroidism</u>: Hypothyroidism can easily mimic PMR by producing an inflammatory myopathy that affects the shoulder muscles and which remits following normalization of thyroid status.
- <u>Rheumatoid arthritis, SLE, vasculitis, or other autoimmune disorder</u>
- <u>Infection</u>: WBC count is normal in GCA/PMR and is generally elevated in patients with severe infection.
- <u>Cervical spondylosis</u>

<u>Clinical assessments</u>:
- **History/subjective**:
  - See clinical presentations
- **Physical examination/objective**:
  - Palpate pulses for strength and symmetry:
    - Carotid artery in the anterior neck
    - Axillary/brachial in the axilla and inner arm, respectively

- Radial pulse at the distal radius
- Aorta in the abdomen
- Femoral pulses in the groin
- Dorsalis pedis and posterior tibial arteries at the ankle/foot
- **Laboratory assessments**:
  - **ESR**: Most patients will have a very high ESR > 50 mm/h.
  - **CBC**: Anemia is common.
  - **Chemistry/metabolic panel**: Hepatic alkaline phosphatase is elevated in 20% of patients.
  - **RF**: generally negative
  - **Muscle enzymes:** are almost always normal.
  - **No evidence of proteinuria or monoclonal gammopathy, as seen in MM.**
- **Imaging**:
  - Not generally indicated except when looking for complications or concomitant disease
- **Establishing the diagnosis**:
  - PMR is a clinical diagnosis based on 1) painful inflammation of the shoulder/neck and hip muscles along with 2) systemic manifestations of fever, malaise, and weight loss and 3) the absence of evidence supporting an alternate diagnosis.[1]
  - GCA is classically diagnosed following biopsy of the temporal artery.
  - Clinical diagnosis:[2] Pattern recognition (proximal muscle pain with no other explanation) and evidence of inflammation in an elderly patient when other diseases have been ruled out.

Complications:
- GCA can lead to blindness.
- Dry cough is seen in some patients and may be the presenting complaint.
- Mononeuritis multiplex may cause (shoulder) paralysis.
- Aneurysms of the thoracic aorta are 17x more common in patients with GCA than the general population

Clinical management:
- Referral if clinical outcome is unsatisfactory or if serious complications are possible/evident.
- Assess for temporal arteritis—educate patient about the significance of the onset of eye symptoms, headache, and jaw claudication.
- A few patients treated with prednisone will have permanent remission within 2 years.

Treatments:

Drug treatments:
1. Prednisone (10-20 mg per day for PMR) should result in "dramatic improvement" within 72 hours.[3] Prednisone dose for GCA is typically 60 mg per day at the start of treatment in order to prevent one of the most feared complications—blindness. Dose is tapered after clinical remission. Low-dose aspirin appears to reduce the risk of blindness and stroke in GCA patients.
2. Methotrexate

- **Presumptive treatment: In comparison with other, more common diseases such as SLE and RA, very little research has been done using non-pharmacologic treatments for PMR/GCA. Thus, patients must be treated and managed on a *patient per patient* basis.**
- Orthoendocrinology: Assess prolactin, cortisol, DHEA, free and total testosterone, serum estradiol, and thyroid status (e.g., TSH, T4, *and* anti-thyroid peroxidase antibodies). Correct as indicated (see Chapter 4). **Prolactin levels are typically elevated in patients with PMR and**

[1] Tierney ML. McPhee SJ, Papadakis MA (eds). Current Medical Diagnosis and Treatment 2006. 45th edition. New York; Lange Medical Books: 2006, pages 486
[2] Tierney ML. McPhee SJ, Papadakis MA. Current Medical Diagnosis and Treatment. 35th edition. Stamford: Appleton and Lange, 1996 page 751
[3] Tierney ML. McPhee SJ, Papadakis MA (eds). Current Medical Diagnosis and Treatment 2006. 45th edition. New York; Lange Medical Books: 2006, pages 487

correlate with clinical symptomatology.[4] Adrenal hypofunction in patients with PR/GCA is suggested by the relative insufficiencies of cortisol and DHEA.[5]

> "Patients with PMR/GCA with new-onset active disease before steroid treatment have inappropriately normal cortisol levels regarding the ongoing inflammation, and **significantly lower levels of DHEAS** compared to the age- and sex-matched healthy control subjects. These data support the existence of a **relative adrenal hypofunction in PMR and GCA**."
>
> Narvaez et al. Low serum levels of DHEAS in untreated polymyalgia rheumatica/giant cell arteritis. *J Rheumatol* 2006;33:1293-8

- o **Assess the testosterone-estrogen balance as discussed in Chapter 4 and intervene (e.g., with Arimidex) as appropriate.**
- o **DHEA (insufficiency and supraphysiologic supplementation):** Patients with autoimmunity should be tested for DHEA insufficiency by measurement of serum DHEA-sulfate; insufficiencies should generally be corrected except in cases of concomitant hormone-responsive cancer such as breast cancer or prostate cancer. Physiologic doses are approximately 15-25 mg for women and 25-50 mg for men. However, many patients with autoimmunity will respond favorably to supraphysiologic doses in the range of 200 mg per day. The rationale for using high-dose DHEA in patients with autoimmune diseases is reviewed in Chapter 4.
- o **Hyperprolactinemia:** Use appropriate and effective treatment as indicated: thyroid hormone, high-dose pyridoxine (250 mg qd-bid with food), *Vitex astus-cagnus*[6,7,8], bromocriptine[9], cabergoline/Dostinex (0.25 mg twice per week[10]).[11]

- Avoidance of pro-inflammatory foods: Pro-inflammatory foods act *directly* and *indirectly* to promote and exacerbate systemic inflammation. *Direct* mechanisms include the activation of Toll-like receptors and NF-kappaB, while *indirect* mechanisms include depleting the body of anti-inflammatory nutrients and dietary displacement of more nutrient-dense anti-inflammatory foods. Arachidonic acid (found in cow's milk, beef, liver, pork, and lamb) is the direct precursor to pro-inflammatory prostaglandins and leukotrienes[12] and pain-promoting isoprostanes.[13] Saturated fats promote inflammation by activating/enabling pro-inflammatory Toll-like receptors, which are otherwise "specific" for inducing pro-inflammatory responses to microorganisms.[14] Consumption of saturated fat in the form of cream creates marked oxidative stress and lipid peroxidation that lasts for at least 3 hours postprandially.[15] Corn oil rapidly activates NF-kappaB (in hepatic Kupffer cells) for a pro-inflammatory effect[16]; similarly, consumption of PUFA and linoleic acid promotes antioxidant depletion and may thus promote oxidation-mediated inflammation via activation of NF-kappaB. Linoleic acid causes intracellular oxidative stress and calcium influx and results in increased NF-kappaB-stimulated transcription

[4] Straub RH, Georgi J, Helmke K, Vaith P, Lang B. In polymyalgia rheumatica serum prolactin is positively correlated with the number of typical symptoms but not with typical inflammatory markers. *Rheumatology* (Oxford). 2002 Apr;41(4):423-9 http://rheumatology.oxfordjournals.org/cgi/content/full/41/4/423

[5] "Patients with PMR/GCA with new-onset active disease before steroid treatment have inappropriately normal cortisol levels regarding the ongoing inflammation, and significantly lower levels of DHEAS compared to the age- and sex-matched healthy control subjects. These data support the existence of a relative adrenal hypofunction in PMR and GCA." Narvaez J, Bernad B, Diaz Torne C, Momplet JV, Montpel JZ, Nolla JM, Valverde-Garcia J. Low serum levels of DHEAS in untreated polymyalgia rheumatica/giant cell arteritis. *J Rheumatol*. 2006 Jul;33(7):1293-8. Epub 2006 Jun 15

[6] "Since AC extracts were shown to have beneficial effects on premenstrual mastodynia serum prolactin levels in such patients were also studied in one double-blind, placebo-controlled clinical study. Serum prolactin levels were indeed reduced in the patients treated with the extract." Wuttke W, Jarry H, Christoffel V, Spengler B, Seidlova-Wuttke D. Chaste tree (Vitex agnus-castus)-- pharmacology and clinical indications. *Phytomedicine*. 2003 May;10(4):348-57

[7] German abstract from Medline: "The prolactin release was reduced after 3 months, shortened luteal phases were normalised and deficits in the luteal progesterone synthesis were eliminated." Milewicz A, Gejdel E, Sworen H, Sienkiewicz K, Jedrzejak J, Teucher T, Schmitz H. [Vitex agnus castus extract in the treatment of luteal phase defects due to latent hyperprolactinemia. Results of a randomized placebo-controlled double-blind study] *Arzneimittelforschung*. 1993 Jul;43(7):752-6

[8] "In conditions such as endometriosis and fibroids, for which a significant estrogen antagonist effect is needed, doses of at least 2 g/day DHE may be required and typically are used by professional herbalists." Bone K. New Insights Into Chaste Tree. *Nutritional Wellness* 2005 November http://www.nutritionalwellness.com/archives/2005/nov/11_bone.php

[9] "...clinical observations and trials support the use of bromocriptine as a nonstandard primary or adjunctive therapy in the treatment of recalcitrant RA, SLE, Reiter's syndrome, and psoriatic arthritis and associated conditions unresponsive to traditional approaches." McMurray RW. Bromocriptine in rheumatic and autoimmune diseases. *Semin Arthritis Rheum*. 2001 Aug;31(1):21-32

[10] Serri O, Chik CL, Ur E, Ezzat S. Diagnosis and management of hyperprolactinemia. *CMAJ*. 2003 Sep 16;169(6):575-81 http://www.cmaj.ca/cgi/content/full/169/6/575

[11] Erb N, Pace AV, Delamere JP, Kitas GD. Control of unremitting rheumatoid arthritis by the prolactin antagonist cabergoline. *Rheumatology* (Oxford). 2001 Feb;40(2):237-9 http://rheumatology.oxfordjournals.org/cgi/content/full/40/2/237

[12] Vasquez A. Reducing Pain and Inflammation Naturally. Part 2: New Insights into Fatty Acid Supplementation and Its Effect on Eicosanoid Production and Genetic Expression. *Nutritional Perspectives* 2005; January: 5-16 www.optimalhealthresearch.com/part2

[13] Evans AR, Junger H, Southall MD, Nicol GD, Sorkin LS, Broome JT, Bailey TW, Vasko MR. Isoprostanes, novel eicosanoids that produce nociception and sensitize rat sensory neurons. *J Pharmacol Exp Ther*. 2000 Jun;293(3):912-20

[14] Lee JY, Sohn KH, Rhee SH, Hwang D. Saturated fatty acids, but not unsaturated fatty acids, induce the expression of cyclooxygenase-2 mediated through Toll-like receptor 4. *J Biol Chem*. 2001 May 18;276(20):16683-9. Epub 2001 Mar 2 http://www.jbc.org/cgi/content/full/276/20/16683

[15] "CONCLUSIONS: Both fat and protein intakes stimulate ROS generation. The increase in ROS generation lasted 3 h after cream intake and 1 h after protein intake. Cream intake also caused a significant and prolonged increase in lipid peroxidation." Mohanty P, Ghanim H, Hamouda W, Aljada A, Garg R, Dandona P. Both lipid and protein intakes stimulate increased generation of reactive oxygen species by polymorphonuclear leukocytes and mononuclear cells. *Am J Clin Nutr*. 2002 Apr;75(4):767-72 http://www.ajcn.org/cgi/content/full/75/4/767

[16] Rusyn I, Bradham CA, Cohn L, Schoonhoven R, Swenberg JA, Brenner DA, Thurman RG. Corn oil rapidly activates nuclear factor-kappaB in hepatic Kupffer cells by oxidant-dependent mechanisms. *Carcinogenesis*. 1999 Nov;20(11):2095-100 http://carcin.oxfordjournals.org/cgi/content/full/20/11/2095

of pro-inflammatory genes.[17]   High glycemic foods cause oxidative stress[18,19] and inflammation via activation of NF-kappaB and other mechanisms—e.g., *white bread causes inflammation*[20] as does *a high-fat high-carbohydrate fast-food-style breakfast.*[21]   High glycemic foods suppress immune function[22,23] and thus promote the perpetuation of infection/dysbiosis. Delivery of a high carbohydrate load to the gastrointestinal lumen promotes bacterial overgrowth[24,25], which is inherently pro-inflammatory[26,27] and which appears to be myalgenic in humans[28] at least in part due to the ability of endotoxin to impair muscle function.[29]   Overconsumption of high-carbohydrate low-phytonutrient grains, potatoes, and manufactured foods displaces phytonutrient-dense foods such as fruits, vegetables, nuts, seeds, and berries which contain more than 8,000 phytonutrients, many of which have antioxidant and thus anti-inflammatory actions.[30,31]

- Supplemented Paleo-Mediterranean diet: The health-promoting diet of choice for the majority of people is a diet based on abundant consumption of fruits, vegetables, seeds, nuts, omega-3 and monounsaturated fatty acids, and lean sources of protein such as lean meats, fatty cold-water fish, soy and whey proteins. This diet obviates overconsumption of chemical preservatives, artificial sweeteners, and carbohydrate-dominant foods such as candies, pastries, breads, potatoes, grains, and other foods with a high glycemic load and high glycemic index. This "Paleo-Mediterranean Diet" is a combination of the "Paleolithic" or "Paleo diet" and the well-known "Mediterranean diet", both of which are well described in peer-reviewed journals and the lay press. (See Chapter 2 and my other publications[32,33] for details). This diet is the most nutrient-dense diet available, and its benefits are further enhanced by supplementation with vitamins, minerals, and the health-promoting fatty acids: ALA, GLA, EPA, DHA.

- Avoidance of allergenic foods: Any patient may be allergic to any food, even if the food is generally considered a health-promoting food. Generally speaking, the most notorious allergens are wheat, citrus (especially juice due to the industrial use of fungal hemicellulases), cow's milk, eggs, peanuts, chocolate, and yeast-containing foods. According to a study in patients with migraine, some patients will have to avoid as many as 10 specific foods in order to become symptom-free.[34]   Celiac disease can present with inflammatory oligoarthritis that resembles rheumatoid arthritis and which remits with avoidance of wheat/gluten. The inflammatory

[17] "Exposing endothelial cells to 90 micromol linoleic acid/L for 6 h resulted in a significant increase in lipid hydroperoxides that coincided wih an increase in intracellular calcium concentrations." Hennig B, Toborek M, Joshi-Barve S, Barger SW, Barve S, Mattson MP, McClain CJ. Linoleic acid activates nuclear transcription factor-kappa B (NF-kappa B) and induces NF-kappa B-dependent transcription in cultured endothelial cells. *Am J Clin Nutr.* 1996 Mar;63(3):322-8 http://www.ajcn.org/cgi/reprint/63/3/322

[18] Mohanty P, Hamouda W, Garg R, Aljada A, Ghanim H, Dandona P. Glucose challenge stimulates reactive oxygen species (ROS) generation by leucocytes. *J Clin Endocrinol Metab.* 2000 Aug;85(8):2970-3 http://jcem.endojournals.org/cgi/content/full/85/8/2970 Glucose/carbohydrate and saturated fat consumption appear to be the two biggest offenders in the food-stimulated production of oxidative stress. The effect by protein is much less. "CONCLUSIONS: Both fat and protein intakes stimulate ROS generation. The increase in ROS generation lasted 3 h after cream intake and 1 h after protein intake. Cream intake also caused a significant and prolonged increase in lipid peroxidation." Mohanty P, Ghanim H, Hamouda W, Aljada A, Garg R, Dandona P. Both lipid and protein intakes stimulate increased generation of reactive oxygen species by polymorphonuclear leukocytes and mononuclear cells. *Am J Clin Nutr.* 2002 Apr;75(4):767-72 http://www.ajcn.org/cgi/content/full/75/4/767

[19] Koska J, Blazicek P, Marko M, Grna JD, Kvetnansky R, Vigas M. Insulin, catecholamines, glucose and antioxidant enzymes in oxidative damage during different loads in healthy humans. *Physiol Res.* 2000;49 Suppl 1:S95-100 http://www.biomed.cas.cz/physiolres/pdf/2000/49_S95.pdf

[20] "Conclusion - The present study shows that high GI carbohydrate, but not low GI carbohydrate, mediates an acute proinflammatory process as measured by NF-kappaB activity." Dickinson S, Hancock DP, Petocz P, Brand-Miller JC..High glycemic index carbohydrate mediates an acute proinflammatory process as measured by NF-kappaB activation. *Asia Pac J Clin Nutr.* 2005;14 Suppl:S120

[21] Aljada A, Mohanty P, Ghanim H, Abdo T, Tripathy D, Chaudhuri A, Dandona P. Increase in intranuclear nuclear factor kappaB and decrease in inhibitor kappaB in mononuclear cells after a mixed meal: evidence for a proinflammatory effect. *Am J Clin Nutr.* 2004 Apr;79(4):682-90 http://www.ajcn.org/cgi/content/full/79/4/682

[22] Sanchez A, Reeser JL, Lau HS, et al. Role of sugars in human neutrophilic phagocytosis. *Am J Clin Nutr.* 1973 Nov;26(11):1180-4

[23] "Postoperative infusion of carbohydrate solution leads to moderate fall in the serum concentration of inorganic phosphate. ... The hypophosphatemia was associated with significant reduction of neutrophil phagocytosis, intracellular killing, consumption of oxygen and generation of superoxide during phagocytosis." Rasmussen A, Segel E, Hessov I, Borregaard N. Reduced function of neutrophils during routine postoperative glucose infusion. *Acta Chir Scand.* 1988 Jul-Aug;154(7-8):429-33

[24] Ramakrishnan T, Stokes P. Beneficial effects of fasting and low carbohydrate diet in D-lactic acidosis associated with short-bowel syndrome. *JPEN J Parenter Enteral Nutr.* 1985 May-Jun;9(3):361-3

[25] Gottschall E. Breaking the Vicious Cycle: Intestinal Health Through Diet. Kirkton Press; Rev edition (August 1, 1994)

[26] Lin HC. Small intestinal bacterial overgrowth: a framework for understanding irritable bowel syndrome. *JAMA.* 2004 Aug 18;292(7):852-8

[27] Lichtman SN, Wang J, Sartor RB, Zhang C, Bender D, Dalldorf FG, Schwab JH. Reactivation of arthritis induced by small bowel bacterial overgrowth in rats: role of cytokines, bacteria, and bacterial polymers. *Infect Immun.* 1995 Jun;63(6):2295-301

[28] Pimentel M, et al. A link between irritable bowel syndrome and fibromyalgia may be related to findings on lactulose breath testing. *Ann Rheum Dis.* 2004 Apr;63(4):450-2

[29] Bundgaard H, Kjeldsen K, Suarez Krabbe K, van Hall G, Simonsen L, Qvist J, Hansen CM, Moller K, Fonsmark L, Lav Madsen P, Klarlund Pedersen B. Endotoxemia stimulates skeletal muscle Na+-K+-ATPase and raises blood lactate under aerobic conditions in humans. *Am J Physiol Heart Circ Physiol.* 2003 Mar;284(3):H1028-34. Epub 2002 Nov 21 http://ajpheart.physiology.org/cgi/reprint/284/3/H1028

[30] "We propose that the additive and synergistic effects of phytochemicals in fruit and vegetables are responsible for their potent antioxidant and anticancer activities, and that the benefit of a diet rich in fruit and vegetables is attributed to the complex mixture of phytochemicals present in whole foods." Liu RH. Health benefits of fruit and vegetables are from additive and synergistic combinations of phytochemicals. *Am J Clin Nutr.* 2003 Sep;78(3 Suppl):517S-520S

[31] Seaman DR. The diet-induced proinflammatory state: a cause of chronic pain and other degenerative diseases? *J Manipulative Physiol Ther.* 2002;25(3):168-79

[32] Vasquez A. A Five-Part Nutritional Protocol that Produces Consistently Positive Results. *Nutritional Wellness* 2005 September Available in the printed version and on-line at http://www.nutritionalwellness.com/archives/2005/sep/09_vasquez.php and http://optimalhealthresearch.com/protocol

[33] Vasquez A. Implementing the Five-Part Nutritional Wellness Protocol for the Treatment of Various Health Problems. *Nutritional Wellness* 2005 November. Available on-line at http://www.nutritionalwellness.com/archives/2005/nov/11_vasquez.php and http://optimalhealthresearch.com/protocol

[34] Grant EC. Food allergies and migraine. *Lancet.* 1979 May 5;1(8123):966-9

arthropathy of celiac disease has preceded bowel symptoms and/or an accurate diagnosis by as many as 3-15 years.[35,36] Clinicians must explain to their patients that celiac disease and wheat allergy are two different clinical entities and that exclusion of one does not exclude the other, and in neither case does mutual exclusion obviate the promotion of intestinal bacterial overgrowth (i.e., pro-inflammatory dysbiosis) by indigestible wheat oligosaccharides.

- Gluten-free vegetarian/vegan diet: Vegetarian/vegan diets have a place in the treatment plan of all patients with autoimmune/inflammatory disorders[37,38,39,40]; this is also true for patients for whom long-term exclusive reliance on a meat-free vegetarian diet is either not appropriate or not appealing. No scientist or clinician familiar with the research literature doubts the antirheumatic power and anti-inflammatory advantages of vegetarian diets, whether used short-term or long term.[41] The benefits of gluten-free vegetarian diets are well documented, and the mechanisms of action are well elucidated, including reduced intake of pro-inflammatory linoleic[42] and arachidonic acids[43], iron[44], common food antigens[45], gluten[46] and gliadin[47,48], pro-inflammatory sugars[49] and increased intake of omega-3 fatty acids, micronutrients[50], and anti-inflammatory and antioxidant phytonutrients.[51] Vegetarian diets also effect subtle yet biologically and clinically important changes—both *qualitative* and *quantitative*—in intestinal flora[52,53] that correlate with clinical improvement.[54] Patients who rely on the Paleo-Mediterranean diet (which is inherently omnivorous) can use vegetarian *meals* on a daily basis or for days at a time—for example, by having a daily vegetarian meal, or one week per month of vegetarianism. Some (not all) patients can use a purely vegetarian diet long-term provided that nutritional needs (especially protein and cobalamin) are consistently met.

- Short-term fasting: Whether the foundational diet is Paleo-Mediterranean, vegetarian, vegan, or a combination of all of these, autoimmune/inflammatory patients will still benefit from periodic fasting, whether on a weekly (e.g., every Saturday), monthly (every first week or weekend of the

[35] "We report six patients with coeliac disease in whom arthritis was prominent at diagnosis and who improved with dietary therapy. Joint pain preceded diagnosis by up to three years in five patients and 15 years in one patient." Bourne JT, Kumar P, Huskisson EC, Mageed R, Unsworth DJ, Wojtulewski JA. Arthritis and coeliac disease. *Ann Rheum Dis.* 1985 Sep;44(9):592-8

[36] "A 15-year-old girl, with synovitis of the knees and ankles for 3 years before a diagnosis of gluten-sensitive enteropathy, is described." Pinals RS. Arthritis associated with gluten-sensitive enteropathy. *J Rheumatol.* 1986 Feb;13(1):201-4

[37] "The immunoglobulin G (IgG) antibody levels against gliadin and beta-lactoglobulin decreased in the responder subgroup in the vegan diet-treated patients, but not in the other analysed groups." Hafstrom I, Ringertz B, Spangberg A, von Zweigbergk L, Brannemark S, Nylander I, Ronnelid J, Laasonen L, Klareskog L. A vegan diet free of gluten improves the signs and symptoms of rheumatoid arthritis: the effects on arthritis correlate with a reduction in antibodies to food antigens. *Rheumatology* (Oxford). 2001 Oct;40(10):1175-9 http://rheumatology.oxfordjournals.org/cgi/content/abstract/40/10/1175

[38] "After four weeks at the health farm the diet group showed a significant improvement in number of tender joints, Ritchie's articular index, number of swollen joints, pain score, duration of morning stiffness, grip strength, erythrocyte sedimentation rate, C-reactive protein, white blood cell count, and a health assessment questionnaire score." Kjeldsen-Kragh J, Haugen M, Borchgrevink CF, Laerum E, Eek M, Mowinkel P, Hovi K, Forre O. Controlled trial of fasting and one-year vegetarian diet in rheumatoid arthritis. *Lancet.* 1991 Oct 12;338(8772):899-902

[39] "During fasting, arthralgia was less intense in many subjects. In some types of skin diseases (pustulosis palmaris et plantaris and atopic eczema) an improvement could be demonstrated during the fast. During the vegan diet, both signs and symptoms returned in most patients, with the exception of some patients with psoriasis who experienced an improvement." Lithell H, Bruce A, Gustafsson IB, Hoglund NJ, Karlstrom B, Ljunghall K, Sjolin K, Venge P, Werner I, Vessby B. A fasting and vegetarian diet treatment trial on chronic inflammatory disorders. *Acta Derm Venereol.* 1983;63(5):397-403

[40] Tanaka T, Kouda K, Kotani M, Takeuchi A, Tabei T, Masamoto Y, Nakamura H, Takigawa M, Suemura M, Takeuchi H, Kouda M. Vegetarian diet ameliorates symptoms of atopic dermatitis through reduction of the number of peripheral eosinophils and of PGE2 synthesis by monocytes. *J Physiol Anthropol Appl Human Sci.* 2001 Nov;20(6):353-61 http://www.jstage.jst.go.jp/article/jpa/20/6/20_353/_article/-char/en

[41] "For the patients who were randomised to the vegetarian diet there was a significant decrease in platelet count, leukocyte count, calprotectin, total IgG, IgM rheumatoid factor (RF), C3-activation products, and the complement components C3 and C4 after one month of treatment." Kjeldsen-Kragh J, Mellbye OJ, Haugen M, Mollnes TE, Hammer HB, Sioud M, Forre O. Changes in laboratory variables in rheumatoid arthritis patients during a trial of fasting and one-year vegetarian diet. *Scand J Rheumatol.* 1995;24(2):85-93

[42] Rusyn I, Bradham CA, Cohn L, Schoonhoven R, Swenberg JA, Brenner DA, Thurman RG. Corn oil rapidly activates nuclear factor-kappaB in hepatic Kupffer cells by oxidant-dependent mechanisms. *Carcinogenesis.* 1999 Nov;20(11):2095-100 http://carcin.oxfordjournals.org/cgi/content/full/20/11/2095

[43] Vasquez A. Reducing Pain and Inflammation Naturally. Part 2: New Insights into Fatty Acid Supplementation and Its Effect on Eicosanoid Production and Genetic Expression. *Nutritional Perspectives* 2005; January: 5-16 http://optimalhealthresearch.com/part2

[44] Dabbagh AJ, Trenam CW, Morris CJ, Blake DR. Iron in joint inflammation. *Ann Rheum Dis.* 1993 Jan;52(1):67-73

[45] Hafstrom I, Ringertz B, Spangberg A, von Zweigbergk L, Brannemark S, Nylander I, Ronnelid J, Laasonen L, Klareskog L. A vegan diet free of gluten improves the signs and symptoms of rheumatoid arthritis: the effects on arthritis correlate with a reduction in antibodies to food antigens. *Rheumatology* (Oxford). 2001 Oct;40(10):1175-9 http://rheumatology.oxfordjournals.org/cgi/reprint/40/10/1175

[46] "The data provide evidence that dietary modification may be of clinical benefit for certain RA patients, and that this benefit may be related to a reduction in immunoreactivity to food antigens eliminated by the change in diet." Hafstrom I, Ringertz B, Spangberg A, von Zweigbergk L, Brannemark S, Nylander I, Ronnelid J, Laasonen L, Klareskog L. A vegan diet free of gluten improves the signs and symptoms of rheumatoid arthritis: the effects on arthritis correlate with a reduction in antibodies to food antigens. *Rheumatology* (Oxford). 2001 Oct;40(10):1175-9

[47] "Despite the increased AGA [antigliadin antibodies] positivity found distinctively in patients with recent-onset RA, none of the RA patients showed clear evidence of coeliac disease." Paimela L, Kurki P, Leirisalo-Repo M, Piirainen H. Gliadin immune reactivity in patients with rheumatoid arthritis. *Clin Exp Rheumatol.* 1995;13(5):603-7

[48] "The median IgA antigliadin ELISA index was 7.1 (range 2.1-22.4) for the RA group and 3.1 (range 0.3-34.9) for the controls (p = 0.0001)." Koot VC, Van Straaten M, Hekkens WT, Collee G, Dijkmans BA. Elevated level of IgA gliadin antibodies in patients with rheumatoid arthritis. *Clin Exp Rheumatol.* 1989 Nov-Dec;7(6):623-6

[49] Seaman DR. The diet-induced proinflammatory state: a cause of chronic pain and other degenerative diseases? *J Manipulative Physiol Ther.* 2002 Mar-Apr;25(3):168-79

[50] Hagfors L, Nilsson I, Skoldstam L, Johansson G. Fat intake and composition of fatty acids in serum phospholipids in a randomized, controlled, Mediterranean dietary intervention study on patients with rheumatoid arthritis. *Nutr Metab* (Lond). 2005 Oct 10;2:26 http://www.nutritionandmetabolism.com/content/2/1/26

[51] Liu RH. Health benefits of fruit and vegetables are from additive and synergistic combinations of phytochemicals. *Am J Clin Nutr* 2003;78(3 Suppl):517S-520S http://www.ajcn.org/cgi/content/full/78/3/517S

[52] "Significant alteration in the intestinal flora was observed when the patients changed from omnivorous to vegan diet. ... This finding of an association between intestinal flora and disease activity may have implications for our understanding of how diet can affect RA." Peltonen R, Kjeldsen-Kragh J, Haugen M, Tuominen J, Toivanen P, Forre O, Eerola E. Changes of faecal flora in rheumatoid arthritis during fasting and one-year vegetarian diet. *Br J Rheumatol.* 1994 Jul;33(7):638-43

[53] Toivanen P, Eerola E. A vegan diet changes the intestinal flora. *Rheumatology* (Oxford). 2002 Aug;41(8):950-1 http://rheumatology.oxfordjournals.org/cgi/reprint/41/8/950

[54] "We conclude that a vegan diet changes the faecal microbial flora in RA patients, and changes in the faecal flora are associated with improvement in RA activity." Peltonen R, Nenonen M, Helve T, Hanninen O, Toivanen P, Eerola E. Faecal microbial flora and disease activity in rheumatoid arthritis during a vegan diet. *Br J Rheumatol.* 1997 Jan;36(1):64-8 http://rheumatology.oxfordjournals.org/cgi/reprint/36/1/64

month, or every other month), or yearly (1-2 weeks of the year) basis. Since consumption of food—particularly unhealthy foods—induces an inflammatory effect[55], abstinence from food provides a relative anti-inflammatory effect. Fasting indeed provides a distinct anti-inflammatory benefit and may help "re-calibrate" metabolic and homeostatic mechanisms by breaking self-perpetuating "vicious cycles"[56] that autonomously promote inflammation independent of pro-inflammatory stimuli. Water-only fasting is completely hypoallergenic (assuming that the patient is not sensitive to chlorine, fluoride, or other contaminants), and subsequent re-introduction of foods provides the ideal opportunity to identify offending foods. Fasting deprives intestinal microbes of substrate[57], stimulates intestinal B-cell immunity[58], improves the bactericidal action of neutrophils[59], reduces lysozyme release and leukotriene formation[60], and ameliorates intestinal hyperpermeability.[61] In case reports and clinical trials, short-term fasting (or protein-sparing fasting) has been documented as safe and effective treatment for SLE[62], RA[63], and non-rheumatic diseases such as chronic severe hypertension[64], moderate hypertension[65], obesity[66,67], type-2 diabetes[68], and epilepsy.[69]

- **Broad-spectrum fatty acid therapy with ALA, EPA, DHA, GLA and oleic acid**: Fatty acid supplementation should be delivered in the form of combination therapy with ALA, GLA, DHA, and EPA. Given at doses of 3,000 – 9,000 mg per day, ALA from flaxseed oil has impressive anti-inflammatory benefits demonstrated by its ability to halve prostaglandin production in humans.[70] Numerous studies have demonstrated the benefit of GLA in the treatment of rheumatoid arthritis when used at doses between 500 mg – 4,000 mg per day.[71,72] Fish oil provides EPA and DHA which have well-proven anti-inflammatory benefits in rheumatoid arthritis[73,74,75] and lupus.[76,77] ALA, EPA, DHA, and GLA need to be provided in the form of supplements; when using high doses of therapeutic oils, *liquid* supplements that can be mixed in juice or a smoothie are

[55] Aljada A, Mohanty P, Ghanim H, Abdo T, Tripathy D, Chaudhuri A, Dandona P. Increase in intranuclear nuclear factor kappaB and decrease in inhibitor kappaB in mononuclear cells after a mixed meal: evidence for a proinflammatory effect. *Am J Clin Nutr.* 2004 Apr;79(4):682-90 http://www.ajcn.org/cgi/content/full/79/4/682

[56] "The ability of therapeutic fasts to break metabolic vicious cycles may also contribute to the efficacy of fasting in the treatment of type 2 diabetes and autoimmune disorders." McCarty MF. A preliminary fast may potentiate response to a subsequent low-salt, low-fat vegan diet in the management of hypertension - fasting as a strategy for breaking metabolic vicious cycles. *Med Hypotheses.* 2003 May;60(5):624-33

[57] Ramakrishnan T, Stokes P. Beneficial effects of fasting and low carbohydrate diet in D-lactic acidosis associated with short-bowel syndrome. *JPEN J Parenter Enteral Nutr.* 1985 May-Jun;9(3):361-3

[58] Trollmo C, Verdrengh M, Tarkowski A. Fasting enhances mucosal antigen specific B cell responses in rheumatoid arthritis. *Ann Rheum Dis.* 1997 Feb;56(2):130-4 http://ard.bmjjournals.com/cgi/content/full/56/2/130

[59] "An association was found between improvement in inflammatory activity of the joints and enhancement of neutrophil bactericidal capacity. Fasting appears to improve the clinical status of patients with RA." Uden AM, Trang L, Venizelos N, Palmblad J. Neutrophil functions and clinical performance after total fasting in patients with rheumatoid arthritis. *Ann Rheum Dis.* 1983 Feb;42(1):45-51

[60] "We thus conclude that a reduced ability to generate cytotaxins, reduced release of enzyme, and reduced leukotriene formation from RA neutrophils, together with an altered fatty acid composition of membrane phospholipids, may be mechanisms for the decrease of inflammatory symptoms that results from fasting." Hafstrom I, Ringertz B, Gyllenhammar H, Palmblad J, Harms-Ringdahl M. Effects of fasting on disease activity, neutrophil function, fatty acid composition, and leukotriene biosynthesis in patients with rheumatoid arthritis. *Arthritis Rheum.* 1988 May;31(5):585-92

[61] "The results indicate that, unlike lactovegetarian diet, fasting may ameliorate the disease activity and reduce both the intestinal and the non-intestinal permeability in rheumatoid arthritis." Sundqvist T, Lindstrom F, Magnusson KE, Skoldstam L, Stjernstrom I, Tagesson C. Influence of fasting on intestinal permeability and disease activity in patients with rheumatoid arthritis. *Scand J Rheumatol.* 1982;11(1):33-8

[62] Fuhrman J, Sarter B, Calabro DJ. Brief case reports of medically supervised, water-only fasting associated with remission of autoimmune disease. *Altern Ther Health Med.* 2002 Jul-Aug;8(4):112, 110-1

[63] "An association was found between improvement in inflammatory activity of the joints and enhancement of neutrophil bactericidal capacity. Fasting appears to improve the clinical status of patients with RA." Uden AM, Trang L, Venizelos N, Palmblad J. Neutrophil functions and clinical performance after total fasting in patients with rheumatoid arthritis. *Ann Rheum Dis.* 1983 Feb;42(1):45-51

[64] "The average reduction in blood pressure was 37/13 mm Hg, with the greatest decrease being observed for subjects with the most severe hypertension. Patients with stage 3 hypertension (those with systolic blood pressure greater than 180 mg Hg, diastolic blood pressure greater than 110 mg Hg, or both) had an average reduction of 60/17 mm Hg at the conclusion of treatment." Goldhamer A, Lisle D, Parpia B, Anderson SV, Campbell TC. Medically supervised water-only fasting in the treatment of hypertension. *J Manipulative Physiol Ther.* 2001 Jun;24(5):335-9 http://www.healthpromoting.com/335-339Goldhamer115263.QXD.pdf

[65] "RESULTS: Approximately 82% of the subjects achieved BP at or below 120/80 mm Hg by the end of the treatment program. The mean BP reduction was 20/7 mm Hg, with the greatest decrease being observed for subjects with the highest baseline BP." Goldhamer AC, Lisle DJ, Sultana P, Anderson SV, Parpia B, Hughes B, Campbell TC. Medically supervised water-only fasting in the treatment of borderline hypertension. *J Altern Complement Med.* 2002 Oct;8(5):643-50 http://www.healthpromoting.com/Articles/articles/study%202/acmpaper5.pdf

[66] Vertes V, Genuth SM, Hazelton IM. Supplemented fasting as a large-scale outpatient program. *JAMA.* 1977 Nov 14;238(20):2151-3

[67] Bauman WA, Schwartz E, Rose HG, Eisenstein HN, Johnson DW. Early and long-term effects of acute caloric deprivation in obese diabetic patients. *Am J Med.* 1988 Jul;85(1):38-46

[68] Goldhamer AC. Initial cost of care results in medically supervised water-only fasting for treating high blood pressure and diabetes. *J Altern Complement Med.* 2002 Dec;8(6):696-7 http://www.healthpromoting.com/Articles/pdf/Study%2032.pdf

[69] "The ketogenic diet should be considered as alternative therapy for children with difficult-to-control seizures. It is more effective than many of the new anticonvulsant medications and is well tolerated by children and families when it is effective." Freeman JM, Vining EP, Pillas DJ, Pyzik PL, Casey JC, Kelly LM. The efficacy of the ketogenic diet-1998: a prospective evaluation of intervention in 150 children. *Pediatrics.* 1998 Dec;102(6):1358-63 http://pediatrics.aappublications.org/cgi/reprint/102/6/1358

[70] Adam O, Wolfram G, Zollner N. Effect of alpha-linolenic acid in the human diet on linoleic acid metabolism and prostaglandin biosynthesis. *J Lipid Res.* 1986 Apr;27(4):421-6 http://www.jlr.org/cgi/reprint/27/4/421

[71] "Other results showed a significant reduction in morning stiffness with gamma-linolenic acid at 3 months and reduction in pain and articular index at 6 months with olive oil." Brzeski M, Madhok R, Capell HA. Evening primrose oil in patients with rheumatoid arthritis and side-effects of non-steroidal anti-inflammatory drugs. *Br J Rheumatol.* 1991 Oct;30(5):370-2

[72] Rothman D, DeLuca P, Zurier RB. Botanical lipids: effects on inflammation, immune responses, and rheumatoid arthritis. *Semin Arthritis Rheum.* 1995 Oct;25(2):87-96

[73] Adam O, Beringer C, Kless T, Lemmen C, Adam A, Wiseman M, Adam P, Klimmek R, Forth W. Anti-inflammatory effects of a low arachidonic acid diet and fish oil in patients with rheumatoid arthritis. *Rheumatol Int.* 2003 Jan;23(1):27-36

[74] Lau CS, Morley KD, Belch JJ. Effects of fish oil supplementation on non-steroidal anti-inflammatory drug requirement in patients with mild rheumatoid arthritis--a double-blind placebo controlled study. *Br J Rheumatol.* 1993 Nov;32(11):982-9

[75] Kremer JM, Jubiz W, Michalek A, Rynes RI, Bartholomew LE, Bigaouette J, Timchalk M, Beeler D, Lininger L. Fish-oil fatty acid supplementation in active rheumatoid arthritis. A double-blinded, controlled, crossover study. *Ann Intern Med.* 1987 Apr;106(4):497-503

[76] Walton AJ, Snaith ML, Locniskar M, Cumberland AG, Morrow WJ, Isenberg DA. Dietary fish oil and the severity of symptoms in patients with systemic lupus erythematosus. *Ann Rheum Dis.* 1991 Jul;50(7):463-6

[77] Duffy EM, Meenagh GK, McMillan SA, Strain JJ, Hannigan BM, Bell AL. The clinical effect of dietary supplementation with omega-3 fish oils and/or copper in systemic lupus erythematosus. *J Rheumatol.* 2004 Aug;31(8):1551-6

generally more convenient and palatable than are *capsules*. For example, at the upper end of oral fatty acid administration, the patient may be consuming as much as one-quarter cup per day of fatty acid supplementation; this same dose administered in the form of pills would require at least 72 capsules to attain the equivalent doses of ALA, EPA, DHA, and GLA. Therapeutic amounts of oleic acid can be obtained from generous use of olive oil, preferably on fresh vegetables. Supplementation with polyunsaturated fatty acids warrants increased intake of antioxidants from diet, from fruit and vegetable juices, and from properly formulated supplements. Since patients with systemic inflammation are generally in a pro-oxidative state, consideration must be given to the timing and starting dose of fatty acid supplementation and the need for antioxidant protection; some patients should start with a low dose of fatty acid supplementation until inflammation and the hyperoxidative state have been reduced; see the final chapter in this text on Therapeutics for more fatty acid details and biochemical pathways. Clinicians must realize that fatty acids are not clinically or biochemically interchangeable and that one fatty acid does not substitute for another; each of the fatty acids must be supplied in order for its benefits to be obtained.[78]

- <u>Vitamin D3 supplementation with physiologic doses and/or tailored to serum 25(OH)D levels</u>: Vitamin D deficiency is common in the general population and is even more common in patients with chronic illness and chronic musculoskeletal pain.[79] Correction of vitamin D deficiency supports normal immune function against infection and provides a clinically significant anti-inflammatory[80] and analgesic benefit in patients with back pain[81] and limb pain.[82] Reasonable daily doses for children and adults are 1,000-2,000 and 4,000 IU, respectively.[83] Deficiency and response to treatment are monitored with serum 25(OH)vitamin D while safety is monitored with serum calcium; inflammatory granulomatous diseases and certain drugs such as hydrochlorothiazide greatly increase the propensity for hypercalcemia and warrant increment dosing and frequent monitoring of serum calcium. Vitamin D2 (ergocalciferol) is not a human nutrient and should not be used in clinical practice.

- <u>Assessment for dysbiosis</u>: Assess patients for multifocal dysbiosis.

- <u>Oral enzyme therapy with proteolytic/pancreatic enzymes</u>: Polyenzyme supplementation is used to ameliorate the pathophysiology induced by immune complexes, such as rheumatoid arthritis.[84]

- <u>Phytonutritional modulation of NF-kappaB</u>: As a stimulator of pro-inflammatory gene transcription, NF-kappaB is almost universally activated in conditions associated with inflammation.[85,86] As we would expect, NF-kappaB plays a central role in the pathogenesis of synovitis and joint destruction seen in RA.[87] Nutrients and botanicals which either directly or indirectly inhibit NF-kappaB for an anti-inflammatory benefit include vitamin D[88,89], curcumin[90]

[78] Vasquez A. Reducing Pain and Inflammation Naturally. Part 2: New Insights into Fatty Acid Supplementation and Its Effect on Eicosanoid Production and Genetic Expression. *Nutritional Perspectives* 2005; January: 5-16 http://optimalhealthresearch.com/part2

[79] Plotnikoff GA, Quigley JM. Prevalence of severe hypovitaminosis D in patients with persistent, nonspecific musculoskeletal pain. *Mayo Clin Proc.* 2003 Dec;78(12):1463-70

[80] Timms PM, Mannan N, Hitman GA, Noonan K, Mills PG, Syndercombe-Court D, Aganna E, Price CP, Boucher BJ. Circulating MMP9, vitamin D and variation in the TIMP-1 response with VDR genotype: mechanisms for inflammatory damage in chronic disorders? *QJM.* 2002 Dec;95(12):787-96 http://qjmed.oxfordjournals.org/cgi/content/full/95/12/787

[81] Al Faraj S, Al Mutairi K. Vitamin D deficiency and chronic low back pain in Saudi Arabia. *Spine.* 2003 Jan 15;28(2):177-9

[82] Masood H, Narang AP, Bhat IA, Shah GN. Persistent limb pain and raised serum alkaline phosphatase the earliest markers of subclinical hypovitaminosis D in Kashmir. *Indian J Physiol Pharmacol.* 1989 Oct-Dec;33(4):259-61

[83] Vasquez A, Manso G, Cannell J. The clinical importance of vitamin D (cholecalciferol): a paradigm shift with implications for all healthcare providers. *Altern Ther Health Med.* 2004 Sep-Oct;10(5):28-36 http://optimalhealthresearch.com/monograph04

[84] Galebskaya LV, Ryumina EV, Niemerovsky VS, Matyukov AA. Human complement system state after wobenzyme intake. *VESTNIK MOSKOVSKOGO UNIVERSITETA. KHIMIYA.* 2000. Vol. 41, No. 6. Supplement. Pages 148-149

[85] Tak PP, Firestein GS. NF-kappaB: a key role in inflammatory diseases. *J Clin Invest.* 2001 Jan;107(1):7-11 http://www.jci.org/cgi/content/full/107/1/7

[86] D'Acquisto F, May MJ, Ghosh S. Inhibition of Nuclear Factor KappaB (NF-B): An Emerging Theme in Anti-Inflammatory Therapies. *Mol Interv.* 2002 Feb;2(1):22-35 http://molinterv.aspetjournals.org/cgi/content/abstract/2/1/22

[87] "NF-B plays a central role in the pathogenesis of synovitis in RA and PsA." Foell D, Kane D, Bresnihan B, Vogl T, Nacken W, Sorg C, Fitzgerald O, Roth J. Expression of the pro-inflammatory protein S100A12 (EN-RAGE) in rheumatoid and psoriatic arthritis. *Rheumatology* (Oxford). 2003 Nov;42(11):1383-9 http://rheumatology.oxfordjournals.org/cgi/content/full/42/11/1383

[88] "1Alpha,25-dihydroxyvitamin D3 (1,25-(OH)2-D3), the active metabolite of vitamin D, can inhibit NF-kappaB activity in human MRC-5 fibroblasts, targeting DNA binding of NF-kappaB but not translocation of its subunits p50 and p65." Harant H, Wolff B, Lindley IJ. 1Alpha,25-dihydroxyvitamin D3 decreases DNA binding of nuclear factor-kappaB in human fibroblasts. *FEBS Lett.* 1998 Oct 9;436(3):329-34

[89] "Thus, 1,25(OH)₂D₃ may negatively regulate IL-12 production by downregulation of NF-kB activation and binding to the p40-kB sequence." D'Ambrosio D, Cippitelli M, Cocciolo MG, Mazzeo D, Di Lucia P, Lang R, Sinigaglia F, Panina-Bordignon P. Inhibition of IL-12 production by 1,25-dihydroxyvitamin D3. Involvement of NF-kappaB downregulation in transcriptional repression of the p40 gene. *J Clin Invest.* 1998 Jan 1;101(1):252-62

[90] "Curcumin, EGCG and resveratrol have been shown to suppress activation of NF-kappa B." Surh YJ, Chun KS, Cha HH, Han SS, Keum YS, Park KK, Lee SS. Molecular mechanisms underlying chemopreventive activities of anti-inflammatory phytochemicals: down-regulation of COX-2 and iNOS through suppression of NF-kappa B activation. *Mutat Res.* 2001 Sep 1;480-481:243-68

(requires piperine for absorption[91]), lipoic acid[92], green tea[93], rosemary[94], grape seed extract[95], propolis[96], zinc[97], high-dose selenium[98], indole-3-carbinol[99,100], N-acetyl-L-cysteine[101], resveratrol[102,103], isohumulones[104], GLA via PPAR-gamma[105] and EPA via PPAR-alpha.[106] I have reviewed the phytonutritional modulation of NF-kappaB later in this text and elsewhere.[107] Several phytonutritional products targeting NF-kappaB are available.

Notes:

_____

_____

_____

_____

_____

_____

_____

_____

_____

_____

_____

_____

_____

_____

_____

[91] Shoba G, Joy D, Joseph T, Majeed M, Rajendran R, Srinivas PS. Influence of piperine on the pharmacokinetics of curcumin in animals and human volunteers. *Planta Med.* 1998 May;64(4):353-6

[92] "ALA reduced the TNF-alpha-stimulated ICAM-1 expression in a dose-dependent manner, to levels observed in unstimulated cells. Alpha-lipoic acid also reduced NF-kappaB activity in these cells in a dose-dependent manner." Lee HA, Hughes DA. Alpha-lipoic acid modulates NF-kappaB activity in human monocytic cells by direct interaction with DNA. *Exp Gerontol.* 2002 Jan-Mar;37(2-3):401-10

[93] "In conclusion, EGCG is an effective inhibitor of IKK activity. This may explain, at least in part, some of the reported anti-inflammatory and anticancer effects of green tea." Yang F, Oz HS, Barve S, de Villiers WJ, McClain CJ, Varilek GW. The green tea polyphenol (-)-epigallocatechin-3-gallate blocks nuclear factor-kappa B activation by inhibiting I kappa B kinase activity in the intestinal epithelial cell line IEC-6. *Mol Pharmacol.* 2001 Sep;60(3):528-33

[94] "These results suggest that carnosol suppresses the NO production and iNOS gene expression by inhibiting NF-kappaB activation, and provide possible mechanisms for its anti-inflammatory and chemopreventive action." Lo AH, Liang YC, Lin-Shiau SY, Ho CT, Lin JK. Carnosol, an antioxidant in rosemary, suppresses inducible nitric oxide synthase through down-regulating nuclear factor-kappaB in mouse macrophages. *Carcinogenesis.* 2002 Jun;23(6):983-91

[95] "Constitutive and TNFalpha-induced NF-kappaB DNA binding activity was inhibited by GSE at doses > or =50 microg/ml and treatments for > or =12 h." Dhanalakshmi S, Agarwal R, Agarwal C. Inhibition of NF-kappaB pathway in grape seed extract-induced apoptotic death of human prostate carcinoma DU145 cells. *Int J Oncol.* 2003 Sep;23(3):721-7

[96] "Caffeic acid phenethyl ester (CAPE) is an anti-inflammatory component of propolis (honeybee resin). CAPE is reportedly a specific inhibitor of nuclear factor-kappaB (NF-kappaB)." Fitzpatrick LR, Wang J, Le T. Caffeic acid phenethyl ester, an inhibitor of nuclear factor-kappaB, attenuates bacterial peptidoglycan polysaccharide-induced colitis in rats. *J Pharmacol Exp Ther.* 2001 Dec;299(3):915-20

[97] "Our results suggest that zinc supplementation may lead to downregulation of the inflammatory cytokines through upregulation of the negative feedback loop A20 to inhibit induced NF-kappaB activation." Prasad AS, Bao B, Beck FW, Kucuk O, Sarkar FH. Antioxidant effect of zinc in humans. *Free Radic Biol Med.* 2004 Oct 15;37(8):1182-90

[98] Note that the patients in this study received a very high dose of selenium: 960 micrograms per day. This is at the top—and some would say over the top—of the safe and reasonable dose for long-term supplementation. In this case, the study lasted for three months. "In patients receiving selenium supplementation, selenium NF-kappaB activity was significantly reduced, reaching the same level as the nondiabetic control group. CONCLUSION: In type 2 diabetic patients, activation of NF-kappaB measured in peripheral blood monocytes can be reduced by selenium supplementation, confirming its importance in the prevention of cardiovascular diseases." Faure P, Ramon O, Favier A, Halimi S. Selenium supplementation decreases nuclear factor-kappa B activity in peripheral blood mononuclear cells from type 2 diabetic patients. *Eur J Clin Invest.* 2004 Jul;34(7):475-81

[99] Takada Y, Andreeff M, Aggarwal BB. Indole-3-carbinol suppresses NF-{kappa}B and I{kappa}B{alpha} kinase activation causing inhibition of expression of NF-{kappa}B-regulated antiapoptotic and metastatic gene products and enhancement of apoptosis in myeloid and leukemia cells. *Blood.* 2005 Apr 5; [Epub ahead of print]

[100] "Overall, our results indicated that indole-3-carbinol inhibits NF-kappaB and NF-kappaB-regulated gene expression and that this mechanism may provide the molecular basis for its ability to suppress tumorigenesis." Takada Y, Andreeff M, Aggarwal BB. Indole-3-carbinol suppresses NF-kappaB and IkappaBalpha kinase activation, causing inhibition of expression of NF-kappaB-regulated antiapoptotic and metastatic gene products and enhancement of apoptosis in myeloid and leukemia cells. *Blood.* 2005 Jul 15;106(2):641-9. Epub 2005 Apr 5.

[101] "CONCLUSIONS: Administration of N-acetylcysteine results in decreased nuclear factor-kappa B activation in patients with sepsis, associated with decreases in interleukin-8 but not interleukin-6 or soluble intercellular adhesion molecule-1. These pilot data suggest that antioxidant therapy with N-acetylcysteine may be useful in blunting the inflammatory response to sepsis." Paterson RL, Galley HF, Webster NR. The effect of N-acetylcysteine on nuclear factor-kappa B activation, interleukin-6, interleukin-8, and intercellular adhesion molecule-1 expression in patients with sepsis. *Crit Care Med.* 2003 Nov;31(11):2574-8

[102] "Resveratrol's anticarcinogenic, anti-inflammatory, and growth-modulatory effects may thus be partially ascribed to the inhibition of activation of NF-kappaB and AP-1 and the associated kinases." Manna SK, Mukhopadhyay A, Aggarwal BB. Resveratrol suppresses TNF-induced activation of nuclear transcription factors NF-kappa B, activator protein-1, and apoptosis: potential role of reactive oxygen intermediates and lipid peroxidation. *J Immunol.* 2000 Jun 15;164(12):6509-19

[103] "Both resveratrol and quercetin inhibited NF-kappaB-, AP-1- and CREB-dependent transcription to a greater extent than the glucocorticosteroid, dexamethasone." Donnelly LE, Newton R, Kennedy GE, Fenwick PS, Leung RH, Ito K, Russell RE, Barnes PJ. Anti-inflammatory Effects of Resveratrol in Lung Epithelial Cells: Molecular Mechanisms. *Am J Physiol Lung Cell Mol Physiol.* 2004 Jun 4 [Epub ahead of print]

[104] Yajima H, Ikeshima E, Shiraki M, Kanaya T, Fujiwara D, Odai H, Tsuboyama-Kasaoka N, Ezaki O, Oikawa S, Kondo K. Isohumulones, bitter acids derived from hops, activate both peroxisome proliferator-activated receptor alpha and gamma and reduce insulin resistance. *J Biol Chem.* 2004 Aug 6;279(32):33456-62. Epub 2004 Jun 3. http://www.jbc.org/cgi/content/full/279/32/33456

[105] "Thus, PPAR gamma serves as the receptor for GLA in the regulation of gene expression in breast cancer cells. " Jiang WG, Redfern A, Bryce RP, Mansel RE. Peroxisome proliferator activated receptor-gamma (PPAR-gamma) mediates the action of gamma linolenic acid in breast cancer cells. *Prostaglandins Leukot Essent Fatty Acids.* 2000 Feb;62(2):119-27

[106] "...EPA requires PPARalpha for its inhibitory effects on NF-kappaB." Mishra A, Chaudhary A, Sethi S. Oxidized omega-3 fatty acids inhibit NF-kappaB activation via a PPARalpha-dependent pathway. *Arterioscler Thromb Vasc Biol.* 2004 Sep;24(9):1621-7. Epub 2004 Jul 1. http://atvb.ahajournals.org/cgi/content/full/24/9/1621

[107] "Indeed, the previous view that nutrients only interact with human physiology at the metabolic/post-transcriptional level must be updated in light of current research showing that nutrients can, in fact, modify human physiology and phenotype at the genetic/pre-transcriptional level." Vasquez A. Reducing pain and inflammation naturally - part 4: nutritional and botanical inhibition of NF-kappaB, the major intracellular amplifier of the inflammatory cascade. A practical clinical strategy exemplifying anti-inflammatory nutrigenomics. *Nutritional Perspectives*, July 2005:5-12. www.OptimalHealthResearch.com/part4

Wegener's Granulomatosis

Description/pathophysiology:

- This inflammatory condition generally begins with granulomatous involvement of the upper or lower respiratory tract and then progresses to systemic vasculitis and glomerulonephritis.
- Biopsy of nasopharyngeal/pulmonary/renal lesions reveals granulomatous/inflammatory tissue.
- Allopathic textbooks generally describe this condition as *idiopathic*, although the condition is increasingly associated with occult sinorespiratory dysbiosis with *Staphylococcus aureus*.[1,2] Additionally, *Klebsiella aerogenes*, *Haemophilus influenzae*, and *Bacillus subtilis* have been implicated.[3]
- Immune complexes contribute to pathophysiology

Clinical presentations:

- Twice as common in males as in females
- Sinorespiratory symptoms:
  - Hemorrhagic rhinorrhea
  - Sinusitis
  - Otitis media
  - Mucosal ulcerations/friability
  - Cough
  - Hemoptosis due to intraalveolar hemorrhage
  - Pleuritis
- Renal complications are inevitable without effective/immunosuppressive treatment
- Typical autoimmune systemic manifestations: fatigue, malaise, low-grade fever, anorexia, and weight loss, polyarthritis.

Major differential diagnoses:

- Extramedullary plasmacytoma of multiple myeloma (typically occurs in the nasopharyngeal region)
- Sinus infection
- Lung cancer
- Tuberculosis
- Septicemia or septic arthritis
- Lymphoma
- Other systemic/inflammatory disorder such as lupus (ANA and low complement)
- Bacterial endocarditis

Clinical assessments:

- **History/subjective:** See clinical presentations.
- **Physical examination/objective:**
  - Examination of oral and nasal mucosa
  - Pulmonary auscultation
  - Dermatologic screen for cutaneous vasculitis

---

[1] Brons RH, Bakker HI, Van Wijk RT, Van Dijk NW, Muller Kobold AC, Limburg PC, Manson WL, Kallenberg CG, Tervaert JW. Staphylococcal acid phosphatase binds to endothelial cells via charge interaction; a pathogenic role in Wegener's granulomatosis? *Clin Exp Immunol.* 2000 Mar;119(3):566-73 http://www.blackwell-synergy.com/doi/abs/10.1046/j.1365-2249.2000.01172.x
[2] Popa ER, Stegeman CA, Kallenberg CG, Tervaert JW. Staphylococcus aureus and Wegener's granulomatosis. *Arthritis Res.* 2002;4(2):77-9 http://arthritis-research.com/content/4/2/77
[3] George J, Levy Y, Kallenberg CG, Shoenfeld Y. Infections and Wegener's granulomatosis--a cause and effect relationship? *QJM.* 1997 May;90(5):367-73 http://qjmed.oxfordjournals.org/cgi/reprint/90/5/367

- **Laboratory assessments**:
  - Urinalysis for assessment of renal status
  - Chemistry/metabolic panel for BUN and creatinine, etc.
  - Comprehensive stool analysis and comprehensive parasitology—mandatory in all autoimmune diseases.
  - Nasal culture for *Staphylococcus aureus*[4] and other bacterial or fungal contaminants
  - Complement levels are normal or elevated
  - ESR/CRP is elevated
  - CBC may reveal leukocytosis and anemia
  - **ANA (antinuclear antibodies) are generally absent**
  - **ANCA are almost always present and strongly support the diagnosis of this condition. The finding of the more specific C-ANCA is 97% specific for the diagnosis of Wegener's granulomatosis.**[5] Interestingly ANCA can also be induced by gastrointestinal parasitic infections.
- **Imaging**: generally not required; only indicated as needed
- **Establishing the diagnosis**: Based on clinical, serologic, and biopsy findings.
  - Respiratory tract symptoms and mucosal lesions
  - C-ANCA: positive C-ANCA result can replace biopsy in a patient with a clinical picture of Wegener's granulomatosis.[6]
  - Biopsy of respiratory tract granulomas

Complications:
- Severe anemia requiring blood transfusion
- Secondary bacterial infections on ulcerated mucosa
- Respiratory and renal failure
- Hypoxic complications due to vasculitis

Clinical management:
- Referral to internist/rheumatologist for additional treatment and defensive management as indicated. Unless you are a specialist, you need to have a specialist as part of the care team who can help you manage acute exacerbations which can occur with any autoimmune/inflammatory disease.

Therapeutic considerations:

Medical treatment routinely includes the following:[7]
- Cyclophosphamide: 1-2 mg/kg/d PO or IV: associated with increased risk for cancer, particularly bladder cancer
- Prednisone: 1 mg/kg/d po; use the lowest dose possible
- Methotrexate: pulse treatment < 20-30 mg per week po
- **Antibiotic treatment: trimeth-sulfa 160/800 up to 480/2400 mg/d po**
- Blood transfusions for anemia

- **Assessment for multifocal dysbiosis: emphasis on gastrointestinal and sinorespiratory dysbiosis**
  - *Staphylococcus aureus* **produces an antigenic acid phosphatase which haptenizes with endothelial cells for the induction of autoimmune vasculitis in Wegener's granulomatosis.**[8] Antimicrobial treatment to eradicate *Staphylococcus aureus* results

[4] Brons RH, Bakker HI, Van Wijk RT, et al. Staphylococcal acid phosphatase binds to endothelial cells via charge interaction; a pathogenic role in Wegener's granulomatosis? *Clin Exp Immunol.* 2000 Mar;119(3):566-73 http://www.blackwell-synergy.com/doi/abs/10.1046/j.1365-2249.2000.01172.x PDF available from this link on November 27, 2005.
[5] Beers MH, Berkow R (eds). The Merck Manual. Seventeenth Edition. Whitehouse Station; Merck Research Laboratories 1999 Page 443
[6] Shojania K. Rheumatology: 2. What laboratory tests are needed? *CMAJ.* 2000 Apr 18;162(8):1157-63 http://www.cmaj.ca/cgi/content/full/162/8/1157
[7] Beers MH, Berkow R (eds). The Merck Manual. Seventeenth Edition. Whitehouse Station; Merck Research Laboratories 1999 Page 443
[8] Brons RH, Bakker HI, Van Wijk RT, et al. Staphylococcal acid phosphatase binds to endothelial cells via charge interaction; a pathogenic role in Wegener's granulomatosis? *Clin Exp Immunol.* 2000 Mar;119(3):566-73 http://www.blackwell-synergy.com/doi/abs/10.1046/j.1365-2249.2000.01172.x PDF available from this link on November 27, 2005.

in clinical remission of the "autoimmune" disease, thus proving the microbe-rheumatic link.[9] Hyperforin from *Hypericum perforatum* is highly effective against *Staphylococcus aureus*[10] and can be used nasally and orally.

- o *Entamoeba histolytica* **induces formation of antineutrophil cytoplasmic antibodies (ANCA).**[11] Stool testing with a specialty laboratory is strongly recommended.
- o **Other microbes such as *Klebsiella aerogenes*, *Haemophilus influenzae* and *Bacillus subtilis*** have also been implicated.[12]

- Supplemented Paleo-Mediterranean diet: The health-promoting diet of choice for the majority of people is a diet based on abundant consumption of fruits, vegetables, seeds, nuts, omega-3 and monounsaturated fatty acids, and lean sources of protein such as lean meats, fatty cold-water fish, soy and whey proteins. (See Chapter 2 for details).

- Broad-spectrum fatty acid therapy with ALA, EPA, DHA, GLA and oleic acid: Fatty acid supplementation should be delivered in the form of combination therapy with ALA, GLA, DHA, EPA as described in this book and elsewhere.[13]

- Vitamin D3 supplementation with physiologic doses and/or tailored to serum 25(OH)D levels: **Since Wegener's *granulomatosis* is obviously a *granulomatous* disease, caution and frequent monitoring must be employed when optimizing vitamin D status to avoid hypercalcemia.** A reasonable clinical approach would be to start with a relatively low dose (1,000 – 2,000 IU cholecalciferol per day following the exclusion of hypercalcemia. Thereafter, serum calcium can be measured at 2 weeks, 4 weeks, 6 weeks, 8 weeks, and monthly thereafter. See Therapeutics section of this text and the review by Vasquez et al[14] for more details.

- Orthoendocrinology: Assess prolactin, cortisol, DHEA, free and total testosterone, serum estradiol, and thyroid status (e.g., TSH, T4, *and* anti-thyroid peroxidase antibodies). Treat effectively as indicated.

- Assess for heavy metals, especially mercury: **Exposure to mercury and lead is associated with increased risk of developing Wegener's granulomatosis.**[15] Consider urine toxic metal assessment following 10-30 mg/kg DMSA as described in Chapter 4 and as described elsewhere for the assessment of heavy metals in patients with autism.[16]

- Proteolytic enzymes: Wegener's granulomatosis is mediated in large part by IgG and IgA immune complexes, which directly contribute to vasculitis and nephritis.[17] Polyenzyme supplementation is used to ameliorate the pathophysiology induced by immune complexes.[18]

- Hepatobiliary stimulation: IgA immune complexes are removed from the serum by hepatocytes and transported intact into the bile.[19,20,21,22,23,24,25] Therefore, stimulating bile flow would be

[9] Popa ER, Stegeman CA, Kallenberg CG, Tervaert JW. Staphylococcus aureus and Wegener's granulomatosis. *Arthritis Res*. 2002;4(2):77-9 http://arthritis-research.com/content/4/2/077

[10] Schempp CM, Pelz K, Wittmer A, Schopf E, Simon JC. Antibacterial activity of hyperforin from St John's wort, against multiresistant Staphylococcus aureus and gram-positive bacteria. *Lancet*. 1999 Jun 19;353(9170):2129

[11] George J, Levy Y, Kallenberg CG, Shoenfeld Y. Infections and Wegener's granulomatosis--a cause and effect relationship? QJM. 1997 May;90(5):367-73 http://qjmed.oxfordjournals.org/cgi/reprint/90/5/367

[12] George J, Levy Y, Kallenberg CG, Shoenfeld Y. Infections and Wegener's granulomatosis--a cause and effect relationship? *QJM*. 1997 May;90(5):367-73 http://qjmed.oxfordjournals.org/cgi/reprint/90/5/367

[13] Vasquez A. Reducing Pain and Inflammation Naturally. Part 2: New Insights into Fatty Acid Supplementation and Its Effect on Eicosanoid Production and Genetic Expression. *Nutritional Perspectives* 2005; January: 5-16 http://optimalhealthresearch.com/part2

[14] Vasquez A, Manso G, Cannell J. The clinical importance of vitamin D (cholecalciferol): a paradigm shift with implications for all healthcare providers. *Altern Ther Health Med*. 2004 Sep-Oct;10(5):28-36 http://optimalhealthresearch.com/monograph04

[15] " Results suggest that mercury and perhaps lead exposure were positively associated with WG as compared with either control group, although the number of patients exposed was small… CONCLUSION: We conclude that heavy metal exposure and a prior history of allergy may play a role in the etiopathogenesis of Wegener's granulomatosis." Albert D, Clarkin C, Komoroski J, Brensinger CM, Berlin JA. Wegener's granulomatosis: Possible role of environmental agents in its pathogenesis. *Arthritis Rheum*. 2004 Aug 15;51(4):656-64

[16] Bradstreet J, Geier DA, Kartzinel JJ, Adams JB, Geier MR. A case-control study of mercury burden in children with autistic spectrum disorders. *Journal of American Physicians and Surgeons* 2003; 8: 76-79 http://www.jpands.org/vol8no3/geier.pdf

[17] "RESULTS: Four of 11 biopsies taken at initial presentation and four of 21 biopsies taken at the onset of a relapse of WG showed IgG and/or IgA containing immune deposits in the subepidermal blood vessels. ...CONCLUSION: A substantial number of skin biopsies showed immune deposits during active disease. These results could support the hypothesis that immune complexes may trigger vasculitic lesions in WG." Brons RH, de Jong MC, de Boer NK, Stegeman CA, Kallenberg CG, Tervaert JW. Detection of immune deposits in skin lesions of patients with Wegener's granulomatosis. Ann Rheum Dis. 2001 Dec;60(12):1097-102 http://ard.bmjjournals.com/cgi/content/full/60/12/1097

[18] Galebskaya LV, Ryumina EV, Niemerovsky VS, Matyukov AA. Human complement system state after wobenzyme intake. *VESTNIK MOSKOVSKOGO UNIVERSITETA. KHIMIYA.* 2000. Vol. 41, No. 6. Supplement. Pages 148-149

[19] Russell MW, Brown TA, Claflin JL, Schroer K, Mestecky J. Immunoglobulin A-mediated hepatobiliary transport constitutes a natural pathway for disposing of bacterial antigens. *Infect Immun*. 1983 Dec;42(3):1041-8 http://www.pubmedcentral.gov/articlerender.fcgi?tool=pubmed&pubmedid=6642659

[20] "The liver therefore appears to be singularly capable of transporting both free and complexed IgA into its secretion, the bile." Russell MW, Brown TA, Mestecky J. Preferential transport of IgA and IgA-immune complexes to bile compared with other external secretions. *Mol Immunol*. 1982 May;19(5):677-82

[21] "These results indicate that mouse hepatocytes are involved in the uptake and hepatobiliary transport of pIgA-IC and pIgA-IC of low mol. wt." Phillips JO, Komiyama K, Epps JM, Russell MW, Mestecky J. Role of hepatocytes in the uptake of IgA and IgA-containing immune complexes in mice. *Mol Immunol*. 1988 Sep;25(9):873-9

[22] "Thus hepatobiliary transport appears to be the major pathway for the clearance of both IgA IC and free IgA from the circulation." Brown TA, Russell MW, Kulhavy R, Mestecky J. IgA-mediated elimination of antigens by the hepatobiliary route. *Fed Proc*. 1983 Dec;42(15):3218-21

expected to expedite the removal of IgA immune complexes from the serum, thus lessening their clinical consequences. Dietary and botanical therapeutics that stimulate bile flow include beets, ginger[26], curcumin/turmeric[27], *Picrorhiza*[28], milk thistle[29], *Andrographis paniculata*[30] and *Boerhaavia diffusa*.[31] Therapeutic enemas safely and effectively stimulate bile flow for 45-60 minutes following administration.[32]

Notes:

_____

_____

_____

_____

_____

_____

_____

_____

_____

_____

_____

_____

_____

_____

_____

_____

_____

_____

_____

_____

_____

_____

[23] "Clearance of IgA immune complexes was delayed after bile duct ligation." Harmatz PR, Kleinman RE, Bunnell BW, McClenathan DT, Walker WA, Bloch KJ. The effect of bile duct obstruction on the clearance of circulating IgA immune complexes. *Hepatology*. 1984 Jan-Feb;4(1):96-100

[24] Lemaitre-Coelho I, Jackson GD, Vaerman JP. High levels of secretory IgA and free secretory component in the serum of rats with bile duct obstruction. *J Exp Med*. 1978 Mar 1;147(3):934-9 http://www.jem.org/cgi/reprint/147/3/934

[25] "CONCLUSIONS: Biliary obstruction secondary to both calculus or malignancy of the hepatobiliary system causes suppression of bile IgA secretion and elevated serum level of secretory IgA. Bile secretory IgA secretion recovers with endoscopic drainage of the obstructed system." Sung JJ, Leung JC, Tsui CP, Chung SS, Lai KN. Biliary IgA secretion in obstructive jaundice: the effects of endoscopic drainage. *Gastrointest Endosc*. 1995 Nov;42(5):439-44

[26] "Further analyses for the active constituents of the acetone extracts through column chromatography indicated that [6]-gingerol and [10]-gingerol, which are the pungent principles, are mainly responsible for the cholagogic effect of ginger." Yamahara J, Miki K, Chisaka T, Sawada T, Fujimura H, Tomimatsu T, Nakano K, Nohara T. Cholagogic effect of ginger and its active constituents. *J Ethnopharmacol*. 1985;13(2):217-25

[27] "On the basis of the present findings, it appears that curcumin induces contraction of the human gall-bladder." Rasyid A, Lelo A. The effect of curcumin and placebo on human gall-bladder function: an ultrasound study. *Aliment Pharmacol Ther*. 1999 Feb;13(2):245-9

[28] "Significant anticholestatic activity was also observed against carbon tetrachloride induced cholestasis in conscious rat, anaesthetized guinea pig and cat. Picroliv was more active than the known hepatoprotective drug silymarin." Saraswat B, Visen PK, Patnaik GK, Dhawan BN. Anticholestatic effect of picroliv, active hepatoprotective principle of Picrorhiza kurrooa, against carbon tetrachloride induced cholestasis. *Indian J Exp Biol*. 1993 Apr;31(4):316-8

[29] "We conclude that SIL counteracts TLC-induced cholestasis by preventing the impairment in both the BS-dependent and -independent fractions of the bile flow." Crocenzi FA, Sanchez Pozzi EJ, Pellegrino JM, Rodriguez Garay EA, Mottino AD, Roma MG. Preventive effect of silymarin against taurolithocholate-induced cholestasis in the rat. *Biochem Pharmacol*. 2003 Jul 15;66(2):355-64

[30] "Andrographolide from the herb Andrographis paniculata (whole plant) per se produces a significant dose (1.5-12 mg/kg) dependent choleretic effect (4.8-73%) as evidenced by increase in bile flow, bile salt, and bile acids in conscious rats and anaesthetized guinea pigs." Shukla B, Visen PK, Patnaik GK, Dhawan BN. Choleretic effect of andrographolide in rats and guinea pigs. *Planta Med*. 1992 Apr;58(2):146-9

[31] "The extract also produced an increase in normal bile flow in rats suggesting a strong choleretic activity." Chandan BK, Sharma AK, Anand KK. Boerhaavia diffusa: a study of its hepatoprotective activity. *J Ethnopharmacol*. 1991 Mar;31(3):299-307

[32] Garbat AL, Jacobi HG. Secretion of Bile in Response to Rectal Installations. *Arch Intern Med* 1929; 44: 455-462

Vasculitides and Vasculitis Syndromes

<u>Description/pathophysiology, and clinical presentations</u>:

- "Vasculitis" refers to a heterogeneous group of inflammatory disorders primarily affecting blood vessels, particularly the arteries and arterioles. Although the underlying pathomechanisms are similar among different disorders, these diseases differ in the location/size and number of affected vessels, and thus the clinical presentations and complications differ accordingly. Polymyalgia rheumatica / giant cell arteritis (Chapter 14), Wegener's granulomatosis (Chapter 15), and Behcet's disease (Chapter 17) are subtypes of vasculitis that are discussed in their respective chapters. As you can see from the table at the right, several subtypes of vasculitis can be categorized based on the size/location of the vessel affected, and whether or not the cause of the vasculitis has been determined. Given the similarities of these disorders and that several are detailed in their respective chapters, only a few vasculopathies will be detailed here.
- Systemic manifestations are comparable to many other autoimmune disorders: insidious onset of fever, malaise, weight loss, generalized aches/pains.

Primary vasculitides
Large vessel diseases
- Takayasu's arteritis
- Giant cell arteritis (Chapter 14)
- Behcet's disease (Chapter 17)

Medium vessel diseases
- Polyarteritis nodosa
- Buerger's disease

Small vessel diseases
Immune-complex mediated
- Cutaneous leukocystoclastic vasculitis
- Henoch-Schonlein purpura
- Cryoglobulinemia

ANCA-associated disorders
- Wegener's granulomatosis (Chapter 15)
- Microscopic polyangiitis
- Churg-Strauss syndrome

Secondary vasculitides
- Infections
- Other autoimmune disease
- Crohn's disease or ulcerative colitis
- Cancer
- Drug reactions

Vasculitis subtype	Unique presentations	Assessment and treatment considerations
Polyarteritis nodosa ▪ 10% of patients have Hepatitis B—testing for hepatitis B is mandatory.[1] ▪ Without treatment, only 20% of patients survive 5 years; with treatment, survival improves to 60-90% at 5 years.	▪ Abdominal pain, nausea, vomiting exacerbated by eating (due to ischemia) ▪ Mononeuritis multiplex, vasculitic neuropathy: foot drop is most common manifestation ▪ Dermal lesions include nodules, erythema, and ulceration ▪ Hypertension due to renal involvement ▪ Pulmonary involvement is rare	▪ Anemia ▪ Elevated ESR ▪ Leukocytosis ▪ Autoantibodies commonly normal or low-positive ▪ Diagnosis is established with biopsy or angiogram ▪ Prednisone: 60 mg/d ▪ Pulsed methylprednisolone: 1 gram IV daily for 3 days ▪ Cyclophosphamide or other immunosuppressant drug ▪ Plasmapheresis ▪ Treatment of underlying hepatitis: must balance immunosuppression with anti-infective treatments
Cryoglobulinemia ▪ Many patients have underlying hepatitis C.	▪ Purpura ▪ Peripheral neuropathy ▪ Glomerulonephritis ▪ Abdominal pain ▪ Hepatitis ▪ May have pulmonary involvement	▪ Diagnosis is based on clinical picture and serology for cryoglobulins ▪ Testing for and treatment of underlying hepatitis is essential ▪ Immunosuppression may exacerbate viral replication ▪ **Avoidance of food allergens is highly beneficial**[2,3]
Henoch-Schonlein purpura	▪ Dermal purpura ▪ Abdominal pain ▪ Arthritis ▪ Hematuria	▪ The disease is generally self-limiting to 1-6 weeks, subsiding without complications if renal involvement is mild ▪ No generally effective allopathic treatment is known

[1] Tierney ML. McPhee SJ, Papadakis MA (eds). <u>Current Medical Diagnosis and Treatment 2006. 45th edition</u>. New York; Lange Medical Books: 2006, pages 844-850
[2] "CONCLUSION: These data show that an LAC diet decreases the amount of circulating immune complexes in MC and can modify certain signs and symptoms of the disease." Ferri C, Pietrogrande M, Cecchetti R, et al. Low-antigen-content diet in the treatment of patients with mixed cryoglobulinemia. *Am J Med.* 1989 Nov;87(5):519-24
[3] Pietrogrande M, Cefalo A, Nicora F, Marchesini D. Dietetic treatment of essential mixed cryoglobulinemia. *Ric Clin Lab.* 1986 Apr-Jun;16(2):413-6

Major differential diagnoses:

- <u>Infection</u>
- <u>Cancer</u>, especially leukemia, lymphoma, and multiple myeloma
- <u>Autoimmunity</u>: Concomitant or independent
- <u>Trauma or abuse</u>: Numerous unexplainable bruises/purpura may indicate abuse

Clinical assessments:

- **History/subjective**:
  - See clinical presentations
- **Physical examination/objective**:
  - General physical examination with emphasis placed on symptomatic regions, circulatory examination, and dermal lesions
- **Laboratory assessments**:
  - <u>Chemistry/metabolic panel</u>: Assess for complications, especially renal insufficiency
  - <u>Urinalysis</u>: Assess for renal involvement
  - <u>CRP/ESR</u>: Generally elevated
  - <u>Serum immune complexes</u>: Most vasculopathies are associated with immune complex deposition
  - <u>Testing for multifocal dysbiosis</u>: As discussed in Chapter 4
  - <u>ANA</u>
  - <u>CH50</u>: Complement levels may be low during exacerbations.
- **Imaging and biopsy**:
  - Angiography is commonly used in the evaluation of vasculitic syndromes
  - Biopsy of dermal lesions, superficial arteries, and other tissues can support the diagnosis
- **Establishing the diagnosis**:
  - Based on clinical, laboratory, and biopsy/imaging findings

Major complications:

- Tissue necrosis: Complications depend on location of hypoxia and can include dermal necrosis, myocardial infarction, stroke, and intestinal infarction
- Infection secondary to immunosuppression
- Renal damage

Clinical management:

- Exacerbations are best managed pharmaceutically with appropriate immunosuppression. Patients may require hospital admission

Treatments:

- <u>Avoidance of allergenic foods</u>: **Hypoallergenic diets can benefit patients with immune-complex-mediated diseases such as mixed cryoglobulinemia[4,5], hypersensitivity vasculitis[6], and leukocystoclastic vasculitis with arthritis.[7]** Any patient may be allergic to any food, even if the food is generally considered a health-promoting food. Generally speaking, the most notorious allergens are wheat, citrus (especially juice due to the industrial use of fungal hemicellulases), cow's milk, eggs, peanuts, chocolate, and yeast-containing foods. According to a study in patients with migraine, some patients will have to avoid as many as 10 specific foods in order to become symptom-free.[8] **The severe wheat allergy** *celiac disease* **can present with inflammatory oligoarthritis[9,10], and celiac disease can also present as cryoglobulinemia and vasculitis[11], cutaneous leukocystoclastic vasculitis[12], including cerebral vasculitis[13] and pediatric stroke.[14]**

---

[4] "CONCLUSION: These data show that an LAC diet decreases the amount of circulating immune complexes in MC and can modify certain signs and symptoms of the disease." Ferri C, Pietrogrande M, Cecchetti R, et al. Low-antigen-content diet in the treatment of patients with mixed cryoglobulinemia. *Am J Med*. 1989 Nov;87(5):519-24

[5] Pietrogrande M, Cefalo A, Nicora F, Marchesini D. Dietetic treatment of essential mixed cryoglobulinemia. *Ric Clin Lab*. 1986 Apr-Jun;16(2):413-6

[6] "In three cases the vasculitis relapsed following the introduction of food additives; in one case with the addition of potatoes and green vegetables (i.e., beans and green peas) and in the last case with the addition of eggs to the diet." Lunardi C, Bambara LM, Biasi D, Zagni P, Caramaschi P, Pacor ML. Elimination diet in the treatment of selected patients with hypersensitivity vasculitis. *Clin Exp Rheumatol*. 1992 Mar-Apr;10(2):131-5

[7] "Described in this report are two children with severe vasculitis caused by specific foods." Businco L, Falconieri P, Bellioni-Businco B, Bahna SL. Severe food-induced vasculitis in two children. *Pediatr Allergy Immunol*. 2002 Feb;13(1):68-71

[8] Grant EC. Food allergies and migraine. *Lancet*. 1979 May 5;1(8123):966-9

[9] "We report six patients with coeliac disease in whom arthritis was prominent at diagnosis and who improved with dietary therapy. Joint pain preceded diagnosis by up to three years in five patients and 15 years in one patient." Bourne JT, Kumar P, Huskisson EC, Mageed R, Unsworth DJ, Wojtulewski JA. Arthritis and coeliac disease. *Ann Rheum Dis*. 1985 Sep;44(9):592-8

[10] "A 15-year-old girl, with synovitis of the knees and ankles for 3 years before a diagnosis of gluten-sensitive enteropathy, is described." Pinals RS. Arthritis associated with gluten-sensitive enteropathy. *J Rheumatol*. 1986 Feb;13(1):201-4

[11] "Immunosuppressive treatment led to a normalization of transaminase levels and resolved the cryoglobulinaemic vasculitis. In addition, the patient exhibited low ferritin and iron levels, which led to the diagnosis of coeliac disease." Biecker E, Stieger M, Zimmermann A, Reichen J. Autoimmune hepatitis, cryoglobulinaemia and untreated coeliac disease: a case report. *Eur J Gastroenterol Hepatol*. 2003 Apr;15(4):423-7

- <u>Avoidance of pro-inflammatory foods</u>: Pro-inflammatory foods act *directly* and *indirectly* to promote and exacerbate systemic inflammation. *Direct* mechanisms include the activation of Toll-like receptors and NF-kappaB, while *indirect* mechanisms include depleting the body of anti-inflammatory nutrients and dietary displacement of more nutrient-dense anti-inflammatory foods. Arachidonic acid (found in cow's milk, beef, liver, pork, and lamb) is the direct precursor to pro-inflammatory prostaglandins and leukotrienes[15] and pain-promoting isoprostanes.[16] Saturated fats promote inflammation by activating/enabling pro-inflammatory Toll-like receptors, which are otherwise "specific" for inducing pro-inflammatory responses to microorganisms.[17] Consumption of saturated fat in the form of cream creates marked oxidative stress and lipid peroxidation that lasts for at least 3 hours postprandially.[18] Corn oil rapidly activates NF-kappaB (in hepatic Kupffer cells) for a pro-inflammatory effect[19]; similarly, consumption of PUFA and linoleic acid promotes antioxidant depletion and may thus promote oxidation-mediated inflammation via activation of NF-kappaB. Linoleic acid causes intracellular oxidative stress and calcium influx and results in increased NF-kappaB-stimulated transcription of pro-inflammatory genes.[20] High glycemic foods cause oxidative stress[21,22] and inflammation via activation of NF-kappaB and other mechanisms—e.g., *white bread causes inflammation*[23] as does *a high-fat high-carbohydrate fast-food-style breakfast*.[24] High glycemic foods suppress immune function[25,26] and thus promote the perpetuation of infection/dysbiosis. Delivery of a high carbohydrate load to the gastrointestinal lumen promotes bacterial overgrowth[27,28], which is inherently pro-inflammatory[29,30] and which appears to be myalgenic in humans[31] at least in part due to the ability of endotoxin to impair muscle function.[32] Overconsumption of high-carbohydrate low-phytonutrient grains, potatoes, and manufactured foods displaces phytonutrient-dense foods such as fruits, vegetables, nuts, seeds, and berries which contain more than 8,000 phytonutrients, many of which have antioxidant and thus anti-inflammatory actions.[33,34]

[12] "A 38 year old female, with chronic uncontrolled coeliac disease, presented with the rare complication of cutaneous leucocytoclastic vasculitis." Meyers S, Dikman S, Spiera H, Schultz N, Janowitz HD. Cutaneous vasculitis complicating coeliac disease. *Gut.* 1981 Jan;22(1):61-4

[13] "A 51-year-old white man with celiac disease presented with seizures unresponsive to medical therapy." Rush PJ, Inman R, Bernstein M, Carlen P, Resch L. Isolated vasculitis of the central nervous system in a patient with celiac disease. *Am J Med.* 1986 Dec;81(6):1092-4

[14] "Because celiac disease is a potentially treatable cause of cerebral vasculopathy, serology-specifically antitissue transglutaminase antibodies-should be included in the evaluation for cryptogenic stroke in childhood, even in the absence of typical gut symptoms." Goodwin FC, Beattie RM, Millar J, Kirkham FJ.Celiac disease and childhood stroke. *Pediatr Neurol.* 2004 Aug;31(2):139-42

[15] Vasquez A. Reducing Pain and Inflammation Naturally. Part 2: New Insights into Fatty Acid Supplementation and Its Effect on Eicosanoid Production and Genetic Expression. *Nutritional Perspectives* 2005; January: 5-16 www.optimalhealthresearch.com/part2

[16] Evans AR, Junger H, Southall MD, Nicol GD, Sorkin LS, Broome JT, Bailey TW, Vasko MR. Isoprostanes, novel eicosanoids that produce nociception and sensitize rat sensory neurons. *J Pharmacol Exp Ther.* 2000 Jun;293(3):912-20

[17] Lee JY, Sohn KH, Rhee SH, Hwang D. Saturated fatty acids, but not unsaturated fatty acids, induce the expression of cyclooxygenase-2 mediated through Toll-like receptor 4. *J Biol Chem.* 2001 May 18;276(20):16683-9. Epub 2001 Mar 2 http://www.jbc.org/cgi/content/full/276/20/16683

[18] "CONCLUSIONS: Both fat and protein intakes stimulate ROS generation. The increase in ROS generation lasted 3 h after cream intake and 1 h after protein intake. Cream intake also caused a significant and prolonged increase in lipid peroxidation." Mohanty P, Ghanim H, Hamouda W, Aljada A, Garg R, Dandona P. Both lipid and protein intakes stimulate increased generation of reactive oxygen species by polymorphonuclear leukocytes and mononuclear cells. *Am J Clin Nutr.* 2002 Apr;75(4):767-72 http://www.ajcn.org/cgi/content/full/75/4/767

[19] Rusyn I, Bradham CA, Cohn L, Schoonhoven R, Swenberg JA, Brenner DA, Thurman RG. Corn oil rapidly activates nuclear factor-kappaB in hepatic Kupffer cells by oxidant-dependent mechanisms. *Carcinogenesis.* 1999 Nov;20(11):2095-100 http://carcin.oxfordjournals.org/cgi/content/full/20/11/2095

[20] "Exposing endothelial cells to 90 micromol linoleic acid/L for 6 h resulted in a significant increase in lipid hydroperoxides that coincided wih an increase in intracellular calcium concentrations." Hennig B, Toborek M, Joshi-Barve S, Barger SW, Barve S, Mattson MP, McClain CJ. Linoleic acid activates nuclear transcription factor-kappa B (NF-kappa B) and induces NF-kappa B-dependent transcription in cultured endothelial cells. *Am J Clin Nutr.* 1996 Mar;63(3):322-8 http://www.ajcn.org/cgi/reprint/63/3/322

[21] Mohanty P, Hamouda W, Garg R, Aljada A, Ghanim H, Dandona P. Glucose challenge stimulates reactive oxygen species (ROS) generation by leucocytes. *J Clin Endocrinol Metab.* 2000 Aug;85(8):2970-3 http://jcem.endojournals.org/cgi/content/full/85/8/2970 Glucose/carbohydrate and saturated fat consumption appear to be the two biggest offenders in the food-stimulated production of oxidative stress. The effect by protein is much less. "CONCLUSIONS: Both fat and protein intakes stimulate ROS generation. The increase in ROS generation lasted 3 h after cream intake and 1 h after protein intake. Cream intake also caused a significant and prolonged increase in lipid peroxidation." Mohanty P, Ghanim H, Hamouda W, Aljada A, Garg R, Dandona P. Both lipid and protein intakes stimulate increased generation of reactive oxygen species by polymorphonuclear leukocytes and mononuclear cells. *Am J Clin Nutr.* 2002 Apr;75(4):767-72 http://www.ajcn.org/cgi/content/full/75/4/767

[22] Koska J, Blazicek P, Marko M, Grna JD, Kvetnansky R, Vigas M. Insulin, catecholamines, glucose and antioxidant enzymes in oxidative damage during different loads in healthy humans. *Physiol Res.* 2000;49 Suppl 1:S95-100 http://www.biomed.cas.cz/physiolres/pdf/2000/49_S95.pdf

[23] "Conclusion - The present study shows that high GI carbohydrate, but not low GI carbohydrate, mediates an acute proinflammatory process as measured by NF-kappaB activity." Dickinson S, Hancock DP, Petocz P, Brand-Miller JC..High glycemic index carbohydrate mediates an acute proinflammatory process as measured by NF-kappaB activation. *Asia Pac J Clin Nutr.* 2005;14 Suppl:S120

[24] Aljada A, Mohanty P, Ghanim H, Abdo T, Tripathy D, Chaudhuri A, Dandona P. Increase in intranuclear nuclear factor kappaB and decrease in inhibitor kappaB in mononuclear cells after a mixed meal: evidence for a proinflammatory effect. *Am J Clin Nutr.* 2004 Apr;79(4):682-90 http://www.ajcn.org/cgi/content/full/79/4/682

[25] Sanchez A, Reeser JL, Lau HS, et al. Role of sugars in human neutrophilic phagocytosis. *Am J Clin Nutr.* 1973 Nov;26(11):1180-4

[26] "Postoperative infusion of carbohydrate solution leads to moderate fall in the serum concentration of inorganic phosphate. ... The hypophosphatemia was associated with significant reduction of neutrophil phagocytosis, intracellular killing, consumption of oxygen and generation of superoxide during phagocytosis." Rasmussen A, Segel E, Hessov I, Borregaard N. Reduced function of neutrophils during routine postoperative glucose infusion. *Acta Chir Scand.* 1988 Jul-Aug;154(7-8):429-33

[27] Ramakrishnan T, Stokes P. Beneficial effects of fasting and low carbohydrate diet in D-lactic acidosis associated with short-bowel syndrome. *JPEN J Parenter Enteral Nutr.* 1985 May-Jun;9(3):361-3

[28] Gottschall E. *Breaking the Vicious Cycle: Intestinal Health Through Diet.* Kirkton Press; Rev edition (August 1, 1994)

[29] Lin HC. Small intestinal bacterial overgrowth: a framework for understanding irritable bowel syndrome. *JAMA.* 2004 Aug 18;292(7):852-8

[30] Lichtman SN, Wang J, Sartor RB, Zhang C, Bender D, Dalldorf FG, Schwab JH. Reactivation of arthritis induced by small bowel bacterial overgrowth in rats: role of cytokines, bacteria, and bacterial polymers. *Infect Immun.* 1995 Jun;63(6):2295-301

[31] Pimentel M, et al. A link between irritable bowel syndrome and fibromyalgia may be related to findings on lactulose breath testing. *Ann Rheum Dis.* 2004 Apr;63(4):450-2

[32] Bundgaard H, Kjeldsen K, Suarez Krabbe K, van Hall G, Simonsen L, Qvist J, Hansen CM, Moller K, Fonsmark L, Lav Madsen P, Klarlund Pedersen B. Endotoxemia stimulates skeletal muscle Na+-K+-ATPase and raises blood lactate under aerobic conditions in humans. *Am J Physiol Heart Circ Physiol.* 2003 Mar;284(3):H1028-34. Epub 2002 Nov 21 http://ajpheart.physiology.org/cgi/reprint/284/3/H1028

[33] "We propose that the additive and synergistic effects of phytochemicals in fruit and vegetables are responsible for their potent antioxidant and anticancer activities, and that the benefit of a diet rich in fruit and vegetables is attributed to the complex mixture of phytochemicals present in whole foods." Liu RH. Health benefits of fruit and vegetables are from additive and synergistic combinations of phytochemicals. *Am J Clin Nutr.* 2003 Sep;78(3 Suppl):517S-520S

[34] Seaman DR. The diet-induced proinflammatory state: a cause of chronic pain and other degenerative diseases? *J Manipulative Physiol Ther.* 2002;25(3):168-79

- <u>Alcohol/ethanol avoidance</u>: Consumption of alcoholic beverages—even in low doses—increases intestinal permeability and can exacerbate inflammatory disorders, particularly those associated with food allergies, gastrointestinal dysbiosis, and/or overproduction of estrogen.

- <u>Supplemented Paleo-Mediterranean diet</u>: The health-promoting diet of choice for the majority of people is a diet based on abundant consumption of fruits, vegetables, seeds, nuts, omega-3 and monounsaturated fatty acids, and lean sources of protein such as lean meats, fatty cold-water fish, soy and whey proteins. This diet obviates overconsumption of chemical preservatives, artificial sweeteners, and carbohydrate-dominant foods such as candies, pastries, breads, potatoes, grains, and other foods with a high glycemic load and high glycemic index. This "Paleo-Mediterranean Diet" is a combination of the "Paleolithic" or "Paleo diet" and the well-known "Mediterranean diet", both of which are well described in peer-reviewed journals and the lay press. (See Chapter 2 and my other publications[35,36] for details). This diet is the most nutrient-dense diet available, and its benefits are further enhanced by supplementation with vitamins, minerals, probiotics, and the health-promoting fatty acids: ALA, GLA, EPA, DHA.

- <u>Gluten-free vegetarian diet</u>: Vegetarian/vegan diets have a place in the treatment plan of all patients with autoimmune/inflammatory disorders[37,38]; this is also true for patients for whom long-term exclusive reliance on a meat-free vegetarian diet is either not appropriate or not appealing. No legitimate scientist or literate clinician doubts the antirheumatic power and anti-inflammatory advantages of vegetarian diets, whether used short-term or long term.[39] The benefits of gluten-free vegetarian diets are well documented, and the mechanisms of action are well elucidated, including reduced intake of proinflammatory linoleic[40] and arachidonic acids[41], iron[42], common food antigens[43], gluten[44] and gliadin[45,46], proinflammatory sugars[47] and increased intake of omega-3 fatty acids and micronutrients[48], and anti-inflammatory and anti-oxidant phytonutrients[49]; vegetarian diets also effect profound changes—both *qualitative* and *quantitative*—in intestinal flora[50,51] that correlate with clinical improvement.[52] Patients who rely on the Paleo-Mediterranean Diet can use vegetarian meals, on a daily basis or for days at a time, for example, by having a daily vegetarian meal, or one week per month of vegetarianism. Of course, some (not all) patients can use a purely vegetarian diet long-term provided that nutritional needs (especially protein and cobalamin) are consistently met.

- <u>Short-term fasting</u>: Whether the foundational diet is Paleo-Mediterranean, vegetarian, vegan, or a combination of all of these, autoimmune/inflammatory patients will still benefit from periodic fasting, whether on a weekly (e.g., every Saturday), monthly (every first week or weekend of the month, or every other month), or yearly (1-2 weeks of the year) basis. Since consumption of

[35] Vasquez A. A Five-Part Nutritional Protocol that Produces Consistently Positive Results. *Nutritional Wellness* 2005 September Available in the printed version and on-line at http://www.nutritionalwellness.com/archives/2005/sep/09_vasquez.php and http://optimalhealthresearch.com/protocol

[36] Vasquez A. Implementing the Five-Part Nutritional Wellness Protocol for the Treatment of Various Health Problems. *Nutritional Wellness* 2005 November. Available on-line at http://www.nutritionalwellness.com/archives/2005/nov/11_vasquez.php and http://optimalhealthresearch.com/protocol

[37] "After four weeks at the health farm the diet group showed a significant improvement in number of tender joints, Ritchie's articular index, number of swollen joints, pain score, duration of morning stiffness, grip strength, erythrocyte sedimentation rate, white blood cell count, and a health assessment questionnaire score." Kjeldsen-Kragh J, Haugen M, Borchgrevink CF, Laerum E, Eek M, Mowinkel P, Hovi K, Forre O. Controlled trial of fasting and one-year vegetarian diet in rheumatoid arthritis. Lancet. 1991 Oct 12;338(8772):899-902

[38] "During the vegan diet, both signs and symptoms returned in most patients, with the exception of some patients with psoriasis who experienced an improvement." Lithell H, Bruce A, Gustafsson IB, Hoglund NJ, Karlstrom B, Ljunghall K, Sjolin K, Venge P, Vessby B. A fasting and vegetarian diet treatment trial on chronic inflammatory disorders. Acta Derm Venereol. 1983;63(5):397-403

[39] "For the patients who were randomised to the vegetarian diet there was a significant decrease in platelet count, leukocyte count, calprotectin, total IgG, IgM rheumatoid factor (RF), C3-activation products, and the complement components C3 and C4 after one month of treatment." Kjeldsen-Kragh J, Mellbye OJ, Haugen M, Mollnes TE, Hammer HB, Sioud M, Forre O. Changes in laboratory variables in rheumatoid arthritis patients during a trial of fasting and one-year vegetarian diet. Scand J Rheumatol. 1995;24(2):85-93

[40] Rusyn I, Bradham CA, Cohn L, Schoonhoven R, Swenberg JA, Brenner DA, Thurman RG. Corn oil rapidly activates nuclear factor-kappaB in hepatic Kupffer cells by oxidant-dependent mechanisms. Carcinogenesis. 1999 Nov;20(11):2095-100 http://carcin.oxfordjournals.org/cgi/content/full/20/11/2095

[41] Vasquez A. Reducing Pain and Inflammation Naturally. Part 2: New Insights into Fatty Acid Supplementation and Its Effect on Eicosanoid Production and Genetic Expression. *Nutritional Perspectives* 2005; January: 5-16 http://optimalhealthresearch.com/part2

[42] Dabbagh AJ, Trenam CW, Morris CJ, Blake DR. Iron in joint inflammation. Ann Rheum Dis. 1993 Jan;52(1):67-73

[43] Hafstrom I, Ringertz B, Spangberg A, von Zweigbergk L, Brannemark S, Nylander I, Ronnelid J, Laasonen L, Klareskog L. A vegan diet free of gluten improves the signs and symptoms of rheumatoid arthritis: the effects on arthritis correlate with a reduction in antibodies to food antigens. Rheumatology (Oxford). 2001 Oct;40(10):1175-9 http://rheumatology.oxfordjournals.org/cgi/reprint/40/10/1175

[44] "The data provide evidence that dietary modification may be of clinical benefit for certain RA patients, and that this benefit may be related to a reduction in immunoreactivity to food antigens eliminated by the change in diet." Hafstrom I, Ringertz B, Spangberg A, von Zweigbergk L, Brannemark S, Nylander I, Ronnelid J, Laasonen L, Klareskog L. A vegan diet free of gluten improves the signs and symptoms of rheumatoid arthritis: the effects on arthritis correlate with a reduction in antibodies to food antigens. Rheumatology (Oxford). 2001 Oct;40(10):1175-9

[45] "Despite the increased AGA [antigliadin antibodies] positivity found distinctively in patients with recent-onset RA, none of the RA patients showed clear evidence of coeliac disease." Paimela L, Kurki P, Leirisalo-Repo M, Piirainen H. Gliadin immune reactivity in patients with rheumatoid arthritis. Clin Exp Rheumatol. 1989 Nov-Dec;7(6):623-6

[46] "The median IgA antigliadin ELISA index was 7.1 (range 2.1-22.4) for the RA group and 3.1 (range 0.3-34.9) for the controls (p = 0.0001)." Koot VC, Van Straaten M, Hekkens WT, Collee G, Dijkmans BA. Elevated level of IgA gliadin antibodies in patients with rheumatoid arthritis. Clin Exp Rheumatol. 1989 Nov-Dec;7(6):623-6

[47] Seaman DR. The diet-induced proinflammatory state: a cause of chronic pain and other degenerative diseases? J Manipulative Physiol Ther. 2002 Mar-Apr;25(3):168-79

[48] Hagfors L, Nilsson I, Skoldstam L, Johansson G. Fat intake and composition of fatty acids in serum phospholipids in a randomized, controlled, Mediterranean dietary intervention study on patients with rheumatoid arthritis. Nutr Metab (Lond). 2005 Oct 10;2:26 http://www.nutritionandmetabolism.com/content/2/1/26

[49] Liu RH. Health benefits of fruit and vegetables are from additive and synergistic combinations of phytochemicals. Am J Clin Nutr 2003;78(3 Suppl):517S-520S http://www.ajcn.org/cgi/content/full/78/3/517S

[50] "Significant alteration in the intestinal flora was observed when the patients changed from omnivorous to vegan diet. ... This finding of an association between intestinal flora and disease activity may have implications for our understanding of how diet can affect RA." Peltonen R, Kjeldsen-Kragh J, Haugen M, Tuominen J, Toivanen P, Forre O, Eerola E. Changes of faecal flora in rheumatoid arthritis during fasting and one-year vegetarian diet. Br J Rheumatol. 1994 Jul;33(7):638-43

[51] Toivanen P, Eerola E. A vegan diet changes the intestinal flora. Rheumatology (Oxford). 2002 Aug;41(8):950-1 http://rheumatology.oxfordjournals.org/cgi/reprint/41/8/950

[52] "We conclude that a vegan diet changes the faecal microbial flora in RA patients, and changes in the faecal flora are associated with improvement in RA activity." Peltonen R, Nenonen M, Helve T, Hanninen O, Toivanen P, Eerola E. Faecal microbial flora and disease activity in rheumatoid arthritis during a vegan diet. Br J Rheumatol. 1997 Jan;36(1):64-8 http://rheumatology.oxfordjournals.org/cgi/reprint/36/1/64

food—particularly unhealthy foods—induces an inflammatory effect[53], abstinence from food provides a relative anti-oxidative and anti-inflammatory benefit[54] with many of the antioxidant benefits beginning within 24 hours of the initiation of the fast.[55] Fasting indeed provides a distinct anti-inflammatory benefit and may help "re-calibrate" metabolic and homeostatic mechanisms by breaking self-perpetuating "vicious cycles"[56] that autonomously promote inflammation independent from proinflammatory stimuli. Of course, water-only fasting is completely hypoallergenic (assuming that the patient is not sensitive to chlorine, fluoride, or other contaminants), and subsequent re-introduction of foods provides the ideal opportunity to identify offending foods. Fasting deprives intestinal microbes of substrate[57], stimulates intestinal B-cell immunity[58], improves the bactericidal action of neutrophils[59], reduces lysozyme release and leukotriene formation[60], and ameliorates intestinal hyperpermeability.[61] In case reports and clinical trials, short-term fasting (or protein-sparing fasting) has been documented as safe and effective treatment for SLE[62], RA[63], and non-rheumatic diseases such as chronic severe hypertension[64], moderate hypertension[65], obesity[66,67], type-2 diabetes[68], and epilepsy.[69]

- <u>Broad-spectrum fatty acid therapy with ALA, EPA, DHA, GLA and oleic acid</u>: **Fish oil provides EPA and DHA which have well-proven anti-inflammatory benefits when used in the treatment of various autoimmune and cardiovascular disorders.** Fatty acid supplementation should be delivered in the form of combination therapy with ALA, GLA, DHA, and EPA. Given at doses of 3,000 – 9,000 mg per day, ALA from flax oil has impressive anti-inflammatory benefits demonstrated by its ability to halve prostaglandin production in humans.[70] Numerous studies have demonstrated the benefit of GLA in the treatment of rheumatoid arthritis when used at doses between 500 mg – 4,000 mg per day.[71,72] Fish oil provides EPA and DHA which have well-proven anti-inflammatory benefits in RA[73,74,75] and SLE.[76,77] ALA, EPA, DHA, and GLA need to be provided in the form of supplements; when using high doses of therapeutic oils, liquid

---

[53] Aljada A, Mohanty P, Ghanim H, Abdo T, Tripathy D, Chaudhuri A, Dandona P. Increase in intranuclear nuclear factor kappaB and decrease in inhibitor kappaB in mononuclear cells after a mixed meal: evidence for a proinflammatory effect. *Am J Clin Nutr.* 2004 Apr;79(4):682-90 http://www.ajcn.org/cgi/content/full/79/4/682

[54] "This is the first demonstration of ...a decrease in reactive oxygen species generation by leukocytes and oxidative damage to lipids, proteins, and amino acids after dietary restriction and weight loss in the obese over a short period." Dandona P, Mohanty P, Ghanim H, Aljada A, Browne R, Hamouda W, Prabhala A, Afzal A, Garg R. The suppressive effect of dietary restriction and weight loss in the obese on the generation of reactive oxygen species by leukocytes, lipid peroxidation, and protein carbonylation. *J Clin Endocrinol Metab.* 2001 Jan;86(1):355-62 http://jcem.endojournals.org/cgi/content/full/86/1/355

[55] "Thus, a 48h fast may reduce ROS generation, total oxidative load and oxidative damage to amino acids." Dandona P, Mohanty P, Hamouda W, Ghanim H, Aljada A, Garg R, Kumar V. Inhibitory effect of a two day fast on reactive oxygen species (ROS) generation by leucocytes and plasma ortho-tyrosine and meta-tyrosine concentrations. *J Clin Endocrinol Metab.* 2001 Jun;86(6):2899-902 http://jcem.endojournals.org/cgi/content/abstract/86/6/2899

[56] "The ability of therapeutic fasts to break metabolic vicious cycles may also contribute to the efficacy of fasting in the treatment of type 2 diabetes and autoimmune disorders." McCarty MF. A preliminary fast may potentiate response to a subsequent low-salt, low-fat vegan diet in the management of hypertension - fasting as a strategy for breaking metabolic vicious cycles. *Med Hypotheses.* 2003 May;60(5):624-33

[57] Ramakrishnan T, Stokes P. Beneficial effects of fasting and low carbohydrate diet in D-lactic acidosis associated with short-bowel syndrome. *JPEN J Parenter Enteral Nutr.* 1985 May-Jun;9(3):361-3

[58] Trollmo C, Verdrengh M, Tarkowski A. Fasting enhances mucosal antigen specific B cell responses in rheumatoid arthritis. *Ann Rheum Dis.* 1997 Feb;56(2):130-4 http://ard.bmjjournals.com/cgi/content/full/56/2/130

[59] "An association was found between improvement in inflammatory activity of the joints and enhancement of neutrophil bactericidal capacity. Fasting appears to improve the clinical status of patients with RA." Uden AM, Trang L, Venizelos N, Palmblad J. Neutrophil functions and clinical performance after total fasting in patients with rheumatoid arthritis. *Ann Rheum Dis.* 1983 Feb;42(1):45-51

[60] "We thus conclude that a reduced ability to generate cytotaxins, reduced release of enzyme, and reduced leukotriene formation from RA neutrophils, together with an altered fatty acid composition of membrane phospholipids, may be mechanisms for the decrease of inflammatory symptoms that results from fasting." Hafstrom I, Ringertz B, Gyllenhammar H, Palmblad J, Harms-Ringdahl M. Effects of fasting on disease activity, neutrophil function, fatty acid composition, and leukotriene biosynthesis in patients with rheumatoid arthritis. *Arthritis Rheum.* 1988 May;31(5):585-92

[61] "The results indicate that, unlike lactovegetarian diet, fasting may ameliorate the disease activity and reduce both the intestinal and the non-intestinal permeability in rheumatoid arthritis." Sundqvist T, Lindstrom F, Magnusson KE, Skoldstam L, Stjernstrom I, Tagesson C. Influence of fasting on intestinal permeability and disease activity in patients with rheumatoid arthritis. *Scand J Rheumatol.* 1982;11(1):33-8

[62] Fuhrman J, Sarter B, Calabro DJ. Brief case reports of medically supervised, water-only fasting associated with remission of autoimmune disease. *Altern Ther Health Med.* 2002 Jul-Aug;8(4):112, 110-1

[63] "An association was found between improvement in inflammatory activity of the joints and enhancement of neutrophil bactericidal capacity. Fasting appears to improve the clinical status of patients with RA." Uden AM, Trang L, Venizelos N, Palmblad J. Neutrophil functions and clinical performance after total fasting in patients with rheumatoid arthritis. *Ann Rheum Dis.* 1983 Feb;42(1):45-51

[64] "The average reduction in blood pressure was 37/13 mm Hg, with the greatest decrease being observed for subjects with the most severe hypertension. Patients with stage 3 hypertension (those with systolic blood pressure greater than 180 mg Hg, diastolic blood pressure greater than 110 mg Hg, or both) had an average reduction of 60/17 mm Hg at the conclusion of treatment." Goldhamer A, Lisle D, Parpia B, Anderson SV, Campbell TC. Medically supervised water-only fasting in the treatment of hypertension. *J Manipulative Physiol Ther.* 2001 Jun;24(5):335-9 http://www.healthpromoting.com/335-339Goldhamer115263.QXD.pdf

[65] "RESULTS: Approximately 82% of the subjects achieved BP at or below 120/80 mm Hg by the end of the treatment program. The mean BP reduction was 20/7 mm Hg, with the greatest decrease being observed for subjects with the highest baseline BP." Goldhamer AC, Lisle DJ, Sultana P, Anderson SV, Parpia B, Hughes B, Campbell TC. Medically supervised water-only fasting in the treatment of borderline hypertension. *J Altern Complement Med.* 2002 Oct;8(5):643-50 http://www.healthpromoting.com/Articles/articles/study%202/acmpaper5.pdf

[66] Vertes V, Genuth SM, Hazelton IM. Supplemented fasting as a large-scale outpatient program. *JAMA.* 1977 Nov 14;238(20):2151-3

[67] Bauman WA, Schwartz E, Rose HG, Eisenstein HN, Johnson DW. Early and long-term effects of acute caloric deprivation in obese diabetic patients. *Am J Med.* 1988 Jul;85(1):38-46

[68] Goldhamer AC. Initial cost of care results in medically supervised water-only fasting for treating high blood pressure and diabetes. *J Altern Complement Med.* 2002 Dec;8(6):696-7 http://www.healthpromoting.com/Articles/pdf/Study%2032.pdf

[69] "The ketogenic diet should be considered as alternative therapy for children with difficult-to-control seizures. It is more effective than many of the new anticonvulsant medications and is well tolerated by children and families when it is effective." Freeman JM, Vining EP, Pillas DJ, Pyzik PL, Casey JC, Kelly LM. The efficacy of the ketogenic diet-1998: a prospective evaluation of intervention in 150 children. *Pediatrics.* 1998 Dec;102(6):1358-63 http://pediatrics.aappublications.org/cgi/reprint/102/6/1358

[70] Adam O, Wolfram G, Zollner N. Effect of alpha-linolenic acid in the human diet on linoleic acid metabolism and prostaglandin biosynthesis. *J Lipid Res.* 1986 Apr;27(4):421-6 http://www.jlr.org/cgi/reprint/27/4/421

[71] "Other results showed a significant reduction in morning stiffness with gamma-linolenic acid at 3 months and reduction in pain and articular index at 6 months with olive oil." Brzeski M, Madhok R, Capell HA. Evening primrose oil in patients with rheumatoid arthritis and side-effects of non-steroidal anti-inflammatory drugs. *Br J Rheumatol.* 1991 Oct;30(5):370-2

[72] Rothman D, DeLuca P, Zurier RB. Botanical lipids: effects on inflammation, immune responses, and rheumatoid arthritis. *Semin Arthritis Rheum.* 1995 Oct;25(2):87-96

[73] Adam O, Beringer C, Kless T, Lemmen C, Adam A, Wiseman M, Adam P, Klimmek R, Forth W. Anti-inflammatory effects of a low arachidonic acid diet and fish oil in patients with rheumatoid arthritis. *Rheumatol Int.* 2003 Jan;23(1):27-36

[74] Lau CS, Morley KD, Belch JJ. Effects of fish oil supplementation on non-steroidal anti-inflammatory drug requirement in patients with mild rheumatoid arthritis--a double-blind placebo controlled study. *Br J Rheumatol.* 1993 Nov;32(11):982-9

[75] Kremer JM, Jubiz W, Michalek A, Rynes RI, Bartholomew LE, Bigaouette J, Timchalk M, Beeler D, Lininger L. Fish-oil fatty acid supplementation in active rheumatoid arthritis. A double-blinded, controlled, crossover study. *Ann Intern Med.* 1987 Apr;106(4):497-503

[76] Walton AJ, Snaith ML, Locniskar M, Cumberland AG, Morrow WJ, Isenberg DA. Dietary fish oil and the severity of symptoms in patients with systemic lupus erythematosus. *Ann Rheum Dis.* 1991 Jul;50(7):463-6

[77] Duffy EM, Meenagh GK, McMillan SA, Strain JJ, Hannigan BM, Bell AL. The clinical effect of dietary supplementation with omega-3 fish oils and/or copper in systemic lupus erythematosus. *J Rheumatol.* 2004 Aug;31(8):1551-6

supplements that can be mixed in juice or a smoothie are generally more convenient and palatable than capsules. Therapeutic amounts of oleic acid can be obtained from generous use of olive oil, preferably on fresh vegetables. Supplementation with polyunsaturated fatty acids warrants increased intake of antioxidants from diet, fruit and vegetable juices, and properly formulated supplements; since patients with systemic inflammation are generally in a pro-oxidative state, consideration must be given to the timing and starting dose of fatty acid supplementation and the need for anti-oxidant protection. See chapter on Therapeutics for more details and biochemical pathways. Clinicians must realize that fatty acids are not clinically or biochemically interchangeable and that one fatty acid does not substitute for another; each of the fatty acids must be supplied in order for its benefits to be obtained.[78]

- **Vitamin D3 supplementation with physiologic doses and/or tailored to serum 25(OH)D levels:** Vitamin D deficiency is common in the general population and is even more common in patients with chronic illness and chronic musculoskeletal pain.[79] Correction of vitamin D deficiency supports normal immune function against infection and provides a clinically significant anti-inflammatory[80] and analgesic benefit in patients with back pain[81] and limb pain.[82] Reasonable daily doses for children and adults are 2,000 and 4,000 IU, respectively, as defined by Vasquez, et al.[83] Deficiency and response to treatment are monitored with serum 25(OH)vitamin D while safety is monitored with serum calcium; inflammatory granulomatous diseases and certain drugs such as hydrochlorothiazide greatly increase the propensity for hypercalcemia and warrant increment dosing and frequent monitoring of serum calcium.

- **Assessment and treatment for dysbiosis:** **Dysbiotic loci should be investigated as discussed previously in Chapter 4.** Each cause—each contributor to disease—may in itself be "clinically insignificant" but when numerous "insignificant" additive and synergistic influences coalesce, we find ourselves confronted with an "idiopathic disease." We must then decide between the only two available options: 1) despair in the failure of our "one cause, one disease, one drug" paradigm, or 2) appreciate that numerous influences work together to disrupt physiologic function and produce the biologic dysfunction that we experience as disease.

- **Orthoendocrinology:** Assess melatonin, prolactin, cortisol, DHEA, free and total testosterone, serum estradiol, and thyroid status (e.g., TSH, T4, *and* anti-thyroid peroxidase antibodies). Treat accordingly as discussed in Chapter 4.

- **Oral enzyme therapy with proteolytic/pancreatic enzymes:** Polyenzyme supplementation is used to ameliorate the pathophysiology induced by immune complexes, such as rheumatoid arthritis.[84]

- **CoQ10 (antihypertensive, renoprotective, and probably immunomodulatory):** CoQ10 is a powerful antioxidant with a wide margin of safety and excellent clinical tolerability. **At least four studies have documented its powerful blood-pressure-lowering ability, which often surpasses the clinical effectiveness of antihypertensive drugs.[85,86,87,88] Furthermore, at least two published papers[89,90] and one case report[91] advocate that CoQ10 has powerful renoprotective benefits.** CoQ10 levels are low in patients with allergies[92], and the symptomatic relief that many allergic patients experience following supplementation with CoQ10 suggests that CoQ10 has an immunomodulatory effect. Common doses start at > 100 mg per day with food; doses of 200 mg per day are not uncommon, and doses up to 1,000 mg per day are clinically well tolerated though the high financial toll resembles that of many pharmaceutical drugs.

[78] Vasquez A. Reducing Pain and Inflammation Naturally. Part 2: New Insights into Fatty Acid Supplementation and Its Effect on Eicosanoid Production and Genetic Expression. *Nutritional Perspectives* 2005; January: 5-16 http://optimalhealthresearch.com/part2
[79] Plotnikoff GA, Quigley JM. Prevalence of severe hypovitaminosis D in patients with persistent, nonspecific musculoskeletal pain. *Mayo Clin Proc.* 2003 Dec;78(12):1463-70
[80] Timms PM, Mannan N, Hitman GA, Noonan K, Mills PG, Syndercombe-Court D, Aganna E, Price CP, Boucher BJ. Circulating MMP9, vitamin D and variation in the TIMP-1 response with VDR genotype: mechanisms for inflammatory damage in chronic disorders? *QJM.* 2002 Dec;95(12):787-96 http://qjmed.oxfordjournals.org/cgi/content/full/95/12/787
[81] Al Faraj S, Al Mutairi K. Vitamin D deficiency and chronic low back pain in Saudi Arabia. *Spine.* 2003 Jan 15;28(2):177-9
[82] Masood H, Narang AP, Bhat IA, Shah GN. Persistent limb pain and raised serum alkaline phosphatase the earliest markers of subclinical hypovitaminosis D in Kashmir. *Indian J Physiol Pharmacol.* 1989 Oct-Dec;33(4):259-61
[83] Vasquez A, Manso G, Cannell J. The clinical importance of vitamin D (cholecalciferol): a paradigm shift with implications for all healthcare providers. *Altern Ther Health Med.* 2004 Sep-Oct;10(5):28-36 http://optimalhealthresearch.com/monograph04
[84] Galebskaya LV, Ryumina EV, Niemerovsky VS, Matyukov AA. Human complement system state after wobenzyme intake. *VESTNIK MOSKOVSKOGO UNIVERSITETA. KHIMIYA.* 2000. Vol. 41, No. 6. Supplement. 148-149
[85] Burke BE, Neuenschwander R, Olson RD. Randomized, double-blind, placebo-controlled trial of coenzyme Q10 in isolated systolic hypertension. *South Med J.* 2001 Nov;94(11):1112-7
[86] Singh RB, Niaz MA, Rastogi SS, Shukla PK, Thakur AS. Effect of hydrosoluble coenzyme Q10 on blood pressures and insulin resistance in hypertensive patients with coronary artery disease. *J Hum Hypertens.* 1999 Mar;13(3):203-8
[87] Digiesi V, Cantini F, Oradei A, Bisi G, Guarino GC, Brocchi A, Bellandi F, Mancini M, Littarru GP. Coenzyme Q10 in essential hypertension. *Mol Aspects Med.* 1994;15 Suppl:s257-63
[88] Langsjoen P, Langsjoen P, Willis R, Folkers K. Treatment of essential hypertension with coenzyme Q10. *Mol Aspects Med.* 1994;15 Suppl:S265-72
[89] Singh RB, Khanna HK, Niaz MA. Randomized, double-blind placebo-controlled trial of coenzyme Q10 in chronic renal failure: discovery of a new role. *J Nutr Environ Med* 2000;10:281-8
[90] Singh RB, Kumar A, Niaz MA, Singh RG, Gujrati S, Singh VP, Singh M, Singh UP, Taneja C, AND Rastogi SS. Randomized, Double-blind, Placebo-controlled Trial of Coenzyme Q10 in Patients with End-stage Renal Failure. *J Nutr Environ Med* 2003; Volume 13, Number 1: 13–22
[91] Singh RB, Singh MM. Effects of CoQ10 in new indications with antioxidant vitamin deficiency. *J Nutr Environ Med* 1999; 9:223-228
[92] Ye CQ, Folkers K, Tamagawa H, Pfeiffer C. A modified determination of coenzyme Q10 in human blood and CoQ10 blood levels in diverse patients with allergies. *Biofactors.* 1988 Dec;1(4):303-6

Behcet's Disease
Behcet's Syndrome

<u>Description/pathophysiology</u>:
- **A relapsing systemic/multiorgan autoimmune disease associated with vasculopathy and ulcerations of the oral and genital mucosa**
- Idiopathic[1]; etiopathogenic associations include:
    - Occult **bacterial**/viral/fungal/parasitic infections with resultant molecular mimicry and stimulation of autoreactive T-cells[2]: as summarized by Verity et al[3], "…the evidence indicates that **the underlying immune events in BD are triggered by a microbial antigen** and subsequently driven by genetic influences which control leukocyte behavior and the coagulation pathways."
    - Associated with HLA-B51 in Japan and Mediterranean areas
- Considered **uncommon in the US**

<u>Clinical presentations</u>:
- Two-fold more common in men than in women
- Age of onset is generally in 20's and 30's; may occur in children
- <u>**Painful oral and genital ulcers:**</u> **resembles recurrent aphthous stomatitis, most commonly the first manifestation of the disease**
- <u>**Ocular complaints:**</u> **pain, photophobia, blurred vision, iridocyclitis**
- <u>**Skin lesions in 80% of patients:**</u> **papules, pustules, vesicles, folliculitis, erythema nodosum-like lesions, "exaggerated" inflammatory reactions to minor skin trauma**
- Joint pain: nondestructive arthritis in 50% of patients
- **Vasculitis** and thrombophlebitis: can affect any organ
- Neurocognitive disturbances and central nervous system involvement
- Abdominal pain and intestinal involvement: some patients have evidence of enteropathy

<u>Major differential diagnoses</u>:
- Crohn's disease
- Acrodermatitis enteropathica (and related zinc deficiency)
- Aphthous stomatitis (DDX: oral herpes)
- Reactive arthritis
- Infection
- AS
- SLE
- Wegener's granulomatosis

<u>Clinical assessments</u>:
- <u>**History/subjective**</u>:
    - See clinical presentations
- <u>**Physical examination/objective**</u>:
    - Oral, ocular, and genital examinations
    - Other examinations as indicated

[1] Beers MH, Berkow R (eds). <u>The Merck Manual. Seventeenth Edition</u>. Whitehouse Station; Merck Research Laboratories 1999 Page 424
[2] Sakane T, Suzuki N, Nagafuchi H. Etiopathology of Behcet's disease: immunological aspects. *Yonsei Med J.* 1997 Dec;38(6):350-8 http://www.eymj.org/1997/pdf/12350.pdf
[3] Verity DH, Wallace GR, Vaughan RW, Stanford MR. Behcet's disease: from Hippocrates to the third millennium. *Br J Ophthalmol.* 2003 Sep;87(9):1175-83 http://bjo.bmjjournals.com/cgi/reprint/87/9/1175

- **Laboratory assessments**:
  - ESR: high
  - CBC: mild leukocytosis
  - HLA-B51: may or may not be positive, but is consistently associated with increased likelihood of the disease
  - Homocysteine: Patients with Behcet's syndrome have elevated homocysteine which exacerbates arterial and venous occlusion which underlies many of the clinical complications of the disease.[4,5]
  - Lactulose/mannitol assay: Patients with Behcet's disease have increased intestinal permeability.[6] Whether this is due in an individual patient to gastrointestinal dysbiosis or is simply a gastrointestinal reflection of systemic inflammation should be determined on a per-patient basis. Dysbiosis is so common in patients with the combination of 1) autoimmunity and 2) "leaky gut" that such patients should be presumed to have dysbiosis until proven otherwise by comprehensive parasitology assessment by a specialty laboratory.
  - Oxidant/antioxidant assessment: Numerous studies have documented increased oxidative stress and decrease antioxidant defenses in patients with Behcet's disease.[7] Vitamin C deficiency has been documented.[8] Broad-spectrum antioxidant therapy with diet and supplements is indicated.
  - Assessment for occult infections and dysbiosis: Research suggests the probability that Behcet's disease is stimulated by occult bacterial/viral/fungal/parasitic infections with resultant molecular mimicry and stimulation of autoreactive T-cells.[9] **Bacteria that have been most consistently associated with this disease are *Streptococcus sanguis*, *Escherichia coli*, *Staphylococcus aureus*[10], and *Chlamydia pneumoniae*,** as discussed in the Treatment section that follows. **The fact that antimicrobial/penicillin administration reduces the severity and frequency of the disease clearly indicates that the disease is perpetuated at least in part by an occult infection.**[11] Additional support for a microbial contribution to the pathogenesis of this disease comes from studies showing **exacerbations of the disease following exposure to streptococcal antigens**.[12] There is no consistent evidence of *B. burgdorferi*[13] (Lyme disease), varicella zoster[14], or viral hepatitis[15] in most patients with Behcet's.
  - Detoxification for xenobiotic accumulation: Impairment in acetylation has been demonstrated[16] and may contribute to the pathogenesis of Behcet's disease by leading to the accumulation of xenobiotics or the haptenization of endogenous antigens by reactive intermediates. Assessment of detoxification with caffeine-benzoate-aspirin-

[4] "CONCLUSION: Homocysteine may play a role in ocular involvement of BD. Chronic inflammation can induce hyperhomocysteinemia, thereby leading to thrombosis in the retinal vascular bed in a way similar to that recently proposed for the pathogenesis of coronary artery disease." Okka M, Ozturk M, Kockar MC, Bavbek N, Rasier Y, Gunduz K. Plasma homocysteine level and uveitis in Behcet's disease. *Isr Med Assoc J*. 2002 Nov;4(11 Suppl):931-4

[5] "CONCLUSION: Hyperhomocysteinaemia may be assumed to be an independent risk factor for venous thrombosis in BD. Unlike the factor V Leiden mutation, hyperhomocysteinaemia is a correctable risk factor. This finding might lead to new avenues in the prophylaxis of thrombosis in BD." Aksu K, Turgan N, Oksel F, Keser G, Ozmen D, Kitapcioglu G, Gumusdis G, Bayindir O, Doganavsargil E. Hyperhomocysteinaemia in Behcet's disease. *Rheumatology* (Oxford). 2001 Jun;40(6):687-90 http://rheumatology.oxfordjournals.org/cgi/reprint/40/6/687

[6] "The intestinal permeability in BS was significantly more than that seen among the healthy controls." Fresko I, Hamuryudan V, Demir M, Hizli N, Sayman H, Melikoglu M, Tunc R, Yurdakul S, Yazici H. Intestinal permeability in Behcet's syndrome. *Ann Rheum Dis*. 2001 Jan;60(1):65-6 http://ard.bmjjournals.com/cgi/reprint/60/1/65

[7] Kose K, Yazici C, Cambay N, Ascioglu O, Dogan P. Lipid peroxidation and erythrocyte antioxidant enzymes in patients with Behcet's disease. *Tohoku J Exp Med*. 2002 May;197(1):9-16 http://www.jstage.jst.go.jp/article/tjem/197/1/9/_pdf

[8] Noyan T, Sahin I, Sekeroglu MR, Dulger H. The serum vitamin C levels in Behcet's disease. *Yonsei Med J*. 2003 Oct 30;44(5):771-4 http://www.eymj.org/2003/pdf/10771.pdf

[9] Sakane T, Suzuki N, Nagafuchi H. Etiopathology of Behcet's disease: immunological aspects. *Yonsei Med J*. 1997 Dec;38(6):350-8 http://www.eymj.org/1997/pdf/12350.pdf

[10] Direskeneli H. Behcet's disease: infectious aetiology, new autoantigens, and HLA-B51. *Ann Rheum Dis*. 2001 Nov;60(11):996-1002 http://ard.bmjjournals.com/cgi/reprint/60/11/996

[11] "CONCLUSION: Penicillin treatment was demonstrated to offer adjunctive benefits in the prevention of arthritis episodes which are not obtainable with colchicine monotherapy. This finding could provide additional evidence for antigen triggering in the pathogenesis of Behcet's disease." Calguneri M, Kiraz S, Ertenli I, Benekli M, Karaarslan Y, Celik I. The effect of prophylactic penicillin treatment on the course of arthritis episodes in patients with Behcet's disease. A randomized clinical trial. *Arthritis Rheum*. 1996 Dec;39(12):2062-5

[12] "Interestingly, the induction of systemic Behcet's disease symptoms was observed after the streptococcus skin test in 15 of 85 cases tested, but no case of induction by the other bacteria was observed. Our study supports the possible pathogenetic role of certain streptococcal antigens in Behcet's disease." [No authors listed] Skin hypersensitivity to streptococcal antigens and the induction of systemic symptoms by the antigens in Behcet's disease--a multicenter study. The Behcet's Disease Research Committee of Japan. *J Rheumatol*. 1989 Apr;16(4):506-11

[13] "CONCLUSION: These results suggest no association between Behcet's disease and B. burgdorferi infection." Onen F, Tuncer D, Akar S, Birlik M, Akkoc N. Seroprevalence of Borrelia burgdorferi in patients with Behcet's disease. *Rheumatol Int*. 2003 Nov;23(6):289-9

[14] "The serological positivity for VZV IgG and IgM antibodies in BD was not statistically different from other skin diseases." Akdeniz S, Harman M, Atmaca S, Akpolat N. The seroprevalence of varicella zoster antibodies in Behcet's and other skin diseases. *Eur J Epidemiol*. 2003;18(1):91-3

[15] "HGV-RNA was detected in two patients with BD and in none of the healthy controls. In conclusion, BD does not seem to be associated with hepatitis viral infections including hepatitis B, C, or G." Ozkan S, Toklu T, Ilknur T, Abacioglu H, Soyal MC, Gunes AT. Is there any association between hepatitis G virus (HGV), other hepatitis viruses (HBV, HCV) and Behcet's disease? *J Dermatol*. 2005 May;32(5):361-4

[16] "As a result of this study we conclude the NAT2 slow acetylator status may be a determinant in susceptibility to Behcet's disease. This finding may have implications for the theories of the pathogenesis of the disease as well as for therapeutic aspects." Tamer L, Tursen U, Eskandari G, Ates NA, Ercan B, Yildirim H, Atik U. N-acetyltransferase 2 polymorphisms in patients with Behcet's disease. *Clin Exp Dermatol*. 2005 Jan;30(1):56-60

acetaminophen challenge may provide therapeutic insight when working with individual patients, particularly those with a history of xenobiotic exposure and/or multiple chemical sensitivity.

- **Imaging**:
  - o Only for monitoring complications and excluding other diseases
- **Establishing the diagnosis**: Clinical assessment based on published criteria[17]

> **1) Recurrent oral/genital mucosal lesions: at least 3 times in one 12-month period**
> *Plus two of the following*:
> - ☐ **Eye lesions: Anterior uveitis, posterior uveitis, or retinal vasculitis**
> - ☐ **Skin lesions: Erythema nodosum, pseudofolliculitis, papulopustular lesions, or acneiform nodules**
> - ☐ **Positive pathergy test: Exaggerated inflammatory skin response 24–48 hours following otherwise benign injury/trauma to the skin**

Diagnosis is additionally supported by:
- ▪ Elevated ESR
- ▪ Systemic/multiorgan relapsing disease, and associated clinical presentations and findings
- ▪ Exclusion of other diseases: this is "relative" rather than "absolute" due to the nonspecific nature of Behcet's disease

Complications:

- **Blindness: patients with ocular involvement are at risk for blindness—urgent/emergency referral/immunosuppression may be necessary**
- Paralysis
- Vena cava obstruction

Clinical management:

- Referral if clinical outcome is unsatisfactory or if serious complications are evident.
- *Medical approach*: "The syndrome is generally chronic and manageable... Symptomatic treatment is relatively successful." [18]

Treatments:

Medical/pharmaceutical treatments:
- Colchicine: 0.5 mg BID or TID for the treatment of oral/genital ulcers[19]
- Topical corticosteroids: for oral and ocular involvement; oral corticosteroid therapy does not alter the course of the disease[20]
- High-dose oral prednisone: 60-80 mg/d is indicated for severe uveitis, CNS involvement, or other urgent complications; cyclosporine immunosuppression is indicated for patients who do not respond to prednisone[21]

- Antioxidant therapy: Such as with mixed tocopherols[22] or Chinese herbal formula called "BG-104"[23] and any combination of antioxidants such as lipoic acid and phytonutrients. Recall that the Paleo-Mediterranean diet is inherently antioxidative due to the low glycemic indexes and

[17] Verity DH, Wallace GR, Vaughan RW, Stanford MR. Behcet's disease: from Hippocrates to the third millennium. *Br J Ophthalmol*. 2003 Sep;87(9):1175-83 http://bjo.bmjjournals.com/cgi/reprint/87/9/1175

[18] Beers MH, Berkow R (eds). The Merck Manual. Seventeenth Edition. Whitehouse Station; Merck Research Laboratories 1999 page 425

[19] Beers MH, Berkow R (eds). The Merck Manual. Seventeenth Edition. Whitehouse Station; Merck Research Laboratories 1999 page 425

[20] Beers MH, Berkow R (eds). The Merck Manual. Seventeenth Edition. Whitehouse Station; Merck Research Laboratories 1999 page 425

[21] Beers MH, Berkow R (eds). The Merck Manual. Seventeenth Edition. Whitehouse Station; Merck Research Laboratories 1999 page 425

[22] Kokcam I, Naziroglu M. Effects of vitamin E supplementation on blood antioxidants levels in patients with Behcet's disease. *Clin Biochem*. 2002 Nov;35(8):633-9

[23] "The treatment with BG-104 and/or vitamin E significantly enhanced the plasma SSA in all disorders studied. Both the erythrocyte sedimentation rates, the absolute number of neutrophils, as well as C-reactive protein levels were significantly lower in patients treated with BG-104 and/or vitamin E than those without these drugs." Pronai L, Arimori S. BG-104 enhances the decreased plasma superoxide scavenging activity in patients with Behcet's disease, Sjogren's syndrome or hematological malignancy. *Biotherapy*. 1991;3(4):365-71

loads and the additive and synergistic effects of phytonutrients from fruits, vegetables, nuts, seeds, and berries.[24]

- Orthoendocrinology: On an individual basis, clinicians and patients may find it valuable to assess prolactin, cortisol, DHEA, free and total testosterone, serum estradiol, and thyroid status (e.g., TSH, T4, *and* anti-thyroid peroxidase antibodies). Some studies have shown that **patients with Behcet's disease have higher levels of proinflammatory prolactin than do normal controls**[25]**, while other groups have contradicted these findings.**[26,27]

- Antimicrobial treatments and assessment for dysbiosis: **Assess for occult infections; treat as indicated.** In patients for whom no specific microbes are detected with specialty testing such as stool testing or mucosal culture, clinicians should treat for presumptive bacterial overgrowth of the small bowel.

  o Orodental dysbiosis: Since **oral infection with variant strains of** *Streptococcus sanguis* **are the most likely and most consistently identified single source of antigenic stimulation in patients with Behcet's disease**[28], all patients should use potent antimicrobial mouthwashes daily. Obviously, extracts from berberine-containing botanicals such as *Hydrastis canadensis* are first-line therapy due to their potency against oral *Streptococcus* species.[29] Since non-berberine constituents—flavonoids—from *Hydrastis* are synergistically antimicrobial and increase the effectiveness of berberine against oral pathogens[30], the ideal antimicrobial in this regard would be a broad-spectrum extract standardized for its content of berberine. Berberine/Hydrastis powder can be used in a "swish, hold, and swallow" mouth rinse—the initial taste is quite bitter but it becomes tolerable; patients may prefer a comparatively better-tasting antimicrobial mouthwash such as 'Listerine' or its generic equivalent. Warm water nasal lavage with Berberine/Hydrastis powder, salt and baking soda (sodium chloride and sodium bicarbonate) can be used twice daily and is well-tolerated. **Patients with orodental/sinus dysbiosis should get into the habit of cleaning their sinuses when they brush their teeth and using antimicrobial mouthwash, a tripartite event that should occur at least twice daily.**

  o Gastrointestinal dysbiosis: Although patients with Behcet's disease appear to have a similar prevalence of *Helicobacter pylori* as the rest of the population, **eradication of gastrointestinal** *H. pylori* **infection leads to clinical improvement and resolution of genital and oral ulcers in these patients, thus showing that gastrointestinal dysbiosis is an underlying pathoetiologic factor in this condition.**[31]

  o Sinorespiratory dysbiosis: **Recent research has clearly demonstrated evidence of chronic** *Chlamydia pneumoniae* **infections in Behcets patients.**[32]

  o Cutaneous dysbiosis: Recent research implicates the skin as a loci of dysbiosis: **pustules of patients with Behcet's disease are not sterile**[33] and are contaminated with bacteria that are distinct from those seen in regular acne and which are productive of antigens

---

[24] Liu RH. Health benefits of fruit and vegetables are from additive and synergistic combinations of phytochemicals. *Am J Clin Nutr*. 2003 Sep;78(3 Suppl):517S-520S http://www.ajcn.org/cgi/content/full/78/3/517S

[25] "The mean prolactin levels in all subgroups of patients with BD were higher than normal, but no statistically significant difference was shown between these subgroups. CONCLUSION: Hyperprolactinemia occurred in a small number of patients with BD and its significance remained unclear. Serum PRL level did not correlate with disease manifestations and activity." Houman H, Ben Ghorbel I, Lamloum M, Feki M, Khanfir M, Mebazaa A, Miled M. Prolactin levels in Behcet's disease: no correlation with disease manifestations and activity. *Ann Med Interne* (Paris). 2001 Apr;152(3):209-11 http://www.masson.fr/

[26] "However, we found no such correlation in Behcet's disease. On the contrary, prolactin levels were lower in attacks than in remissions." Apaydin KC, Duranoglu Y, Ozgurel Y, Saka O. Serum prolactin levels in Behcet's disease. *Jpn J Ophthalmol*. 2000 Jul-Aug;44(4):442-5

[27] "We found that mean PRL levels in patients with clinically active BS, were not significantly higher than patients with clinically inactive BS and healthy controls." Keser G, Oksel F, Ozgen G, Aksu K, Doganavsargil E. Serum prolactin levels in Behcet's Syndrome. *Clin Rheumatol*. 1999;18(4):351-2

[28] Direskeneli H. Behcet's disease: infectious aetiology, new autoantigens, and HLA-B51. *Ann Rheum Dis*. 2001;60(11):996-1002 http://ard.bmjjournals.com/cgi/content/full/60/11/996#B26

[29] "Thus, berberine sulfate interferes with the adherence of group A streptococci by two distinct mechanisms: one by releasing the adhesin lipoteichoic acid from the streptococcal cell surface and another by directly preventing or dissolving lipoteichoic acid-fibronectin complexes." Sun D, Courtney HS, Beachey EH. Berberine sulfate blocks adherence of Streptococcus pyogenes to epithelial cells, fibronectin, and hexadecane. *Antimicrob Agents Chemother*. 1988 Sep;32(9):1370-4 http://www.pubmedcentral.gov/articlerender.fcgi?tool=pubmed&pubmedid=3058020

[30] "Berberine (3) exhibited an additive antimicrobial effect when tested against S. mutans in combination with 1." Hwang BY, Roberts SK, Chadwick LR, Wu CD, Kinghorn AD. Antimicrobial constituents from goldenseal (the Rhizomes of Hydrastis canadensis) against selected oral pathogens. *Planta Med*. 2003 Jul;69(7):623-7

[31] "In 13 patients with BD, the number and size of oral and genital ulcers diminished significantly and various clinical manifestations regressed after the eradication of HP. CONCLUSION: HP may be involved in the pathogenesis of BD." Avci O, Ellidokuz E, Simsek I, Buyukgebiz B, Gunes AT. Helicobacter pylori and Behcet's disease. *Dermatology*. 1999;199(2):140-3

[32] "These finding provide serological evidence of chronic C. pneumoniae infection in association with Behcet's disease." Ayaslioglu E, Duzgun N, Erkek E, Inal A. Evidence of chronic Chlamydia pneumoniae infection in patients with Behcet's disease. *Scand J Infect Dis*. 2004;36(6-7):428-30

[33] "At least one type of microorganism was grown from each pustule. Staphylococcus aureus (41/70, 58.6%, p = 0.008) and Prevotella spp (17/70, 24.3%, p = 0.002) were significantly more common in pustules from BS patients, and coagulase negative staphylococci (17/37, 45.9%, p = 0.007) in pustules from acne patients. CONCLUSIONS: The pustular lesions of BS are not usually sterile." Hatemi G, Bahar H, Uysal S, Mat C, Gogus F, Masatlioglu S, Altas K, Yazici H. The pustular skin lesions in Behcet's syndrome are not sterile. *Ann Rheum Dis*. 2004 Nov;63(11):1450-2

and superantigens that are capable of perpetuating the disease via proinflammatory immunodysregulation. Furthermore, there is **a direct relationship between number of pustules and the severity of arthritis**[34] which suggests that proinflammatory immunodysregulation may result from microbial antigens and superantigens from cutaneous dysbiosis.

- o Clinical implementation: In patients with established Behcet's disease, clinicians may be faced with the task of simultaneously treating numerous dysbiotic loci—mouth and gastrointestinal tract, sinus and lungs, and skin. Indeed, treatment should be orchestrated to address different loci with as few treatments as possible and as broadly as possible—**all loci should be treated simultaneously**. This may require co-administration of botanical and pharmaceutical antimicrobials, with the latter chosen for their systemic bioavailability. Patients should generally implement the alkalinizing supplemented Paleo-Mediterranean diet (with broad-spectrum fatty acid supplementation, probiotics, vitamin D, etc.) to effect a down-regulation of inflammation for the purpose of gaining some stability before facing aggressive antimicrobial treatment, from which the development of a "die off" Herxheimer-type reaction is possible and may not be benign.[35] Since the treatment of large or systemic bacterial infections can lead to a dramatic increase in endotoxin release[36], prophylactic treatment with NF-kappaB inhibitors (discussed in the chapter on Therapeutics), or other potent anti-inflammatory treatments (such as single-dose prednisone) should be considered.

- • Treatments to lower homocysteine: Patients with Behcet's syndrome have elevated homocysteine which exacerbates arterial and venous occlusion which underlies many of the clinical complications of the disease.[37,38] Doses given here for various treatments are for adults:
  - o Folic acid: 5-10 mg, should be used with high-dose vitamin B-12
  - o Hydroxocobalamin: 2,000-6,000 mcg/d orally, or 1,000-4,000 mcg/wk by injection
  - o Pyridoxine: 250 mg/day with meals, co-administered with magnesium (e.g., >200 mg/d)
  - o NAC: 600 mg tid
  - o Betaine: 1-2 grams tid
  - o Lecithin: 2.6 g choline/d (as phosphatidylcholine) decreased mean fasting plasma homocysteine by 18%.[39] Attaining this high dose might require as many as 45 capsules of commercially available supplements; an equivalent dose in the form of powdered lecithin granules delivered in a smoothie may be better tolerated than the capsules.
  - o Thyroid hormone: as indicated

- • *Ginkgo biloba*: Ginkgo may be of therapeutic value due to its anticoagulant, vasodilating, antioxidant, and anti-inflammatory actions. *In vitro* studies demonstrate an antioxidant benefit of ginkgo in erythrocytes of Behcets patients.[40]

- • Avoidance of proinflammatory foods: Proinflammatory foods act *directly* or *indirectly*; direct mechanisms include activating Toll-like receptors or NF-kappaB or inducing oxidative stress, while indirect mechanisms include depleting the body of anti-inflammatory nutrients and displacing more nutritious anti-inflammatory foods. Arachidonic acid (found in beef, liver, pork,

---

[34] Diri E, Mat C, Hamuryudan V, Yurdakul S, Hizli N, Yazici H. Papulopustular skin lesions are seen more frequently in patients with Behcet's syndrome who have arthritis: a controlled and masked study. *Ann Rheum Dis.* 2001 Nov;60(11):1074-6 http://ard.bmjjournals.com/cgi/reprint/60/11/1074

[35] "There is clear experimental evidence that antibiotics increase the bioavailability of endotoxin from Gram-negative bacteria." Hurley JC. Antibiotic-induced release of endotoxin. A therapeutic paradox. *Drug Saf.* 1995 Mar;12(3):183-95

[36] "A three- to 20-fold increase in the total concentration of endotoxin occurs as a consequence of antibiotic action on gram-negative bacteria both in vitro and in vivo." Hurley JC. Antibiotic-induced release of endotoxin: a reappraisal. *Clin Infect Dis.* 1992 Nov;15(5):840-54

[37] "CONCLUSION: Homocysteine may play a role in ocular involvement of BD. Chronic inflammation can induce hyperhomocysteinemia, thereby leading to thrombosis in the retinal vascular bed in a way similar to that recently proposed for the pathogenesis of coronary artery disease." Okka M, Ozturk M, Kockar MC, Bavbek N, Rasier R, Gunduz K. Plasma homocysteine level and uveitis in Behcet's disease. *Isr Med Assoc J.* 2002 Nov;4(11 Suppl):931-4

[38] "CONCLUSION: Hyperhomocysteinaemia may be assumed to be an independent risk factor for venous thrombosis in BD. Unlike the factor V Leiden mutation, hyperhomocysteinaemia is a correctable risk factor. This finding might lead to new avenues in the prophylaxis of thrombosis in BD." Aksu K, Turgan N, Oksel F, Keser G, Ozmen D, Kitapcioglu G, Gumusdis G, Bayindir O, Doganavsargil E. Hyperhomocysteinaemia in Behcet's disease. *Rheumatology* (Oxford). 2001 Jun;40(6):687-90 http://rheumatology.oxfordjournals.org/cgi/reprint/40/6/687

[39] Olthof MR, Brink EJ, Katan MB, Verhoef P. Choline supplemented as phosphatidylcholine decreases fasting and postmethionine-loading plasma homocysteine concentrations in healthy men. *Am J Clin Nutr.* 2005 Jul;82(1):111-7

[40] "These data indicate that an oxidative damage is present in erythrocytes obtained from Behcet's patients, and EGb 761 [Ginkgo biloba extract], which may strengthen the antioxidant defense system, may contribute to the treatment of BD." Kose K, Dogan P, Ascioglu M, Ascioglu O. In vitro antioxidant effect of Ginkgo biloba extract (EGb 761) on lipoperoxidation induced by hydrogen peroxide in erythrocytes of Behcet's patients. *Jpn J Pharmacol.* 1997 Nov;75(3):253-8

and cow's milk) is the direct precursor to proinflammatory prostaglandins and leukotrienes[41] and pain-promoting isoprostanes.[42] Saturated fats promote inflammation by activating/enabling proinflammatory Toll-like receptors.[43] Consumption of saturated fat in the form of cream creates marked oxidative stress and lipid peroxidation that lasts for at least 3 hours postprandially.[44] Corn oil rapidly activates NF-kappaB (in hepatic Kupffer cells) for a proinflammatory effect[45]; similarly, consumption of PUFA and linoleic acid promotes antioxidant depletion and may thus promote oxidation-mediated inflammation via activation of NF-kappaB; linoleic acid causes intracellular oxidative stress and calcium influx and results in increased transcription of NF-kappaB activated pro-inflammatory genes.[46] High glycemic foods cause oxidative stress[47,48] and inflammation via activation of NF-kappaB and other mechanisms—*white bread causes inflammation*.[49] High glycemic foods suppress immune function[50,51] and thus perpetuate and promote infection/dysbiosis. Delivery of a high carbohydrate load to the gastrointestinal lumen promotes bacterial overgrowth[52,53], which is inherently proinflammatory[54,55] and which appears to be myalgenic in humans.[56] Consumption of grains, potatoes, and manufactured foods displaces phytonutrient-dense foods such as fruits, vegetables, nuts, seeds, and berries which in sum contain more than 8,000 phytonutrients, many of which have anti-oxidant and thus anti-inflammatory actions.[57,58]

- <u>Avoidance of allergenic foods</u>: Any patient may be allergic to any food, even if the food is generally considered a health-promoting food. Generally speaking, the most notorious allergens are wheat, citrus (especially juice due to the industrial use of fungal hemicellulases), cow's milk, eggs, peanuts, chocolate, and yeast-containing foods; according to a study in patients with migraine, some patients will have to avoid as many as 10 specific foods in order to become symptom-free.[59]

- <u>Supplemented Paleo-Mediterranean diet</u>: The health-promoting diet of choice for the majority of people is a diet based on abundant consumption of fruits, vegetables, seeds, nuts, omega-3 and monounsaturated fatty acids, and lean sources of protein such as lean meats, fatty cold-water fish, soy and whey proteins. This diet obviates overconsumption of chemical preservatives, artificial sweeteners, and carbohydrate-dominant foods such as candies, pastries, breads,

---

[41] Vasquez A. Reducing Pain and Inflammation Naturally. Part 2: New Insights into Fatty Acid Supplementation and Its Effect on Eicosanoid Production and Genetic Expression. *Nutritional Perspectives* 2005; January: 5-16 www.optimalhealthresearch.com/part2

[42] Evans AR, Junger H, Southall MD, Nicol GD, Sorkin LS, Broome JT, Bailey TW, Vasko MR. Isoprostanes, novel eicosanoids that produce nociception and sensitize rat sensory neurons. *J Pharmacol Exp Ther*. 2000 Jun;293(3):912-20

[43] Lee JY, Sohn KH, Rhee SH, Hwang D. Saturated fatty acids, but not unsaturated fatty acids, induce the expression of cyclooxygenase-2 mediated through Toll-like receptor 4. *J Biol Chem*. 2001 May 18;276(20):16683-9. Epub 2001 Mar 2 http://www.jbc.org/cgi/content/full/276/20/16683

[44] "CONCLUSIONS: Both fat and protein intakes stimulate ROS generation. The increase in ROS generation lasted 3 h after cream intake and 1 h after protein intake. Cream intake also caused a significant and prolonged increase in lipid peroxidation." Mohanty P, Ghanim H, Hamouda W, Aljada A, Garg R, Dandona P. Both lipid and protein intakes stimulate increased generation of reactive oxygen species by polymorphonuclear leukocytes and mononuclear cells. *Am J Clin Nutr*. 2002 Apr;75(4):767-72 http://www.ajcn.org/cgi/content/full/75/4/767

[45] Rusyn I, Bradham CA, Cohn L, Schoonhoven R, Swenberg JA, Brenner DA, Thurman RG. Corn oil rapidly activates nuclear factor-kappaB in hepatic Kupffer cells by oxidant-dependent mechanisms. *Carcinogenesis*. 1999 Nov;20(11):2095-100 http://carcin.oxfordjournals.org/cgi/content/full/20/11/2095

[46] "Exposing endothelial cells to 90 micromol linoleic acid/L for 6 h resulted in a significant increase in lipid hydroperoxides that coincided wih an increase in intracellular calcium concentrations." Hennig B, Toborek M, Joshi-Barve S, Barger SW, Barve S, Mattson MP, McClain CJ. Linoleic acid activates nuclear transcription factor-kappa B (NF-kappa B) and induces NF-kappa B-dependent transcription in cultured endothelial cells. *Am J Clin Nutr*. 1996 Mar;63(3):322-8 http://www.ajcn.org/cgi/reprint/63/3/322

[47] Mohanty P, Hamouda W, Garg R, Aljada A, Ghanim H, Dandona P. Glucose challenge stimulates reactive oxygen species (ROS) generation by leucocytes. *J Clin Endocrinol Metab*. 2000 Aug;85(8):2970-3 http://jcem.endojournals.org/cgi/content/full/85/8/2970 Glucose/carbohydrate and saturated fat consumption appear to be the two biggest offenders in the food-stimulated production of oxidative stress. The effect by protein is much less. "CONCLUSIONS: Both fat and protein intakes stimulate ROS generation. The increase in ROS generation lasted 3 h after cream intake and 1 h after protein intake. Cream intake also caused a significant and prolonged increase in lipid peroxidation." Mohanty P, Ghanim H, Hamouda W, Aljada A, Garg R, Dandona P. Both lipid and protein intakes stimulate increased generation of reactive oxygen species by polymorphonuclear leukocytes and mononuclear cells. *Am J Clin Nutr*. 2002 Apr;75(4):767-72 http://www.ajcn.org/cgi/content/full/75/4/767

[48] Koska J, Blazicek P, Marko M, Grna JD, Kvetnansky R, Vigas M. Insulin, catecholamines, glucose and antioxidant enzymes in oxidative damage during different loads in healthy humans. *Physiol Res*. 2000;49 Suppl 1:S95-100 http://www.biomed.cas.cz/physiolres/pdf/2000/49_S95.pdf

[49] "Conclusion - The present study shows that high GI carbohydrate, but not low GI carbohydrate, mediates an acute proinflammatory process as measured by NF-kappaB activity." Dickinson S, Hancock DP, Petocz P, Brand-Miller JC..High glycemic index carbohydrate mediates an acute proinflammatory process as measured by NF-kappaB activation. *Asia Pac J Clin Nutr*. 2005;14 Suppl:S120

[50] Sanchez A, Reeser JL, Lau HS, et al. Role of sugars in human neutrophilic phagocytosis. *Am J Clin Nutr*. 1973 Nov;26(11):1180-4

[51] "Postoperative infusion of carbohydrate solution leads to moderate fall in the serum concentration of inorganic phosphate. ... The hypophosphatemia was associated with significant reduction of neutrophil phagocytosis, intracellular killing, consumption of oxygen and generation of superoxide during phagocytosis." Rasmussen A, Segel E, Hessov I, Borregaard N. Reduced function of neutrophils during routine postoperative glucose infusion. *Acta Chir Scand*. 1988 Jul-Aug;154(7-8):429-33

[52] Ramakrishnan T, Stokes P. Beneficial effects of fasting and low carbohydrate diet in D-lactic acidosis associated with short-bowel syndrome. *JPEN J Parenter Enteral Nutr*. 1985 May-Jun;9(3):361-3

[53] Gottschall E. Breaking the Vicious Cycle: Intestinal Health Through Diet. Kirkton Press; Rev edition (August 1, 1994)

[54] Lin HC. Small intestinal bacterial overgrowth: a framework for understanding irritable bowel syndrome. *JAMA*. 2004 Aug 18;292(7):852-8

[55] Lichtman SN, Wang J, Sartor RB, Zhang C, Bender D, Dalldorf FG, Schwab JH. Reactivation of arthritis induced by small bowel bacterial overgrowth in rats: role of cytokines, bacteria, and bacterial polymers. *Infect Immun*. 1995 Jun;63(6):2295-301

[56] Pimentel M, et al. A link between irritable bowel syndrome and fibromyalgia may be related to findings on lactulose breath testing. *Ann Rheum Dis*. 2004 Apr;63(4):450-2

[57] "We propose that the additive and synergistic effects of phytochemicals in fruit and vegetables are responsible for their potent antioxidant and anticancer activities, and that the benefit of a diet rich in fruit and vegetables is attributed to the complex mixture of phytochemicals present in whole foods." Liu RH. Health benefits of fruit and vegetables are from additive and synergistic combinations of phytochemicals. *Am J Clin Nutr*. 2003 Sep;78(3 Suppl):517S-520S

[58] Seaman DR. The diet-induced proinflammatory state: a cause of chronic pain and other degenerative diseases? *J Manipulative Physiol Ther*. 2002;25(3):168-79

[59] Grant EC. Food allergies and migraine. *Lancet*. 1979 May 5;1(8123):966-9

potatoes, grains, and other foods with a high glycemic load and high glycemic index. This "Paleo-Mediterranean Diet" is a combination of the "Paleolithic" or "Paleo diet" and the well-known "Mediterranean diet", both of which are well described in peer-reviewed journals and the lay press. (See Chapter 2 for details). **Habitual avoidance of refined sugars and other immunosuppressing foods is essential when treating chronic systemic infections**.

- Short-term fasting: Whether the foundational diet is Paleo-Mediterranean, vegetarian, vegan, or a combination of all of these, autoimmune/inflammatory patients will still benefit from periodic fasting, whether on a weekly (e.g., every Saturday), monthly (every first week or weekend of the month, or every other month), or yearly (1-2 weeks of the year) basis. Since consumption of food—particularly unhealthy foods—induces an inflammatory effect[60], abstinence from food provides a relative anti-inflammatory effect. Fasting indeed provides a distinct anti-inflammatory benefit and may help "re-calibrate" metabolic and homeostatic mechanisms by breaking self-perpetuating "vicious cycles"[61] that autonomously promote inflammation independent from pro-inflammatory stimuli. Of course, water-only fasting is completely hypoallergenic (assuming that the patient is not sensitive to chlorine, fluoride, or other contaminants), and subsequent re-introduction of foods provides the ideal opportunity to identify offending foods. Fasting deprives intestinal microbes of substrate[62], stimulates intestinal B-cell immunity[63], improves the bactericidal action of neutrophils[64], reduces lysozyme release and leukotriene formation[65], and ameliorates intestinal hyperpermeability.[66] In case reports and/or clinical trials, short-term fasting (or protein-sparing fasting) has been documented as safe and effective treatment for SLE[67], RA[68], and non-rheumatic diseases such as chronic severe hypertension[69], moderate hypertension[70], obesity[71,72], type-2 diabetes[73], and epilepsy.[74]

- Broad-spectrum fatty acid therapy with ALA, EPA, DHA, GLA and oleic acid: Fatty acid supplementation should be delivered in the form of combination therapy with ALA, GLA, DHA, and EPA. Given at doses of 3,000 – 9,000 mg per day, ALA from flax oil has impressive anti-inflammatory benefits demonstrated by its ability to halve prostaglandin production in humans.[75] Numerous studies have demonstrated the benefit of GLA in the treatment of rheumatoid arthritis

---

[60] Aljada A, Mohanty P, Ghanim H, Abdo T, Tripathy D, Chaudhuri A, Dandona P. Increase in intranuclear nuclear factor kappaB and decrease in inhibitor kappaB in mononuclear cells after a mixed meal: evidence for a proinflammatory effect. *Am J Clin Nutr.* 2004 Apr;79(4):682-90 http://www.ajcn.org/cgi/content/full/79/4/682

[61] "The ability of therapeutic fasts to break metabolic vicious cycles may also contribute to the efficacy of fasting in the treatment of type 2 diabetes and autoimmune disorders." McCarty MF. A preliminary fast may potentiate response to a subsequent low-salt, low-fat vegan diet in the management of hypertension - fasting as a strategy for breaking metabolic vicious cycles. *Med Hypotheses.* 2003 May;60(5):624-33

[62] Ramakrishnan T, Stokes P. Beneficial effects of fasting and low carbohydrate diet in D-lactic acidosis associated with short-bowel syndrome. *JPEN J Parenter Enteral Nutr.* 1985 May-Jun;9(3):361-3

[63] Trollmo C, Verdrengh M, Tarkowski A. Fasting enhances mucosal antigen specific B cell responses in rheumatoid arthritis. *Ann Rheum Dis.* 1997 Feb;56(2):130-4 http://ard.bmjjournals.com/cgi/content/full/56/2/130

[64] "An association was found between improvement in inflammatory activity of the joints and enhancement of neutrophil bactericidal capacity. Fasting appears to improve the clinical status of patients with RA." Uden AM, Trang L, Venizelos N, Palmblad J. Neutrophil functions and clinical performance after total fasting in patients with rheumatoid arthritis. *Ann Rheum Dis.* 1983 Feb;42(1):45-51

[65] "We thus conclude that a reduced ability to generate cytotaxins, reduced release of enzyme, and reduced leukotriene formation from RA neutrophils, together with an altered fatty acid composition of membrane phospholipids, may be mechanisms for the decrease of inflammatory symptoms that results from fasting." Hafstrom I, Ringertz B, Gyllenhammar H, Palmblad J, Harms-Ringdahl M. Effects of fasting on disease activity, neutrophil function, fatty acid composition, and leukotriene biosynthesis in patients with rheumatoid arthritis. *Arthritis Rheum.* 1988 May;31(5):585-92

[66] "The results indicate that, unlike lactovegetarian diet, fasting may ameliorate the disease activity and reduce both the intestinal and the non-intestinal permeability in rheumatoid arthritis." Sundqvist T, Lindstrom F, Magnusson KE, Skoldstam L, Stjernstrom I, Tagesson C. Influence of fasting on intestinal permeability and disease activity in patients with rheumatoid arthritis. *Scand J Rheumatol.* 1982;11(1):33-8

[67] Fuhrman J, Sarter B, Calabro DJ. Brief case reports of medically supervised, water-only fasting associated with remission of autoimmune disease. *Altern Ther Health Med.* 2002 Jul-Aug;8(4):112, 110-1

[68] "An association was found between improvement in inflammatory activity of the joints and enhancement of neutrophil bactericidal capacity. Fasting appears to improve the clinical status of patients with RA." Uden AM, Trang L, Venizelos N, Palmblad J. Neutrophil functions and clinical performance after total fasting in patients with rheumatoid arthritis. *Ann Rheum Dis.* 1983 Feb;42(1):45-51

[69] "The average reduction in blood pressure was 37/13 mm Hg, with the greatest decrease being observed for subjects with the most severe hypertension. Patients with stage 3 hypertension (those with systolic blood pressure greater than 180 mg Hg, diastolic blood pressure greater than 110 mg Hg, or both) had an average reduction of 60/17 mm Hg at the conclusion of treatment." Goldhamer A, Lisle D, Parpia B, Anderson SV, Campbell TC. Medically supervised water-only fasting in the treatment of hypertension. *J Manipulative Physiol Ther.* 2001 Jun;24(5):335-9 http://www.healthpromoting.com/335-339Goldhamer115263.QXD.pdf

[70] "RESULTS: Approximately 82% of the subjects achieved BP at or below 120/80 mm Hg by the end of the treatment program. The mean BP reduction was 20/7 mm Hg, with the greatest decrease being observed for subjects with the highest baseline BP." Goldhamer AC, Lisle DJ, Sultana P, Anderson SV, Parpia B, Hughes B, Campbell TC. Medically supervised water-only fasting in the treatment of borderline hypertension. J Altern Complement Med. 2002 Oct;8(5):643-50 http://www.healthpromoting.com/Articles/articles/study%202/acmpaper5.pdf

[71] Vertes V, Genuth SM, Hazelton IM. Supplemented fasting as a large-scale outpatient program. *JAMA.* 1977 Nov 14;238(20):2151-3

[72] Bauman WA, Schwartz E, Rose HG, Eisenstein HN, Johnson DW. Early and long-term effects of acute caloric deprivation in obese diabetic patients. *Am J Med.* 1988 Jul;85(1):38-46

[73] Goldhamer AC. Initial cost of care results in medically supervised water-only fasting for treating high blood pressure and diabetes. J Altern Complement Med. 2002 Dec;8(6):696-7 http://www.healthpromoting.com/Articles/pdf/Study%2032.pdf

[74] "The ketogenic diet should be considered as alternative therapy for children with difficult-to-control seizures. It is more effective than many of the new anticonvulsant medications and is well tolerated by children and families when it is effective." Freeman JM, Vining EP, Pillas DJ, Pyzik PL, Casey JC, Kelly LM. The efficacy of the ketogenic diet-1998: a prospective evaluation of intervention in 150 children. *Pediatrics.* 1998 Dec;102(6):1358-63 http://pediatrics.aappublications.org/cgi/reprint/102/6/1358

[75] Adam O, Wolfram G, Zollner N. Effect of alpha-linolenic acid in the human diet on linoleic acid metabolism and prostaglandin biosynthesis. *J Lipid Res.* 1986 Apr;27(4):421-6 http://www.jlr.org/cgi/reprint/27/4/421

when used at doses between 500 mg – 4,000 mg per day.[76,77] Fish oil provides EPA and DHA which have well-proven anti-inflammatory benefits in rheumatoid arthritis[78,79,80] and lupus.[81,82] ALA, EPA, DHA, and GLA need to be provided in the form of supplements; when using high doses of therapeutic oils, liquid supplements that can be mixed in juice or a smoothie are generally more convenient and palatable than capsules. Therapeutic amounts of oleic acid can be obtained from generous use of olive oil, preferably on fresh vegetables. Supplementation with polyunsaturated fatty acids warrants increased intake of antioxidants from diet, fruit and vegetable juices, and properly formulated supplements; since patients with systemic inflammation are generally in a pro-oxidative state, consideration must be given to the timing and starting dose of fatty acid supplementation and the need for anti-oxidant protection. See chapter on Therapeutics for more details and biochemical pathways. Clinicians must realize that fatty acids are not clinically or biochemically interchangeable and that one fatty acid does not substitute for another; each of the fatty acids must be supplied in order for its benefits to be obtained.[83]

Additional notes:

_____

_____

_____

_____

_____

_____

_____

_____

_____

_____

_____

_____

_____

_____

_____

_____

_____

_____

_____

_____

_____

[76] "Other results showed a significant reduction in morning stiffness with gamma-linolenic acid at 3 months and reduction in pain and articular index at 6 months with olive oil." Brzeski M, Madhok R, Capell HA. Evening primrose oil in patients with rheumatoid arthritis and side-effects of non-steroidal anti-inflammatory drugs. *Br J Rheumatol*. 1991 Oct;30(5):370-2
[77] Rothman D, DeLuca P, Zurier RB. Botanical lipids: effects on inflammation, immune responses, and rheumatoid arthritis. *Semin Arthritis Rheum*. 1995 Oct;25(2):87-96
[78] Adam O, Beringer C, Kless T, Lemmen C, Adam A, Wiseman M, Adam P, Klimmek R, Forth W. Anti-inflammatory effects of a low arachidonic acid diet and fish oil in patients with rheumatoid arthritis. *Rheumatol Int*. 2003 Jan;23(1):27-36
[79] Lau CS, Morley KD, Belch JJ. Effects of fish oil supplementation on non-steroidal anti-inflammatory drug requirement in patients with mild rheumatoid arthritis--a double-blind placebo controlled study. *Br J Rheumatol*. 1993 Nov;32(11):982-9
[80] Kremer JM, Jubiz W, Michalek A, Rynes RI, Bartholomew LE, Bigaouette J, Timchalk M, Beeler D, Lininger L. Fish-oil fatty acid supplementation in active rheumatoid arthritis. A double-blinded, controlled, crossover study. *Ann Intern Med*. 1987 Apr;106(4):497-503
[81] Walton AJ, Snaith ML, Locniskar M, Cumberland AG, Morrow WJ, Isenberg DA. Dietary fish oil and the severity of symptoms in patients with systemic lupus erythematosus. *Ann Rheum Dis*. 1991 Jul;50(7):463-6
[82] Duffy EM, Meenagh GK, McMillan SA, Strain JJ, Hannigan BM, Bell AL. The clinical effect of dietary supplementation with omega-3 fish oils and/or copper in systemic lupus erythematosus. *J Rheumatol*. 2004 Aug;31(8):1551-6
[83] Vasquez A. Reducing Pain and Inflammation Naturally. Part 2: New Insights into Fatty Acid Supplementation and Its Effect on Eicosanoid Production and Genetic Expression. *Nutritional Perspectives* 2005; January: 5-16 http://optimalhealthresearch.com/part2

Iron Overload
Primary/Genetic Hemochromatosis
Secondary Hemochromatosis

> Iron overload and genetic hemochromatosis are not systemic autoimmune diseases, but are included in this text because they are very common in clinical practice and can mimic both osteoarthritis and systemic inflammatory arthritis.

<u>Description/pathophysiology</u>:

- **Hereditary iron overload disorders are now recognized as being among the most common genetic diseases in the human population.**[1,2,3,4,5,6,7]

- Iron overload is a phenotypic state to which a patient arrives by either genetic or environmental/iatrogenic routes. The severity of iron overload can range from moderate to severe.

- Excess iron catalyses oxidative stress which damages body tissues and structures in which the iron is stored. In patients with genetic hemochromatosis, two problems exist simultaneously: 1) a disproportionately large amount of iron is absorbed from the gastrointestinal tract (i.e., these patients' iron absorption is "too efficient"), and 2) iron is preferentially deposited in parenchymal tissues such as the heart, liver, pancreas, pituitary gland, and joints rather than being stored safely within the reticuloendothelial system. The deposition of excess iron in parenchymal tissues promotes destruction of these organs/tissues via oxidative mechanisms and subsequent tissue necrosis and fibrosis, leading to the protean manifestations of the disease dependent upon which organs are most affected in the individual patient: heart failure, hepatic fibrosis, hypoinsulinemic diabetes, hypopituarism, and hemochromatoic arthropathy.[8]

- Iron overload can be defined as a state of "iron toxicity" similar to mercury toxicity or poisoning with any other heavy metal or toxin, except that the mechanism is more related to the *quantity* of the iron rather than the unique characteristics or *quality* of iron itself. In other words, whereas the toxicity of mercury can be seen even when only small amounts of the metal are present, the toxicity of iron is directly related to the amount of the excess iron, rather than the inherent toxicity of the iron itself.

Conditions associated with iron overload

Primary/genetic disorders
1. Homozygous genetic hemochromatosis
2. Heterozygous genetic hemochromatosis
3. African iron overload
4. African-American hemochromatosis (African-American iron overload)
5. Non-HLA-linked hemochromatosis
6. Juvenile hemochromatosis
7. Neonatal hemochromatosis

Secondary and metabolic disorders
8. Dietary excess of iron
9. Parenteral administration of iron in the form of iron injections and blood transfusions
10. Porphyria cutanea tarda
11. Portacaval shunt
12. Hepatic cirrhosis, portal hypertension, and splenomegaly
13. AIDS
14. Sudden infant death syndrome
15. Alcoholism
16. Metabolic syndrome

Inherited red blood cell abnormalities ("iron-loading anemias", hemoglobinopathies)
17. Alpha-thalassemia
18. Beta-thalassemia
19. Thalassemia intermedia
20. Sideroblastic anemia
21. Aplastic anemia
22. Anemia associated with pyruvate kinase deficiency
23. AC hemoglobinopathy
24. AS hemoglobinopathy
25. X-linked hypochromic anemia
26. Pyridoxine-responsive anemia
27. Atransferrinemia

[1] Olynyk JK, Bacon BR. Hereditary hemochromatosis: detecting and correcting iron overload. *Postgrad Med* 1994; 96: 151-65
[2] Phatak PD, Cappuccio JD. Management of hereditary hemochromatosis. *Blood Rev* 1994; 8: 193-8
[3] Rouault TA. Hereditary hemochromatosis. *JAMA* 1993; 269: 3152-4
[4] Crosby WH. Hemochromatosis: current concepts and management. Hosp Pract 1987; 22:173-92
[5] Bloom PD, Gordeuk VR, MacPhail AP. HLA-linked hemochromatosis and other forms of iron overload. *Dermatol Clin* 1995; 13: 57-63
[6] Barton JC, Bertoli LF. Hemochromatosis: the genetic disorder of the twenty-first century. *Nat Med* 1996; 2: 394-5
[7] Lauffer, RB. <u>Iron and Your Heart</u>. New York: St. Martin's Press, 1991
[8] **Vasquez A. Musculoskeletal disorders and iron overload disease: comment on the American College of Rheumatology guidelines for the initial evaluation of the adult patient with acute musculoskeletal symptoms.** *Arthritis Rheum* **1996 Oct;39(10):1767-8**

Clinical presentations:

- Many patients are asymptomatic.
- Most patients eventually present with a problem that is attributed to another disorder:
  - Patients may present with diabetes, which is erroneously attributed to metabolic syndrome or type-2 diabetes.[9]
  - Patients may present with joint pain that is erroneously attributed to osteoarthritis[10], rheumatoid arthritis[11], or some other musculoskeletal syndrome.[12]
  - Patients may present with heart failure that is written off as "idiopathic cardiomyopathy."[13]
- Fatigue, lethargy, weakness
- Chronic abdominal pain
- Liver damage: hepatomegally, elevated serum levels of liver enzymes and alkaline phosphatase, fibrosis and cirrhosis, hepatocellular carcinoma, or other findings such as hematemesis and melena, ascites, hyperbilirubenemia and jaundice, hypoalbuminemia, hepatic encephalopathy, clotting dysfunction, anemia, liver abscess, increased incidence of esophageal carcinoma.
- Abnormal glucose metabolism or diabetes mellitus: elevated glucose levels. Usually asymptomatic, yet can cause weight loss, polyuria, polyphagia, polydypsia.
- Musculoskeletal disorders: arthritis and arthralgia, generalized osteoporosis, bone pain, myalgia. Especially arthropathy of the hands and wrists, hips, and knees.
- Cardiac dysfunction: cardiomyopathy, arrhythmia, fibrillation, congestive heart failure; shortness of breath or dyspnea on exertion, fatigue.
- Cutaneous manifestations: 'slate-gray' or ashen coloration, increased pigmentation ('tan') of the skin, atrophy of the skin, ichthyosis, koilonychia, loss of body hair, increased incidence of malignant melanoma.
- Endocrine disorders: hypogonadotrophic hypogonadism, (autoimmune) hypothyroidism, hyperthyroidism; manifest as decreased libido, impotence, testicular atrophy, or sterility in males, amenorrhea or difficulty conceiving in females, loss of body hair.
- Susceptibility to increased frequency and severity of infections, especially infections due to *Yersinia enterocolitica*, *Vibrio vulnificus*, *HIV*, and *Mycobacterium tuberculosis*.
- Neurologic symptoms: blurred vision, sensorineural hearing loss, hyperactivity, dementia, attention deficit disorder, ataxia, lightheadedness, dizziness, anxiety, depression, tinnitus, confusion, lethargy, memory loss, disorientation, headaches and migraine headaches, personality changes, hallucinations, paranoia, chronic treatment-resistant psychiatric illness such as schizophrenia, compulsive disorders, bipolar affective disorder.

Musculoskeletal manifestations of iron overload

Clinical findings may include:
- **Joint pain**
- **Bone pain**
- Joint swelling
- Loss of motion
- Bursitis
- Tendonitis
- Tenosynovitis
- Subcutaneous nodules

Sites of involvement
- **Metacarpophalangeal joints**
- **Wrist**
- **Hip**
- **Knee**
- Shoulder
- Ankle
- Metatarsophalangeal joints
- Elbow
- Spine
- Symphysis pubis
- Achilles tendon
- Plantar fascia

Radiographic findings
- **Joint space narrowing**
- **Sclerosis**
- Cysts
- Pseudocysts
- Osteophytes
- **Hook-like osteophytes at the metacarpal heads (high specificity)**
- Flattened or "squared-off" metacarpal heads
- Generalized osteopenia
- Generalized osteoporosis
- Chondrocalcinosis
- Subchondral cysts
- Carpal erosions
- Calcific tendonitis

---

[9] "Most of the patients (95%) had one or more of the following conditions; obesity, hyperlipidaemia, abnormal glucose metabolism, or hypertension. INTERPRETATION: We have found a new non-HLA-linked iron-overload syndrome which suggests a link between iron excess and metabolic disorders." Moirand R, Mortaji AM, Loreal O, Paillard F, Brissot P, Deugnier Y. A new syndrome of liver iron overload with normal transferrin saturation. *Lancet*. 1997 Jan 11;349(9045):95-7

[10] Axford JS, Bomford A, Revell P, Watt I, Williams R, Hamilton EBD. Hip arthropathy in genetic hemochromatosis: radiographic and histologic features. *Arthritis Rheum* 1991; 34: 357-61

[11] Bensen WG, Laskin CA, Little HA, Fam AG. Hemochromatoic arthropathy mimicking rheumatoid arthritis. A case with subcutaneous nodules, tenosynovitis, and bursitis. *Arthritis Rheum* 1978; 21: 844-8

[12] Olynyk J, Hall P, Ahern M, Kwiatek R, Mackinnon M. Screening for genetic hemochromatosis in a rheumatology clinic. *Australian and New Zealand Journal of Medicine* 1994; 24: 22-25

[13] [No authors listed] Case records of the Massachusetts General Hospital. Weekly clinicopathological exercises. Case 31-1994. A 25-year-old man with the recent onset of diabetes mellitus and congestive heart failure. *N Engl J Med*. 1994 Aug 18;331(7):460-6

- 'Alcoholism': Alcoholism can cause elevated liver enzymes and liver damage, and many iron overload patients are erroneously diagnosed as alcoholics despite their abstinence from alcohol when the clinician fails to consider iron overload as the cause for the hepatopathy.
- Any race, nationality, or ethnic background: Hereditary iron overload conditions have been identified in people of all ethnic backgrounds and nationalities. Secondary iron overload conditions can occur irrespective of genetic predisposition.
- Either gender: Iron overload conditions occur in both men and women
- A family history of, or suggestive of, a hereditary iron overload condition: family history of iron overload, hereditary anemia or iron-loading anemia, cardiac disorders or "heart disease", arthritis, diabetes, neurologic disorders, liver disease, impotence, amenorrhea, sterility.

Differential diagnoses:
- Diabetes mellitus: Remember that the classic presentation of hemochromatosis is "bronze diabetes with cirrhosis." **All patients with diabetes should be tested for iron overload.**[14,15]
- Cardiomyopathy:
- Hepatopathy: **Iron overload is one of the most important rule-outs in patients with liver disease.**[16] Liver biopsy is often indicated to assess condition and disease co-existence.
- Musculoskeletal disorders: **Patients with polyarthropathy should be tested for iron overload.**[17,18]
  - o Degenerative arthritis or osteoarthritis
  - o Pseudogout, calcium pyrophosphate dihydrate deposition disease
  - o Rheumatoid arthritis[19]
  - o Ankylosing spondylitis: The resemblance here is only superficial, related primarily to calcification of the intervertebral discs and ligaments.[20]
- Hypogonadotrophic hypogonadism: impotence in men, subfertility in women[21]
- Hyperthyroidism and hypothyroidism[22,23]
- Porphyria cutanea tarda: "Virtually all patients have increased iron stores; serum iron, iron saturation, and ferritin values."[24] **All patients with porphyria cutanea tarda must be tested for iron overload.**

Clinical assessment:
- **History/subjective**:
  - o The manifestations of the condition are so protean that history is generally non-sensitive and non-specific for the disorder. Rarely, a patient will mention that a relative was diagnosed with iron overload or that a relative had an unusual heart or liver disease, and this clue may lead to a diagnosis of iron overload in unsuspecting family members.

> **Rationale for screening all patients**:
> 1. Hereditary iron-accumulation disorders occur in a large percentage of the population.
> 2. Persons with the disease usually have no symptoms.
> 3. Clinical manifestations are often indicative of irreversible organ damage or organ failure.
> 4. Iron overload can cause death if not treated early.
> 5. Early treatment ensures normal life expectancy.
> 6. **Therefore, early detection (before the onset of symptoms and organ damage) requires screening asymptomatic patients.**
>
> **Test of choice: serum ferritin**, because it shows the best correlation with body iron stores and thus prognosis and need for treatment

---

[14] Czink E, Tamas G. Screening for idiopathic hemochromatosis among diabetic patients. *Diabetes Care* 1991; 14: 929-30
[15] Phelps G, Chapman I, Hall P, Braund W, Mackinnon M. Prevalence of genetic haemochromatosis among diabetic patients. *Lancet* 1989; 2: 233-4
[16] Herrera JL. Abnormal liver enzyme levels: clinical evaluation in asymptomatic patients. *Postgrad Med* 1993; 93: 119-32
[17] M'Seffar AM, Fornasier VL, Fox IH. Arthropathy as the major clinical indicator of occult iron storage disease. *JAMA* 1977; 238: 1825-8
[18] Vasquez A. Musculoskeletal disorders and iron overload disease: comment on the American College of Rheumatology guidelines for the initial evaluation of the adult patient with acute musculoskeletal symptoms [letter/ comment]. *Arthritis Rheum* 1996;39:1767-8
[19] Bensen WG, Laskin CA, Little HA, Fam AG. Hemochromatoic arthropathy mimicking rheumatoid arthritis. A case with subcutaneous nodules, tenosynovitis, and bursitis. *Arthritis Rheum* 1978; 21: 844-8
[20] Bywaters EGL, Hamilton EBD, Williams R. The spine in idiopathic hemochromatosis. *Ann Rheum Dis* 1971; 30: 453-65
[21] Tweed MJ, Roland JM. Haemochromatosis as an endocrine cause of subfertility. *BMJ*. 1998 Mar 21;316(7135):915-6 http://bmj.bmjjournals.com/cgi/content/full/316/7135/915
[22] Edwards CQ, Kelly TM, Ellwein G, Kushner JP. Thyroid disease in hemochromatosis. Increased incidence in homozygous men. *Arch Intern Med* 1983 Oct;143(10):1890-3
[23] Phillips G Jr, Becker B, Keller VA, Hartman J 4th. Hypothyroidism in adults with sickle cell anemia. *Am J Med* 1992 May;92(5):567-70
[24] "Virtually all patients have increased iron stores; serum iron, iron saturation, and ferritin values." Rich MW. Porphyria cutanea tarda. Don't forget to look at the urine. *Postgrad Med*. 1999;105: 208-10, 213-4

- **Physical examination/objective**:
  - The classic presentation of the fully developed disease is "bronze diabetes with arthritis and cirrhosis."
  - Physical examination should be specific for the patient's complaint(s) of arthritis, cardiomyopathy, diabetes, etc.
- **Imaging & laboratory assessments**:
  - **Routine screening with serum ferritin for iron overload among all patients should be the standard of care in clinical practice**.
    - "In view of the high prevalence of hereditary hemochromatosis, its dire consequences when untreated, and its treatability, screening for the disorder should be performed routinely."[25]
    - "Screening for hemochromatosis is both feasible and cost-effective, and we recommend its use in patients seeking medical care."[26]
    - "The high gene frequency in the general population warrants routine screening tests in asymptomatic healthy young adults."[27]
    - "CONCLUSIONS: Primary iron overload occurs in African Americans... Clinicians should look for this condition."[28]
  - Imaging: The radiographic findings are nearly identical to those of osteoarthritis, except more joints are typically involved and that the distribution is typically symmetric (both due to the systemic/metabolic nature of the disease). Hook-like osteophytes at the metacarpal heads—with the "hooks" pointing proximally (rather than distally, as in rheumatoid arthritis) may be the only finding that could be called pathognomonic. Flattened or "squared-off" metacarpal heads are also seen. See previous table labeled *"Musculoskeletal manifestations of iron overload"* for more details.
  - Laboratory evaluation: Serum ferritin is the test of choice when looking for primary iron overload, secondary iron overload, and/or iron deficiency and should be a component of each new patient's evaluation, just as are CBC and the chemistry/metabolic panel.
    - **Ferritin: Routine use of serum ferritin is the most reasonable and cost-effective means for diagnosing this condition in symptomatic and asymptomatic patients.** Elevations of ferritin (i.e., >200 mcg/L in women and >300 mcg/L in men) need to be retested along with CRP (to rule out false elevation due to excessive inflammation) before making the presumptive diagnosis of iron overload. **In the absence of significant inflammation, ferritin values >200 mcg/L in women and >300 mcg/L in men indicate iron overload and the need for treatment/phlebotomy regardless of the absence of symptoms or end-stage complications.**[29] Another benefit to the use of serum ferritin is the frequent detection of iron deficiency.
    - Transferrin saturation: good test for detecting genetic hemochromatosis before iron overload has occurred; values greater than 40% should be repeated *in conjunction with a measurement of serum ferritin*.
    - CRP: should be relatively normal as iron overload is not inflammatory, per se. If the ferritin is elevated and the CRP is markedly elevated, then inflammatory and hepatocentric diseases must be considered, namely advanced cancer, viral hepatitis or other hepatopathy, and alcoholic liver disease. If the ferritin is elevated and the CRP is normal, then the most likely diagnosis is iron overload, which should be confirmed either with liver biopsy or diagnostic/therapeutic phlebotomy.
    - CBC: may show anemia, but the findings here are nonspecific
    - Chemistry panel: may show evidence of diabetes and hepatopathy

[25] Fairbanks VF. Laboratory testing for iron status. *Hosp Pract* (Off Ed) 1991 Suppl 3:17-24
[26] Balan V, Baldus W, Fairbanks V, Michels V, Burritt M, Klee G. Screening for hemochromatosis: a cost-effectiveness study based on 12, 258 patients. *Gastroenterology* 1994; 107: 453-9
[27] Gushusrt TP, Triest WE. Diagnosis and management of precirrhotic hemochromatosis. *W Virginia Med J* 1990; 86: 91-5
[28] Wurapa RK, Gordeuk VR, Brittenham GM, Khiyami A, Schechter GP, Edwards CQ. Primary iron overload in African Americans. *Am J Med.* 1996 Jul;101(1):9-18
[29] Barton JC, McDonnell SM, Adams PC, Brissot P, Powell LW, Edwards CQ, Cook JD, Kowdley KV. Management of hemochromatosis. Hemochromatosis Management Working Group. *Ann Intern Med.* 1998 Dec 1;129(11):932-9

- **Thyroid assessment**: may show hyperthyroidism or hypothyroidism, both of which are more common in patients with iron overload.
- **Bone marrow biopsy**: unnecessary and archaic in this setting, now that serum ferritin is widely available.
- **Liver biopsy**: traditionally considered the "gold standard" for diagnosing iron overload but is now clearly unnecessary for the diagnosis, which can be established by monitoring the response to therapeutic phlebotomy, which is the treatment of choice.[30] **Life-saving diagnostic and therapeutic phlebotomy should never be denied or delayed for lack of liver biopsy in patients with laboratory indicators of iron overload.**[31]
- **Genetic testing, such as for the HFE mutation** is a waste of time and money in most clinical situations; these tests should be reserved for research purposes. The only value these tests may have in clinical practice is that of supporting a diagnosis in a patient with elevated serum ferritin who refuses biopsy, liver MRI, or phlebotomy; however, a negative result is meaningless if the ferritin is high and the clinical picture is compatible with iron overload. If the diagnosis is established, genetic relatives must be tested.

Guide to Patient Management Based on Iron Status

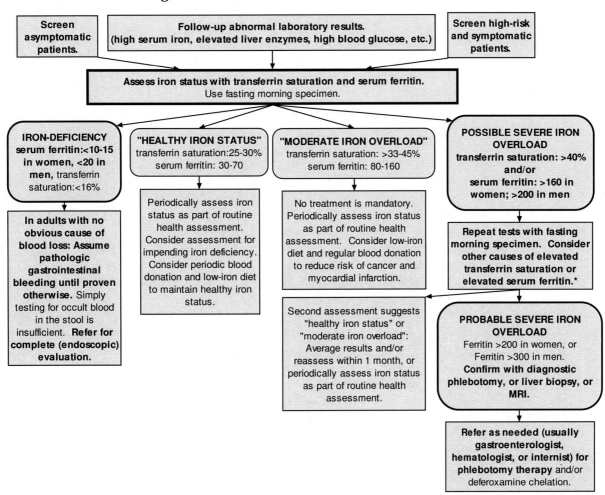

---

[30] "Therapeutic phlebotomy is used to remove excess iron and maintain low normal body iron stores, and it should be initiated in men with serum ferritin levels of 300 microg/L or more and in women with serum ferritin levels of 200 microg/L or more, regardless of the presence or absence of symptoms." Barton JC, McDonnell SM, Adams PC, Brissot P, Powell LW, Edwards CQ, Cook JD, Kowdley KV. Management of hemochromatosis. Hemochromatosis Management Working Group. *Ann Intern Med.* 1998 Dec 1;129(11):932-9

[31] Sullivan JL, as quoted in Crawford R, ed. "The debate." In: *Ironic Blood: information on iron overload.* West Palm Beach: Iron Overload Diseases Association, Inc. 1996; 16 (2)

- **Establishing the diagnosis**: Any *one* of the following three is sufficient:
  - Diagnostic liver biopsy shows heavy iron deposits
  - Characteristic laboratory findings (ferritin >200 in women or >300 in men) *and* the ability to resist intractable anemia with serial/weekly phlebotomies
  - Characteristic MRI of liver *and* the ability to tolerate serial/weekly phlebotomies

Complications:
- Patients diagnosed *and effectively treated* before the onset of signs and symptoms have normal life expectancy.
- The most common causes of premature mortality in undiagnosed and untreated patients are related to heart failure, liver failure, infections and/or complications of diabetes.

Clinical management:
- Treatment for severe iron overload is iron-removal therapy. Since blood is high in iron, the removal of blood—therapeutic phlebotomy—is the treatment of choice. Deferoxamine chelation can be administered to patients who refuse or cannot withstand phlebotomy (i.e., patients with cardiomyopathy, severe anemia, hypoproteinemia) but is much less effective, much more expensive, and with side effects such as neurotoxicity. Adjunctive nutritional and lifestyle modifications are no substitute for iron-removal therapy, and weekly phlebotomy is the treatment of choice.

Treatments:
- *Medical standard*: Iron-removal is accomplished by weekly phlebotomy of 1-2 units (250-500 mL of blood, each of which removes 250 mg of iron), and deferoxamine chelation is used in patients who cannot tolerate phlebotomy. Complications of the disease, such as arthritis, heart failure, hypogonadism, and diabetes are treated appropriately. Cirrhotic patients must be monitored for hepatoma with twice-yearly liver ultrasound and measurement of serum alpha-fetoprotein. Always, when a hereditary iron overload disorder is diagnosed, all (first-degree) blood relatives must be screened for iron overload.
- Diet modifications: These are no substitute for iron-removal therapy with phlebotomy and are weak in their effectiveness by comparison.
  - Decrease consumption of foods and nutritional supplements which are significant sources of iron: Iron supplements, iron-fortified foods and supplements, liver, beef, pork, lamb.
  - Increase consumption of foods that will decrease intestinal absorption of iron from ingested food: tannins in tea, phytates (in whole-grain products, bran, legumes, nuts, and seeds), soy protein, egg, calcium supplements.
  - Ensure adequate protein intake to replace protein lost during phlebotomy.
  - Decrease consumption of excess ascorbic acid (vitamin C); high-dose vitamin C supplementation is clearly contraindicated.[32]
  - Alcohol consumption should be avoided because ethanol exacerbates liver damage and increases iron absorption from the gut.
- Silymarin: Milk thistle has proved benefit in an animal model of iron overload[33] and is probably suitable for use in patients with iron overload, particularly given its ability to reverse cirrhosis.[34]
- Antioxidant supplementation (excluding high-dose ascorbate): Oxidative stress is increased and antioxidant reserves are decreased in patients with iron overload.
- Coenzyme Q10: CoQ-10 probably has a role in the treatment of hemochromatoic cardiomyopathy given its safety and efficacy in other cardiomyopathies.[35,36,37,38,39,40,41,42]

[32] Mclarlan CJ, et al. Congestive cardiomyopathy and hemochromatosis: rapid progression possibly accelerated by excessive ingestion of ascorbic acid. *Aust NZ J Med* 1982; 12: 187-8
[33] "CONCLUSIONS: Oral administration of silybin protects against iron-induced hepatic toxicity in vivo. This effect seems to be caused by the prominent antioxidant activity of this compound." Pietrangelo A, Borella F, Casalgrandi G, et al. Antioxidant activity of silybin in vivo during long-term iron overload in rats. *Gastroenterology*. 1995 Dec;109(6):1941-9
[34] Salmi HA, Sarna S. Effect of silymarin and chemical, functional, and morphological alterations of the liver. A double-blind controlled study. *Scand J Gastroenterol* 1982; 17: 517-21
[35] Greenberg S, Frishman WH. Co-enzyme Q-10: a new drug for cardiovascular disease. *J Clin Pharmacol* 1990; 30: 596-608
[36] Langsjoen PH, Langsjoen PH, Folkers K. Long-term efficacy and safety of coenzyme Q-10 therapy for idiopathic dilated cardiomyopathy. *Am J Cardiol* 1990; 65: 521-3
[37] Manzoli U, Rossi E, Littarru GP, et al. Coenzyme Q-10 in dilated cardiomyopathy. *Int J Tiss Reac* 1990; 12: 173-8
[38] Langsjoen PH, Folkers K, Lyson K, Muratsu K, Lyson T, Langsjoen P. Pronounced increase of survival of patients with cardiomyopathy when treated with coenzyme Q-10 and conventional therapy. *Int J Tiss Reac* 1990; 12: 163-8
[39] Folkers K. Heart failure is a dominant deficiency of coenzyme Q-10 and challenges for future clinical research on CoQ-10. *Clin Investig* 1993; 71: s51-s54
[40] Folkers K, Langsjoen P, Langsjoen PH. Therapy with coenzyme Q-10 of patients in heart failure who are eligible or ineligible for a transplant. *Biochem Biophys Res Commun* 1992;182:247-53
[41] Mortensen SA, et al. Coenzyme Q-10: clinical benefits with biochemical correlates suggesting a scientific breakthrough.... *Int J Tiss Reac* 1990;12:155-62
[42] Langsjoen PH, Langsjoen PH, Folkers K. A six-year clinical study of therapy of cardiomyopathy with coenzyme Q-10. *Int J Tiss Reac* 1990; 12: 169-71

<u>Topics</u>:
- **Fatty acid supplementation and modulation of eicosanoid metabolism and genetic expression**
- **NF-kappaB and its phytonutritional modulation**
- **Selected nutritional and botanical therapeutics**
    - Flaxseed oil: Alpha-linolenic acid (ALA)
    - Fish oil: Eicosapentaenoic acid (EPA), Docosahexaenoic acid (DHA)
    - Gamma-linolenic acid (GLA)
    - Vitamin D3: Cholecalciferol
    - Vitamin E: Alpha-tocopherol, beta-tocopherol, delta-tocopherol, gamma-tocopherol
    - Niacinamide
    - Glucosamine sulfate and Chondroitin Sulfate
    - Pancreatin, bromelain, papain, trypsin and alpha-chymotrypsin: "proteolytic enzymes" and "pancreatic enzymes"
    - *Zingiber officinale*, Ginger
    - *Uncaria tomentosa, Uncaria guianensis*, "Cat's claw", "una de gato"
    - *Salix alba*, Willow Bark
    - *Capsicum annuum, Capsicum frutescens*, Cayenne pepper, hot chili pepper
    - *Boswellia serrata*, Frankincense, Salai guggal
    - *Harpagophytum procumbens*, Devil's claw
    - *Curcuma longa,* Turmeric
    - Avocado/soybean unsaponifiabiles
- **Piezoelectric properties of the human body and clinical implications**
- **Physiotherapy notes: available on-line**
- **Review of major vitamins and minerals**

Fatty Acid Supplementation and Modulation of Eicosanoid Metabolism and Genetic Expression

Despite their tremendous importance for a wide range of conditions seen in clinical practice, the basics of fatty acid metabolism are unfamiliar to many practicing clinicians. Add to this misinformation on behalf of the lay press and from researchers and professors with financial interests in inferior products and concepts and we can easily see how students and clinicians alike misunderstand and underutilize the clinical applications of fatty acid supplementation and eicosanoid modulation. An accurate and detailed understanding of fatty acid metabolism is important for the complete and effective management of many clinical conditions including mental depression, coronary artery disease, hypertension, diabetes, other inflammatory and autoimmune disorders[1] and many of the musculoskeletal conditions described in this text. The practical application of this information is relatively straightforward, and with a detailed understanding of precursors and modulators of fatty acid, prostaglandin, and leukotriene metabolism, clinicians can facilitate or restrict the production of bioactive chemicals to promote the desired clinical result.

The section that follows is compiled from the research literature and from biochemistry and nutrition textbooks. It is noteworthy that none of the primary sources[2,3] or textbooks[4,5] contained a complete description or biochemical flow diagram of the fatty acid and eicosanoid cascade. Furthermore, there were occasionally discrepancies between the information contained in well-known texts and articles from respected authorities.

[1] Simopoulos AP. Essential fatty acids in health and chronic disease. *Am J Clin Nutr.* 1999 Sep;70(3 Suppl):560S-569S

[2] Horrobin DF. Ascorbic acid and prostaglandin synthesis. *Subcell Biochem.* 1996;25:109-15

[3] Horrobin DF. Interactions between n-3 and n-6 essential fatty acids (EFAs) in the regulation of cardiovascular disorders and inflammation. *Prostaglandins Leukot Essent Fatty Acids.* 1991 Oct;44(2):127-31

[4] McGlivery RW. <u>Biochemistry: A Functional Approach. Third Edition.</u> Philadelphia: WB Saunders, 1983. Pages 747-750

[5] Delvin TM. <u>Textbook of Biochemistry with Clinical Correlations.</u> New York: Wiley-Liss, 1997. Pages 431-441

The Major Fatty Acids and End-products of Clinical Significance

The fatty acids of major importance and the ones discussed here are all polyunsaturated fatty acids, meaning that they have *several* carbon-to-carbon double bonds (i.e., C=C), which are vulnerable to oxidation, rancidification, and/or hydrogenation. Therefore, these fatty acids must be protected from oxygen, heat, light, and prolonged storage. Once structurally altered by oxygen, heat, or light, these fatty acids lose some or all of their biologic value, and they take on disease-promoting properties by interfering with fatty acid metabolism, altering cell membrane dynamics, and/or by having direct/indirect inflammatory and carcinogenic actions.

Fatty acids serve three primary biologic functions: 1) as cell membrane components that modulate membrane pliability and receptor sensitivity, 2) as precursors to potent biologic regulators such as prostaglandins and leukotrienes, and 3) as modulators of gene expression. Each fatty acid must be either provided by diet or manufactured from enzymatic conversion of its predecessor in order to carry out its physiologic role. Deficiency of any fatty acid results in impairment of physiologic function. These impairments begin subtly and often go unrecognized by clinicians who may then erroneously employ pharmacologic and surgical interventions to alleviate *diseases* that originate from *deficiencies* of fatty acids and other nutrients.

Polyunsaturated fatty acids (PUFA) are categorized based on the location of the first carbon-to-carbon double bond from the methyl group, which is located at the opposite end from the carboxyl carbon.[6] The major categories from a biological and nutritional standpoint are the omega-3 fatty acids (having the first carbon-to-carbon double bond starting at the third carbon from the methyl group) and the omega-6 fatty acids (having the first carbon-to-carbon double bond starting at the sixth carbon from the methyl group). The most commonly known member of the omega-9 group is oleic acid from olive oil; but it is of lesser biologic importance than the omega-3 and omega-6 fatty acids, which are the key determinants of the biologically powerful thromboxanes, leukotrienes, prostaglandins, and isoprostanes. The term "omega" is commonly represented as either "Ω" or "w" or "ω" or "n". For the sake of consistency and readability, I will use either the word "omega" or the symbol "n" in this text.

The general term "eicosanoids" is used to describe the various metabolic end products of 20-carbon fatty acid metabolism, including thromboxanes (TX), leukotrienes (LT), and prostaglandins (PG). Produced in minute quantities of approximately 1 milligram per day[7], prostaglandins are produced by nearly all mammalian cells; their production is not confined to leukocytes even though they are often associated with immune activation. Since they are produced and act locally at the site of metabolic activation, they are autocrine and paracrine rather than endocrine.[8] These chemicals have short half-lives, with thromboxanes existing only for a few seconds after production[9] while leukotrienes persist for as long as four hours.[10] While specific enzymes transform one fatty acid into another (within the same family, n-3 or n-6, respectively), the production of eicosanoids is *initiated by enzymes* but often *completed by non-specific, random interactions* dependent on free radicals and/or random conformational changes in enzymes and substrates.[11]

The two main families of bioactive fatty acids are the omega-3 and omega-6 families. These families have generally *opposing* effects to each other and therefore the quantitative balance of these fatty acids serves to dictate the body's ability to establish and retain homeostasis with regard to the modulation of cellular function in general and the production of thromboxanes, leukotrienes, and prostaglandins in particular.[12] With an excess of n-6 fatty acids and a deficiency of n-3 fatty acids, the human body fails to function optimally and the clinical result is an increase in the prevalence and severity of clinical diseases associated with imbalanced gene expression, cell membrane function, and eicosanoid production—namely cancer, heart disease, diabetes, arthritis, allergy, autoimmune diseases, depression, bipolar disorder, schizophrenia, and the long list of "diseases of Western civilization."[13]

---

[6] Erasmus U. Fats that heal, fats that kill. British Columbia Canada: Alive Books, 1993 Page 15-16
[7] Delvin TM. Textbook of Biochemistry with Clinical Correlations. New York: Wiley-Liss, 1997. Pages 431-441
[8] McGlivery RW. Biochemistry: A Functional Approach. Third Edition. Philadelphia: WB Saunders, 1983. Pages 747-750
[9] McGlivery RW. Biochemistry: A Functional Approach. Third Edition. Philadelphia: WB Saunders, 1983. Pages 747-750
[10] Delvin TM. Textbook of Biochemistry with Clinical Correlations. New York: Wiley-Liss, 1997. Pages 431-441
[11] Thuresson ED, Lakkides KM, Smith WL. Different catalytically competent arrangements of arachidonic acid within the cyclooxygenase active site of prostaglandin endoperoxide H synthase-1 lead to the formation of different oxygenated products. J Biol Chem. 2000 Mar 24;275(12):8501-7 Available on-line at http://www.jbc.org/cgi/reprint/275/12/8501 as of December 28, 2003.
[12] Tapiero H, Ba GN, Couvreur P, Tew KD. Polyunsaturated fatty acids (PUFA) and eicosanoids in human health and pathologies. Biomed Pharmacother. 2002;56(5):215-22
[13] Price WA. Nutrition and Physical Degeneration. Santa Monica: Price-Pottinger Nutrition Foundation, 1945

Omega-3 fatty acids:
- **General properties**
    - The first double bond is at third carbon from the methyl group
    - **Primarily from flax seed and cold-water aquatic animals ("antifreeze" for deep water fish, seal, whale) and game animals, also from some leafy green vegetables in small amounts**
    - Maintain cell membrane fluidity and tissue flexibility and elasticity due to markedly curved structure (maintains space between molecules) compared to saturated fatty acids (straight molecules are closely packed with less room for motion)
    - N-3 fatty acids consistently lower serum triglycerides levels in contrast to n-6 fatty acids, which generally cause serum triglycerides to increase.[14]
    - **Causes of n-3 deficiency include:**
        1. Low-fat diets (in general)
        2. Decreased intake of omega-3 (specifically)
        3. Increased intake of omega-6 (such as "to lower cholesterol")
        4. Intake of unnatural *trans*-fatty acids versus natural *cis*-fatty acids. *Trans*-fatty acids are found in hydrogenated oils (hydrogenation makes oil thicker, prevents oxidation, and "improves" taste), fried foods. *Trans*-PUFA increase LDL and reduce HDL.[15]
        5. Alteration of feed for farm animals (substitution of grasses, plants, insects with grains, which are high in n-6 FA), this is why wild game animals have more n-3
        6. High-fat diets if fats are imbalanced with excess of n-6 and trans-FA's
        7. Maldigestion and/or malabsorption
        8. Primary or secondary defects in enzyme function for the conversion of dietary precursors to the end-stage biologically-active fatty acids
    - **Clinical manifestations of deficiency of omega-3 fats are far more subtle than those associated with omega-6 deficiency: (in animal studies) reduced learning, impaired vision, polydypsia.** Given the importance of n-3 fatty acids in health and disease and the relative deficiency state which is the norm in America, we could also argue that deficiency of n-3 fatty acids predispose to the chronic degenerative diseases of cancer, diabetes, cardiovascular disease and to the more subtle functional problems of dermatitis and the epidemic of neurocognitive and neuropsychiatric disorders.
    - **Tissue levels are measurably changed within one week of supplementation and are restored to constant levels in 12 weeks of supplementation (in monkeys).** Not all manifestations of deficiency are corrected with supplementation, indicating that fatty acid deficiencies may leave permanent residual effects, particularly if deficiency occurs early in life during the time of rapid growth and development, especially of the brain.
- **Alpha-linolenic acid, linolenic acid, ALA, α-LNA, ALNA, 18:3n3**
    - **Essential fatty acid:** ALA is the parent fatty acid of the omega-3 class; it is the "first in line."
    - Sources include **flax seed oil** (57% ALA) and canola (rape seed) oil (9% ALA), soy oil, breast milk, English/black walnuts, soybeans, pine nuts, green vegetables, and beans.
    - ALA may theoretically be converted to EPA and DHA but this should not be expected to occur sufficiently in all patients at all times due to interindividual variations in enzyme activity and inadequate nutritional/cofactor status. To attain a measurable increase in EPA from ALA supplementation, approximately eleven-times (11x) the amount of ALA must be consumed to achieve a proportional response to that which can be achieved with direct supplementation of EPA.[16] No increase in DHA has been observed in humans after supplementation of ALA; in fact, supplementation with flax seed oil has actually been shown to reduce DHA levels in humans.[17,18]

[14] Simopoulos AP. Essential fatty acids in health and chronic disease. *Am J Clin Nutr.* 1999 Sep;70(3 Suppl):560S-569S
[15] Tapiero H, Ba GN, Couvreur P, Tew KD. Polyunsaturated fatty acids (PUFA) and eicosanoids in human health and pathologies. *Biomed Pharmacother.* 2002;56(5):215-22
[16] "Indu and Ghafoorunissa showed that while keeping the amount of dietary LA constant, 3.7 g ALA appears to have biological effects similar to those of 0.3 g long-chain n-3 PUFA with conversion of 11 g ALA to 1 g long-chain n-3 PUFA." Simopoulos AP. Essential fatty acids in health and chronic disease. *Am J Clin Nutr.* 1999 Sep;70(3 Suppl):560S-569S
[17] Saldeen T. Health Effects of Fish Oil with a Focus on Natural, Stable, Fish Oil. Buxton Road, New Mills, High Peak: Nutri Ltd. [Date unknown] page 33
[18] "Linear relationships were found between dietary alpha-LA and EPA in plasma fractions and in cellular phospholipids. … There was an inverse relationship between dietary alpha-LA and docosahexaenoic acid concentrations in the phospholipids of plasma, neutrophils, mononuclear cells, and platelets." Mantzioris E, James MJ, Gibson RA, Cleland LG. Differences exist in the relationships between dietary linoleic and alpha-linolenic acids and their respective long-chain metabolites. *Am J Clin Nutr.* 1995 Feb;61(2):320-4

- o Lipid-lowering effects are not seen with ALA supplementation and are only attained with the use of EPA and DHA; however ALA can reduce blood pressure.[19]
- o **ALA has potent anti-inflammatory benefits independent of its conversion to EPA or DHA.**[20] The mechanism of action appears to be downregulation of NF-KappaB rather than the direct modulation of eicosanoid biosynthesis. One study using flax oil as a source of ALA to treat rheumatoid arthritis found no clinical or biochemical benefit (i.e., no change in Hgb, CRP, ESR).[21]

- **Stearidonic acid, 18:4n3, octadecatetraenoic acid**
  - o Small amount found in black currant oil
  - o Human studies have found that stearidonic acid increases EPA 2x more efficiently than does ALA but does not increase DHA.[22]
  - o Inhibits 5-lipoxygenase.[23]

- **N-3 Eicosatetraenoic acid, 20:4n3**
  - o 20:4n-3 is eicosatetraenoic acid.[24,25]
  - o The term "eicosatetraenoic acid" applies to both 20:4n6 (arachidonic acid) of the omega-6 fatty acid family[26] and 20:4n3 of the omega-3 fatty acid family.[27,28] Therefore, to avoid the confusion that would result from the use of the term "eicosatetraenoic acid" by itself, "n-6 eicosatetraenoic acid" should be used when referring to 20:4n6 (arachidonic acid) and "n-3 eicosatetraenoic acid" should be used when referring to 20:4n3.

- **Eicosapentaenoic acid, EPA, 20:5n3**
  - o Effectively absent in vegan diets; the major dietary source is fish oil.
  - o EPA can decrease production of DGLA.[29]
  - o EPA doses of at least 4 grams per day are needed to increase bleeding time.[30]
  - o EPA–derived eicosanoids have anti-inflammatory properties, including a reduction in the production of pro-inflammatory eicosanoids such as LT-B4, PAFs, and cytokines such as TNF-alpha and IL-1, and a large reduction in PG-E2 and TX-B2.[31]
  - o Animal studies suggest that vitamin B-6 deficiency can reduce the function of delta-6-desaturase by 64% and lead to a reduction in EPA and DHA.[32]
  - o Children with allergies show altered fatty acid metabolism[33] that is not caused by impaired delta-6-desaturase activity and which results reduced EPA levels.[34]
  - o N-6 fatty acids facilitate elongation of EPA to n-3 DPA.[35] Thus, anti-inflammatory EPA is depleted by consumption of proinflammatory n-6 fatty acids.
  - o Evidence suggests that EPA must be incorporated into cell membrane phospholipids for its beneficial effects on eicosanoid metabolism to be realized. Administration of n-6 fatty acids removes EPA from cell membranes and relocates EPA from phospholipids into triacylglycerols. Therefore the benefits of EPA are mitigated by n-6 fatty acids, and thus

[19] Simopoulos AP. Essential fatty acids in health and chronic disease. *Am J Clin Nutr.* 1999 Sep;70(3 Suppl):560S-569S
[20] "CONCLUSIONS: Dietary supplementation with ALA for 3 months decreases significantly CRP, SAA and IL-6 levels in dyslipidaemic patients. This anti-inflammatory effect may provide a possible additional mechanism for the beneficial effect of plant n-3 polyunsaturated fatty acids in primary and secondary prevention of coronary artery disease." Rallidis LS, Paschos G, Liakos GK, Velissaridou AH, Anastasiadis G, Zampelas A. Dietary alpha-linolenic acid decreases C-reactive protein, serum amyloid A and interleukin-6 in dyslipidaemic patients. *Atherosclerosis.* 2003 Apr;167(2):237-42
[21] "Thus, 3-month's supplementation with alpha-LNA did not prove to be beneficial in rheumatoid arthritis." Nordstrom DC, Honkanen VE, Nasu Y, Antila E, Friman C, Konttinen YT. Alpha-linolenic acid in the treatment of rheumatoid arthritis. A double-blind, placebo-controlled and randomized study: flaxseed vs. safflower seed. *Rheumatol Int.* 1995;14(6):231-4
[22] "RESULTS: Dietary SDA increased EPA and docosapentaenoic acid concentrations but not DHA concentrations in erythrocyte and in plasma phospholipids. The relative effectiveness of the tested dietary fatty acids in increasing tissue EPA was 1:0.3:0.07 for EPA:SDA:ALA." James MJ, Ursin VM, Cleland LG. Metabolism of stearidonic acid in human subjects: comparison with the metabolism of other n-3 fatty acids. *Am J Clin Nutr.* 2003 May;77(5):1140-5
[23] Guichardant M, Traitler H, Spielmann D, Sprecher H, Finot PA. Stearidonic acid, an inhibitor of the 5-lipoxygenase pathway. A comparison with timnodonic and dihomogammalinolenic acid. *Lipids.* 1993 Apr;28(4):321-4
[24] Tapiero H, Ba GN, Couvreur P, Tew KD. Polyunsaturated fatty acids (PUFA) and eicosanoids in human health and pathologies. *Biomed Pharmacother.* 2002;56(5):215-22
[25] Erasmus U. Fats that heal, fats that kill. British Columbia Canada: Alive Books, 1993 Page 276
[26] "5,8,11,14-eicosatetraenoic (20:4(n-6))" Mimouni V, Christiansen EN, Blond JP, Ulmann L, Poisson JP, Bezard J. Elongation and desaturation of arachidonic and eicosapentaenoic acids in rat liver. Effect of clofibrate feeding. *Biochim Biophys Acta.* 1991 Nov 27;1086(3):349-53
[27] Tapiero H, et al. Polyunsaturated fatty acids (PUFA) and eicosanoids in human health and pathologies. *Biomed Pharmacother.* 2002 Jul;56(5):215-22
[28] Erasmus U. Fats that heal, fats that kill. British Columbia Canada: Alive Books, 1993 Page 276
[29] Horrobin DF. Interactions between n-3 and n-6 essential fatty acids (EFAs) in the regulation of cardiovascular disorders and inflammation. *Prostaglandins Leukot Essent Fatty Acids.* 1991 Oct;44(2):127-31
[30] "A dose of 1.8 g EPA/d did not result in any prolongation in bleeding time, but 4 g/d increased bleeding time and decreased platelet count with no adverse effects. In human studies, there has never been a case of clinical bleeding…" Simopoulos AP. Essential fatty acids in health and chronic disease. *Am J Clin Nutr.* 1999 Sep;70(3 Suppl):560S-569S
[31] Tapiero H, et al. Polyunsaturated fatty acids (PUFA) and eicosanoids in human health and pathologies. *Biomed Pharmacother.* 2002 Jul;56(5):215-22
[32] Tsuge H, Hotta N, Hayakawa T. Effects of vitamin B-6 on (n-3) polyunsaturated fatty acid metabolism. *J Nutr.* 2000 Feb;130(2S Suppl):333S-334S
[33] Yu G, Bjorksten B. Serum levels of phospholipid fatty acids in mothers and their babies in relation to allergic disease. *Eur J Pediatr.* 1998 Apr;157(4):298-303
[34] Yu G, Bjorksten B. Polyunsaturated fatty acids in school children in relation to allergy and serum IgE levels. *Pediatr Allergy Immunol.* 1998 Aug;9(3):133-8
[35] "The major findings of this study were: 1) n-6 fatty acids markedly stimulated the elongation of EPA to 22:5..." Rubin D, Laposata M. Cellular interactions between n-6 and n-3 fatty acids: a mass analysis of fatty acid elongation/desaturation, distribution among complex lipids, and conversion to eicosanoids. *J Lipid Res.* 1992 Oct;33(10):1431-40

"…dietary therapies designed to increase the EPA content of tissue phospholipids may need to focus on limiting n-6 fatty acid intake in addition to increasing EPA intake." [36]

- **DPA: n-3 docosapentaenoic acid, 22:5n3**
    - Production is increased slightly with consumption of the n-3 precursor ALA. [37]
    - Production can be increased with consumption of n-6 fatty acids. [38] The clinical implications of this finding are significant, because it implies that concomitant administration of n-6 fatty acids such as ALA and arachidonate with EPA would preferentially shuttle EPA to DPA, and therefore the formation of the beneficial EPA-derived eicosanoids would be reduced.
    - The term "docosapentaenoic acid" can apply to both 22:5n3 of the omega-3 fatty acid family [39,40] and 22:5n6 of the omega-6 fatty acid family. [41,42,43] Because to use the term "docosapentaenoic acid" may be ambiguous, the terms "n-3 docosapentaenoic acid" should be used when discussing 22:5n3 and "n-6 docosapentaenoic acid" should be used when discussing 22:5n6.

- **DHA: docosahexaenoic acid, 22:6n-3**
    - Found only in plants of the sea, phytoplankton/microalgae, and consumers of microalgae (such as fish)
    - Essential for neural function, effectively absent in vegan diets, present in breast milk (low in vegetarians); major n-3 in tissues; component of phosphatidylethanolamine and phosphatidylserine; deficiency is associated with inadequate intake of DHA and/or deficient conversion from ALA or EPA.
    - Animal studies have shown that induction of DHA deficiency causes memory deficits and a reduction in hippocampal cell size. [44]
    - DHA is an important component of cell membranes and generally appears to improve cell membrane function via improving receptor function and signal transduction.
    - DHA levels are reduced by ethanol consumption. [45]
    - Animal studies suggest that vitamin B-6 deficiency can reduce the function of delta-6-desaturase by 64% and lead to a reduction in EPA and DHA. [46]
    - Supplementation with EPA+DHA is generally safe and reduces all-cause mortality. [47]
    - In late 2003, bioactive metabolites of DHA were discovered. Previous to the publication of this research, production of bioactive metabolites of DHA via lipoxygenase and cyclooxygenase was unsuspected and/or unproved, and the anti-inflammatory biochemical and clinical effects of DHA were mostly thought to be due to alterations in membrane/receptor function and retroconversion to EPA. We now know that DHA is converted by several mechanisms (lipoxygenase, cyclooxygenase, random reactions, and cell-to-cell interactions) into docosatrienes and resolvins, which are described below. [48]

[36] Rubin D, Laposata M. Cellular interactions between n-6 and n-3 fatty acids: a mass analysis of fatty acid elongation/desaturation, distribution among complex lipids, and conversion to eicosanoids. *J Lipid Res.* 1992 Oct;33(10):1431-40

[37] Tarpila S, Aro A, Salminen I, Tarpila A, Kleemola P, Akkila J, Adlercreutz H. The effect of flaxseed supplementation in processed foods on serum fatty acids and enterolactone. *Eur J Clin Nutr.* 2002 Feb;56(2):157-65

[38] Rubin D, Laposata M. Cellular interactions between n-6 and n-3 fatty acids: a mass analysis of fatty acid elongation/desaturation, distribution among complex lipids, and conversion to eicosanoids. *J Lipid Res.* 1992 Oct;33(10):1431-40

[39] "docosapentaenoic acid (22:5n-3)" Williard DE, Harmon SD, Kaduce TL, Preuss M, Moore SA, Robbins ME, Spector AA. Docosahexaenoic acid synthesis from n-3 polyunsaturated fatty acids in differentiated rat brain astrocytes. *J Lipid Res.* 2001 Sep;42(9):1368-76

[40] "…docosapentaenoic acid (22:5n-3)…" Takahashi R, Nassar BA, Huang YS, Begin ME, Horrobin DF. Effect of different ratios of dietary N-6 and N-3 fatty acids on fatty acid composition, prostaglandin formation and platelet aggregation in the rat. *Thromb Res.* 1987 Jul 15;47(2):135-46

[41] Retterstol K, Haugen TB, Christophersen BO. The pathway from arachidonic to docosapentaenoic acid (20:4n-6 to 22:5n-6) and from eicosapentaenoic to docosahexaenoic acid (20:5n-3 to 22:6n-3) studied in testicular cells from immature rats. *Biochim Biophys Acta.* 2000 Jan 3;1483(1):119-31

[42] "docosapentaenoic acid (DPAn-6)" Ahmad A, Murthy M, Greiner RS, Moriguchi T, Salem N Jr. A decrease in cell size accompanies a loss of docosahexaenoate in the rat hippocampus. *Nutr Neurosci.* 2002 Apr;5(2):103-13

[43] "The desaturation of adrenic acid to n-6 docosapentaenoic acid was decreased in the normo- and hyperglycemic diabetic rats." Mimouni V, Narce M, Huang YS, Horrobin DF, Poisson JP. Adrenic acid delta 4 desaturation and fatty acid composition in liver microsomes of spontaneously diabetic Wistar BB rats. *Prostaglandins Leukot Essent Fatty Acids.* 1994 Jan;50(1):43-7

[44] Ahmad A, Murthy M, Greiner RS, Moriguchi T, Salem N Jr. A decrease in cell size accompanies a loss of docosahexaenoate in the rat hippocampus. *Nutr Neurosci.* 2002 Apr;5(2):103-13

[45] Pawlosky RJ, Bacher J, Salem N Jr. Ethanol consumption alters electroretinograms and depletes neural tissues of docosahexaenoic acid in rhesus monkeys: nutritional consequences of a low n-3 fatty acid diet. *Alcohol Clin Exp Res.* 2001 Dec;25(12):1758-65

[46] Tsuge H, Hotta N, Hayakawa T. Effects of vitamin B-6 on (n-3) polyunsaturated fatty acid metabolism. *J Nutr.* 2000 Feb;130(2S Suppl):333S-334S

[47] "The recent GISSI (Gruppo Italiano per lo Studio della Sopravvivenza nell'Infarto miocardico)-Prevention study of 11,324 patients showed a 45% decrease in risk of sudden cardiac death and a 20% reduction in all-cause mortality in the group taking 850 mg/d of omega-3 fatty acids." O'Keefe JH Jr, Harris WS. From Inuit to implementation: omega-3 fatty acids come of age. *Mayo Clin Proc.* 2000 Jun;75(6):607-14

[48] "These results indicate that DHA is the precursor to potent protective mediators generated via enzymatic oxygenations to novel docosatrienes and 17S series resolvins that each regulate events of interest in inflammation and resolution." Hong S, Gronert K, Devchand PR, Moussignac RL, Serhan CN. Novel docosatrienes and 17S-resolvins generated from docosahexaenoic acid in murine brain, human blood, and glial cells. Autacoids in anti-inflammation. *J Biol Chem.* 2003 Apr 25;278(17):14677-87

Bioactive and Clinically Significant End-products of Omega-3 Fatty Acids

End-products from n-3 fatty acids generally have what are considered "health-promoting effects" which are generally weaker than and opposite to the end-products of the major n-6 fatty acid, arachidonate. Additionally, since n-3 fatty acids compete with the same metabolizing enzymes as do the n-6 family of fatty acids, a major portion of the "clinical effectiveness" of n-3 fatty acids comes not from the production of n-3 end-products but rather from the *impairment of the n-6 cascade*.

- **Prostaglandin E-3 (PG-E3)**
  - PG-E3 and EPA both reduce formation of arachidonate-derived eicosanoids[49]
- **Prostaglandin G-3 (PG-G3)**
  - Formed from EPA by cyclooxygenase (COX)
- **Prostaglandin H-3 (PG-H3)**
  - Formed from PG-G3 by peroxidase
- **Prostaglandin I-3 (PG-I3)**
  - Decreases platelet aggregation[50]
  - Causes vasodilation[51]
  - Possibly antiarrhythmic
  - Probably contributes to the hypotensive effect of fish oil[52]
- **Thromboxane A-3 (TX-A3)**
  - Biologically inert
- **Leukotriene B-5 (LT-B5)**
  - Significantly weaker than LT-B4; "functionally attenuated"[53]
  - May possess mild anti-inflammatory activity either directly or by reducing production of the more powerful arachidonate-derived LT-B4. [54]
- **Plasminogen activator inhibitor-1 (PAI-1)**
  - Increased with fish oil supplementation to maintain hemostasis
- **Docosatrienes**
  - Formed by (12-, 15-, 17-) lipoxygenase and cyclooxygenase-2 from DHA
  - Potent inhibitors of TNFa
  - Downregulate gene expression for proinflammatory IL-1
  - Reduce neutrophil entry to sites of inflammation
- **Resolvins**
  - Downregulate cytokine expression
  - Reduce neutrophil entry to sites of inflammation

[49] Erasmus U. Fats that heal, fats that kill. British Columbia Canada: Alive Books, 1993 Page 278
[50] Horrobin DF. Ascorbic acid and prostaglandin synthesis. *Subcell Biochem.* 1996;25:109-15
[51] Horrobin DF. Ascorbic acid and prostaglandin synthesis. *Subcell Biochem.* 1996;25:109-15
[52] Du Plooy WJ, Venter CP, Muntingh GM, Venter HL, Glatthaar II, Smith KA. The cumulative dose response effect of eicosapentaenoic and docosahexaenoic acid on blood pressure, plasma lipid profile and diet pattern in mild to moderate essential hypertensive black patients. *Prostaglandins Leukot Essent Fatty Acids* 1992 Aug;46(4):315-21
[53] Rubin D, Laposata M. Cellular interactions between n-6 and n-3 fatty acids: a mass analysis of fatty acid elongation/desaturation, distribution among complex lipids, and conversion to eicosanoids. *J Lipid Res.* 1992 Oct;33(10):1431-40
[54] Rubin D, Laposata M. Cellular interactions between n-6 and n-3 fatty acids: a mass analysis of fatty acid elongation/desaturation, distribution among complex lipids, and conversion to eicosanoids. *J Lipid Res.* 1992 Oct;33(10):1431-40

Metabolism of Omega-3 Fatty Acids and Related Eicosanoids

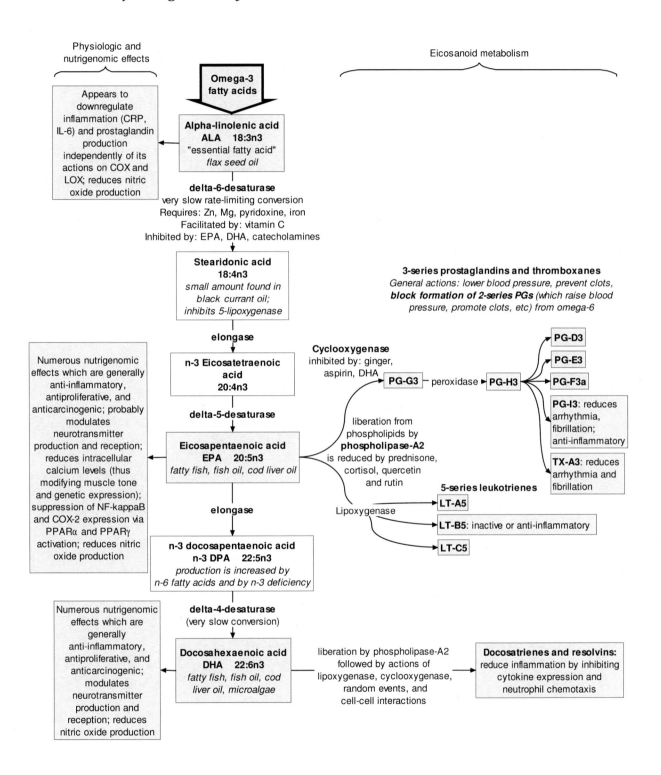

OMEGA-6—first double bond at 6th carbon from the methyl group

- **linoleic acid, LA, 18:2n6, linoleate**
    - <u>Essential fatty acid</u> from nut, seed, and vegetable oils, especially safflower oil, sunflower oil, corn oil, walnut oil, sesame seed oil, LA is the parent fatty acid of the omega-6 class,
    - EPA and DHA decrease conversion of linoleate to arachidonate; high doses of LA inhibit conversion of alpha-LNA to EPA and DHA due to competition for delta-6 desaturase
    - Hydrogenated "trans" forms are common in processed and fried foods,
    - LA favors oxidative modification of LDL cholesterol, increases platelet response to aggregation, and suppresses the immune system.[55] Adipose LA levels are positively correlated with CVD.
    - Promotes metastasis and inflammation.
    - LA is the predominant PUFA in US diets. Daily intake of linoleic acid is approximately 10 grams, only a small amount of which is converted to arachidonate.[56]
    - LA effectively lowers cholesterol, but otherwise this fatty acid is consistently associated with exacerbation of cancer and inflammation and thus should be avoided.
    - LA undergoes oxidative metabolism by 15-lipoxygenase-1 to form 13-S-HODE[57], and this is discussed in greater detail later in this section.

- **gamma (γ)-linolenic acid, GLA, 18:3n6, gamma-linolenate**
    - Formation is increased from linoleic acid by vitamin C[58]
    - Found in evening primrose oil, borage seed oil, hemp seed oil, and black currant seed oil
    - GLA restores action of delta-6-desaturase (D6D) in aging animals, suggesting that GLA intake should increase in older rats and humans
    - Useful in eczema for improvement in skin health and in diabetes especially for improvement in nerve function
    - GLA may facilitate the conversion of ALA to EPA and perhaps to DHA.
    - In patients who respond to GLA supplementation, we can reasonably hypothesize that they have impaired D-6-Desaturase activity since most patients have adequate dietary intake of LA. Therefore, by extension, we can suppose that their conversion of ALA to EPA is likewise impaired and that they may benefit from EPA supplementation.
    - Formation of GLA from LA is inhibited by EPA and other n-3 EFAs[59]
    - Overall, the weight of the research suggests that supplementation with GLA *does* lead to modest increases in arachidonate, despite the slow conversion of DGLA to arachidonate by delta-5 desaturase. Coadministration of EPA with GLA prevents any rise in arachidonate, as discussed later in this section.

- **Dihomo-gamma-linolenic acid, 20:3n6, DGLA, eicosatrienoic acid, eicosatrienoate**
    - DGLA eicosanoids have benefits for the cardiovascular system and have anti-inflammatory effects
    - Generally speaking, metabolites of DGLA are fewer in number and weaker in physiologic effect than the metabolites of arachidonic acid.
    - Vitamin C "has a significant effect in stimulating the conversion of DGLA into its metabolites…" at doses which are "…clinically relevant."[60]
    - DGLA levels are 34% lower than normal in patients with magnesium deficiency.[61]
    - Production is decreased with supplementation of ALA[62] and EPA and other n-3 EFAs except when GLA is provided directly[63]
    - Low levels of DGLA are associated with increased risk for stroke and myocardial infarction.[64] We could speculate that low levels of DGLA may be associated with pyridoxine or magnesium deficiency, of which are associated with cardiovascular disease.

[55] Simopoulos AP. Essential fatty acids in health and chronic disease. *Am J Clin Nutr.* 1999 Sep;70(3 Suppl):560S-569S
[56] Delvin TM. <u>Textbook of Biochemistry with Clinical Correlations.</u> New York: Wiley-Liss, 1997. Pages 431-441
[57] Shureiqi I, Lippman SM. Lipoxygenase modulation to reverse carcinogenesis. *Cancer Res.* 2001 Sep 1;61(17):6307-12
[58] Horrobin DF. Ascorbic acid and prostaglandin synthesis. *Subcell Biochem* 1996;25:109-15
[59] Horrobin DF. Interactions between n-3 and n-6 essential fatty acids (EFAs) in the regulation of cardiovascular disorders and inflammation. *Prostaglandins Leukot Essent Fatty Acids* 1991 Oct;44(2):127-31
[60] Horrobin DF. Ascorbic acid and prostaglandin synthesis. *Subcell Biochem.* 1996;25:109-15
[61] "…dihomogamma linoleic acid (20:3 n-6) was 34% lower..." Galland L. Impaired essential fatty acid metabolism in latent tetany. *Magnesium* 1985;4(5-6):333-8
[62] Simopoulos AP. Essential fatty acids in health and chronic disease. *Am J Clin Nutr.* 1999 Sep;70(3 Suppl):560S-569S
[63] Horrobin DF. Interactions between n-3 and n-6 essential fatty acids (EFAs) in the regulation of cardiovascular disorders and inflammation. *Prostaglandins Leukot Essent Fatty Acids.* 1991 Oct;44(2):127-31

- o DGLA metabolites reduce the formation of the arachidonate-derived 2-series prostaglandins, 4-series leukotrienes and platelet-activating factor.[65]
- **Arachidonic acid, 20:4n6, n-6 eicosatetraenoic acid, AA, ARA**
  - o Arachidonic acid is the predominant fatty acid in most tissues (diet-dependent!) acted upon by cyclooxygenase (to form prostaglandins and thromboxanes) and lipoxygenase (to form leukotrienes); it is the major n-6 in cell membranes and body tissues
  - o Liberated from phospholipids by phospholipase enzymes, most notably phospholipase A2.
  - o Most end-products of arachidonate metabolism are pro-inflammatory and are "in general harmful"[66] although arachidonate itself is a necessary component of phospholipids and sphingolipids in cell membranes.
  - o Arachidonate and its metabolites are referred to as eicosanoids.[67] Arachidonic acid is the predominant fatty acid in membrane phospholipids and is the preferred substrate for eicosanoid production relative to EPA.[68] Given that arachidonate's eicosanoids are biologically more powerful than those of EPA, we can accurately generalize that arachidonate and its respective prostaglandins and leukotrienes dominate the fatty acid and eicosanoid playground in both *quantitative* and *qualitative* respects. Therefore, successful intervention against arachidonate metabolism must consider 1) the quantity of arachidonate, 2) the balance of n-3 to n-6, and also 3) specific measures to hinder the production of the harmful arachidonate metabolites.
  - o Arachidonic acid is the direct precursor to the isoprostanes 8-iso prostaglandin-E2 (8-iso-PG-E2) and 8-iso prostaglandin-F2-alpha (8-iso-PG-F2-alpha), mediators that possess **inflammatory and hyperalgesic** properties and which are produced by the radical-mediated non-enzymatic peroxidation of arachidonate.[69] Inhibition of cyclooxygenase and/or lipoxygenase does not decrease the inflammatory and pain-producing effects of isoprostanes. Production of 8-iso-PG-F2-alpha is increased by and is a marker of oxidative stress. Obviously, inhibition of isoprostane formation is part of the biochemical and therefore clinical justification for antioxidant therapy in the treatment of painful orthopedic and rheumatic disorders. Supplemental ascorbic acid, tocopherols, and EPA have been shown to lower isoprostane levels in humans.
  - o Formation of arachidonate from DGLA is inhibited by EPA.[70]
  - o Formation of arachidonic metabolites is not increased by vitamin C.[71]
  - o The term "eicosatetraenoic acid" can apply to both 20:4n6 (arachidonic acid) of the omega-6 fatty acid family[72] and to 20:4n3 of the omega-3 fatty acid family. [73,74] Therefore, to avoid the confusion that would result from the use of the term "eicosatetraenoic acid" by itself, "n-6 eicosatetraenoic acid" should be used when referring to 20:4n6 (arachidonic acid) and "n-3 eicosatetraenoic acid" should be used when referring to 20:4n3.
  - o Liberation of arachidonic acid from membrane phospholipids phosphatidylcholine and phosphatidylinositol is increased by contact with IgE.[75] This finding presumably helps explain why inflammatory conditions are generally exacerbated by allergen exposure and why allergy elimination and anti-allergy immunomodulatory treatments result in a reduction in pain and inflammation.

[64] Horrobin DF. Interactions between n-3 and n-6 essential fatty acids (EFAs) in the regulation of cardiovascular disorders and inflammation. *Prostaglandins Leukot Essent Fatty Acids* 1991 Oct;44(2):127-31

[65] Fan YY, Chapkin RS. Importance of dietary gamma-linolenic acid in human health and nutrition. *J Nutr*. 1998 Sep;128(9):1411-4

[66] Horrobin DF. Ascorbic acid and prostaglandin synthesis. *Subcell Biochem*. 1996;25:109-15

[67] Delvin TM. Textbook of Biochemistry with Clinical Correlations. New York: Wiley-Liss, 1997. Pages 431-441

[68] Rubin D, Laposata M. Cellular interactions between n-6 and n-3 fatty acids: a mass analysis of fatty acid elongation/desaturation, distribution among complex lipids, and conversion to eicosanoids. *J Lipid Res*. 1992 Oct;33(10):1431-40

[69] Evans AR, Junger H, Southall MD, Nicol GD, Sorkin LS, Broome JT, Bailey TW, Vasko MR. Isoprostanes, novel eicosanoids that produce nociception and sensitize rat sensory neurons. *J Pharmacol Exp Ther*. 2000 Jun;293(3):912-20

[70] Horrobin DF. Interactions between n-3 and n-6 essential fatty acids (EFAs) in the regulation of cardiovascular disorders and inflammation. *Prostaglandins Leukot Essent Fatty Acids* 1991 Oct;44(2):127-31

[71] Horrobin DF. Ascorbic acid and prostaglandin synthesis. *Subcell Biochem*. 1996;25:109-15

[72] "5,8,11,14-eicosatetraenoic (20:4(n-6))" Mimouni V, Christiansen EN, Blond JP, Ulmann L, Poisson JP, Bezard J. Elongation and desaturation of arachidonic and eicosapentaenoic acids in rat liver. Effect of clofibrate feeding. *Biochim Biophys Acta*. 1991 Nov 27;1086(3):349-53

[73] Tapiero H, Ba GN, Couvreur P, Tew KD. Polyunsaturated fatty acids (PUFA) and eicosanoids in human health and pathologies. *Biomed Pharmacother*. 2002 Jul;56(5):215-22

[74] Erasmus U. Fats that heal, fats that kill. British Columbia Canada: Alive Books, 1993 Page 276

[75] McGlivery RW. Biochemistry: A Functional Approach. Third Edition. Philadelphia: WB Saunders, 1983. Pages 747-750

- o Elevated ARA may lead to altered binding of hormones, growth factors, neurotransmitters, and common food antigen peptides.
  - o Dietary ARA works synergistically with proinflammatory genotypes such as the variant 5-lipoxygenase alleles which are common in the general population: Africans (24%), Asians and Pacific Islanders (19.4%), other racial/ethnic groups (18.2%), Hispanics (3.6%), whites (3.1%), and the atherogenic effect of dietary arachidonic acid in these patients can be mitigated by dietary EPA.[76]
- **Adrenic acid, 22:4n6, docosatetraenoic acid**
  - o Little is known about this fatty acid.
  - o Concentrated in and may have a regulatory role in the adrenal glands.[77]
- **N-6 docosapentaenoic acid, 22:5n6**
  - o 22:5n6 is increased by n-3 fatty acid deficiency, especially in the brain cortex.[78]
  - o The term "docosapentaenoic acid" can apply to both 22:5n3 of the omega-3 fatty acid family[79,80] and to 22:5n6 of the omega-6 fatty acid family.[81,82,83] Therefore, because to use the term "docosapentaenoic acid" may be ambiguous, the terms "n-3 docosapentaenoic acid" should be used when discussing 22:5n3 and "n-6 docosapentaenoic acid" should be used when discussing 22:5n6.

DGLA metabolites formed by cyclooxygenase
- **Prostaglandin E-1 (PG-E1)**
  - o The main metabolite from DGLA.[84]
  - o Production is increased by vitamin C.[85]
  - o Decreases platelet aggregation.[86]
  - o Causes vasodilation.[87]
  - o Lowers blood pressure.[88]
  - o Inhibits cholesterol biosynthesis and lowers cholesterol levels in animals.[89]
  - o "A potent anti-inflammatory agent."[90]
  - o Probably the most potent PG with respect to bronchodilation.[91]
  - o Production is decreased by n-3 fatty acids.[92]
  - o May have a mood elevating effect insofar as levels are elevated in patients with mania, reduced in patients with depression, and are elevated by ethanol intake.[93]
  - o Certain biological properties of PG-E1 are 20 times stronger than those of PG-E2.[94]
  - o PG-E1 inhibits vascular smooth muscle cell proliferation in vitro.[95]

---

[76] Dwyer JH, Allayee H, Dwyer KM, Fan J, Wu H, Mar R, Lusis AJ, Mehrabian M. Arachidonate 5-lipoxygenase promoter genotype, dietary arachidonic acid, and atherosclerosis. *N Engl J Med.* 2004 Jan 1;350(1):29-37

[77] Horrobin DF. Ascorbic acid and prostaglandin synthesis. *Subcell Biochem.* 1996;25:109-15

[78] Retterstol K, Woldseth B, Christophersen BO. The metabolism of 22:5(-6) and of docosahexaenoic acid [22:6(-3)] compared in rat hepatocytes. *Biochim Biophys Acta.* 1996 Oct 18;1303(3):180-6

[79] "docosapentaenoic acid (22:5n-3)" Williard DE, Harmon SD, Kaduce TL, Preuss M, Moore SA, Robbins ME, Spector AA. Docosahexaenoic acid synthesis from n-3 polyunsaturated fatty acids in differentiated rat brain astrocytes. *J Lipid Res.* 2001 Sep;42(9):1368-76

[80] "…docosapentaenoic acid (22:5n-3)…" Takahashi R, Nassar BA, Huang YS, Begin ME, Horrobin DF. Effect of different ratios of dietary N-6 and N-3 fatty acids on fatty acid composition, prostaglandin formation and platelet aggregation in the rat. *Thromb Res.* 1987 Jul 15;47(2):135-46

[81] Retterstol K, Haugen TB, Christophersen BO. The pathway from arachidonic to docosapentaenoic acid (20:4n-6 to 22:5n-6) and from eicosapentaenoic to docosahexaenoic acid (20:5n-3 to 22:6n-3) studied in testicular cells from immature rats. *Biochim Biophys Acta.* 2000 Jan 3;1483(1):119-31

[82] "docosapentaenoic acid (DPAn-6)" Ahmad A, Murthy M, Greiner RS, Moriguchi T, Salem N Jr. A decrease in cell size accompanies a loss of docosahexaenoate in the rat hippocampus. *Nutr Neurosci.* 2002 Apr;5(2):103-13

[83] "The desaturation of adrenic acid to n-6 docosapentaenoic acid was decreased in the normo- and hyperglycemic diabetic rats." Mimouni V, Narce M, Huang YS, Horrobin DF, Poisson JP. Adrenic acid delta 4 desaturation and fatty acid composition in liver microsomes of spontaneously diabetic Wistar BB rats. *Prostaglandins Leukot Essent Fatty Acids.* 1994 Jan;50(1):43-7

[84] Horrobin DF. Ascorbic acid and prostaglandin synthesis. *Subcell Biochem* 1996;25:109-15

[85] Horrobin DF. Ascorbic acid and prostaglandin synthesis. *Subcell Biochem.* 1996;25:109-15

[86] Horrobin DF. Interactions between n-3 and n-6 essential fatty acids (EFAs) in the regulation of cardiovascular disorders and inflammation. *Prostaglandins Leukot Essent Fatty Acids* 1991 Oct;44(2):127-31

[87] Tapiero H, Ba GN, Couvreur P, Tew KD. Polyunsaturated fatty acids (PUFA) and eicosanoids in human health and pathologies. *Biomed Pharmacother.* 2002 Jul;56(5):215-22

[88] Horrobin DF. Interactions between n-3 and n-6 essential fatty acids (EFAs) in the regulation of cardiovascular disorders and inflammation. *Prostaglandins Leukot Essent Fatty Acids* 1991 Oct;44(2):127-31

[89] Horrobin DF. Interactions between n-3 and n-6 essential fatty acids (EFAs) in the regulation of cardiovascular disorders and inflammation. *Prostaglandins Leukot Essent Fatty Acids* 1991 Oct;44(2):127-31

[90] Horrobin DF. Ascorbic acid and prostaglandin synthesis. *Subcell Biochem.* 1996;25:109-15

[91] Horrobin DF. Ascorbic acid and prostaglandin synthesis. *Subcell Biochem.* 1996;25:109-15

[92] Rubin D, Laposata M. Cellular interactions between n-6 and n-3 fatty acids: a mass analysis of fatty acid elongation/desaturation, distribution among complex lipids, and conversion to eicosanoids. *J Lipid Res.* 1992 Oct;33(10):1431-40

[93] Horrobin DF, Manku MS. Possible role of prostaglandin E1 in the affective disorders and in alcoholism. *Br Med J.* 1980 Jun 7;280(6228):1363-6

[94] Fan YY, Chapkin RS. Importance of dietary gamma-linolenic acid in human health and nutrition. *J Nutr.* 1998 Sep;128(9):1411-4

[95] Fan YY, Chapkin RS. Importance of dietary gamma-linolenic acid in human health and nutrition. *J Nutr.* 1998 Sep;128(9):1411-4

DGLA metabolites formed by 15-lipoxygenase

- **15-hydroxy-eicosatrienoic acid, 15-OH-DGLA, 15-OH-20:3n-6, 15-HETrE**
  - Potent anti-inflammatory action and inhibition of arachidonic acid cascade via inhibition of 5-lipoxygenase and 12-lipoxygenase.[96,97]

Arachidonic acid metabolites formed by cyclooxygenase

- **Thromboxane A-2 (TX-A2)**
  - Causes platelet aggregation[98] and vasoconstriction.[99]
  - Promotes cardiac arrhythmias and hypertension.
  - Considered much more powerful than the thromboxanes derived from EPA and DGLA.
  - Precursor to TX-B2.
- **Thromboxane B2**
  - Inactive[100]
- **Prostaglandin I2,PG-I2, prostacyclin**
  - Commonly considered one of the only desirable/beneficial end-products of arachidonic acid metabolism[101] despite the little known fact that increases nociception and thus promotes hyperalgesia.[102]
  - Production is increased by vitamin C.[103]
  - Decreases platelet aggregation.
  - Causes vasodilation[104] and lowers blood pressure.[105,106]
  - Formed from PG-H2 via prostacyclin synthase.[107]
- **Prostaglandin D2, PG-D2**
  - Causes bronchoconstriction, smooth muscle contraction, and hypotension and is the major arachidonate-cyclooxygenase product produced in mast cells.[108]
  - Accentuates production of histamine and can trigger release of histamine from mast cells in the absence of IgE binding.
- **Prostaglandin E2, PG-E2**
  - Produced from arachidonic acid by cyclooxygenase. PG-E2 increases expression of cyclooxygenase and IL-6; thus inflammation manifested by an increase in PG-E2 leads to additive expression of cyclooxygenase, which further increases inflammation.[109]
  - Suppresses lymphocyte proliferation and natural killer cell activity[110]; appears to cause stimulation of "suppressor cells"
  - Released by tumor cells and suppressor cells
  - Promotes chemotaxis
  - Increases platelet aggregation
  - Causes relaxation of bronchus and uterus smooth muscle in nonpregnant animals and uterine contractions in pregnant animals[111]
  - PG-E2 causes pain and also but increases the intensity and duration of pain sensations that are mediated by other triggers such as histamine and bradykinin[112]

[96] Horrobin DF. Interactions between n-3 and n-6 essential fatty acids (EFAs) in the regulation of cardiovascular disorders and inflammation. *Prostaglandins Leukot Essent Fatty Acids* 1991 Oct;44(2):127-31
[97] Fan YY, Chapkin RS. Importance of dietary gamma-linolenic acid in human health and nutrition. *J Nutr.* 1998 Sep;128(9):1411-4
[98] Delvin TM. Textbook of Biochemistry with Clinical Correlations. New York: Wiley-Liss, 1997. Pages 431-441
[99] Horrobin DF. Ascorbic acid and prostaglandin synthesis. *Subcell Biochem* 1996;25:109-15
[100] Delvin TM. Textbook of Biochemistry with Clinical Correlations. New York: Wiley-Liss, 1997. Pages 431-441
[101] Horrobin DF. Ascorbic acid and prostaglandin synthesis. *Subcell Biochem.* 1996;25:109-15
[102] Evans AR, Junger H, Southall MD, Nicol GD, Sorkin LS, Broome JT, Bailey TW, Vasko MR. Isoprostanes, novel eicosanoids that produce nociception and sensitize rat sensory neurons. *J Pharmacol Exp Ther.* 2000 Jun;293(3):912-20
[103] Horrobin DF. Ascorbic acid and prostaglandin synthesis. *Subcell Biochem.* 1996;25:109-15
[104] Horrobin DF. Ascorbic acid and prostaglandin synthesis. *Subcell Biochem.* 1996;25:109-15
[105] Delvin TM. Textbook of Biochemistry with Clinical Correlations. New York: Wiley-Liss, 1997. Pages 431-441
[106] Tapiero H, Ba GN, Couvreur P, Tew KD. Polyunsaturated fatty acids (PUFA) and eicosanoids in human health and pathologies. *Biomed Pharmacother.* 2002 Jul;56(5):215-22
[107] "Prostacyclin synthase catalyzes an intramolecular redox reaction in which prostaglandin endoperoxide, PGH2, is converted to prostacyclin." http://www.oxfordbiomed.com/pg61prossyn.html on September 6, 2006
[108] Peters SP, Schleimer RP, Kagey-Sobotka A, Naclerio RM, MacGlashan DW Jr, Schulman ES, Adkinson NF Jr, Lichtenstein LM. The role of prostaglandin D2 in IgE-mediated reactions in man. *Trans Assoc Am Physicians.* 1982;95:221-8
[109] Bagga D, Wang L, Farias-Eisner R, Glaspy JA, Reddy ST. Differential effects of prostaglandin derived from omega-6 and omega-3 polyunsaturated fatty acids on COX-2 expression and IL-6 secretion. *Proc Natl Acad Sci U S A.* 2003 Feb 18;100(4):1751-6. Available at http://www.pnas.org/cgi/reprint/100/4/1751.pdf
[110] Calder PC. Long-chain n-3 fatty acids and inflammation: potential application in surgical and trauma patients. *Braz J Med Biol Res.* 2003 Apr;36(4):433-46
[111] McGlivery RW. Biochemistry: A Functional Approach. Third Edition. Philadelphia: WB Saunders, 1983. Pages 747-750
[112] Calder PC. Long-chain n-3 fatty acids and inflammation: potential application in surgical and trauma patients. *Braz J Med Biol Res.* 2003 Apr;36(4):433-46

- o Increases IgE production[113]
- o Increases vascular permeability and vasodilation thus enhancing edema[114]
- o Promotes action of epidermal growth factor[115]
- o Production is decreased by n-3 fatty acids[116]
- **Prostaglandin F2-alpha, PG-F2a, PG-F2α**
  - o Promotes bronchoconstriction and uterine contractions
  - o Increased levels associated with dysmenorrhea
  - o Increased production with vitamin C deficiency, formation is reduced by vitamin C, and low levels of vitamin C are seen in women with dysmenorrhea.[117]
  - o Promotes formation of MMP-2 and other collagenases that promote joint destruction in various types of arthritis and are required by metastasizing cancer cells to penetrate basement membranes
- **Prostaglandin G2 (PG-G2)**
  - o Induces rapid and irreversible platelet aggregation[118]
- **Prostaglandin H2 (PG-H2)**
  - o Induces rapid and irreversible platelet aggregation[119]

Linoleic acid metabolites formed by lipoxygenases
- **13-S-HODE, 13-S-hydroxyoctadecadienoic acid**
  - o 13-S-HODE is formed from linolenic acid by 15-LOX-1 and is generally considered to have anticancer actions[120]
  - o 13-S-HODE inhibits ornithine decarboxylase[121]

Arachidonic acid metabolites formed by lipoxygenases
- **5-hydroperoxyeicosatetraenoic acid, 5-HPETE**
  - o HPETEs are converted to their respective HETEs either spontaneously or by peroxidases.[122]
  - o 5-hydroxyeicosatetraenoic acid is known to reduce the depolarization threshold of primary afferent neurons and may thus lead to pain
  - o Reinforces activation of 5-lipoxygenase
  - o May be directly cytotoxic
  - o Necessary for the formation of MMP-2 and other collagenases that promote joint destruction in various types of arthritis and are required by metastasizing cancer cells to penetrate basement membranes; formation is inhibited by the lipoxygenase inhibitors esculetin and caffeic acid[123]
  - o 5-HPETE is the major lipoxygenase product in inflamed tissues and promotes chemotaxis and neutrophil degranulation of lysosomal hydrolytic enzymes[124]
  - o 5-HPETE is considered to have pro-cancer actions and facilitates production of proteolytic enzymes that promote joint destruction and tumor invasiveness[125]
- **5-HETE, 5-S-HETE**
  - o 5-HETE is considered to have pro-cancer actions by blocking apoptosis in cancer cells and promoting tumor growth[126]
- **8-S-HETE**
  - o 8-S-HETE is genotoxic and promotes cancer development[127]

[113] Calder PC. Long-chain n-3 fatty acids and inflammation: potential application in surgical and trauma patients. *Braz J Med Biol Res.* 2003 Apr;36(4):433-46
[114] Calder PC. Long-chain n-3 fatty acids and inflammation: potential application in surgical and trauma patients. *Braz J Med Biol Res.* 2003 Apr;36(4):433-46
[115] Tapiero H, Ba GN, Couvreur P, Tew KD. Polyunsaturated fatty acids (PUFA) and eicosanoids in human health and pathologies. *Biomed Pharmacother.* 2002;56(5):215-22
[116] Rubin D, Laposata M. Cellular interactions between n-6 and n-3 fatty acids: a mass analysis of fatty acid elongation/desaturation, distribution among complex lipids, and conversion to eicosanoids. *J Lipid Res.* 1992 Oct;33(10):1431-40
[117] Horrobin DF. Ascorbic acid and prostaglandin synthesis. *Subcell Biochem* 1996;25:109-15
[118] McGlivery RW. Biochemistry: A Functional Approach. Third Edition. Philadelphia: WB Saunders, 1983. Pages 747-750
[119] McGlivery RW. Biochemistry: A Functional Approach. Third Edition. Philadelphia: WB Saunders, 1983. Pages 747-750
[120] Shureiqi I, Lippman SM. Lipoxygenase modulation to reverse carcinogenesis. *Cancer Res.* 2001 Sep 1;61(17):6307-12
[121] Shureiqi I, Lippman SM. Lipoxygenase modulation to reverse carcinogenesis. *Cancer Res.* 2001 Sep 1;61(17):6307-12
[122] Delvin TM. Textbook of Biochemistry with Clinical Correlations. New York: Wiley-Liss, 1997. Pages 431-441
[123] Reich R, Martin GR. Identification of arachidonic acid pathways required for the invasive and metastatic activity of malignant tumor cells. *Prostaglandins* 1996 Jan;51(1):1-17
[124] Delvin TM. Textbook of Biochemistry with Clinical Correlations. New York: Wiley-Liss, 1997. Pages 431-441
[125] "Specific metabolites of each pathway, i.e. PGF2 alpha and 5-HPETE, are able to transcend the block and restore collagenase production, invasiveness in vitro and metastatic activity in vivo." Reich R, Martin GR. Identification of arachidonic acid pathways required for the invasive and metastatic activity of malignant tumor cells. *Prostaglandins* 1996 Jan;51(1):1-17
[126] Shureiqi I, Lippman SM. Lipoxygenase modulation to reverse carcinogenesis. *Cancer Res.* 2001 Sep 1;61(17):6307-12
[127] Shureiqi I, Lippman SM. Lipoxygenase modulation to reverse carcinogenesis. *Cancer Res.* 2001 Sep 1;61(17):6307-12

- **12-HPETE, 12-hydroperoxyeicosatetraenoic acid, 12-hydroperoxyeicosatetraenoate,**
  - 12-HPETE is the major lipoxygenase product in platelets and the pancreas[128]
- **12-R-HETE**
  - 12-R-HETE is produced by 12-R-LOX and promotes proliferation of colon cancer cells[129]
- **12-S-HETE**
  - 12-S-HETE promotes tumor growth by several mechanisms, including 1) "up-regulating adhesion molecules and increasing the adhesion of tumor cells to the microvessel endothelium," 2) "…promoting tumor spread,"" and 3) inhibiting apoptosis[130]
  - Expression of 12-S-LOX and presumably therefore production of 12-S-HETE is directly correlated with aggressiveness, stage, and grade in human prostate cancer[131]
- **15-hydroperoxyeicosatetraenoic acid, 15-HPETE, 15-hydroperoxyeicosatetraenoate**
  - 15-HPETE is the major lipoxygenase product in eosinophils, T-lymphocytes, and the trachea[132]
- **15-S-HETE**
  - 15-S-HETE is formed from arachidonic acid by the action of 15-LOX-2 and appears to have anticancer action, yet the data on this are conflicting[133]
- **Leukotriene B4: LT-B4**
  - Promotes immunosuppression via inhibition of CD4 cells and promotion of proliferation of CD8 cells.[134]
  - Promotes edema: increases vascular permeability, enhances local blood flow, is a potent chemotactic agent for leukocytes,
  - Exacerbates tissue damage: induces release of lysosomal enzymes, increases production of reactive oxygen species, TNF-a, IL-1, and IL-6[135]
  - Associated with accelerated atherosclerosis in patients with proinflammatory variants of 5-lipoxygenase[136]
  - Production is increased by dietary arachidonic acid and production is reduced by EPA.[137]
  - LT-B4 inhibits apoptosis in cancer cells and is generally considered procarcinogenic.[138]
- **LT-C4 and LT-D4 and LT-E4:**
  - Promote muscle contraction, bronchoconstriction, intestinal muscle contraction,
  - Promote increased capillary permeability which results in edema
  - More powerful than histamine in promotion of "allergic" symptoms[139]
  - Patients with severe asthma have elevated levels of LT-E4 that are not reduced with steroid treatment.[140]

---

[128] Delvin TM. <u>Textbook of Biochemistry with Clinical Correlations</u>. New York: Wiley-Liss, 1997. Pages 431-441
[129] Shureiqi I, Lippman SM. Lipoxygenase modulation to reverse carcinogenesis. *Cancer Res.* 2001 Sep 1;61(17):6307-12
[130] Shureiqi I, Lippman SM. Lipoxygenase modulation to reverse carcinogenesis. *Cancer Res.* 2001 Sep 1;61(17):6307-12
[131] Shureiqi I, Lippman SM. Lipoxygenase modulation to reverse carcinogenesis. *Cancer Res.* 2001 Sep 1;61(17):6307-12
[132] Delvin TM. <u>Textbook of Biochemistry with Clinical Correlations</u>. New York: Wiley-Liss, 1997. Pages 431-441
[133] Shureiqi I, Lippman SM. Lipoxygenase modulation to reverse carcinogenesis. *Cancer Res.* 2001 Sep 1;61(17):6307-12
[134] Delvin TM. <u>Textbook of Biochemistry with Clinical Correlations</u>. New York: Wiley-Liss, 1997. Pages 431-441
[135] Calder PC. Long-chain n-3 fatty acids and inflammation: potential application in surgical and trauma patients. *Braz J Med Biol Res.* 2003 Apr;36(4):433-46
[136] Dwyer JH, Allayee H, Dwyer KM, Fan J, Wu H, Mar R, Lusis AJ, Mehrabian M. Arachidonate 5-lipoxygenase promoter genotype, dietary arachidonic acid, and atherosclerosis. *N Engl J Med.* 2004 Jan 1;350(1):29-37
[137] Dwyer JH, Allayee H, Dwyer KM, Fan J, Wu H, Mar R, Lusis AJ, Mehrabian M. Arachidonate 5-lipoxygenase promoter genotype, dietary arachidonic acid, and atherosclerosis. *N Engl J Med.* 2004 Jan 1;350(1):29-37
[138] Shureiqi I, Lippman SM. Lipoxygenase modulation to reverse carcinogenesis. *Cancer Res.* 2001 Sep 1;61(17):6307-12
[139] Delvin TM. <u>Textbook of Biochemistry with Clinical Correlations</u>. New York: Wiley-Liss, 1997. Pages 431-441
[140] Vachier I, Kumlin M, Dahlen SE, Bousquet J, Godard P, Chanez P. High levels of urinary leukotriene E4 excretion in steroid treated patients with severe asthma. *Respir Med.* 2003 Nov;97(11):1225-9

Metabolism of Omega-6 Fatty Acids and Related Eicosanoids

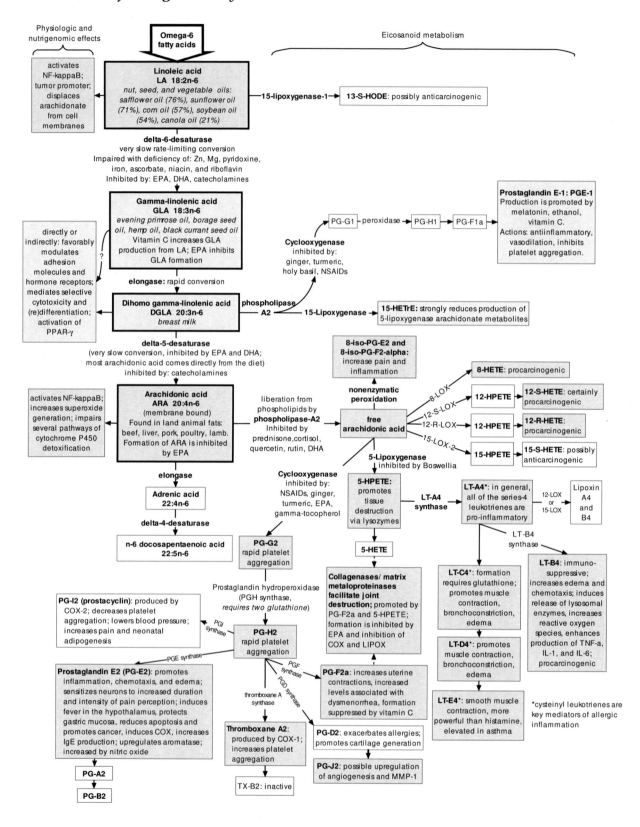

Important Enzymes in Fatty Acid Metabolism

Fatty acids are converted to other fatty acids in the same family by the desaturase and elongase enzymes. The major "direction" of these reactions is depicted in the diagrams; however these reactions, like nearly all enzymatic reactions, are reversible to a limited extent. Fatty acids are converted to biologically active end-products by enzymes such as the cyclooxygenases, lipoxygenases, cytochrome P-450 enzymes and by nonenzymatic conversion. Four important concepts need to be understood in relation to the enzymes that interconvert fatty acids:

1) **These enzymes do not work with equal efficiency**, and thus their end-products may not be produced in sufficient amounts to be biologically or clinically significant. Therefore, *on paper*, the cascade of fatty acid metabolism appears to flow easily from one fatty acid to its downstream progeny; in reality however, this process is often slow and therefore not immediately reliable when one is looking for rapid and reliable clinical results. The desaturase enzymes are slow and rate limiting, whereas the elongase enzymes function efficiently and rapidly. For example, Horrobin noted, "Because the 6-desaturation step is so rate-limiting, it is impossible to produce any significant elevation of DGLA levels in humans by increasing linoleic acid intake."[141]

2) **These enzymes are subject to significant interpatient variability** due to inherited and acquired factors that can reduce enzyme activity. For example, many patients (especially those with eczema and diabetes) have extreme reductions in the activity of delta-6-desaturase, the rate-limiting enzyme in the fatty acid cascades from ALA and LA. When delta-6-desaturase is slow to perform its conversions, synthesis of all downstream fatty acids is greatly reduced.

3) **These enzymes, like all enzymes, require cofactors.** If the patient is deficient in cofactors, the efficiency of enzymatic conversions is greatly impaired. Since micronutrient deficiencies are common even in developed countries, and since people can have clinically significant micronutrient deficiencies (i.e., "marginal malnutrition"[142]) yet still be "apparently healthy", a wise clinical strategy is to ensure that the patient's micronutrient status is adequate by encouraging the patient to consume a nutritious organic[143] whole foods diet along with a high-potency broad-spectrum multivitamin and multimineral supplement. Patients with magnesium deficiency show impaired fatty acid metabolism because desaturase enzymes are unable to function properly without sufficient magnesium.[144] Animal studies suggest that vitamin B-6 deficiency can reduce the function of delta-6-desaturase by 64% and lead to a reduction in EPA and DHA.[145]

4) **Substrates compete for enzymatic conversion.** In several instances, the same enzyme must act upon two different fatty acids in two different omega families. For example, delta-6-desaturase converts the omega-3 linolenic acid to stearidonic acid, yet this same enzyme also converts the omega-6 linoleic acid to gamma-linolenic acid. If the diet contains an absolute or relative excess of linoleic acid, then on a molecular and functional level, this excess linoleic acid will disproportionately utilize delta-6-desaturase and conversion of available linoleic acid to gamma-linolenic acid will be reduced. As reviewed by Dupont[146], "A competitive interaction between fatty acids exists so that those of the [alpha-linolenic acid, omega-3] family suppress the metabolism of those of the [linoleic acid, omega-6] family, and the [linoleic acid, omega-6] family suppress metabolism of the [linolenic acid, omega-3] family although less strongly. Both the [linoleic acid, omega-6] and [alpha-linolenic acid, omega-3] fatty acids suppress metabolism of the [oleic acid, omega-9] fatty acids." Stated more plainly by Pizzorno[147], "...a relative excess of one fatty acid will tend to hog an enzyme system, resulting in decreased conversion of the other fatty acids." In reviewing clinical evidence that EPA

[141] Horrobin DF. Interactions between n-3 and n-6 essential fatty acids (EFAs) in the regulation of cardiovascular disorders and inflammation. *Prostaglandins Leukot Essent Fatty Acids*. 1991 Oct;44(2):127-31
[142] Allen LH. The nutrition CRSP: what is marginal malnutrition, and does it affect human function? *Nutr Rev*. 1993 Sep;51(9):255-67
[143] Bob Smith. *Journal of Applied Nutrition* 1993; 45: 35-39
[144] Galland L. Impaired essential fatty acid metabolism in latent tetany. *Magnesium*. 1985;4(5-6):333-8
[145] Tsuge H, Hotta N, Hayakawa T. Effects of vitamin B-6 on (n-3) polyunsaturated fatty acid metabolism. *J Nutr*. 2000 Feb;130(2S Suppl):333S-334S
[146] Dupont J. Lipids. In: Brown ML (ed). Present Knowledge in Nutrition. Sixth Edition. Washington DC: International Life Sciences Institute Nutrition Foundation;1990page 62
[147] Pizzorno JE. Total Wellness. Rocklin: Prima; 1996 page 170

supplementation leads to significant reductions (50%) in DGLA levels, Horrobin[148] noted, "However, the n-3 EFAs are much more effective in inhibiting n-6 EFA metabolism than vice versa." A practical example: in a patient who is deficient in both omega-3 and omega-6 fatty acids, supplementation exclusively with flax oil will exacerbate the deficiency of gamma-linolenic acid.

- **Delta-6-desaturase (D6D):**
  - In omega-3 fatty acid metabolism, D6D converts linolenic acid to stearidonic acid. In omega-6 fatty acid metabolism, D6D converts linoleic acid to gamma-linolenic acid. D6D is the rate-limiting enzyme in fatty acid metabolism, meaning that it is the slowest functioning enzyme in the cascade of fatty acid conversions. Recall that in biochemistry the first enzyme in a series of biochemical reactions tends to be the rate-limiting enzyme for the sake of avoiding unnecessary downstream conversions. D6D is inhibited by trans fatty acids.[149] Action of this enzyme is increased during essential fatty acid deficiency.[150] Patients with eczema and diabetes have been noted to have defects in the function of D6D.[151]
  - Efficient function of D6D requires iron, magnesium, zinc, pyridoxine, niacin, and riboflavin. Administration of supraphysiologic doses of enzyme cofactors can improve function of defective or mutated enzymes.[152]
  - The catecholamines epinephrine and norepinephrine inhibit D5D and D6D.[153]
- **Delta-5-desaturase (D5D):**
  - In omega-6 fatty acid metabolism, D5D converts DGLA to arachidonic acid. However, this enzyme is slow, so that virtually all arachidonic acid found in body tissues originated from the consumption of land animal fats/meats[154] such as beef, liver, pork, lamb, and poultry. Additionally, some people (such as those with X-linked retinitis pigmentosa[155]) have reduced action of D5D and therefore have low levels of DHA. D5D is inhibited by EPA.[156] Released in increased amounts during stress and anxiety, the catecholamines epinephrine and norepinephrine inhibit D5D and D6D.[157]
- **Delta-4-desaturase**
  - Action of this enzyme is increased during essential fatty acid deficiency.[158]
- **Elongase**: These enzymes efficiently add carbon groups to the fatty acid chain.
- **Prostaglandin synthase complex (PGS)**: This is the major enzyme system that is responsible for prostaglandin biosynthesis. PGS includes phospholipase A2 and cyclooxygenase.[159]
- **Phospholipase-A2**
  - Crucial to the arachidonic acid cascade since cyclooxygenase can act only on free arachidonate (i.e., after arachidonate has been liberated from membrane phospholipids); this is the rate-limiting step in the formation of arachidonate-derived prostaglandins.[160]
  - Contact of IgE with mast cells stimulates the release of arachidonate, which must occur via phospholipase A2[161]
  - Inhibited by adrenal steroids (cortisol) and prednisone

[148] Horrobin DF. Interactions between n-3 and n-6 essential fatty acids (EFAs) in the regulation of cardiovascular disorders and inflammation. *Prostaglandins Leukot Essent Fatty Acids.* 1991 Oct;44(2):127-31
[149] Simopoulos AP. Essential fatty acids in health and chronic disease. *Am J Clin Nutr.* 1999 Sep;70(3 Suppl):560S-569S
[150] "The delta 4 desaturase activity is increased in essential fatty acid deficiency similar to delta 6 desaturase." Christophersen BO, Hagve TA, Christensen E, Johansen Y, Tverdal S. Eicosapentaenoic- and arachidonic acid metabolism in isolated liver cells. *Scand J Clin Lab Invest Suppl.* 1986;184:55-60
[151] "This concept is illustrated by atopic eczema and diabetes, which may represent inherited and acquired examples of inadequate delta-6-desaturation." Horrobin DF. Fatty acid metabolism in health and disease: the role of delta-6-desaturase. *Am J Clin Nutr.* 1993 May;57(5 Suppl):732S-736S
[152] Ames BN, Elson-Schwab I, Silver EA. High-dose vitamin therapy stimulates variant enzymes with decreased coenzyme binding affinity (increased K(m)): relevance to genetic disease and polymorphisms. *Am J Clin Nutr.* 2002 Apr;75(4):616-58
[153] Mamalakis G, Kafatos A, Tornaritis M, Alevizos B. Anxiety and adipose essential fatty acid precursors for prostaglandin E1 and E2. *J Am Coll Nutr.* 1998 Jun;17(3):239-43
[154] Pizzorno JE. Total Wellness. Rocklin: Prima; 1996 page 169
[155] Hoffman DR, DeMar JC, Heird WC, Birch DG, Anderson RE. Impaired synthesis of DHA in patients with X-linked retinitis pigmentosa. *J Lipid Res* 2001 Sep;42(9):1395-401 This article is available on-line at http://www.jlr.org/cgi/reprint/42/9/1395.pdf as of December 26, 2003
[156] Barham JB, Edens MB, Fonteh AN, Johnson MM, Easter L, Chilton FH. Addition of eicosapentaenoic acid to gamma-linolenic acid-supplemented diets prevents serum arachidonic acid accumulation in humans. *J Nutr.* 2000 Aug;130(8):1925-31
[157] Mamalakis G, Kafatos A, Tornaritis M, Alevizos B. Anxiety and adipose essential fatty acid precursors for prostaglandin E1 and E2. *J Am Coll Nutr.* 1998 Jun;17(3):239-43
[158] "The delta 4 desaturase activity is increased in essential fatty acid deficiency similar to delta 6 desaturase." Christophersen BO, Hagve TA, Christensen E, Johansen Y, Tverdal S. Eicosapentaenoic- and arachidonic acid metabolism in isolated liver cells. *Scand J Clin Lab Invest Suppl.* 1986;184:55-60
[159] Delvin TM. Textbook of Biochemistry with Clinical Correlations. New York: Wiley-Liss, 1997. Pages 431-441
[160] Delvin TM. Textbook of Biochemistry with Clinical Correlations. New York: Wiley-Liss, 1997. Pages 431-441
[161] McGlivery RW. Biochemistry: A Functional Approach. Third Edition. Philadelphia: WB Saunders, 1983. Pages 747-750

- **Cyclooxygenase (COX) (also called "prostaglandin synthase" or "PGS" or "prostaglandin endoperoxide synthase")**
    - o COX-1 is "constitutive" and is found in all cells, while COX-2 is inducible by stimulation from monocytes/macrophages following stimulation by PAF, IL-1, or bacterial lipopolysaccharide; its induction is inhibited by glucocorticoids.[162]
    - o COX is irreversibly inhibited following acetylation by aspirin.
    - o The expression of COX is inhibited by glucocorticoids,[163] which also inhibit phospholipase A2.
    - o **COX forms TXs and PGs, while LIPOX form LTs.**
    - o The COX metabolite PG-F2alpha is necessary for the formation of matrix metalloproteinase-2 and other collagenases which are utilized for the destruction of connective tissue[164]
    - o **COX is apparently activated by either n-6 fatty acids or the oxidized metabolites of n-6 fatty acids.[165] Therefore, consumption of n-6 fatty acids alone—*without trauma or inflammatory stimuli*—is sufficient for the increased production of the harmful arachidonate-derived prostaglandins and leukotrienes.** Thus, by definition, a diet high in n-6 fatty acids may subtly yet significantly promote pain, inflammation, joint destruction, and cancer.
    - o A well-established consequence of inhibiting COX is that of increasing LIPOX metabolites. Inhibiting COX will decrease COX metabolites, yet will cause an increase in LIPOX metabolites because of increased substrate levels; i.e., the liberated arachidonate that is not metabolized by COX is now available to be metabolized by LIPOX. Thus, inhibiting COX produces a "metabolic shunt" effect that increases production of inflammatory mediators such as HETE and the leukotrienes. Additionally, inhibition of COX inhibits formation of the beneficial anti-inflammatory DGLA metabolites.
    - o Arachidonate metabolites from COX function for the most part to increase inflammation and pain.[166]
    - o Increased expression of COX-2 increases production of PG-E2 and has been associated with increased production of anti-apoptotic proteins and a reduction in pro-apoptotic proteins in cultured rat intestinal cells.[167]
    - o The activity of lipoxygenase and cyclooxygenase produces reactive oxygen species (ROS) intermediates.
    - o The paradox of how a single enzyme such as cyclooxygenase can produce such a wide array of metabolites from a single substrate such as arachidonic acid is solved by recognizing that arachidonate is three-dimensionally rearranged once within the cyclooxygenase enzyme and that these random arrangements favor the production of different metabolites by the preferential molecular modification of the original arachidonate.[168] Additionally, cyclooxygenase may become slightly rearranged as well, thus further promoting the heterogeneity of progeny.
- **Lipoxygenases**: a family of enzymes that form leukotrienes
    - o Corneal lipoxygenase is inhibited by vitamin C[169]
    - o The activity of lipoxygenase and cyclooxygenase produce ROS intermediates
    - o **5-lipoxygenase, 5-LOX**

---

[162] Delvin TM. <u>Textbook of Biochemistry with Clinical Correlations</u>. New York: Wiley-Liss, 1997. Pages 431-441

[163] Tapiero H, Ba GN, Couvreur P, Tew KD. Polyunsaturated fatty acids (PUFA) and eicosanoids in human health and pathologies. *Biomed Pharmacother*. 2002;56(5):215-22

[164] "Specific metabolites of each pathway, i.e. PGF2 alpha and 5-HPETE, are able to transcend the block and restore collagenase production, invasiveness in vitro and metastatic activity in vivo." Reich R, Martin GR. Identification of arachidonic acid pathways required for the invasive and metastatic activity of malignant tumor cells. *Prostaglandins* 1996 Jan;51(1):1-17

[165] "…due to activation of cyclooxygenase either by oxygenated metabolites of n-6 fatty acids or by the n-6 fatty acids themselves." Rubin D, Laposata M. Cellular interactions between n-6 and n-3 fatty acids: a mass analysis of fatty acid elongation/desaturation, distribution among complex lipids, and conversion to eicosanoids. *J Lipid Res*. 1992 Oct;33(10):1431-40

[166] Tapiero H, Ba GN, Couvreur P, Tew KD. Polyunsaturated fatty acids (PUFA) and eicosanoids in human health and pathologies. *Biomed Pharmacother*. 2002;56(5):215-22

[167] Tapiero H, Ba GN, Couvreur P, Tew KD. Polyunsaturated fatty acids (PUFA) and eicosanoids in human health and pathologies. *Biomed Pharmacother*. 2002;56(5):215-22

[168] Thuresson ED, Lakkides KM, Smith WL. Different catalytically competent arrangements of arachidonic acid within the cyclooxygenase active site of prostaglandin endoperoxide H synthase-1 lead to the formation of different oxygenated products. *J Biol Chem*. 2000 Mar 24;275(12):8501-7 Available on-line at http://www.jbc.org/cgi/reprint/275/12/8501 on March 16, 2004

[169] Horrobin DF. Ascorbic acid and prostaglandin synthesis. *Subcell Biochem* 1996;25:109-15

- This is a pro-inflammatory enzyme that has different basal levels of activity in different people and in different disease conditions. Proinflammatory variances of this enzyme are seen in Africans (24%), Asians and Pacific Islanders (19.4%), other racial/ethnic groups (18.2%), Hispanics (3.6%) and whites (3.1%) and are associated with accelerated atherosclerosis and elevations in CRP especially when the diet is high in arachidonic acid and low in EPA.[170]
- 5-LOX has been described as "procarcinogenic" due to its role in producing LT-B4 which has mitogenic and anti-apoptotic actions[171]
- The 5-LOX metabolite 5-HPETE is necessary for the formation of matrix metalloproteinase-2 and other collagenases which are utilized for the destruction of connective tissue[172]
  - **8-lipoxygenase, 8-LOX**
    - 8-LOX is upregulated in animal models of cancer and has been described as "procarcinogenic" due to its role in producing 8-HETE, which has genotoxic effects and which is found in humans[173]
  - **12-R-lipoxygenase, 12-R-LOX**
    - 12-R-LOX has been described as "procarcinogenic" due to its role in producing 12-R-HETE[174]
  - **12-S-lipoxygenase, 12-S-LOX**
    - 12-S-LOX has been described as "procarcinogenic" due to its role in producing 12-S-HETE[175]
    - Expression of 12-S-LOX is directly correlated with aggressiveness, stage, and grade in human prostate cancer[176]
  - **15-lipoxygenase-1, 15-LOX-1**
    - 15-LOX-1 metabolizes n-6 linoleic acid into 13-S-HODE, which appears to have *anti*cancer actions[177]
  - **15-lipoxygenase-2, 15-LOX-2**
    - 15-LOX-2 metabolizes n-6 arachidonic acid into 15-S-HETE, which appears to have *anti*cancer actions[178]

Notes:

_____

_____

_____

_____

_____

_____

_____

_____

_____

_____

[170] Dwyer JH, Allayee H, Dwyer KM, Fan J, Wu H, Mar R, Lusis AJ, Mehrabian M. Arachidonate 5-lipoxygenase promoter genotype, dietary arachidonic acid, and atherosclerosis. *N Engl J Med*. 2004 Jan 1;350(1):29-37

[171] "These targets include procarcinogenic lipoxygenases (LOXs), including 5-, 8-, and 12-LOX, and anticarcinogenic LOXs, including 15-LOX-1 and possibly 15-LOX-2." Shureiqi I, Lippman SM. Lipoxygenase modulation to reverse carcinogenesis. *Cancer Res*. 2001 Sep 1;61(17):6307-12

[172] "Specific metabolites of each pathway, i.e. PGF2 alpha and 5-HPETE, are able to transcend the block and restore collagenase production, invasiveness in vitro and metastatic activity in vivo." Reich R, Martin GR. Identification of arachidonic acid pathways required for the invasive and metastatic activity of malignant tumor cells. *Prostaglandins* 1996 Jan;51(1):1-17

[173] Shureiqi I, Lippman SM. Lipoxygenase modulation to reverse carcinogenesis. *Cancer Res*. 2001 Sep 1;61(17):6307-12

[174] Shureiqi I, Lippman SM. Lipoxygenase modulation to reverse carcinogenesis. *Cancer Res*. 2001 Sep 1;61(17):6307-12

[175] Shureiqi I, Lippman SM. Lipoxygenase modulation to reverse carcinogenesis. *Cancer Res*. 2001 Sep 1;61(17):6307-12

[176] Reich R, Martin GR. Identification of arachidonic acid pathways required for the invasive and metastatic activity of malignant tumor cells. *Prostaglandins* 1996 Jan;51(1):1-17

[177] Shureiqi I, Lippman SM. Lipoxygenase modulation to reverse carcinogenesis. *Cancer Res*. 2001 Sep 1;61(17):6307-12

[178] Shureiqi I, Lippman SM. Lipoxygenase modulation to reverse carcinogenesis. *Cancer Res*. 2001 Sep 1;61(17):6307-12

NF-kappaB and Its Phytonutritional Modulation

Nuclear transcription factor kappaB (NF-kappaB) is one of several transcription factors which act as "facilitators" for the elaboration and amplification of specific gene products. In the case of NF-kappaB, most of the genes that appear to be influenced are those that increase the production of pro-inflammatory mediators such as IL-2 (which increases production of collagen-digesting proteases), IL-6 (which then increases production of C-reactive protein), cyclooxygenase-2 (which then increases production of prostaglandins), lipoxygenase (which produces leukotrienes), and inducible nitric oxide synthase (for the production of nitric oxide), etc. Inhibition of NF-kappaB is increasingly considered a major therapeutic goal in the treatment and prevention of a wide range of illnesses, including cancer, arthritis, autoimmune diseases, neurologic illnesses such as Alzheimer's and Parkinson's disease, and other "inflammatory" diseases.[179] [180] While we as holistic clinicians work to address the underlying cause of the problem in a given patient, I believe that some degree of "suppression" of NF-kappaB is therapeutically appropriate for at least two reasons: 1) it helps to limit tissue damage and to improve patient outcomes, and 2) suppression of NF-kappaB helps to *break the vicious cycle* of positive feedback wherein *inflammation promotes more inflammation* by the NF-kappaB stimulating effect of several of the products of NF-kappaB activation: NF-kappaB increases the production of IL-1, PG-E2, oxidative stress, TNF-a, and CRP—all of which work additively and synergistically to increase activation of NF-kappaB. Therefore, regardless of the underlying cause, which may have already been addressed and eradicated, it is conceivable that some patients will suffer from inflammatory disorders simply because of the positive feedback that mediators have on the activation of NF-kappaB, which then promotes more inflammation.

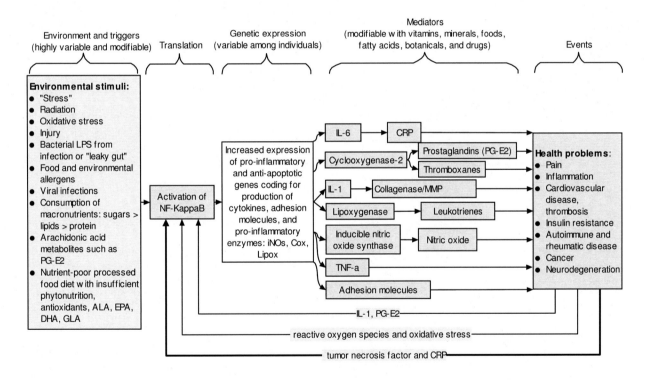

Pharmaceutical companies are currently scrambling to develop clinically useful synthetic inhibitors of NF-kappaB. These companies will eventually be successful in this endeavor, and we can also confidently predict that the pharmaceutical version of NF-kappaB suppression will arrive with a plethora of adverse effects, most likely <u>because of</u> *the potency and specificity* of the drug. NF-kappaB plays an important role in a wide range of normal, healthy physiologic processes, including the immune response to infectious diseases. We should therefore seek to *modulate* its function rather than sophomorically *suppress* its function. Fortunately, we can do

---

[179] D'Acquisto F, May MJ, Ghosh S. Inhibition of Nuclear Factor Kappa B (NF-B): An Emerging Theme in Anti-Inflammatory Therapies. *Mol Interv.* 2002 Feb;2(1):22-35 http://molinterv.aspetjournals.org/cgi/content/full/2/1/22
[180] Tak PP, Firestein GS. NF-kappaB: a key role in inflammatory diseases. *J Clin Invest.* 2001 Jan;107(1):7-11 http://www.jci.org/cgi/content/full/107/1/7

this with several natural interventions, not the least of which are vitamin D[181,182], curcumin[183] (requires piperine for absorption[184]), lipoic acid[185], green tea[186], rosemary[187], grape seed extract[188], propolis[189], zinc[190], high-dose selenium[191], indole-3-carbinol[192,193], N-acetyl-L-cysteine[194], and resveratrol.[195,196] Other nutrients such as isohumulones from *Humulus lupulus*[197] and fatty acids inhibit NF-kappaB *indirectly* via activation of peroxisome proliferator-activated receptors alpha (PPAR-ά) and gamma (PPAR-γ). GLA activates PPAR-gamma and thereby inhibits NF-kappaB[198], while (oxidized) EPA activates PPAR-alpha and thus inhibits NF-kappaB[199]; these latter findings reflect a quantum leap in our understanding of the mechanisms of diet-induced anti-inflammation (i.e., anti-inflammatory nutrigenomics, or anti-inflammatory immunonutrigenomics) since they show that food constituents modify human physiology and phenotype at the genetic/pre-transcriptional level and not only at the metabolic/post-transcriptional level as was previously thought.[200]

I believe that future research will elucidate that the proposed anti-inflammatory benefits of plant-based diets[201] are partially resultant from the downregulation of NF-kappaB by dietary phytonutrients, of which more than 5,000 exist.[202] Notice that the above-mentioned suppressors of NF-kappaB are mostly phenolic compounds that are naturally occurring in fruits, vegetables, herbs, and spices. A diet based upon fruits and vegetables would be naturally high in these compounds and would be likely to provide an anti-inflammatory influence on genetic expression. Indeed, this dietary and phytonutritional environment would be consistent with that in which human physiology evolved, to which it adapted, and upon which it thereby became dependent.[203,204] Relatedly, our epidemic of vitamin D deficiency[205] resultant from our artificial, indoor, clothed lifestyles unquestionably contributes to our modern pro-inflammatory tendency, and vitamin D supplementation has already proven to be immunomodulating and anti-inflammatory in human clinical trials.[206,207,208]

---

181 "1Alpha,25-dihydroxyvitamin D3 (1,25-(OH)2-D3), **the active metabolite of vitamin D, can inhibit NF-kappaB activity** in human MRC-5 fibroblasts, targeting DNA binding of NF-kappaB but not translocation of its subunits p50 and p65." Harant H, Wolff B, Lindley IJ. 1Alpha,25-dihydroxyvitamin D3 decreases DNA binding of nuclear factor-kappaB in human fibroblasts. *FEBS Lett.* 1998 Oct 9;436(3):329-34

182 "Thus, 1,25$(OH)_2D_3$ may negatively regulate IL-12 production by downregulation of NF-kB activation and binding to the p40-kB sequence." D'Ambrosio D, Cippitelli M, Cocciolo MG, Mazzeo D, Di Lucia P, Lang R, Sinigaglia F, Panina-Bordignon P. Inhibition of IL-12 production by 1,25-dihydroxyvitamin D3. Involvement of NF-kappaB downregulation in transcriptional repression of the p40 gene. *J Clin Invest.* 1998 Jan 1;101(1):252-62

183 "Curcumin, EGCG and resveratrol have been shown to suppress activation of NF-kappa B." Surh YJ, Chun KS, Cha HH, Han SS, Keum YS, Park KK, Lee SS. Molecular mechanisms underlying chemopreventive activities of anti-inflammatory phytochemicals: down-regulation of COX-2 and iNOS through suppression of NF-kappa B activation. *Mutat Res.* 2001 Sep 1;480-481:243-68

184 Shoba G, Joy D, Joseph T, Majeed M, Rajendran R, Srinivas PS. Influence of piperine on the pharmacokinetics of curcumin in animals and human volunteers. *Planta Med.* 1998 May;64(4):353-6

185 "ALA reduced the TNF-alpha-stimulated ICAM-1 expression in a dose-dependent manner, to levels observed in unstimulated cells. Alpha-lipoic acid also reduced NF-kappaB activity in these cells in a dose-dependent manner." Lee HA, Hughes DA.Alpha-lipoic acid modulates NF-kappaB activity in human monocytic cells by direct interaction with DNA. *Exp Gerontol.* 2002 Jan-Mar;37(2-3):401-10

186 "In conclusion, EGCG is an effective inhibitor of IKK activity. This may explain, at least in part, some of the reported anti-inflammatory and anticancer effects of green tea." Yang F, Oz HS, Barve S, de Villiers WJ, McClain CJ, Varilek GW. The green tea polyphenol (-)-epigallocatechin-3-gallate blocks nuclear factor-kappa B activation by inhibiting I kappa B kinase activity in the intestinal epithelial cell line IEC-6. *Mol Pharmacol.* 2001 Sep;60(3):528-33

187 "These results suggest that carnosol suppresses the NO production and iNOS gene expression by inhibiting NF-kappaB activation, and provide possible mechanisms for its anti-inflammatory and chemopreventive action." Lo AH, Liang YC, Lin-Shiau SY, Ho CT, Lin JK. Carnosol, an antioxidant in rosemary, suppresses inducible nitric oxide synthase through down-regulating nuclear factor-kappaB in mouse macrophages. *Carcinogenesis.* 2002 Jun;23(6):983-91

188 "Constitutive and TNFalpha-induced NF-kappaB DNA binding activity was inhibited by GSE at doses > or =50 microg/ml and treatments for > or =12 h." Dhanalakshmi S, Agarwal R, Agarwal C. Inhibition of NF-kappaB pathway in grape seed extract-induced apoptotic death of human prostate carcinoma DU145 cells. *Int J Oncol.* 2003 Sep;23(3):721-7

189 "Caffeic acid phenethyl ester (CAPE) is an anti-inflammatory component of propolis (honeybee resin). CAPE is reportedly a specific inhibitor of nuclear factor-kappaB (NF-kappaB)." Fitzpatrick LR, Wang J, Le T. Caffeic acid phenethyl ester, an inhibitor of nuclear factor-kappaB, attenuates bacterial peptidoglycan polysaccharide-induced colitis in rats. *J Pharmacol Exp Ther.* 2001 Dec;299(3):915-20

190 "Our results suggest that zinc supplementation may lead to downregulation of the inflammatory cytokines through upregulation of the negative feedback loop A20 to inhibit induced NF-kappaB activation." Prasad AS, Bao B, Beck FW, Kucuk O, Sarkar FH. Antioxidant effect of zinc in humans. *Free Radic Biol Med.* 2004 Oct 15;37(8):1182-90

191 Note that the patients in this study received a very high dose of selenium: 960 micrograms per day. This is at the top—and some would say over the top—of the safe and reasonable dose for long-term supplementation. In this case, th study lasted for three months. "In patients receiving selenium supplementation, selenium NF-kappaB activity was significantly reduced, reaching the same level as the nondiabetic control group. CONCLUSION: In type 2 diabetic patients, activation of NF-kappaB measured in peripheral blood monocytes can be reduced by selenium supplementation, confirming its importance in the prevention of cardiovascular diseases." Faure P, Ramon O, Favier A, Halimi S. Selenium supplementation decreases nuclear factor-kappa B activity in peripheral blood mononuclear cells from type 2 diabetic patients. *Eur J Clin Invest.* 2004 Jul;34(7):475-81

192 Takada Y, Andreeff M, Aggarwal BB. Indole-3-carbinol suppresses NF-{kappa}B and I{kappa}B{alpha} kinase activation causing inhibition of expression of NF-{kappa}B-regulated antiapoptotic and metastatic gene products and enhancement of apoptosis in myeloid and leukemia cells. *Blood.* 2005 Apr 5; [Epub ahead of print]

193 "Overall, our results indicated that indole-3-carbinol inhibits NF-kappaB and NF-kappaB-regulated gene expression and that this mechanism may provide the molecular basis for its ability to suppress tumorigenesis." Takada Y, Andreeff M, Aggarwal BB. Indole-3-carbinol suppresses NF-kappaB and IkappaBalpha kinase activation, causing inhibition of expression of NF-kappaB-regulated antiapoptotic and metastatic gene products and enhancement of apoptosis in myeloid and leukemia cells. *Blood.* 2005 Jul 15;106(2):641-9. Epub 2005 Apr 5.

194 "CONCLUSIONS: Administration of N-acetylcysteine results in decreased nuclear factor-kappa B activation in patients with sepsis, associated with decreases in interleukin-8 but not interleukin-6 or soluble intercellular adhesion molecule-1. These pilot data suggest that antioxidant therapy with N-acetylcysteine may be useful in blunting the inflammatory response to sepsis." Paterson RL, Galley HF, Webster NR. The effect of N-acetylcysteine on nuclear factor-kappa B activation, interleukin-6, interleukin-8, and intercellular adhesion molecule-1 expression in patients with sepsis. *Crit Care Med.* 2003 Nov;31(11):2574-8

195 "Resveratrol's anticarcinogenic, anti-inflammatory, and growth-modulatory effects may thus be partially ascribed to the inhibition of activation of NF-kappaB and AP-1 and the associated kinases." Manna SK, Mukhopadhyay A, Aggarwal BB. Resveratrol suppresses TNF-induced activation of nuclear transcription factors NF-kappa B, activator protein-1, and apoptosis: potential role of reactive oxygen intermediates and lipid peroxidation. *J Immunol.* 2000 Jun 15;164(12):6509-19

196 "Both resveratrol and quercetin inhibited NF-kappaB-, AP-1- and CREB-dependent transcription to a greater extent than the glucocorticosteroid, dexamethasone." Donnelly LE, Newton R, Kennedy GE, Fenwick PS, Leung RH, Ito K, Russell RE, Barnes PJ.Anti-inflammatory Effects of Resveratrol in Lung Epithelial Cells: Molecular Mechanisms. *Am J Physiol Lung Cell Mol Physiol.* 2004 Jun 4 [Epub ahead of print]

197 Yajima H, Ikeshima E, Shiraki M, Kanaya T, Fujiwara D, Odai H, Tsuboyama-Kasaoka N, Ezaki O, Oikawa S, Kondo K. Isohumulones, bitter acids derived from hops, activate both peroxisome proliferator-activated receptor alpha and gamma and reduce insulin resistance. *J Biol Chem.* 2004 Aug 6;279(32):33456-62. Epub 2004 Jun 3. http://www.jbc.org/cgi/content/full/279/32/33456

198 "Thus, PPAR gamma serves as the receptor for GLA in the regulation of gene expression in breast cancer cells. " Jiang WG, Redfern A, Bryce RP, Mansel RE. Peroxisome proliferator activated receptor-gamma (PPAR-gamma) mediates the action of gamma linolenic acid in breast cancer cells. *Prostaglandins Leukot Essent Fatty Acids.* 2000 Feb;62(2):119-27

199 "...EPA requires PPARalpha for its inhibitory effects on NF-kappaB." Mishra A, Chaudhary A, Sethi S. Oxidized omega-3 fatty acids inhibit NF-kappaB activation via a PPARalpha-dependent pathway. *Arterioscler Thromb Vasc Biol.* 2004 Sep;24(9):1621-7. Epub 2004 Jul 1. http://atvb.ahajournals.org/cgi/content/full/24/9/1621

200 "Indeed, the previous view that nutrients only interact with human physiology at the metabolic/post-transcriptional level must be updated in light of current research showing that nutrients can, in fact, modify human physiology and phenotype at the genetic/pre-transcriptional level." Vasquez A. Reducing pain and inflammation naturally - part 4: nutritional and botanical inhibition of NF-kappaB, the major intracellular amplifier of the inflammatory cascade. A practical clinical strategy exemplifying anti-inflammatory nutrigenomics. *Nutritional Perspectives*, July 2005:5-12. www.OptimalHealthResearch.com/part4

201 Seaman DR. The diet-induced proinflammatory state: a cause of chronic pain and other degenerative diseases? *J Manipulative Physiol Ther.* 2002;25(3):168-79

202 "We propose that the additive and synergistic effects of phytochemicals in fruit and vegetables are responsible for their potent antioxidant and anticancer activities, and that the benefit of a diet rich in fruit and vegetables is attributed to the complex mixture of phytochemicals present in whole foods." Liu RH. Health benefits of fruit and vegetables are from additive and synergistic combinations of phytochemicals. *Am J Clin Nutr.* 2003 Sep;78(3 Suppl):517S-520S

203 **Heaney RP. Long-latency deficiency disease: insights from calcium and vitamin D. *Am J Clin Nutr.* 2003 Nov;78(5):912-9**

204 **O'Keefe JH Jr, Cordain L. Cardiovascular disease resulting from a diet and lifestyle at odds with our Paleolithic genome: how to become a 21st-century hunter-gatherer. *Mayo Clin Proc.* 2004 Jan;79(1):101-8**

205 Thomas MK, Lloyd-Jones DM, Thadhani RI, Shaw AC, Deraska DJ, Kitch BT, Vamvakas EC, Dick IM, Prince RL, Finkelstein JS. Hypovitaminosis D in medical inpatients. *N Engl J Med.* 1998 Mar 19;338(12):777-83

206 Van den Berghe G, Van Roosbroeck D, Vanhove P, Wouters PJ, De Pourcq L, Bouillon R. Bone turnover in prolonged critical illness: effect of vitamin D. *J Clin Endocrinol Metab.* 2003 Oct;88(10):4623-32

207 Hypponen E, Laara E, Reunanen A, Jarvelin MR, Virtanen SM. Intake of vitamin D and risk of type 1 diabetes: a birth-cohort study. *Lancet.* 2001 Nov 3;358(9292):1500-3

208 Mahon BD, Gordon SA, Cruz J, Cosman F, Cantorna MT. Cytokine profile in patients with multiple sclerosis following vitamin D supplementation. *J Neuroimmunol.* 2003;134(1-2):128-32

Basic Physiology of NF-kappaB: A Simplified Conceptual Model

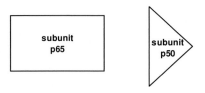

NF-kappaB is made from two subunit proteins: p65 and p50.

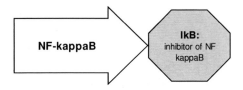

In the cytosol, inhibitor KappaB binds to NF-kappaB and makes it inactive.

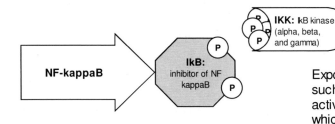

Exposure to 'stressful stimuli' such as LPS or oxidative stress, activates "inhibitory kappaB kinase", which phosphorylates IkB for destruction.

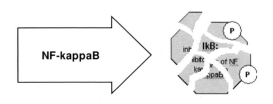

Once IkB is destroyed, then NF-kappaB is free to enter the nucleus and bind with DNA.

NF-kappaB enters the nucleus and binds with DNA to activate genes which encode for the increased production of inflammatory mediators.

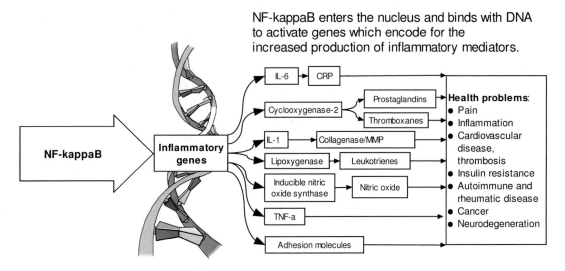

Increased production of inflammatory mediators - such as cytokines, prostaglandins, leukotrienes - promotes cellular dysfunction and tissue destruction.

Selected Nutritional and Botanical Therapeutics: Brief Clinical Monographs

The following pages emphasize clinically relevant concise reviews of **selected nutritional and botanical therapeutics** that are commonly considered in the treatment of musculoskeletal pain and for the promotion of tissue healing. Future editions of this book will contain a broader compendium. However, the power of natural medicine lies not in the size of our pharmacopoeia; it is rather to be found in the completeness of our approach and in the conceptual and philosophical underpinnings which support our assessments and interventions.

By now, the concept of "holistic treatment" as advocated in this text should be clear to the reader. While the medical model of disease treatment continues to seek a single "silver bullet" to treat each disease, the advantage of holistic medicine is that we consider and address a wide range of therapeutics—each of which addresses a particular aspect of the patient's complex pathophysiologic phenomena. For example, in the treatment of low-back pain, rather than relying on a single treatment/drug to effect 100% benefit (100% "cure" is almost never attained with single interventions, especially with drugs), we seek a 20% improvement from EPA+DHA supplementation, 40% improvement from proprioceptive retraining and exercise, 30% improvement with anti-inflammatory botanical medicines, and at least another 10% improvement with vitamin C. In the end, my experience in using this style of *multiple intervention therapy* is that the majority of patients are not only effectively "cured" of their former health problem(s), but that they enjoy a higher level of overall health as a result of dietary improvements, nutritional supplementation, exercise, and the other biochemical and behavioral modifications that I have prescribed, such as described in this text.

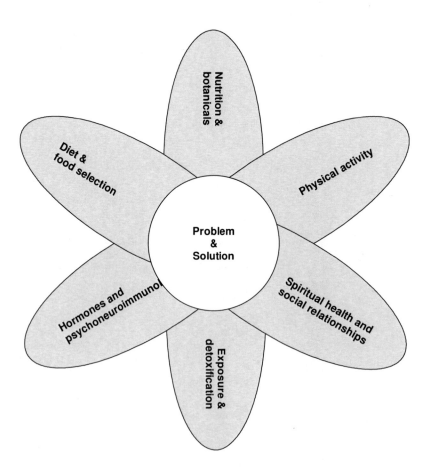

Nutrient:	***Alpha-linolenic acid (ALA)***
Common name:	**Flaxseed oil (57% ALA)**

Applications and mechanisms of action:	▪ <u>Anti-inflammatory, modulation of gene transcription, and several other benefits</u>: ALA clearly has anti-inflammatory benefits as consistently demonstrated in human studies. In a study of men with metabolic syndrome, ALA was shown to have anti-inflammatory benefits independent of its conversion to EPA or DHA.[209] The mechanism of action appears to be downregulation of NF-KappaB (the main "amplifier" for the expression of proinflammatory gene products[210]) rather than the direct modulation of eicosanoid biosynthesis. One study using flaxseed oil as a source of ALA to treat rheumatoid arthritis found no clinical or biochemical benefit (i.e., no change in Hgb, CRP, ESR)[211]; however, the poor results of this study may have been due to the inferior quality of the flaxseed oil product that was used which only supplied 32% ALA compared with the much higher concentration of 57% found in most products. **Moderate intakes of ALA from flaxseed oil profoundly reduce production of proinflammatory prostaglandins (e.g., PG-E2, measured by urinary excretion) by 52% to 85% in humans.**[212] This level of prostaglandin inhibition is greater than the 42% reduction induced by rofecoxib/Vioxx.[213] However, since the reduction in prostaglandin formation by ALA is more generalized (rather than specific for the Cox-2 enzyme), the anti-inflammatory benefit occurs without adverse cardiovascular effects caused by Cox-2 inhibitors.
Toxicity and contraindications:	▪ None that are generally known. ▪ Overconsumption or imbalanced intake of ALA is known to cause reductions in DHA, and this reduction would be expected to have adverse effects on neurological performance, cognition, and vision.
Dosage and administration:	▪ One to two tablespoons of flaxseed oil contain 6,200 mg or 12,400 mg of ALA, respectively. ▪ Fatty acids should always be supplemented in balanced combination rather than in isolation.[214]
Additional information:	▪ Conversion of ALA to the more biologically active EPA and DHA does not reliably or efficiently occur in humans.[215] No increase in DHA has been consistently observed in humans after supplementation of ALA[216]; in fact, supplementation with flax seed oil has actually been shown to reduce DHA levels in humans.[217]

---

[209] "CONCLUSIONS: Dietary supplementation with ALA for 3 months decreases significantly CRP, SAA and IL-6 levels in dyslipidaemic patients. This anti-inflammatory effect may provide a possible additional mechanism for the beneficial effect of plant n-3 polyunsaturated fatty acids in primary and secondary prevention of coronary artery disease." Rallidis LS, Paschos G, Liakos GK, Velissaridou AH, Anastasiadis G, Zampelas A. Dietary alpha-linolenic acid decreases C-reactive protein, serum amyloid A and interleukin-6 in dyslipidaemic patients. *Atherosclerosis.* 2003 Apr;167(2):237-42

[210] Tak PP, Firestein GS. NF-kappaB: a key role in inflammatory diseases. *J Clin Invest.* 2001 Jan;107(1):7-11

[211] "Thus, 3-month's supplementation with alpha-LNA did not prove to be beneficial in rheumatoid arthritis." Nordstrom DC, Honkanen VE, Nasu Y, Antila E, Friman C, Konttinen YT. Alpha-linolenic acid in the treatment of rheumatoid arthritis. A double-blind, placebo-controlled and randomized study: flaxseed vs. safflower seed. *Rheumatol Int.* 1995;14(6):231-4

[212] Adam O, Wolfram G, Zollner N. Effect of alpha-linolenic acid in the human diet on linoleic acid metabolism and prostaglandin biosynthesis. *J Lipid Res.* 1986 Apr;27(4):421-6

[213] Van Hecken A, Schwartz JI, Depre M, De Lepeleire I, Dallob A, Tanaka W, Wynants K, Buntinx A, Arnout J, Wong PH, Ebel DL, Gertz BJ, De Schepper PJ. Comparative inhibitory activity of rofecoxib, meloxicam, diclofenac, ibuprofen, and naproxen on COX-2 versus COX-1 in healthy volunteers. *J Clin Pharmacol.* 2000 Oct;40(10):1109-20

[214] **Vasquez A. Reducing Pain and Inflammation Naturally. Part 2: New Insights into Fatty Acid Supplementation and Its Effect on Eicosanoid Production and Genetic Expression. *Nutritional Perspectives* 2005; January: 5-16 www.optimalhealthresearch.com/part2**

[215] "Indu and Ghafoorunissa showed that while keeping the amount of dietary LA constant, 3.7 g ALA appears to have biological effects similar to those of 0.3 g long-chain n-3 PUFA with conversion of 11 g ALA to 1 g long-chain n-3 PUFA." Simopoulos AP. Essential fatty acids in health and chronic disease. *Am J Clin Nutr.* 1999 Sep;70(3 Suppl):560S-569S

[216] Francois CA, Connor SL, Bolewicz LC, Connor WE. Supplementing lactating women with flaxseed oil does not increase docosahexaenoic acid in their milk. *Am J Clin Nutr.* 2003 Jan;77(1):226-33

[217] "Linear relationships were found between dietary alpha-LA and EPA in plasma fractions and in cellular phospholipids. ... There was an inverse relationship between dietary alpha-LA and docosahexaenoic acid concentrations in the phospholipids of plasma, neutrophils, mononuclear cells, and platelets." Mantzioris E, James MJ, Gibson RA, Cleland LG. Differences exist in the relationships between dietary linoleic and alpha-linolenic acids and their respective long-chain metabolites. *Am J Clin Nutr.* 1995 Feb;61(2):320-4

Nutrients:	*Eicosapentaenoic acid (EPA)*
	Docosahexaenoic acid (DHA)
Common name:	**Fish oil**

Applications and
mechanisms of action:

- <u>Anti-inflammatory, modulation of gene transcription, and many other benefits</u>: Fish oil has a wide range of applications, proven effectiveness, and record of safety that is second to none; no other single treatment is as effective for such a wide range of conditions. Positive results have been documented in clinical trials in patients with hypertension, hypercholesterolemia, various types of joint pain, mental depression, diabetes, bipolar illness, ulcerative colitis, Crohn's disease, schizophrenia and various other conditions, particularly inflammatory and neurologic diseases. Rather than being specific for any one disease, the provision of EPA and DHA via supplementation with fish oil quite simply *makes the body work better* by supplying the long-chain omega-3 fatty acids that are necessary for proper physiologic function but which are commonly deficient in our modern diets. Benefits include reduction in harmful 2-series pro-inflammatory and pain-enhancing eicosanoids, increased production of 3-series eicosanoids, modulation of gene transcription, and enhancement of cell membranes with the general result of increased receptor sensitivity and thus improved intercellular communication and improved efficiency of cell membrane signal transduction.

- <u>Clinical benefits</u>: **EPA supplementation has proven beneficial for patients with lupus,[218] cancer[219], borderline personality disorder[220], mental depression[221,222,223], schizophrenia[224], and osteoporosis (when used with GLA).[225]** DHA appears essential for optimal cognitive function in infants and adults, and DHA in fish oil provides some protection against thrombosis, arrhythmia, cardiovascular death, Alzheimer's disease[226], otitis media (when used with nutritional supplementation[227]), and coronary restenosis following angioplasty.[228] Supplementation with DHA (often in the form of fish oil, which includes EPA) has been shown to benefit patients with bipolar disorder[229], Crohn's disease[230],

[218] Duffy EM, Meenagh GK, McMillan SA, Strain JJ, Hannigan BM, Bell AL. The clinical effect of dietary supplementation with omega-3 fish oils and/or copper in systemic lupus erythematosus. *J Rheumatol*. 2004 Aug;31(8):1551-6

[219] Wigmore SJ, Barber MD, Ross JA, Tisdale MJ, Fearon KC. Effect of oral eicosapentaenoic acid on weight loss in patients with pancreatic cancer. *Nutr Cancer*. 2000;36(2):177-84

[220] Zanarini MC, Frankenburg FR. omega-3 Fatty acid treatment of women with borderline personality disorder: a double-blind, placebo-controlled pilot study. *Am J Psychiatry*. 2003 Jan;160(1):167-9

[221] Nemets B, Stahl Z, Belmaker RH. Addition of omega-3 fatty acid to maintenance medication treatment for recurrent unipolar depressive disorder. *Am J Psychiatry*. 2002 Mar;159(3):477-9

[222] Puri BK, Counsell SJ, Hamilton G, Richardson AJ, Horrobin DF.Eicosapentaenoic acid in treatment-resistant depression associated with symptom remission, structural brain changes and reduced neuronal phospholipid turnover. *Int J Clin Pract*. 2001 Oct;55(8):560-3

[223] Peet M, Horrobin DF.A dose-ranging study of the effects of ethyl-eicosapentaenoate in patients with ongoing depression despite apparently adequate treatment with standard drugs. *Arch Gen Psychiatry*. 2002 Oct;59(10):913-9

[224] Emsley R, Myburgh C, Oosthuizen P, van Rensburg SJ. Randomized, placebo-controlled study of ethyl-eicosapentaenoic acid as supplemental treatment in schizophrenia. *Am J Psychiatry*. 2002 Sep;159(9):1596-8

[225] Kruger MC, Coetzer H, de Winter R, Gericke G, van Papendorp DH. Calcium, gamma-linolenic acid and eicosapentaenoic acid supplementation in senile osteoporosis. *Aging* (Milano). 1998 Oct;10(5):385-94

[226] Horrocks LA, Yeo YK. Health benefits of docosahexaenoic acid (DHA). *Pharmacol Res*. 1999 Sep;40(3):211-25

[227] Linday LA, Dolitsky JN, Shindledecker RD, Pippenger CE. Lemon-flavored cod liver oil and a multivitamin-mineral supplement for the secondary prevention of otitis media in young children: pilot research. *Ann Otol Rhinol Laryngol*. 2002 Jul;111(7 Pt 1):642-52

[228] Bairati I, Roy L, Meyer F. Double-blind, randomized, controlled trial of fish oil supplements in prevention of recurrence of stenosis after coronary angioplasty. *Circulation*. 1992 Mar;85(3):950-6

[229] Stoll AL, Severus WE, Freeman MP, Rueter S, Zboyan HA, Diamond E, Cress KK, Marangell LB. Omega 3 fatty acids in bipolar disorder: a preliminary double-blind, placebo-controlled trial. *Arch Gen Psychiatry*. 1999 May;56(5):407-12

[230] Belluzzi A, Brignola C, Campieri M, Pera A, Boschi S, Miglioli M. Effect of an enteric-coated fish-oil preparation on relapses in Crohn's disease. *N Engl J Med*. 1996 Jun 13;334(24):1557-60

[231] Adam O, Beringer C, Kless T, Lemmen C, Adam A, Wiseman M, Adam P, Klimmek R, Forth W. Anti-inflammatory effects of a low arachidonic acid diet and fish oil in patients with rheumatoid arthritis. *Rheumatol Int*. 2003 Jan;23(1):27-36

[232] Lau CS, Morley KD, Belch JJ. Effects of fish oil supplementation on non-steroidal anti-inflammatory drug requirement in patients with mild rheumatoid arthritis--a double-blind placebo controlled study. *Br J Rheumatol*. 1993 Nov;32(11):982-9

[233] Kremer JM, Jubiz W, Michalek A, Rynes RI, Bartholomew LE, Bigaouette J, Timchalk M, Beeler D, Lininger L. Fish-oil fatty acid supplementation in active rheumatoid arthritis. A double-blinded, controlled, crossover study. *Ann Intern Med*. 1987 Apr;106(4):497-503

[234] Walton AJ, Snaith ML, Locniskar M, Cumberland AG, Morrow WJ, Isenberg DA. Dietary fish oil and the severity of symptoms in patients with systemic lupus erythematosus. *Ann Rheum Dis*. 1991 Jul;50(7):463-6

[235] "The recent GISSI (Gruppo Italiano per lo Studio della Sopravvivenza nell'Infarto miocardico)-Prevention study of 11,324 patients showed a 45% decrease in risk of sudden cardiac death and a 20% reduction in all-cause mortality in the group taking 850 mg/d of omega-3 fatty acids." O'Keefe JH Jr, Harris WS. From Inuit to implementation: omega-3 fatty acids come of age. *Mayo Clin Proc*. 2000 Jun;75(6):607-14

[236] Bittiner SB, Tucker WF, Cartwright I, Bleehen SS. A double-blind, randomised, placebo-controlled trial of fish oil in psoriasis. *Lancet*. 1988;1(8582):378-80

[237] Gogos CA, Ginopoulos P, Salsa B, Apostolidou E, Zoumbos NC, Kalfarentzos F. Dietary omega-3 polyunsaturated fatty acids plus vitamin E restore immunodeficiency and prolong survival for severely ill patients with generalized malignancy: a randomized control trial. *Cancer*. 1998 Jan 15;82(2):395-402

[238] Hamazaki T, Itomura M, Sawazaki S, Nagao Y. Anti-stress effects of DHA. *Biofactors*. 2000;13(1-4):41-5

[239] Sawazaki S, Hamazaki T, Yazawa K, Kobayashi M. The effect of docosahexaenoic acid on plasma catecholamine concentrations and glucose tolerance during long-lasting psychological stress: a double-blind placebo-controlled study. *J Nutr Sci Vitaminol* (Tokyo). 1999 Oct;45(5):655-65

[240] O'Keefe JH Jr, Harris WS. From Inuit to implementation: omega-3 fatty acids come of age. *Mayo Clin Proc*. 2000 Jun;75(6):607-14

rheumatoid arthritis[231,232,233], lupus[234], cardiovascular disease[235], psoriasis[236], and cancer.[237] DHA appears to have an "anti-stress" benefit manifested by 30% reductions in norepinephrine and improved resilience to psychoemotional stress.[238,239] Supplementation with EPA+DHA in fish oil is extremely safe and reduces all-cause mortality.[240]

Toxicity and contraindications:

- EPA and DHA have been used in relatively high doses with little or no evidence of adverse effects. In one study, 10,000 mg per day of EPA did not cause adverse effects[241]; this dose is equivalent to approximately 6-7 tablespoons of cod-liver oil per day—much more than is commonly prescribed for long-term use. Another study found that administration of 13.1 g of eicosapentaenoic acid + docosahexaenoic acid resulted only in gastrointestinal effects such as diarrhea and abdominal discomfort.[242]

- Anticoagulant medications, surgery, and bleeding: Although EPA+DHA doses of at least 4 grams per day may be necessary to increase bleeding time[243], I routinely recommend dose reduction or discontinuation of EPA+DHA supplementation for patients who are thrombocytopenic or otherwise at risk for hemorrhage due to illness or upcoming surgery. Fish oil can potentate anticoagulant medication such as warfarin/coumadin.[244]

- Vitamin D: High doses of cod-liver oil—4 tablespoons per day (one-quarter cup)—provide approximately 6,000 IU of vitamin D, an amount which is much less than the 10,000 IU of vitamin D that is synthesized following a few minutes of full-body sun exposure and which appears safe according to the extensive review by Vieth.[245] For patients consuming cod-liver oil at one tablespoon per day (long-term use) or up to one-quarter cup (four tablespoons per day for short-term use), the risk of vitamin D toxicity appears to be nonexistent. Interestingly, vitamin D *deficiency* appears to be endemic among people with persistent, nonspecific musculoskeletal pain.[246]

- Vitamin A: Cod-liver oil typically contains up to 1,250 IU of vitamin A per teaspoon, which is 3,750 IU per tablespoon. **Thus, a quarter-cup of cod-liver oil contains 15,000 IU vitamin A—this is a safe dose for several months of supplementation in most adult patients**, but this modest dose is too high for women who are pregnant or might become pregnant because of the theoretical and controversial association between birth defects and vitamin A intakes greater than 10,000 IU per day. Other brands of liquid fish oil contain 1,950 IU vitamin A per teaspoon, or 5,850 IU vitamin A per tablespoon, which totals 23,400 IU per quarter cup of oil—this dose is too high for multi-year consumption, but is safe for short-term use in most patients. Vitamin A toxicity is seen with chronic ingestion of therapeutic doses (for example: **25,000 IU per day for 6 years**, or 100,000 IU per day for 2.5 years[247]). Manifestations of vitamin A toxicity

---

[241] " eicosapentaenoic acid (EPA) and docosahexaenoic acid (DHA) were given in a cumulative manner, every 6 weeks, starting with 10 mg, then 100 mg, 1000 mg and 10,000 mg EPA daily to mild to moderate essential hypertensive black patients. The corresponding DHA doses were 3, 33, 333 and 3333 mg." Du Plooy WJ, Venter CP, Muntingh GM, Venter HL, Glatthaar II, Smith KA. The cumulative dose response effect of eicosapentaenoic and docosahexaenoic acid on blood pressure, plasma lipid profile and diet pattern in mild to moderate essential hypertensive black patients. *Prostaglandins Leukot Essent Fatty Acids* 1992 Aug;46(4):315-21

[242] "This means that a 70-kg patient can generally tolerate up to 21 1-g capsules/day containing 13.1 g of eicosapentaenoic acid + docosahexaenoic acid, the two major omega-3 fatty acids" Burns CP, Halabi S, Clamon GH, Hars V, Wagner BA, Hohl RJ, Lester E, Kirshner JJ, Vinciguerra V, Paskett E. Phase I clinical study of fish oil fatty acid capsules for patients with cancer cachexia: cancer and leukemia group B study 9473. *Clin Cancer Res.* 1999 Dec;5(12):3942-7

[243] "... EPA/d ... 4 g/d increased bleeding time and decreased platelet count with no adverse effects. In human studies, there has never been a case of clinical bleeding, even in patients undergoing angioplasty, while the patients were taking fish oil supplements." Simopoulos AP. Essential fatty acids in health and chronic disease. *Am J Clin Nutr.*1999;70(3 Suppl):560S-569S

[244] "Although controversial, this case report illustrates that fish oil can provide additive anticoagulant effects when given with warfarin. CONCLUSIONS: This case reveals a significant rise in INR after the dose of concomitant fish oil was doubled." Buckley MS, Goff AD, Knapp WE. Fish oil interaction with warfarin. *Ann Pharmacother.* 2004 Jan;38(1):50-2

[245] "Total-body sun exposure easily provides the equivalent of 250 microg (10,000 IU) vitamin D/d. ...Published cases of vitamin D toxicity ...all involve intake of > or = 1000 microg (40000 IU)/d. ... no observed adverse effect limit of 50 microg (2000 IU)/d is too low by at least 5-fold." Vieth R. Vitamin D supplementation, 25-hydroxyvitamin D concentrations, and safety. *Am J Clin Nutr* 1999 May;69(5):842-56

[246] "CONCLUSION: All patients with persistent, nonspecific musculoskeletal pain are at high risk for the consequences of unrecognized and untreated severe hypovitaminosis D. This risk extends to those considered at low risk for vitamin D deficiency: nonelderly, nonhousebound, or nonimmigrant persons of either sex." Plotnikoff GA, Quigley JM. Prevalence of severe hypovitaminosis D in patients with persistent, nonspecific musculoskeletal pain. *Mayo Clin Proc.* 2003 Dec;78(12):1463-70

[247] Geubel AP, De Galocsy C, Alves N, Rahier J, Dive C. Liver damage caused by therapeutic vitamin A administration: estimate of dose-related toxicity in 41 cases. *Gastroenterology.* 1991 Jun;100(6):1701-9

(hypervitaminosis A) include dry skin, chapped or split lips, skin rash (erythematous dermatitis), hair loss, joint pain, bone pain, headaches (pseudotumor cerebri), anorexia (loss of appetite), fatigue, elevated liver enzymes, and increased serum calcium. Women who are pregnant or might become pregnant and who are planning to carry the baby to full term delivery should not ingest more than 10,000 IU of vitamin A per day. Most patients should probably not consume more than 20,000 IU of vitamin A per day for more than 2 months without express supervision by a healthcare provider. **Vitamin A is present in some multivitamin supplements, in cod-liver oil, and in other supplements—patients and doctors are advised to read labels to ensure that the total daily intake is not greater than 20,000 IU per day for long-term use unless it is being used for a specific indication**

Dosage and administration:

- In my clinical practice, **I routinely recommend one tablespoon of cod-liver oil per day for essentially all adult patients**. One tablespoon of fish oil provides 3,000 mg of EPA+DHA, which is consistent with the amounts used in the research literature to provide clinical benefit.[248] Further justification for this recommendation is found in the literature documenting that the provision of EPA and DHA reduces the risk of death and "all-cause mortality" particularly cardiovascular disease, that these two fatty acids have health-promoting and anti-inflammatory effects, and that the risk for adverse effects is minimal to clinically nonexistent. The dose of vitamin A per tablespoon of cod-liver oil is 3,750 IU per day—clearly this is safe for long-term use. Vitamin D at 1,500 IU per day is safe and appears to have antidepressant, immunomodulatory, and anticancer effects.

- Periodically, I start patients at one-quarter cup of fish oil per day for five to ten days, and then reduce the dose to one tablespoon per day thereafter for maintenance. This technique can provide clinical benefit even for patients whom have supplemented fish oil at lower doses for long periods of time without benefit. The probable mechanism of action is primarily the more rapid exchange of fatty acids in cell membranes, with the resultant benefits in eicosanoid production and cell membrane receptor function.

Dosage and administration:

Clinical application	Approximate daily dosage range for combined EPA and DHA (i.e., mg of EPA + mg of DHA)
General preventive medicine for adults and dosage for children	1,000 mg
Therapeutic dose and assertive prevention	3,000 mg
High-dose supplementation (adult dose for short-term or aggressive therapy only)	Up to approximately 12,000 mg

---

[248] "…clinical benefits of the n-3 fatty acids were not apparent until they were consumed for > or =12 wk. It appears that a minimum daily dose of 3 g eicosapentaenoic and docosahexaenoic acids is necessary to derive the expected benefits [in patients with rheumatoid arthritis]." Kremer JM. n-3 fatty acid supplements in rheumatoid arthritis. *Am J Clin Nutr.* 2000 Jan;71(1 Suppl):349S-51S

Dosage and administration (continued):

- Coadminister GLA when using fish oil: Since EPA and other n-3 EFAs inhibit formation of GLA from LA[249] [250] and since administration of GLA will increase levels of arachidonic acid unless EPA is coadministered[251], **the most reasonable clinical approach to improving eicosanoid metabolism in favor of reducing inflammation is to always combine GLA supplementation with EPA/DHA supplementation.** Coadministration of EPA or fish oil will prevent the rise in arachidonate that might occur with supplementation with GLA alone[252], and using GLA when using fish oil and EPA will prevent the reduction in GLA that occurs with administration of EPA alone.[253]

Additional information:

- Given the low cost, high safety, and tremendous benefits of omega-3 fats in general and EPA and DHA in particular, I believe that all adult patients should supplement with one teaspoon to one tablespoon of fish oil per day, providing that they do not have disturbances of hemostasis or of vitamin D or vitamin A metabolism. Failure to address the underlying fatty acid imbalances in the majority of patients is one of the main reasons why otherwise appropriate treatment plans fail.

- Liquid fish oil supplements are easily consumed in a morning smoothie, mixed in tomato or orange juice, or taken straight from the bottle. Liquid supplements are much less expensive per dose than are capsule supplements. To obtain an equivalent dose of EPA and DHA found in one tablespoon of cod-liver oil would require the consumption of 6-21 capsules, depending on the brand and concentration of the capsule fish oil supplement.

- Although the data are inconclusive on the need for vitamin E supplementation to prevent the depletion of antioxidants induced by consumption of polyunsaturated fatty acids, I generally recommend 800-1,200 IU of vitamin E taken as mixed tocopherols with an emphasis on high concentrations of gamma-tocopherol, which has biologic benefits beyond its antioxidant function. For patients with cancer however, I do not use tocopherols because they have consistently been shown to abrogate the anticancer benefits of polyunsaturated fatty acids.[254]

[249] Horrobin DF. Interactions between n-3 and n-6 essential fatty acids (EFAs) in the regulation of cardiovascular disorders and inflammation. *Prostaglandins Leukot Essent Fatty Acids* 1991 Oct;44(2):127-31

[250] Rubin D, Laposata M. Cellular interactions between n-6 and n-3 fatty acids: a mass analysis of fatty acid elongation/desaturation, distribution among complex lipids, and conversion to eicosanoids. *J Lipid Res*. 1992 Oct;33(10):1431-40

[251] "The decrease in serum eicosapentaenoic acid and the increase in arachidonic acid concentrations induced by evening primrose oil may not be favourable effects in patients with rheumatoid arthritis in the light of the roles of these fatty acids as precursors of eicosanoids." Jantti J, Nikkari T, Solakivi T, Vapaatalo H, Isomaki H. Evening primrose oil in rheumatoid arthritis: changes in serum lipids and fatty acids. *Ann Rheum Dis*. 1989 Feb;48(2):124-7

[252] "This study revealed that a GLA and EPA supplement combination may be utilized to reduce the synthesis of proinflammatory AA metabolites, and importantly, not induce potentially harmful increases in serum AA levels." Barham JB, Edens MB, Fonteh AN, Johnson MM, Easter L, Chilton FH. Addition of eicosapentaenoic acid to gamma-linolenic acid-supplemented diets prevents serum arachidonic acid accumulation in humans. *J Nutr*. 2000 Aug;130(8):1925-31

[253] "...intake of fish oil caused a significant depression in the content of DGLA... Since DGLA is the precursor of PGE1, which has been shown to be anti-inflammatory, our findings suggest that the anti-inflammatory effects of fish oil consumption could be mitigated by an associated reduction in DGLA." Cleland LG, Gibson RA, Neumann M, French JK. The effect of dietary fish oil supplement upon the content of dihomo-gammalinolenic acid in human plasma phospholipids. *Prostaglandins Leukot Essent Fatty Acids*. 1990 May;40(1):9-12

[254] See my forthcoming ***The Scientific Basis for the Natural Treatment of Cancer in Humans*** for information on natural cancer treatments:OptimalHealthResearch.com

| Nutrient: | **_Gamma-linolenic acid_** |
| Common name: | **GLA** |

Applications and mechanisms of action:

- Anti-inflammatory effects: As described previously in the section detailing fatty acid metabolism, GLA is efficiently converted to DGLA and is then preferentially converted to the anti-inflammatory prostaglandin PG-E1. While GLA/DGLA have manifold effects, most of the benefits appear to be attributable to increased production of PG-E1. DGLA helps reduce the formation of the arachidonate-derived 2-series prostaglandins, 4-series leukotrienes and platelet-activating factor.[255] GLA is proven to be clinically effective in reducing inflammation and manifestations of disease activity in patients with **rheumatoid arthritis**[256,257,258], eczema[259], and respiratory distress syndrome (when used with EPA)[260]

- Additional clinical benefits: GLA supplementation benefits patients with breast cancer (when used with tamoxifen[261]), premenstrual syndrome[262], diabetic neuropathy[263], and migraine headaches (when used with ALA[264])

Toxicity and contraindications:

- GLA is very safe: In general, no toxicity has been noted using GLA in doses up to 4 grams per day in several long-term studies. Remarkably, one study used 3 grams (3,000 mg per day) of GLA in infants of age < 12 months and found no adverse effects[265] thus testifying to the non-existent toxicity of GLA. As with all dietary oils, some patients note belching and loose stools[266] but this is not an indication of toxicity

- Temporal lobe epilepsy: According to a small trial, GLA administration appears to worsen temporal lobe epilepsy[267]

Dosage and administration:

- Approximately 500 mg per day is the common anti-inflammatory dose: Studies have used 540 mg per day[268] and up to 2.8 grams per day in rheumatoid arthritis[269]

- Coadminister ascorbate: The conversion of DGLA to its bioactive metabolites is expedited by coadministration of vitamin C[270]

[255] Fan YY, Chapkin RS. Importance of dietary gamma-linolenic acid in human health and nutrition. *J Nutr.* 1998 Sep;128(9):1411-4

[256] "CONCLUSION: GLA at doses used in this study is a well-tolerated and effective treatment for active RA." Zurier RB, Rossetti RG, Jacobson EW, DeMarco DM, Liu NY, Temming JE, White BM, Laposata M. gamma-Linolenic acid treatment of rheumatoid arthritis. A randomized, placebo-controlled trial. *Arthritis Rheum.* 1996 Nov;39(11):1808-17

[257] "GLA treatment is associated with clinical improvement in patients with RA, as evaluated by duration of morning stiffness, joint pain and swelling, and ability to reduce other medications." Rothman D, DeLuca P, Zurier RB. Botanical lipids: effects on inflammation, immune responses, and rheumatoid arthritis. *Semin Arthritis Rheum.* 1995 Oct;25(2):87-96

[258] "Forty patients with rheumatoid arthritis and upper gastrointestinal lesions due to non-steroidal anti-inflammatory drugs entered a prospective 6-month double-blind placebo controlled study of dietary supplementation with gamma-linolenic acid 540 mg/day... Other results showed a significant reduction in morning stiffness with gamma-linolenic acid at 3 months..." Brzeski M, Madhok R, Capell HA. Evening primrose oil in patients with rheumatoid arthritis and side-effects of non-steroidal anti-inflammatory drugs. *Br J Rheumatol.* 1991 Oct;30(5):370-2

[259] Fiocchi A, Sala M, Signoroni P, Banderali G, Agostoni C, Riva E. The efficacy and safety of gamma-linolenic acid in the treatment of infantile atopic dermatitis. *J Int Med Res.* 1994 Jan-Feb;22(1):24-32

[260] Pacht ER, DeMichele SJ, Nelson JL, Hart J, Wennberg AK, Gadek JE. Enteral nutrition with eicosapentaenoic acid, gamma-linolenic acid, and antioxidants reduces alveolar inflammatory mediators and protein influx in patients with acute respiratory distress syndrome. *Crit Care Med.* 2003 Feb;31(2):491-500

[261] Kenny FS, Pinder SE, Ellis IO, Gee JM, Nicholson RI, Bryce RP, Robertson JF. Gamma linolenic acid with tamoxifen as primary therapy in breast cancer. *Int J Cancer.* 2000 Mar 1;85(5):643-8

[262] Puolakka J, Makarainen L, Viinikka L, Ylikorkala O. Biochemical and clinical effects of treating the premenstrual syndrome with prostaglandin synthesis precursors. *J Reprod Med.* 1985 Mar;30(3):149-53

[263] Jamal GA, Carmichael H. The effect of gamma-linolenic acid on human diabetic peripheral neuropathy: a double-blind placebo-controlled trial. *Diabet Med.* 1990 May;7(4):319-23

[264] Wagner W, Nootbaar-Wagner U. Prophylactic treatment of migraine with gamma-linolenic and alpha-linolenic acids. *Cephalalgia.* 1997 Apr;17(2):127-30

[265] "The children (mean age, 11.4 months) with atopic dermatitis (mean duration, 8.56 months) were openly treated with 3 g/day gamma-linolenic acid, for 28 days... A gradual improvement in erythema, excoriations and lichenification was seen; .... No side-effects were recorded." Fiocchi A, Sala M, Signoroni P, Banderali G, Agostoni C, Riva E. The efficacy and safety of gamma-linolenic acid in the treatment of infantile atopic dermatitis. *J Int Med Res.* 1994 Jan-Feb;22(1):24-32

[266] "With regard to safety, dietary sources of GLA appear to be completely nontoxic. Although limited cases of soft stools, belching and abdominal bloating have been reported ... long-term GLA administration may be feasible." Fan YY, Chapkin RS. Importance of dietary gamma-linolenic acid in human health and nutrition. J Nutr. 1998 Sep;128(9):1411-4

[267] "Three long-stay, hospitalised schizophrenics who had failed to respond adequately to conventional drug therapy were treated with gamma-linolenic acid and linoleic acid in the form of evening primrose oil. They became substantially worse and electroencephalographic features of temporal lobe epilepsy became apparent." Vaddadi KS. The use of gamma-linolenic acid and linoleic acid to differentiate between temporal lobe epilepsy and schizophrenia. *Prostaglandins Med.* 1981 Apr;6(4):375-9

[268] "Forty patients with rheumatoid arthritis and upper gastrointestinal lesions due to non-steroidal anti-inflammatory drugs entered a prospective 6-month double-blind placebo controlled study of dietary supplementation with gamma-linolenic acid 540 mg/day..." Brzeski M, Madhok R, Capell HA. Evening primrose oil in patients with rheumatoid arthritis and side-effects of non-steroidal anti-inflammatory drugs. *Br J Rheumatol.* 1991 Oct;30(5):370-2

[269] Zurier RB, Rossetti RG, Jacobson EW, DeMarco DM, Liu NY, Temming JE, White BM, Laposata M. gamma-Linolenic acid treatment of rheumatoid arthritis. A randomized, placebo-controlled trial. *Arthritis Rheum.* 1996 Nov;39(11):1808-17

[270] Horrobin DF. Ascorbic acid and prostaglandin synthesis. *Subcell Biochem.* 1996;25:109-15

- <u>Coadminister fish oil (EPA) and GLA</u>: Since EPA and other n-3 EFAs inhibit formation of GLA from LA[271] [272] and since administration of GLA will probably increase levels of arachidonic acid unless EPA is coadministered[273], **the most reasonable clinical approach to improving eicosanoid metabolism in favor of reducing inflammation is to always combine GLA supplementation with EPA/DHA supplementation**. Coadministration of EPA or fish oil will prevent the rise in arachidonate that might occur with supplementation with GLA alone[274], and using GLA when using fish oil and EPA will prevent the reduction in GLA that occurs with administration of EPA alone[275]

Additional information:

- In my clinical practice, I only recommend GLA when I am already using fish oil. No patient has ever noted adverse effects even with doses as high as 4 grams per day of GLA for periods of months or years

Notes:

[271] Horrobin DF. Interactions between n-3 and n-6 essential fatty acids (EFAs) in the regulation of cardiovascular disorders and inflammation. *Prostaglandins Leukot Essent Fatty Acids* 1991 Oct;44(2):127-31

[272] Rubin D, Laposata M. Cellular interactions between n-6 and n-3 fatty acids: a mass analysis of fatty acid elongation/desaturation, distribution among complex lipids, and conversion to eicosanoids. *J Lipid Res.* 1992 Oct;33(10):1431-40

[273] "The decrease in serum eicosapentaenoic acid and the increase in arachidonic acid concentrations induced by evening primrose oil may not be favourable effects in patients with rheumatoid arthritis in the light of the roles of these fatty acids as precursors of eicosanoids." Jantti J, Nikkari T, Solakivi T, Vapaatalo H, Isomaki H. Evening primrose oil in rheumatoid arthritis: changes in serum lipids and fatty acids. *Ann Rheum Dis.* 1989 Feb;48(2):124-7

[274] "This study revealed that a GLA and EPA supplement combination may be utilized to reduce the synthesis of proinflammatory AA metabolites, and importantly, not induce potentially harmful increases in serum AA levels." Barham JB, Edens MB, Fonteh AN, Johnson MM, Easter L, Chilton FH. Addition of eicosapentaenoic acid to gamma-linolenic acid-supplemented diets prevents serum arachidonic acid accumulation in humans. *J Nutr.* 2000 Aug;130(8):1925-31

[275] "...intake of fish oil caused a significant depression in the content of DGLA... Since DGLA is the precursor of PGE1, which has been shown to be anti-inflammatory, our findings suggest that the anti-inflammatory effects of fish oil consumption could be mitigated by an associated reduction in DGLA." Cleland LG, Gibson RA, Neumann M, French JK. The effect of dietary fish oil supplement upon the content of dihomo-gammalinolenic acid in human plasma phospholipids. *Prostaglandins Leukot Essent Fatty Acids.* 1990 May;40(1):9-12

Vitamin:	**Vitamin D3**
Common name:	**Vitamin D, Cholecalciferol**

Applications and mechanisms of action:	▪ <u>Musculoskeletal Pain</u>: Vitamin D deficiency causes dull, achy musculoskeletal pain that is incompletely responsive to both pharmacologic and manual treatments. The pain may be widespread or confined to a particular area, most commonly the low-back and lumbar spine. The mechanism by which this pain is produced has been clearly elucidated by Holick[276]: 1) vitamin D deficiency causes a reduction in calcium absorption, 2) production of parathyroid hormone (PTH) is increased to maintain blood calcium levels, 3) PTH results in increased urinary excretion of phosphorus, which leads to hypophosphatemia, 4) insufficient calcium phosphate results in deposition of unmineralized collagen matrix on the endosteal (inside) and periosteal (outside) of bones, 5) when the collagen matrix hydrates and swells, it causes pressure on the sensory-innervated periosteum resulting in pain. Several clinical investigations have recently shown that vitamin D deficiency is particularly common among people with musculoskeletal pain.[277,278,279] Most importantly, the finding that musculoskeletal pain can be eliminated in a high proportion (>95%) of patients with vitamin D deficiency proves the cause-and-effect relationship between vitamin D deficiency and musculoskeletal pain; among patients who are deficient in vitamin D, their pain levels can be tremendously reduced within 3 months of high-dose vitamin D supplementation[280,281] ▪ **<u>Anti-inflammatory effect</u>**: Vitamin D has shown a modest anti-inflammatory benefit in two recent studies that used insufficient doses of vitamin D for insufficient durations[282,283]
Toxicity and contraindications:	▪ Vitamin D has a wide range of safety according to an extensive review of the literature performed by Vieth.[284] ▪ Doses of 2,000 IU per day of vitamin D3 have been given to children starting at one year of age and were not associated with toxicity but lead to a reduction in the incidence of type 1 diabetes by 80%.[285] ▪ **Vitamin D hypersensitivity syndromes are seen with primary hyperparathyroidism, granulomatous diseases (such as sarcoidosis, Crohn's disease, and tuberculosis), adrenal insufficiency, hyperthyroidism, hypothyroidism, various forms of cancer, as well as adverse drug effects, particularly with thiazide diuretics. When these patients require vitamin D supplementation, additional vigilance must be employed—1) starting with a lower dose of supplementation, and 2) more frequent monitoring of serum calcium.** ▪ Thiazide diuretics are known to potentiate hypercalcemia.
Dosage and administration:	▪ **Vitamin D deficiency and sufficiency are defined by analysis of serum 25(OH) vitamin D levels.** Serum 25(OH)D levels must be above 40 ng/mL (100 nmol/L) in order to sufficiently suppress any rise in PTH levels according to Zittermann[286], Dawson-Hughes et al[287] and Kinyamu et al[288]. Based on the current literature, in our

[276] Holick MF. Vitamin D deficiency: what a pain it is. *Mayo Clin Proc*. 2003 Dec;78(12):1457-9

[277] Al Faraj S, Al Mutairi K. Vitamin D deficiency and chronic low back pain in Saudi Arabia. *Spine*. 2003 Jan 15;28(2):177-9

[278] Plotnikoff GA, Quigley JM. Prevalence of severe hypovitaminosis D in patients with persistent, nonspecific musculoskeletal pain. *Mayo Clin Proc*. 2003 Dec;78(12):1463-70

[279] Masood H, Narang AP, Bhat IA, Shah GN. Persistent limb pain and raised serum alkaline phosphatase the earliest markers of subclinical hypovitaminosis D in Kashmir. *Indian J Physiol Pharmacol*. 1989 Oct-Dec;33(4):259-61

[280] Al Faraj S, Al Mutairi K. Vitamin D deficiency and chronic low back pain in Saudi Arabia. *Spine*. 2003 Jan 15;28(2):177-9

[281] Masood H, Narang AP, Bhat IA, Shah GN. Persistent limb pain and raised serum alkaline phosphatase the earliest markers of subclinical hypovitaminosis D in Kashmir. *Indian J Physiol Pharmacol*. 1989 Oct-Dec;33(4):259-61

[282] Mahon BD, Gordon SA, Cruz J, Cosman F, Cantorna MT. Cytokine profile in patients with multiple sclerosis following vitamin D supplementation. *J Neuroimmunol*. 2003;134(1-2):128-32

[283] Van den Berghe G, et al. Bone turnover in prolonged critical illness: effect of vitamin D. *J Clin Endocrinol Metab*. 2003 Oct;88(10):4623-32

[284] Vieth R. Vitamin D supplementation, 25-hydroxyvitamin D concentrations, and safety. *Am J Clin Nutr*. 1999 May;69(5):842-56

[285] Hypponen E, Laara E, Reunanen A, Jarvelin MR, Virtanen SM. Intake of vitamin D and risk of type 1 diabetes: a birth-cohort study. *Lancet*. 2001 Nov 3;358(9292):1500-3

[286] Zittermann A. Vitamin D in preventive medicine: are we ignoring the evidence? *Br J Nutr*. 2003 May;89(5):552-72

[287] Dawson-Hughes B, Harris SS, Dallal GE. Plasma calcidiol, season, and serum parathyroid hormone concentrations in healthy elderly men and women. *Am J Clin Nutr*. 1997 Jan;65(1):67-71

recent review of the literature[289], we proposed that **optimal vitamin D status is defined as 40 – 65 ng/mL (100 - 160 nmol/L).** This proposed optimal range is compatible with other published recommendations: Zittermann[290] states that serum levels of 40 - 80 ng/mL (100 - 200 nmol/L) are "adequate", and Mahon *et al*[291] recently advocated an optimal range of 40 - 100 ng/mL (100 - 250 nmol/L) for patients with multiple sclerosis. There are no acute or subacute risks associated with the 25(OH)D levels suggested here. Conversely, there is clear evidence of long-term danger associated with vitamin D levels that are *insufficient*.

- In our recent review article[292], we concluded, "Until proven otherwise, the balance of the research clearly indicates that oral supplementation in the range of 1,000 IU per day for infants, 2,000 IU per day for children and 4,000 IU per day for adults is safe and reasonable to meet physiologic requirements, to promote optimal health, and to reduce the risk of several serious diseases. Safety and effectiveness of supplementation are assured by periodic monitoring of serum 25(OH)D and serum calcium."

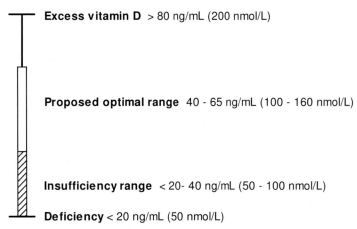

Excess vitamin D > 80 ng/mL (200 nmol/L)

Proposed optimal range 40 - 65 ng/mL (100 - 160 nmol/L)

Insufficiency range < 20- 40 ng/mL (50 - 100 nmol/L)

Deficiency < 20 ng/mL (50 nmol/L)

Proposed normal and optimal ranges for serum 25(OH)D levels based on current research.

Additional information:

- Exposure to sunlight can produce the equivalent of more than 10,000 IU vitamin D3 per day and can produce serum levels of 25(OH)D greater than 80 ng/mL (200 nmol/L).[293,294] No one has ever become vitamin D toxic from sun exposure.
- Patients with hypercalcemia should discontinue vitamin D supplementation and receive a thorough diagnostic evaluation to determine the cause of the problem.
- **Summary: vitamin D supplementation in the doses recommended here is generally very safe. However, safety *in a particular patient* is determined by periodic monitoring of serum calcium (perhaps weekly at first, then monthly until a steady state and confidence are attained). Routine vitamin D supplementation and testing for vitamin D insufficiency should become standard, day-to-day components of patient care. Caution must be used in patients predisposed to hypercalcemia ("vitamin D hypersensitivity syndromes") and patients taking drugs that affect calcium metabolism.**
- For additional research on the importance and safety of vitamin D, see the articles by Vieth[295], Heaney et al[296], Holick[297], and Vasquez, Manso, and Cannell.[298]

[288] Kinyamu HK, Gallagher JC, Rafferty KA, Balhorn KE. Dietary calcium and vitamin D intake in elderly women: effect on serum parathyroid hormone and vitamin D metabolites. *Am J Clin Nutr.* 1998 Feb;67(2):342-8

[289] Vasquez A, Manso G, Cannell J. The Clinical Importance of Vitamin D (Cholecalciferol): A Paradigm Shift with Implications for All Healthcare Providers. *Alternative Therapies in Health and Medicine* 2004; 10: 28-37. Also published in *Integrative Medicine: A Clinician's Journal* 2004; 3: 44-54. See optimalhealthresearch.com/monograph04

[290] Zittermann A. Vitamin D in preventive medicine: are we ignoring the evidence? *Br J Nutr.* 2003 May;89(5):552-72

[291] Mahon BD, Gordon SA, Cruz J, Cosman F, Cantorna MT. Cytokine profile in patients with multiple sclerosis following vitamin D supplementation. *J Neuroimmunol.* 2003;134(1-2):128-32

[292] Vasquez A, Manso G, Cannell J. The Clinical Importance of Vitamin D (Cholecalciferol): A Paradigm Shift with Implications for All Healthcare Providers. *Alternative Therapies in Health and Medicine* 2004; 10: 28-37. Also published in *Integrative Medicine: A Clinician's Journal* 2004; 3: 44-54. See optimalhealthresearch.com/monograph04

[293] Vieth R. Vitamin D supplementation, 25-hydroxyvitamin D concentrations, and safety. *Am J Clin Nutr.* 1999 May;69(5):842-56

[294] Holick MF. Calcium and Vitamin D. Diagnostics and Therapeutics. *Clin Lab Med.* 2000 Sep;20(3):569-90

Vitamin: **Alpha-tocopherol, beta-tocopherol, delta-tocopherol, gamma-tocopherol**

Common name: **Vitamin E**

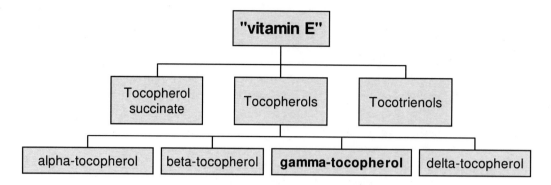

Applications and mechanisms of action:

- <u>Antioxidant</u>: vitamin E is a tremendously important fat-soluble antioxidant vitamin that is generally non-toxic in doses up to 3,200 IU per day.[299] Given that increased oxidative stress is associated with nearly every known disease including the aging process itself, common sense provides us with sufficient justification for the use of vitamin E as a matter of course in nearly all patients, including those who are asymptomatic.

- <u>Anti-inflammatory and analgesic</u>: The gamma form of vitamin E inhibits cyclooxygenase and thus has anti-inflammatory activity.[300] Patients with **rheumatoid arthritis** treated with methotrexate, oral sulfasalazine, and indomethacin show significant subjective and objective improvements when antioxidants and vitamin E are added to the treatment plan.[301] Another study of patients with RA showed no biochemical evidence of improvement, but patients reported a reduction in pain.[302] An abstract from the foreign medical research found that patients with **spondylosis and back pain** had lower levels of vitamin E than did the control group, and that administration of vitamin E lead to "complete pain relief" and "cure" of spondylosis.[303] German research abstracts state that vitamin E is able to reduce the pain and swelling associated with **osteoarthritis**[304] and that higher serum levels of vitamin E following supplementation correlated with improved clinical outcome.[305] Indeed the majority of research suggests a mild-moderate analgesic and anti-inflammatory effect of vitamin E in patients with arthritis.[306] The noteworthy research by Ayres and

[295] Vieth R. Vitamin D supplementation, 25-hydroxyvitamin D concentrations, and safety. *Am J Clin Nutr.* 1999 May;69(5):842-56

[296] Heaney RP, Davies KM, Chen TC, Holick MF, Barger-Lux MJ. Human serum 25-hydroxycholecalciferol response to extended oral dosing with cholecalciferol. *Am J Clin Nutr.* 2003 Jan;77(1):204-10

[297] Holick MF. Vitamin D: importance in the prevention of cancers, type 1 diabetes, heart disease, and osteoporosis. *Am J Clin Nutr.* 2004 Mar;79(3):362-71

[298] Vasquez A, Manso G, Cannell J. The Clinical Importance of Vitamin D (Cholecalciferol): A Paradigm Shift with Implications for All Healthcare Providers. *Alternative Therapies in Health and Medicine* 2004; 10: 28-37. Also published in *Integrative Medicine: A Clinician's Journal* 2004; 3: 44-54. See optimalhealthresearch.com/monograph04

[299] Meydani M. Vitamin E. *Lancet.* 1995 Jan 21;345(8943):170-5

[300] Jiang Q, Christen S, Shigenaga MK, Ames BN. gamma-tocopherol, the major form of vitamin E in the US diet, deserves more attention. *Am J Clin Nutr* 2001;74(6):714-22

[301] Helmy M, Shohayeb M, Helmy MH, el-Bassiouni EA. Antioxidants as adjuvant therapy in rheumatoid disease. A preliminary study. *Arzneimittelforschung.* 2001;51(4):293-8

[302] Edmonds SE, Winyard PG, Guo R, Kidd B, Merry P, Langrish-Smith A, Hansen C, Ramm S, Blake DR. Putative analgesic activity of repeated oral doses of vitamin E in the treatment of rheumatoid arthritis. Results of a prospective placebo controlled double blind trial. *Ann Rheum Dis.* 1997 Nov;56(11):649-55

[303] Mahmud Z, Ali SM. Role of vitamin A and E in spondylosis. *Bangladesh Med Res Counc Bull.* 1992 Apr;18(1):47-59

[304] Blankenhorn G. [Clinical effectiveness of Spondyvit (vitamin E) in activated arthroses. A multicenter placebo-controlled double-blind study] [Article in German] *Z Orthop Ihre Grenzgeb.* 1986 May-Jun;124(3):340-3

[305] Scherak O, Kolarz G, Schodl C, Blankenhorn G. [High dosage vitamin E therapy in patients with activated arthrosis] [Article in German] *Z Rheumatol.* 1990 Nov-Dec;49(6):369-73

[306] Machtey I, Ouaknine L. Tocopherol in Osteoarthritis: a controlled pilot study. *J Am Geriatr Soc.* 1978 Jul;26(7):328-30

[307] Ayres S Jr, Mihan R. Is vitamin E involved in the autoimmune mechanism? *Cutis.* 1978 Mar;21(3):321-5

[308] Ayres S Jr, Mihan R. Lupus erythematosus and vitamin E: an effective and nontoxic therapy. *Cutis.* 1979 Jan;23(1):49-52, 54

[309] Killeen RN, Ayres S Jr, Mihan R. Polymyositis: response to vitamin E. *South Med J.* 1976 Oct;69(10):1372-4

Mihan[307] has suggested that vitamin E may have efficacy in the treatment of **autoimmune diseases** via its antioxidant and membrane-stabilizing effects; the authors state, "Among the diseases that were successfully controlled were a number in the autoimmune category, including **scleroderma**, **discoid lupus erythematosus**[308], **porphyria cutanea tarda**, several types of **vasculitis**, and **polymyositis**.[309] Since vitamin E is a physiologic stabilizer of cellular and lysosomal membranes, and since some autoimmune diseases respond to vitamin E, we suggest that a relative deficiency of vitamin E damages lysosomal membranes, thus initiating the autoimmune process."

- <u>Other uses</u>: In dialysis patients who suffer from leg cramps, vitamin E is just as effective but less toxic that quinine.[310]

Toxicity and contraindications:

- <u>Anticoagulant medications, surgery, and bleeding</u>: Vitamin E has some weak ability to impair coagulation. Therefore it should be used advisedly in patients taking other "blood thinners" such as aspirin, fish oil, and ginkgo. Particular care and attention are needed when coadministering vitamin E with coumadin/warfarin. Any clinically significant increase in bleeding or bruising associated with vitamin E supplementation indicates the need for dosage reduction.

Dosage and administration:

- <u>400 IU BID-TID</u>: "Vitamin E" should be administered in a mixed tocopherol combination that provides a high percentage (i.e., ~40%) of gamma-tocopherol. Common doses are 400 IU BID-TID. While consumption of sesame seeds raises gamma-tocopherol levels[311], all researchers agree that consumption of vitamin E supplements is necessary to obtain the high doses necessary to achieve clinical benefit in severe illnesses.

Additional information:

- The term "vitamin E" applies to several different chemicals, each with its own biochemical and clinical effects. Generally speaking, regarding the tocopherols, alpha- and gamma- are the most important, with gamma-appearing to provide the greatest degree of benefit. Most multivitamin products contain only the alpha-form of the vitamin, which unfavorably impairs gamma-tocopherol function and creates the illusion that one is obtaining sufficient vitamin E supplementation despite the lack of the most important form of vitamin E: gamma-tocopherol.
- The "dl" forms of vitamin E are synthetic and should be avoided; adverse effects from this type of vitamin E include transient hypertension and headache.
- Many of the clinical trials with vitamin E, especially those reporting negative effects have used either 1) the synthetic "dl" form of the vitamin, 2) exclusively alpha-tocopherol, rather than the blend of all tocopherols, or 3) have used insufficient doses to achieve clinical benefit. Thus the "failure of vitamin E" in these studies is directly related to the failure by these researchers to understand the basic pharmacodynamics of the agent they were testing, namely that vitamin E comes in different forms with different effects and that the commonly used alpha-tocopherol does not possess the stronger anti-inflammatory, antiproliferative, and analgesic effects of gamma-tocopherol. Furthermore, in conditions such as rheumatoid arthritis and other inflammatory conditions that are characterized by greatly increased oxidative stress, low doses of antioxidant supplementation are barely sufficient for creating a state of *normal* redox potential and are thus unable to provide clinical "supranutritional" or pharmacologic benefit.

---

[310] Roca AO, Jarjoura D, Blend D, Cugino A, Rutecki GW, Nuchikat PS, Whittier FC. Dialysis leg cramps. Efficacy of quinine versus vitamin E. *ASAIO J*. 1992 Jul-Sep;38(3):M481-5
[311] Cooney RV, Custer LJ, Okinaka L, Franke AA. Effects of dietary sesame seeds on plasma tocopherol levels. *Nutr Cancer*. 2001;39(1):66-71

Vitamin:	**Niacinamide**
Common name:	**Niacinamide, Nicotinamide, Vitamin B3**

Applications and mechanisms of action:

- <u>Joint pain and inflammation</u>: The credit for discovering the effectiveness of niacinamide in the treatment of arthritis goes to Kaufman, whose studies published in 1949 documented the safety and efficacy in hundreds of patients with **rheumatoid arthritis** and **osteoarthritis**. While the mechanism of action is probably multifaceted, inhibition of joint-destroying nitric oxide appears to be an important benefit.[312] A recent double-blind placebo-controlled study found that niacinamide therapy improved joint mobility, reduced objective inflammation as assessed by ESR, reduced the impact of the arthritis on the activities of daily living, and allowed a reduction in medication use.[313]

Toxicity and contraindications:

- The treatment is generally safe
- <u>Liver damage</u>: Given that a small risk for liver damage exists, liver enzymes should be assessed before and after the first month of treatment and periodically thereafter in patients receiving more than 2,000 mg per day. Patients are advised to discontinue treatment with the onset of abdominal pain, jaundice or nausea.

Dosage and administration:

- <u>Doses have ranged from 1,000 mg per day to 4,000 mg per day. 500 mg 4-6 times per day is a common dosing regimen.</u>
- The most important clinical pearl for improving the effectiveness of niacinamide in the treatment of osteoarthritis is found in the timing and distribution of the dosing. The treatment must be administered several times per day in small doses rather than a few times per day in large doses. As Gaby and Wright[314] point out, "500 mg taken 3 times a day is about half as effective as 250 mg taken every 3 hours for 6 doses, even though the total daily dose is the same."
- Treatment must be maintained for a minimum of 4 weeks before beneficial subjective and objective improvements can be expected. The general trend is rapid improvement in joint mobility and a reduction in pain in the first 1-2 months followed by slower improvement which may continue for the next 1-3 years.
- Improved results may be seen with concomitant administration of other vitamins, particularly thiamine and riboflavin.

Additional information:

- To refer to niacinamide as "vitamin B-3" is accurate, but to refer to "vitamin B-3" as niacinamide is somewhat incomplete since vitamin B-3 represents a family of related compounds including 1) niacinamide, 2) NADH, 2) plain niacin, 3) time-released niacin (hepatotoxic), 4) prescription strength sustained-release niacin ("Niaspan"), and 5) inositol hexaniacinate. Each form of niacin has its form, function, clinical applications, risk and safety.

---

[312] McCarty MF, Russell AL. Niacinamide therapy for osteoarthritis--does it inhibit nitric oxide synthase induction by interleukin 1 in chondrocytes? *Med Hypotheses*. 1999 Oct;53(4):350-60
[313] Jonas WB, Rapoza CP, Blair WF. The effect of niacinamide on osteoarthritis: a pilot study. *Inflamm Res* 1996 Jul;45(7):330-4
[314] Gaby AR, Wright JV. <u>Nutritional therapy in medical practice. Reference manual and study guide. 1996 edition</u>. Wright/Gaby Seminars 1996. page 102

Nutrient:

Glucosamine Sulfate
Chondroitin Sulfate

Applications and mechanisms of action:

- <u>Promotion of cartilage regeneration</u>: Glucosamine and chondroitin stimulate the synthesis of glycosaminoglycan, proteoglycan and hyaluronic acid, which are the "building blocks" of joint cartilage. The goal with supplementation with glucosamine/chondroitin is to shift the anabolic:catabolic ratio in favor of cartilage formation rather than cartilage destruction. Thus, the classic application for glucosamine/chondroitin is the treatment of joint degeneration and joint pain seen with osteoarthritis.[315,316,317] A recent study showed that glucosamine sulfate 500 mg TID was nearly as effective as and much safer than ibuprofen 400 mg TID for the relief of knee pain.[318] Glucosamine sulfate 500 mg TID is superior to ibuprofen 400 mg TID for the treatment of TMJ osteoarthritis.[319]

Toxicity and contraindications:

- <u>Allergy</u>: Immediate allergy to glucosamine sulfate has been reported, as has another case involving exacerbation of asthma in a patient following supplementation with glucosamine and chondroitin.[320] Since glucosamine is commonly sourced from shells of shrimp, crab, or lobster, it is conceivable that people with **hypersensitivity to shellfish or seafood** might have an allergic response to the ingestion of glucosamine. Such people should either avoid glucosamine supplementation or use glucosamine from a synthetic/hypoallergenic source.

- Glucosamine is safe in patients with diabetes, as it does not alter blood glucose or HgbA1c levels.[321]

Dosage and administration:

- <u>Glucosamine 1500 mg and/or chondroitin 1000-1,500 mg in divided doses</u>: Can be taken with or without food.

- Treatment must be continued for at least eight weeks before significant results can be expected. Long-term treatment for several years is both safe and effective in treating joint pain and reducing progression of joint destruction.[322]

Additional information:

- To improve results, glucosamine can be coadministered with niacinamide and botanical antiinflammatories, particularly *Uncaria*.

- Chondroitin sulfate is cardioprotective and ameliorates atherosclerosis.[323,324,325,326]

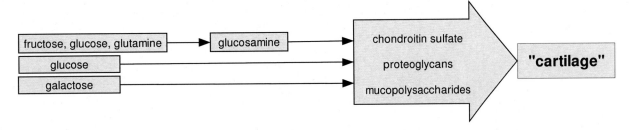

---

[315] Braham R, Dawson B, Goodman C. The effect of glucosamine supplementation on people experiencing regular knee pain. *Br J Sports Med*. 2003;37(1):45-9

[316] Nguyen P, Mohamed SE, Gardiner D, Salinas T. A randomized double-blind clinical trial of the effect of chondroitin sulfate and glucosamine hydrochloride on temporomandibular joint disorders: a pilot study. *Cranio*. 2001 Apr;19(2):130-9

[317] "...oral glucosamine therapy achieved a significantly greater improvement in articular pain score than ibuprofen, and the investigators rated treatment efficacy as 'good' in a significantly greater proportion of glucosamine than ibuprofen recipients. In comparison with piroxicam, glucosamine significantly improved arthritic symptoms after 12 weeks of therapy..." Matheson AJ, Perry CM. Glucosamine: a review of its use in the management of osteoarthritis. *Drugs Aging*. 2003; 20(14): 1041-60

[318] Muller-Fassbender H, Bach GL, Haase W, Rovati LC, Setnikar I. Glucosamine sulfate compared to ibuprofen in osteoarthritis of the knee. *Osteoarthritis Cartilage*. 1994 Mar;2(1):61-9

[319] "...patients taking GS had a significantly greater decrease in TMJ pain with function, effect of pain, and acetaminophen used between Day 90 and 120 compared with patients taking ibuprofen." Thie NM, Prasad NG, Major PW. Evaluation of glucosamine sulfate compared to ibuprofen for the treatment of temporomandibular joint osteoarthritis: a randomized double blind controlled 3 month clinical trial. *J Rheumatol*. 2001 Jun;28(6):1347-55

[320] Tallia AF, Cardone DA. Asthma exacerbation associated with glucosamine-chondroitin supplement. J Am Board Fam Pract. 2002 Nov-Dec;15(6):481-4 Available at http://www.jabfp.org/cgi/reprint/15/6/481.pdf on March 21, 2004

[321] Scroggie DA, Albright A, Harris MD. The effect of glucosamine-chondroitin supplementation on glycosylated hemoglobin levels in patients with type 2 diabetes mellitus: a placebo-controlled, double-blinded, randomized clinical trial. *Arch Intern Med*. 2003 Jul 14;163(13):1587-90

[322] "Long-term treatment with glucosamine sulfate retarded the progression of knee osteoarthritis, possibly determining disease modification." Pavelka K, Gatterova J, Olejarova M, Machacek S, Giacovelli G, Rovati LC. Glucosamine sulfate use and delay of progression of knee osteoarthritis: a 3-year, randomized, placebo-controlled, double-blind study. *Arch Intern Med*. 2002 Oct 14;162(18):2113-23

[323] Morrison LM. Treatment of coronary arteriosclerotic heart disease with chondroitin sulfate-A: preliminary report. *J Am Geriatr Soc*. 1968;16(7):779-85

[324] Morrison LM, Branwood AW, Ershoff BH, Murata K, Quilligan JJ Jr, Schjeide OA, Patek P, Bernick S, Freeman L, Dunn OJ, Rucker P. The prevention of coronary arteriosclerotic heart disease with chondroitin sulfate A: preliminary report. *Exp Med Surg*. 1969;27(3):278-89

[325] Morrison LM, Bajwa GS. Absence of naturally occurring coronary atherosclerosis in squirrel monkeys (Saimiri sciurea) treated with chondroitin sulfate A. *Experientia*. 1972 Dec 15;28(12):1410-1

[326] Morrison LM, Enrick N. Coronary heart disease: reduction of death rate by chondroitin sulfate A. *Angiology*. 1973 May;24(5):269-87

| *Nutrients:* | *Pancreatin, bromelain, papain, trypsin and alpha-chymotrypsin* |

| *Common name:* | *"Proteolytic enzymes"*   *"Pancreatic enzymes"* |

Applications and mechanisms of action:

- <u>Actions and mechanisms</u>: Orally administered proteolytic enzymes are well absorbed from the gastrointestinal tract into the systemic circulation[327,328] and that the anti-tumor, anti-metastatic, anti-infectious, anti-inflammatory , analgesic, and anti-edematous actions result from synergism between a variety of mechanisms of action, including the dose-dependent stimulation of reactive oxygen species production and anti-cancer cytotoxicity in human neutrophils[329], a pro-differentiative effect[330], reduction in PG-E2 production[331], reduction in substance P production[332], modulation of adhesion molecules and cytokine levels[333], fibrinolytic effects and a anti-thrombotic effect mediated at least in part by a reduction in 2-series thromboxanes.[334]

- <u>Acute injuries</u>: Reporting from the Tulane University Health Service Center, Trickett[335] reported that a papain-containing preparation benefited 40 patients with various injuries (e.g., contusions, sprains, lacerations, strains, fracture, surgical repair, and muscle tears); no adverse effects were seen. Bromelain also attenuates experimental contraction-induced skeletal muscle injury[336] and reduces production of hyperalgesic PG-E2 and substance P[337],

- <u>Osteoarthritis</u>: Walker et al[338] found a dose-dependent reduction in pain and disability as well as a significant improvement in psychological well-being in patients consuming bromelain orally. Most of the bromelain studies reviewed by Brien et al[339] were suggestive of a positive benefit in patients with knee osteoarthritis, but inadequate dosing clearly prohibited the attainment of optimal results.

- <u>Sinusitis</u>: In a double-blind placebo-controlled trial with 59 patients, Taub[340] documented that oral administration of bromelain significantly promoted the resolution of congestion, inflammation, and edema in patients with acute and chronic refractory sinusitis; no adverse effects were seen in any patient.

- <u>Anti-cancer benefit</u>: One of the first experimental studies was published by Beard in 1906 in the *British Medical Journal* wherein he showed that proteolytic enzymes significantly inhibited tumor growth in mice with implanted tumors[341], and a year later in that same journal, Cutfield[342] reported tumor regression and other objective improvements in a patient treated with proteolytic enzymes. In the American research literature, anti-cancer effects of proteolytic enzymes were reported during this same time in the *Journal of the American Medical Association* in anecdotal case reports of patients with fibrosarcoma[343], breast cancer[344], and head and neck malignancy[345]—all of whom responded positively to the administration of proteolytic

[327] Gotze H, Rothman SS. Enteropancreatic circulation of digestive enzymes as a conservative mechanism. *Nature* 1975; 257(5527): 607-609
[328] Liebow C, Rothman SS. Enteropancreatic Circulation of Digestive Enzymes. *Science* 1975; 189(4201): 472-474
[329] Zavadova E, Desser L, Mohr T. Stimulation of reactive oxygen species production and cytotoxicity in human neutrophils in vitro and after oral administration of a polyenzyme preparation. *Cancer Biother.* 1995;10(2):147-52
[330] Maurer HR, Hozumi M, Honma Y, Okabe-Kado J. Bromelain induces the differentiation of leukemic cells in vitro: an explanation for its cytostatic effects? *Planta Med.* 1988;54(5):377-81
[331] Brien S, Lewith G, Walker A, Hicks SM, Middleton D. Bromelain as a Treatment for Osteoarthritis: a Review of Clinical Studies. *Evidence-based Complementary and Alternative Medicine.* 2004;1(3)251–257
[332] Gaspani L, Limiroli E, Ferrario P, Bianchi M. In vivo and in vitro effects of bromelain on PGE(2) and SP concentrations in the inflammatory exudate in rats. *Pharmacology.* 2002;65(2):83-6
[333] Leipner J, Saller R. Systemic enzyme therapy in oncology: effect and mode of action. *Drugs.* 2000 Apr;59(4):769-80
[334] Vellini M, Desideri D, Milanese A, Omini C, Daffonchio L, Hernandez A, Brunelli G. Possible involvement of eicosanoids in the pharmacological action of bromelain. *Arzneimittelforschung.* 1986;36(1):110-2
[335] Trickett P. Proteolytic enzymes in treatment of athletic injuries. *Appl Ther.* 1964;30:647-52
[336] Walker JA, Cerny FJ, Cotter JR, Burton HW. Attenuation of contraction-induced skeletal muscle injury by bromelain. *Med Sci Sports Exerc.* 1992 Jan;24(1):20-5
[337] Gaspani L, Limiroli E, Ferrario P, Bianchi M. In vivo and in vitro effects of bromelain on PGE(2) and SP concentrations in the inflammatory exudate in rats. *Pharmacology.* 2002;65(2):83-6
[338] Walker AF, Bundy R, Hicks SM, Middleton RW. Bromelain reduces mild acute knee pain and improves well-being in a dose-dependent fashion in an open study of otherwise healthy adults.*Phytomedicine.*2002;9:681-6
[339] Brien S, Lewith G, Walker A, Hicks SM, Middleton D. Bromelain as a Treatment for Osteoarthritis: a Review of Clinical Studies. *Evidence-based Complementary and Alternative Medicine.* 2004;1(3)251–257
[340] Taub SJ. The use of bromelains in sinusitis: a double-blind clinical evaluation. Eye Ear Nose Throat Mon. 1967 Mar;46(3):361-5
[341] Beard J. The action of trypsin upon the living cells of Jensen's mouse-tumour. *Br Med J* 1906; 4 (Jan 20): 140-1
[342] Cutfield A. Trypsin Treatment in Malignant Disease. *Br Med J.* 1907; 5: 525
[343] Wiggin FH. Case of Multiple Fibrosarcoma of the Tongue, With Remarks on the Use of Trypsin and Amylopsin in the Treatment of Malignant Disease." *Journal of the American Medical Association* 1906; 47: 2003-8
[344] Goeth RA. Pancreatic treatment of cancer, with report of a cure. *Journal of the American Medical Association* 1907; (March 23) 48: 1030
[345] Campbell JT. Trypsin Treatment of a Case of Malignant Disease. *Journal of the American Medical Association* 1907; 48: 225-226

enzymes; no adverse effects were seen. Nearly a century would pass before Beard's study and results were replicated with modern techniques[346,347], and modern controlled clinical trials in cancer patients have established the value of enzyme therapy, which produces important clinical benefit (e.g., symptom reduction and prolonged survival) for little cost and with negligible adverse effects.[348,349,350]

Toxicity and contraindications:

- Allergy: As with all treatments—dietary, nutritional, botanical, and pharmaceutical—allergy is generally a manifestation of immune dysfunction which requires specific and personalized treatment. In the meanwhile, or when normalization of immune function is not achieved, then of course the "offending agent" should be avoided. Allergy to proteolytic enzymes is rare; but some patients manifest allergy as rectal itching following the oral administration of enzymes, particularly bromelain.

- Theoretical contraindications: Most doctors are aware of a potential anticoagulant effect and therefore proceed cautiously when using proteolytic enzymes in patients on anticoagulant medications. It is reasonable to discontinue supplements that have an anticoagulant effect for at least one week before any surgical procedures. Likewise, since safety during pregnancy has not been conclusively demonstrated, doctors would be wise to avoid use in patients who are pregnant; lactation is probably not a legitimate reason to withhold use of proteolytic/pancreatic enzymes.

Dosage and administration:

- Although bromelain may be used in isolation, enzyme therapy is generally delivered in the form of polyenzyme preparations containing pancreatin, bromelain, papain, amylase, lipase, trypsin and alpha-chymotrypsin.

- Dosage is determined per product and obviously tailored per patient. The therapeutic margin is exceedingly large, and therefore overdose/toxicity is unlikely with any reasonable dosage regimen.

Additional information:

- Most of the early studies in humans were done with a German-made formulation called "Wobenzym" which no longer exists and which is commonly confused with a product called "Wobenzym-N" which is not chemically or clinically identical to the original formulation. The closest formulation to the original "Wobenzym" is "Intenzyme Forte" from Biotics Research Corporation. I commonly use 8 tablets 3 times per day in patients with cancer, marked inflammation, or infection since the effectiveness of proteolytic/pancreatic enzymes is dose-dependent[351] up to approximately the dose I have described here. Since each tablet contains 50 mg of bromelain, then only 4 tablets per day would be required to produce relief from osteoarthritis according to the study by Walker et al[352] even if there were no other components in the product.

- The anticancer benefits of proteolytic/pancreatic enzymes are augmented by the use of thymus extract. Some studies that emphasize the use of "oral enzymes" in their title and abstract actually use enzymes *with thymus extract* according to the details in the methodology section of the printed paper.[353] Proteolytic/pancreatic enzymes by themselves have anticancer benefits, and thymus extract is immunosupportive — indeed immunostimulatory — especially in elderly and severely ill patients.

[346] Saruc M, Standop S, Standop J, Nozawa F, Itami A, Pandey KK, Batra SK, Gonzalez NJ, Guesry P, Pour PM. Pancreatic enzyme extract improves survival in murine pancreatic cancer. *Pancreas.* 2004;28(4):401-12

[347] Batkin S, Taussig SJ, Szekerezes J. Antimetastatic effect of bromelain with or without its proteolytic and anticoagulant activity. *J Cancer Res Clin Oncol.* 1988;114(5):507-8

[348] Gonzalez NJ, Isaacs LL. Evaluation of pancreatic proteolytic enzyme treatment of adenocarcinoma of the pancreas, with nutrition and detoxification support. *Nutr Cancer.* 1999;33(2):117-24

[349] Sakalova A, Bock PR, Dedik L, Hanisch J, Schiess W, Gazova S, Chabronova I, Holomanova D, Mistrik M, Hrubisko M. Retrolective cohort study of an additive therapy with an oral enzyme preparation in patients with multiple myeloma. *Cancer Chemother Pharmacol.* 2001 Jul;47 Suppl:S38-44

[350] Popiela T, Kulig J, Hanisch J, Bock PR. Influence of a complementary treatment with oral enzymes on patients with colorectal cancers--an epidemiological retrolective cohort study. *Cancer Chemother Pharmacol.* 2001;47 Suppl:S55-63

[351] Zavadova E, Desser L, Mohr T. Stimulation of reactive oxygen species production and cytotoxicity in human neutrophils in vitro and after oral administration of a polyenzyme preparation. *Cancer Biother.* 1995 Summer;10(2):147-52

[352] Walker AF, Bundy R, Hicks SM, Middleton RW. Bromelain reduces mild acute knee pain and improves well-being in a dose-dependent fashion in an open study of otherwise healthy adults.*Phytomedicine.*2002;9:681-6

[353] Sakalova A, Bock PR, Dedik L, Hanisch J, Schiess W, Gazova S, Chabronova I, Holomanova D, Mistrik M, Hrubisko M. Retrolective cohort study of an additive therapy with an oral enzyme preparation in patients with multiple myeloma. *Cancer Chemother Pharmacol.* 2001 Jul;47 Suppl:S38-44

Botanical Medicine:	*Zingiber officinale*

Common name: **Ginger**

Applications and mechanisms of action:	• <u>Anti-inflammatory and analgesic actions</u>: Ginger is a well known spice and food with a long history of use as an anti-inflammatory, anti-nausea, and gastroprotective agent.[354] Components of ginger have been shown to reduce production of the leukotriene LTB4 by inhibiting 5-lipoxygenase and to reduce production of the prostaglandin PG-E2 by inhibiting cyclooxygenase.[355,356] With its dual reduction in the formation of inflammation-promoting prostaglandins and leukotrienes, ginger has been shown to safely reduce **musculoskeletal pain in general**[357,358] and to provide relief from **osteoarthritis** of the knees[359] and **migraine headaches**.[360]
Toxicity and contraindications:	• Doses up to one gram of ginger per day have been safely used during pregnancy to reduce the nausea and vomiting of pregnancy[361] and the more severe hyperemesis gravidarum.[362] • The pungent principles of ginger often create a warm or burning sensation in the stomach that is mild, reducible with food consumption, and not indicative of tissue irritation.
Additional information:	• Ginger can be consumed as a root or in capsule or powder form. Most capsules are standardized for the concentration of gingerols.

Notes:

_____

_____

_____

_____

_____

_____

_____

_____

_____

_____

_____

_____

_____

_____

_____

_____

_____

_____

_____

[354] Langner E, Greifenberg S, Gruenwald J. Ginger: history and use. *Adv Ther* 1998 Jan-Feb;15(1):25-44

[355] Kiuchi F, Iwakami S, Shibuya M, Hanaoka F, Sankawa U. Inhibition of prostaglandin and leukotriene biosynthesis by gingerols and diarylheptanoids. *Chem Pharm Bull* (Tokyo) 1992 Feb;40(2):387-91

[356] Tjendraputra E, Tran VH, Liu-Brennan D, Roufogalis BD, Duke CC. Effect of ginger constituents and synthetic analogues on cyclooxygenase-2 enzyme in intact cells. *Bioorg Chem* 2001 Jun;29(3):156-63

[357] Srivastava KC, Mustafa T. Ginger (Zingiber officinale) in rheumatism and musculoskeletal disorders. *Med Hypotheses.* 1992 Dec;39(4):342-8

[358] Srivastava KC, Mustafa T. Ginger (Zingiber officinale) and rheumatic disorders. *Med Hypotheses.* 1989 May;29(1):25-8

[359] Altman RD, Marcussen KC. Effects of a ginger extract on knee pain in patients with osteoarthritis. *Arthritis Rheum.* 2001 Nov;44(11):2531-8

[360] Mustafa T, Srivastava KC. Ginger (Zingiber officinale) in migraine headache. *J Ethnopharmacol.* 1990 Jul;29(3):267-73

[361] Vutyavanich T, Kraisarin T, Ruangsri R. Ginger for nausea and vomiting in pregnancy: randomized, double-masked, placebo-controlled trial. *Obstet Gynecol* 2001 Apr;97(4):577-82

[362] Fischer-Rasmussen W, Kjaer SK, Dahl C, Asping U. Ginger treatment of hyperemesis gravidarum. *Eur J Obstet Gynecol Reprod Biol.* 1991 Jan 4;38(1):19-24

Botanical Medicine:	### *Uncaria tomentosa, Uncaria guianensis*
Common names:	### "Cat's claw" "una de gato"

Applications and mechanisms of action:

- Osteoarthritis: 30 patients with osteoarthritis of the knees benefited from highly-concentrated freeze-dried aqueous extraction of *U. guianensis* dosed at 1 capsule of 100 mg daily. Reduction in pain was approximately 36% at 4 weeks. No major adverse effects were noted; however headache and dizziness were more common in the treatment group. *Uncaria* inhibits NF-κB, TNFα, COX-2, and thus PGE-2 production.[363]
- Rheumatoid arthritis: A year-long study of patients with active rheumatoid arthritis (RA) treated with sulfasalazine or hydroxychloroquine showed "relative safety and modest benefit" of *Uncaria tomentosa* (UT).[364]

Toxicity and contraindications:

- No major adverse effects were noted; however headache and dizziness were more common in the treatment group.
- This herb should probably not be used during pregnancy based on its historical use as a contraceptive.

Dosage and administration:

- High-quality extractions from reputable manufacturers used according to directions are recommended. Most products contain between 250-500 mg and are standardized to 3.0% alkaloids and 15% total polyphenols; QD-TID po dosing should be sufficient as *part* of a comprehensive plan.

Additional information:

- Other studies with *Uncaria tomentosa* have shown enhancement of post-vaccination immunity[365] and enhancement of DNA repair in humans.[366] Traditional uses have included the use of the herb as a contraceptive and as treatment for gastrointestinal ulcers.

Notes:

_____

_____

_____

_____

_____

_____

_____

_____

_____

_____

_____

[363] Piscoya J, Rodriguez Z, Bustamante SA, Okuhama NN, Miller MJ, Sandoval M.Efficacy and safety of freeze-dried cat's claw in osteoarthritis of the knee: mechanisms of action of the species Uncaria guianensis. *Inflamm Res.* 2001 Sep;50(9):442-8

[364] "This small preliminary study demonstrates relative safety and modest benefit to the tender joint count of a highly purified extract from the pentacyclic chemotype of UT in patients with active RA taking sulfasalazine or hydroxychloroquine." Mur E, Hartig F, Eibl G, Schirmer M. Randomized double blind trial of an extract from the pentacyclic alkaloid-chemotype of uncaria tomentosa for the treatment of rheumatoid arthritis. *J Rheumatol.* 2002 Apr;29(4):678-81

[365] "C-Med-100 is a novel nutraceutical extract from the South American plant Uncaria tomentosa or Cat's Claw which is known to possess immune enhancing and antiinflammatory properties in animals. However, statistically significant immune enhancement for the individuals on C-Med-100 supplement was observed..." Lamm S, Sheng Y, Pero RW. Persistent response to pneumococcal vaccine in individuals supplemented with a novel water soluble extract of Uncaria tomentosa, C-Med-100. *Phytomedicine.* 2001 Jul;8(4):267-74

[366] "There was a statistically significant decrease of DNA damage and a concomitant increase of DNA repair in the supplement groups (250 and 350 mg/day) when compared with non-supplemented controls (p < 0.05)." Sheng Y, Li L, Holmgren K, Pero RW. DNA repair enhancement of aqueous extracts of Uncaria tomentosa in a human volunteer study. *Phytomedicine.* 2001 Jul;8(4):275-82

Botanical Medicine:	## *Salix alba, Salix* species
Common names:	## "Willow bark"

Applications and mechanisms of action:

- <u>Musculoskeletal pain, osteoarthritis, low-back pain</u>: Clinical studies in humans with musculoskeletal pain have consistently demonstrated safety and effectiveness of willow bark. In a double-blind placebo-controlled clinical trial in 210 patients with moderate/severe low-back pain (20% of patients had positive straight-leg raising test), extract of willow bark showed a dose-dependent analgesic effect with benefits beginning in the first week of treatment.[367] In a head-to-head study of 228 patients comparing willow bark (standardized for 240 mg salicin) with Vioxx (rofecoxib), treatments were equally effective yet willow bark was safer and 40% less expensive.[368] Because willow bark's salicylates were the original source for the chemical manufacture of acetylsalicylic acid (aspirin), researchers and clinicians have erroneously mistaken willow bark to be synonymous with aspirin; this is certainly inaccurate and therefore clarification of willow's mechanism of action will be provided here. Aspirin has two primary effects via three primary mechanisms of action: 1) anticoagulant effects mediated by the acetylation and permanent inactivation of thromboxane-A synthase, which is the enzyme that makes the powerful proaggregatory thromboxane-A2; 2) antiprostaglandin action via acetylation of both isoforms of cyclooxygenase (COX-1 inhibition 25-166x more than COX-2) with widespread inhibition of prostaglandin formation, and 3) antiprostaglandin formation via "retroconversion" of acetylsalicylate into salicylic acid which then inhibits cyclooxygenase-2 gene transcription.[369] Notice that the acetylation reactions are specific to aspirin and thus actions #1 and #2 are not seen with willow bark; whereas #3—inhibition of COX-2 transcription by salicylates—appears to be the major mechanism of action of willow bark extract. Proof of this principle is supported by the lack of adverse effects associated with willow bark in the research literature. If willow bark were pharmacodynamically synonymous with aspirin, then we would expect case reports of gastric ulceration, hemorrhage, and Reye's syndrome to permeate the research literature; this is not the case and therefore—with the exception of possible allergic reactions in patients previously allergic to aspirin and salicylates—extensive "warnings" on willow bark products[370] are unnecessary.[371] Salicylates are widely present in fruits, vegetables, herbs and spices and are partly responsible for the anti-cancer, anti-inflammatory, and health-promoting benefits of plant consumption.[372,373]

Toxicity and contraindications:

- <u>Allergy</u>: There is one single case report of serious anaphylaxis following use of willow bark in a patient previously sensitized to aspirin.[374]

Dosage and administration:

- The daily dose should not exceed 240 mg of salicin, and products should include other components of the whole plant. Of course, we would expect that lower doses will be effective in our clinical practices because we always use willow bark with other anti-inflammatory diet and nutritional interventions, particularly EPA/DHA and ALA—each of which has been shown to lower prostaglandin formation.

---

[367] Chrubasik S, Eisenberg E, Balan E, Weinberger T, Luzzati R, Conradt C. Treatment of low-back pain exacerbations with willow bark extract: a randomized double-blind study. *Am J Med.* 2000;109:9-14

[368] Chrubasik S, Kunzel O, Model A, Conradt C, Black A. Treatment of low-back pain with a herbal or synthetic anti-rheumatic: a randomized controlled study. Willow bark extract for low-back pain. *Rheumatology* (Oxford). 2001;40:1388-93

[369] Hare LG, Woodside JV, Young IS. Dietary salicylates. *J Clin Pathol* 2003 Sep;56(9):649-50

[370] Clauson KA, Santamarina ML, Buettner CM, Cauffield JS. Evaluation of Presence of Aspirin-Related Warnings with Willow Bark (July/August). *Ann Pharmacother.* 2005 May 31; [Epub ahead of print]

[371] **Vasquez A, Muanza DN. Evaluation of Presence of Aspirin-Related Warnings with Willow Bark: Comment on the Article by Clauson et al. *Ann Pharmacotherapy* 2005 Oct;39(10):1763**

[372] Lawrence JR, Peter R, Baxter GJ, Robson J, Graham AB, Paterson JR. Urinary excretion of salicyluric and salicylic acids by non-vegetarians, vegetarians, and patients taking low dose aspirin. *J Clin Pathol.* 2003 Sep;56(9):651-3

[373] Paterson JR, Lawrence JR. Salicylic acid: a link between aspirin, diet and the prevention of colorectal cancer. *QJM.* 2001 Aug;94(8):445-8

[374] Boullata JI, McDonnell PJ, Oliva CD. Anaphylactic reaction to a dietary supplement containing willow bark. *Ann Pharmacother.* 2003 Jun;37(6):832-5

Botanical Medicine:	**Capsicum annuum, Capsicum frutescens**
Common names:	**Cayenne pepper, hot chili pepper**

Applications and mechanisms of action:	• <u>Pain relief</u>: Controlled clinical trials have conclusively demonstrated capsaicin's ability deplete sensory fibers of the neuropeptide substance P to thus reduce pain. Capsaicin also blocks transport and de-novo synthesis of substance P. Topical capsaicin is proven effective in relieving the pain associated with **diabetic neuropathy**[375], **chronic low back pain**[376], **chronic neck pain**[377], **osteoarthritis**[378], **rheumatoid arthritis**[379], **notalgia paresthetica**[380], **reflex sympathetic dystrophy** and **cluster headache** (intranasal application).[381] Surprisingly, capsaicin was shown to be ineffective in the treatment of pain associated with temporomandibular dysfunction.[382]
Toxicity and contraindications:	• Do not get into eyes. • Transient burning, sneezing, and coughing are common following intranasal application. • Topical application of capsaicin during pregnancy has not been evaluated but is almost certain to be safe.
Dosage and administration:	• Capsaicin creams are available OTC at strengths of 0.025% and 0.075%. The stronger creams have a more powerful analgesic effect but result in more initial burning, which abates with continued use. The cream is generally not applied to areas of skin that are broken or bleeding.
Additional information:	• Since the cream reduces sensitivity to pain, patients should not use a heating pad at the site where the capsaicin is applied, as the capsaicin may induce insensitivity to local overheating.

Notes:

_____

_____

_____

_____

_____

_____

_____

_____

_____

_____

[375] Treatment of painful diabetic neuropathy with topical capsaicin. A multicenter, double-blind, vehicle-controlled study. The Capsaicin Study Group. [No authors listed] *Arch Intern Med.* 1991 Nov;151(11):2225-9

[376] Keitel W, Frerick H, Kuhn U, Schmidt U, Kuhlmann M, Bredehorst A. Capsicum pain plaster in chronic non-specific low back pain. *Arzneimittelforschung.* 2001 Nov;51(11):896-903

[377] Mathias BJ, Dillingham TR, Zeigler DN, Chang AS, Belandres PV. Topical capsaicin for chronic neck pain. A pilot study. *Am J Phys Med Rehabil* 1995 Jan-Feb;74(1):39-44

[378] McCarthy GM, McCarty DJ. Effect of topical capsaicin in the therapy of painful osteoarthritis of the hands. *J Rheumatol.* 1992;19(4):604-7

[379] Deal CL, Schnitzer TJ, Lipstein E, Seibold JR, Stevens RM, Levy MD, Albert D, Renold F. Treatment of arthritis with topical capsaicin: a double-blind trial. *Clin Ther.* 1991 May-Jun;13(3):383-95

[380] Leibsohn E. Treatment of notalgia paresthetica with capsaicin. *Cutis* 1992 May;49(5):335-6

[381] Hautkappe M, Roizen MF, Toledano A, Roth S, Jeffries JA, Ostermeier AM. Review of the effectiveness of capsaicin for painful cutaneous disorders and neural dysfunction. *Clin J Pain* 1998 Jun;14(2):97-106

[382] Winocur E, Gavish A, Halachmi M, Eli I, Gazit E. Topical application of capsaicin for the treatment of localized pain in the temporomandibular joint area. *J Orofac Pain.* 2000 Winter;14(1):31-6

Botanical Medicine:	*Boswellia serrata*
Common names:	**Frankincense, Salai guggal**

Applications and mechanisms of action:

- <u>Anti-inflammatory, via inhibition of 5-lipoxygenase[383] with no apparent effect on cyclooxygenase[384]</u>: A recent clinical study showed that *Boswellia* was able to reduce pain and swelling while increasing joint flexion and walking distance in patients with **osteoarthritis of the knees**.[385] While reports from clinical trials published in English are relatively rare, a recent abstract from the German medical research[386] stated, "In clinical trials promising results were observed in patients with rheumatoid arthritis, chronic colitis, ulcerative colitis, Crohn's disease, bronchial asthma and peritumoral brains edemas." Additional recent studies have confirmed the effectiveness of *Boswellia* in the treatment of **asthma**[387] and **ulcerative colitis**.[388] A German study showing that *Boswellia* was ineffective for rheumatoid arthritis[389] was poorly conducted, with inadequate follow-up, inadequate controls, and abnormal dosing of the herb.

Toxicity:

- Minor gastrointestinal upset has been reported.

Dosage and administration:

- Products are generally standardized to contain 37.5–65% boswellic acids, which are currently considered the active constituents with clinical benefit. The target dose is approximately 150 mg of boswellic acids TID; dose and number of capsules/tablets will vary depending upon the concentration found in differing products.

Additional information:

- Even though *Boswellia* is an effective anti-inflammatory, its use should not preclude searching for and addressing the underlying cause of the inflammatory problem.

Notes:

_____

_____

_____

_____

_____

_____

_____

_____

_____

_____

_____

_____

_____

[383] Wildfeuer A, Neu IS, Safayhi H, Metzger G, Wehrmann M, Vogel U, Ammon HP. Effects of boswellic acids extracted from a herbal medicine on the biosynthesis of leukotrienes and the course of experimental autoimmune encephalomyelitis. *Arzneimittelforschung* 1998 Jun;48(6):668-74

[384] Safayhi H, Mack T, Sabieraj J, Anazodo MI, Subramanian LR, Ammon HP. Boswellic acids: novel, specific, nonredox inhibitors of 5-lipoxygenase. *J Pharmacol Exp Ther* 1992 Jun;261(3):1143-6

[385] Kimmatkar N, Thawani V, Hingorani L, Khiyani R. Efficacy and tolerability of Boswellia serrata extract in treatment of osteoarthritis of knee--a randomized double blind placebo controlled trial. *Phytomedicine*. 2003 Jan;10(1):3-7

[386] Ammon HP. [Boswellic acids (components of frankincense) as the active principle in treatment of chronic inflammatory diseases] [Article in German] *Wien Med Wochenschr*. 2002;152(15-16):373-8

[387] Gupta I, Gupta V, Parihar A, Gupta S, Ludtke R, Safayhi H, Ammon HP. Effects of Boswellia serrata gum resin in patients with bronchial asthma: results of a double-blind, placebo-controlled, 6-week clinical study. *Eur J Med Res*. 1998 Nov 17;3(11):511-4

[388] Gupta I, Parihar A, Malhotra P, Singh GB, Ludtke R, Safayhi H, Ammon HP. Effects of Boswellia serrata gum resin in patients with ulcerative colitis. *Eur J Med Res*. 1997 Jan;2(1):37-43

[389] Sander O, Herborn G, Rau R. [Is H15 (resin extract of Boswellia serrata, "incense") a useful supplement to established drug therapy of chronic polyarthritis? Results of a double-blind pilot study] [Article in German] *Z Rheumatol*. 1998 Feb;57(1):11-6

Botanical Medicine:	# Harpagophytum procumbens
Common name:	# Devil's claw

Applications and mechanisms of action:

- <u>Analgesic and weak anti-inflammatory</u>: Safety and moderate effectiveness of *Harpagophytum* has been demonstrated in patients with **hip pain, low back pain**, and **knee pain**.[390] An abstract from the German research literature showed that *Harpagophytum* is safe and effective for the treatment of **muscle pain and muscle tension of the low back, shoulders, and neck**.[391] In a study of patients with **osteoarthritis of the hip and knee**, *Harpagophytum* was found to be just as effective yet safer and better tolerated than the drug diacerhein.[392,393] While anti-inflammatory effects have been reported, the anti-inflammatory effects are weak[394] and appear secondary to the analgesic benefits. Administration of *Harpagophytum* to healthy volunteers does not alter eicosanoid production.[395] In a study involving 183 patients with low back pain, *Harpagophytum* was found to be safe and moderately effective in patients with **"severe and unbearable pain" and radiating pain with neurologic deficit**.[396] Most recently, *Harpagophytum* was studied in a head-to-head clinical trial with the popular but dangerous selective Cox-2 inhibitor Vioxx (rofecoxib); the data clearly indicate that *Harpagophytum* was safer and at least as effective.[397]

Toxicity and contraindication:

- Treatment is generally considered very safe. About 8% of patients may experience diarrhea or other mild gastrointestinal effects. A few patients may experience dizziness. Long-term multi-year safety data is not available.

Dosage and administration:

- Treatment should be continued for at least 4 weeks, and many patients will continue to improve after 8 weeks from the initiation of treatment.[398]
- Products are generally standardized for the content of harpagosides, with a target dose of 60 mg harpagoside per day.[399] However, the whole plant is considered to contain effective constituents, not only the iridoid glycosides.
- The results of one laboratory study suggest that the active components are reduced following exposure to acid[400], and therefore the product might be consumed between meals, perhaps with Alka Seltzer or sodium bicarbonate.

Additional information:

- Immediately before the revision of this monograph in August 2004, I was in communication with Dr. Sigrun Chrubasik who shared with me her most recent article[401] in which she reviewed the clinical trials to date. In her 2004 review published in *Phytotherapy Research*, she states that while *Harpagophytum* appears to be safe and moderately effective for the treatment musculoskeletal pain, different proprietary products show significant variances in potency and clinical effectiveness. She states that additional research is necessary before the clinical value of *Harpagophytum* can be firmly established. However, if one reviews the data presented in Table 1 of her 2003 review article published in *Phytomedicine*[402], then one is entitled to conclude that *Harpagophytum* does indeed consistently show clinical benefit that is better than no treatment (open trials), better than placebo (placebo-controlled trials), and at least as good as the pharmaceutical drugs diacerhein and rofecoxib (head-to-head comparisons). Since therapeutic efficacy of *Harpagophytum* is at least as good as commonly used NSAIDs, *Harpagophytum* should be clinically preferred over NSAIDs due to its lower cost and apparently greater safety.[403]

---

[390] Chrubasik S, Thanner J, Kunzel O, Conradt C, Black A, Pollak S. Comparison of outcome measures during treatment with the proprietary Harpagophytum extract doloteffin in patients with pain in the lower back, knee or hip. *Phytomedicine* 2002 Apr;9(3):181-94

[391] Gobel H, Heinze A, Ingwersen M, Niederberger U, Gerber D. [Effects of Harpagophytum procumbens LI 174 (devil's claw) on sensory, motor und vascular muscle reagibility in the treatment of unspecific back pain] [Article in German] *Schmerz* 2001 Feb;15(1):10-8

[392] Chantre P, Cappelaere A, Leblan D, Guedon D, Vandermander J, Fournie B. Efficacy and tolerance of Harpagophytum procumbens versus diacerhein in treatment of osteoarthritis. *Phytomedicine* 2000 Jun;7(3):177-83

[393] Leblan D, Chantre P, Fournie B. Harpagophytum procumbens in the treatment of knee and hip osteoarthritis. Four-month results of a prospective, multicenter, double-blind trial versus diacerhein. *Joint Bone Spine* 2000;67(5):462-7

[394] Whitehouse LW, Znamirowska M, Paul CJ. Devil's Claw (Harpagophytum procumbens): no evidence for anti-inflammatory activity in the treatment of arthritic disease. *Can Med Assoc J* 1983 Aug 1;129(3):249-51

[395] Moussard C, Alber D, Toubin MM, Thevenon N, Henry JC. A drug used in traditional medicine, harpagophytum procumbens: no evidence for NSAID-like effect on whole blood eicosanoid production in human. *Prostaglandins Leukot Essent Fatty Acids* 1992 Aug;46(4):283-6

[396] "...subgroup analyses suggested that the effect was confined to patients with more severe and radiating pain accompanied by neurological deficit. ...a slightly different picture, with the benefits seeming, if anything, to be greatest in the H600 group and in patients without more severe pain, radiation or neurological deficit." Chrubasik S, Junck H, Breitschwerdt H, Conradt C, Zappe H. Effectiveness of Harpagophytum extract WS 1531 in the treatment of exacerbation of low back pain: a randomized, placebo-controlled, double-blind study. *Eur J Anaesthesiol* 1999 Feb;16(2):118-29

[397] Chrubasik S, Model A, Black A, Pollak S. A randomized double-blind pilot study comparing Doloteffin and Vioxx in the treatment of low back pain. *Rheumatology* (Oxford). 2003 Jan;42(1):141-8

[398] Chrubasik S, Thanner J, Kunzel O, Conradt C, Black A, Pollak S. Comparison of outcome measures during treatment with the proprietary Harpagophytum extract doloteffin in patients with pain in the lower back, knee or hip. *Phytomedicine* 2002 Apr;9(3):181-94

[399] "They took an 8-week course of Doloteffin at a dose providing 60 mg harpagoside per day... Doloteffin is well worth considering for osteoarthritic knee and hip pain and nonspecific low back pain." Chrubasik S, Thanner J, Kunzel O, Conradt C, Black A, Pollak S. Comparison of outcome measures during treatment with the proprietary Harpagophytum extract doloteffin in patients with pain in the lower back, knee or hip. *Phytomedicine* 2002 Apr;9(3):181-94

[400] Lanhers MC, Fleurentin J, Mortier F, Vinche A, Younos C. Anti-inflammatory and analgesic effects of an aqueous extract of Harpagophytum procumbens. *Planta Med* 1992 Apr;58(2):117-23

[401] Chrubasik S, Conradt C, Roufogalis BD. Effectiveness of Harpagophytum extracts and clinical efficacy. *Phytother Res.* 2004 Feb;18(2):187-9

[402] Chrubasik S, Conradt C, Black A. The quality of clinical trials with Harpagophytum procumbens. *Phytomedicine.* 2003;10(6-7):613-23

[403] Chrubasik S, Junck H, Breitschwerdt H, Conradt C, Zappe H. Effectiveness of Harpagophytum extract WS 1531 in the treatment of exacerbation of low back pain: a randomized, placebo-controlled, double-blind study. *Eur J Anaesthesiol* 1999 Feb;16(2):118-29

Botanical Medicine:	*Curcuma longa*
Common names:	**Turmeric**

Applications and
mechanisms of action:

- Anti-inflammatory *in vitro*: Turmeric is a common spice and food additive, providing foods with antioxidant/preservative benefit, as well as the characteristic golden yellow color which is characteristic of curry and mustard. The anti-inflammatory effects of turmeric have been well established in many *in vitro* studies and studies in animals involving *intraperitoneal* administration. Many researchers and supplement companies have interpreted this to mean that turmeric would also have strong clinical effectiveness in humans with conditions such as arthritis, and thus turmeric is marketed as an anti-inflammatory botanical medicine. The problem with this approach is that the active components of turmeric are only minimally absorbed from oral dosing and therefore the systemic and intraarticular concentrations of the active components are only minimally increased or not increased at all with oral dosing in humans.[404] Nearly all studies that show potential relevance for clinical use of turmeric in treating arthritis, cancer, and other human illnesses have been performed either *in vitro* or *in vivo with intraperitoneal administration* to achieve cellular levels of the active constituents that could never be achieved with oral administration. However, a single report that turmeric administered as a hydroalcoholic extract could reduce the serum levels of the acute phase reactant fibrinogen does suggest that turmeric, when processed or coadministered with alcohol, might be absorbed and possess a systemic anti-inflammatory effect.[405] **To my knowledge, no human studies exist showing that pure curcumin/turmeric when used alone (i.e., not with other herbs, drugs, or piperine) has effectiveness in the treatment of joint pain or inflammation in humans following oral administration.[406]**

Toxicity and
contraindications:

- Turmeric is generally considered non-toxic
- No drug interactions are commonly known

Dosage and
administration:

- Doses of up to eight grams per day have been used with moderate clinical effectiveness on local oral and gastrointestinal tissues with no evidence of toxicity[407]
- Coadministration with 10 of piperine increases bioavailability of curcuminoids to humans by 2,000%[408]—thus, coadministration of curcumin with piperine appears to be the best and perhaps the only way to increase bioavailability of the active components of the spice and obtain systemic benefits

Notes:
_____

_____

_____

_____

_____

---

[404] "…curcumin is absorbed poorly by the gastrointestinal tract and/or underlies presystemic transformation. Systemic effects therefore seem to be questionable after oral application except that they occur at very low concentrations of curcumin. This does not exclude a local action in the gastrointestinal tract." Ammon HP, Wahl MA. Pharmacology of Curcuma longa. *Planta Med* 1991 Feb;57(1):1-7

[405] Ramirez Bosca A, Soler A, Carrion-Gutierrez MA, Pamies Mira D, Pardo Zapata J, Diaz-Alperi J, Bernd A, Quintanilla Almagro E, Miquel J. An hydroalcoholic extract of Curcuma longa lowers the abnormally high values of human-plasma fibrinogen. *Mech Ageing Dev.* 2000 Apr 14;114(3):207-10

[406] **Vasquez A, Muanza DN. Accolades and Addenda for "Use of Botanicals in Osteoarthritis and Rheumatoid Arthritis": Comment on Article by Ahmed et al.** *Evidence-based Complementary and Alternative Medicine.* **2005 published on-line December 15** http://ecam.oxfordjournals.org/cgi/eletters/2/3/301#19

[407] "In conclusion, this study demonstrated that curcumin is not toxic to humans up to 8,000 mg/day when taken by mouth for 3 months." Cheng AL, Hsu CH, Lin JK, Hsu MM, Ho YF, Shen TS, Ko JY, Lin JT, Lin BR, Ming-Shiang W, Yu HS, Jee SH, Chen GS, Chen TM, Chen CA, Lai MK, Pu YS, Pan MH, Wang YJ, Tsai CC, Hsieh CY. Phase I clinical trial of curcumin, a chemopreventive agent, in patients with high-risk or pre-malignant lesions. *Anticancer Res.* 2001 Jul-Aug;21(4B):2895-900

[408] Shoba G, Joy D, Joseph T, Majeed M, Rajendran R, Srinivas PS. Influence of piperine on the pharmacokinetics of curcumin in animals and human volunteers. *Planta Med.* 1998;64(4):353-6

Botanical Medicine:	### *Avocado/soybean unsaponifiables*
Common name:	## ASU

Applications and mechanisms of action:

- <u>Osteoarthritis</u>: The use of avocado/soybean unsaponifiables (ASU) has been shown to improve joint function and reduce the need for NSAIDs/analgesic medication in patients with osteoarthritis.[409,410] A study of patients with **hip osteoarthritis** suggested that ASU may retard the progression of joint space narrowing.[411] A study of patients with **knee osteoarthritis** showed that patients receiving ASU were able to reduce the use of NSAIDs and analgesics by 60% compared to only a 36% reduction by the patients receiving placebo.[412] The mechanism of action of ASU appears to be the stimulation of collagen/cartilage synthesis in addition to a modest anti-inflammatory effect via reduction in nitric oxide, PG-E2, and other mediators.[413]

Toxicity:

- None known.

Dosage and administration:

- Common doses are 300 mg per day or 600 mg per day, with a slight increase in efficacy with the 600 mg per day dose, according to a study of patients with knee osteoarthritis.[414]

Additional information:

- ASU products are generally not available in the United States.
- Due to the reduced clinical efficacy of ASU compared to other natural therapeutics as reported in the research, I would consider ASU a "last resort" treatment for osteoarthritis after using glucosamine sulfate, fish oil, vitamin E, niacinamide, and *Uncaria* and *Boswellia*.
- Be sure to rule out iron overload in any patient with osteoarthritis, especially osteoarthritis that is polyarticular or resistant to treatment.[415]
- The unsaponifiable fraction of vegetable oils includes plant sterols, or phytosterols, which have documented benefit in hypercholesterolemia and prostate hyperplasia.

Notes:

_____

_____

_____

_____

_____

_____

_____

_____

[409] Blotman F, Maheu E, Wulwik A, Caspard H, Lopez A. Efficacy and safety of avocado/soybean unsaponifiables in the treatment of symptomatic osteoarthritis of the knee and hip. A prospective, multicenter, three-month, randomized, double-blind, placebo-controlled trial. *Rev Rhum Engl Ed.* 1997 Dec;64(12):825-34

[410] Maheu E, Mazieres B, Valat JP, Loyau G, Le Loet X, Bourgeois P, Grouin JM, Rozenberg S. Symptomatic efficacy of avocado/soybean unsaponifiables in the treatment of osteoarthritis of the knee and hip: a prospective, randomized, double-blind, placebo-controlled, multicenter clinical trial with a six-month treatment period and a two-month followup demonstrating a persistent effect. *Arthritis Rheum.* 1998;41(1):81-91

[411] Lequesne M, Maheu E, Cadet C, Dreiser RL. Structural effect of avocado/soybean unsaponifiables on joint space loss in osteoarthritis of the hip. *Arthritis Rheum.* 2002 Feb;47(1):50-8

[412] Appelboom T, Schuermans J, Verbruggen G, Henrotin Y, Reginster JY. Symptoms modifying effect of avocado/soybean unsaponifiables (ASU) in knee osteoarthritis. A double blind, prospective, placebo-controlled study. *Scand J Rheumatol.* 2001;30(4):242-7

[413] Henrotin YE, Sanchez C, Deberg MA, Piccardi N, Guillou GB, Msika P, Reginster JY. Avocado/soybean unsaponifiables increase aggrecan synthesis and reduce catabolic and proinflammatory mediator production by human osteoarthritic chondrocytes. *J Rheumatol.* 2003 Aug;30(8):1825-34

[414] Appelboom T, Schuermans J, Verbruggen G, Henrotin Y, Reginster JY. Symptoms modifying effect of avocado/soybean unsaponifiables (ASU) in knee osteoarthritis. A double blind, prospective, placebo-controlled study. *Scand J Rheumatol.* 2001;30(4):242-7

[415] Vasquez A. Musculoskeletal disorders and iron overload disease: comment on the American College of Rheumatology guidelines for the initial evaluation of the adult patient with acute musculoskeletal symptoms. *Arthritis Rheum* 1996;39: 1767-8

Piezoelectric Properties of the Human Body and Clinical Implications

"...pyroelectric [and piezoelectric] behavior constitutes a basic physical property of all living organisms." [416]

Piezoelectricity has been defined as "the generation of electricity or of electric polarity in dielectric crystals subjected to mechanical stress, or the generation of stress in such crystals subjected to an applied voltage."[417] When we are discussing the piezoelectric properties of the human body, we are discussing the translation/transformation of mechanical energy into and out of electric energy. Relatedly, **pyroelectricity is defined as "the electrical potential created in certain materials when they are heated."**[418] Therefore, we can schematize a relationship between the tissues of living organisms (plants, animals, humans), mechanical stress, electrical energy, and heat. Clinically relevant questions/issues then become those of qualifying/quantifying these pyroelectric and piezoelectric properties of the human body, and determining whether and/or how these are clinically relevant.

All living tissue—namely plant and animal tissues— have both pyroelectric and piezoelectric properties. Since these properties are seen in the tissues, they are of course seen in the organisms themselves. With regard to physical medicine in general and spinal manipulation in particular, we note that bone, collagen, and the spinal cord are notably pyroelectric/piezoelectric, as detailed in the *Annals of the*

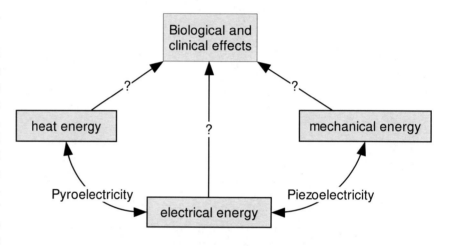

New York Academy of Sciences monograph by Athenstaedt in 1974. Other tissues and molecules with pyroelectric/piezoelectric and "semiconductive" properties include wood, silk, skin, nucleic acids, fibrin, hyaluronic acid, actin and myosin.[419] This electrophysiologic property is based not on the inherent "electrical" and ionic properties of the nervous system or the cell membranes, but rather upon the alignment of the molecules within the tissues. **When linear, organic molecules of varying length are aligned in parallel along a longitudinal axis, the resultant microscopic and therefore macroscopic structure will have a permanent dipole moment.**[420]

Indeed, as Athenstaedt notes in *American Journal of Physiology*[421], "The existence of an inherent electric dipole moment has been established throughout the entire length of the spinal cord of humans, horses, and cows." This is illustrated in the diagram to the right.

Clinical relevance: In 1977, Lipiski from Tufts University School of Medicine[422] summarized the current research of the day and speculated on the effects of spinal manipulation, osteopathic manipulation, yoga, and acupuncture as mediated via the body's inherent pyroelectric and piezoelectric properties. Lipinski's literature

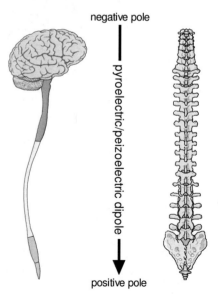

---

[416] Athenstaedt H. Pyroelectric and piezoelectric properties of vertebrates. *Ann N Y Acad Sci.* 1974;238:68-94
[417] American Heritage Dictionary
[418] http://www.free-definition.com/Pyroelectricity.html on October 3, 2004
[419] Lipinski B. Biological significance of piezoelectricity in relation to acupuncture, Hatha Yoga, osteopathic medicine and action of air ions. *Med Hypotheses.* 1977 Jan-Feb;3(1):9-12
[420] Athenstaedt H. Pyroelectric and piezoelectric properties of vertebrates. *Ann N Y Acad Sci.* 1974;238:68-94
[421] Athenstaedt H. "Functional polarity" of the spinal cord caused by its longitudinal electric dipole moment. *Am J Physiol.* 1984 Sep;247(3 Pt 2):R482-7
[422] Lipinski B. Biological significance of piezoelectricity in relation to acupuncture, Hatha Yoga, osteopathic medicine and action of air ions. *Med Hypotheses.* 1977 Jan-Feb;3(1):9-12

review (particularly including the work of Bassett[423]) suggests that **"...piezoelectricity present in many biological systems may theoretically control cell nutrition, local pH, enzyme activation and inhibition, orientation of intra-and extra-cellular macromolecules, migratory and proliferative activity of cells, contractility of permeability of cell membranes, and energy transfer."** With these concepts and possibilities considered, we can construct a conceptual model that allows an understanding of the interconnectedness of *mechanical stimuli* such as massage, manipulation, stretching/exercise, and yoga with *"energetic" stimuli such as acupuncture, meditation, "prayer" and intentionality* with their possible biochemical/physiological effects which then translate into clinical effects. This integrated model helps to explain the nonbiochemical nonpharmacologic effects of "energetic" therapeutics such as moxibustion, acupuncture, and yoga that may be mediated by nonlinear/nonbiochemical physiologic mechanisms. This model also helps us to understand the observed but hitherto unexplainable clinical effects of phenomena such as the well-reported sensitivity that some people display in relation to changes in the weather and the positioning of their bodies in relation to electromagnetic fields of the planet and electrical equipment and power lines, the effect of "distance healing" via prayer[424,425] and intentionality[426], and the clinical benefits of grounding/earthing the human body for the resultant improvements in sleep, normalization of cortisol rhythms, and reduction in somatic pain.[427]

Speculative model for the interconnectedness and biologic effects of heat, mechanical and electrician energies and their clinical effects as mediated physiologically and biochemically via the pyroelectric-piezoelectric and "superconductive" properties of body tissues and organ systems: modified from the discussion by Lipinski[428]

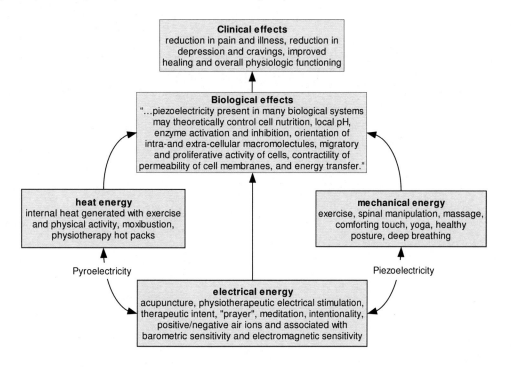

[423] Bassett CA. Biologic significance of piezoelectricity. *Calcif Tissue Res.* 1968 Mar;1(4):252-72

[424] "The control patients required ventilatory assistance, antibiotics, and diuretics more frequently than patients in the IP group. These data suggest that intercessory prayer to the Judeo-Christian God has a beneficial therapeutic effect in patients admitted to a CCU." Byrd RC. Positive therapeutic effects of intercessory prayer in a coronary care unit population. *South Med J.* 1988 Jul;81(7):826-9

[425] "CONCLUSIONS: In-person intercessory prayer may be a useful adjunct to standard medical care for certain patients with rheumatoid arthritis. Supplemental, distant intercessory prayer offers no additional benefits." Matthews DA, Marlowe SM, MacNutt FS. Effects of intercessory prayer on patients with rheumatoid arthritis. *South Med J.* 2000 Dec;93(12):1177-86

[426] "CONCLUSIONS: Remote, intercessory prayer was associated with lower CCU course scores. This result suggests that prayer may be an effective adjunct to standard medical care." Harris WS, Gowda M, Kolb JW, Strychacz CP, Vacek JL, Jones PG, Forker A, O'Keefe JH, McCallister BD. A randomized, controlled trial of the effects of remote, intercessory prayer on outcomes in patients admitted to the coronary care unit. *Arch Intern Med.* 1999 Oct 25;159(19):2273-8

[427] "Results indicate that grounding the human body to earth ("earthing") during sleep reduces night-time levels of cortisol and resynchronizes cortisol hormone secretion ... Furthermore, subjective reporting indicates that grounding the human body to earth during sleep improves sleep and reduces pain and stress." Ghaly M, Teplitz D. The biologic effects of grounding the human body during sleep as measured by cortisol levels and subjective reporting of sleep, pain, and stress. *J Altern Complement Med.* 2004 Oct;10(5):767-76

[428] Lipinski B. Biological significance of piezoelectricity in relation to acupuncture, Hatha Yoga, osteopathic medicine and action of air ions. *Med Hypotheses.* 1977 Jan-Feb;3(1):9-12

Physiotherapy—notes available on-line

Commonly utilized physiotherapeutic interventions include the following:

1. **Constitutional Hydrotherapy**
2. **Ultrasound**
3. **Contrast hydrotherapy**
4. **Heating compress,**
5. **Wet sock treatments**
6. **Cold friction rub**
7. **Immersion bath**
8. **Cold compress**
9. **Hyperthermia**
10. **Hot pack**
11. **Ice pack**
12. **Interferential**
13. **Tens—transcutaneous electrical nerve stimulation**
14. **Infrared**
15. **Electrical muscle stimulation**
16. **Bipolar for muscle contraction (using interferential machine)**
17. **Ionophoresis, ion transfer**
18. **Uni/mono-polar motor point stimulation of denervated muscle with electrical muscle stimulation**
19. **Short wave diathermy**

Since I do not consider this an area that I specialize in nor necessarily advocate, I have provided a draft of my physiotherapy notes at the website where you can download and print 20 pages of notes for free by accessing the page at http://OptimalHealthResearch.com/physiotherapy. One of the main reasons I've decided to forgo detailing these treatments here is particularly relevant to the use of the physiotherapy electronic equipment: with so many different brands and machines, detailing the settings and use for each type of machine would prove impossible. See the notes for general concepts and ideas.

Appendix A: Brief Overview of Clinical Considerations of Vitamins and Minerals

Nutrients	Physiology, toxicity, and contraindications	Clinical applications (adult doses)
Vitamin A	◆ Vitamin A comes in different forms with different characteristics; of these, all-*trans* retinol is the most common, and retinol palmitate is one of the least toxic. The richest dietary source of vitamin A is liver. Vitamin A has little or no antioxidant activity; rather, the antioxidant action commonly attributed to vitamin A is more accurately ascribed to its carotenoid precursor. Vitamin A is necessary for proper immune function, vision, and cell growth and differentiation (especially in epithelial tissue). Insufficiency of vitamin A causes epithelial tissue to produce excess keratin; hence the keratinization of the eye and skin in patients with vitamin A deficiency. ◆ Because of the risks of toxicity even with modest doses in the range of 25,000 IU per day[429] , most patients should consume <10,000-20,000 IU per day unless they are aware of the warning signs of toxicity and/or are under the care of a nutrition-knowledgeable doctor. This is particularly true for women who might get pregnant while supplementing with vitamin A, as an association between an increased risk of birth defects in association with daily intake ≥10,000 has been published and generally accepted, controversy notwithstanding. ◆ Vitamin A is present in some multivitamins, in cod liver oil, and in other supplements—read labels to ensure that the total daily intake is not greater than 10,000-20,000 IU per day. Approximately 200 cases of vitamin A toxicity are reported worldwide each year. ◆ Manifestations of vitamin A deficiency are "night blindness" (more properly termed "flash blindness" since vitamin A deficiency impairs ability of photoreceptors to recover following light exposure), follicular hyperkeratosis, frequent infections, and poor wound healing. Tissue damage (i.e., burns and trauma) and infections greatly increase the requirement for and tolerability of vitamin A supplementation.	◆ Short-term (few days) prescription of 100,000 – 200,000 IU per day is common for children and adults, especially during acute viral infections and the initial treatment of acne. ◆ Vitamin A toxicity is seen with chronic ingestion of therapeutic doses, for example: 25,000 IU per day for 6 years, or 100,000 IU per day for 2.5 years.[430] Because of the possible increased risk of hepatotoxicity, do not administer high doses of vitamin A to patients on numerous medications or with liver disease. ◆ Doses of vitamin A ≥ 10,000 IU are controversially associated with an increased risk for birth defects; therefore women who are pregnant or might soon become pregnant should keep their daily intake of vitamin A below 10,000 IU from all sources. ◆ **Clinical applications for supraphysiologic doses in the range of 100,000-300,000 IU per day of vitamin A include: adult acne, menorrhagia, and viral infections, especially measles.** ◆ **Medicolegal considerations: Any time high-dose vitamin A (i.e., greater than 25,000-50,000 IU per day) is used, the doctor must clearly define the time limit of this treatment *in writing* so that the patient will not mistakenly continue taking the vitamin and end up with vitamin A toxicity.** ◆ Patients must be advised of limited duration of use (e.g., 1-4 weeks) and to reduce or stop supplementation if signs of toxicity occur such as skin problems (dry skin, flaking skin, chapped or split lips, red skin rash, hair loss), joint pain, bone pain, headaches, anorexia (loss of appetite), edema (water retention, weight gain, swollen ankles, difficulty breathing), fatigue, and/or liver damage.

---

[429] "At 25,000 IU vitamin A per day, although elevated liver enzymes may be seen, hepatotoxicity is rare. We report a case of severe hepatotoxicity associated with the habitual daily ingestion of 25,000 IU of vitamin A bought as an over-the-counter dietary supplement." Kowalski TE, Falestiny M, Furth E, Malet PF. Vitamin A hepatotoxicity: a cautionary note regarding 25,000 IU supplements. *Am J Med.* 1994 Dec;97(6):523-8
[430] Geubel AP, De Galocsy C, Alves N, Rahier J, Dive C. Liver damage caused by therapeutic vitamin A administration: estimate of dose-related toxicity in 41 cases. *Gastroenterology.* 1991 Jun;100(6):1701-9

Nutrients	Physiology, toxicity, and contraindications	Clinical applications (adult doses)
Carotenoids	♦ Carotenoids are antioxidants and have additional specific functions. Fewer than 10% of carotenoids can serve as precursors to vitamin A; of these, beta-, alpha-, and gamma-carotene are the most efficient. Provitamin carotenoids are converted to all-*trans* retinal which is then converted to retinyl ester. ♦ Carotenoids are generally administered in microgram doses and should be delivered in a broad-spectrum combination including: beta carotene, alpha carotene, zeaxanthin, cryptoxanthin, and lutein. Due to competitive absorption, the use of high doses of a single carotenoid will tend to induce a deficiency of the other carotenoids; this mechanism probably explains the adverse effects associated with long-term high dose supplementation with beta-carotene, especially when the synthetic ♦ Virtually non-toxic when administered in rational doses from natural sources and in balanced combination. Conversion of carotenes to vitamin A is impaired in patients with diabetes and hypothyroidism.	♦ **Antioxidant** ♦ **Immunosupportive (e.g., in HIV)** ♦ **Eye protection (especially lutein)** ♦ **Prostate protection (especially lycopene)**

Vitamin E	♦ Deficiency of vitamin E is rarely recognized but can present as ataxia and neurologic dysfunction, especially in patients with malabsorption. Best dietary sources are seed and nut oils, especially sesame seeds, almonds, sunflower seeds, and wheat germ oil.
	♦ A reasonable preventive dose is 200-800 IU per day. Doses up to 3,200 IU per day are generally considered nontoxic.[431]
	♦ Vitamin E is commonly described as a "chain breaking antioxidant" with special importance in protecting cell membranes and lipoproteins from oxidative damage.
		♦ "Vitamin E" is a family of related chemicals including:
		  ▪ DL-tocopherol: This is synthetic and should not be used clinically; can cause headache and hypertension.
		  ▪ Alpha-tocopherol: commonly used but it depletes the body of the more important gamma-tocopherol.[432]
		  ▪ Beta-tocopherol:
		  ▪ Delta-tocopherol:
		  ▪ Gamma-tocopherol: this is the most important form of vitamin E and should be provided at approximately 40% when "mixed tocopherols" are consumed.
		  ▪ Tocopherol succinate: specific for improving mitochondrial function and for its anti-cancer effect.[433]
		  ▪ Tocotrienols: appear protective against breast cancer

---

[431] Meydani M. Vitamin E. *Lancet*. 1995 Jan 21;345(8943):170-5
[432] Jiang Q, Christen S, Shigenaga MK, Ames BN. gamma-tocopherol, the major form of vitamin E in the US diet, deserves more attention. *Am J Clin Nutr*. 2001 Dec;74(6):714-22

Appendix A: Brief Overview of Clinical Considerations of Vitamins and Minerals—*continued*

Nutrients	Physiology, toxicity, and contraindications	Clinical applications (adult doses)
Vitamin D3 (cholecalciferol)	♦ Vitamin D deficiency is well documented to be extremely common: ~40% of the general population and >90% of patients with musculoskeletal pain. ♦ The physiologic requirement for vitamin D3 is approximately 4,000 IU per day in adult men. [Data not yet collected in women; but is probably about the same, and higher during pregnancy and lactation.] Clinical guidelines for supplementation are as follows: 1,000 – 2,000 IU for infants; 2,000 IU for children and adolescents; 2,000-4,000 IU for adults, may go up to 10,000 IU per day for adults for up to 6 months and/or with periodic laboratory supervision (starting weekly). Dietary sources of vitamin D are insufficient to meet physiologic needs—vitamin D needs can only be met by sun exposure (full-body, without sunscreen, less than latitude 35 degrees from the equator, near noon, for 15-45 minutes) or by high-dose vitamin D supplementation. ♦ Physiologic doses are non-toxic except in patients with vitamin D hypersensitivity or those taking certain medications that induce hypercalcemia. ♦ The thiazide class of diuretics (including hydrochlorothiazide) can induce hypercalcemia. Correction of underlying hypovitaminosis D may precipitate hypercalcemia. ♦ "Vitamin D hypersensitivity" is seen in granulomatous diseases including tuberculosis, sarcoidosis, Crohn's disease, and some types of cancer; also adrenal failure, hypothyroidism and hyperthyroidism.	♦ Implement vitamin D replacement in all patients unless contraindicated. Vitamin D assessment and administration is becoming the standard of care and failure to implement vitamin D therapy when clinically indicated may be grounds for malpractice.[434] ♦ **Assess vitamin D status with serum 25-OH-vitamin D.** ♦ **Monitor for vitamin D toxicity by measuring serum calcium.** **Conditions Associated with Vitamin D Deficiency:** ♦ Rickets (children) and osteomalacia (adults) ♦ Osteoporosis ♦ Diabetes mellitus ♦ Osteoarthritis ♦ **Hypertension** ♦ Cardiovascular disease ♦ **Metabolic syndrome** ♦ **Depression** ♦ Multiple sclerosis ♦ Rheumatoid arthritis ♦ Grave's disease ♦ Ankylosing spondylitis ♦ Systemic lupus erythematosus ♦ Cancers of the breast, prostate, and colon ♦ Polycystic ovary syndrome ♦ **Musculoskeletal pain**[435] ♦ Epilepsy ♦ Migraine headaches ♦ **Chronic low-back pain** ♦ **Inflammation**

[433] Prasad KN, Kumar B, Yan XD, Hanson AJ, Cole WC. Alpha-tocopheryl succinate, the most effective form of vitamin E for adjuvant cancer treatment: a review. *J Am Coll Nutr.* 2003 Apr;22(2):108-17
[434] Heaney RP. Vitamin D, nutritional deficiency, and the medical paradigm. *J Clin Endocrinol Metab.* 2003 Nov;88(11):5107-8
[435] Al Faraj S, Al Mutairi K. Vitamin D deficiency and chronic low back pain in Saudi Arabia. *Spine.* 2003 Jan 15;28(2):177-9

Nutrients	Physiology, toxicity, and contraindications	Clinical applications (adult doses)
Vitamin K1 (phylloquinone): from plants **Vitamin K2 (menaquinone):** from animals and bacteria **Vitamin K3 (menadione):** synthetic	♦ **Vitamin K1 (phylloquinone)**—this is the form of vitamin K found in plants ♦ **Vitamin K2 (menaquinone)**—found in animal tissues and synthesized by bacteria ♦ **Vitamin K3 (menadione)**—synthetic form that must be alkylated in the body prior to use; this form of vitamin K is difficult to obtain and is generally not used for nutritional supplementation. ♦ 500-1000 mcg is a common supplemental dose. ♦ Vitamin K must not be taken by patients needing anticoagulation and taking coumadin-warfarin-heparin. Vitamin K is necessary for the production of clotting factors: factor II (prothrombin), factor VII, factor IX, and factor X. ♦ Vitamin K is also necessary for the formation of osteocalcin—a calcium-binding protein in bone	♦ Vitamin K is necessary for bone formation and blood clotting, thus obvious clinical applications include osteoporosis/osteopenia and menorrhagia/ecchymosis. ♦ **Vitamin K1 (phylloquinone)**—doses of at least 1,000 IU per day of K1 are needed in order to optimize carboxylation of osteocalcin.[436] ♦ **Vitamin K2 (menaquinone)**—A recent study with 21 patients in the treatment group published in JAMA used 45 mg/d (forty five milligrams per day = 45,000 mcg per day) of vitamin K2 for an 80% reduction in liver cancer in patients with viral cirrhosis: *"Compliance with vitamin K2 in the treatment group was good; no patient had adverse reactions or dropped out of the study."*[437]
B-1 (thiamine)	♦ Classic deficiency is dry beriberi (central and peripheral neurologic dysfunction, dementia, psychosis, weakness, neuropathy) and wet beriberi (congestive heart failure). The classic CNS manifestations of thiamine/magnesium deficiency seen in alcoholics is Wernecke-Korsakoff syndrome. ♦ Conversion from the inactive form to the active form of the vitamin requires magnesium. ♦ Functions include: enzyme cofactor, aldehyde transfer, modulates chloride ion channels in the CNS, energy production in hexose monophosphate shunt, phagocytic respiratory burst, neurotransmitter synthesis and release. ♦ Anaphylaxis to parenteral thiamine has been reported	♦ 20-100 mg is a common supplemental dose; one study used 5,000 mg to find evidence of a cholinergic effect.[438] The densest food source of thiamine is brewer's yeast. ♦ Thiamine insufficiency is common in patients with **cardiomyopathy**.[439,440] Alleviates congestive heart failure in some patients, especially when used with CoQ10 and magnesium.[441] ♦ Deficiency is common in the demented elderly; alleviates "Alzheimer's disease" in some patients
B-2 (riboflavin)	♦ Classic deficiency: angular stomatitis ♦ 20-200 mg is a common supplemental dose. The richest dietary sources are yeast and liver. ♦ Several studies have used 400 mg per day in patients with migraine and have not reported any serious adverse effects. ♦ Functions include: enzyme cofactor (especially for energy production as FAD in the electron transport chain), drug/xenobiotic detoxification via support of Cy-P450, antioxidant functions via glutathione reductase.	♦ 400 mg per morning is safe and effective for the alleviation of **migraine**.[442]

[436] Binkley NC, Krueger DC, Kawahara TN, Engelke JA, Chappell RJ, Suttie JW. A high phylloquinone intake is required to achieve maximal osteocalcin gamma-carboxylation. *Am J Clin Nutr.* 2002 Nov;76(5):1055-60

[437] Habu D, Shiomi S, Tamori A, Takeda T, Tanaka T, Kubo S, Nishiguchi S. Role of vitamin K2 in the development of hepatocellular carcinoma in women with viral cirrhosis of the liver. *JAMA.* 2004 Jul 21;292(3):358-61

[438] Meador KJ, Nichols ME, Franke P, Durkin MW, Oberzan RL, Moore EE, Loring DW. Evidence for a central cholinergic effect of high-dose thiamine. *Ann Neurol.* 1993 Nov;34(5):724-6

[439] da Cunha S, Albanesi Filho FM, da Cunha Bastos VL, Antelo DS, Souza MM. Thiamin, selenium, and copper levels in patients with idiopathic dilated cardiomyopathy taking diuretics. *Arq Bras Cardiol.* 2002 Nov;79(5):454-65

[440] Wohl MG, Brody M, Shuman CR, Turner R, Brody J. Thiamine and cocarboxylase concentration in heart, liver and kidney, of patients with heart failure. *J Clin Invest.* 1954;33(11):1580-6

[441] Shimon I, Almog S, Vered Z, Seligmann H, Shefi M, Peleg E, Rosenthal T, Motro M, Halkin H, Ezra D. Improved left ventricular function after thiamine supplementation in patients with congestive heart failure receiving long-term furosemide therapy. *Am J Med.* 1995 May;98(5):485-90

[442] Boehnke C, Reuter U, Flach U, Schuh-Hofer S, Einhaupl KM, Arnold G. High-dose riboflavin treatment is efficacious in migraine prophylaxis: an open study in a tertiary care centre. *Eur J Neurol.* 2004 Jul;11(7):475-7

Appendix A: Clinical and Physiologic Considerations of Vitamins and Minerals—*continued*

Nutrients	*Physiology, toxicity, contraindications*	*Clinical applications (adult doses)*
B-3: niacin	♦ Classic deficiency is pellagra: depression, dermatitis, dementia, diarrhea, death. Endogenous production requires 60 mg tryptophan to make 1 mg niacin. Richest dietary sources are yeast, rice bran, wheat bran, liver, and poultry breast meat. ♦ 20-100 mg is a common supplemental dose; doses up to 2,000 mg per day in divided doses are used for the treatment of hypercholesterolemia and must be monitored with lab tests to assess for possible liver dysfunction. Up to 6 grams (6,000 mg) per day in divided doses has been used safely. ♦ Liver damage has been seen with doses > 2,000 mg per day. Patients on high doses must be monitored with periodic measurements of liver enzymes; not to be used in patients with liver disease. "Time-release niacin" is the most hepatotoxic form of niacin.	♦ **Dyslipidemia**: Niacin at 2000-3000 mg per day in divided doses can lower total and LDL cholesterol, fibrinogen, triglyceride levels, and raise HDL. In a head-to-head study 2,000 mg niacin was more powerful than 1,200 mg gemfibrozil for favorably modifying lipids.[443]
B-3: niacinamide	♦ 20-100 mg is a common supplemental dose. ♦ 500 mg 4-6 times per day for 2,000 – 3,000 mg per day is safe and effective for osteoarthritis. ♦ Toxicity is rare; however monitoring liver enzymes at 1 and 4 months and yearly thereafter is encouraged when doses ≥ 2000 mg are used.	♦ anti-aging (reversal of aging phenotypes via histone acetylation) ♦ **osteoarthritis**
B-3: inositol hexaniacinate ("no-flush niacin")	♦ This is a slow release form of vitamin B3 that allows supplementation with niacin at high doses without the flushing and hepatotoxicity seen with plain niacin. However, despite one enthusiastic article stating that this is the preferred form of B3 for treating lipid disorders, inositol hexaniacinate appears clinically ineffective for the treatment of dyslipidemia.	♦ 2000 mg per day in divided doses of 500-1000 mg each is common. ♦ 4,000 mg per day safely improves circulation in patients with **Raynaud's phenomenon**[444]
B-5 (pantothenic acid)	♦ Deficiency is generally unrecognized, but may include depression, acne, anemia, and weight gain; richest dietary sources are yeast and liver. ♦ Main physiologic functions include its structural role in the formation of the Coenzyme A molecule.	♦ 20-100 mg is a common supplemental dose, and doses of 10,000 mg calcium pantothenate have been used safely; it is virtually non-toxic. ♦ May help alleviate **fatigue** in some patients. ♦ May alleviate **acne** in some patients.

[443] Sprecher DL. Raising high-density lipoprotein cholesterol with niacin and fibrates: a comparative review. *Am J Cardiol.* 2000 Dec 21;86(12A):46L-50L
[444] Sunderland GT, Belch JJ, Sturrock RD, Forbes CD, McKay AJ. A double blind randomised placebo controlled trial of hexopal in primary Raynaud's disease. *Clin Rheumatol.* 1988 Mar;7(1):46-9

Nutrients	Physiology, toxicity, and contraindications	Clinical applications (adult doses)
B-6 Pyridoxine	♦ Deficiency can cause widespread—subtle or severe—problems and manifestations since this cofactor is used in more than 100 enzymatic reactions. Modest dietary sources are yeast, sunflower seeds, and wheat germ. Deficiency of B6 can be induced by the drug Isoniazid. ♦ 20-100 mg is a common supplemental dose; 250 mg per day with breakfast is safe and reasonable when higher doses are needed; this should be co-administered with a multivitamin/multimineral supplement that supplies other vitamins and minerals, especially replacement doses (200-600 mg) of magnesium. Very high doses of vitamin B6 (600-900 mg) are supported by the literature for the treatment of specific conditions, and doses ≤ 1,000 mg per day have been used safely with doctor supervision.[445] ♦ Peripheral sensory (and motor) neuropathy has been reported in patients taking gram doses for several years. Most of these reports appear associated with synthetic pyridoxine HCl and the toxicity is likely due to untreated magnesium deficiency which impairs conversion of neurotoxic pyridoxine HCl into the safe and active pyridoxal 5' phosphate. Doses of B6 greater than 150 mg may suppress prolactin and lactation.	♦ Pyridoxine HCl is synthetic and somewhat neurotoxic until it is converted to pyridoxal 5' phosphate which requires magnesium. Pyridoxine HCl must always be coadministered with magnesium. ♦ **Clinical applications: carpal tunnel syndrome, autism, epilepsy, PMS, calcium oxalate nephrolithiasis, nausea/vomiting of pregnancy.** ♦ Vitamin B6 is commonly used to promote various forms of detoxification; however high doses may paradoxically inhibit the sulfotransferase aspect of detoxification.
B-12 (cobalamin) "Active" and biologically useful forms of this vitamin: ♦ Hydroxy-cobalamin also called hydroxo-cobalamin ♦ Adenosyl-cobalamin ♦ Methyl-cobalamin ♦ Cyanocobala min contains cyanide, which is poisonous at high doses[446]	♦ Classic deficiency manifests as megaloblastic anemia, dorsal column lesions (i.e., loss of pedal vibration and proprioception), mental depression, fatigue, peripheral neuropathy. "Pernicious anemia" is a type of B12 deficiency caused by autoimmune atrophic gastritis wherein parietal cells are destroyed, leaving the host without intrinsic factor. Best dietary sources are liver, clams, and kidneys—vegetarian diets are notoriously deficient in B12. ♦ 100 – 2,000 mcg is a common supplemental dose; at least 2,000 mcg per day is required to increase blood levels in patients with B12 deficiency and malabsorption ♦ essentially non-toxic ♦ cyanocobalamin contains cyanide and should be avoided; anaphylaxis to parenteral b12 has been reported	♦ Cyanocobalamin contains cyanide and should be avoided as it can contribute to chronic cyanide toxicity and loss of vision (tobacco-alcohol amblyopia)—the treatment for the latter problem is administration of nutrients with an emphasis on hydroxocobalamin ♦ "active" forms include methylcobalamin and hydroxocobalamin ♦ At least 2,000 mcg per day is required to increase blood levels in patients with B12 deficiency to the same levels that can be obtained with standard regimens of parenteral/intramuscular administration.[447] ♦ **Vitamin B12 in high doses appears to help alleviate low-back pain[448]: this study used intramuscular administration, but high-dose oral supplementation should be superior if doses >2,000 mcg are used.** ♦ Can alleviate fatigue, especially neurogenic fatigue in patients with chronic infections.

[445] Ames BN, Elson-Schwab I, Silver EA. High-dose vitamin therapy stimulates variant enzymes with decreased coenzyme binding affinity (increased K(m)): relevance to genetic disease and polymorphisms. *Am J Clin Nutr*. 2002 Apr;75(4):616-58

[446] Reidenberg MM. Cyanocobalamin--a case for withdrawal. *J R Soc Med*. 1993 May;86(5):309

[447] Kuzminski AM, Del Giacco EJ, Allen RH, Stabler SP, Lindenbaum J. Effective treatment of cobalamin deficiency with oral cobalamin. *Blood*. 1998 Aug 15;92(4):1191-8

[448] Mauro GL, Martorana U, Cataldo P, Brancato G, Letizia G. Vitamin B12 in low back pain: a randomised, double-blind, placebo-controlled study. *Eur Rev Med Pharmacol Sci*. 2000 May-Jun;4:53-8

Appendix A: Clinical and Physiologic Considerations of Vitamins and Minerals—*continued*

Nutrients	Physiology, toxicity, and contraindications	Clinical applications (adult doses)
Biotin	◆ Necessary for fatty acid metabolism and mitochondrial function. Deficiency can include hyperlactatemia, ataxia, seizures, hypotonia, seborrheic dermatitis, and hair loss. Richest dietary source is brewer's yeast. Deficiency is uncommon in the general population however it is commonly seen in patients taking inadequate parenteral nutrition. ◆ **Virtually non-toxic**: In 2001, the Food and Nutrition Board (FNB) reported that no adverse effects had been documented due to either dietary or supplemental consumption of biotin, and this document was still presented as accurate/current as of September 2005.[449] ◆ Avidin in raw egg whites irreversibly binds to biotin and prevents absorption	◆ 50 – 3,000 mcg is a common supplemental dose. ◆ **May provide benefit to diabetics, especially for the treatment/prevention of peripheral neuropathy[450]** ◆ **Biotin deficiency during pregnancy is common may result in birth defects; supplementation of pregnant women with ~300 mcg is warranted[451]**
Folic acid	◆ Found in low doses in foliage. Numerous functions include the transfer of methyl groups, necessary for the formation of myelin, neurotransmitters, and for the protection of DNA. Brewer's yeast is clearly the densest dietary source of folic acid. Deficiency causes macrocytic anemia, fatigue, depression, and hyperhomocysteinemia. B12 and folic acid should be coadministered. ◆ 800 mcg is a reasonable supplemental dose and should be considered the minimal supplemental dose. Doses of 5, 10, and 20 mg (i.e., up to 20,000 mcg) are commonly used and are generally safe. ◆ Use folic acid cautiously in patients with a history of seizure or those who are taking anti-seizure medications. Anti-seizure medications induce deficiency of folate, and if folate is replaced, then anti-seizure protection may be lost.	◆ Always use with B-12 and other B-vitamins ◆ **Potentiates antidepressants by addressing the previously undiagnosed folic acid deficiency** ◆ **Improves efficacy and reduces toxicity of methotrexate** ◆ **Lowers homocysteine levels, may also require B12, B6, NAC, etc.**
Vitamin C **Ascorbic acid**	◆ Classic deficiency is scurvy: bleeding gums, subcutaneous bleeding (ecchymoses, petechiae), weak and friable skin and mucus membranes, reduced immunity, corkscrew hairs, and follicular hyperkeratosis. Vitamin C has some function as an antioxidant, in immune support, and in (dopaminergic) neurotransmission. The best dietary sources are fresh fruits and vegetables, which also contain the phytochemicals necessary to optimize the function of vitamin C. ◆ 500-1,000 mg is a reasonable daily dosage for preventive healthcare; ◆ High doses cause benign loose stools; this varies from patient to patient and time to time; some patients get loose stools with 500 mg while others can tolerate 10,000 mg with no problems. ◆ Intravenous ascorbate can induce hemolysis in patients with G6PD deficiency ◆ Oral supplementation can exacerbate cardiac complications of iron overload[452]	◆ **Anti-allergy benefits in high doses due to mechanisms including ~40% reductions in serum histamine** ◆ **6,000 mg/d in divided doses has been shown to have anti-stress benefits.[453]** ◆ **Anticancer effects may require bowel-tolerance dosing or intravenous administration.** ◆ **High doses benefit autistic children via a dopaminergic mechanism[454]**

[449] Food and Nutrition Board (FNB). Dietary Reference Intakes-Vitamins. http://www.nal.usda.gov/fnic/etext/000105.html http://www.iom.edu/Object.File/Master/7/296/0.pdf   Sept 6, 2005

[450] Koutsikos D, Agroyannis B, Tzanatos-Exarchou H. Biotin for diabetic peripheral neuropathy. *Biomed Pharmacother.* 1990;44(10):511-4

[451] Mock DM, Quirk JG, Mock NI. Marginal biotin deficiency during normal pregnancy. *Am J Clin Nutr.* 2002 Feb;75(2):295-9

[452] McLaran CJ, Bett JH, Nye JA, Halliday JW. Congestive cardiomyopathy and haemochromatosis--rapid progression possibly accelerated by excessive ingestion of ascorbic acid. *Aust N Z J Med.* 1982 Apr;12(2):187-8

Nutrients	Physiology, toxicity, and contraindications	Clinical applications (adult doses)
Calcium	◆ 500 - 1,500 mg is the common supplemental dose ◆ 1,000 - 1,500 mg is the recommended supplemental dose in patients with osteopenia ◆ may promote constipation, especially if not balanced with magnesium, supplementation should provide a 1:2 to 1:1 ratio of calcium to magnesium ◆ Do not administer with certain medications, especially antibiotics such as tetracycline, due to the binding effect which renders the drug systemically unavailable and can result in death in patients with life-threatening infections like pneumonia	◆ **can promote constipation** ◆ **always use with magnesium** ◆ **alleviates bruxism** ◆ **alleviates PMS** ◆ **significantly lowers blood pressure in hypertensive patients when used with vitamin D**
Magnesium	◆ Magnesium deficiency is clearly one of the most common nutritional deficiencies in all populations. ◆ 200 -800 mg is a common supplemental dose; high doses cause loose stools. ◆ Do not administer high doses to patients with severe constipation or with renal failure due to potential for hypermagnesemia. ◆ Do not administer with certain medications, especially antibiotics such as tetracycline, due to the binding effect; spironolactone is a magnesium-sparing diuretic that can potentiate hypermagnesemia	◆ **alleviates bruxism** ◆ **alleviates PMS** ◆ **alleviates migraine headaches** ◆ **alleviates constipation** ◆ **alleviates muscle spasm and hypertonicity** ◆ **helps with asthma, hypertension, insomnia, irritability, anxiety, detoxification,**
Zinc	◆ 10 – 25 mg per day is common in supplements; ◆ Doses up to 150 mg can be used therapeutically, preferably for short-term only or balanced with 2-4 mg copper ◆ Excess or imbalanced zinc supplementation can promote copper deficiency by competition for absorption ◆ Do not use high-dose zinc in patients with Alzheimer's disease[455] ◆ Must be administered with food in order to avoid stomach irritation	◆ **Improves mucosal integrity in patients with Crohn's disease when used at 150 mg per day** ◆ **Promotes tissue healing: trauma, diabetic ulcers**
Copper	◆ 2 mg is the most common supplemental dose ◆ Excess or imbalanced copper supplementation can promote zinc deficiency by competition for absorption ◆ Wilson's disease is a type of copper toxicity associated with liver disease and neuropsychiatric disorder	◆ A good multivitamin should have enough so that you don't have to use a separate supplement. ◆ **up to 4 mg per day can be used in patients with connective tissue disorders such as Marfan's syndrome and/or to promote healing**

[453] Brody S, Preut R, Schommer K, Schurmeyer TH. A randomized controlled trial of high dose ascorbic acid for reduction of blood pressure, cortisol, and subjective responses to psychological stress. *Psychopharmacology* (Berl). 2002 Jan;159(3):319-24

[454] Dolske MC, Spollen J, McKay S, Lancashire E, Tolbert L. A preliminary trial of ascorbic acid as supplemental therapy for autism. *Prog Neuropsychopharmacol Biol Psychiatry.* 1993 Sep;17(5):765-74

[455] Vasquez A. A brief review of two potential adverse effects of zinc supplementation: cognitive deterioration in patients with Alzheimer's disease, and copper deficiency. *Nutritional Perspectives* 1995; 18: 11, 19

Appendix A: Clinical and Physiologic Considerations of Vitamins and Minerals—*continued*

Nutrients	Physiology and contraindications	Clinical applications (adult doses)
Chromium	♦ Appears to have a homeostatic effect on glucose-insulin metabolism ♦ may potentiate diabetic medications; start slowly and with 6x daily glucose monitoring in severe diabetics	♦ 200 mcg is the most common supplemental dose ♦ 500 mcg is commonly used in diabetics ♦ doses up to 1,000 mcg have been used safely in diabetics ♦ Quality multivitamin-multimineral supplements will contain at least 200 mcg of chromium ♦ Can alleviate diabetes mellitus and hypoglycemia
Iodide And Iodine	♦ Necessary for the formation of thyroid hormone ♦ May beneficially modulate estrogen metabolism in women ♦ Thins mucus ♦ May have antimicrobial benefits, especially in the stomach and upper intestine ♦ Iodine is the natural elemental diatomic form of this element, consisting of two iodide molecules; **both iodine and iodine have beneficial properties and one does not necessarily substitute for the other—supplementation should include both forms** ♦ A few patients appear allergic to iodine-iodide and should avoid supplementation until their immune function is normalized	♦ **Several experts in iodine/iodide nutrition—namely Wright, Abraham, and Brownstein—are now advocating iodine-iodide supplementation with daily doses as high as 12 milligrams (12,000 micrograms) since these doses provide benefit, are without acute toxicity, and are very comparable to the average daily Japanese intake at 13.8 milligrams per day**[456] ♦ High doses of iodine 3-6 mg per day can reduce breast pain during 6 months of treatment[457] ♦ Lecithin-bound iodine modulates cytokine release and may improve symptoms in patients with asthma[458] ♦ Daily doses greater than 750 mcg iodide can contribute to exacerbation of hypothyroidism in patients with *pre-existing* thyroid disorders or borderline thyroid function[459]; the combination of iodine-iodide may actually improve thyroid function in patients with thyroid disease[460] ♦ Abraham[461] has advocated the use of high-dose iodine supplementation ("orthoiodosupplementation") and has used short-term doses as high as 50 mg per day (fifty milligrams per day). He reports that the toxicity associated with iodine-containing drugs (Amiodarone: antiarrhythmic) is due to the drug itself and not the iodine. Rationale for "high dose" iodine supplementation is suggested by the increased prevalence of halogenated/brominated pesticides/herbicides and other pollutants in our environment which are known to have adverse health effects
Potassium	♦ Get potassium from fruits and vegetables, not from supplements ♦ High-normal intake of potassium from fruits and vegetables can cause fatal hyperkalemia in patients with renal failure such as due to diabetes	♦ lowers blood pressure ♦ reduces risk of stroke independently from its ability to lower blood pressure ♦ promotes urinary alkalinization, which is important for mineral retention and increased excretion of most xenobiotics
Selenium	♦ 200 mcg is considered the standard supplemental and therapeutic dose ♦ Daily doses should be kept below 800-1,000 mcg, and high doses are generally used for a limited time only, such as a few days to a maximum of 3 months at a time	♦ antioxidant ♦ protects against cancer and heart disease ♦ immunosupportive; powerfully inhibits risk of serious infection in patients with HIV ♦ highly effective for relieving lymphedema

[456] Wright JV. Why you need 83 times more of this essential, cancer-fighting nutrient than the 'experts' say you do. *Nutrition and Healing* 2005; 12: 1

[457] "Patients recorded statistically significant decreases in pain by month 3 in the 3.0 and 6.0 mg/day treatment groups, but not the 1.5 mg/day or placebo group; more than 50% of the 6.0 mg/day treatment group recorded a clinically significant reduction in overall pain. All doses were associated with an acceptable safety profile." Kessler JH. The effect of supraphysiologic levels of iodine on patients with cyclic mastalgia. *Breast J*. 2004 Jul-Aug;10(4):328-36

[458] "Also, a longer course of treatment with LBI may markedly improve the clinical conditions of the asthmatic children, because even a period of just 8 weeks LBI therapy improved the cough and reduced the severity of the asthmatic attacks in two out of the nine patients enrolled in this study." Kawano Y, Saeki T, Noma T. Effect of lecithin-bound iodine on the patients with bronchial asthma. *Int Immunopharmacol*. 2005 Apr;5(4):805-10

[459] Chow CC, Phillips DI, Lazarus JH, Parkes AB. Effect of low dose iodide supplementation on thyroid function in potentially susceptible subjects: are dietary iodide levels in Britain acceptable? *Clin Endocrinol* (Oxf). 1991 May;34(5):413-6

[460] Brownstein D. Clinical Experience with Inorganic Non-radioactive Iodine/Iodide. http://www.optimox.com/pics/Iodine/IOD-09/IOD_09.htm Accessed January 15, 2007

[461] Abraham GE. Serum inorganic iodide levels following ingestion of a tablet form of Lugol solution: evidence for an enterohepatic circulation of iodine. *The Original Internist*. 2004; 11: 29-35

Nutrients	Physiology, toxicity, and contraindications	Clinical applications (adult doses)
Iron	♦ Iron supplementation should not be used in patients unless their iron levels are low, and this is determined by measuring serum ferritin—not by performing a CBC which can show anemia that is unrelated to iron deficiency and which may be associated with iron overload. ♦ The finding of iron deficiency in any adult patient requires that the patient be referred to a gastroenterologist for endoscopic evaluation. Failure to make a timely referral for any adult patient with iron deficiency is grounds for malpractice litigation. ♦ Iron promotes the formation of "free radicals" and is thus implicated in several diseases, such as infections, cancer, liver disease, diabetes, and cardiovascular disease. Iron supplements should not be consumed except by people who have been definitively diagnosed with iron deficiency by measurement of serum ferritin. For a simplistic review, see http://vix.com/menmag/alexiron.htm	♦ **Never use iron supplementation without first testing serum ferritin.**[462,463] ♦ **Replacement dose for iron deficiency is 60-180 mg of iron per day. 40-60 mg 3x per day is reasonable for correcting iron deficiency; may promote constipation and stomach upset; consume with food, especially meat;** ♦ **All adult patients with iron deficiency have a gastrointestinal lesion such as cancer until proven otherwise. CLINICIANS MUST REFER THESE PATIENTS TO A GASTROENTEROLOGIST.**[464]

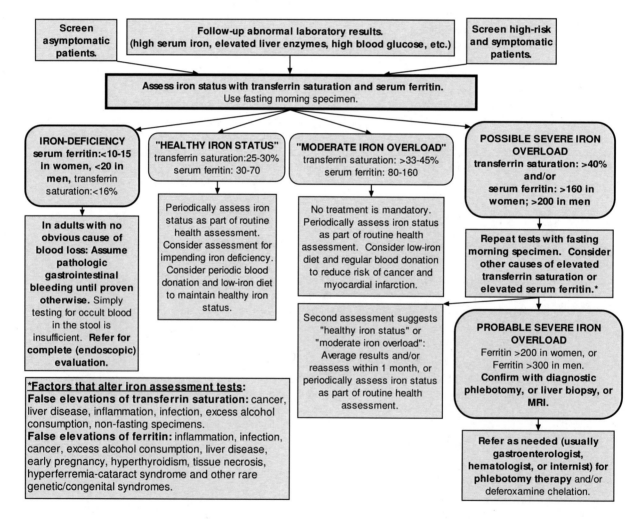

[462] Vasquez A. Integrative Orthopedics: Concepts, Algorithms, and Therapeutics. The art of creating wellness while effectively managing acute and chronic musculoskeletal disorders. Natural Health Consulting Corporation: www.OptimalHealthResearch.com 2004, Revised edition August 2004

[463] Hollan S, Johansen KS. Adequate iron stores and the 'Nil nocere' principle. *Haematologia* (Budap). 1993;25(2):69-84

[464] Green BT, Rockey DC. Gastrointestinal endoscopic evaluation of premenopausal women with iron deficiency anemia. *J Clin Gastroenterol*. 2004 Feb;38(2):104-9

Core Competencies and Standards of Clinical Excellence:

1) You must know how to diagnose developmental dysplasia of the hip in a newborn.

2) What is the proper management of stress fractures of the proximal femur?

3) Define atlantoaxial instability and os odontoidium and list their presentations, complications and management.

4) How do you diagnose and manage slipped capital femoral epiphysis, avascular necrosis, and septic arthritis?

5) How do you differentially diagnose and manage meralgia paresthetica from femoral neuropathy?

6) Since differentiation based on physical examination and history is impossible, you must know which lab tests are used to distinguish hip osteoarthritis from hemochromatoic arthropathy and how the tests are correlatively interpreted.

7) You must know how to diagnose by cauda equina syndrome *by history and physical examination alone* (e.g., without CT or MRI results).

8) You must know how to diagnose and manage vertebral osteomyelitis and infectious discitis.

9) Be able to explain the mechanism by which vitamin D deficiency causes low back pain; know the indications, contraindications, dosing, and monitoring involved with vitamin D supplementation.

10) Name five inflammatory disorders that can affect the lumbar spine and sacroiliac joints. Provide the diagnostic criteria and management strategy of each.

11) List at least five ways to improve proprioceptive/sensorimotor function in patients with low-back pain.

12) Differentially diagnose a bladder infection from a kidney infection; describe appropriate management strategies for both problems.

13) Be able to explain why "fibromyalgia" is an overused diagnosis and be able to provide a list of treatable conditions that are often misdiagnosed as fibromyalgia.

14) Name the proper angle for obtaining an anteroposterior radiograph of the knee to demonstrate osteoarthritis.

15) List the characteristics of migraine headaches and the proper administration of six nutritional treatments.

16) Differentiate a benign headache from one that is potentially life-threatening.

17) Name the two best and most commonly used tests for assessing the anterior cruciate ligament. Which test is better and why?

18) McMurray's test is one of the most commonly used tests for assessing menisci. How is the test performed, and what is the sensitivity and specificity of a positive finding?

19) You must know how to identify and manage acute compartment syndrome.

20) If you think your patient may have a meniscus injury, how do you decide for or against ordering an MRI?

21) Describe the clinical manifestations of spinal cord compression.

22) Your patient is a cyclist and presents with knee pain under the patella on the lateral aspect. What is the most likely diagnosis and your treatment?

23) Why must you examine the *hip* of an adolescent patient who presents with *knee* pain? Provide the specific anatomic basis.

24) You must know how to distinguish *benign* sacroiliac and pelvic pain from that which results from rheumatic diseases such as the spondyloarthropathies and infections.

25) You must know the wrist/hand manifestations of hemochromatosis and how to differentiate this potentially life-threatening condition from benign osteoarthritis. Compare and contrast the physical examination, laboratory, and treatment differences.

26) You must know how to differentially diagnose and treat rheumatoid arthritis, osteoarthritis, and hemochromatosis.

27) You must know how to properly administer high-dose pyridoxine as a component of the treatment plan for a patient with carpal tunnel syndrome.

28) You must know how to diagnose and manage fracture of the scaphoid.

29) You must know how to manage a hand/bone injury that has been contaminated with human saliva, such as a hand injury resulting from a fist fight.

30) You must know how to diagnose and manage supracondylar fractures of the humerus.

31) You must know how to diagnose and manage lateral epicondylitis.

32) Differentially diagnose and treat rotator cuff tendonitis from proximal biceps tendonitis.

33) Differentially diagnose overuse bursitis from septic bursitis.

34) Differentiate thoracic outlet syndrome from fibromyalgia and the musculoskeletal manifestations of hypothyroidism.

35) You must know how to grade reflexes and muscle strength and know the implications and management of abnormal findings

36) You must know how to rapidly diagnose and effectively manage the following musculoskeletal emergencies: Neuropsychiatric lupus, Giant cell arteritis, Temporal arteritis, Acute red eye, including acute iritis and scleritis, Atlantoaxial subluxation & instability, Myelopathy, spinal cord compression, Cauda equina syndrome, Septic arthritis, Osteomyelitis, Acute nontraumatic monoarthritis

37) Following a joint aspiration for acute monoarthritis, which analyses are used to differentiate septic arthritis from inflammatory arthritis and gout?

38) Demonstrate competency in the interpretation and correlative interpretation of the following commonly performed tests: CRP, ESR, CBC, Chemistry/metabolic panel, Ferritin, Serum 25(OH)-vitamin D, TSH, ANA, CCP.

39) For example, what is the important difference between "elevated CRP with a normal ferritin" and "elevated CRP with elevated ferritin."

40) *Bonus*: If the lactulose-mannitol assay is abnormal (elevated lactulose-to-mannitol ratio) and the comprehensive stool analysis and comprehensive parasitology results are normal, what are the two most likely diagnoses, assuming that your patient does not overconsume alcohol or NSAIDs.

41) If your patient's serum 25(OH)-vitamin D is low but the serum calcium level is elevated, what are three possible underlying diseases and what single blood test is most indicated?

42) Describe how to clinically distinguish fibromyalgia from polymyalgia rheumatica.

43) How are nondisplaced clavicle fractures managed?

44) Provide one example from each letter of the "p.r.i.c.e. a. t.u.r.n." and "b.e.n.d. s.t.e.m.s." mnemonic acronyms for holistic acute care for musculoskeletal injuries.

45) List the two most common clinical findings associated with myofascial trigger points and describe appropriate physical/manual and nutritional treatments.

46) Describe a plan for proproceptive retraining/rehabilitation for a patient who has no exercise equipment.

47) Describe the effects of stereotypic NSAIDs on chrondrocyte metabolism and the long-term effects on joint structure.

48) Name four biochemical/physiologic mechanisms by which COX-2 inhibiting drugs predispose to cardiovascular death.

49) Name the only absolute contraindication to the use of willow bark extract.

50) In a patient with fever and focal back pain exacerbated by spinal percussion, what is the most likely diagnosis?

51) How do you differentiate chest/back pain resulting from a "benign" musculoskeletal condition from pain that is a manifestation of intrathoracic pathology?

52) Briefly and generally describe how to administer the following relative to the treatment of musculoskeletal pain; you must know the treatments by their commonly used names and abbreviations: ALA, EPA, DHA, GLA, D3, Niacinamide, Glucosamine sulfate and Chondroitin Sulfate, proteolytic enzymes, *Zingiber*, Cat's claw, *Salix*, topical *Capsicum annuum*, *Boswellia*, Devil's claw, *Curcuma longa*

The following questions are derived from the midterm and final exam questions that I created when I taught Orthopedics at Bastyr University in 2000. The emphasis of the exam is on clinical synthesis—combining history, physical examination, lab and imaging, along with basic knowledge of therapeutics such as manipulation, botanical medicine, nutrition, physiotherapy, and other subjects taught and tested in other courses. "Core competencies" represent the information that every student and doctor must know; missing even one of these questions meant failure for the entire examination. An answered version of first edition of this assessment is available on-line at: www.OptimalHealthResearch.com/tests/**musculoskeletal**. Questions in **bold** were added in March 2007.

PART ONE

List and provide one example of the **4 general categories** that need to be assessed during the history and physical when a patient presents with a musculoskeletal complaint:

1. _____ Example: _____

2. _____ Example: _____

3. _____ Example: _____

4. _____ Example: _____

Your patient presents with a complex history and examination picture that suggests the possibility of organic disease as a cause of his/her complaints, but you are not sure what disease might be present. **List the combination of lab tests that represent a safe and reasonably inexpensive means of laboratory investigation that allows you to objectively screen for several different diseases**:

1. (essential) _____

2. (essential) _____

3. (essential) _____

4. (optional) _____

5. (optional) _____

What percentage range of "trauma-related" injuries
are actually associated with organic disease? _____

A 50-year-old woman presents with generalized stiffness and pain in the shoulder for 2 months duration; she recalls no trauma. On examination she exhibits severe loss of internal and external rotation and abduction at the shoulder.

What is the most likely diagnosis? _____

What two endocrine conditions must she be assessed for with a blood test? _____

A 60-year-old man presents with diffuse pain in the left shoulder region for 4-weeks duration; he recalls no trauma and notes that the pain is worse at night. His health history reveals that he follows a typical American diet, walks for exercise, is right-handed, is a house painter by profession, and that he no longer smokes. Physical examination reveals the following:

- Shoulder ROM is full and generally painless except for what you consider to be mild age-related stiffness that is symmetric
- Provocative maneuvers are negative
- He is afebrile, and blood pressure, pulse, and peripheral capillary refill are normal
- Lab tests performed by his MD last week show slight anemia, normal ferritin, and slightly elevated Hgb-A1c

What condition should he be assessed for? _____

What additional physical examination procedures should be performed? _____

If the above test is positive, what is your next step? _____

Mark the 1 (one) best answer for each of the following questions.

1) Which of the following are characteristics of "cancer pain:"
   A. Vague, diffuse pain
   B. Worse at night
   C. Increasing severity
   D. Unrelieved by rest, unresponsive to standard musculoskeletal treatment
   E. All of the above.

2) Your patient is over age 50 and has back pain, which he cannot ascribe to any recent injury, motions, or positions. The ESR is 40 and ferritin is 8. Which of the following is the best next step?
   A. High-dose proteolytic enzymes
   B. *Boswellia* tincture dosed per body weight
   C. Topical capsaicin
   D. Radiographs
   E. A 2-week trial of spinal manipulation

3) Your 55-year-old patient presents with left-sided shoulder pain, wrist weakness, miosis, ptosis of the left eyelid, and anhidrosis (decreased sweating) of the left side of the face. The condition for which you must assess is:
   A. Cauda equina syndrome
   B. Thoracic outlet syndrome
   C. Pancoast syndrome
   D. Chronic fatigue syndrome
   E. Frozen shoulder syndrome

4) Which of the following are causes of shoulder pain:
   A. Apical lung tumor
   B. Cervical radiculopathy
   C. Impingement syndrome
   D. Biceps tendonitis
   E. All of the above

5) Your 25-year-old patient presents to you following a car accident that occurred earlier that morning. He has neck pain, and requests that you treat him homeopathically and with herbs for the tingling he now has in his arms and legs. You should:
   A. Immediately perform the Sotto-Hall neck-flexion test to assess him for cervical instability.
   B. Take a complete homeopathic history and send him home with a remedy after telling him to avoid coffee and mint. Follow-up visit is scheduled for 2 weeks.
   C. Prescribe high-dose bromelain.
   D. Perform a cautious physical examination to determine which is more appropriate: radiographs or hospital referral.
   E. Begin treatment with manipulation.

6) Your 42-year-old patient presents with "shoulder pain" and "insomnia." History reveals that she has difficulty getting to sleep due to the shoulder pain. During physical examination, you find that ROM is full and does not exacerbate her pain, and that there is slight swelling in the supraclavicular fossa. The best choice from the selection below is:
   A. Order radiographs or CT scan
   B. Request a diet diary
   C. Request a urinalysis
   D. Recommend that she get a new pillow
   E. Valerian tincture to help her sleep

7) Your new 20-year-old patient presents with chief complaints of "back pain" and "the flu." The onset of both complaints was yesterday with a slight fever and now the back pain is rated 7 on a scale of 1-10 with 10 being severe pain. Lungs are clear to auscultation, and the lower back is stiff and painful to percussion. Your main concern is:
   A. Pancoast syndrome
   B. Myofascial trigger points
   C. Costochondritis
   D. Osteomyelitis
   E. Pneumonia

8) **Your diabetic adult male patient has CRP of 5, ESR of 5, and ferritin of 600. He is asymptomatic. The most likely cause to explain these findings is:**
   A. **Diabetes mellitus**
   B. **Osteochondritis**
   C. **Behcet's disease**
   D. **Hepatitis**
   E. **Hemochromatosis**

9) Rust's sign, whereby the patient needs to support head/neck during normal motions and positions to prevent pain, is considered indicative of:
   A. Cervical instability
   B. Cervical radiculopathy
   C. Tietze's syndrome
   D. Myofascial trigger points in the sternocleidomastoid
   E. Impingement syndrome

10) **Your elderly adult female patient presents with subacute back pain and has ESR of 40, CRP of 28, and ferritin of 5. She is afebrile and has no cardiac or intestinal complaints. Your next action is:**
    A. **Referral to a rheumatologist for immunosuppression**
    B. **Lumbar radiographs**
    C. **Referral to a gastroenterologist**
    D. **Joint aspiration**
    E. **Treat conservatively and repeat labs in 2 months**

11) Cervical radiculopathy is characterized by:
    A. Babinski reflex
    B. Upper extremity motor deficits with dermatomal sensory abnormalities
    C. Lower extremity hyperreflexia
    D. Bowel and bladder dysfunction
    E. Delayed Achilles' reflex return

12) In a patient with neck pain and dermatomal sensory changes in the arm, associated onset of which of the following suggests the need for additional investigation and/or referral to a surgeon?
    A. Asymmetric biceps weakness
    B. Babinski reflex
    C. Lower extremity clonus
    D. Incontinence
    E. All of the above

13) Recent trauma-related onset of myelopathy indicates the need for treatment, specifically with methylprednisolone, within:
    A. 8 hours
    B. 10 days
    C. 12 weeks
    D. The first 30 days of treatment

14) Which of the following are causes of torticollis?
    A. Cancer
    B. Infection
    C. Injury at birth
    D. Neuromuscular disease
    E. All of the above

15) **Your patient was in a severe car accident 2 days ago. Now she feels sleepy during the day, despite sleeping 10 hours each night, and has recent onset clonus. Proper management for this patient includes:**
    A. **Adrenergic agonist treatment, either with drugs or amino acid therapy**
    B. **Dopamine agonist, either with drugs or botanical medicines**
    C. **Laboratory assessment for anti-myelin antibodies**
    D. **CT scan**
    E. **Sotto-Hall test**

16) Pain in the C5 dermatome, with biceps strength +5
   A. Bicipital tendonitis—conservative treatment, no need for referral
   B. Cervical myelopathy—urgent referral
   C. Cervical radiculitis—conservative treatment, no need for referral
   D. Cervical radiculopathy—conservative treatment, no need for referral
   E. Supraspinatus tendonitis—conservative treatment, no need for referral

17) Pain in the C5 dermatome, with biceps strength +3
   A. Bicipital tendonitis—consider conservative treatment, PAR
   B. Cervical myelopathy—urgent referral
   C. Cervical radiculitis—consider conservative treatment, PAR
   D. Cervical radiculopathy—consider conservative treatment, PAR, recommend referral
   E. Supraspinatus tendonitis—consider conservative treatment, no need for referral

18) Pain in the C5 dermatome, lower extremity weakness, patellar and Achilles reflexes +4
   A. Bicipital tendonitis—conservative treatment, PAR
   B. Cervical myelopathy—urgent referral
   C. Cervical radiculitis—conservative treatment, PAR
   D. Cervical radiculopathy—conservative treatment, PAR, recommend referral
   E. Supraspinatus tendonitis—conservative treatment, no need for referral

19) Positive Speed's test and Yergason's test, sensory testing WNL, with biceps strength +4
   A. Bicipital tendonitis—conservative treatment, no need for referral
   B. Cervical myelopathy—urgent referral
   C. Cervical radiculitis—conservative treatment
   D. Cervical radiculopathy—recommend referral
   E. Supraspinatus tendonitis—conservative treatment, no need for referral

20) Pain with 90° shoulder abduction and internal rotation, pain with "empty can" test
   A. Bicipital tendonitis—conservative treatment, no need for referral
   B. Cervical myelopathy—urgent referral
   C. Cervical radiculitis—conservative treatment
   D. Cervical radiculopathy—recommend referral
   E. Supraspinatus tendonitis—conservative treatment, no need for referral

21) Your patient presents with neck pain following trauma. Your clinical assessment needs to evaluate for which of the following:
   A. Myelopathy
   B. Radiculopathy
   C. Fracture
   D. Instability
   E. All of the above

22) Tom is a 47-year-old right-handed male who presents to your office with a chief complaint of "chest pain" on the right that he first noticed this morning when he was finishing a tennis match with his son. He has anterior peristernal chest pain with point tenderness, increased pain with hyperabduction of the ipsilateral arm, increased pain with deep inspiration, increased pain with palpation-provocation of the peristernal structures. Cardiopulmonary assessments are WNL. Tom most likely has:
   A. Costochondritis
   B. Pancoast syndrome
   C. Horner's syndrome
   D. Intercostal neuralgia
   E. Cardiovascular disease

23) Bob is a 47-year-old right-handed male who presents to your office with a chief complaint of "chest pain" on the left that he first noticed this morning when he was finishing a tennis match with his son. He experienced anterior peristernal chest pain with diffuse tenderness, and your clinical assessment finds no increased pain with hyperabduction of the ipsilateral arm, no increased pain with deep inspiration, and no increased pain with palpation-provocation of the thoracic structures. Bob most likely has:
   A. Costochondritis (Tietze's syndrome)
   B. Pancoast syndrome
   C. Horner's syndrome
   D. Intercostal strain
   E. Cardiovascular disease

24) Mary is a 47-year-old right-handed female who presents to your office with a chief complaint of "chest pain" on the right that she first noticed this morning when she was finishing a tennis match with her son. She experienced anterior-lateral chest pain with sharp tenderness, and your clinical assessment finds increased pain with hyperabduction of the ipsilateral arm, increased pain with deep inspiration, and increased pain with deep palpation of the space between her 8th and 9th ribs. Mary most likely has:
   A. Costochondritis (Tietze's syndrome)
   B. Pancoast syndrome
   C. Horner's syndrome
   D. Intercostal muscle strain
   E. Cardiovascular disease

25) Suggested by signs of myelopathy with flexion and diagnosed with lateral radiographs demonstrating dens abnormities or increased atlantodental interval; may be seen in a patient with rheumatoid arthritis or ankylosing spondylitis:
   A. Atlantoaxial instability
   B. Cervical radiculitis
   C. Cervical radiculopathy
   D. Supraspinatus tendonitis
   E. De Quervain's syndrome

26) Common in patients with Down's syndrome, contraindication to cervical spine manipulation
   A. Atlantoaxial instability
   B. Foraminal encroachment
   C. Cervical radiculopathy
   D. Supraspinatus tendonitis
   E. Lesion of the subscapularis

27) Inability of the patient to lift the dorsum of the hand from the sacrum
   A. Atlantoaxial instability
   B. Bicipital tendonitis
   C. Cervical myelopathy
   D. Supraspinatus tendonitis
   E. Lesion of the subscapularis

28) Any patient diagnosed with adhesive capsulitis (and/or frozen shoulder) needs to be assessed with which of the following tests:
   A. Phalen's test
   B. Serum glucose
   C. Adson's test
   D. Soto-Hall test
   E. Serum CK-Mb

29) Elbow extended or flexed, forearm pronated, wrist extended, patient resists wrist flexion force by doctor
   A. Speed's test
   B. Lift-off test
   C. Codman's test
   D. Yergason's test
   E. Cozen's test

30) Elbow extended, passive wrist flexion to stretch the wrist extensors
   A. Phalen's test
   B. Mill's test
   C. Adson's test
   D. Soto-Hall test
   E. Varus testing

31) Inability to elevate the dorsum of the hand from the sacrum
   A. "Empty can" test, supraspinatus isolation test—supraspinatus tendonitis
   B. Speed's test—biceps tendonitis
   C. Lift-off test—subscapularis lesion
   D. Codman's test, arm drop test—supraspinatus tendonitis
   E. Yergason's test—biceps tendonitis

32) Weakness and pain when patient resists downward force applied to the distal forearm when shoulder is 90° abducted, internally rotated, with the arm in the scapular plane, with the elbow extended.
    A. "Empty can" test, supraspinatus isolation test—supraspinatus tendonitis
    B. Speed's test—biceps tendonitis
    C. Lift-off test—subscapularis pathology
    D. Codman's test, arm drop test—supraspinatus tendonitis
    E. Yergason's test—biceps tendonitis

33) Which of the following problems is potentially serious and requires immediate assessment for neurovascular injury?
    A. Supracondylar fracture of the humerus
    B. Carpal tunnel syndrome
    C. Rotator cuff tear
    D. Costochondritis
    E. De Quervain's syndrome

34) Following trauma or overuse of the brachioradialis or the wrist extensors; positive Cozen's test, positive Mill's test
    A. Supraspinatus tendonitis
    B. Lateral epicondylitis
    C. Medial epicondylitis
    D. Lesion of the subscapularis
    E. De Quervain's syndrome

35) Positive Finkelstein's test
    A. Pancoast syndrome
    B. Lateral epicondylitis
    C. Medial epicondylitis
    D. Lesion of the subscapularis
    E. De Quervain's syndrome

36) Reproduction of carpal tunnel syndrome manifestations with forced wrist flexion, may be held for 1 minute
    A. Phalen's test
    B. Mill's test
    C. Codman's test
    D. Yergason's test
    E. Cozen's test

37) Your patient presents with pain at the "anatomic snuff box" following a fall on the palm with an extended wrist. While your evaluation should include assessment of neighboring regions, which condition is most likely in this patient:
    A. Fracture of the dens
    B. Medial epicondylitis
    C. Fracture of the scaphoid
    D. Supraspinatus tendonitis
    E. Supracondylar fracture of the humerus

38) Flexion deformities of the fingers, usually 3rd and 4th fingers and/or a tender nodule in the ulnar palm suggests which of the following problems:
    A. De Quervain's
    B. Dupuytren's
    C. Finkelstein's
    D. Phalen's
    E. Normal finding—no need for additional investigation

39) Spinal percussion causes deep dull pain that disappears slowly. Choose the best single answer.
    A. Atlantoaxial instability
    B. Spinal fracture
    C. Bilateral pneumothorax
    D. Spinal tumor or vertebral osteomyelitis
    E. Normal finding—no need for additional investigation

40) Spinal percussion causes acute pain that rapidly subsides
   A. Desiccated intervertebral disc
   B. Recent joint or ligament injury
   C. Normal finding—no need for additional investigation
   D. Supracondylar fracture
   E. Acute compartment syndrome

41) **Your patient is a 15-yo male with progressive scoliosis for the past 6 months. Which of the following is inconsistent with early benign idiopathic scoliosis?**
   A. **Platelet abnormalities**
   B. **Morphologic changes in the cerebellum**
   C. **Pain**
   D. **Proprioceptive defects**
   E. **Compensatory lateral curvature of the spine**

42) **Your patient presents with ESR of 30, CRP of 25, negative rheumatoid factor, negative HLA-B27, ferritin of 150, and positive cyclic citrullinated peptide antibodies. What is this patient's clinical status?**
   A. **Early iron overload**
   B. **Severe lupus**
   C. **Probable early rheumatoid arthritis**
   D. **Seronegative spondyloarthropathy**
   E. **Klippel-Feil syndrome**

43) **Which of the following is consistent with occult gastrointestinal dysbiosis?**
   A. **Increased lactulose-mannitol ratio**
   B. **Upregulated phase 1 of detoxification/biotransformation**
   C. **Inhibited phase 1 of detoxification/biotransformation**
   D. **Systemic immune activation**
   E. **All of the above**

44) Which of the following characteristics places a patient in a higher risk category when associated with musculoskeletal pain and suggests the need for additional assessment?
   A. Age greater than 50 years, or diabetes
   B. Drug or alcohol use
   C. Low-grade fever
   D. Elevated WBC, ESR, or CRP; anemia
   E. All of the above.

45) Your 12-year-old gymnast patient presents with non-traumatic elbow pain in her dominant arm associated with stiffness, locking, and crepitus. Cozen's and Mill's tests are negative, and neurologic screening examination is normal. Regional assessments of neighboring regions are unremarkable. Your clinical concern and means of assessment are:
   A. Fracture of the olecranon—radiographs
   B. Supracondylar fracture of the humerus—radiographs
   C. Osteochondritis dissecans or osteochondrosis—radiographs
   D. Dislocation of the ulna—radiographs
   E. Fracture of the scaphoid—radiographs

46) Your 55-year-old patient presents with left-sided shoulder pain, wrist weakness, miosis, ptosis of the left eyelid, and anhidrosis on the left side of the face. The condition for which you must assess is:
   A. Cauda equina syndrome
   B. Thoracic outlet syndrome
   C. Pancoast syndrome
   D. Chronic fatigue syndrome
   E. Frozen shoulder syndrome

47) Which of the following are causes of shoulder pain:
   A. Apical lung tumor
   B. Cervical radiculopathy
   C. Impingement syndrome
   D. Biceps tendonitis
   E. All of the above

48) Your new 20-year-old patient presents with chief complaints of "back pain" and "the flu." The onset of both complaints was yesterday with a slight fever and now the back pain is rated 7 on a scale of 1-10 with 10 being severe pain. Lungs are clear to auscultation, and the lower back is stiff and painful to percussion. Your main concern is:
   A. Pancoast syndrome
   B. Myofascial trigger points
   C. Costochondritis
   D. Osteomyelitis
   E. Pneumonia

49) **Elevated ferritin with elevated CRP correlates with:**
   A. **Cancer**
   B. **Iron overload**
   C. **Systemic inflammation**
   D. **Acute infection**
   E. **All of the above**

50) Acute onset of pain in the C5 dermatome, lower extremity strength +3, patellar and Achilles reflexes +4
   A. Bicipital tendonitis—conservative treatment, PAR
   B. Cervical myelopathy—urgent referral
   C. Cervical radiculitis—conservative treatment, PAR
   D. Cervical radiculopathy—conservative treatment, PAR, recommend referral
   E. Supraspinatus tendonitis—conservative treatment, no need for referral

51) Positive Speed's test and Yergason's test, sensory testing WNL, with biceps strength +4
   A. Bicipital tendonitis—conservative treatment, no need for referral
   B. Cervical myelopathy—urgent referral
   C. Cervical radiculitis—conservative treatment
   D. Cervical radiculopathy—recommend referral
   E. Supraspinatus tendonitis—conservative treatment, no need for referral

52) Billy Bob is a 51-year-old right-handed male who presents to your office with a chief complaint of "chest pain" on the right that he first noticed this morning when he was finishing a tennis match with his daughter. He has anterior peristernal chest pain with point tenderness, increased pain with hyperabduction of the ipsilateral arm, increased pain with deep inspiration, increased pain with palpation-provocation of the peristernal structures. Heart and lung auscultation are WNL. Billy Bob most likely has:
   A. Costochondritis
   B. Pancoast syndrome
   C. Horner's syndrome
   D. Intercostal neuralgia
   E. Cardiovascular disease

53) Your patient presents with pain at the "anatomic snuff box" following trauma. Which condition is most likely in this patient?
   A. Fracture of the dens
   B. Medial epicondylitis
   C. Fracture of the scaphoid
   D. Supraspinatus tendonitis
   E. Supracondylar fracture of the humerus

54) Which of the following conditions can predispose your patient to atlantoaxial instability?
   A. Down syndrome
   B. Inflammatory arthropathy, such as rheumatoid arthritis
   C. Congenital agenesis of the dens, os odontoidium
   D. Trauma
   E. All of the above

55) Patient seated with flexion of spine, patient then extends knee; a test for lumbar discogenic radiculopathy:
    A. Bechterew's test
    B. Sotto-Hall test
    C. Empty can test
    D. Kemp's test
    E. Cozen's test

56) Patient seated, then lumbar spine is passively moved into rotation, extension, lateral flexion:
    A. Bechterew's test
    B. Braggard's test
    C. Empty can test
    D. Kemp's test
    E. Cozen's test

57) Dorsiflexion of ankle with straight leg raising, confirms the radicular nature of a positive straight leg raising test
    A. Bechterew's test
    B. Braggard's test
    C. Empty can test
    D. Kemp's test
    E. Cozen's test

58) Your patient is a 60-year-old male who presents with back pain and slight nausea of 1-month duration. During your comprehensive low back examination, your abdominal examination reveals a large midline pulsatile abdominal mass, and the femoral and dorsalis pedis pulses are weak. Your main concern and method of assessment are:
    A. Ovarian cancer—assess with ultrasound
    B. Aneurysm of the abdominal aorta—assess with ultrasound
    C. Lymphoma—assess with CBC
    D. Testicular torsion—assess with palpation and transillumination
    E. Meralgia paresthetica—assess with MRI

59) Which of the following are general categories of causes of low back pain:
    A. Serious organic diseases
    B. Serious musculoskeletal disorders requiring immediate attention
    C. Psychogenic
    D. Benign musculoskeletal disorders requiring conservative treatment and monitoring
    E. All of the above

60) Patient age 30-50 years with a history of chronic/recurrent low back pain notices an exacerbation of low back pain or the onset of leg pain associated with a bending and/or twisting motion; leg pain predominates over the severity of the low back pain. This is the classic presentation for:
    A. Atlantoaxial instability
    B. Meralgia paresthetica
    C. Osteochondrosis dissecans
    D. Lumbar disc herniation
    E. De Quervain's syndrome

61) Low back and leg pain exacerbated by spinal extension and relieved by flexion suggests which of the following differential diagnoses:
    A. Lumbar disc herniation or De Quervain's syndrome
    B. Meralgia paresthetica or cauda equina syndrome
    C. Sacroiliac joint dysfunction or scoliosis
    D. Spinal stenosis or facet syndrome
    E. Atlantoaxial instability or Tietze's syndrome

62) Results from rupture/laxity of the soft tissues at the symphysis pubis; associated with pregnancy and/or vaginal delivery in women or repetitive overuse in men; conservative management with a trochanteric-SIJ support belt is appropriate:
    A. Symphysis pubis diastasis or osteitis pubis
    B. SIJ sprain
    C. SIJ functional subluxation and/or dysfunction
    D. SIJ infection
    E. All of the above

63) Supine infant with flexed and abducted hip, the physician gently pulls the femur anteriorly while palpating at the trochanter for hints of anterior glide/dislocation
   A. Ortolani test
   B. Barlow test
   C. Allis's sign
   D. Thomas test
   E. Ober's test

64) Supine infant with flexed and adducted hip; physician gently pushes the femur posteriorly while palpating at the gluteus maximus for hints of posterior glide/dislocation
   A. Ortolani test
   B. Barlow test
   C. Allis's sign
   D. Thomas test
   E. Ober's test

65) Management of infants with congenital hip dysplasia minimally includes:
   A. Antiinflammatories
   B. Calcium supplementation
   C. Bromelain
   D. Manipulation
   E. Orthopedic referral

66) Children and adolescents with afebrile hip pain are evaluated by which of the following:
   A. Applied kinesiology
   B. Urinalysis
   C. Food allergy elimination and provocation
   D. Radiographs
   E. Assessing response to a 3-week trail of manipulation

67) Which of the following are causes of hip pain in children?
   A. Avascular necrosis of the femoral head
   B. Apophysitis
   C. Slipped capital femoral epiphysis
   D. Transient synovitis
   E. All of the above

68) In your office, what procedure(s) allows you do you differentiate septic arthritis from transient synovitis (assume classic location and presentation)?
   A. Observation and "vitals"
   B. Patrick's test
   C. Lift-off test confirmed by active internal rotation
   D. Sotto-Hall test
   E. Spinal percussion and lung auscultation

69) Your patient is a 40-year-old woman who presents with pain of the right hip. She recalls no trauma; and the onset of pain and limited motion has been gradual over the past week. She is obese, diabetic, smokes, and drinks a 6-pack of beer per day. Except for her prednisone to treat her asthma, she is not on any other medications. Physical examination of her right hip reveals painful limited ROM, and pain with compressive circumduction. Otherwise, she is in no acute distress, and vitals are normal, except for hypertension of 150/95. This patient most likely has:
   A. Transient synovitis
   B. Slipped femoral capital epiphysis
   C. Avascular necrosis of the femoral head
   D. Septic arthritis
   E. Meralgia paresthetica

70) Your management of the above patient includes:
   A. Radiographs of the hip
   B. Immediate referral for joint aspiration
   C. Immediate referral to the emergency room
   D. Urinalysis
   E. Ultrasound of the abdomen

71) You are a student clinician at the Bastyr clinic, and your supervising doctor assesses the 35-year-old patient with osteoarthritis of both hips and knees. Since you are well educated and since you care enough about your patient to ensure that he/she gets a proper evaluation, you tactfully remind your clinician that this patient needs to be assessed with which of the following lab tests?
   - A. Lipoprotein(a)
   - B. Urinalysis
   - C. Blood pH
   - D. Creatine phosphokinase
   - E. Serum ferritin

72) Positive McMurray's test, positive bounce test, pain and limited motion with waddling, negative Lachman's test, negative patellar ballottement test, negative patellar grinding test:
   - A. Joint effusion
   - B. Meniscus injury
   - C. Patellofemoral arthralgia
   - D. Meralgia paresthetica
   - E. None of the above

73) Which of the following suggest the need for knee radiographs following trauma:
   - A. Local tenderness at the head of fibula or patella
   - B. Inability to flex the knee to 90°
   - C. Inability to walk >4 steps
   - D. Blunt trauma or fall with one of the following: Age <12 years or >50 years
   - E. All of the above

74) Your 14-year-old overweight male patient presents with knee pain and a limp. Clinical assessment reveals the following: negative McMurray's test, negative bounce test, negative Lachman's test, negative patellar ballottement test, negative patellar grinding test, and pain and hesitancy with the following assessments: Patrick's (FABER) test, Thomas test, circumduction. He is afebrile. This patient most likely has _____ and needs to be assessed with _____.
   - A. Meniscus injury—MRI of the knee
   - B. Congenital hip dysplasia—ultrasound of both hips
   - C. Slipped femoral capital epiphysis—radiographs of both hips
   - D. Osteochondritis dissecans of the knee—radiographs of both knee
   - E. Osteoarthritis--radiographs

75) **Which of the following is the most consistent finding associated with compartment syndrome?**
   - **A. Elevated troponin and positive Rovsing's sign**
   - **B. Painful passive stretch and elevated serum haptoglobin**
   - **C. Proximal pallor, arterial hypotension, low TSH**
   - **D. Pulselessness with elevated urobilinogen**
   - **E. Sensory deficit, distal pulselessness, elevated CK**

76) Which of the following are nerve root tension tests for the assessment of lumbar radiculopathy?
   - A. Straight leg raising
   - B. Bechterew's test
   - C. Braggard's test
   - D. All of the above
   - E. Only two of the above answers (A, B, or C) are correct

77) Regarding the management of what appears to be mechanical low back pain, failure to produce significant resolution of pain and symptoms after _____ indicates the need for additional evaluation, imaging, and/or referral to a specialist.
   - A. 2 days
   - B. 1 week
   - C. 2 weeks
   - D. 4 weeks
   - E. 10 weeks

78) **Leg weakness, bladder/bowel incontinence, and perineal numbness suggests:**
   A. **Klippel-Feil syndrome**
   B. **Turner syndrome**
   C. **Acute compartment syndrome**
   D. **Cauda equina syndrome**
   E. **Pelvic inflammatory disease**

79) **Your patient is an overweight 55-year-old woman who presents to your office after a recent diagnosis of meralgia paresthetica. A doctor at her HMO, who saw her for 5 minutes and performed essentially no physical examination, made the diagnosis. She would like you to treat her for this condition, and to help her modify her lifestyle so that she can loose weight, get off her blood pressure meds, stop smoking, and reduce her risk for ovarian cancer, which was the cause of death in her mother and sister. After your physical examination confirms that she has meralgia paresthetica and excludes radiculopathy, which of the following should you perform?**
   A. **Hemoglobin A1c**
   B. **Lumbosacral radiographs**
   C. **Diagnostic ultrasound**
   D. **Electromyography**
   E. **Joint aspiration**

Match the following.

   A. Tibial stress fracture
   B. Shin splints
   C. Compressive compartment syndrome
   D. Jones fracture
   E. Metatarsal stress fracture
   E. Metatarsalgia

80) Overuse strain of the compartmentalized muscles of the lower leg and/or inflammation of the tibial periosteum

81) Localized leg pain in an endurance or overtrained athlete; exacerbation of pain with static weight-bearing

82) Diffuse pain in a novice overtrained athlete; clinical findings include: painful passive stretch, pallor, pulselessness

83) Pain at the 2nd or 3rd metatarsal head in a runner or obese patient;

84) Pain at the middle inferior lateral aspect of the foot following a "twisted ankle"; exacerbation of pain with weight-bearing and walking

85) Pain in the metatarsal shaft in a runner or obese patient

Mark "A" for true and "B" for false for the remaining questions.

86) Generally speaking, any patient with a history of cancer who presents with a complaint of pain or loss of function needs to be carefully clinically evaluated for metastatic disease and should be assessed with laboratory tests (e.g., ESR, CRP, alk phos) and imaged with radiographs, ultrasound, CT, or MRI, as indicated.

87) Trauma to the thoracolumbar region mandates a urinalysis to assess for kidney damage.

88) Any patient with a recent head injury who demonstrates depressed sensorium must be evaluated with CT to assess for possible subdural hematoma or other intracranial pathology.

89) Any woman over the age of 40 who presents with chronic or recalcitrant neck, chest, shoulder, or arm pain which is not definitively ascribed to another condition must be assessed for breast cancer: history, family history, physical examination (breast exam, lymph nodes, regional exam, and mammography if appropriate).

90) Patients with recent trauma and the possibility of serious bleeding such as subdural hematoma or internal bleeding are not treated with medications/nutrients/botanicals that significantly impair coagulation.

91) Physical examination of a painful region also requires examination of neighboring regions and organs.

92) Differentiating viscerosomatic referral from mechanical causes of musculoskeletal pain, depends upon 1) the doctor's taking a complete patient history, 2) the doctor's performing a complete examination, 3) the doctor's obtaining proper laboratory tests, 4) the doctor's effective and appropriate use of imaging studies.

93) "Osteoarthritis" is a diagnosis of exclusion, and one of the diseases that must be ruled out before osteoarthritis can be diagnosed is hemochromatosis, which must be screened for with the laboratory tests serum ferritin and transferrin saturation.

CORE COMPETENCIES

Provide the standard grading and description of MUSCLE STRENGTH.

Grade	Description

Provide the standard grading and description of REFLEXES.

Grade	Description

Verbal assessment for myelopathy, cauda equina syndrome, and radiculopathy includes the following:

1) _____

2) _____

3) _____

List the **4 general categories** that need to be assessed during the history and physical when a patient presents with **any musculoskeletal complaint**:

1.	2.
3.	4.

5. Describe the clinical management of the patient with cauda equina syndrome—be specific with regard to <u>what you will do</u> and <u>what the patient will do</u>:

_____

_____

_____

Your patient presents with a complex history and examination picture that suggests the possibility of organic disease as a cause of his/her complaints. A safe and reasonably inexpensive means of laboratory investigation that allows you to objectively screen for several different diseases includes (essential tests only):

6.	7.	8.

9. Your patient is sick and presents with recent onset of severe back pain, a rigid back, fever, and a raised WBC and sedimentation rate. The most likely diagnosis and your method for managing this patient are: _____

_____

Your patient is a 46-year-old woman whom you have been treating for various complaints including low back and neck pain, which she has had for several years following two car accidents. Today she presents to you with some concern because her low-back pain is worse, and she mentions that she has recently noticed a decrease in sensitivity of the regions around her anus and genitals. She denies pain or sensory changes in her legs and arms. Vital signs and routine neurologic examination of the upper and lower extremities are normal.

10. What is the most serious and likely diagnosis that you must consider? _____

11. What key question must you ask? _____

12. If your clinical suspicion of #10 is high, and #11 is positive/abnormal, how will you manage this patient? What needs to happen? _____

_____

_____

13. What is the approximate time frame for implementing the management plan that you have described in #12?_____

Two causes of knee joint locking:

14.	15.

4 musculoskeletal conditions that can typically cause low back pain with thigh pain:

16.	17.
18.	19.

20. Proper method of evaluation for **acute febrile non-traumatic monoarthritis** is (provide at least 3 specific answers, at least one of which must be the "gold standard"): _____

_____

_____

_____

Phrases coined by the author during the development of this text and other recent projects:

- **Antibiologic**: Although I am not the first to use this word (as of January 2006, only eight international websites used this word), I am the first to use it "medically" since the term is not listed in Medline (as of January 2006). My use of the word describes misused pharmaceutical drugs—most of which are enzyme *inhibitors* and thus work *against* physiology—and/or drugs which are used to mask an underlying problem that could have been identified and addressed to provide the patient an opportunity for *cure* rather than *codependence* upon lifelong medicalization. Most pharmaceutical drugs can be accurately described as antibiologic (against the logic of life) because they interfere with normal *eu*biologic functions or because they serve as a detour away from effective intervention. For example, as generally used, HMG-CoA reductase cholesterol-lowering drugs are antibiologic to the extent that they dysfunctionally enable patients to continue their destructive lifestyles by continuing to overeat and underexercise. Such a co-dependent enabling of dysfunctional behavior is **anti-health**, even if it does prolong life for patients unable to self-regulate. Proof of the superfluous overutilization of these drugs was demonstrated by O'Keefe, Cordain, et al[1] in their article noting that in healthy and active cultures, the average serum cholesterol level is approximately 100-150 mg/dL whereas in so-called industrialized nations such as the US the average serum cholesterol level is > 205 mg/dL, a level which "requires" drug intervention according to the pharmaceutical model. A more glaring example of the antibiologic use of drugs is the overuse of so-called antidepressant medications, which detour patients away from dealing with their internal emotional issues thanks to a corporate-driven "healthcare" paradigm that pushes medications for problems that *originate emotionally* and then later *manifest biochemically*.[2] Admittedly, some enzyme inhibitors such as Anastrozole (Arimidex®) clearly do have a place in healthcare and medicine, since for many patients this drug provides the only means by which to effectively lower their estrogen levels. Similarly, a statin HMG-CoA reductase inhibiting drug might be eubiologic in a patient with hypercholesterolemia who has already optimized diet and lifestyle but continues to have hypercholesterolemia. Thus, "antibiologic" relates more to the use of a given drug or treatment, rather than the treatment or drug itself. Forcing a patient to use a drug rather than empowering the patient toward disease resolution when available is against the inherent logic of life and can thus be described as antibiologic. Using that same drug to prolong life and maximize function in a patient who has earnestly exhausted other natural *primary* interventions could very well be eubiologic. Obviously, analyzing an intervention as *antibiologic* or *eubiologic* is best performed within a framework that appreciates the importance of a "hierarchy of therapeutics" such as outlined in Chapter 1 in the section on Naturopathic Medicine.

- **Anticausative**: Anticausative is a word used in the field of linguistics to describe "an intransitive verb that shows an event affecting its subject, while giving no semantic or syntactic indication of the cause of the event.[3] My use of the word implies **treatments that intentionally avoid addressing the underlying cause of the disease so that the patient experiences incomplete improvement yet must continue using the treatment (generally a drug) in order to avoid complications from the disease**. In other words, **anticausative treatments are detours** *away from effective healthcare* **under the guise of "healthcare."** Hypercholesterolemic drugs are the best example, since they are so often used to mask the cause of the problem (unhealthy diet and lifestyle) by addressing the manifestation of the problem (hypercholesterolemia) while the real metabolic problem (nutritional deficiencies, sarcopenia, insulin resistance) are left unaddressed.

- **Antidysbiotic**: (*adjective*) Describes anything that counteracts dysbiosis by elimination of microbes.

- **Dietary haptenization**: The binding of dietary moieties to body tissues for the formation of an immunogenic neoantigen.

- **Disease identification**: When a patient uses his/her disease as a source of personal identity.

- **Dysbiotic arthropathy, dysbiotic autoimmunity:** Arthritis, arthropathy, systemic inflammation, and "autoimmunity" that results from unifocal or multifocal dysbiosis.

- **Envirosociogenomics**: The phenomenon by which our social, economic, and political environments shape our biology by shaping our lifestyles and experiences for the induction of a specific phenotype. A recent example is the epidemic of diabetic obesity triggered by the impoverishment of the populace due to political manipulations that enrich the few at the expense of the many. America's trend toward increased concentration of wealth—rather than equitable and democratic distribution of resources—is a nonmedical contributor to the problems of hypertension, depression, insulin resistance, and obesity. See the recent article by McCarthy[4] for an excellent and concise review.

- **Idiopathicization**: The intentional action of attempting to convince doctors and patients that a disease or group of diseases are "of unknown origin" and that therefore—since the cause of the disease is not known and cannot therefore be treated—both doctor and patient must turn their hopes *away from health* and *toward medicalization in general and pharmaceuticalization in particular*. The cause(s) of many diseases is known and can be treated; however, those who benefit from *selling drugs* and from *keeping the population dependent on drugs* work to convince us that nutrition is ineffective, that proactive strategies are futile, and that drugs and surgery are the best answers to our problems, even

---

[1] O'Keefe JH, Cordain L, Harris, WH, Moe RM, Vogel R. Optimal low-density lipoprotein is 50 to 70 mg/dl. Lower is better and physiologically normal. *J Am Coll Cardiol* 2004;43: 2142-6 http://www.thepaleodiet.com/published_research/

[2] Miller A. The truth will set you free: overcoming emotional blindness and finding your true adult self. [Translated from German]. New York: Basic Books; 2001

[3] http://en.wikipedia.org/wiki/Anticausative_verb

[4] McCarthy M. The economics of obesity. *Lancet*. 2004 Dec 18-31;364(9452):2169-70

those within our control which are easily addressed with intentional action.[5] See my 2006 Editorial for further explication: http://www.naturopathydigest.com/archives/2006/mar/idiopathic.php

- **Immunonutrigenomics**: The phenomenon by which nutrients influence genetic expression to modulate immune function either toward or away from inflammation, toward or away from immune dysfunction.

- **Intracellular hypercalcinosis**: I coined this phrase in 2004 following the publication of my vitamin D monograph[6] and reading a brief but very important paper in which Fujita[7] noted, in essence, that vitamin D deficiency and/or calcium deficiency resulted in a secondary hyperparathyroidism which essentially drove excess calcium into the intracellular compartment. Since excess intracellular calcium acts to stimulate and disrupt a wide range of intracellular *and therefore systemic* processes, this condition, which I have labeled as "intracellular hypercalcinosis" appears, as suggested by Fujita, to contribute to the development of hypertension, arteriosclerosis, diabetes mellitus, neurodegenerative diseases, malignancy, and degenerative joint disease. Beyond deficiencies of 1) vitamin D and 2) calcium (both of which increase intracellular calcium by stimulating release of parathyroid hormone), other nutritional and lifestyle contributors to this phenomenon are likely to include 3) the epidemic of magnesium deficiency, 4) the Western style of eating which promotes loss of magnesium and calcium in the urine to due the net acid load placed on the kidneys[8,9] and consumption of foods and beverages with 5) caffeine, 6) sugar, and/or 7) alcohol/ethanol, and 6) fatty acid imbalances—namely insufficient intake of the omega-3 fatty acids in general and EPA in particular, particularly in a setting of excess arachidonic acid.[10] No doubt that 8) psychoemotional/physical stress also plays a role here due to the induced renal hyperexcretion of calcium and/or magnesium occurs following stressful events.[11] The concept of intracellular hypercalcinosis is supported by the medical use of "calcium channel blocking drugs" for example in the treatment of hypertension, which also responds to 1) vitamin D supplementation, 2) calcium supplementation, 3) magnesium supplementation, 4) an un-Western style of eating which promotes alkalinization, 5) caffeine avoidance, 6) sugar avoidance, 7) alcohol/ethanol avoidance, 6) n-3 fatty acid supplementation, and 8) stress reduction. For further discussion, please see http://www.naturopathydigest.com/archives/2006/sep/vasquez.php

- **Multifocal dysbiosis**: Dysbiosis occurring in more than one location at the same time in the same patient. Each locus may be subtle and "subclinical" however the effects are at least **additive** and are more often **synergistic**. See the most current edition of *Integrative Rheumatology* for details, clinical implications, and interventions; for a superficial overview, see my article on-line: http://www.naturopathydigest.com/archives/2006/jun/vasquez.php

- **Multifocal polydysbiosis**: See *polydysbiosis* below.

- **Myalgenic**: (adjective) Producing muscle pain.

- **NeoHeroic Medicine**: I coined this phrase in November 2006 to connote the similarities between the *passé* Heroic medicine and modern allopathic medicine

- **Naturogenomics**: I coined this phrase on October 29, 2006 while writing the third part of an Editorial for *Naturopathy Digest*—see http://www.naturopathydigest.com/archives/2006/dec/editor.php. I define it as the study and clinical application of the modulation of gene expression with "naturopathic" and "natural" interventions such as diet, nutritional supplementation, botanical medicines, spinal and musculoskeletal manipulation, exercise, and other non-surgical non-pharmacologic interventions.

- **Orthoendocrinology**: Optimization of hormonal status by assessing and correcting levels of all major hormones, particularly those with inflammatory/anti-inflammatory actions—thyroid, prolactin, Cortisol, DHEA, estrogen(s), testosterone. This is detailed in *Integrative Rheumatology*.

- **Pharmacopathic**: Disease caused by drugs; pharmaceutical iatrogenesis

- **Pharmacoeconomic**: Describes the link between drugs and money, such as the financial interests that push drugs on the American people.

- **Polydysbiosis**: I coined this term in May 2006 during a discussion on the IFM Forum (FunctionalMedicine.org) to connote that gastrointestinal dysbiosis is generally multi-/poly-microbial in nature, rather than due to a single dysbiotic microbe. Thus, the probability is that many dysbiotic patients have **multifocal polydysbiosis**—dysbiosis in more than one location caused by the presence of more than one dysbiotic microbe or overgrowth of otherwise benign microbes.

- **Xenobiotic diabetogenesis**: Induction of diabetes mellitus by persistent organic pollutants and toxic metals, see my articles at http://www.naturopathydigest.com/archives/2007/apr/diabetes.php and http://optimalhealthresearch.com/archives/toxins-diabetes.html

---

[5] van der Steen WJ, Ho VK. Drugs versus diets: disillusions with Dutch health care. *Acta Biotheor.* 2001;49(2):125-40

[6] Vasquez A, Manso G, Cannell J. The Clinical Importance of Vitamin D (Cholecalciferol): A Paradigm Shift with Implications for All Healthcare Providers. *Alternative Therapies in Health and Medicine* 2004; 10: 28-37 http://www.optimalhealthresearch.com/monograph04

[7] "Such intracellular paradoxical Ca overload as a consequence of nutritional calcium deficiency may give rise to a number of diseases common in old age: hypertension, arteriosclerosis, diabetes mellitus, neurodegenerative diseases, malignancy, and degenerative joint disease." Fujita T. Calcium paradox: consequences of calcium deficiency manifested by a wide variety of diseases. *J Bone Miner Metab.* 2000;18(4):234-6

[8] Maurer M, Riesen W, Muser J, Hulter HN, Krapf R. Neutralization of Western diet inhibits bone resorption independently of K intake and reduces cortisol secretion in humans. *Am J Physiol Renal Physiol.* 2003 Jan;284(1):F32-40 http://ajprenal.physiology.org/cgi/content/full/284/1/F32

[9] "Acid loading resulted in massive calciuria in both groups, with significantly higher urinary calcium excretion rates in the stone-formers compared to the healthy subjects. ... Acid loading (i.e. protein ingestion) may contribute to disturbed bone metabolism in idiopathic calcium nephrolithiasis as well as calcium stone formation." Osther PJ. Effect of acute acid loading on acid-base and calcium metabolism. *Scand J Urol Nephrol.* 2006;40(1):35-44

[10] "The Ca(2+) influx rate varied from 0.5 to 3 nM Ca(2+)/s in the presence of AA and from 0.9 to 1.7 nM Ca(2+)/s with EPA." Soldati L, Lombardi C, Adamo D, Terranegra A, Bianchin C, Bianchi G, Vezzoli G. Arachidonic acid increases intracellular calcium in erythrocytes. *Biochem Biophys Res Commun.* 2002 May 10;293(3):974-8

[11] "Our study shows that noise induces significant increases of serum calcium and magnesium, with a borderline increase of serum phosphorus; this in turn is reflected in a significantly increased urinary excretion of magnesium and phosphate after exposure, which lasts for the following 2 days." Mocci F, Canalis P, Tomasi PA, Casu F, Pettinato S. The effect of noise on serum and urinary magnesium and catecholamines in humans. *Occup Med* (Lond). 2001 Feb;51(1):56-61 http://occmed.oxfordjournals.org/cgi/reprint/51/1/56